D1278705

Clinical Urography

ASSOCIATE EDITORS

Marc P. Banner, M.D.

Joshua A. Becker, M.D.

Morton A. Bosniak, M.D.

Peter L. Choyke, M.D.

Alan J. Davidson, M.D.

Richard M. Friedenberg, M.D.

Gerald W. Friedland, M.D., F.R.C.P., F.R.C.R.

David S. Hartman, M.D.

Glen W. Hartman, M.D.

Robert R. Hattery, M.D.

Bruce J. Hillman, M.D.

Erich K. Lang, M.D., M.S.

Bruce L. McClennan, M.D.

Richard C. Pfister, M.D.

Lee B. Talner, M.D.

David M. Witten, A.B., M.D., M.S., F.A.C.R.

UROLOGIC CONSULTANTS

John W. Duckett, Jr., M.D.

A. Richard Kendall, M.D.

Andrew C. Novick, M.D.

Martin I. Resnick, M.D.

Keith N. Van Arsdalen, M.D.

Alan J. Wein, M.D.

Volume 1

Edited by

Howard M. Pollack, M.D.

Professor of Radiology and Urology
University of Pennsylvania School of Medicine
Chief, Section of Uroradiology
Department of Radiology
Hospital of the University of Pennsylvania
Philadelphia, Pennsylvania

Clinical Urography

An Atlas and Textbook of Urological Imaging

1990

W. B. SAUNDERS COMPANY
Harcourt Brace Jovanovich, Inc.

Philadelphia   London   Toronto
Montreal   Sydney   Tokyo

W. B. SAUNDERS COMPANY
Harcourt Brace Jovanovich, Inc.

The Curtis Center
Independence Square West
Philadelphia, PA 19106

Library of Congress Cataloging-in-Publication Data

Clinical urography/[edited by] Howard M. Pollack.
p. cm.
ISBN 0–7216–1555–4 (set)

1. Genitourinary organs—Diseases—Diagnosis.
  2. Genitourinary organs—Imaging.
  3. Genitourinary organs—Diseases—Diagnosis—Atlases.
  4. Genitourinary organs—Imaging—Atlases.
  I. Pollack, Howard M, 1928–
[DNLM: 1. Urography.   WJ 141 C641]

RC874.C55   1990

616.6′07572—dc19   88-39682

Editor: Lisette Bralow
Developmental Editor: Kathleen McCullough
Designer: Terri Siegel
Production Manager: Peter Faber
Manuscript Editor: Leslie Fenton, Mimi McGinnis, Amy Eckenthal
Illustration Coordinator: Walt Verbitski and Alexis O'Hare
Permissions Coordinator: Christy Hurst
Indexer: Alexandra Nickerson
Cover Designer: Denise Pollack

Clinical Urography

Volume 1 0–7216–1556–2
Volume 2 0–7216–1557–0
Volume 3 0–7216–1558–9
Three Volume set 0–7216–1555–4

Copyright © 1990 by W. B. Saunders Company. All rights reserved. No part of this publication may be reproduced or transmitted in any form or by any means, electronic or mechanical, including photocopy, recording, or any information storage and retrieval system, without permission in writing from the publisher.

Printed in the United States of America.

Last digit is the print number: 9   8   7   6   5   4   3   2   1

WJ
141
C6412
1990
v.1

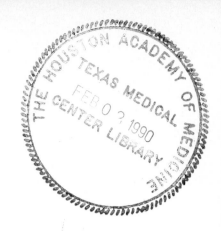

To my loving wife, Shanlee.
Every day I count my blessings.

Contributors

E. WILLLIAM AKINS, M.D.
Assistant Professor, University of Florida; Assistant Professor, Shands Teaching Hospital, Gainesville, Florida
Percutaneous Retrograde Nephrostomy

MARCO A. AMENDOLA, M.D.
Professor of Radiology, University of Pennsylvania School of Medicine and Hospital, Philadelphia, Pennsylvania
Amyloidosis of the Urinary Tract

E. STEPHEN AMIS, Jr., M.D.
Associate Professor of Radiology, College of Physicians and Surgeons of Columbia University; Chief of Uroradiology and Associate Attending in Radiology, Columbia-Presbyterian Medical Center, New York, New York
Cysts of the Renal Sinus

YONG HO AUH, M.D.
Professor and Chairman, Department of Radiology, Ulsan University Medical School, Seoul, Korea
Computed Tomography of the Lower Urinary Tract and Pelvis

HISHAM BADAWY, M.D.
Fellow in Urology, Division of Urology, Harvard Medical School, Boston, Massachusetts; Urologist, University of Cairo, Cairo, Egypt
Radiology of Specific Neuromuscular Diseases Affecting the Urinary Tract: Diseases of the Spinal Cord

GOPAL H. BADLANI, M.D.
Assistant Professor of Urology, Albert Einstein College of Medicine; Chief, Division of Neurourology and Prosthetics, Department of Urology, Long Island Jewish Medical Center; Chief of Urology, Queens Hospital Center, Long Island Jewish Medical Center, New York, New York
Endoscopy of the Ureter and Renal Pelvis

ROBERT R. BAHNSON, M.D.
Assistant Professor of Urology and Chief of Urologic Oncology, Division of Urologic Surgery and Renal Transplantation, University of Pittsburgh School of Medicine; Presbyterian University Hospital; Veterans Administration Hospital of Pittsburgh; Children's Hospital of Pittsburgh; Montefiore Hospital, Pittsburgh, Pennsylvania
Inflammation of the Bladder

DENNIS M. BALFE, M.D.
Associate Professor of Radiology, Washington University School of Medicine; Associate Radiologist, Barnes Hospital, Children's Hospital of St. Louis, St. Louis, Missouri
Genitourinary Manifestations of Gastrointestinal Disease

MARC P. BANNER, M.D.
Professor of Radiology and Urology, University of Pennsylvania School of Medicine and Hospital, Philadelphia, Pennsylvania
Associate Editor, Part III, Section 7: Calculous Disease
Calculous Disease of the Urinary Tract: General Considerations; Radiological Characteristics of Urolithiasis; Nephrocalcinosis; Causes of Upper Urinary Tract Urolithiasis and Medullary Nephrocalcinosis; Roentgen Evaluation of Upper Tract Urolithiasis; Complications of Upper Urinary Tract Urolithiasis; The Recently Passed Ureteral Calculus; Urolithiasis During Pregnancy; Expectant Management of Ureteral Calculi; Lower Urinary Tract Calculi and Calcifications

ZORAN L. BARBARIC, M.D.
Professor of Radiology, University of California Los Angeles School of Medicine, Los Angeles, California
Abdominal Plain Radiography

CLYDE BARKER, M.D.
Professor of Surgery, University of Pennsylvania School of Medicine and Hospital; Chairman of Surgery, Hospital of the University of Pennsylvania, Philadelphia, Pennsylvania
Renal Transplantation: Clinical Considerations

DAVID M. BARRETT, M.D.
Professor of Urology, Mayo Medical School; Consultant, Department of Urology, Mayo Clinic and Mayo Foundation, Rochester, Minnesota
Radiology of Prostheses for Urinary Incontinence

JOSHUA A. BECKER, M.D.
Professor and Chairman, Department of Radiology, State University of New York Health Science Center at Brooklyn; Director of Diagnostic Radiology, Kings County Hospital Center, Brooklyn, New York
Associate Editor, Part VII: Renal Failure, Dialysis, and Transplantation
Imaging of Renal Failure; Dialysis and Its Complications; Imaging the Transplanted Kidney

WALTER E. BERDON, M.D.
Professor of Radiology, Columbia College of Physicians and Surgeons; Director of Pediatric Radiology, Columbia Presbyterian Medical Center; Director of Radiology, Babies Hospital, New York, New York
Diseases of the Adrenal in Infancy and Childhood

LAWRENCE R. BIGONGIARI, M.D.
Clinical Associate Professor, University of Kansas School of Medicine; Staff Radiologist, St. Francis Regional Medical Center, Wichita, Kansas; Susan B. Allen Memorial Hospital, El Dorado, Kansas
Dilatation of Urinary Tract Obstructions

JERRY G. BLAIVAS, M.D.
Associate Professor and Vice-Chairman, Department of Urology, College of Physicians and Surgeons, Columbia University; Attending Urologist, The Presbyterian Hospital in the City of New York, New York, New York
Evaluation of the Effects of Neuromuscular Disease of the Urinary Tract: The Neurourological Evaluation; Urodynamic and Videourodynamic Examination

M. DONALD BLAUFOX, M.D., Ph.D.
Professor of Medicine and Nuclear Medicine, Albert Einstein College of Medicine; Chairman, Department of Nuclear Medicine, Albert Einstein College of Medicine; Attending Physician at Montefiore Medical Center; Bronx Municipal Hospital Center; Weiker Hospital of the Albert Einstein College of Medicine, Bronx, New York
Urological Applications of Radionuclides

JOSEPH J. BOOKSTEIN, M.D.
Professor of Radiology, University of California at San Diego; Chief, Cardiovascular Radiology, University of California at San Diego Hospital, San Diego, California
Angiography of the Genitourinary Tract: Techniques and Applications; Disorders of the Renal Arterial Circulation and Renal Vascular Hypertension: Significance of Angiographic Findings

MORTON A. BOSNIAK, M.D.
Professor of Radiology, New York University School of Medicine; Director of Abdominal Radiology, New York University Medical Center, New York, New York
Associate Editor, Part IV: The Adrenal Glands Introduction; Neoplasms of the Adrenal Medulla; Metastatic Neoplasms to the Adrenal Glands and Adrenal Lymphoma; Miscellaneous Conditions of the Adrenals and Adrenal Pseudotumors

JAMES G. BOVA, D.O.
Associate Professor of Radiology, Ohio State University College of Medicine; Attending Radiologist, The University Hospitals, Ohio State University College of Medicine, Columbus, Ohio
Genitourinary Manifestations of Gastrointestinal Disease

EAMANN S. BREATNACH, M.B., M.R.C.P., F.R.C.R.
Consultant Radiologist, Mater Misericordiae Hospital, Dublin, Ireland
Renal Inflammation: Chronic Inflammation; Pyonephrosis

ANNE C. BROWER, M.D., F.A.C.R.
Professor of Radiology, Uniformed Services University of the Health Sciences; Consultant, Bethesda Naval Hospital, National Institutes of Health, Walter Reed Army Medical Center, Armed Forces Institute of Pathology, Bethesda, Maryland
Systemic Manifestations of Renal Failure: Renal Osteodystrophy

PETER N. BURNS, Ph.D.
Associate Professor of Radiology, Jefferson Medical College; Director of Ultrasound Physics, Thomas Jefferson University Hospital, Philadelphia, Pennsylvania
Ultrasonography of the Urinary Tract

LEONID CALENOFF, M.D.
Professor of Radiology, Northwestern University Medical School; Chief, Outpatient Diagnostic Radiology, Northwestern Memorial Hospital, Chicago, Illinois
Radiology of Urinary Tract Complications in Neuromuscular Disorders

JOHN F. CARDELLA, M.D.
Clinical Assistant Professor, University of Minnesota; Attending Radiologist at Metropolitan Medical Center, Minneapolis; St. Paul-Ramsey Medical Center, St. Paul, Minnesota
Percutaneous Management of Upper Urinary Tract Calculi; Complications of Percutaneous Stone Removal

C. HUMBERTO CARRASCO, M.D.
Associate Professor of Radiology, University of Texas at Houston, Medical School; Associate Radiologist, M. D. Anderson Cancer Center, Houston, Texas
Embolization of Malignant Renal Tumors; Intraarterial Chemotherapy of Genitourinary Tumors

MARK CARVLIN, Ph.D.
Assistant Professor of Radiology, Georgetown University; Georgetown University Hospital, Washington, District of Columbia
Imaging of Renal Failure

WILFRIDO R. CASTAÑEDA-ZUÑIGA, M.D.
Professor of Radiology, University of Minnesota; Attending Radiologist, University of Minnesota Hospital, Minneapolis, Minnesota
Percutaneous Management of Upper Urinary Tract Calculi; Complications of Percutaneous Stone Removal

RONALD A. CASTELLINO, M.D.
Professor of Radiology, Stanford Medical School; Director, Diagnostic Radiology, Chairman (Acting), Department of Diagnostic Radiology and Director, Medical Diagnostic Radiology and Nuclear Medicine, Stanford, California
Lymphography

CHUSILP CHARNSANGAVEJ, M.D.
Professor of Radiology, University of Texas at Houston Medical School; Radiologist, M. D. Anderson Cancer Center, Houston, Texas
Embolization of Malignant Renal Tumors; Intraarterial Chemotherapy of Genitourinary Tumors

CHRISTIAN G. CHAUSSY, M.D.
Stadt. Krankenhaus Harlaching, Department of Urology, University of Munich, Munich, West Germany
Extracorporeal Shock Wave Lithotripsy for the Treatment of Urinary Calculi

HUMBERTO CHIANG, M.D.
Assistant Professor, Universidad de Chile; Attending Staff, Associate, Clínica Los Condes and Hospital Mutual de Seguridad, Santiago, Chile
Radiology of Urinary Incontinence

KYUNG J. CHO, M.D.
Professor of Radiology and Director of the Division of Cardiovascular Radiology, Department of Radiology, University of Michigan, Ann Arbor, Michigan
Abnormalities in Position and Number of the Renal Arteries; Renal Venous Abnormalities

PETER L. CHOYKE, M.D.
Associate Professor of Radiology Georgetown University Medical Center; Staff Radiologist, National Institutes of Health, Warren G. Magnuson Clinical Center, Bethesda, Maryland
Associate Editor, Part VII: Renal Failure, Dialysis, and Transplantation
Imaging of Renal Failure; Dialysis and Its Complications; Imaging the Transplanted Kidney

ROBERT J. CHURCHILL, M.D.
Professor of Radiology, University of Missouri School of Medicine; Chairman Department of Radiology, University of Missouri Hospital and Clinics, Columbia, Missouri
Computed Tomography of the Upper Urinary Tract

RICHARD L. CLARK, M.D.
Professor of Radiology and Associate Chairman, Department of Radiology, University of North Carolina School of Medicine; Department of Radiology, North Carolina Memorial Hospital, Chapel Hill, North Carolina
The Normal Vasculature of the Genitourinary Tract: Embryology, Anatomy, and Hemodynamics

RALPH V. CLAYMAN, M.D.
Associate Professor of Urologic Surgery and Radiology; Washington University Affiliated Hospitals, St. Louis, Missouri
Inflammation of the Bladder; Nephroscopy and Intrarenal Surgery

RONALD COHEN, M.D.
Clinical Assistant Professor of Radiology, University of California, Davis; Staff Radiologist, Children's Hospital, Oakland, California
Congenital Anomalies of the Urinary Tract

CONSTANTIN COPE, M.D.
Professor of Radiology, University of Pennsylvania; Section of Vascular and Interventional Radiology, Hospital of the University of Pennsylvania; Philadelphia, Pennsylvania
Exchanging Nephrostomy Tubes: Insertion and Maintenance of Long-Term Nephrostomy Drainage; Exchanging Nephrostomy Tubes: Replacement of Occluded or Dislodged Nephrostomy Tubes

BRYAN J. CREMIN, M.D. (Cape Town) F.R.C.R., F.R.A.C.R.
Professor of Radiology, University of Cape Town; Head of Radiology, Red Cross Children's War Memorial Hospital, Cape Town, South Africa
Pediatric Urological Neoplasms

JOHN J. CRONAN, M.D.
Clinical Associate Professor, Department of Radiation Medicine, Brown University Program in Medicine; Radiologist, Associate Departmental Director, Department of Diagnostic Imaging, Rhode Island Hospital, Providence, Rhode Island
Percutaneous Renal Biopsy

NANCY S. CURRY, M.D.
Associate Professor and Director of Uroradiology, Medical University of South Carolina, Charleston, South Carolina
Hernias of the Urinary Tract

JOHN T. CUTTINO, Jr., M.D.
Associate Professor, Department of Radiology, University of North Carolina School of Medicine, Chapel Hill, North Carolina; Lahey Clinic Medical Center, Department of Radiology, Burlington, Massachusetts
The Normal Vasculature of the Genitourinary Tract: Embryology, Anatomy, and Hemodynamics

DONALD DAFOE, M.D.
Associate Professor of Surgery, University of Pennsylvania School of Medicine and Hospital; Chief, Transplantation Division, Hospital of the University of Pennsylvania, Philadelphia, Pennsylvania
Renal Transplantation: Clinical Considerations

ALAN J. DAVIDSON, M.D.
Senior Scientist, Armed Forces Institute of Pathology, Washington, District of Columbia
Associate Editor, Part III, Section 10: Parenchymal Disease
A Systematic Approach to the Radiological Diagnosis of Renal Parenchymal Disease; Acute Parenchymal Disease; Chronic Parenchymal Disease

CHARLES J. DAVIS, M.D.
Associate Chairman, Department of Genitourinary Pathology, Armed Forces Institute of Pathology, Washington, District of Columbia
Multicystic Dysplastic Kidney

GEORGE E. DESHON, Jr., M.D.
Assistant Clinical Professor of Urology, University of California; Co-Director, Urology Residency Program, Letterman Army Medical Center, San Francisco, California
Radiology of Vesical and Supravesical Urinary Diversions

PIETER A. deVRIES, M.D.
Chief of Pediatric Surgery, Santa Clara Kaiser Permanente Hospital, Santa Clara, California
Congenital Anomalies of the Urinary Tract

DAVID J. DiSANTIS, M.D.
Assistant Professor of Radiology, Eastern Virginia Medical School; Attending Radiologist, DePaul Hospital, Norfolk, Virginia
Urethral Inflammation

JOHN L. DOPPMAN, M.D.
Professor of Radiology, Georgetown University Medical Center, Washington, District of Columbia; Director of Radiology, National Institutes of Health, Bethesda, Maryland
Diseases of the Adrenal Cortex (Causing Hypofunction)

JOHN W. DUCKETT, Jr., M.D.
Professor of Urology, University of Pennsylvania School of Medicine; Chief, Department of Urology, Children's Hospital of Philadelphia, Philadelphia, Pennsylvania
Consultant, Part III, Section 1: Developmental and Congenital Disorders

J. SCOTT DUNBAR, M.D.
Clinical Professor of Radiology, University of California, San Francisco, California
Excretory Urography in Infants and Children

N. REED DUNNICK, M.D.
Professor of Radiology, Duke University Medical School; Director, Division of Diagnostic Imaging, Duke University Medical Center, Durham, North Carolina
Diseases of the Adrenal Cortex: Hyperfunctioning and Nonfunctioning Neoplasms

DOUGLAS EGGLI, M.D.
Associate Professor of Radiology; Director of Nuclear Medicine, Milton S. Hershey Medical Center, Pennsylvania State University, Hershey, Pennsylvania
Imaging of Renal Failure

KATHLEEN DUNNE EGGLI, M.D.
Assistant Professor of Radiology; Staff Pediatric Radiologist, Milton S. Hershey Medical Center, Pennsylvania State University, Hershey, Pennsylvania
Autosomal Recessive Polycystic Kidney Disease

LEIF EKELUND, M.D., Ph.D.
Professor of Diagnostic Radiology, University of Umeå; Chairman, Department of Diagnostic Radiology, University Hospital, Umeå, Sweden
Complications of Percutaneous Nephrostomy

MILTON ELKIN, M.D.
Professor of Radiology and University Professor, Albert Einstein College of Medicine; Attending Radiologist, Bronx Municipal Hospital Center, Bronx, New York
Urogenital Tuberculosis

MAJID ESHGHI, M.D.
Assistant Professor, New York Medical College, Valhalla, New York; Chief, Section of Endourology, Department of Urology, New York Medical College and Westchester Medical Center, New York, New York
Endoscopy of the Ureter and Renal Pelvis

WILLIAM R. FAIR, M.D.
Professor of Surgery, Cornell University School of Medicine; Chief, Urology Service, Memorial Sloan-Kettering Cancer Center; Attending Surgeon and Chief, Urology Memorial Hospital; Attending Surgeon, The New York Hospital, New York, New York
Urinary Tract Inflammation: An Overview

MICHAEL P. FEDERLE, M.D.
Professor of Radiology, University of California, San Francisco; Chief of Radiology, San Francisco General Hospital, San Francisco, California
Evaluation of Renal Trauma

INGMAR FERNSTRÖM, M.D.
Professor in Radiology, Karolinska Hospital, Stockholm, Sweden
Preface: Interventional Procedures

IRWIN FEUERSTEIN, M.D.
Assistant Professor, Georgetown University Hospital and Medical School, Washington, District of Columbia; Staff Radiologist, National Institutes of Health, Bethesda, Maryland
Systemic Complications of Renal Transplantation

EUGENE J. FINE, M.D., M.S.
Assistant Professor of Nuclear Medicine, Albert Einstein College of Medicine; Chief, Department of Nuclear Medicine, Bronx Municipal Hospital Center; Assistant Attending Physician at Montefiore Medical Center, Weiler Hospital of the Albert Einstein College of Medicine, Bronx, New York
Urological Applications of Radionuclides

ALEX E. FINKBEINER, M.D.
Professor of Urology, University of Arkansas for Medical Sciences, Little Rock, Arkansas
Radiology of Specific Neuromuscular Diseases Affecting the Urinary Tract: Diseases of the Brain

RICHARD M. FRIEDENBERG, M.D.
Professor and Chairman, Department of Radiological Sciences, University of California; Director, Department of Radiology, University of California Irvine Medical Center, Irvine, California
Associate Editor, Part II: Techniques and Applications of Urological Imaging
Excretory Urography in the Adult

GERALD W. FRIEDLAND, M.D., F.R.C.P. (EDINBURGH), F.R.C.R.
Professor of Radiology, Stanford University, San Francisco; Chief of Radiology, Palo Alto Veterans Administration Medical Center, Palo Alto, California
Associate Editor, Part III, Section 1: Developmental and Congenital Disorders
Congenital Anomalies of the Urinary Tract; Evaluation of the Effects of Neuromuscular Disease of the Urinary Tract: Ultrasonographic Evaluation in Neurourology

PEGGY FRITZSCHE, M.D.
Professor of Radiology, Loma Linda University School of Medicine; Director of Uroradiology, Loma Linda University Medical Center, Loma Linda, California
Fistulas of the Genitourinary Tract; Stenting of the Ureter: Antegrade and Retrograde Techniques

GERHARD J. FUCHS, M.D.
Associate Professor Surgery/Urology, University of California at Los Angeles School of Medicine; Director, University of California at Los Angeles Stone Center, University of California at Los Angeles, Los Angeles, California
Extracorporeal Shock Wave Lithotripsy for the Treatment of Urinary Calculi

OLGA M. B. GATEWOOD, M.D.
Associate Professor of Radiology, Johns Hopkins University School of Medicine; Radiologist, Johns Hopkins Hospital; Director, GU Radiology and Co-Director, Mammography, Johns Hopkins Hospital, Baltimore, Maryland
Neoplasms of the Renal Collecting System, Pelvis, and Ureters

SIDNEY GLANZ, M.D.
Professor of Radiology, Director of Cardiovascular and Interventional Radiology, State University of New York, Downstate Medical Center, Brooklyn, New York
Dialysis and Its Complications; Angiography and Interventional Techniques in Renal Transplants

MARK GLASS-ROYAL, M.S., M.D.
Instructor, Department of Radiology, Georgetown University Hospital, Washington, District of Columbia
Systemic Manifestations of Renal Failure: Nonosseous Manifestations

RICHARD PALMER GOLD, M.D.
Associate Professor of Radiology, Columbia University College of Physicians and Surgeons; Senior Attending Radiologist, St. Luke's-Roosevelt Hospital Center, New York, New York
Renal Inflammation: Acute Infections of the Renal Parenchyma

STANFORD M. GOLDMAN, M.D.
Professor of Radiology, Johns Hopkins University School of Medicine; Professor of Urology, James Buchanan Brady Urological Institute, Johns Hopkins University; Adjunct Professor of Diagnostic Radiology, University of Maryland School of Medicine; Clinical Professor of Radiology and Nuclear Medicine, University Services, University of the Health Sciences School of Medicine; Radiologist-in-Chief, Francis Scott Key Medical Center; Co-Director, Uroradiology, Johns Hopkins Hospital, Baltimore, Maryland
The Simple Renal Cyst; Autosomal Dominant Polycystic Kidney Disease; Medullary Sponge Kidney; Neoplasms of the Renal Collecting System, Pelvis, and Ureters

IRWIN GOLDSTEIN, M.D.
Associate Professor of Urology, Boston University School of Medicine; Co-Director, New England Male Reproductive Center, The University Hospital, Boston, Massachusetts
Seminal Vesiculography and Vasography; Vascular Diseases of the Penis: Impotence and Priapism

ROY L. GORDON, M.D.
Visiting Professor of Radiology, Department of Radiology, University of California at San Francisco, San Francisco, California
Renal and Adrenal Embolization for Functional Ablation

JAN H. GÖTHLIN, M.D., Ph.D.
Professor and Chairman, Institute of Radiology; Director, Oncological Research Laboratory, University of Bergen; Professor and Chairman, Department of Diagnostic Radiology, Haukeland University Hospital, Bergen, Norway
Aspiration Biopsy of Renal Masses

EDWARD G. GRANT, M.D.
Professor of Radiological Sciences, University of California at Los Angeles; Director of Ultrasound, University of California at Los Angeles Medical Center, Los Angeles, California
Dialysis and Its Complications

ALAN J. GREENFIELD, M.D.
Associate Professor of Radiology, Boston University School of Medicine; Chief, Interventional Radiology, Department of Radiology, Boston University Medical Center, Boston, Massachusetts
Seminal Vesiculography and Vasography; Vascular Diseases of the Penis: Impotence and Priapism; Interventional Procedures for Management of Impotence and Priapism

MILTON D. GROSS, M.D.
Associate Professor, Division of Nuclear Medicine, Department of Internal Medicine, University of Michigan Medical School; Chief, Nuclear Medicine Service, Veterans Administration Medical Center, Ann Arbor, Michigan
Scintigraphic Localization of Adrenal Disease

ROLF W. GÜNTHER, M.D.
Professor and Chairman, Department of Diagnostic Radiology, Klinikum Aachen, University of Technology, Aachen, Federal Republic of Germany
Therapeutic Occlusion of the Ureter; Retrieval of Foreign Bodies from the Kidney and Ureter

DIETBERT HAHN, M.D.
Professor of Radiology, University of Munich, Munich, German Federal Republic
Neoplasms of the Urinary Bladder

WILLIAM HALDEN, M.D.
Staff Radiologist, Reston Hospital, Reston, Virginia
Imaging of Renal Failure

JOHN HALE, Ph.D.
Professor Emeritus of Radiologic Physics, Department of Radiology, Hospital of the University of Pennsylvania, Philadelphia, Pennsylvania
Radiation Protection

WILLIAM S. C. HARE, M.D., B.S., D.D.R., F.R.C.R., F.R.A.C.R., F.R.A.C.P., D.D.V.
Professor of Radiology, The University of Melbourne; Director of Radiology, The Royal Melbourne Hospital, Victoria, Australia
The Role of Interventional Radiology in the Lower Urinary Tract

DAVID S. HARTMAN, M.D.
Professor of Radiology, Uniformed Services, University of the Health Sciences; Chairman, Department of Radiology, Bethesda Naval Hospital, Bethesda, Maryland
Associate Editor, Part III, Section 3: Cystic Disease
Overview of Renal Cystic Disease; The Simple Renal Cyst; Autosomal Dominant Polycystic Kidney Disease; Autosomal Recessive Polycystic Kidney Disease; Renal Cystic Disease Associated with Renal Neoplasms; Multicystic Dysplastic Kidney; Medullary Sponge Kidney; Medullary Cystic Disease of the Kidney

GLEN W. HARTMAN, M.D.
Professor of Diagnostic Radiology, Mayo Medical School; Rochester Methodist Hospital, Saint Mary's Hospital, Rochester, Minnesota
Associate Editor, Part III, Section 4: Neoplastic Disease

ROBERT R. HATTERY, M.D.
Professor of Radiology, Mayo Medical School; Consultant in Radiology, Mayo Clinic and Mayo Foundation, Rochester, Minnesota
Associate Editor, Part III, Section 4: Neoplastic Disease

IRVIN F. HAWKINS, Jr., M.D.
Professor and Chief, Angio/Interventional Radiology, University of Florida; Professor, Shands Teaching Hospital, Gainesville, Florida
Percutaneous Retrograde Nephrostomy

JAY P. HEIKEN, M.D.
Associate Professor of Radiology and Co-Director, Computed Body Tomography, Mallinckrodt Institute of Radiology, Washington University School of Medicine; Attending Staff, Barnes Hospital and St. Louis Children's Hospital, St. Louis, Missouri
Tumors of the Testis and Testicular Adnexae

MARJORIE HERTZ, M.D.
Professor of Radiology, Sackler School of Medicine, Tel Aviv University; Head, Division of Uroradiology, Department of Imaging, The Chaim Sheba Medical Center, Tel Hashomer, Affiliated to the Tel Aviv University, Sackler School of Medicine, Israel
Cystourethrography

MICHAEL HILL, M.B.
Professor of Radiology, George Washington University Medical Center; Chief, Cross-Sectional Imaging Section, George Washington University Medical Center, St. Louis, Missouri
Imaging the Transplanted Kidney

BRUCE J. HILLMAN, M.D.
Professor of Radiology, University of Arizona College of Medicine; Vice-Chairman, Department of Radiology, University Medical Center, Tucson, Arizona
Associate Editor, Part III, Section 9: Vascular Disease
Digital Subtraction Angiography; Disorders of the Renal Arterial Circulation and Renal Vascular Hypertension

HEDVIG HRICAK, M.D.
Professor of Radiology and Urology, University of California, San Francisco Medical School; Chief, Uroradiology Section, University Hospitals: Moffitt and Long Hospitals, San Francisco, California
Neoplasms of the Prostate Gland

THOMAS J. IMRAY, M.D.
Professor and Chairman, Department of Radiology, University of Nebraska Medical Center; Omaha, Nebraska
Retrograde Pyelography

SAID KARMI, M.D.
Professor of Urology and Surgery, George Washington University Medical Center, Washington, District of Columbia
Imaging the Transplanted Kidney

BARRY T. KATZEN, M.D.
Clinical Professor, University of Miami School of Medicine; Director, Miami Vascular Institute, Baptist Hospital of Miami, Miami, Florida
Thrombectomy and Thrombolytic Therapy of Renovascular Disease

ELIAS KAZAM, M.D.
Professor of Radiology, Cornell University Medical Center; Attending Radiologist, The New York Hospital—CUMC, Head, Division of Ultrasound and Computed Body Tomography, New York, New York
Computed Tomography of the Lower Urinary Tract and Pelvis

MICHAEL A. KEATING, M.D.
Assistant Professor of Urology in Surgery, University of Pennsylvania School of Medicine; Staff Surgeon, Children's Hospital of Philadelphia, Division of Urology, Philadelphia, Pennsylvania
Radiology of Specific Neuromuscular Diseases Affecting the Urinary Tract: Myelomeningocele and Related Myelodysplasias

FREDERICK S. KELLER, M.D.
Professor of Radiology and Surgery, Department of Diagnostic Radiology; Chief, Angiography and Interventional Radiology, University of Alabama at Birmingham, Birmingham, Alabama
Renal and Adrenal Embolization for Functional Ablation

A. RICHARD KENDALL, M.D.
Professor and Chairman, Department of Urology, Temple University School of Medicine and Health Sciences Center, Philadelphia, Pennsylvania
Consultant, Part III, Section 2: Inflammatory Disease

PHILIP J. KENNEY, M.D.
Associate Professor of Radiology, University of Alabama School of Medicine; University of Alabama Hospital, Birmingham, Alabama
Renal Inflammation: Chronic Inflammation; Pyonephrosis

RANDOLPH J. KNIFIC, M.D.
Attending Staff, Southwest Florida Regional Medical Center, Fort Meyers, Florida
Perinephric Inflammation

MELVYN KOROBKIN, M. D.
Clinical Professor of Radiology, Wayne State University School of Medicine; Director of Computed Tomography, Department of Diagnostic Imaging/Radiology, Sinai Hospital of Detroit, Detroit, Michigan
Pheochromocytoma

ROBERT J. KRANE, M.D.
Professor and Chairman, Department of Urology, Boston University School of Medicine; Urologist-in-Chief, Boston University Hospital, Boston, Massachusetts
Seminal Vesiculography and Vasography; Vascular Diseases of the Penis: Impotence and Priapism

HERBERT Y. KRESSEL, M.D.
Professor of Radiology, University of Pennsylvania School of Medicine and Hospital; Director, David W. Devon Medical Imaging Center, Hospital of the University of Pennsylvania, Philadelphia, Pennsylvania
Magnetic Resonance Imaging

ALFRED B. KURTZ, M.D.
Professor of Radiology and Obstetrics and Gynecology, Division of Diagnostic Ultrasound, Department of Radiology, Jefferson University Hospital and Jefferson Medical College, Philadelphia, Pennsylvania
Fetal Obstructive Uropathy: Theoretical Aspects and Practical Applications in the Use of Antenatal Intervention

ERICH K. LANG, M.D., M.S.
Professor and Chairman, Department of Radiology, Louisiana State University Medical Center; Professor of Urology, Louisiana State University Medical Center; Professor of Radiology, Tulane School of Medicine; Director, Department of Radiology, Charity Hospital, New Orleans, Louisiana
Associate Editor, Part III, Section 5: Trauma Ureteral Injuries; Fistulas of the Genitourinary Tract; Stenting of the Ureter: Antegrade and Retrograde Techniques; Transcatheter Radioactive Seed Therapy of Advanced Renal Cell Carcinoma

ELLIOTT C. LASSER, M.D.
Professor of Radiology, University of California at San Diego; Staff, University of California at San Diego Medical Center, San Diego, California
Contrast Media for Urography

ROBERT L. LEBOWITZ, M.D.
Professor of Radiology, Harvard Medical School; Director of Uroradiology, The Children's Hospital, Boston, Massachusetts
Renal Inflammation: Reflux Nephropathy; Postoperative Uroradiological Appearances in the Child

JOSEPH K. T. LEE, M.D.
Professor of Radiology, Washington University School of Medicine; Director, Magnetic Resonance Imaging, Mallinckrodt Institute of Radiology; Attending Physician, Barnes Hospital, Consulting Physician, St. Louis Children's Hospital, St. Louis, Missouri
Perinephric Inflammation

ANDREW J. LeROY, M.D.
Associate Professor of Diagnostic Radiology, Mayo Clinic and Mayo Medical School; Consultant in Diagnostic Radiology, Mayo Clinic, Rochester, Minnesota
Brucellosis; Percutaneous Nephrostomy: Techniques and Instrumentation

ERROL LEVINE, M.D., Ph.D.
Professor of Diagnostic Radiology; Chief, Sections of Uroradiology, Computed Body Tomography, and Magnetic Resonance Imaging, University of Kansas Medical Center, Kansas City, Kansas
Renal Cystic Disease Associated with Renal Neoplasms; Malignant Renal Parenchymal Tumors in Adults

ROBERT P. LIEBERMAN, M.D.
Associate Professor of Radiology, University of Nebraska Medical Center, Omaha, Nebraska
Retrograde Pyelography

ERIC LINDSTEDT, M.D., Ph.D.
Associate Professor of Urology, University of Lund; Chairman, Department of Urology, University Hospital, Lund, Sweden
Complications of Percutaneous Nephrostomy

L. KEITH LLOYD, M.D
Professor of Surgery (Urology), University of Alabama in Birmingham; Director of the Urological Rehabilitation and Research Center, Spain Rehabilitation Center, University Hospital, Veterans Administration Hospital, Birmingham, Alabama
Evaluation of the Effects of Neuromuscular Disease of the Urinary Tract: Isotopic Evaluation

CHRISTOPHER LOGOTHETIS, M.D.
Associate Professor of Medicine, University of Texas at Houston Medical School; Chief, Section of Genitourinary Oncology; Internist, M. D. Anderson Cancer Center, Houston, Texas
Intra-arterial Chemotherapy of Genitourinary Tumors

LEON LOVE, M.D.
Professor of Radiology; Attending Radiologist, Loyola University Medical Center, Maywood, Illinois; Consultant Radiologist, Hines Veterans Administration Hospital, Hines, Illinois
Computed Tomography of the Upper Urinary Tract

SCOTT N. LURIE, M.D.
House Officer, Department of Psychiatry, Duke University Medical Center, Durham, North Carolina
Physiology of the Adrenal Gland

JOHN A. MARKISZ, M.D., Ph.D.
Assistant Professor of Radiology; Head, Division of Magnetic Resonance Imaging, Cornell University Medical Center; Assistant Attending Radiologist, The New York Hospital, New York, New York
Computed Tomography of the Lower Urinary Tract and Pelvis

MURRAY J. MAZER, B.Sc., M.D., F.R.C.P.(C)
Associate Professor of Radiology and Radiological Sciences and Assistant Professor of Surgery, Vanderbilt University School of Medicine; Director of Cardiovascular and Interventional Radiology, Vanderbilt University Medical Center, Nashville, Tennessee
Vascular Abnormalities of the Lower Urinary Tract

RONALD W. McCALLUM, M.D., Ch.B., F.R.C.P.(C.), F.A.C.R.
Professor of Radiology, University of Toronto; Radiologist-in-Chief, Department of Diagnostic Imaging, St. Michael's Hospital, Toronto, Ontario, Canada
Urethral Neoplasms; Injuries of the Urethra; Calculous Disease of the Urinary Tract: Lower Urinary Tract Calculi and Calcifications

BRUCE L. McCLENNAN, M.D.
Professor of Radiology, Washington University Medical School; Attending Radiologist, Barnes Hospital, St. Louis, Missouri
Associate Editor, Part III, Section 2: Inflammatory Disease; Renal Inflammation: Acute Infections of the Renal Parenchyma

EDWARD J. McGUIRE, M.D.
Professor and Head, Section of Urology, The University of Michigan, Ann Arbor, Michigan
Radiology of Urinary Incontinence: Urethral Sphincter Mechanisms and the Evaluation of Incontinence

HARRY Z. MELLINS, M.D., A.B., M.S. in Rad., A.M. (Hon.)
Professor of Radiology, Harvard Medical School; Director of Radiological Education and Training, Brigham and Women's Hospital, Boston, Massachusetts
Anomalies of the Inferior Vena Cava; Inferior Vena Cava Obstruction; Renal Vein Obstruction; Abdominal Aortic Aneurysm Affecting the Ureter; Hypogastric Artery Aneurysm; Gonadal Vein Thrombophlebitis; Portal Hypertension

HOWARD J. MINDELL, M.D., F.A.C.R.
Professor of Radiology, University of Vermont College of Medicine; Director, Division of Diagnostic Radiology; Head, Section of Uroradiology; Medical Center Hospital of Vermont, Burlington, Vermont
Postoperative Uroradiological Appearances in the Adult

HAROLD A. MITTY, M.D.
Professor of Radiology and Urology, The Mount Sinai School of Medicine of the City University of New York; Attending Radiologist and Director of Interventional Radiology and Uroradiology, The Mount Sinai Hospital, New York
Adrenal Embryology, Anatomy, and Imaging Techniques

JOHN B. NANNINGA, M.D.
Associate Professor of Urology, Northwestern University Medical School; Attending Urologist, Northwestern Memorial Hospital; Consultant in Urology, Rehabilitation Institute of Chicago, Chicago, Illinois
Radiological Appearances Following Surgery for Neuromuscular Diseases Affecting the Urinary Tract

FRANCIS A. NEELON, M.D.
Associate Professor of Medicine, Duke University Medical School; Duke University Medical Center, Durham, North Carolina
Physiology of the Adrenal Gland

JEFFREY H. NEWHOUSE, M.D.
Professor of Radiology, Columbia University College of Physicians and Surgeons; Chief, Abdominal Radiology, Presbyterian Hospital, New York, New York
Antegrade Pyelography

MATILDE NINO-MURCIA, M.D.
Assistant Professor of Radiology, Stanford University; Assistant Chief of Radiology, Palo Alto Veterans Administration Medical Center, Palo Alto, California
Congenital Anomalies of the Urinary Tract

JØRGEN NORDLING, D.M.Sc.
Assistant Professor, University of Copenhagen; Chief Urologist, Department of Urology, Herlev Hospital, Herlev, Denmark
Evaluation of the Effects of Neuromuscular Disease of the Urinary Tract: Basic Urographic and Cystourethrographic Patterns

ANDREW C. NOVICK, M.D.
Chairman, Department of Urology, Cleveland Clinic Foundation, Cleveland, Ohio
Consultant, Part III, Section 9: Vascular Disease

ROBERT A. OLDER, M.D.
Associate Clinical Professor of Radiology, University of North Carolina at Chapel Hill School of Medicine, Chapel Hill; Head, Section of Uroradiology, Department of Radiology, Durham County General Hospital, Durham, North Carolina
Endometriosis of the Genitourinary Tract

KNUD P. OLESEN, D.M.Sc.
Assistant Professor, University of Copenhagen; Chief Radiologist, Department of Radiology, Bispebjerg Hospital, Copenhagen, Denmark
Evaluation of the Effects of Neuromuscular Disease of the Urinary Tract: Basic Urographic and Cystourethrographic Patterns

OLLE OLSSON, M.D.
Professor and Chairman; Consulting Radiologist, Department of Diagnostic Radiology, University Hospital, Lund, Sweden
An Overview of Uroradiology

HARIN PADMA-NATHAN, M.D., F.R.C.S.(C.)
Assistant Professor, Department of Urology, University of Southern California School of Medicine; Staff Urologist, USC Consultation Center, White Memorial Medical Center, Hospital of The Good Samaritan, LAC-USC County Hospital, and The Norris Cancer Hospital and Research Center, Los Angeles, California
Vascular Diseases of the Penis: Impotence and Priapism

PHILIP E. S. PALMER, M.D., F.R.C.P., F.R.C.R.
Professor of Radiology, University of California; Professor and Chairman, Department of Radiology, University of California, Davis Medical Center, Sacramento, California
Parasitic Disease of the Urinary Tract

BHALCHANDRA G. PARULKAR, M.B., B.S., M.S., M.Ch.
Special Fellow in Urodynamics and Genitouri-

nary Prosthetics, Mayo Graduate School of Medicine, Rochester, Minnesota
Radiology of Prostheses for Urinary Incontinence

SURESH K. PATEL, M.D.
Associate Professor of Radiology, Rush Medical College; Senior Attending Physician, Department of Diagnostic Radiology and Nuclear Medicine, Rush–Presbyterian–St. Luke's Medical Center, Chicago, Illinois
Retroperitoneal Tumors and Cysts

INDER PERKASH, M.D., F.R.C.S.(Engl.), F.R.C.S.(Edin.), F.A.C.S.
The Paralyzed Veterans of America Professor of Spinal Cord Injury, Stanford University, San Francisco; Chief, The Spinal Cord Injury Service, Palo Alto Veterans Administration Medical Center, Palo Alto, California
Evaluation of the Effects of Neuromuscular Disease of the Urinary Tract: Ultrasonographic Evaluation in Neurourology

RICHARD C. PFISTER, M.D.
Associate Professor of Radiology, Harvard Medical School; Chief, Division of Uroradiology, Massachusetts General Hospital, Boston, Massachusetts
Associate Editor, Part VIII: Interventional Uroradiology
Antegrade Pyelography; Drainage of Abscesses and Fluid Collections; Percutaneous Sclerotherapy of Symptomatic Renal Cysts and Lymphoceles; Percutaneous Chemolysis of Renal Stones

THOMAS G. PICKERING, M.D.
Professor of Medicine, Cornell University Medical College; Associate Director of Cardiovascular Center, The New York Hospital–Cornell University Medical Center, New York, New York
Percutaneous Transluminal Angioplasty in Renal Artery Stenosis

HOWARD M. POLLACK, M.D.
Professor of Radiology and Urology, University of Pennsylvania School of Medicine and Hospital; Chief, Section of Uroradiology, Department of Radiology, Hospital of the University of Pennsylvania, Philadelphia, Pennsylvania
Associate Editor, Part I: Introduction to Urological Imaging
Associate Editor, Part II: Techniques and Applications of Urological Imaging
Associate Editor, Part VI: Miscellaneous Disorders of the Urinary Tract
Abdominal Plain Radiography; Brush Biopsy of the Upper Urinary Tract

ANITA PRICE, M.D.
Associate Professor of Radiology, State University of New York Health Science Center at Brooklyn; Kings County Hospital Center, Brooklyn, New York
The Imaging of Renal Failure and Transplantation in Children

THELMA QUIOGUE, M.D.
Assistant Professor of Radiology, Milton S. Hershey Medical Center, Hershey, Pennsylvania
Postoperative Uroradiological Appearances in the Child

SHLOMO RAZ, M.D.
Professor of Surgery/Urology, University of California at Los Angeles School of Medicine; Center for the Health Sciences, Los Angeles, California
Radiology of Urinary Incontinence

MAURICE M. REEDER, M.D.
Professor and Chairman, Department of Radiology, University of Hawaii School of Medicine; Radiologist, Fronk Clinic, Honolulu, Hawaii
Parasitic Disease of the Urinary Tract

JACK S. RESNICK, M.D.
Formerly Staff Radiologist, Naval Hospital, San Diego, California, Captain USNR; Staff Radiologist, Sharp REES Stealy Medical Group, Inc., San Diego, California
Medullary Cystic Disease of the Kidney

MARTIN I. RESNICK, M.D.
Professor and Chairman, Division of Urology, Case Western Reserve University School of Medicine; Chief of Urology, University Hospitals of Cleveland; Consulting Urologist, Cleveland Veterans Administration Hospital and Cleveland Metropolitan General Hospital, Cleveland, Ohio
Calculus Disease of the Urinary Tract: General Considerations
Consultant, Part III, Section 4: Neoplastic Disease

STEWART R. REUTER, M.D., J.D.
Professor of Radiology; Chairman, Department of Radiology, The University of Texas Health Science Center at San Antonio, San Antonio, Texas
Medical-Legal Issues in Uroradiology

MATTHEW D. RIFKIN, M.D.
Professor of Radiology and Urology, Jefferson Medical College, Thomas Jefferson University; Staff Radiologist, Director, Division of Magnetic Resonance Imaging; Director of Research, Department of Radiology, Thomas Jefferson University Hospital, Philadelphia, Pennsylvania
Congenital Anomalies of the Urinary Tract; Inflammation of the Lower Genitourinary Tract: The Prostate, Seminal Vesicles, and Scrotum

CHRISTOPHER M. RIGSBY, M.D.
Attending Radiologist, Fairfax Hospital, Falls Church, Virginia
Ultrasonography of the Urinary Tract

ERNEST J. RING, M.D.
Professor of Radiology, University of California, San Francisco; Chief, Interventional Section University of California at San Francisco; University of California Hospitals, San Francisco, California
Embolization of Benign Lesions of the Urinary Tract

ROBERTO ROMERO, M.D.
Associate Professor of Obstetrics and Gynecology; Director of Perinatal Research, Yale University School of Medicine, New Haven, Connecticut; Attending Physician, Yale-New Haven Hospital, New Haven, Connecticut
Ultrasonography of the Urinary Tract

ARTHUR T. ROSENFIELD, M.D.
Professor of Diagnostic Radiology and Surgery (Urology); Head, Section of Computed Tomography, Yale University, School of Medicine, New Haven, Connecticut; Attending Radiologist, Yale-New Haven Hospital, New Haven, Connecticut
Ultrasonography of the Urinary Tract

ALLEN J. ROVNER, M.D.
Associate Professor of Radiology, Northeastern Ohio Universities College of Medicine; Chairman, Department of Radiology, Aultman Hospital, Canton, Ohio
Genitourinary Involvement in AIDS

WILLIAM A. RUBENSTEIN, M.D.
Associate Professor of Radiology, Cornell University Medical Center; Associate Attending Radiologist, The New York Hospital, Cornell Medical Center, New York, New York
Computed Tomography of the Lower Urinary Tract and Pelvis

WILLIAM M. RUMANCIK, M.D.
Associate Professor of Clinical Radiology, State University of New York Health Sciences Center at Brooklyn; Attending Radiologist, and Director, Magnetic Resonance, The Long Island College Hospital, Brooklyn, New York
Metastatic Neoplasms to the Adrenal Glands and Adrenal Lymphoma; Miscellaneous Conditions of the Adrenals and Adrenal Pseudotumors

ERICH SALOMONOWITZ, M.D.
Associate Professor of Radiology, University of Vienna; Attending Radiologist, University of Vienna Hospitals, Vienna, Austria
Percutaneous Management of Upper Urinary Tract Calculi

CARL M. SANDLER, M.D.
Professor of Radiology and Surgery (Urology), University of Texas Medical School at Houston; Attending Radiologist, Chief of Genitourinary Radiology, Hermann Hospital, Houston, Texas
Bladder Trauma; Injuries of the Urethra

HUGH M. SAXTON, F.R.C.P., F.R.C.R.
Consultant Radiologist, Guy's Hospital, London, England
Pelvic Lipomatosis

CHRISTIAN P. SCHMIDBAUER, M.D.
Associate Professor of Urology, University of Vienna; Staff Urologist, Department of Urology, Allgemeine Poliklinik, Vienna, Austria
Radiology of Urinary Incontinence

MARK SCHWIMMER, M.D.
Attending Radiologist, Memorial Hospital, Hollywood, Florida; Attending Radiologist, Pembroke Pines Medical Center, Pembroke Pines, Florida; Vice Chief, Department of Radiology, Hollywood Medical Center, Hollywood, Florida
Gynecological Inflammatory Disease

ARTHUR J. SEGAL, M.D.
Clinical Associate Professor of Radiology and Urology, University of Rochester School of Medicine and Dentistry; Director, Section of Uroradiology, Rochester General Hospital, Rochester, New York
Calculous Disease of the Urinary Tract: Radiological Characteristics of Urolithiasis

JOSEPH W. SEGURA, M.D.
Carl Rosen Professor of Urology, Mayo Medical School; Staff Consultant at Mayo Clinic, St. Mary's Hospital and Rochester Methodist Hospital, Rochester, Minnesota
Percutaneous Ultrasonic Lithotripsy

BRAHM SHAPIRO, M.B., Ch.B., Ph.D.
Professor, Division of Nuclear Medicine, Department of Internal Medicine, University of Michigan Medical School, Ann Arbor, Michigan
Scintigraphic Localization of Adrenal Disease

THOMAS SHERWOOD, M.B., F.R.C.P., F.R.C.R.
Professor of Radiology and Clinical Dean, University of Cambridge; Honorary Consultant Radiologist, Addenbrooke's Hospital, Cambridge, England
Percutaneous Pyeloureterodynamics (Whitaker Test)

JAMES G. SMIRNIOTOPOULOS, M.D.
Assistant Professor of Radiology, Uniformed Services University of the Health Sciences, Bethesda, Maryland; Department of Radiologic Pathology, Armed Forces Insitute of Pathology, Washington, District of Columbia
Renal Cystic Disease Associated with Renal Neoplasms

ARTHUR D. SMITH, M.D.
Professor, Department of Urology, Albert Einstein College of Medicine; Chairman, Department of Urology, Long Island Jewish Medical Center, New Hyde Park, New York
Endoscopy of the Ureter and Renal Pelvis

THOMAS A. SOS, M.D.
Professor of Radiology, Cornell University Medical College; Director, Division of Cardiovascular and Interventional Radiology, The New York Hospital–Cornell University Medical Center, New York, New York
Percutaneous Transluminal Angioplasty in Renal Artery Stenosis

ROBERT F. SPATARO, M.D.
Associate Professor of Radiology and Urology, University of Rochester School of Medicine and Dentistry; Radiologist, The Genesse Hospital, Rochester, New York
Inflammatory Conditions of the Renal Pelvis and Ureter; Abnormalities in Position and Number of the Renal Arteries; Renal Venous Abnormalities; Renal Hemorrhage and Renal Complications of Hemorrhagic Hypotension

J. PATRICK SPIRNAK, M.D.
Assistant Professor, Division of Urologic Surgery, Case Western Reserve University; Director, Department of Urology, Metrohealth Medical Center, Cleveland, Ohio
Calculous Disease of the Urinary Tract: General Considerations

DAVID B. SPRING, M.D.
Associate Clinical Professor of Radiology, University of California, San Francisco; Staff Radiologist, Kaiser Permanente Medical Center, Oakland, California
Radiology of Vesical and Supravesical Urinary Diversions; Fungal Diseases of the Urinary Tract

ROBERT J. STANLEY, M.D.
Professor and Chairman, Department of Radiology, University of Alabama School of Medicine; Staff, University of Alabama Hospital, Birmingham, Alabama
Renal Inflammation: Chronic Inflammation; Renal Inflammation: Pyonephrosis

DAVID R. STASKIN, M.D.
Assistant Professor of Urology, Boston University Medical Center; Staff, University Hospital, Boston, Massachusetts
Cavernosography

DAVID A. SWANSON, B.A., M.D.
Associate Professor of Urology, University of Texas at Houston Medical School; Deputy Chairman of Department of Urology, M. D. Anderson Cancer Center, Houston, Texas
Embolization of Malignant Renal Tumors

LEE B. TALNER, M.D.
Professor of Radiology, University of California, San Diego; Chief of Diagnostic Radiology, University of California San Diego Medical Center, San Diego, California
Associate Editor, Part III, Section 6: Obstructive Uropathy
Urinary Obstruction; Specific Causes of Obstruction

DAVID THICKMAN, M.D.
Assistant Professor of Radiology, University of Colorado Health Sciences Center; Director of

Ultrasound, University of Colorado Health Sciences Center, Denver, Colorado
Imaging of Renal Failure

RUEDI F. THOENI, M.D.
Associate Professor, University of California, San Francisco; Chief, CT/GI Section, University Hospitals: Moffitt and Long Hospitals, San Francisco, California
Neoplasms of the Prostate Gland

JOHN R. THORNBURY, M.D.
Professor of Radiology, University of Wisconsin; Active Medical Staff, University of Wisconsin Hospitals and Clinics, Madison, Wisconsin
Abnormalities in Position and Number of the Renal Arteries; Renal Venous Abnormalities; Renal Hemorrhage and Renal Complications of Hemorrhagic Hypotension; Foreign Bodies in the Urinary Tract

CORITO S. TOLENTINO, M.D.
Assistant Professor of Radiology, University of California at San Francisco; San Francisco General Hospital, San Francisco, California
Embolization of Benign Lesions of the Urinary Tract

KEITH N. Van ARSDALEN, M.D.
Associate Professor of Surgery (Urology), University of Pennsylvania School of Medicine and Hospital, Philadelphia, Pennsylvania
Consultant, Part VIII: Interventional Uroradiology

ARINA van BREDA, M.D.
Associate Professor of Radiology, George Washington University Medical School, Washington, District of Columbia; Director, Cardiovascular/ Interventional Radiology, Alexandria Hospital, Alexandria, Virginia; Consultant, Children's Hospital, National Medical Centers, Washington, District of Columbia; Reston Hospital, Reston, Virginia
Thrombectomy and Thrombolytic Therapy of Renovascular Disease

SIDNEY WALLACE, M.D.
Professor of Radiology, The University of Texas at Houston; Radiologist and Deputy Department Chairman, Department of Diagnostic Radiology, M. D. Anderson Cancer Center, Houston, Texas
Embolization of Malignant Renal Tumors; Intraarterial Chemotherapy of Genitourinary Tumors

RONALD J. WAPNER, M.D.
Associate Professor of Obstetrics and Gynecology, Jefferson Medical College; Director, Division of Maternal-Fetal Medicine of the Department of Obstetrics and Gynecology, Thomas Jefferson University Hospital, Philadelphia, Pennsylvania
Fetal Obstructive Uropathy: Theoretical Aspects and Practical Applications in the Use of Antenatal Intervention

ALAN J. WEIN, M.D.
Professor and Chairman, Division of Urology, University of Pennsylvania School of Medicine; Chief of Urology, Hospital of the University of Pennsylvania, Philadelphia, Pennsylvania

Associate Editor, Part III, Section 8: Neuromuscular Disorders (Neurourology)
Overview of Voiding Function and Dysfunction: Relevant Anatomy, Physiology, Pharmacology, Classification, Definitions
Consultant, Part III, Section 5: Trauma

PHILIP J. WEYMAN, M.D.
Clinical Associate Professor of Radiology, Washington University School of Medicine; Barnes Hospital, St. Luke's Hospital, St. Louis, Missouri
Inflammation of the Bladder

ROBERT I. WHITE, Jr., M.D.
Professor and Chairman, Department of Diagnostic Radiology, Yale University School of Medicine; Chairman, Department of Diagnostic Imaging, Yale New Haven Hospital, New Haven, Connecticut
Embolotherapy of Varicocele

BYRN WILLIAMSON, Jr., M.D.
Associate Professor of Radiology, Mayo Medical School, Rochester, Minnesota
Benign Neoplasms of the Renal Parenchyma

ALAN C. WINFIELD, M.D., F.A.C.R.
Professor of Radiology and Radiological Sciences and Assistant Professor of Urology, Vanderbilt University School of Medicine; Chief, Abdominal Section, Chief, Breast Imaging Section, Department of Radiology, and Co-Director, Breast Diagnostic Center, The Vanderbilt Clinic, Vanderbilt University Medical Center, Nashville, Tennessee
Vascular Abnormalities of the Lower Urinary Tract

DAVID M. WITTEN, A.B., M.D., M.S. (Radiology), F.A.C.R.
Professor Emeritus, Department of Radiology, University of Missouri, Columbia, Missouri
Associate Editor, Part V: Other Retroperitoneal Diseases
Retroperitoneal Fibrosis

JEFFREY R. WOODSIDE, M.D., M.B.A.
Professor of Urology, University of Texas Medical School at Houston; Director, University of Texas Center for Incontinence and Urodynamics; Medical Staff, Hermann Hospital and Shriners Hospital for Crippled Children, Houston, Texas
Radiology of Specific Neuromuscular Diseases Affecting the Urinary Tract: Diseases of the Peripheral Nervous System

SUBBARAO V. YALLA, M.D.
Associate Professor of Surgery (in Urology), Harvard Medical School; Chief of Urology, Brockton–West Roxbury Veterans Administration Medical Center; Associate Surgeon, Division of Urology, Brigham and Women's Hospital, Boston, Massachusetts
Radiology of Specific Neuromuscular Diseases Affecting the Urinary Tract: Diseases of the Spinal Cord

ISABEL C. YODER, M.D.
Assistant Professor of Radiology, Harvard Medical School; Radiologist, Division of Uroradiology, Massachusetts General Hospital, Boston, Massachusetts
Drainage of Abscesses and Fluid Collections

HARVEY A. ZEISSMAN, M.D.
Associate Professor of Radiology, Georgetown University Medical Center, Washington, District of Columbia
Imaging of Renal Failure; Imaging the Transplanted Kidney

KENNETH ZIRINSKY, M.D.
Assistant Professor of Radiology, Cornell University Medical Center; Assistant Attending Radiologist, The New York Hospital, New York, New York
Computed Tomography of the Lower Urinary Tract and Pelvis

JESUS ZORNOZA, M.D.
Radiologist, Danbury Hospital, Danbury, Connecticut
Fine-Needle Biopsy of Lymph Nodes, Adrenal Glands, and Periureteral Tissues

Preface

This book had its beginnings in a suggestion made by Suzanne Boyd Enright, a medical editor at W. B. Saunders Company, that there was a serious need for a new, definitive textbook on urinary tract radiology. Advances in both diagnostic and interventional radiology, as well as in clinical urology, were happening at a rapid rate, and wholesale changes in traditional concepts of urological imaging occurred almost daily. Existing texts were either out-of-date or fast becoming so, and the need for a new publication seemed incontrovertible. But formidable challenges loomed.

Although uroradiology is one of the newest radiological subspecialties, it has grown, in only a few short years, into a unique discipline, with its own professional organization (The Society of Uroradiology) and a medical journal. Could one book still cover this subject in an authoritative way? If so, could it be kept within reasonable size limits? How many experts would be required to produce such a work? With the publisher's assurances that, first, this task was indeed a realistic one, and second, that they would do everything reasonably possible to facilitate its completion, we were persuaded to undertake the job. The result now lies at the reader's fingertips. One hopes that the product fulfills the promise.

Every publication has a purpose, but not necessarily one that is easy to define or abide by. If the raison d'être of this text can be stated briefly, our goal is to provide under one set of bindings a work that comprehensively covers the field of uroradiology in its broadest context, and one that literally defines the specialty. To reach this end requires, of course, an atlas of outstanding urinary tract images, but in addition, a detailed text that not only supplements the illustrations but is also thorough enough to stand as an independent clinical sourcebook. Since today's radiologist must also be an astute clinician, this work is heavily oriented toward the clinical aspects of uroradiology. A concerted effort has been made to include, where appropriate, newer imaging modalities such as magnetic resonance imaging, transrectal ultrasonography, and dynamic cavernosography, as well as other modern and traditional methods. The text has been embellished with more than 6000 carefully selected illustrations. The references are numerous and as up-to-date as possible. Thus, although the stated goals of this work are lofty, it is hoped that they have been, in great measure, met by the efforts noted here.

Although the scope of this work is vast, it is a mistake to think of it solely or even primarily as a reference book. The text has been written as much to satisfy the needs of practicing physicians faced with a clinical problem as to fulfill the bibliographic requirements of the researcher. Physicians in training will also find the book valuable for conference preparation, systematic study, augmentation of daily clinical experiences, and preparation for certifying examinations.

Although of interest mainly to radiologists and urologists, nephrologists, obstetrician/gynecologists, pediatricians, oncologists, transplant surgeons, and others will also find within these covers material germane to their practices. The radiologic orientation of the book is obvious, but there has been an intense effort to make it above reproach as a source of urological information as well. An editorial staff of six internationally known urologists reviewed the entire text to verify the accuracy, completeness, and relevance of the clinically related material. Wherever possible, a close balance has been struck between what the radiologist wants to know and what the urologist needs to know. A pragmatic guide to imaging that emphasizes the needs of the patient has therefore been one of the underpinnings of this book. In the final analysis, it should be quite useful to all physicians wishing to have current, detailed information on the available techniques of genitourinary imaging and their role in diagnosis, management, and intervention.

There are many ways to organize a text such as this. After considerable thought, we decided that the purpose of the book would best be served by a disease-oriented approach rather than an anatomy- or symptom-oriented one. Even so, a few deviations from this format are unavoidable (e.g., Diseases of the Adrenal Glands). Accordingly, the text is divided into eight parts.

Part I is a general introduction to the subject of urological imaging and includes in-depth reviews of radiation protection and medical-legal issues as applied to uroradiology. Part II describes the various imaging techniques used in the urinary tract. It begins with an extensive review of the chemistry, physiology, toxicity, and utilization of contrast media, followed by separate chapters dedicated to the more common studies such as excretory urography, retrograde pyelography, cystourethrography, ultrasonography, computed tomography, magnetic resonance imaging, radionuclide imaging, and angiography, as well as the less frequently employed examinations such as cavernosography, lymphography, digital subtraction angiography, seminal vesiculography, and the imaging of urinary tract diversions.

Discussion of particular problems seen in the urinary tract is initiated in Part III with a remarkably thorough treatment of urinary tract development and congenital disorders. This is followed by equally superb presentations of inflammatory, cystic, neoplastic, traumatic, obstructive, calculous, vascular, and parenchymal diseases. Also included is a section on neurourology authored by some of the leading urologists in the world. Special consideration is given to the pediatric aspects of genitourinary imaging in these chapters as well as throughout the book. Each of the more than 60 chapters in Part III contains basic information on etiology, physiology, pathology, bacteriology, epidemiology, clinical presentations, treatment, and prognosis, as well as a complete discussion of all imaging modalities that might be employed in the evaluation of a given urological disorder in both adults and children.

Abnormalities affecting the adrenal glands are covered in Part IV. Other retroperitoneal diseases are discussed in Part V, and Part VI is devoted to a variety of other urinary tract disorders.

Part VII is concerned with the imaging of renal failure, dialysis, and renal transplantation, and the text closes on a strong note with Part VIII, a spectral treatment of interventional uroradiology comprising 34 chapters and describing all procedures considered useful and clinically relevant.

This compendium could not have been written by one or even a handful of persons. To cover as broad and diverse a field as modern uroradiology requires the services of numerous experts. We were very fortunate indeed to have assembled what can only be termed an all-star cast of contributors, each an acknowledged expert in his or her own sphere of interest, and each an experienced teacher, lecturer, and author.

As in any multiauthored work, a certain fluctuation of writing style and diversity of viewpoints is found in this text. We have strived mightily to see that these differences have not affected the integrity of the book; and besides, there is something to be said for variety. So, although many editorial changes were effected to enhance readability and understanding, none was made merely to ensure conformity to a uniform writing style or point of view. Each contributor's opinion was respected even if it varied from or conflicted with that of others.

Another bête noir of a multiauthored text is duplication of both text and illustrations. To a great extent this is unavoidable in a book of this size. On the other hand, is overlap necessarily bad? It is unlikely that the reader will peruse the text from first page to last in order, and some purpose is served by having information where it is needed rather than forcing a busy practitioner to search through various chapters for material. Nonetheless, every attempt has been made to delete annoying redundancies when they seemed to serve no purpose. In many instances, however, our blue pencil was stayed when it appeared that rigid pruning would constitute a disservice to the reader. Often these apparent duplications represent a slightly different emphasis, especially with regard to illustrations.

If, after all is said and done, this work has met its goals and fulfilled its mission, the kudos belongs to the many contributors who, after all, did most of the work and whose efforts speak for themselves. Brickbats, however, belong squarely on the shoulders of the editor-in-chief, whose authority provided him with all the opportunities and tools as well

as the responsibility to put things right, regardless of the measures required. To the extent that this was not accomplished, he is solely accountable.

One text cannot be all things to all people. It is, however, the hope of the contributors, the associate editors, and the editor-in-chief that insofar as one book can fill the role, this work will become the standard working and reference text of urological imaging for the 1990s and perhaps even beyond.

HOWARD M. POLLACK, M.D.
Philadelphia, Pennsylvania
August 1989

Acknowledgments

The organization, preparation, writing, and publishing of a 3100-page textbook requires the collaboration of many persons. I should like to thank the following individuals for their contributions to this work:

The contributors, whose uniformly sterling efforts make up the essence of this book. Without their writings, these pages would be blank. I express my gratitude to all of them for the countless hours they have expended in behalf of this project and for their willingness to accept editorial changes.

The associate editors, who helped me in outlining the text, selecting the authors, and editing the manuscripts. Their collective knowledge and experience were indispensable to the success of this work.

The editorial staff of W. B. Saunders Company, beginning with Suzanne Boyd Enright, the medical editor who started it all, through the chain of acquisitions, manuscript, copy, proof, and development editors, designers, production managers, indexers, and layout and marketing specialists who compose the production line of any large publishing house: to them my sincerest thanks for a most professional job. In particular, I wish to acknowledge the invaluable guidance of Lisette Bralow, who served as my mother hen, and Kitty McCullough, my trouble-shooter. In addition, William J. Lamsback, Leslie Fenton, Mimi McGinnis, Wynette Kommer, Amy Eckenthal, Bob Butler, Peter Faber, Patti Maddaloni, and Carol Trumbold were most understanding and helpful. I especially appreciate the support (as well as the indulgence) of Lewis Reines, president of W. B. Saunders Company. At great inconvenience and not inconsiderable corporate expense, he ensured that his company stood by its promise to allow corrections and additions to already edited manuscripts, galleys, and even page proofs—almost to the last moment— thus assuring a work that was as up-to-date as any three-volume tome could possibly be. The fact that this textbook is unusually fresh and timely can be ascribed in great measure to his forbearance and the fact that not once was a complaint heard about 11th-hour changes.

The many house officers and visiting physicians who uncomplainingly reviewed galleys and page proofs—often on very short notice and at times convenient only to me—for content, accuracy, and photographic layout. They are Richard A. Baum, M.D., Jeffrey M. Boorstein, M.D., Mark P. Bryer, M.D., Teresa W. Chan, M.D., Thomas M. Davis, Jr., M.D., Pragnesh Desai, D.O., Barbara J. Dinsmore, M.D., Louis George, M.D., Timothy J. Greenan, M.D., Manuel E. Grinburg, M.D., John F. Hiehle, Jr., M.D., Elizabeth A. Holland, M.D., Jeffrey G. Jarvik, M.D., Cheryl L. Kirby, M.D., Jill E. Langer, M.D., Larry A. LeCavalier, M.D., Elliot J. Lerner, M.D., Robert A. Lipman, M.D., Barry J. Menick, M.D., Wallace T. Miller, Jr., M.D., Robert L. Mittl, Jr., M.D., Rodney S. Owen, M.D., Jeffrey S. Pollak, M.D., Michael V. Rocco, M.D., Bruce N. Schlakman, M.D., Mitchell D. Schnall, M.D., Ph.D., Martin E. Sheline, M.D., David Sussman, D.O., Joseph C. Tsai, M.D., Charles N. Witten, M.D., and Ching-Jiunn Wu, M.D.

My daughter-in-law, Denise Pollack, who took time from her busy schedule as a graphic arts designer to create the elegant cover design. After contending with my unreasonable demands, I am sure she is grateful that her husband has not inherited his father's stubbornness.

Linda A. DiSandro, my valued secretary for many years, was literally the glue that held this book together throughout its many phases. Her many talents were never more brightly displayed than when called upon to solve a last-minute crisis, of which there were many, and which she never failed to do with consummate skill and grace. Loyal coworker,

tactful diplomat, exceedingly competent office manager, and secretary par excellence, she resisted numerous opportunities to move on to positions of greater responsibility and prestige, pending completion of this book. Now that the task is finished, her absence will be accompanied by a sense of irreplaceable loss.

Richard A. Levy, M.D., for his meticulously drawn, clear, and detailed illustrations, carried out while he was a resident in radiology at the University of Vermont School of Medicine.

Milne B. Hewish, Steven Strommer, and Juanita James for their superb photographic craftsmanship. There were times when, I know, I taxed the collective patience of these three with requests for "reshoots," but in retrospect, I hope that they realize that I have nothing but the greatest admiration for their professional abilities.

Peter de Vries, M.D., whose yeoman-like efforts in providing the embryological basis for Chapter 19 went far beyond the call of duty. Dr. de Vries spent weeks personally examining and re-examining hundreds of human embryos from collections both within and outside of the United States to ensure that his descriptions were verifiably accurate, consistent with modern and not outdated embryological concepts, and fresh rather than repetitious, oft-copied material from the past. Such a level of dedication has, I am sure, few parallels among contributors to textbooks.

One of my greatest regrets is that Dr. C. John Hodson did not live to see the publication of this book. Dr. Hodson, who was one of the founding fathers of uroradiology, was originally one of the associate editors of the text, and he had looked forward to contributing to it. Unfortunately, he died before he could set pen to paper, but his memory lives on in the indelible stamp he left on our current understanding of so many facets of renal physiology and renal disease. His influence is felt in many pages of this book.

The unsung heroine of this book is, without a doubt, my wife, Shanlee. Although the lot of any author's spouse is a lonely one, it seems to me that, in this case, the burden was unusually onerous. (Imagine, if you will, kitchen and dining room tables both so full of manuscripts, books, reprints, and the like that for the better part of 4 years there was barely room for one person to eat, let alone two. Innumerable other patience-trying episodes could be cited.) Yet, throughout it all, I received only the staunchest support and the most gratifying encouragement. (Yes, there were occasional requests to "hurry it up," but these were invariably good-natured, and after all, who could blame her?) Even when it must have seemed that a hermit's life by comparison would have been far more cheerful and lively, she rarely complained and never wavered in her enthusiasm for this project. Without her understanding and acquiescence, it would have been doomed from the start. A more patient and devoted partner could not be imagined.

> Words are but empty thanks.
> Women's Wit, Act V
> Colley Cibber

Contents

Volume 1

Volume 2

Volume 3

I INTRODUCTION TO UROLOGICAL IMAGING

HOWARD M. POLLACK
Editor

1 An Overview of Uroradiology

OLLE OLSSON

Diagnostic radiology has an important position in diagnostic and therapeutic procedures in the specialties of urology and nephrology. From the beginning of the clinical use of x-rays, the kidneys have attracted interest, first in the diagnosis of renal stones, and later to demonstrate calcified tuberculous lesions.

As the techniques of diagnostic radiology have developed, their use has been extended to an increasing number of areas. Anatomical views wider than those previously obtained by plain films were opened by pyelography and cystourethrography. The introduction of urography made morphological studies less invasive and led to very important physiological trends. Angiography was given an important role in the study of the renal arterial system, the inferior caval and renal veins, and also the renal parenchyma. In addition, by using angiography, it became possible to translate indirect, nonspecific roentgenological signs into direct, unequivocal signs, for instance in the diagnosis and differential diagnosis of renal tumor. Before the angiographic era, expansive renal lesions were diagnosed, in most cases, by changes in the shape of the kidney and the kidney pelvis. These mainly indirect approaches offered less definitive diagnoses; for example, different types of tumefactions could cause the same type of deformity. Angiography made it possible to demonstrate direct diagnostic signs, such as pathological vessels in tumors. These diagnostic possibilities were refined through the use of selective renal angiography as a method per se or as a complement to abdominal renal angiography. The introduction of image amplifiers facilitated and improved these procedures.

The extremely rapid development of computed tomography (CT), ultrasound, magnetic resonance imaging (MRI), digital radiography, and—the latest—digitization of the entire radiologic department, has made imaging increasingly important. Therapeutic procedures in diagnostic radiology (so-called interventional radiology) have expanded the field. These procedures include nephrostomy for emptying a dilated kidney pelvis, catheterization for drainage of abscesses and urinomas, nephrostomy for injection of stone-resolving agents, dilatation of stenoses

in ureters and arteries, embolization of tumors, and, perhaps most importantly, percutaneous extraction of renal and ureteral stones.

The rapid development and the technical demands of imaging procedures continuously underline the need for specialists to use these procedures responsibly. Specialists are also required to be proficient because of the versatility of the imaging procedures and, still more so, because of cost-benefit factors. For many of these techniques, a certain number of examinations per doctor per year are necessary to maintain an acceptable level of experience, and therefore certain of these procedures should be centralized in larger hospitals.

Many imaging procedures can replace one another, and the radiologist must have enough experience to decide which should be the basic procedure for each patient.

Close cooperation between the radiologist and the urologist and other referring colleagues is necessary. Contributing to this cooperation are daily conferences in the x-ray department at well-defined times, in order to demonstrate examinations, discuss results, consider the need for further examinations, and decide on interventions and controls.

All roentgen examinations should be made on requisition only. The requisition should contain all information necessary to plan the examination correctly. It should always be performed by, or under the supervision of, a radiologist. Examinations should not be conducted in a standardized manner, but should be varied according to the information desired regarding the particular patient and the specific problems that are known or that arise in the course of the examination.

The films should document the results of a competent examination. Diagnostic roentgenology does not mean studying schematically produced films. Although the film reading is important, more important is the actual production of films or other images that demonstrate characteristic changes leading to a single diagnosis. The examination thus must be performed in such a way that the various techniques result in *one* diagnosis and not in films that require guess work.

In a technical and technicological specialty such as diagnostic radiology, there is a risk that all interest will be concentrated on the equipment and performance and that the patient will be neglected or forgotten. This must *never* happen. The radiologist and other staff must have the patient at the center of their attention at every moment. Although it is understood that the films, being a translation of the patient, necessarily attract great interest, this does not excuse paying too little attention to the patient.

Certain personnel not directly involved with the patients, such as secretaries and viewing room assistants, should clearly understand that behind every film and every direct report is an unhappy and anxious fellow human being.

Priority should always be given to the parts of the procedure that reduce the time spent in the x-ray department and return the patient to the referring doctor with definite results. In certain procedures, such as CT and MRI, the patient is alone for a period of time, more or less "encapsulated" in the machinery. Under those circumstances every effort should be made to maintain good communication with the patient, who should be thoroughly informed of what will occur. For certain procedures, the best way to inform the patient is to have the radiologist, who is going to perform the procedure, see the patient in the hospital room the day before the examination. At this visit, the radiologist and the patient can get to know each other and discuss how and why the procedure is to be performed. This discussion will also facilitate the procedure itself. In many cases, however, the information can be given in the x-ray department in connection with the procedure.

It is also important to remember that patients must not be left alone during protracted procedures such as angiography or left lying on the examination table under ureteral compression. Furthermore, personnel talking and laughing outside the examination room, well within earshot of the patient, cannot be accepted within the bounds of medical ethics.

If these basic points are well considered, uroradiology will be an excellent example for all subspecialties in diagnostic radiology. If, besides these considerations, enormous amounts of knowledge and experience are added, the specialist will be a person in whom the patient can have confidence.

2

Medical–Legal Issues in Uroradiology

STEWART R. REUTER

Uroradiologists practice under the same legal rules as all other radiologists and most other physicians. However, some aspects of that general body of law, more than others, affect uroradiologists and other physicians who perform uroradiological procedures, and this chapter concentrates on the particular issues that have been of interest to uroradiologists. These include problems related to the standard of care, such as missed diagnoses; who should perform uroradiological procedures; some special problems of the interventional uroradiologist; and problems of informed consent, specifically, consent for intravenous injections of contrast agents.

STANDARD OF CARE

In this country, little attempt has been made to dictate what type of medicine physicians practice. In fact, physicians graduating from medical schools generally obtain unlimited licenses from State Boards of Medical Examiners to practice medicine and surgery. Thus, a physician possessing a state license may practice surgery, radiology, or urology, or any other form of medical care, without further training. A physician trying to do so may run into some external constrictions, such as the credentials committee of a hospital, but as long as he stays in an office setting, which may itself restrict the type of procedures that can be performed, physicians themselves determine, to a great extent, the level at which they practice their profession. If family practitioners or urologists feel comfortable interpreting radiographs and performing intravenous urograms, their practices will certainly include these procedures. They will bill for them and will be reimbursed by third-party carriers. Few restrictions have been placed on the type of medical care physicians in the United States can practice relative to their training, and at least one deterrent that keeps physicians from practicing beyond their level of skill and training is the fear of malpractice litigation. A malpractice action caused by a family practitioner missing a renal tumor or a urologist missing a bone lesion on an intravenous urogram may cause them to send their patients to radiologists in the future.

The Duty of the Physician Providing Care in Uroradiology and the Standard by Which the Care is to be Measured

The duty of the physician grows primarily out of the physician–patient relationship. For the radiologist this begins when the patient is accepted for an examination. The radiologist must exercise the same level of skill and care as other physicians performing or interpreting uroradiographic procedures under the same or similar circumstances. Legal negligence (also known as malprac-

tice), which may lead to a malpractice suit and a judgment against the physician, results from failure to meet this duty and when the failure is the proximate cause of an injury to the patient.

A physician is not a guarantor of the results of the treatment. Therefore, a bad result, although usually the starting point for a medical malpractice suit, does not prove that the physician has been negligent. The patient-plaintiff must show that the physician has not practiced to the level of acceptable standards of care in the community and that the physician's failure to do so was the cause of the maloccurrence. An exception to this rule occurs when the injury falls under the doctrine of *res ipsa loquitur*. If the injury is one that usually does not occur in the absence of negligence and the instrumentality that causes the injury is under the control of the defendant, the burden of proof shifts to the defendant to show that he or she was not negligent. Such situations occur occasionally in the surgical setting, for example, when a sponge or a broken needle is left in a patient. It is unlikely that the doctrine has application to procedures performed in the uroradiological setting.

Although this is all rather straightforward and well known to most physicians, special problems of interest to radiologists and nonradiologists alike occur in three particular areas: the missed diagnosis, the question of who is adequately trained to perform uroradiological procedures, and whether to proceed with a urogram on the patient who has had previous reactions to contrast agents.

The Missed Diagnosis

All physicians miss diagnoses. No one is perfect. However, if the missed diagnosis causes an injury to the patient, a lawsuit may well result. At the trial of the suit, the jury will attempt to determine whether or not the miss was negligent: that is, whether or not the physician was acting reasonably at the time he missed the diagnosis and if not, whether his failure to do so injured the patient. In general, the more complex the thought processes entering into a diagnosis, the more difficulty the jury has determining that the physician was negligent. Since lay jurors do not have the knowledge and experience to make judgments about medical procedures, expert witnesses are presented by both the plaintiff and the defendant to help the jury understand the medical questions. The jury takes this information into the jury room and uses it to determine whether or not the physician practiced according to an acceptable standard of care. However, the easier it is for the jurors themselves to understand the thought processes, the more likely they will use their own knowledge in making a decision. For example, contrast the internist who incorrectly diagnoses the cause of vague, intermittent abdominal pain with the radiologist who misses a hip fracture. Without dwelling on the obvious

3

difficulties for a juror in the former situation, a juror who can easily see the fracture line, particularly after the film has been magnified three or four times by the plaintiff's attorney, will have difficulty understanding how a radiologist, with years of training, could miss such an obvious diagnosis.

One must distinguish between a misdiagnosis and a missed diagnosis. With a misdiagnosis, the physician correctly visualizes the abnormality on the radiograph, but his or her mental processes lead to an erroneous conclusion as to the cause. With the missed diagnosis, the physician simply does not see the abnormality on the radiograph. The latter is the major problem for radiologists. Misdiagnosis involves a great deal of decision making and judgment, and the jurors must depend to a great extent on the opinion of the expert witnesses. With the missed diagnosis, the jury can generally see the abnormality once it has been pointed out to them, and if the finding is obvious, they will tend to disregard expert testimony that a reasonable physician, studying the radiograph, might have missed the abnormality. As observed by Berlin,[1] the diagnostic radiologist is more vulnerable to retrospective review of his work than other physicians. All jurors, knowing that pain and other symptoms come and go, may be willing to give the physician the benefit of a doubt in deciding whether an abnormality was present or absent at the time the physician recorded the examination and diagnosis. The presence or absence of a radiological abnormality is usually etched on the film for all time and for all to see.

All radiologists know that a significant number of diagnoses are missed.[2, 3] All radiologists should spend more time with each radiograph, should obtain as much clinical information about the patient as possible, and should work to develop effective search patterns to decrease the number of diagnoses that are missed. Beyond this, the American College of Radiology is working to educate the courts to realize that radiologists are not infallible[4] and is helping to provide expert witnesses to testify that missing some diagnoses on radiographs is not below the standard of reasonable care. Recently, two radiologists have been found by juries not to be negligent for having missed diagnoses.[5] Nonetheless, as a general rule, the more obvious the lesion missed or the more obvious the diagnosis missed, the more likely negligence will be found.

Who is Adequately Trained to Perform Uroradiological Procedures?

From a philosophical or "turf" point of view, the answer to this question depends very much upon who supplies it. However, from a legal point of view, anyone who has the skill, knowledge, training, or experience to meet the standard of care in the community for the performance or interpretation of uroradiological examinations may do so. In this sense the *community* is a legal term meaning the physicians who perform such procedures. Note that the above list of qualifications does not require a residency or a fellowship program in radiology. One can acquire the requisite training in a urology or other training program, or may simply acquire the experience over a number of years of performing such examinations. Many physicians are self-trained, progressing from simple to more complex procedures throughout their careers. Stated conversely, physicians who cannot meet the community standard of care should not perform or interpret uroradiological examinations, regardless of their specialty.

However, as a general rule of negligence law, persons must hold to the same experience, skill, and training as the group that they purport to represent. Thus, a family practitioner practicing plastic surgery will be held to the standard of the plastic surgeon; a urologist interpreting radiographs, to the standard of the radiologist. A family practitioner or urologist cannot escape an allegation of negligence for having missed a diagnosis by claiming inadequate training in that field. In fact, they may well find that the expert witness for the plaintiff in the case is a radiologist. Similarly, a radiologist may find that the plaintiff's expert witness is a urologist, if the judge decides the urologist has adequate experience in the interpretation of radiographs and that the individual's knowledge will help the jury. During the battle of the experts, the defense attorney for the radiologist will attempt to discredit the urologist's qualifications to interpret uroradiographs. However, a definite trend has developed in recent years to allow minimally qualified experts to testify in malpractice trials and allow the jury to decide the merit of the expert's testimony. This has resulted from the difficulty many plaintiffs have obtaining well-qualified expert witnesses. With a few exceptions, if the plaintiffs cannot find expert witnesses to testify as to the standard of medical care, they will not prevail.*[7]

The Patient Who Has Had a Previous Reaction to Contrast Agents

All physicians performing intravenous contrast studies are faced with this problem several times a year. Basically, this is also a "standard-of-care" question. Did the physician meet the standard of care of the community in making a decision to proceed with a repeat injection of contrast agent? Did that individual take appropriate precautions to mitigate the effects of a repeat reaction? Did he or she act within the standard of care of the community in treating any reaction that occurred? In deciding whether or not to proceed with a second intravenous injection of contrast agent, the physician must have knowledge of the nature of the first reaction and the current standard of practice nationwide regarding the amount and type of premedication generally used to prevent or ameliorate subsequent reactions. The reader is referred to Chapter 4 for a comprehensive discussion of contrast medium reactions and the standard of care in dealing with them.

The subject of contrast medium reactions raises the question of skin testing prior to the intravascular use of contrast medium. Unfortunately, the results of pretesting with subcutaneous injections of contrast agent have shown

---

*Expert witnesses are supposed to be completely objective, regardless of whether they are testifying for the plaintiff or defendant. However, the legal system is clearly adversarial and the parties to the suit are going to pick those expert witnesses whose testimony coincides most closely to their theory of the case, whether on the issue of negligence or on the issue of informed consent.

no significant correlation with the subsequent occurrence of a major reaction to the contrast medium. Therefore, no legal liability arises for failure to use skin testing. Certainly, there is no deviation from the standard of care in the community, because no one today uses skin testing. However, if a simple, effective, inexpensive, and reliable test were developed that might identify patients who might have severe reactions to contrast agents, a few state supreme courts would require that the tests be performed, regardless of the standard of the community. In such a situation, some courts reason—erroneously in the opinion of the author—that even nonphysicians can decide that the risk is so small and the benefit so great that the tests must be done as a matter of law.[6]

The availability of low osmolar and nonionic contrast agents has also changed the manner in which patients who have had previous reactions to contrast agents are treated. Although exact statistics are not yet available, it is clear that these new contrast agents cause a significantly lower level of reaction than conventional contrast agents and are therefore safer to use in patients who have had previous reactions. In a recent article on the legal aspects of contrast agents, I recommended that low osmolar and nonionic contrast agents should be used in patients who are at a higher risk of having a reaction than the general population.[6a] This group includes the patients who have had previous reactions. The recommendation was made that the at-risk group be defined liberally, that the radiologists and hospital formulate a policy statement related to the use of contrast agents in high-risk patients, and that the written policy be followed religiously. Because of the high cost of low osmolar and nonionic contrast agents, I do not recommend the use of these agents in all patients at this time. Although the courts may mandate this in the future, statistical information and the legal precedent to mandate such a change at this time are inadequate. Similar opinions have been expressed by others.[6b]

Radiologists who give an intravenous injection of contrast medium to a patient who has had a previous reaction may increase their exposure to a suit, but this does not necessarily increase their legal liability. That is, the very fact that an increased number of repeat reactions to contrast medium will occur in previous reactors indicates that these patients have a greater risk when they receive subsequent contrast agents. However, if the examination is definitely indicated, if the patient is given adequate doses of steroids and histamine blockers prior to the examination, if the appropriate equipment and drugs are available to take care of a reaction, and if the patient is appropriately treated following a reaction, no deviation from the acceptable standard of care has occurred and no legal liability should result. Although informed consent is discussed in the next section, it should be mentioned at this point that the radiologist's burden of disclosure increases in patients who have had previous contrast reactions, and the patient must be made aware of the increased chance of an anaphylactic reaction and death.

While on the subject of contrast agents and the standard of care, the author is impressed with the number of times a suit results because a contrast reaction occurs while the patient is unattended. This takes place because the radiologist or other physician injects a bolus of contrast medium, watches the patient for several seconds, and then leaves the room. The radiographer exposes the radiograph and leaves to develop the film. Then the patient has a hypotensive episode and is found unconscious when the technologist returns to take the next film. Delayed reactions to intravenous injections of contrast agents may occur up to 20 minutes after injection of the contrast medium and a reasonable standard of care should probably require that someone be present with the patient throughout the examination.

INFORMED CONSENT FOR URORADIOLOGICAL PROCEDURES

The bottom line of informed consent is simple consent.[25] Regardless of any state's specific rules concerning the information a patient must be given in order to allow an informed consent to a proposed procedure or treatment, all states require that the physician obtain the patient's simple consent before proceeding. This consent may be express or implied. Thus, patients may state that it is all right to proceed with the procedure, or, by some action such as holding out an arm for the injection of intravenous contrast medium, they may imply their consent. Because almost all uroradiological procedures are performed on conscious patients, it would be unusual to find a patient who has not, by some act, implied consent to the procedure.

The above rule requiring consent has an exception. All states have an implied consent doctrine to allow emergency treatment of patients who are unconscious or otherwise unable to give consent. If the patient is in a true emergency and delay would cause a deterioration in condition, and if a reasonable person under the same or similar circumstances would have given consent, consent will be implied. Thus, when we discuss consent, we are talking about nonemergent situations. If a true emergency exists, the physician is protected by the implied consent doctrine.

There are two settings in which consent must be obtained, but it need not be informed consent. The first occurs when the patient states that he or she does not want to know the complications. This is known as waiver and the physician can simply make a note in the chart to this effect, preferably cosigned by the patient, and no further information need be given. The second exception is known as the therapeutic privilege. If the information to be divulged about the procedure would be harmful to the patient, the physician need not provide such information. This is a reasonably narrow exception, however, and probably is limited to extremely severe mental anguish. Moreover, the use of such a defense in a malpractice trial sounds self serving, particularly if the plaintiff insists that, if he had been adequately informed of the risks and complications, he would have refused the procedure.

Physicians tend to use the therapeutic privilege when they fear that full disclosure of the risks and complications may frighten the patient from undergoing a needed elective procedure. In fact, the author has even heard physicians state that if a patient refused a needed procedure because they provided too much information about the risks, they might be liable. This is not the law in any state, and it is unlikely to ever become such. A court ruling in favor of the plaintiff in this situation would undermine the basic principle of informed consent, which encourages physicians to share as much knowledge as possible with the patient so that the patients can participate actively in decisions regarding their health care. On the other hand, courts have held that a physician's knowledge that an adequately informed consent would have caused the patient to reject the needed procedure is inadequate justification for the use of the therapeutic privilege. In a national survey of radiologists, Spring and colleagues found that less than 1% of patients refused contrast injections after being fully informed of the risks.[26, 27]

When a procedure or treatment is given to a patient without consent, this action constitutes civil battery, and the physician becomes liable for all of the damages that occur because of that battery. Most states have retained the battery theory for nonconsent to medical procedures, and a few states have retained the theory of battery for defective consents (such as lack of informed consent or consent from a patient who does not have the mental capacity to give consent). However, courts have never been comfortable with the legal theory of battery for lack of informed consent, because the stigma that attaches to an intentional tort should not apply to a physician who has negligently failed to give the patient adequate information about a procedure. Therefore, almost all states have moved to a negligence standard for evaluating the adequacy of the informed consent, some by statute, most by case law.

An interesting case illustrating how a radiologist can be trapped by not obtaining simple consent is *Gragg v. Neurological Associates*.[11] In *Gragg*, a neurologist was performing a cerebral arteriogram in the radiology department. Having a problem manipulating the catheter into the carotid artery, he requested help from the neuroradiologist, who came to the angiography room, put the catheter in the proper position, and left. The neurologist then injected the carotid artery, and the patient had a stroke. The patient sued the neurologist for negligence in performing the injection and the neuroradiologist for lack of consent.

The trial court found in favor of both defendants; for the neurologist because the plaintiff could not find an expert witness to testify that he had not met the standard of care, and for the radiologist because the judge accepted the radiologist's defense of the Good Samaritan statute.

The plaintiff appealed to the Georgia Court of Appeals, claiming that the court's use of the Good Samaritan statute to release the radiologist from liability was in error. The Court of Appeals agreed. Reversing the trial court judgment, the appellate court held that the difficulties experienced by the neurologist during the performance of the angiogram were not the type of emergency that the Good Samaritan statute was intended to cover. After the Court of Appeals decision, Mr. Gragg again filed his suit against the neuroradiologist, and the neuroradiologist moved for summary judgment. This time, the trial court denied his motion on the issue of consent.

Although the decision sounds "unjust" on the surface, it is technically correct from a legal point of view. Many of us have been in the neuroradiologist's shoes; however, it is important to remember that when a radiologist agrees to assist another physician who has obtained an appropriate consent for the procedure, the radiologist must introduce himself to the patient, request permission to assist, and place a note in the chart that such permission was granted.

Before moving to a more detailed discussion of the ramifications of informed consent to uroradiologists, a list of the elements of an action for negligent failure to obtain informed consent, all of which must be satisfied for the plaintiff to prevail, should be given. The actual information that must be transmitted to the patient varies from state to state but, in general, includes a description of the procedure to be done, the risks and complications of the procedure, alternative procedures that are available, and the risk to the patient of not having the procedure performed at all. These tend to be the material facts a patient should have in order to balance the pros and cons and decide whether or not to accept the procedure. If the patient-plaintiff can show that the information given was inadequate for a reasonable person to make a decision, the physician has breached his duty. However, remember that the plaintiff must also show causation, and this requirement may frequently be more difficult than showing the breach of the duty. The patient must show that if the information that was negligently omitted had been known, the patient would have rejected the procedure. Finally, the plaintiff must show that acceptance of the procedure without adequate knowledge resulted in an injury.

Several states require that consent to medical procedures be obtained in writing, signed by the patient, and witnessed by a neutral observer. In states without such requirements, a verbal consent and a written consent are equally valid. However, the physician, for his or her own protection, should make a note on the chart that the risks and complications and alternative procedures were explained to the patient. In fact, some attorneys prefer a vague description of the consent process in the chart signed by the physician because juries tend to believe the information written in patients' charts, unless it is clearly fraudulent. At the time of the trial, the physician's attorney can ask what risks and alternative procedures are usually divulged to the patient. Of course, the complication that occurred will likely be given. On the other hand, if a detailed listing of the complications does not include the complication that occurred, the physician faces a presumption that that specific complication was not revealed.

If the plaintiff can prove absence of informed consent, the defendant will be liable for the damages that flow from that lack of informed consent, including the injuries caused by the alleged, even if unproven, medical negligence in performing the procedure.

The Standards for Negligent Failure to Obtain Adequately Informed Consent

The various states have chosen among three legal standards for judging whether or not the amount of information given the patient was negligently inadequate. In increasing order of the amount of information required to be disclosed to the patient, these standards are: the reasonable physician standard, the reasonable patient standard, and the subjective patient standard. In addition, several states have passed statutes that regulate the information to be obtained; most of these are codifications of one of the preceding standards.

The reasonable physician standard focuses upon what information reasonable physicians under the same or similar circumstances would tell their patients about the procedures to be done. This requires expert testimony, since the lay juror has no idea about the standard of care of the physicians in the community. However, when a jurisdiction moves to the reasonable person standard, the focus becomes what a reasonable person would want to know under the same or similar circumstances to make a decision as to whether or not to accept a procedure. Under this standard expert testimony is generally not required, because the jury knows what a reasonable person would want to know, all jurors assuming they are reasonable persons themselves.

In recent years, informed consent has become an important part of medical malpractice litigation, more because of technical than substantive reasons. As pointed out in a recent Rand Corporation Report,[8] the progressive move away from the reasonable physician approach toward the reasonable patient approach for deciding whether or not consent obtained was negligently uninformed allows a plaintiff to get the case before a jury without an expert witness.

Oklahoma[9] uses the subjective patient standard. In most states the jury is asked to focus on what an abstract, objective patient-plaintiff would want to know to decide whether to accept or reject a procedure. In a subjective patient state, the jury focuses on what the specific patient would want to know. This is, in effect, an unworkable rule and places an unacceptable burden on the physician, since the plaintiff, at the time of the trial, will consider whatever piece of information that was missing from the physician's informed consent to be material. Physicians in these states must inform the patients of all potential risks and complications of the proposed procedure.

Each radiologist or other physician performing urora-diological procedures should be familiar with rules of that particular state regarding the amount and type of information that they must give the patients. Some 23 states now have consent statutes and, at the very minimum, every physician should be aware of the requirements of the appropriate state statute.

Consent for Intravenous Injections of Contrast Agent

One of the major questions facing uroradiologists is whether or not informed consent need be obtained for the intravenous injection of contrast agents and, if so, what complications must be disclosed.[26] Since we have little guidance from the courts or the legislatures to give a definitive answer, the answer to this question must be speculative. In the author's opinion, the answer depends upon the type of jurisdiction in which one practices. In the jurisdictions that use the reasonable physician approach, the physician should inquire as to whether or not his colleagues are informing patients about the risks and complications of intravenous injections and, if they are, what complications are being disclosed. In this type of jurisdiction the physicians, to a great extent, set their own standards, and if some physicians are giving the

patient information about the complications of intravenous injection of contrast agents, all should probably do so.

In the reasonable patient type of jurisdiction, all patients should be informed of the approximately 1 in 40,000 chance of death that accompanies the injection of ionic intravenous contrast agents, because every reasonable person would probably consider the chance of death to be material, even when its occurrence is low. What information is divulged beyond the possibility of death depends upon what the uroradiologist or physician determines would be material to an informed decision. As a general rule, materiality = incidence × severity. Therefore, the patient should probably be informed of all very common complications, such as the common allergic reactions, as well as death. As a practical procedural matter, patients who accept an intravenous contrast agent, knowing about the risk of death, should have a more difficult time showing that they would have rejected the procedure if they had been informed of a less severe complication.

In a recent case in Washington, a state that uses the reasonable person standard, an injection of contrast medium for an intravenous urogram resulted in thrombo-phlebitis.[12] Although this is an unusual complication in intravenous urography, it is listed as one of the complications that might be expected in the *Physician's Desk Reference (PDR)*.[13] In fact, some 11 complications of intravenous injection of contrast agent are listed in the *PDR*. The *PDR* has become as important to lawyers as it is to physicians, and every plaintiff's attorney has a copy in his office bookcase. The plaintiff claimed at the trial that the very fact that thrombophlebitis is listed as a potential complication in the *PDR* indicated that it should have been disclosed to the patient. At the trial, the jury found that the complication was not particularly severe and that its incidence was uncommon enough that a reasonable person would not necessarily want to know about it in making a decision to have an intravenous urogram. On appeal, the Washington Supreme Court agreed, stating that the *PDR*, although helpful to the physician in deciding what to tell the patient, is not determinative of what must be revealed.

In jurisdictions using the subjective standard,[9] the physician is in a difficult position and must reveal all potential risks and complications of intravenous urography. For the physicians in these states, the list in the *PDR* is a very useful guide as to what should be disclosed. Texas has codified informed consent for all radiological procedures and, by statute, the physicians need not inform the patients of the risks of intravenous injections of contrast agent, unless the patient asks.[14]

Who Can Give Consent to Medical Procedures?

The basic rule in all jurisdictions is that a competent adult patients or their legal representatives can consent to or reject medical procedures to be performed on themselves or their legal wards. Besides competent adult patients, however, physicians are frequently faced with minors or incompetent adult patients who do not have legal representatives. Almost all states have statutes that allow parents, adult brothers and sisters, and a list of other near relatives to give consent for the treatment of minors. However, few states have such statutes for incompetent adults. The definition of incompetency and the mental level required for a person to be competent varies from one type of decision making to another. In the informed consent context, however, competence requires the ability to understand the nature of the consent process and the ability to balance the pros and cons of the procedure and come to a rational decision as to whether or not to accept the procedure. This is a relatively high level of mentation and physicians are faced frequently with patients who do not have this level of mental capacity, particularly physicians who practice in public hospitals.

Who can give consent for such patients? In a few enlightened states, including Arkansas, Idaho, Maine, Maryland, Mississippi, North Carolina, and Utah, consent may be obtained from the spouse or specified near relatives by statute.[15] In Georgia and Louisiana the statutes allow substituted consent by spouses.[16] In all states, consent may be obtained from a legal representative, that is, a person who has the legal power to act on behalf of others. This includes guardians, conservators, and persons with a valid, durable power of attorney. In most states no statute exists to grant spouses or near relatives the legal right to give consent, although these are usually the persons to whom the physician commonly turns if a legal representative is not readily available. In a few jurisdictions, including the District of Columbia, California, Kentucky, Massachusetts, Missouri, Oklahoma, Tennessee, and Washington, courts have stated that spouses or near relatives can give substituted consent.[17] However, in Texas the Supreme Court has stated that the spousal relationship, in and of itself, does not confer the appropriate agency relationship to make such consent valid,[18] and New Mexico has invalidated a consent by an adult daughter.[19] If a state has no statutory or case law that gives a spouse or near relative the right to consent on behalf of an incompetent patient, the physician is best advised not to obtain substituted consent for such individuals. Rather, the physician should request that the hospital attorney get a court order or have a guardian ad litem appointed by the court of appropriate jurisdiction in the community. This usually can be done quickly.

Detailed Consent Forms

Another aspect of informed consent that has interested radiologists is the use of detailed consent forms. These forms give the patient, in writing, the necessary information about risks, alternative procedures, and so forth. They are certainly an excellent record of the information provided to the patient. They allow patients to read the information and formulate questions that they may want to ask the physician before consenting to the procedure. The patient's witnessed signature on the form indicates agreement to have the procedure performed with the knowledge of the complications, risks, and alternative procedures that are listed on the form. Unfortunately, however, the printed form indicates equally well the risks and complications about which the patient was not informed. This may become a problem if the patient develops one of those complications. Although the courts have not reviewed the validity of detailed consent forms in a radiological context, they have done so in other phases of medical practice. In these cases the courts have upheld the validity of the consent form as a documentation of what information the patient was given. In one case involving the experimental use of an artificial heart the detailed consent forms were a central part of the court's decision that the consent was an informed consent.[20]

Detailed consent forms are probably most useful in states using the reasonable person or subjective person standard. In the former type of jurisdiction, they should describe the procedures to be done in lay language and list all *material* risks, complications, and alternative procedures; in the subjective patient type of state they should probably list *all* complications and risks. The incidence of the complication should be supplied, if it is known. The consent should have a paragraph that invites the patient to ask the physician any further questions and should include a clause stating that the patient has read and understands the nature of the risks and complications. The signature should be witnessed by a disinterested party.

If detailed consent forms are used, they should not replace a discussion between the physician performing the procedure and the patient. Courts have been consistent in holding that the responsibility for obtaining the consent lies with the physician performing the procedure or treatment.[21] Therefore, the physician should have a discussion with the patient about the procedure, elaborating on the information on the detailed consent form. The consent form should be used simply as a documentation of what the patient was told, in case a complication or other problem related to the procedure leads to a lawsuit. The detailed written consent form should remove informed consent as an issue at the time of litigation if the complication that occurred was listed on the signed consent form.

LIABILITY OF RADIOLOGISTS FOR THE ACTS OF OTHERS INVOLVED IN URORADIOLOGICAL PROCEDURES

As the complexity of the procedure increases, the more technologists, nurses, and other personnel become involved in helping the radiologist perform the procedure. It is important that radiologists who receive the help of nurses and technologists recognize that, if they are present and supervising the nurses and technologists during the course of a radiological procedure, they may become the nurse or technologist's employer for that procedure.[22] This occurs under the rules of respondeat superior and the borrowed servant rule, even though the hospital hires the employees, fires them, and pays their salary. Without entering a long discussion of the legal theories behind such a rule, which certainly seems strange to most physicians, this is long established law. Therefore, just as the angiographer has the responsibility for checking that the technologist has loaded the appropriate contrast medium into the injector and set the appropriate injection factors, it is equally important that radiologists and physicians performing uroradiological interventional procedures understand and carefully control the activities of the technologists and nurses assisting them. A negligent act on the part of one of the nurses or technologists that occurs in the physician's presence may well be imputed to the physician.

The ultimate extension of this principle was embodied in the captain of the ship doctrine,[23] which held an operating surgeon liable for all of the negligent acts of hospital employees working in the operating room during the course of the operation. Although many jurisdictions have retreated from an express captain of the ship doctrine approach in the hospital, some have retained the rule. An appellate court in California recently reaffirmed the rule for that jurisdiction.*[24] Despite the general retreat from the arbitrary harshness of the captain of the ship doctrine, the rule that most jurisdictions have retained still places a great responsibility upon the supervising physician for acts of negligence by hospital employees that are committed in his presence.

Whether or not a physician is liable for a negligent injection of contrast medium by a nurse, technologist or other hospital employee in the physician's absence depends upon whether or not an agreement exists between the physician and the hospital. As a general rule, a physician can expect that hospital nurses and technologists will carry out the duties that are assigned by the hospital in a non-negligent manner. However, if an agreement, expressed or implied, allocates responsibility for supervision of the nurse or technologist in the performance of intravenous injections or any other procedures within the department to the physician, the hospital will likely be able to shift its liability to the physician under the borrowed servant rule. In other words, the physician has borrowed the nurse from the hospital and the nurse is that physician's employee for that procedure, even though the hospital pays the salary and has the power to hire and fire the nurse.

From the physician's point of view, the most important document to which the courts have looked to determine whether or not an agreement exists is the departmental Policies and Procedures Manual. Radiologists should actively participate in the formulation of departmental policies and procedures and should be careful not to accept the supervisory responsibility over hospital employee acts that they, in fact, cannot actively supervise. In general, courts have considered a detailed description of how the employee is to carry out a given act or procedure in the Policies and Procedures Manual as evidence that the hospital intended to retain control over that act.

References

1. Berlin L: Is a radiologic "miss" malpractice? An ominous example. AJR, 140:1031–1034, 1983.
2. Yerushalmy J: The statistical assessment of the variability in observer perception and description of roentgenographic pulmonary shadows. Radiol Clin North Am 7:381–392, 1969.
3. Lehr JL, Lodwick GS, Farrell C, et al: Direct measurement of film miniaturization on diagnostic accuracy. Radiology 118:257–263, 1976.
4. Resolution #13, approved at the 1983 annual meeting of the American College of Radiology.
5. Moses v Gaba, 435 So 2d 58 (Ala, 1983), Sawka v Prokopowycz, 306 NW 2d 354 (Mich App, 1981), reversed on other grounds.
6. Helling v Carey, 519 P 2d 981 (Wash, 1974).
6a. Reuter SR: The use of conventional vs. low-osmolar contrast agents: A legal analysis. AJR 151:529–531, 1988.
6b. Jacobson PD, Rosenquist CJ: The introduction of low-osmolar contrast agents in radiology: Medical, economic, legal and public policy issues. JAMA 260:1586, 1988.
7. Brent RL: The irresponsible expert witness: A failure of biomedical graduate education and professional accountability. Pediatrics 70:754–762, 1982.
8. Danzon PM: The Frequency and Severity of Medical Malpractice Claims. Santa Monica, The Rand Corporation, 1982, p 28.
9. Scott v Bradford, 606 P 2d 554 (Okla, 1983).
10. Simpson v Dickson, 306 SE 2d 404 (Ga App, 1983), Ga Code §31-9-6.
11. Gragg v Neurological Associates, 263 SE 2d 496 (Ga App, 1979).
12. Smith v Shannon, 666 P 2d 351 (Wash, 1983).
13. Physicians Desk Reference. Oradell, Medical Economics, Inc, 1983, p 3031.
14. Tex Rev Civ Stat Ann, art 4590i §6.01 to 6.07 (Vernon, 1983).
15. Ark Stat §§82-363 (h)(i)(j)(k), Idaho Code, §39-4303, Me Rev Stat Ann, tit 24, §2905 (1), Md Ann Code, Health—General §20-107 (d)(e), Miss Code Ann §41-41-3, NC Gen Stat §90-21.13(a), Utah Code Ann §78-14-5(4)(b)(d).
16. Ga Code Ann §31-9-2(a)(3), La Rev Stat §40:1299.53(c) (West).
17. Canterbury v Spence, 464 F 2d 772, 789 n 92 (DC Cir, 1972), Cobbs v Grant, 502 P 2d 1, 10 (Cal, 1972), Haywood v Allen, 406 SW 2d 721, 722 (Ky App, 1968), In the Matter of Spring, 399 NE 2d 493, 497 n 5 (Mass, 1979), Steele v Woods, 327 SW 2d 187, 198 (Mo, 1959), Murray v Van Devander, 522 P 2d 302, 304 (Okl App, 1974), Campbell v Oliva, 424 F 2d 1244, 1251 (6th Cir, 1970), Grannum v Berard, 422 P 2d 812, 814 (Wash, 1967).
18. Gravis v Physicians and Surgeons Hosp of Alice, 427 SW 2d 310, 311 (Tex, 1968).
19. Eis v Chestnut, 627 P 2d 1244, 1247 (NM App, 1981).
20. Karp v Cooley, 493 F 2d 408 (5th Circ, 1974), rehearing denied, 1974.
21. Halley v Birbiglia, 458 NE 2d 710, 716 (Mass, 1983), Nelson v Patrick, 293 SE 2d 829, 832 (NC App, 1982).
22. Davis v Potter, 2 P 2d 318 (Idaho, 1931), Gray v McLaughlin, 179 SW 2d 686 (Ark, 1944).
23. McConnell v Williams, 65 A 2d 243 (Pa, 1949).
24. Schultz v Mutch, 211 Cal Rptr 445 (Cal App, 1985).
25. Reuter, SR: An overview of informed consent for radiologists. AJR 148:219, 1987.
26. Spring DB, Akin JR, Margulis AR: Informed consent for intravenous contrast-enhanced radiography; a national survey of practice and opinion. Radiology 152:609–613, 1984.
27. Spring DB, Winfield AC, Friedland GW, et al: Written informed consent for IV contrast-enhanced radiography: Patients' attitudes and common limitations. AJR 151:1243, 1988.

---

*Note that this opinion is by a court of appeals and that another California Court of Appeals, using a more thoughtful and more contemporary analysis, has expressly rejected the doctrine [Truhitt v French Hospital, 180 Cal Rptr 152 (Cal App, 1982)]. If *Schultz* is appealed, the California Supreme Court must decide what the rule for the state will be.

Radiation Protection

JOHN HALE

In uroradiology, as in any discipline that uses radiation as an agent in diagnostic studies or in therapy, the possible deleterious effect of radiation should be kept in mind and methods for minimizing the radiation dose should be pursued.

Two classes of individuals are at risk in a radiological procedure: the patients and the members of the staff performing the examination. There are several useful review papers on this subject, especially in regard to uroradiology.[20, 31, 38] The issue of patient protection in diagnostic radiology has been specially addressed by the International Commission on Radiological Protection.[25] In addition, the National Council on Radiation Protection and Measurement has published a handbook on medical radiation exposure of pregnant and potentially pregnant women.[33]

In this chapter, methods for estimating pertinent organ dose consequent to radiation exposure will be considered for patients and staff. First, however, we must review the concepts of radiation exposure and dose.

DEFINITIONS

Radiation exposure is the parameter that is most often measured to quantify the attributes of an x-ray beam. Photons comprising an x-ray beam passing through air can transfer energy to the air molecules by the classical photoelectric effect or Compton interactions. In the photoelectric effect, the entire photon energy is transferred to a photoelectron. In a Compton interaction, part of the photon energy is transferred to a Compton electron, and the remainder is transferred to a Compton scattered photon. These high-speed electrons produce ionized air molecules in a device called an ionization chamber. When this chamber is connected to an electronic device called an exposure meter, the charge carried by these ions can be measured. This quantity is called *exposure*. To quantify this concept, a unit called the roentgen (abbreviated R) has been defined. One roentgen is the release of 2.54×10^4 coulombs of electrical charge per kilogram of air.

The second characteristic of an x-ray beam that is important in radiation protection is the penetrating power of the beam. This is usually measured by interposing sheets of metal called filters, which are ordinarily made of aluminum, in the x-ray beam between the x-ray tube and the ionization chamber. The response of the exposure meter is noted as the filtration is increased, and a plot is made to estimate the thickness of aluminum necessary to reduce the meter response to one-half of its initial value. This is called the half value layer (HVL), and in diagnostic radiology it is usually specified in millimeters of aluminum.

When an x-ray beam enters the body, the same physical processes already described govern the interactions of the x-ray photons with the cell molecules to transfer energy

from the photons to the cells. A measure of the amount of energy transferred to the body is called *dose*. Dose is measured in rads (1 rad = 0.01 joules of energy absorbed from the x-ray beam per kilogram of tissue) or grays (1 gray [Gy] = 1.0 joule/kg). The biological effect of the radiation beam is related to the distribution of dose in the body of the individual.

The ability of an x-ray beam to form an image also depends on the absorption mechanism. Compared with soft tissue, the x-ray beam will interact more strongly with bone (because it has a high density and atomic number) and less strongly with lung tissue (because it is less dense). The spatial pattern of the x-ray beam emerging from the patient will reflect this differential attenuation of the relatively few photons (1% for the abdomen to 10% for the chest) that travel through the patient without an atomic interaction. When this spatial distribution of photons interacts with an image recorder, such as film in an x-ray cassette or the input phosphor of an image intensifier tube, the pattern, when suitably processed, forms a visual image that can provide useful diagnostic information about the patient, if it is interpreted correctly.

A direct and straightforward relationship exists between exposure (R) and dose (rads). This derivation is contained in elementary textbooks. The conversion factor, rads/R, depends on the atomic number and density of the absorbing tissue and on the effective energy of the photon beam. For muscle and conventional diagnostic x-ray beams, the conversion factor is 0.92 rad/R.

In some situations—for workers in nuclear power reactors, who receive their dose from neutrons, for example—account must be taken of dose from radiation other than photons. A new concept is introduced called dose equivalent (H). Dose equivalent is measured in rems, the dose in rads times a quality factor (Q), or in sieverts (Sv), the dose in grays times the quality factor. For medical x-ray beams Q is defined as 1, so that the dose in rads is numerically equivalent to the dose equivalent in rems. The reports from companies that process film badges are stated in rems.

ESTIMATING PATIENT ORGAN DOSE: RADIOGRAPHIC MACHINES

Use of "Typical Examination Data"

A fairly large number of reports are available in the literature on patient organ doses for typical examination techniques. A review of data relevant to uroradiological procedures is shown in Tables 3–1 and 3–2. The organs of concern regarding possible genetic deleterious effect are the gonads. For somatic deleterious effects, the principal worry is induction of leukemia, so the bone marrow is the organ of concern.

These various compilations are useful for giving students, for instance, examples of the gonadal and bone marrow dose consequent to "typical" technical factors, patient sizes, film/screen combinations, and examination procedures. These data, however, cannot be applied to a particular installation because of the wide variation of these technical factors. Shrimpton and colleagues[47] studied patient doses in a sample of 25 hospitals in England and showed a standard deviation amounting to almost 200% in some studies. For intravenous urograms, for example, they report these organ doses: ovaries, 0.358 rad ± 95%; testes 0.434 rad ± 184%; and red bone marrow, 0.19 rad ± 81%. Maillie and associates[29] showed that entrance exposure must be varied over wide limits to compensate for changes in patient thickness, because the exit exposure must be kept about the same to produce appropriate film densities. Also these variations depend on the operating potential of the x-ray tube. Many of the older dosage estimates were arrived at before the development of rare earth screens. Because of this and other technological developments the more recent publications no doubt reflect a truer picture of current radiation exposure than do older studies.

Frequently, a more accurate and specific estimate of organ doses is required. If a patient discovers that she was pregnant at the time of a recent examination, for example, it is incumbent on the institution to make a reasonably accurate estimate of the fetal dose for that patient.

To make these estimates, data are needed about the entrance surface exposure and the consequent dose to organs of interest.

Entrance Surface Exposure (ESE)

Typical exposures at skin surface for a variety of diagnostic examinations have been tabulated, for example, by Rogers[40] and the United Nations Scientific Committee on the Effects of Atomic Radiation. These may also be calculated by data provided by Edmonds.[8]

Obtaining Data for Calculating Entrance Surface Exposure

It is preferable to use data specific to each radiographic unit. The annual calibration of each radiographic unit, which is required by the Joint Commission on Accreditation of Hospitals (JCAH), provides the first part of the experimental data required to estimate patient organ doses from procedures on patients for which a particular x-ray machine was used. In particular, the specific exposure rate (SER), in mR/mAs at 1 meter from the focal spot, should be measured at an established x-ray tube potential: 100 kV peak is recommended. The tube current station chosen for this measurement should be the one ordinarily used for patient studies with this unit. Then the HVL (and probably the tenth-value layer) should be measured. By knowing the SER and the HVL, it is possible to use published data[17, 30, 33] to (1) estimate the total filtration in the x-ray beam and (2) to estimate SER and HVL at any other tube potential.

From these data, the ESE rate for any patient thickness can be calculated by using the inverse square law.

Measuring the Exposure Time

A few installations may still use exposure technique systems that specify the combination of tube potential (kVp), tube current (mA), and the exposure time (seconds, s) as a function of patient thickness for a variety of different radiographic studies. In calculating ESE for these installations it is necessary only to multiply the ESE rate by the radiographic exposure specified, as a function of patient thickness.

For most contemporary units, however, the exposure system is determined by the automatic exposure control (AEC) system. For these units, a minimal calibration protocol must include calibration of the AEC.

We have found that a convenient way to calibrate the AEC is to simulate the attenuation and scattering of a phantom patient with aluminum filters placed in good geometry near the x-ray tube. The exposure that the AEC requires is measured with an ionization chamber; its required exposure time can be measured with some ionization chambers or, alternatively, with an independent detector. We use a lithium drifted silicon semiconductor detector and measure the exposure time with a storage oscilloscope having a calibrated time base.[1]

These measurements should be made under conditions simulating clinical use, and because of the difference in atomic number in geometry, it is essential to calibrate carefully the relationship between the aluminum filter and a soft-tissue phantom. In 1973, we published conversion data for single-phase generators.[14] In 1984, we published data for three-phase generators.[18]

Some of the newer solid-state generators indicate directly the exposure time used for various patient-simulating filters and AEC timed patient exposures.

Calculating the ESE

Finally, the ESE for the examination of a patient with a particular radiographic machine is found by multiplying the ESE rate by the exposure time appropriate for that patient.

Estimating Patient Organ Dose Using Entrance Surface Exposure

Use of Organ Dose Tables

Organ dose tables for number of radiographic projections have been calculated by Rosenstein using Monte Carlo techniques for both adults[41] and children.[42] The tables for adults have been verified experimentally by Gray and coworkers.[15] Tables for projections of interest in uroradiology are shown in Table 3–2 and 3–3.

The input data required are the ESE and the HVL of the x-ray beam. The tables give the ratio of the organ dose (in rads) to the ESE (in mR) for a variety of target organs and projections.

These tables apply only to "average-size" patients.

Use of Tissue–Air Ratio Tables

When data are available for the geometrical factors appropriate to a particular patient, it is preferable to

Table 3–1. Typical Organ Doses for Uroradiological Examinations

Date of Report	Examination	Patients	Mean Dose (rad) or Exposure (R) FEMALE GONADS	MALE GONADS	BONE MARROW	Reference Number	Technical Factors
		Children	94% <0.2	95% <0.3		11(a)	Summary of 10 reports 1957 to 1969.
1970	IVU	500 children	0.04 to 0.06	0.025 to 0.04		11(b)	70 kVp, 2-mm Al filter, 2.3 films/exam. Recommends gonadal shield for boys.
	VCU	51 children	0.20 to 0.30	0.03 to 0.04		11(c)	II exposure rate 5 μR/s; 4.1 spot films/exam; 3.2 minutes fluoro time.
1974	VCU	30 children 23 F, 7M	2 to 4 yr 0.6 / 10 to 14 yr 1.5	2 to 4 yr 0.49 / 10 to 14 yr 1.0		9	Thermoluminescent dosimeter (TLD) measurements in rectum (F) or scrotum (M); 4.5 minutes fluoro time, 10 films.
1975	IVP	50 children	2 to 4 yr 0.13 / 10 to 14 yr 0.20	2 to 4 yr 0.05 / 10 to 14 yr 0.035		10	Fluoro used for 38 of 50 studies 60 kVp, 0.4 mA, 1 to 1.5 minutes; 6 large films; 70 kVp, AEC. Gonadal shields for boys. Fluoro made small contribution.
1976	VCU	53 children	0.4	0.04	0.04	44	TLD measurements. Cine 7.5 frames/s or 70 mm spot films. A risk/benefit analysis.
1980	VCU	50 children	2 to 4 yr 0.18 / 12 to 18 yr 0.62	2 to 4 yr 0.08 / 12 to 18 yr 0.08		27	TLD surface measurements; surface/organ from phantom measurements. Radiographic, 70 to 85 kVp; AEC fluoro, 50 to 100 kVp; 0.5 to 3 mA; 0.5-minute spot films, 73 to 78 kVp, AEC.
1981	IVU	Average 5-yr-old / 11-yr-old	0.034 / 0.034	0.010 / 0.035	0.019 / 0.037	16	TLD measurements; 70 kVp, 3-mm Al total filter; 14 × 17-in films. 1977: Primary = 4.9 films/exam; control = 3.2 films/exam. Gonadal shields for boys. Bone dose calculated. 1977–78 data shown here. Authors demonstrate a 60% to 80% dose reduction from a similar study in 1973 with a 100 speed film/screen system. A risk/benefit analysis.
	VCU	Primary 5-yr-old	0.025	0.077	0.015		
		11-yr-old	0.025	0.21	0.036		
		Control 5-yr-old	0.010	0.028	0.008		
		11-yr-old	0.90	0.072	0.015		

Table 3–1. Typical Organ Doses for Uroradiological Examinations *Continued*

Date of Report	Examination	Patients	Mean Dose (rad) or Exposure (R)			Reference Number	Technical Factors
			FEMALE GONADS	MALE GONADS	BONE MARROW		
1970	IVU	Adults	80% <0.3	80% <0.2		11(d)	Summary of 32 reports, 1937 to 1968.
1984	Percutaneous Nephrostolithotomy	60 adults 42M, 18F	0.58 Surface	0.16		4	C-arm fluoroscopy 2.7 to 5.0 rad/minute, 24-minute fluoro time.
1984	KUB	1970 nationwide evaluation of x-ray trends	0.26	0.016	0.048	13(a)	KUB 1.7 films, IVU 5.5 films.
	IVU	Exposure data	0.64	0.049	0.12		
	KUB		0.22	0.10	0.15	13(b)	KUB 1.6 films, IVU 5.3 films.
	IVU		0.59	0.21	0.42		
1986	IVU	357 adults	0.36	0.43	0.19	47	Survey of 20 hospitals; 8.2 radiographs/study; 27% of exams included tomography; 3.2 minutes fluoro. Large variation among hospitals.
1986	VCU		0.013	—	—	55	TLD intrarectal and intravaginal measurements from fluoroscopy (4.25 min) plus 100-mm films (ave. 26 films). Fluoro dose rate 1.3 mr/min. At 90 kV, dose from one 100-mm exposure equaled dose from 13.1 sec of fluoroscopy at 100 kV, midline measurements.

Note: According to the calculations of Rosenstein[41, 42]:

	Examination	HVL mm Al	Projection	Ratio Bone Marrow Dose/Ovary Dose
Adult	Pelvis	3.0	A–P	0.17
			Lateral	0.45
	Abdomen	3.0	A–P	0.19
			Lateral	0.67
Child, 1 yr	Abdomen	2.5	A–P	0.38
Child, 5 yr	Abdomen	2.5	A–P	0.27

Table 3–2. Organ Dose (mrad) for 1000 mR Entrance Skin Exposure (Free-in-Air)[41]

Pelvis; Lumbopelvic

Conditions:
SID—102 cm (40 in)
Film size = field size—see projection
Entrance exposure (free-in-air)—1000 mR

Projection:
Pelvis, lumbopelvic
43.2 cm × 35.6 cm (17 in × 14 in) AP
35.6 cm × 43.2 cm (14 in × 17 in) LAT

BEAM QUALITY		DOSE, mRAD					
HLV (mm A1) ⟶		1.5	2.0	2.5	3.0	3.5	4.0
Testes	AP	41	60	78	94	109	123
	LAT	9.6	16	23	30	39	47
Ovaries	AP	98	151	206	262	318	374
	LAT	19	34	52	73	97	123
Thyroid	AP	*	*	*	*	*	*
	LAT	*	*	*	*	*	*
Active bone marrow	AP	12	20	32	47	66	88
	LAT	9.4	16	23	33	44	57
Embryo (uterus)	AP	142	212	283	353	421	486
	LAT	13	25	39	56	75	97

Abdominal

Conditions:
SID—102 cm (40 inches)
Film size = field size—35.6 cm × 43.2 cm
14 in × 17 in
Entrance exposure (free-in-air)—1000 mR

Projection:
Retrograde pyelogram, KUB, barium enema, lumbosarcral spine, IVU, renal arteriogram

BEAM QUALITY		DOSE, mRAD					
HVL (mm A1) ⟶		1.5	2.0	2.5	3.0	3.5	4.0
Testes	AP	6.5	11	16	22	28	34
	PA	2.7	4.9	7.9	12	16	22
	LAT	0.8	1.7	2.9	4.3	6.0	8.0
Ovaries	AP	97	149	203	258	313	367
	PA	60	100	146	198	255	317
	LAT	18	33	50	70	93	118
Thyroid	AP	*	*	*	*	*	*
	PA	0.02	0.06	0.1	0.2	0.4	0.5
	LAT	*	*	*	*	*	*
Active bone marrow	AP	13	22	33	48	66	88
	PA	50	74	102	134	170	209
	LAT	8.9	15	22	31	41	54
Embryo (uterus)	AP	133	199	265	330	392	451
	PA	56	90	130	174	222	273
	LAT	13	23	37	54	71	91

*< 0.01 mrad.

Table 3–3. A–P Abdomen—Organ Dose (mrad) for 1 R Entrance Exposure (Free-in-Air)

		Source-to-Image Receptor Distance (SID) and Field Size					
		NEWBORN		1-YEAR OLD		5-YEAR OLD	
Source-to-image receptor distance (SID) (centimeters [inches])		102 [40]		102 [40]		102 [40]	
Field size at image receptor (centimeters [inches])							
Collimated to body part		13 × 13 [5.1 × 5.1]		18 × 21 [7.1 × 8.3]		23 × 30 [9.1 × 11.8]	
Collimated to film size		20 × 25 [8 × 10]		25 × 30 [10 × 12]		28 × 36 [11 × 14]	

Organ Dose (mrad/R)

Beam quality (HVL, mm Al) ⟶		2.0		2.5		3.0	
		BODY PART	FILM SIZE	BODY PART	FILM SIZE	BODY PART	FILM SIZE
Collimation ⟶							
Testes	Newborn	86	910	144	1000	152	1120
	1-year	(105)	(1070)	(105)	(1070)	(105)	(1070)
	5-year	(125)	(1070)	(125)	(1070)	(125)	(1070)
Ovaries	Newborn	390	390	560	560	580	580
	1-year	270	270	370	370	400	400
	5-year	270	270	370	370	400	400
Thyroid	Newborn	(5)	(25)	(5)	(25)	(5)	(25)
	1-year	+	(9)	+	(9)	+	(9)
	5-year	+	(3)	+	(3)	+	(3)
Active Bone	Newborn	91	159	127	211	137	225
Marrow	1-year	69	99	100	140	112	151
	5-year	55	69	83	101	90	112
Lungs	Newborn	49	439	66	497	67	498
	1-year	35	227	48	255	55	290
	5-year	39	102	47	123	54	135
Total	Newborn	186	375	212	419	226	440
Body	1-year	167	263	196	305	210	323
	5-year	158	202	188	239	202	256

+ Indicates <0.01 mrad.

calculate the dose to the organ of interest using the tissue–air ratio (TAR) method. This approach to dosimetry is well described by Schulz and Gignac,[46] who also provide an example of applying the method to a problem of estimating fetal dose. It now appears that the best TAR data are those provided by Harrison.[22] The necessary input information is the target-film distance, the patient thickness, and the depth of the point of interest at which the dose determination is to be made from the entrance surface of the patient. The necessary radiological data are the exposure rate (mR/mAs), the current station (mA), and the exposure time (s) at a defined distance from the target of the x-ray tube. From these data and the geometry of the examination, the exposure in air at the level of the point of interest in the patient can be determined. The TAR tables, then, are appropriately entered to determine the dose (rads) at the point of interest in the patient.

ESTIMATING PATIENT ORGAN DOSE: FLUOROSCOPIC MACHINES

Review of the Literature

Little information about organ doses to patients undergoing fluoroscopic examinations with spot films is available. The classic papers from the Atomic Bomb Casualty Commission[49] give useful information about patient organ doses from upper gastrointestinal series and barium enemas. Tole[50] has attempted to measure doses

with TLD dosimeters and concludes "The problem of assessing organ doses from fluoroscopic examinations with a degree of accuracy comparable with that of radiographic dose remains unsolved. Uncertainties attributed to current method are probably greater than believed."

Hale and coworkers[19] have suggested another approach. They recommend making "free-in-air" measurements of the exposure rate from the fluoroscope and exposure from spot films. Because of the confined space between the table top of the fluoroscope and the image intensifier tower, and because it is necessary to use large field sizes for spot films, patient attenuation and scatter are simulated with very thin lead absorbers set just under the tower.

An ionization chamber can then be placed 20 cm above the table top, and when appropriate small corrections are made for forward scatter from the table top, a close approximation to a free-in-air measurement can be obtained. The foil thickness is changed to simulate varying patient sizes. The exposure times required by the AEC for spot films are measured at the same time.

The data obtained are used to estimate patient organ dose using the TAR approach that has previously been discussed. So far, however, this method has only been applied to double-contrast barium enema studies.

Extracorporeal Shock Wave Lithotripsy (ESWL)

Saunders and colleagues[45] have published a letter describing their results in measuring surface dose from a

Dornier lithotriptor using thermoluminescent dosimeters. For a series of 33 patients, they report a mean dose of 12 cGy (rad) for an average fluoroscopy time of 3.6 min and an average of 22 "snapshots" (a radiographic spot film resulting in a video image). They believe that these doses are comparable to those received from other high-dose x-ray procedures, such as cardiac catheterization. These results have been confirmed by others.[5a, 28, 52] An excellent review of the subject has been provided by Glaze and associates,[12] while Pollack describes some practical suggestions to improve visualization and reduce radiation exposure during ESWL.[37]

Percutaneous Nephrostolithotomy (PCNL)

Using a mobile C-arm fluoroscope, Bush and co-workers[4] determined the radiation doses to patients undergoing PCNL and found them to be as follows (average): testis, 120 mrem; ovary, 440 mrem; dorsolumbar skin (small field), 25 rem. They concluded that the gonadal and skin doses were comparable to those delivered during excretory urography or angiography.[4, 5]

ESTIMATING PATIENT ORGAN DOSE: COMPUTED TOMOGRAPHY AND CONVENTIONAL TOMOGRAPHY

Computed Tomography (CT)

Wagner and coworkers[54] made measurements of dose on the axis and near the anterior surface of reasonable anthropomorphic phantoms representing average and heavy patients. They used state-of-the-art CT machines to put upper and lower limits of dose to the conceptus for a variety of slice thicknesses and number of slices. Typical results are 5.0 rad (surface) to 3.3 rad (axis) for an average-size patient (25 × 30 cm) examined with 10 contiguous 1-cm slices at 120 kVp and 400 mAs. Conceptus dose depends strongly, of course, on patient size and the location of the conceptus in the pelvis. The authors caution that their results should only be used as guidelines for patient management.

Each CT machine, however, must be calibrated at least once a year to comply with the recommendation of the JCAH. Currently, the preferred measuring technique is to use an ionization chamber designed to measure the multiple scan average exposure (MSAE),[26, 29a] using plastic phantoms to simulate the abdomen and head. This machine and specific data should be used with Wagner's data[54] to better estimate the conceptus dose for a particular patient.

Conventional Tomography

There is little information in the literature providing organ doses that are consequent to conventional tomographic studies. The experimental problem is difficult to generalize, because added to the usual physical factors

related to exposure are the tomographic parameters of fulcrum level and tube travel pattern and length. The thorough investigation of Stieve[48] should be consulted for further information.

PERSONNEL EXPOSURE AND ORGAN DOSE

Regulatory Guides

Many agencies have established what are called "maximum permissible dose" limits. The Nuclear Regulatory Commission (NRC) requires observance of these limits as a condition of receiving a license to use radioactive materials.[7] In the United States, the National Council on Radiation Protection and Measurements (NCRP) has published somewhat more detailed advisory recommendations.[34] The International Commission on Radiation Protection (ICRP) uses the same numerical values and extends its concern to the assessment of risks consequent to exposure.[23] In addition, many states have enacted radiation control regulations.

Fortunately, the basic dose-limiting recommendations and rules are nearly all the same. A summary of the levels of immediate concern in medical radiology is shown in Table 3–4. It seems appropriate to follow the Federal Radiation Council and to refer to these as Radiation Protection Guides (RPG). The intent of these agencies was to set advisory dose limits for radiation workers that would carry an "acceptable" level of risk of deleterious effect to the individual (somatic risk) or to future generations (genetic risk).[24]

Exposure Patterns from Patients Being Examined Radiologically

Basic Physics

Exposure to operating personnel during radiological examinations is from Compton scattered x-rays. Scattered x-rays produce two deleterious effects in radiology: Those that emerge sideways from the patient cause exposure to operating personnel; those that are only slightly deflected may travel on to interact with the image-detecting apparatus, where they reduce contrast because they do not

Table 3–4. Current NCRP Dose Limits

Maximum Permissible Dose Equivalent for Occupational Exposure	
Combined whole body occupational exposure	
Prospective annual limit	5 rems in any 1 year
Retrospective annual limit	10 to 15 rems in any 1 year
Long-term accumulation	(N − 18) × 5 rems, where N is age in years
Skin	15 rems in any 1 year
Hands	75 rems in any 1 year (25/qtr)
Forearms	30 rems in any 1 year (10/qtr)
Other organs, tissues, and organ systems	15 rems in any 1 year (5/qtr)
Fertile women (with respect to fetus)	0.5 rem in gestation period

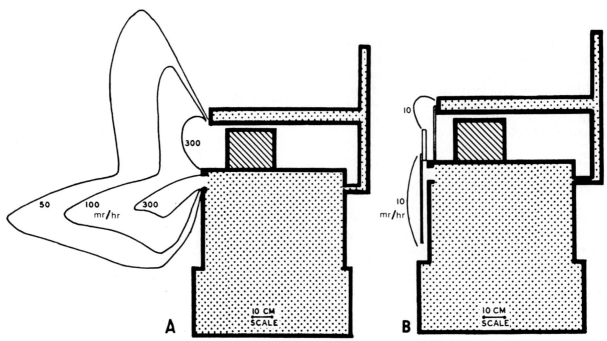

Figure 3–1. *A,* Isoexposure curves (mR/hr) in transverse plane through fluorescent screen of typical fluoroscope. Factors are 85 kVp, 5 mA, HVL 3 mmAl. Field area is 10 × 10 cm. Phantom is 20 × 20 × 20 cm. *B,* Isoexposure curves of same fluoroscope showing reduction of scattered radiation after addition of lead rubber curtain and Bucky slot cover.

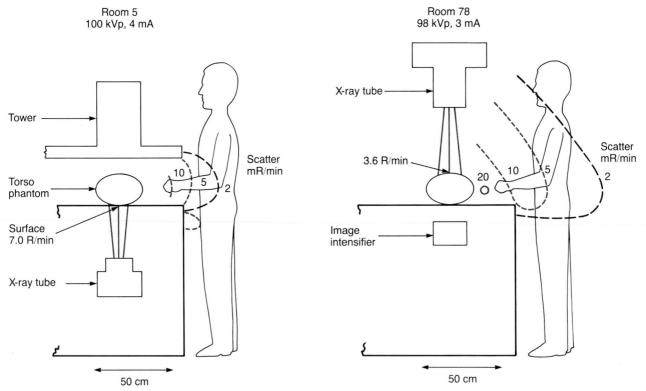

Figure 3–2. *A,* Isoexposure curves from a conventional under-the-table tube fluoroscope (mR/min). Phantom is a Rando torso phantom. Factors are as shown. *B,* Isoexposure curves from a fluoroscope designed with an over-the-table tube. Note the increased exposure to the hands, the torso, and especially the head and neck.

provide information about patient anatomy and tend to fog the image. Thus, using the smallest feasible x-ray field reduces the dose to the patient and personnel and, at the same time, improves image quality.

The magnitude of the x-rays emitted laterally from vertical x-ray beams is drastically reduced, however. Typically, the radiation scattered from a patient at right angles to the useful x-ray beam produces an exposure at 1 m from the central axis of the x-ray beam that is about 0.1% of the ESE.

A typical examination of the pelvis, for example, might have an ESE of 1000 mR. The exposure to an individual at 1 m, then, would be about 1 mR. The inverse square law applies remarkably well. If the individual were to step three paces backwards just before the exposure, so that he was 3.2 m from the central ray of the x-ray beam, the exposure would be reduced by an additional factor of 10 to 0.1 mR.

Ordinarily, however, operating personnel should observe the radiographic procedure from behind the structural protective barrier that must be provided for all fixed x-ray installations.

Consider an example in fluoroscopy, in which the typical ESE rate for an abdominal examination is about 3000 mR/min. Exposure at the table side, approximately 0.5 m from the central ray of the x-ray beam, would be about

$$3000 \times 0.001 \times (1/0.5)^2 = 12 \text{ mR/min}$$

The attenuation of the x-ray beam by the lead apron that the fluoroscopist must wear will reduce the exposure to the individual's trunk by another factor of approximately 10 to about 1 mR/min, even if the lead drape on the image intensifier tower has been removed.

In the section on personnel monitoring, we will discuss how to convert surface exposures, which are recorded on monitor badges, to organ doses of interest in the individual.

Description of Exposure Patterns

Two-dimensional patterns of exposure rates in the vicinity of fluoroscopes have been measured and published by many authors. Usually these patterns are in a plane perpendicular to the floor and to the fluoroscopic table through the vertical axis of the x-ray beam. These patterns are useful for illustrative and teaching purposes. However, they cannot be used quantitatively in radiation protection work, because for each examination it is also necessary to know the average number of minutes of fluoroscopic-beam on-time.

Some examples of exposure patterns are shown here. In Figure 3–1, for instance, the effect on reducing the exposure rate that results from the lead fabric drape on the image intensifier tower and the cover on the Bucky slot is dramatically shown. Clearly, these radiation shielding devices should be used whenever possible during fluoroscopic examinations.

Figure 3–2 contrasts the exposure rate patterns from a typical, traditional under-table tube fluoroscope (A) with an over-table tube fluoroscope (B). The exposure rates from the over-table installation are much higher, especially to the head and neck, because considerable shielding is provided by the structural steel in the table when the x-ray tube is below. Units of this type, which were designed primarily for use as remote control installations, are provided with most cystoscopic-fluoroscopic units: their use should be accompanied by careful attention to the precepts of radiation protection.

It is interesting to note that published exposure rate patterns do not provide information about the additional exposure to personnel that results from spot film, cine radiographic, or digital radiographic examinations. This additional information can easily be obtained. Figure 3–3, for example, shows the exposure rates from a fluoroscope, in mR/min and the exposure, in mR/image from a fluoroscopic/digital radiographic unit with an under-table tube design.

These data, however, are not immediately useful in radiation protection calculations. It is also necessary to have information about the average size of the patients

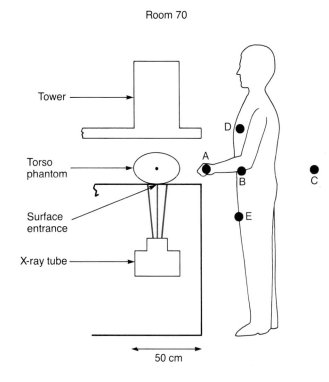

Room 70

	Fluoro	Digital image
X-ray tube	120 kVp 2 mA	77 kVp 800 mA 0.22 s
Surface entrance	1.8 R/min mR/min	0.72 R/image mR/image
A	10.7	2.3
B	2.3	0.5
C	0.8	0.2
D	0.9	0.2
E	1.4	0.3

Figure 3–3. Scattered radiation data from an installation used for fluoroscopy and digital radiography.

and the average number of images recorded per examination.

Personnel Monitoring

All "radiation workers" must be issued a monthly film badge. According to regulations, radiation workers are workers who are reasonably likely to be exposed to as much as 25% of the levels recommended in the Radiation Protection Guide. In our department, there are no exposures of this magnitude, except to the hands of interventional radiologists. We believe, however, that it is important, for morale and for legal reasons, to issue film badges to all individuals who work in the vicinity of x-ray apparatus. Accordingly, we issue film badges to everyone except office workers and file room personnel. These "body" badges are worn either at waist level or are attached to the collar.

Furthermore, individuals who must work in fluoroscopy rooms when the tube current is turned on are issued a second "collar" badge. These individuals are required to wear lead protective garments. Their body badges are worn underneath the lead protective garment at waist level to monitor bone marrow and gonadal dose. The collar badge is worn at the collar to monitor thyroid dose.

Finally, nuclear medicine technologists and radiologists performing special procedures when it is not possible for them to wear lead protective gloves are issued thermoluminescent dosimeter (TLD) monitor ring badges.

In our department, about 200 individuals are issued radiation monitor badges in nine quite separate and individual sections. Because of the considerable personnel turnover expected in a large teaching hospital and because of the continuous "horizontal" transfer of technical personnel between sections, it is not feasible to use the facility of the monitor badge supplier for keeping track of accumulated monitor badge dose. Each person has a cumulative file sheet that is maintained by the department physics group. Each month, the supplier returns the computer printout of the reported monitor badge doses, and these are transferred to each worker's cumulative file sheet. Each dose record is reviewed at this time by a professional radiation safety physicist to ensure that the dose report approximates that anticipated for the individual.

We believe that it is important to supply each individual with an annual summary and evaluation of his/her reported monitor badge reports.

Table 3–5 shows a form that we have developed for the annual summary. For example, data obtained from a staff uroradiologist for a 12-month period are shown. During that time, the radiologist was heavily involved in percutaneous nephroureteral manipulations performed on a standard fluoroscopic-radiographic table with an undertable x-ray tube. This often required insertion of nephrostomy catheters, antegrade catheterization of the ureter, dilatation of a nephrostomy track, insertion of ureteral stents, extraction of renal and ureteral calculi, and dilatation of ureteral stenoses as well as many other procedures. Other studies performed included diagnostic uroradiological evaluations such as retrograde pyelograms, nephrostograms, cystograms, urethrograms, and video-urodynamic studies.

The radiologist fluoroscopically examined an average of 43 patients per month during this time period, and his average fluoroscopic-beam on-time was 8.2 minutes per

Table 3–5. Sample Form for Annual Summary

Monitoring Badges Report Summary, Mar 1987–Feb 1988

Section: Uroradiology
Name: Staff physician

Type monitor:	Body	Collar	Ring L	R
Number of monitor badges				
Issued	12	12	10	10
Returned with reading	10	12	10	10
Returned "M"	1	0	0	0
Total yearly monitor dose, mrem	320	2690	16,290	18,430
Average monthly monitor dose, mrem	29.1	224	1629	1842

Organ Dose/Monitor Dose					**Radiation Protection Guide Levels**			
Bone marrow	Gonads m	f	Thyroid	Extremities	Monitor Type	Target organ	Dose mrem/yr	Dose mrem/mo
0.10	0.45	0.25	0.6	1.0	Body	Bone marrow, gonads	5000	417
					Collar	Thyroid*	15000	1250
					Ring	Extremities	75000	6250

	Bone Marrow	Gonads	Thyroid	Extremities L	R
Per cent of radiation protection guide level	0.7	3.1	10.8	26.1	29.5

Notes:

Monitor badge report M (Minimal) is less than 10 mrem. This may indicate minimal personnel exposure, or it may indicate that the badge had not been worn.

Average monthly doses were calculated by using data from months badges were returned and assuming that M badges were correct. It was assumed that badges not returned would have received the same dose as the average monthly dose.

The percent of Radiation Protection Guide levels were calculated by multiplying the average monthly dose by the ratio organ dose/monitor dose and dividing by the appropriate monthly Radiation Protection Guide level.

Note: the symbol "<" means "less than."

*The Committee on the Biological Effects of Radiation of the National Academy of Science in 1980 (BEIR III) considered that cataract formation is a nonstochastic process with a threshold for chronic exposure of about 1,000,000 mrem.

patient. This fluoroscope was equipped with a Bucky slot cover, but the lead drape on the image intensifier tower had been removed. The organ dose/monitor dose ratios are taken from Wohni and Stranden.[56]

While these figures are well under the NCRP guidelines, they do indicate that a significant radiation burden—especially to the operator—may be accumulated during urological fluoroscopy. For example, estimated doses to the eye during PCNL range from 0.010 to 0.027 rad and to the hands, from 0.027 to 0.136 rad.[5, 38] Whether it is necessary for radiologists and urologists performing procedures guided by fluoroscopy to wear, in addition to the standard lead apron, a thyroid shield and radiation-attenuating eyeglasses is arguable. Radiation induced thyroid carcinoma in adults is a rarity. Unfortunately, attenuating gloves have proved cumbersome and difficult to use, and they are not practical. The responsibility for performing these procedures should be shared, if possible, so that no individual is constantly exposed to radiation in excess of NCRP guidelines, especially in a busy service. Rao and colleagues measured radiation exposure to operators during PCNL and found the dose to be within acceptable limits as long as the total number of procedures performed by any one physician remained within reasonable bounds (e.g., five procedures per week for radiologists; 15 procedures per week for urologists[39]). While radiation is not usually a significant hazard to urologists during ESWL, sound radiation protection practices should be followed with this procedure also, since indiscriminate use of fluoroscopy may inadvertently subject nurses, technologists, and anesthesiologists to significant levels of radiation. With proper technique, physician dose during ESWL can be kept under 2 mrem per case.[5a]

We believe that it is also desirable to monitor trends in organ doses for groups of technologists who work in fluoroscopic rooms. Table 3–6, for example, shows data accumulated for our uroradiographic technologists from 1982 to 1986. These figures reflect a progressive increase in the number of interventional procedures, but show doses well below 10% of the Guide levels.

Pregnant Individuals

Radiation Workers. It is important to establish administrative procedures so that the person responsible for radiation safety in the department is notified as soon as possible when a radiation worker knows that she is pregnant.

An interview should be arranged, then, between the worker and the radiation safety supervisor. The first step is to complete a form that evaluates the past radiation exposure of the individual and determines whether any

Table 3–6. Yearly Monitor Summaries Section—Uroradiology: Technologists

| Year | Number Persons | Return Rate (%) | Per Cent of RPG* Levels | | |
			BONE MARROW	GONADS	THYROID
1982	4	90	0.1	0.2	0.1
1983	3	93	0.1	0.2	0.1
1984	4	90	0.3	0.8	2.9
1985	4	93	0.3	0.9	1.8
1986	3	96	0.3	0.9	2.5

*Radiation Protection Guide

Table 3–7. Sample Form for Evaluating Radiation Exposure History of Pregnant Workers

Radiation Protection Surveillance for Pregnant Personnel

I To: Radiation Safety Office
  1. _____ who works in _____ has advised of pregnancy as follows:
  ___ Known: expected delivery date: _____
  ___ Suspected
  ___ Planned
  2. This individual incurs occupational radiation exposures as follows:
  ___ Nuclear medicine ___ Medical x-ray ___ Dental x-ray
  ___ Other x-ray, specify:
  ___ Other radionuclide. Specify nuclide(s), max. amount(s) handled at one time, estimated total amount(s) handled in 1 month.

  _____   _____
  Signed   Date

II Evaluation of Exposure Potential
  1. Personnel monitoring records if applicable
    (a) Average monthly dose during past year: _____ mrem/_____ mos.
    (b) Maximum single month's dose _____ mrem _____ . date
    (c) Conclusion as to exposure potential.
  2. Other, and conclusion as to maximum exposure potential.
  3. Precautions and/or monitoring surveillance required as follows:
  4. Individual notified of conclusions per (3) _____ . date

  by _____ letter, _____ in person.

  _____   _____
  RSO signature   date

special precautions are needed during the pregnancy. Table 3–7 shows a form that has been developed by the Radiation Safety Office of the University of Pennsylvania to evaluate exposure potential to pregnant personnel. A form such as that shown in Table 3–5 is then filled out to evaluate the gonadal dose that the worker has received during the 9 months prior to the interview.

At this time, it is appropriate to review with the worker the risks of pregnancy that are possible consequent to radiation exposure and also to review the normal and natural risks of pregnancy. Table 3–8 shows a summary of the pertinent radiobiological literature that we have assembled for this purpose.

In our department, pregnant radiation workers understand, after the interview with the radiation safety supervisor, that there is no need for special precautions to ensure that the conceptus dose does not exceed a few per cent of the Radiation Protection Guide level. However, pregnant radiation workers are given the option to transfer to a nonradiation area for the duration of their pregnancy, if they choose to do so. Many individuals, however, continue working during their pregnancy.

The special problem for pregnant radiologists has been considered by Wagner and Hayman.[53] They reviewed the literature and found that, even for fluoroscopic procedures, the risk to the conceptus is extremely small.

In our department, we assign a TLD body badge to each pregnant radiation worker, regardless of where she is stationed. These badges are furnished by the University Radiation Safety Office, and the turn-around time for the results of the previous month to be read out is only a few days. Typically, from 4 to 6 weeks later we receive the parallel reading for the body film badge from the film badge supplier. We now have 12 women-months of ex-

Table 3–8. Risk of In Utero Irradiation

Effect	Reference
During the first 8 to 10 (preimplantation) days: 1 rad leads to about five chances in 1000 of death of the conceptus. No effect on survivors.	International Commission on Radiological Protection[24]
During the first 3 months: With dose less than 5 rads there is no teratological effect, growth retardation, or fetal death.	Brent RL, Gorsen RO[3]
During the final 6 months: In utero dose from obstetrical radiography may increase incidence of childhood leukemia by a factor of about 1.4. Normal incidence is 48/100,000. Increase would be to 67/100,000, an excess of 19/100,000. This is controversial. In 13 retrospective studies, 7 showed no effect. In four prospective studies, three showed no effect. There was no excess leukemia in irradiated Japanese children. Six cases were expected if the risk factor is 1.4. The chance of observing none when the average is six is 2/1000.	Calenoff L and associates[6]
The "normal" incidence of physical and mental defects in childhood of about 4%. The normal incidence of "genetic defects" is 10.5%.	New York Times[36] United Nations Scientific Committee on the Effects of Atomic Radiation[51b]
It would appear that the hazards of exposure in the range of diagnostic radiology (0.02 rad to 5 rads) present an extremely low risk to the embryo, when compared with the spontaneous mishaps that can befall the human embryo. Approximately 25% of human embryos abort spontaneously.	Brent RL[2]
The probability of termination of pregnancy due to fetal death is 9/1000.	Calenoff L and associates[6]

perience in monitoring doses at waist level under the lead apron of radiologists who continued their normal fluoroscopy assignments during their pregnancies. The average reported dose equivalences (mrem/month) were as follows: TLD, 0.5; body film badge, M (minimal or less than 10 mrem); film collar badge, 89.

Patients Who May Be Pregnant. The Department should have a set administrative procedures for technologists preparing to perform a radiological examination of a young woman, if an image of the pelvis will appear on the radiograph.

The procedure that is followed in our department is shown in Table 3–9. Occasionally, a woman who knows that she is pregnant must undergo a radiological examination that does not involve irradiating the pelvis with the useful beam. In these cases, we place a TLD on the anterior abdomen. It is explained to the patient that this is an extra precaution to ensure that the conceptus does not receive a significant radiation dose. The report of the TLD dose produces a legal record that this precaution has been taken, which is entered in the patient's record.

A few times a year, it happens that a woman is examined in our department, not knowing that she was pregnant at the time of the examination. For these patients, it is essential to calculate the estimated concep-

tus dose, using the methods that have been described in this chapter. In our experience, the average conceptus dose in these patients, usually from barium enemas or intravenous urograms, is about 2 rad. We have never had a patient with a calculated conceptus dose greater than 4 rad.

For these patients, a letter should be written to the referring physician reporting the relevant dose. It is also useful to briefly discuss the possible risks from the radiation and the normal risks of pregnancy, using data from Table 3–8. Brent[2] summarizes: "it would appear that the hazards of exposure in the range of diagnostic radiology (0.2 rad to 5 rad) present an extremely low risk to the embryo, when compared with the spontaneous mishaps that can befall the human embryo."

Currently, most departments are not following the "10-day rule" procedure in questioning patients about to receive radiological examinations. This procedure (i.e., limiting x-ray studies to the first 10 days of the menstrual cycle) and a clear discussion of the arguments against the rule are given by Russell.[43] When in doubt, it is possible to obtain a rapid laboratory test that will quickly, and with reasonable accuracy, establish whether the patient is pregnant. An excellent review of the radiation risks in pregnancy has been published by Mossman and Hill.[32]

Table 3–9. Procedures for the Radiological Technologist to Follow Before a Radiological Examination of a Patient in a Reproductive Age Group

A. If the examination is of a woman and if an image of the pelvis will appear on the radiograph, ask the patient if she thinks she may be pregnant.
  1. If the answer is *no*, proceed with the examination.
  2. If the answer is *yes*, call a staff radiologist. The radiologist will decide whether the benefit of the examination outweighs the risk. If that decision is affirmative, the radiologist will explain the situation to the patient, reassure her that the risk involved is very small, and obtain her permission to proceed with the examination. The radiologist will make a note of this consultation on the request slip.
B. If the examination does *not* involve radiation of the pelvis, do not ask the patient about her reproductive status: As an added precaution, drape the pelvic region of either male or female patients with leaded fabric when the patient is recumbent on the x-ray table or seated in a chair. In erect examinations, use lead shields on wheels or fasten a half lead apron about the waist of the patient.

References

1. Bloch P, Worrilow C: Portable radiation and light detector using a p-i-n silicon diode. Phys Med Biol 14:277–281, 1969.
2. Brent RL: Radiation teratogenesis: Fetal risk and abortion. *In* Fullerton GD, Kopp DT, Waggener RG, Webster EW (eds): Biological Risks of Medical Irradiations. New York, American Institute of Physics, 1980.
3. Brent RL, Gorsen RO: Radiation exposure in pregnancy. Cur Prob Radiol, vol 2, 1972.
4. Bush WH, Brannen GW, Gibbons RP, et al: Radiation exposure to patient and urologist during percutaneous nephrostolithotomy. J Urol 132:1148, 1984.
5. Bush WH, Jones D, Brannen GE: Radiation dose to personnel during percutaneous renal calculus removal. AJR 145:1261, 1985.
5a. Bush WH, Jones D, Gibbons RP: Radiation dose to patient and personnel during extracorporeal shock wave lithotripsy. J Urol 138:716, 1987.
6. Calenoff L, Lin P-J, Ward WF: Radiology in obstetrical practice.

In Almadgem S (ed): Obstetrical Practice. St. Louis, CV Mosby, 1980.

7. Code of Federal Regulations Part 20, par 20.101.

8. Edmonds IR: Calculation of patient skin dose from diagnostic x-ray procedures. Br J Radiol 57:733–734, 1984.

9. Engblad M, Berg O, Gottlieb E: Radiation dose measurements in micturation cystourethrography. Ann Radiol 17:423–425, 1974.

10. Engblad M, Gottlieb E: Radiation dose measurements in intravenous pyelography. Ann Radiol 18:321–324, 1975.

11. Fendel H: Radiation exposure due to urinary tract disease. *In* Kaufmann H (ed): Prog. Pediat. Radiol., Vol III: Genito-Urinary Tract. Year Book, Chicago, 1970.

12. Glaze S, Le Blanc AD, Bushong SC, Giffith DP: Patient and personnel exposure during extracorporeal lithotripsy. Health Phys 53:623, 1987.

13. Gorson RO, Lassen M, Rosenstein M: Patient dosimetry in diagnostic radiology. *In* Waggener RG, Kereiakes JG, Shalek RD (eds): CRC Handbook of Medical Physics, Vol II. Boca Raton, CRC Press, 1984.

14. Gould RG, Hale J: Use of aluminum to simulate attenuation in diagnostic x-ray beams. Acta Radiol (Diagn) 14:193–195, 1973.

15. Gray JE, Ragozzino MW, Van Lysel MS, Burke TM: Normalized organ doses for various diagnostic radiology procedures. Am J Radiol 137:463–470, 1981.

16. Gustafssen M, Mortensson W: Radiation doses to children at urologic radiography. Acta Radiol (Diagn) 22:337–348, 1981.

17. Hale J: Physical characteristics of radiation from 2-pulse, 12-pulse, and 1000-pulse x-ray equipment. Health Phys 37:419–422, 1979.

18. Hale J: A method for testing automatic exposure controls in diagnostic radiology: Three phase generators. Health Phys 46:1143–1145, 1984.

19. Hale J, O'Riordan D: Toward estimating fetal dose during barium enema examinations. Med Phys 12:502, 1985.

20. Hale J: X-ray protection. *In* Tavares JM (ed): Radiology, Vol I. Philadelphia, JB Lippincott, 1986.

21. Harrison RM, Clayton CB, Day MJ, et al: A survey of radiation doses to patients in five common diagnostic examinations. Br J Radiol 56:383–395, 1983.

22. Harrison RM: Tissue-air ratios and scatter-air ratios for diagnostic radiology (1–4 mmA1 HVL). Phys Med Biol 28:1–18, 1983.

23. International Commission on Radiation Protection: Publication 26. Recommendations of the International Commission on Radiological Protection. Oxford, Pergamon Press, 1977.

24. International Commission on Radiological Protection: Publication 27. Problems Involved in Developing and Index of Harm, 1977.

25. International Commission on Radiation Protection: Publication 34. Protection of the Patient in Diagnostic Radiology. Oxford, Pergamon Press, 1982.

26. Jucius RA, Kambic GX: Measurement of computed tomography x-ray fields utilizing the partial volume effect. Med Phys 7:379, 1980.

27. Liebovic SJ, Lebowitz RL: Reducing patient dose in voiding cystourethrography. Urol Radiol 2:103–107, 1980.

28. Lin P-J, Hrejsa AF: Patient exposure and radiation environment of extracorporeal shockwave lithotripsy. J Urol 138:712, 1987.

29. Maillie HO, Segal A, Lemkin J: Effect of patient size on doses received by patients in diagnostic radiology. Health Phys 42:665–670, 1982.

29a. McCrohan JL, Patterson JF, Gagne RH, Goldstein HA: Average radiation doses in a standard head examination for 250 CT systems. Radiology 163:263, 1987.

30. Medical Physics Data Book. Padikal TN (ed): National Bureau of Standards Handbook 138. Washington, DC, US Government Printing Office, 1981.

31. Morin RL: Radiation protection in endourology. *In* Smith AD (ed): Principles and Practice. New York, Thieme, 1986.

32. Mossman KL, et al: Radiation risks in pregnancy. Obstet Gynecol 60:237, 1982.

33. National Council on Radiation Protection and Measurements: Report No. 54. Medical radiation exposure of pregnant and potentially pregnant women. Washington, DC, NCRP, 1977.

34. National Council on Radiation Protection and Measurements: Report No. 39. Basic radiation protection criteria. Washington, DC, NCRP, 1971.

35. National Council on Radiation Protection and Measurements: Report No. 43. Review of the current state of radiation protection philosophy. Washington, DC, NCRP, 1975.

36. Lyons RD: Physical and mental disabilities in newborns doubled in 25 years. New York Times, July 18, 1983.

37. Pollack HM: Radiation exposure and extracorporeal shock wave lithotripsy. J Urol 138:850, 1987.

38. Preminger GM, Fulgham PF, Curry T: Fluoroscopic safety for the urologist. AUA Update Series. Lesson 29, Vol V. American Urological Association, 1986.

39. Rao PN, Faulkner K, Sweenery JK, et al: Radiation dose to patient and staff during percutaneous nephrostomy. Br J Urol 59:508, 1987.

40. Rogers RT: Radiation dose to the skin in diagnostic radiography. Br J Radiol 42:511–518, 1969.

41. Rosenstein M: Handbook of Selected Organ Doses for Projections Common in Diagnostic Radiology. HEW Publication (FDA) 76–8031. Washington, DC, US Government Printing Office, 1976.

42. Rosenstein M, et al: Handbook of Selected Organ Doses for Projections Common in Pediatric Radiology. HEW Publication (FDA) 79–8079. Washington, DC, US Government Printing Office, 1979.

43. Russell, JCB: The rise and fall of the ten-day rule. Brit J Radiol 59:3–6, 1986.

44. Saenger EL, Kereiakes JG, Cavanaugh DJ, et al: Cystourethrography procedures in children: Evaluation of benefits versus dose. Radiology 118:123–128, 1976.

45. Saunders JE, Early DJ, Porter JC, Coleman AJ: Radiation dose to patients from extracorporeal shock wave lithotripsy. Br Med J 292:958, 1986.

46. Schulz RJ, Gignac MS: Application of tissue-air ratios for diagnostic radiology. Radiology 120:687–690, 1976.

47. Shrimpton PC, Wall BF, Jones DG, et al: Doses to patients from routine diagnostic x-ray examinations in England. Br J Radiol 59:749–758, 1986.

48. Stieve FE: Radiation exposure in body section radiography. Acta Radiol 55:465–485, 1961.

49. Takeshita K, Shigetoshi A, Sawada SD: Exposure pattern, surface, bone marrow integral and gonadal dose from fluoroscopy. Br J Radiol 45:53–58, 1972.

50. Tole NM: Some observations on skin and organ dose during x-ray fluoroscopic examinations. Br J Radiol 58:381–383, 1985.

51. United Nations Scientific Committee on the Effects of Atomic Radiation, 1977 Report. New York, United Nations Publication, 1977, p 539.

52. Van Swearingen FL, McCullough DL, Dyer R, Appel B: Radiation exposure to patients during extracorporeal shockwave lithotripsy. J Urol 138:18, 1987.

53. Wagner LK, Hayman LA: Pregnant woman radiologists. Radiology 145:559–562, 1982.

54. Wagner LK, Archer BR, Zeck OF: Conceptus dose from two state-of-the-art CT scanners. Radiology 159:787–792, 1986.

55. Westby M, Sandbu J, Jahren R, Asmussen M: Ovarian radiation dose during dynamic cystourethrography using video recording and photofluorography. Acta Radiol (Diagn) 27:55, 1986.

56. Whoni T, Stranden E: The new ICRP concept of person-dose related to the film badge exposures for some geometrics and radiation qualities used in medical x-ray. Health Phys 36:71–73, 1979.

4

Contrast Media for Urography

ELLIOTT C. LASSER

Intravascular contrast media can be processed and/or excreted through the following four pathways: (1) the kidney, (2) the biliary system, (3) the reticuloendothelial system, and (4) the gastrointestinal mucosa.

Excretion from the gastrointestinal tract, under normal circumstances, is so minimal that it is rarely recognized. Excretion via the reticuloendothelial system occurs when the injected contrast material is formulated as a suspension. Excretion via the biliary system occurs when there is sufficient binding of the contrast media to plasma proteins.[1] Lesser degrees of binding will direct contrast media to the kidney, where structure visualization may occur via vascular opacification, extravascular accumulation, and glomerular filtration.

HISTORY

The history of intravascular contrast media development has been well documented in recent years by Wallingford,[2] Strain,[3] Grainger,[4] and Almén.[5] The original observation of urinary tract opacification was made by a young dermatologist working with syphilitic patients at the Mayo Clinic. Osborne and associates, in a 1923 report,[6] noted that films of the abdomen made on some of the patients undergoing treatment with large intravenous or oral doses of sodium iodide displayed an opacified urinary bladder. Purposeful attempts to exploit this finding, however, were unsuccessful because of dose constraints related to the relatively high toxicity of this substance when utilized in quantities necessary to dependably opacify the urinary collecting system. Nevertheless, this first recognition of the key element, iodine, set the stage for all future developments in contrast material for radiographic imaging. Subsequent developments might simply be viewed as additional chapters in the "taming of iodine."

The first of these developments occurred, serendipi-

tously, just 2 years after Osborne's observation. Binz and Rath,[159] working on chemotherapeutic drugs at the agricultural college in Berlin, noted that iodine attached to a pyridine ring was considerably less toxic than simple iodide salts. As elegantly recorded by Grainger,[4] this development led to the subsequent collaboration of an American urologist, Moses Swick, with Binz and Rath, in the introduction of Uroselectan (5-iodo-2-pyridone-n-acetic acid), marketed as Iopax in the United States. Swick, who had just completed a medical internship, changed the focus on the use of the drug, from a potential therapeutic agent to a potential diagnostic agent. He also foresaw the advantage of utilizing a more soluble form of the iodinated pyridones previously synthesized by Binz. Uroselectan, in the form of the sodium salt, could be utilized for clinical intravenous urography.

The important subsequent developments can be briefly summarized. They chronicle the introduction of two, rather than one, iodine atoms into the pyridine ring (iodopyracet [Diodrast]; sodium iodomethamate [Neo-Iopax]), the amination of the benzene ring by the introduction, by V. H. Wallingford,[2] of an acetyl-amino group and the addition of a third iodine atom acetrizoate (Urokon), and, finally, the introduction of a second acetyl-amino group (diatrizoate), which is attributed to J. O. Hoppe (Fig. 4–1).[160]

These completely substituted tri-iodinated benzoic acid compounds, formulated as either the sodium or meglumine salts, or as a mixture of both, have been utilized in intravenous urography by most of the world through a 30-year period. These compounds are described today as ionic monomeric tri-iodinated ratio-1.5 media, since the ratio between the number of iodine atoms and the number of particles in an ideal solution is 1.5 (3 iodine atoms; 2 particles).[5]

In 1968, Almén, a Swedish radiologist, determined to find a contrast material that would produce less pain in arteriography than the available substances, conceived

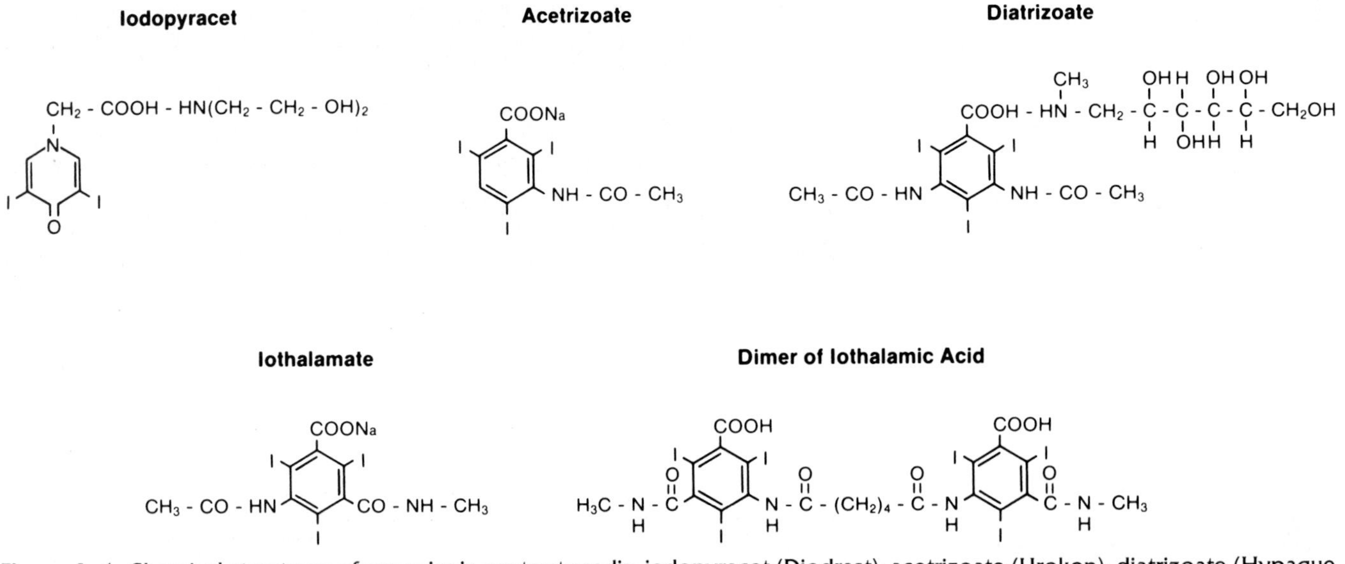

Figure 4—1. Chemical structures of some ionic contrast media: iodopyracet (Diodrast); acetrizoate (Urokon); diatrizoate (Hypaque, Renografin); iothalamate (Conray); dimer of iothalamic acid (iocarmate, Dimer-X). With the development of diatrizoate, a third iodine atom was available on the organic ring. The development of a completely substituted ring (diatrizoate and iothalamate) considerably reduced the toxicity.

the development of a contrast material with lower osmotic effects. This could be accomplished by (1) increasing the number of iodine atoms per particle in solution, (2) producing dimers, trimers, or polymers of the existing anions, or (3) avoiding the use of cations by including a sufficient number of hydrophilic hydroxyl groups to increase the water solubility. Almén decided on the latter approach, and, in conjunction with chemists of the Nyegaard Pharmaceutical Company in Norway, developed the first of the new generation of ratio-3 contrast media (metrizamide).[5] At the time of this writing, metrizamide and three other ratio-3 contrast media (3 iodine atoms; 1 particle) have been produced commercially (iohexol, iopamidol, ioxaglate) (Fig. 4–2). Ioxaglate differs from the other ratio-3 media, since it is formulated as a dimeric monoacidic substance. Each of the nonionics is composed of three elements: The iodinated aromatic moiety, a coupler group, and a polyhydroxylic group.[39] The coupler

groups utilized in these substances and in other experimental media developed thus far are amides, reversed amides, peptides, glycosides, ureides, carbamates, and esters. Hoey and Smith have noted that these couplers have increasing toxicity in the order listed (amides being least toxic).[40]

The new generation of contrast media for radiographic visualization appears to represent a level of development that is unlikely to be surpassed in the near future; hence, it is probable that research in this area will reach a plateau. Since the first generation of nonionic contrast media are almost prohibitively expensive (15 to 25 times the cost of conventional media), a major effort to produce similar but less expensive agents is predictable. Meanwhile, controversies over prioritizing the use of these costly pharmaceuticals will continue.[147–149, 161, 165] Future investigation will undoubtedly focus on the creation of new and novel media to be used in conjunction with

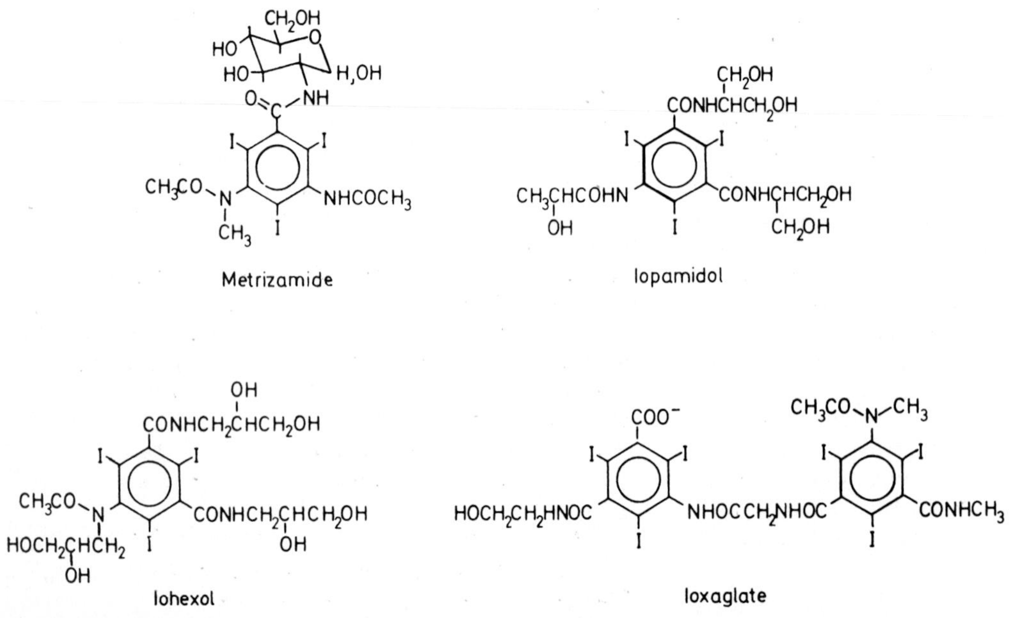

Figure 4—2. Chemical structures of the first four nonionic contrast media produced commercially. Metrizamide is also known as Amipaque, iopamidol as Isovue, iohexol as Omnipaque, and ioxaglate as Hexabrix. Note the three important elements of each of these agents: the iodinated aromatic moiety, a coupler group, and a polyhydroxylic group.

magnetic resonance imaging. These efforts are already under way.[8-11]

CHEMISTRY

General Considerations

From the standpoint of iodine delivery, the tri-iodinated ionic media are only slightly inferior to the nonionics. The more hypertonic media may induce dilutional factors that slightly reduce iodine concentrations. From a practical standpoint, however, a slight dilutional effect would be relevant only in certain excretory urograms, and in any given instance this effect may be obscured by the influence of endogenous dilutional or concentrating factors.[12] Most studies comparing the diagnostic quality of excretory urograms performed with nonionic media to those carried out with ionic agent have given the "edge" to the former, but the results of such investigations have not been consistent.[154, 164] Notwithstanding the major advances in contrast material chemistry, then, are those related to safety and to acceptance by the patient. These features will be reviewed in the paragraphs that follow.

Chemistry and Chemotoxicity

Contrast media toxicity can be best discussed under the general headings of "chemotoxicity" and "systemic toxicity" (or anaphylaxis). Chemotoxicity refers to adverse effects engendered by the injection of a high concentration of a contrast material into a vessel leading to a critical organ or tissue (i.e., arteries leading to the central nervous system, heart, or kidneys). Systemic toxicity may occur when any concentration of a contrast material is injected into any vessel. In an experimental situation, it is far easier to reproducibly assay chemotoxic effects than systemic effects; hence, much more is known about the correlation of chemical structure and chemotoxicity than of chemical structure and anaphylaxis. In fact, there is still no good animal model for contrast-induced human systemic toxicity. The incidence of severe systemic reactions is so low that it will be some time before data on the use of nonionics in humans that are sufficient to competently address this issue are accumulated.

In early work, it was shown that LD_{50} levels in various species correlated reasonably well with the binding of specific contrast material molecules to the serum albumin of the individual animals.[13] The higher the affinity, the greater was the toxicity. Since, empirically, LD_{50} levels correlated with chemotoxic parameters, but not with the incidence of anaphylaxis, the protein-binding index appeared to be an indicator of chemotoxicity. For the contrast media available at that time, the presence or absence of acetamide radicals at positions 3 and 5 on the tri-iodinated benzene ring, and the presence or absence of an aliphatic bridge between benzene rings (in the case of dimers) were the factors that influenced protein binding; incompletely substituted rings and aliphatic bridges increased protein-binding affinities (Fig. 4–1).[14]

Subsequently, it was found that all contrast media had the potential to nonspecifically inhibit enzyme systems and that this characteristic correlated closely with the protein-binding potential of individual molecules.[15] These

characteristics, it was concluded, represented an application of the general principle established by Hansch,[17] which stated that the hydrophobicity/hydrophilicity ratio of a drug, as determined by the partition of the drug in an oily/aqueous milieu, largely determined the expected degree of toxicity. Compounds with a higher hydrophilicity can form extensive hydrogen bonds in aqueous solutions. Charged groups increase hydrophilicity, but their net effect is to increase toxicity by disrupting critical electrolyte balances and increasing the conductivity of body fluids. Segments of the contrast molecule that contain hydrophilic substituents, however, are fully integrated into the aqueous phase and are unable to form bonds with biological macromolecules. Hydrophobic segments can form such bonds, and these segments are then in a position to produce potential perturbations of the intended function of the macromolecule (usually a protein).[18, 19]

Hypertonicity

The contrast media for urography that have been available in the United States for the past 4 decades are ionic monomers that have osmolalities five to six times higher than plasma. The high osmolalities were empirically conceived to supply appropriate iodine concentrations per unit of time to blood vessels, organ parenchyma, and the components of the renal collecting system. These hyperosmolar media have been shown to produce certain harmful cellular effects, which appear to be largely independent of other molecular characteristics. These include disruption of endothelial surfaces, the opening of the junctions between endothelial cells, and induced changes in the conductivity of body fluids and tissues.

The osmolality of a compound in an aqueous solution depends on the number of particles in solution. The development of the ratio-3 media diminished the osmolality of existing media by 50%, and these compounds were approximately twice as safe when administered intravenously to animals.[20] Endothelial cell disruption for equivalent iodine loads[21] was diminished, and subjective patient tolerance in peripheral arteriography was increased.[22]

Renal Toxicity

Theoretical Considerations

Contrast media may be delivered to the kidneys in high concentration via aortography, nonrenal arteriography, selective renal arteriography, or intravenous urography. In appropriate circumstances, all forms of delivery can damage the kidneys.

Potential mechanisms of injury from contrast media include (1) induced diminution in renal perfusion, (2) injury to the glomeruli, and (3) injury to the renal tubules. Diminutions in renal perfusion can occur from a fall in systemic pressure or as a consequence of focal renal factors. The latter include the direct vasoconstrictive effect known to follow renal angiography,[28] hyperosmotic effects in a closed space that result in compression of the capillary loops,[29] and a potential hyperosmolar-triggered tubular-glomerular feedback system that is presumed to induce contraction of modified smooth muscle in glomerular capillary loops.[30] In experimental studies, intravenous dosages of contrast media, chosen to produce an increase of serum creatinine of more than 50% in at least 10% of the animals (rabbits) injected, failed to produce any abnormalities detectable by microangiography in excised kidney vasculature.[31] Nevertheless, direct injuries to the renal glomeruli via chemotoxic and/or osmotic effects of contrast media are theoretically possible, and in experimental studies they have been monitored by assaying proteinuria.[32-33] No significant correlation between proteinuria and the degree of exposure to contrast media could be found, and there was no significant correlation between the osmolality of the media and protein excretion.[32]

Proteinuria, whether idiopathic or due to contrast-induced glomerular injury with increased escape of plasma proteins, may lead to protein precipitates within the tubules. Contrast-induced chemotoxic effects on the tubular epithelium have also been thought to be responsible for some cases of oliguria or anuria. An attempt has been made to evaluate the tubular injury that follows contrast injections by quantifying the resulting enzymuria.[32] This effect is considerably greater after nephroangiography than after intravenous urography, but, as in the case of glomerular injury, no conclusive correlations with clinical findings have been established. In experimental animals, the damage produced by ratio-3 media is not different from that produced by ratio-1.5 media.[32]

Two specific proteins have been thought to play a role in the tubular cast formation identified in several cases of renal failure after contrast injection. The first of these is a glycoprotein (Tamm-Horsfall protein), and the second is a low-molecular-weight globulin (Bence Jones protein). The latter is present in the urine of about 40% of patients with multiple myeloma.

Tamm-Horsfall protein is a major constituent of tubular casts. Berdon and coworkers reported an increased precipitation of this substance on incubation with contrast media in vitro, and an increased excretion of this material in patients recovering from contrast-induced renal failure.[34] Others, however, have pointed out that following intravenous urography in normal individuals, there is no increase in the rate of Tamm-Horsfall clearance, and, in fact, the concentration of this protein in urine and its aggregatability decreased markedly.[35] Thus, the role of Tamm-Horsfall protein in contrast-induced renal failure remains obscure. The role of Bence Jones protein is correspondingly unclear. Although myeloma patients are thought to be at higher risk of renal failure following contrast injections than normal individuals, in vitro studies of contrast material incubated with Bence Jones proteins suggested that urographic media will not produce precipitation of these proteins at the pH values attainable in urine.[36] An argument could be made, therefore, that pre-existing renal failure, rather than Bence Jones proteinuria, accounts for the increased risk of renal failure thought to be present in myeloma patients. Current thinking suggests that urography can be carried out safely in patients with myeloma if a period of rigorous hydration precedes the study.

In summary although precise pathogenic mechanisms have not been conclusively identified, contrast media may produce chemotoxic effects in the kidney. Transient renal failure (characterized by slight increases in serum creatinine or urea values) and varying degrees of oliguria, may occur in as many as 10% of high-risk patients.[37] Chronic renal failure following contrast injections, however, is distinctly uncommon. Pre-existing renal damage appears to be the major contributing factor to contrast-induced renal toxicity.[158]

Clinical Considerations

A major problem in all discussions of contrast-induced renal injury is the lack of agreement on parameters that delineate toxicity. The unit of measurement in this situation is renal failure; however, the indices of renal failure are not tightly circumscribed. The parameters most often utilized are blood urea nitrogen, serum creatinine, creatinine clearance, and diminished urinary output. Hayman and Migliore,[41] mindful of the fact that serum creatinine values reported from 5330 laboratories showed a standard deviation of 0.4 mg/dl,[42] point out that serum creatinine must increase by at least 1.66 SD or 0.7 mg/dl to attain a 95% confidence level regarding the significance of the induced change. Teruel and associates,[47] have made the observation that the combination of an enema, a laxative, and overnight fluid restriction produced an average rise in serum creatinine (prior to contrast material challenge) of 0.5 mg/dl in individuals without renal insufficiency, and 0.9 mg/dl in those with such insufficiency.

Misson and Cutler,[43] in an excellent review summarizing the data from seven retrospective and eight prospective studies between 1972 and 1983, noted that the criteria for contrast-induced renal failure varied widely. For the most widely utilized index, induced elevations of serum creatinine values ranged from 0.2 mg/dl to 1.0 mg/dl and from 12% to 50%.

Despite intensive attempts to understand the factors involved in clinical cases of contrast-induced renal toxicity, the precise mechanisms of the disorder remain elusive. Dawson has recently summarized the pertinent literature.[23] Pre-existing renal disease, diabetes mellitus, and dehydration are thought to be risk factors, although renal disease is the only one that has been repeatedly validated, and even this has been inconsistent.[24-27, 162] Adequately hydrated patients with relatively normal renal function appear to tolerate even very large doses of contrast medium well and exhibit no consistent change in renal function with increasing contrast dosage.[27, 153]

VanZee and associates[44] have highlighted the effects of pre-existing renal disease on contrast-induced renal failure in nondiabetics undergoing intravenous urography. Defining "renal injury" as an abrupt increase in serum creatinine of more than 1.0 mg/dl, with or without oliguria, they found that 5 of 161 nondiabetic patients (3%) with pre-existing renal disease and serum creatinines less than 4.5 mg/dl developed contrast-induced renal injury, whereas 5 of 16 (31%) with pre-existing serum creatinines greater than 4.5 mg/dl developed such injuries. Only 1 of 169 (0.6%) patients without pre-existing renal disease showed any evidence of renal injury following the urogram. Diabetics without pre-existing renal disease incur no greater threat of contrast-induced renal damage than do nondiabetics[45]; however, in diabetics with pre-existing renal disease, the incidence of contrast-induced renal injury may be greater than in nondiabetics with similar impairment.[46, 162] The mechanisms that cause the additional insult are not yet defined. Although the precise role of dehydration in contrast-induced renal injury is still under debate,[43] there appears to be no reason at this point to impose a dehydration regimen on patients with any degree of pre-existing renal disease. At the present time, there has been insufficient clinical experience with nonionics in renal angiography or intravenous urography to determine whether their utilization might be advantageous in high-risk patients.[32, 151, 163, 167]

Systemic Reactions

The severity of systemic reactions may range from merely annoying to life threatening. To better understand the influence on the likelihood of reactions of such variables as the rate of contrast administration and the nature of cations, the Multi-Institutional Contrast Material Study Group divided reactions into three categories. Grade I included nausea, a single episode of emesis, sneezing, and vertigo. Grade II included urticaria, emesis occurring more than once, fever, or chills. Any reaction more severe than these fell into Grade III. All anaphylactic reactions fell into this category. The following were all associated with an increase in Grade I type or Grade II type reactions: rapid intravenous injection of contrast medium, as opposed to drip infusion; the use of sodium salts; the diatrizoate anion, as opposed to iothalamate; and youth as opposed to middle age. Only a history of general allergies or of reaction to previously administered contrast medium, however, were linked to an increase in the more severe (Grade III) reactions.[51]

The severe anaphylactic reactions that occur with current urographic media may be characterized by some of the following symptoms and signs: alterations in blood pressure, bronchospasm, laryngospasm, cardiac arrhythmias, angioedema, loss of consciousness, convulsions, diffuse erythema or urticaria, pulmonary edema, angina, and incontinence. Commonly, one or two of these will characterize the reaction.

According to the literature, severe reactions can be expected to occur, in some selected groups, at an incidence of 1 in 750 (0.13%).[48] More commonly, these reactions are reported to vary in incidence between 1 in 1000[49] to 1 in 2000 patients (0.05% to 0.10%).[49–50] Using the criteria listed above, however, in a double-blinded multi-institutional prospective study of patients with no history of a previous severe reaction, the incidence of severe reactions* was found to be 1 in 191 (0.5%).[51] In the same study, utilizing the criterion of "needed antihistamine therapy in the judgment of the attending radiologist," an incidence of almost 2.0% was noted.

Meaningful statistical data on mortality are even harder to attain. In two different surveys, Ansell reported an overall mortality rate of 1 in 40,000 (0.002%),[48, 52] but in patients over 60 he found the death rate to be four times as high. Hartman and colleagues, in an 18-year prospective study of death resulting from intravenous pyelography in a single institution with a limited number of high-risk patients, reported an incidence of 1 in 75,000 (0.001%).[53] This is approximately the same risk as reported for penicillin.[54]

In all reported series, the incidence of reactions and

deaths is significantly higher in individuals with a history of hypersensitivity of some kind and/or asthma.[52, 53, 55–57] From the historical standpoint, only the history of a previous reaction to contrast material serves as a more reliable predictor index. In the multi-institutional study mentioned earlier,[51] the history of a nonsevere previous reaction increased the likelihood of a severe current reaction, or a reaction that increased the need for antihistamine therapy by approximately threefold. The history of an allergy of any kind resulted in an approximately twofold increase in the likelihood of a current reaction. At the present time, no large-scale double-blind study speaks to the incidence of systemic reactions with the ratio-3 contrast media. Thorough reviews of the literature on adverse reactions to contrast media have recently been presented.[150, 164]

The Pathogenesis of Systemic Reactions

The precise pathogenesis of systemic reactions to contrast media is still incompletely understood. Nevertheless, considerable information bearing on these reactions has been accumulated over the past 2 decades. Histamine, bradykinin, and leukotrienes are well-accepted mediators of anaphylaxis, and vasoactive prostaglandins and the complement factors C3a and C5a are considered likely mediators. Ionic contrast media have been reported to liberate or activate all of these with the exception of the leukotrienes.[62–75] In addition, contrast media have been reported to activate the coagulation and fibrinolysin systems in some reactions[67, 72, 76–78] and to form complexes with circulating antibodies.[79] Most of these contrast-induced changes have been demonstrated both in vitro and in vivo. Because there are complex interrelationships between the complement, contact, coagulation, and immune systems, and since the complement and contact systems may produce activated proteases that can potentiate mediator release by some cells, including mast cells, basophils, platelets, neutrophils, and eosinophils, it is easy to understand why it is so difficult to isolate critical or unique initiating and sequential activation factors.

Nevertheless, speculation and directed research in recent years has tended to focus on three areas. These are (1) the role of mast cells and basophils, (2) the role of acute activation systems, particularly the complement and contact systems, and (3) the role of psychogenic and neurogenic factors. Although such factors as disruption of the blood–brain barrier and cardiac and renal toxicity may be a prominent feature of some systemic reactions, they are more commonly encountered in chemotoxic reactions, as suggested earlier.

THE ROLE OF MAST CELLS AND BASOPHILS

Systemic reactions occurring after intravascular injections of contrast media have been variously termed anaphylactic, anaphylactoid, allergic, hypersensitivity, and idiosyncratic.

Anaphylaxis is the term used for the immediate homeostatic disassembly that follows antigen-IgE–mediated release of mediators from mast cells or basophils.[80] Non–IgE-mediated reactions, however, may result in the release of identical mediators with similar end-organ responses. As pointed out by Sheffer,[81] such reactions are

---

*Excludes cases with diffuse urticaria or erythema as sole abnormality.

often termed *anaphylactoid*, but because the clinical features (and the induced biochemical alterations) are indistinguishable, it now seems most appropriate to expand the application of the term *anaphylaxis* to include all of the pathophysiological events that are governed principally by mediator release, regardless of the initiating factors. I endorse this concept and believe it is particularly applicable to contrast material reactions for which mediator release is well documented,[62-76] but precise triggering mechanisms have yet to be firmly identified.

Of the known mediators, histamine has received the most intensive study, and it is understandable that early investigations of the pathogenesis of contrast material reaction focused on a potential role for histamine. It was widely recognized that this substance, when injected experimentally, could produce vasodilatation with resulting fall in blood pressure, alterations in capillary permeability permitting the egress of fluid, and, occasionally, spasm of the bronchial musculature. These, along with dermatological changes, are certainly the most common manifestations of severe anaphylaxis induced by contrast material.

In early studies, it was demonstrated both in vitro and in vivo[62-67, 84, 86] that contrast material could result in the release of histamine. In both circumstances, contrast material appeared to function as a direct histamine releaser, possibly via hyperosmolarity,[82, 83] rather than working through an IgE-mediated mechanism. Kaliner and associates[87] analyzed urinary histamine values in specimens collected 30 to 45 minutes after contrast challenge and found mean values to be significantly elevated in patients experiencing some combination of wheezing, itching, and hives, compared with asymptomatic patients. The urinary histamine level in the "reactor" group was almost identical to that in individuals having mild reactions to immunotherapy but was considerably less than in individuals with idiopathic anaphylaxis or systemic mastocytosis. Littner and coworkers noted that, despite a dominant role of methylglucamine salts in in vitro and in vivo histamine-release studies, bronchospasm following administration of contrast material was equally frequent in patients receiving sodium diatrizoate and those receiving methylglucamine diatrizoate.[56, 88] Cogen and coworkers[63] found that samples of aortic root blood in patients undergoing pulmonary angiography demonstrated high but transient levels of histamine and that these were not accompanied by symptoms, suggesting that sustained infusions may be necessary to produce symptoms. Thus, overall experimental findings suggest that histamine release, although it occurs in individuals given contrast material, could explain some, but not all, symptoms encountered in anaphylactic reactions.

In addition to histamine, mast cells and/or basophils contain other vasoactive and smooth-muscle–active mediators, chemotactic mediators, enzyme mediators, and proteoglycans.[85] Of these, histamine, leukotrienes, and kallikrein have most often been considered potential agents in human anaphylaxis. Other agents will undoubtedly be recognized with further study.

DOES IgE PLAY A ROLE IN MEDIATOR RELEASE?

Up to this point, we have been discussing mediator release resulting from nonimmunological mechanisms. It is appropriate now to consider whether classical immunological mechanisms play a role.[90] At least two clinical observations point in this direction: (1) The signs and symptoms of contrast material anaphylaxis closely mimic those of IgE-triggered immediate anaphylaxis, and (2) on occasion, very small doses of contrast material may elicit a severe reaction. On the other hand, several theoretical considerations appear to minimize the likelihood of IgE involvement: (1) Patients who have not previously received contrast material may nevertheless suffer a reaction, and (2) the ionic contrast media are highly nonreactive chemically and would not be likely candidates for hapten formation (contrast material, unless combined with proteins to form a hapten, would have no antigenic potential).

Brasch and coworkers have conducted the most extensive studies of the potential role of immunologically mediated hypersensitivity in contrast material anaphylaxis.[61, 79, 91-94] In their papers, they determined that analogues of contrast material, chemically coupled with proteins, could be used to produce IgG-class antibodies in rabbits and that mean IgG antibody levels were higher in human reactor sera than in controls.[92] They also noted that antibodies believed to be of the IgE class were present in the skin of rabbits that demonstrated passive cutaneous anaphylaxis following challenge with contrast material conjugated with gamma globulin or serum albumin[92] after the animals had been sensitized with serum obtained from other rabbits inoculated with conjugated contrast material and protein. Antibodies, also believed to be of the IgE class, were detected in the pooled serum from four contrast reactors by means of a technique involving the immobilization of antibodies on an affinity column containing contrast material conjugated to bovine serum albumin.[61] The same workers found that when using the guinea pig sensitized with conjugated contrast material and protein as a model for contrast material–induced anaphylaxis, they could elicit anaphylaxis on iodipamide challenge, but not on challenge with urographic contrast media.[94]

Siegle and colleagues[71] injected a complex of contrast material and beef serum albumin into rabbits to produce antibodies that bound diatrizoate as detected by an enzyme-linked immunospecific assay system. Three reports in the literature have pointed to the presence of circulating antibodies in patients exhibiting systemic reactions to injected contrast material.[95-97] In two of these, however, the antibodies were of the IgM class, and one of the two received ioglycamic acid (a biliary contrast material). In the third case, the patient was also injected with ioglycamic acid and suffered a true anaphylactic reaction; a passive cutaneous anaphylaxis study was positive.[97] In other reported studies, patients having either no reactions, mild reactions, or severe reactions failed to disclose the presence of serum antibodies.[98, 99]

In the context of the data cited above, how should the role of IgE in contrast material anaphylaxis be regarded? IgE antibodies capable of interacting with unbound contrast molecules in patients exhibiting contrast material reactions have been demonstrated in vivo in only a single instance. That patient was injected with a cholangiographic material that may function as a divalent hapten.[97] The IgE-type antibodies in human sera demonstrated by Brasch and coworkers were conjugated to a contrast material covalently bound to albumin on the column.[61] No one has been able to demonstrate antibodies of *any* class that have been produced in animals or humans by injections of urographic contrast material alone.[98, 99] This is not unexpected, since all experimental work done with the urographic media has shown them to be extremely nonreactive chemically. Even noncovalent binding of these substances to proteins is difficult to demonstrate with any accuracy,[13] and yet the concept that the covalent binding of a simple drug with proteins of the host is mandatory for the induction of an immunological response rests on strong experimental evidence.[100] Furthermore, hapten-specific immediate-type allergic reactions due to serum antibodies have been demonstrated in experimental animals only when the injected antigen possessed several antigenic determinants on the same molecule (i.e., was pleurivalent).[100] Pleurivalent antigens are mandatory, because monovalent antigens lack the mechanics necessary to bridge adjacent IgE molecules and, hence, to initiate the cascade of events that begin in the target cell membrane following such bridging.

Other Potential Mechanisms of Mediator Release

In our discussion thus far, we have attempted to evaluate the role that mast cell or basophil granule release engendered either directly by contrast material or by the formation of contrast material-IgE complexes might play in contrast material anaphylaxis. Now we will expand the discussion to consider potential non–mast cell, non–basophil-derived mediators, and mast cell/basophil effects exclusive of granule release.

In an earlier section, we alluded to the fact that the complement factors C3a and C5a are included in the list of mediators believed to play a role in anaphylaxis. These physiologically active peptides, known as anaphylatoxins, can bring about a wide variety of reactions in vivo, including increased capillary permeability, release of histamine from mast cells or basophils, directed attraction of white blood cells, and release of hydrolases from white blood cells. Furthermore, tiny amounts of these substances can produce a wheal and flare response when injected into the skin. In 1974, it was reported that contrast material appeared to activate serum complement, as demonstrated by a fall in total hemolytic complement levels after a 37°C incubation of sera and contrast media.[101] This was subsequently confirmed in vitro and in vivo.[63, 67, 69–71, 73, 74, 78, 104] In later studies, it was reported

that (1) various contrast media activated complement in the same order of effectiveness in which they bound to serum albumin and in which they produced enzyme inhibition[68]; (2) in addition to the whole complement depletion, depletion of individual complement components, with the exception of C6, C8, and C9, occurred after exposure to contrast media[102]; (3) C3 cleavage could be demonstrated, which along with whole-complement activation appeared to be engendered by contrast media in a fashion other than by the known classic and alternative pathways.[102]

Despite the temptation, based on the above data, to ascribe systemic reactions to contrast material–induced production of C3a and C5a anaphylatoxins in vivo, both experimental[78] and clinical[72, 103] observations dictate otherwise.

These considerations led to an examination of other acute activation pathways that might contribute to consumption of the C1 esterase inhibitor and thus potentiate complement activation (and depletion) in the prechallenge period.[103] Because this protein is the sole inhibitor of activated Factor XII, the initiating protease of the intrinsic coagulation and contact system cascades, and is the most significant inhibitor of kallikrein (another protease in the contact system), an assay was devised to evaluate plasma contact system dynamics.[60] Further impetus for the development of the assay could be found in the role played by kinins in diverse forms of anaphylaxis.[105–108]

The assay that was developed involved using dextran sulfate of 500,000 molecular weight as a soluble contact system "surface," at 0°C to down-regulate contact system plasma inhibitors, and a chromogenic substrate to quantify the amount of kallikrein formed after variable incubations of plasmas in the contact activators.[60] By means of this assay system, it was found that the prechallenge plasmas of reactors, on the average, exhibited a significantly increased rate of kallikrein production when exposed to an exogenous contact activator (Fig. 4–3). Because kallikrein releases bradykinin from high-molecular-weight kininogen when formed (from the plasma zymogen prekallikrein), a faster rate of kallikrein formation in contrast material reactors implies a faster rate of kinin production in these individuals. Although the assay is carried out at 0°C and the C1 esterase inhibitor is significantly more effective at 37°C,[109] thermodynamic considerations dictate that, regardless of the temperature, reactors will exhibit a faster rate of prekallikrein trans-

Figure 4–3. Rate of kallikrein formation at various time periods, when the prechallenge plasmas of contrast material reactors are incubated at 0°C with a soluble contact system activator (dextran sulfate). Contact system dynamics are accelerated in contrast material reactors, compared with controls.

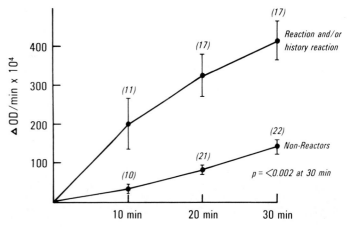

formation (and putative kinin production) than controls. What is the implied significance of these findings? While dextran sulfate, the contact activator utilized in these studies, does not exist endogenously, a number of biological molecules have been shown to have the properties of contact activators.[110–113]

Because the incidence of contrast material reactions is known to be higher in individuals with allergy, particularly those with asthma, it is interesting to note that the baseline plasma levels of atopic asthmatics, compared with controls, showed an acceleration of prekallikrein transformation in the dextran-sulfate–catalyzed assay that closely mimicked that noted for contrast material reactors (Fig. 4–4).

Finally, some contrast material reactors and some asthmatics displayed elevated baseline plasma levels of an anticoagulant having the fundamental inhibitory properties of commercial heparin when tested against Factor Xa or thrombin in the presence of antithrombin III (heparin cofactor).[108, 113, 114] This anticoagulant substance, like commercial heparin, may initiate,[115] and/or potentiate[108] contact system activity in vitro and therefore, when present, could play a meaningful role in such activity in the patient. For various reasons, it is believed that the acute mobilization of this substance involves endothelial and/or plasma and blood cell sources rather than mast cell sources.[113] Thus, it seems reasonable to postulate that a physicochemical (contrast-material modulated) event could trigger contact system activity in vivo.

Assuming that bradykinin is formed after a triggering event at a rate greater in contrast-material reactors or asthmatics than in normal individuals, what is its potential role? Bradykinin can mimic all of the significant pathophysiological effects of histamine but is considerably more potent than histamine in these activities.[116–117] In addition, bradykinin is known to activate phospholipase A_2, the enzyme in cell membranes that is responsible for hydrolyzing surface membrane phospholipids of mast cells and other cells into lysolecithin and arachidonic acid. The latter substance can subsequently be catalyzed into either vasoactive prostaglandins or leukotrienes (leukotriene C4, D4, and E4 constitute what was earlier referred to as slow-reacting substance of anaphylaxis).[85] Recently, it has been shown that contrast media can inhibit angiotensin-converting enzyme, the substance that hydrolyzes bradykinin and limits its systemic effects.[152]

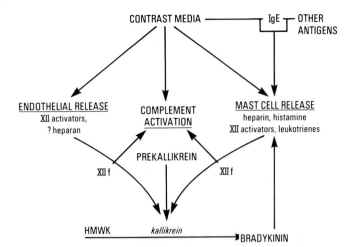

Figure 4–5. Working model to demonstrate the interrelationships of the contact, coagulation, and complement systems in contrast material anaphylaxis. (See text for details.)

To summarize, then, it appears that non-IgE mechanisms can be invoked to account for many, if not all, events involved in contrast-material anaphylaxis. The demonstrated similarity in prekallikrein transformation rates and in the mobilization of endogenous heparin in contrast-material reactors and asthmatics, may help to explain why the incidence of contrast material reactions is increased in asthmatic subjects. It is hoped that future studies will further clarify these issues. Meanwhile, I would propose that the interrelationships of the contact, coagulation, and complement systems, depicted in Figure 4–5, be considered as a simplified state-of-the-art working model for the hypotheses considered in this chapter.

What about anxiety? The thesis that central nervous system events, particularly anxiety, play a key triggering role in contrast material anaphylaxis has been advanced by Lalli.[118] Although there is no doubt that in some individuals classic vago-vasal or vago-vagal mechanisms come into play and that in some anxiety could even promote the release of circulating mediators,[119] neither clinical nor experimental findings support the concept that all contrast-material reactions are related to activation of the limbic portion of the central nervous system.[59]

Pretreatment to Prevent or Diminish Intensity of Contrast Material Anaphylactic Reactions

There is general agreement that patients with a previous history of contrast material reactions and those with a history of severe allergy and/or asthma constitute a population that is at increased risk of contrast material reactions for any subsequent intravascular challenge. This has been addressed in earlier sections. At the present time, thorough history-taking is superior to any available in vitro or in vivo test to identify this high-risk population. When faced with a patient of this type, the radiologist has an obligation to check and double check the indications for the procedure and to unequivocally determine that no alternative procedure entailing less risk might be substituted. At the present time, data are insufficient to appropriately assess the benefits of substituting a nonionic contrast substance for the ionic media in these circumstances, but preliminary observations suggest that the potential benefit might outweigh the increased cost.[146, 168] It is recognized that patients who have not been previ-

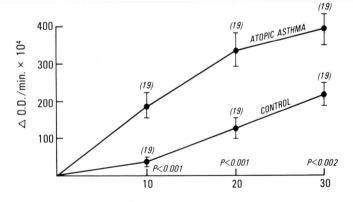

Figure 4–4. Contact system dynamics are accelerated in patients with atopic asthma, compared with controls. (See legend for Fig. 4–3.)

ously exposed to contrast media and who have no history of allergy or asthma may suffer severe contrast material reactions on their first exposure. Thus, it is imperative that any physician injecting contrast media be aware of the composite literature focusing on (1) potential steps that can be taken to minimize the risk for patients with positive histories and (2) the efficacy and risk associated with tested pretreatment regimens.

Only a limited number of papers deal with these subjects. The relatively low incidence of severe reactions in untreated (control) populations imposes a burden on investigators that is not easily overcome.

As a result, studies have generally fallen into one of three categories: (1) Patients in a high-risk group are premedicated with a given regimen and show moderate or severe reactions compared with historical controls. This strategy is selected because withholding premedication could be potentially harmful. (2) Patients with no known risk factors are pretreated and compared with controls. Treated or untreated, severe reactions occur with an incidence so low that individual studies usually contain sufficient numbers to evaluate only mild or moderate reactions. (3) Anecdotal patient reports are kept. Although there are obvious problems with studies in any of these categories, some useful information has been generated.[120–124]

Pretreatment has most commonly included a combination of corticosteroids and antihistamines administered either parenterally or orally.[121] Few reports of treatment with antihistamines alone,[122, 124] or corticosteroids alone,[120] are available. In general, these reports suggest that protection appears to be conferred by each of these three regimens, but strict comparisons with appropriate controls to test statistical validity are not forthcoming for the reasons cited earlier. Some representative data from these studies, nevertheless, can be cited and will indicate the protective trends suggested.

Zweiman and associates in 1975[120] reported that 150 mg of prednisone given orally over a period beginning 18 hours prior to injection with contrast material, and continuing for 12 hours after the procedure, resulted in "rash" reactions in 3 of 37 patients (8%) who expressed previous contrast material rash reactions, and mild mucosal swelling in one of nine patients who experienced previous anaphylactoid reactions. Greenberger and coworkers[121] in 1980 reported that, of 143 patients with a previous history of an immediate generalized reaction to intravascular media (mostly urticaria and/or angioedema), only ten experienced reactions (7.0%, all mild) after pretreatment with 50 mg of oral prednisone given three times over an 18-hour period prior to contrast material challenge, plus 50 mg diphenhydramine, intramuscularly, 1 hour prior to the study. Small and associates,[122] in 1982, divided 220 consecutive patients who were to undergo intravenous pyelography into three approximately equal groups. One group received no premedication, the second group received 10 mg of chlorpheniramine, subcutaneously, and the third group received a subcutaneous injection of saline. Each injection was given approximately 15 minutes prior to challenge. Allergic reactions (hives and pruritus) occurred at an incidence of 15% in the no-medication group, 7% in the saline pretreated group, and 1% in the antihistamine-treated group. In a 1984 report, Greenberger and associates[123] added another element to their combined steroid and antihistamine regimen. In this new approach, they added 25 mg of ephedrine, orally, 1

hour before challenge. At that time, they had 401 patients (with a previous history of reactions) treated with their older regimen, and among these patients the reaction rate was 10%. In 147 patients with a previous reaction receiving ephedrine, in addition to steroids and antihistamines, there was a repeat intravascular reaction rate of 4%; all reactions were minimal.

The only double-blind, randomized study of preventive pretreatment is by Lasser and associates and cites the collected experiences of 27 institutions.[51] In this multi-institutional study that excluded patients who had a previous severe* reaction, patients receiving 32 mg of methylprednisolone (Medrol) twice (24 hours and 2 hours prior to contrast material challenge) or once (2 hours prior to contrast material challenge) were compared with similar placebo groups. As of this writing, 2513 patients had received the two-dose steroid regimen, 1759 the one-dose regimen, and 2491 the one- or two-dose placebo regimens. In earlier comparisons in the study, it was found that the two-dose regimen was significantly better than the other three regimens for all reactions, for reactions necessitating antihistamine therapy in the judgment of the consulting radiologist; the two-dose regimen approached significance for severe reactions. In this preliminary analysis, it was found that the one-dose regimen was, in fact, indistinguishable from the placebo regimens. Therefore, the study was narrowed to two regimens: the two-dose steroid and the two-dose placebo. Table 4–1 summarizes the results of the study as of the analysis of July 1986. When the two-dose regimen was compared with the other three regimens (combined), it was found to be significantly superior for patients experiencing any type of reaction (mild, moderate, or severe) and for reactions necessitating antihistamine therapy in the judgment of the consultant radiologist. For severe reactions (excluding those with solely dermatological manifestations), the two-dose regimen was superior at the $p = .05$ level. No consequential reactions were experienced with the methylprednisolone pretreatment itself in 4272 patients. These preliminary analyses suggest that corticoste-

---

*Severe reactions include shock, bronchospasm, laryngospasm, convulsions, loss of consciousness, fall in blood pressure, increase in blood pressure, cardiac arrhythmias, angina, angioedema, pulmonary edema, oliguria, and anuria.

Table 4–1. National Study of Contrast Material Reactions Data Run–July 1986: 6062 Cases

	Two-dose	One-dose	Two-placebo	One-placebo
All reactions	163/2513 (6.5%) $p = 0.0001$	166/1750 (9.5%)	145/1603 (9.0%)	88/883 (10%)
Antihistamine therapy	24/2513 (0.9%) $p = 0.003$	33/1750 (1.9%)	28/1603 (1.7%)	18/883 (2.0%)
Severe*	5/2513 (0.2%) $p = 0.05$	9/1750 (0.5%)	11/1603 (0.7%)	2/883 (0.2%)

*Excludes patients with diffuse urticaria or erythema as sole abnormality.

Comparison of the effects of the two-dose methylprednisolone (Medrol) regimen to the placebo regimens and the one-dose methylprednisolone regimen. The effects of these regimens were compared for composite mild and severe reactions (all reactions), for reactions necessitating therapy in the judgment of the attending radiologist, and for severe reactions, excluding those manifest solely by dermatological manifestations. This is part of a preliminary report of data accumulated in a multi-institutional double-blind study of the effects of corticosteroid pretreatment on contrast material reactions.

roids appear to confer protection against contrast material anaphylaxis, provided that they are administered over a period of time preceding the challenge. (An alternative explanation might be that 32 mg of methylprednisolone is an insufficient dose, but studies utilizing corticosteroids in other forms of anaphylaxis indicate that the time prior to challenge is an important parameter in conferring protection.)

Only one study has been published, thus far, on the potential protective effects of combined H_1 and H_2 receptor antagonists.[124] In this prospective, randomized, single-blind study, 800 patients were divided into four approximately equal groups. Each group received premedication intravenously, 5 minutes prior to intravenous pyelography. The four pretreatment groups were (1) prednisolone—250 mg, (2) clemastine, an H_1 blocker—0.03 mg/kg, (3) clemastine plus cimetidine—0.03 mg/kg plus 5 mg/kg, and (4) saline. The combined H_1 and H_2 receptor-antagonist regimen was significantly superior to the other three groups for nausea, flush, and urticaria. More severe symptoms did not occur in their series, and therefore the potential protective effects of these regimens in such reactions could not be evaluated.

Finally, it should be noted that a process of desensitization, although time-consuming and expensive, may be considered in special circumstances. Agardh and associates[125] reported on such a procedure applied to 12 patients having previous contrast material reactions manifested by urticaria, angioedema, bronchospasm, cardiovascular collapse, or some combination of these. Desensitization was carried out in graduated steps (approximately every 2 hours) over several days, starting with 1 ml of a 1:100 dilution, and gradually working up to 50 ml of a 1:1 solution on the third day. In 10 of the 12 patients, the definitive contrast study was carried out within 5 days of the end of the desensitization program, and only two of these had a reaction (milder than the original in each case). Studies carried out in periods greater than 5 days after desensitization were less successful.

Some General Principles Regarding the Treatment of Contrast Material Reactions

Every radiologist injecting contrast material will encounter, and must be prepared to deal with, acute systemic reactions. The relative infrequency of severe and particularly life-threatening reactions has both positive and negative aspects. The positive aspect is obvious; the negative is that the infrequent occurrence of these events places the radiologist at a disadvantage, both experientially and emotionally, to respond optimally to crises. More disheartening, however, is that not even the most experienced immunology, anesthesia, or emergency medicine group has had sufficient experience with human anaphylaxis of any origin in a controlled situation.[126, 139] Perhaps the most glaring evidence of this is the fact that the precise role, route of administration, and dose of epinephrine, which is the drug regarded by almost everyone as the first line of defense in anaphylactic reactions, is quite unsettled.[126, 127]

In the light of these considerations, we will consider in this section only general principles and guidelines for administration of contrast material. Readers desiring a detailed course of action are referred to the pamphlet published by the American College of Radiology in 1977, entitled "Prevention and Management of Adverse Reactions to Intravascular Contrast Media."[128] It is telling that a pamphlet published almost a decade earlier, appears to contain most of the available information on "how to." More recently, Cohan and colleagues have reviewed the principles underlying the treatment of reactions to contrast media.[156]

Certain general principles are self-evident. Rooms in which contrast material injections will be done must have all the first-line emergency drugs and equipment either in the room or in an immediately accessible area, and these must be routinely checked. A list of suggested drugs and equipment that should be maintained on a crash cart in the vicinity of the radiology examining rooms is contained in Table 4–2. Established emergency lines of communication should be available among the radiology and anesthesia, and/or the cardiac resuscitation groups. Radiologists must be trained and periodically retrained in cardiopulmonary resuscitation. Contrast examinations should not be conducted outside the institutions unless appropriate support groups are immediately available and/or the radiologists themselves are trained and in all ways properly prepared to assume the role of the support physician groups available in institutions.[166]

No patient should be injected who has not been screened for significant historical factors by both the referring physician and the radiologist. The radiologist should remain in or near the procedure room for at least the first critical 4 to 5 minutes following injection and should stay in the immediate vicinity for the next 30 to 45 minutes. The patient should remain under the watchful eye of an experienced technician or a suitable substitute throughout the entire period that he or she remains in the examination room. All intravenous contrast injections should be made through a short needle-catheter assembly, and this should be left in place (with periodic saline flushes) to ensure access to a vessel in the event of anaphylaxis. (In an emergency, when superficial vessels seem to defy access via the customary approaches, it may be worthwhile to consider the utilization of the femoral vein or intraosseous channels.)

The primary approach to most mild-to-moderate reactions (flush, vertigo, nausea, limited urticaria) is simple reassurance. For more severe reactions, immediate assurance of an open airway with oxygen supplementation, if available, initiation of intravascular physiological fluids, and monitoring of blood pressure and heart rate should be undertaken.

For drug therapy, six categories of drugs have been utilized.[129] They are (1) adrenergic agonists, (2) methylxanthines, (3) anticholinergics, (4) antihistamines, (5) steroids, (6) anticonvulsants. Categories 2, 4, 5, and 6 are noncontroversial and can be easily addressed. Utilization of a methylxanthine such as aminophylline in instances where bronchospasm threatens to limit oxygen exchange and/or does not respond to epinephrine should always be considered. It should be remembered that because overly rapid infusion may result in dysrrhythmias and tachycardia, ECG monitoring should be utilized, if it is available. Antihistamines (H_1 receptor antagonists) are, far and away, the most frequent drugs used by radiologists for treatment of reactions.[51] Goldberg[129] points out that, in fact, antihistamines are probably of little value during severe contrast material reactions. Specific receptors

Table 4–2. Drugs and Equipment to be Near Radiology Examining Rooms

Drugs for Emergency Cart*

Metaraminol (Aramine)	Sodium bicarbonate	Norphine
Diphenhydramine hydrochloride (Benadryl)	Hydrocortisone 21-sodium succinate (Solu-Cortef)	Meperidine (Demerol) Phentolamine (Regitine)
Norepinephrine (Levophed)	Pentobarbital sodium (Nembutal)	Isoproterenol
Atropine	Diazepam (Valium)	Dopamine
Epinephrine (Adrenalin)	Oxygen	Lidocaine
Aminophylline	Nitroglycerin	
Calcium chloride		

Equipment for Emergency Cart*

AMBU bag or equivalent units with adult and child's masks
Oxygen cylinder, reducing valve, face mask, and tubing
Suction apparatus with catheters and tubing
Sphygmomanometer and stethoscope
Tourniquets
Syringes: 2, 5, 10, and 50 ml
Plastic or rubber oral airways (Safar or Brook)
Padded tongue depressors
Dextrose 5% in water
Dextrose 5% in saline with intravenous infusion sets
Tracheostomy tray
"Cutdown" tray
Needles: 19- and 21-gauge, standard length; 20-gauge, 4-inch length for intracardiac injections; 13- and 15-gauge for tracheotomy;
A defibrillator, ECG, a laryngoscopy and various sizes of intratracheal tubes should be accessible for use by personnel knowledgeable about their use.

*Modified from American College of Radiology. Committee on Drugs: Prevention and Management of Adverse Reactions to Intravascular Contrast Media (monograph). July, 1977; Hattery RR, Williamson B Jr, Hartman GW, et al: Intravenous urographic technique. Radiology 167:593, 1988.

blocked by antihistamines may have already been activated. The very weak bronchodilating action of these drugs may be insufficient if they are not supplemented. In an earlier section, we have indicated that experimental evidence downplays a significant role for histamine in severe forms of anaphylaxis. Nevertheless, because these drugs have few significant side-effects of their own, and controlled experimental therapy data are nonexistent, neither we, nor most others writing in this field, are prepared to abandon their use. The utilization of high doses of steroids in severe anaphylaxis does not rest on a secure experimental background. The data available suggest that the most likely mechanism of glucocorticoid protection in these instances involves the production of a protein, now known as lipocortin[130–132] that inhibits a cellular pathway leading to the production of vasoactive prostaglandins and leukotrienes (formerly S-RSA), substances that are generally believed to play a significant role in severe anaphylactic reactions.[90, 133–135] The time necessary to induce this protective protein would preclude a role for steroids in acute reactions. Our own experience[51] and that of others[124] supports this conclusion, because, in humans, steroids given in customary dosages shortly before contrast material challenge failed to confer any protection against reactions. Finally, it should be noted that patients given steroids for the treatment of acute asthmatic attacks did not gain any appreciable help until 4 to 6 hours after steroid administration.[136] Nevertheless, as in the case of antihistamines, it may be imprudent to recommend withholding steroids in treating acute reactions, since it is conceivable that these substances may forestall prolonged reactions, or potential recurrences some hours after the acute episode. The utilization of an anticonvulsant such as IV nembutal or diazepam to control seizures may be indicated in some instances—particularly when seizure activity is prolonged.

The two remaining categories of drugs that have been recommended for the therapy of anaphylaxis demand more thoughtful consideration. Although epinephrine has long been considered the first line of defense in acute anaphylactic reactions, no complete regimen for its utilization in these circumstances is forthcoming.[126] The α-agonist effects of epinephrine increase blood pressure and reverse peripheral vasodilitation. These vasoconstrictor changes may also decrease angioedema and urticaria.[126] The β-agonist actions of the drug reverse bronchoconstriction, produce positive inotropic and chronotropic cardiac effects and may increase intracellular cyclic AMP. Increments in baseline cyclic AMP levels are generally considered to inhibit mediator release from inflammatory cells, whereas decrements presumably have the opposite effect.[137, 138] Epinephrine, however, may have effects of its own, sufficiently untoward that in some situations the pro and con indications for its utilization merit careful consideration. For example, in individuals with a fragile intracerebral or coronary circulation, the α-agonist effects may invoke a hypertensive crisis that could produce a stroke or myocardial ischemia with resultant angina, arrhythmias, or even infarction.[126] Beta-receptor sites ordinarily respond to lower doses of epinephrine than α-sites, but if a patient is on β-blockers the refractory response that might occur when epinephrine is administered could encourage the treating radiologist to increase the dose to the point that unwanted α-effects would be generated. Patients with asthma may simulate patients receiving β-blockers since a β-adrenergic hyporesponsiveness in this disease has long been appreciated.[136, 139, 140] If the degree of β-responsiveness, either drug-induced or by virtue of disease, is sufficiently low, there will be a dominance of cholinergic activity and possibly a secondary bradycardia.[141] In such circumstances, we believe that patients undergoing anaphylaxis refractory to increased doses of epinephrine should be given isoproterenol, a β-agonist. Although there are no specific case reports of contrast material anaphylaxis to buttress this suggestion, we can point to parallel circumstances in the literature in which patients suffering insect sting anaphylaxis have received immediate beneficial effects from isoproterenol infusions.[142]

The effective use of atropine in a number of patients

suffering contrast material anaphylaxis with bradycardia has been reported.[143] Anticholinergics may also stimulate bronchodilatation and decrease bronchial secretions. Because acetylcholine, if present in sufficiently high concentration, has been shown to produce mediator release from mast cells,[144] anticholinergics, in appropriate circumstances, might diminish such release. The precise role of atropine in patients suffering contrast material anaphylaxis with associated bradycardia remains to be defined, as does the relative effectiveness of this drug as compared with that of isoproterenol.

Finally, it should be stressed that appropriate fluid replacement alone has been reported to be an effective treatment for contrast material anaphylaxis,[145] and, hence, the earlier injunction to begin intravenous physiological fluids before resort is taken to drug therapy should be re-emphasized as an axiomatic principle of high priority.

References

1. Sokoloff J, Berk RN, Lang JH, Lasser EC: The role of the Y and Z hepatic proteins in the excretion of radiographic contrast materials. Radiology 106:519–523, March 1973.
2. Wallingford VH: General aspects of contrast media research. Ann NY Acad Sci 78:707–719, 1959.
3. Strain WH: Historical development of radiocontrast agents. *In* Knoefel PK (ed): Encyclopedia of Pharmacological Therapeutics. New York, Pergamon, 1971, p 1–22.
4. Grainger RG: Intravascular contrast media—the past, the present, and the future. Br J Radiol 55:1–18, 1982.
5. Almén T: Development of nonionic contrast media. Invest Radiol (Suppl)20:S2–S9, 1985.
6. Osborne ED, Sutherland CG, Scholl AJ, Rowntree LG: Roentgenography of urinary tract during excretion of sodium iodide. JAMA 80:368–373, 1923.
7. Grainger RG: Intravascular contrast media (Letter to the Editor) Br J Radiol 55:544, 1982.
8. Brasch RC, Wesbey GE, Doemeny J, et al: Contrast media for nuclear magnetic resonance imaging. Invest Radiol (Suppl) 19:S148, 1984.
9. Wolf GL: Tissue-specific nuclear magnetic resonance contrast agents. Invest Radiol (Suppl)19:S148–S149, 1984.
10. Caille JM, Kien P, Lemanceau B, Bonnemain B: Contrast media in nuclear magnetic resonance. Invest Radiol (Suppl)19:S149, 1984.
11. Hoey GB, Adams MD, Robbins MS, et al: Factors in the design of nuclear magnetic resonance imaging agents. Invest Radiol (Suppl)19:S150, 1984.
12. Thompson W: A comparison of Iopamidol and meglumine diatrizoate. Invest Radiol (Suppl)19:S229–S233, 1984.
13. Lasser EC, Farr RS, Fujimagari T, Tripp WM: The significance of protein-binding of contrast media in roentgen diagnosis. Am J Roentgenol Rad Ther Nucl Med 87:338–360, 1962.
14. Lasser EC, Lang JH: The binding of roentgenographic contrast media to serum albumin. Invest Radiol 2:396–400, 1967.
15. Lang JH, Lasser EC: Nonspecific inhibition of enzymes by organic contrast media. J Med Chem 14:233–236, 1971.
16. Levitan H, Rappaport SI: Contrast media: quantitative criteria for designing compounds with low toxicity. Acta Radiologica Diagn 17:81–92, 1975.
17. Hansch C: The use of substituent constants in drug modification. Farmaco (Sci) 23:293–320, 1968.
18. Sovak M: Introduction: State-of-the-art and design principles of contrast media. *In* Sovak M (ed): Radiocontrast Agents. Springer-Verlag, New York, 1985, p 12.
19. Sovak M: Introduction: State-of-the-art and design principles of contrast media. *In* Sovak M (ed): Radiocontrast Agents. Springer-Verlag, New York, 1985, pp 13–17.
20. Hoey GB, Smith KR: Chemistry of x-ray contrast media. *In* Sovak M (ed): Radiocontrast Agents. Springer-Verlag, New York, 1985, p 55.
21. Laerum F: Injurious effects of contrast media on human vascular endothelium. Invest Radiol (Suppl)20:S98–S99, 1985.
22. Reidy JF: Iopamidol in peripheral angiography. Invest Radiol (Suppl)19:S206–S209, 1984.
23. Dawson P: Contrast agent nephrotoxicity on appraisal. Br J Radiol 58:121–124, 1985.
24. Cochran ST, Wong WS, Roe DJ: Predicting angiography–induced acute renal function impairment: Clinical risk model. AJR 141:1027–1033, 1983.
25. D'Elia JA, Gleason RE, Alday M, et al: Nephrotoxicity from angiograpic contrast material—a prospective study. Am J Med 72:719–725, 1982.
26. Ansari Z, Baldwin DS: Acute renal failure due to radio-contrast agents. Nephron 17:28–40, 1976.
27. Hayman LA, Evans RA, Fahr LM, Hinck VC: Renal consequences of rapid high-dose contrast CT. AJR 134:553–555, 1980.
28. Mudge GH: Some questions on nephrotoxicity. Invest Radiol 5:407–412, 1970.
29. Katzberg RW, Pabico RC, Morris TW, Hayakawa K: Mechanisms of contrast medium effects on the kidney. Invest Radiol (Suppl)19:S122, 1984.
30. Caldicott WJH: Discussion—genitourinary radiology session. Invest Radiol (Suppl)19:S128, 1984.
31. Golman K, Salvesen S, Hegedus V, Winding O: Acute renal failure after contrast media injection. Invest Radiol (Suppl) 19:S125, 1984.
32. Golman K, Almén T: Urographic contrast media and methods of investigative uroradiology. *In* Sovak M (ed): Radiocontrast Agents. Springer-Verlag, New York, 1985, p 156.
33. Golman K, Holtas S: Proteinuria produced by urographic contrast media. Invest Radiol 15:61–67, 1980.
34. Berdon WE, Shwartz RH, Becker J, Baker DH: Tamm-Horsfall proteinuria. Its relationship to prolonged nephrogram in infants and children and to renal failure following intravenous urography in adults with with multiple myeloma. Radiology 92:714–722, 1969.
35. Dawnay AB StJ, Thornley C, Nockler I, et al: Tamm-Horsfall glycoprotein excretion and aggregation during intravenous urography. Relevance to acute renal failure. Invest Radiol 20:53–57, 1985.
36. Lasser EC, Lang JH, Zawadski Z: Contrast media—myeloma protein precipitates in urography. JAMA 198:945–947, 1966.
37. Golman K, Almén T: Urographic contrast media and methods of investigative uroradiology. *In* Sovak M (ed): Radiocontrast Agents. Springer-Verlag, New York, 1985, p 153.
38. Hoey GB, Smith KR: Chemistry of x-ray contrast media. *In* Sovak M (ed): Radiocontrast Agents. Springer-Verlag, New York, 1985, p 54.
39. Hoey GB, Smith KR: Chemistry of x-ray contrast media. *In* Sovak M (ed): Radiocontrast Agents. Springer-Verlag, New York, 1985, p 55.
40. Hoey GB, Smith KR: Chemistry of x-ray contrast media. *In* Sovak M (ed): Radiocontrast Agents. Springer-Verlag, New York, 1985, p 56.
41. Hayman LA, Migliore PJ: Contrast-induced renal failure (Letter to the Editor). Radiology 3:867, 1980.
42. Chinn EK, Batsakis JG, Pilon H, Daelbecg K: Serum creatinine. A CAP survey. Am J Clin Pathol (Suppl)70:503–507, 1978.
43. Misson RT, Cutler RE: Radiocontrast-induced renal failure. West J Med 142:657–664, 1985.
44. VanZee BE, Hoy WE, Talley TE, Jaenike JR: Renal injury associated with intravenous pyelography in non-diabetic and diabetic patients. Ann Intern Med 89:51–54, 1978.
45. Harkonen S, Kjellstrand DC: Intravenous pyelography in non-uremic diabetic patients. Nephron 24:268–270, 1979.
46. Harkonen S, Kjellstrand CM: Exacerbation of diabetic renal failure following intravenous pyelography. Am J Med 63:939–946, 1977.
47. Teruel JL, Marcen R, Onaindia JM, et al: Renal function impairment caused by intravenous urography. A prospective study. Arch Int Med 141:1271–1274, 1981.
48. Ansell G, Tweedie MCK, West CR, et al: The current status of reactions to intravenous contrast media. Invest Radiol 15:S32–S39, 1980.
49. Witten DN, Hirsch FD, Hartman GW: Acute reactions to urographic contrast media: Incidence, clinical characteristics in relationship to history of hypersensitivity states. AJR 119:832–840, 1973.
50. Hobbs DB: Adverse reactions to intravenous contrast agents in Ontario, 1975–1979. J Can Assoc Radiol 31:8–10, 1981.
51. Lasser EC, Berry CC, Talner LB: Pretreatment with cortical steroids to alleviate reactions to intravenous contrast material. N Engl J Med 317:845, 1987.
52. Ansell G: Adverse reactions to contrast agents. Scope of problem. Invest Radiol 5:374–384, 1970.
53. Hartman GW, Hattery RR, Witten DM, Williamson B: Mortality

during excretory urography: Mayo Clinic experience. AJR 139:919–922, 1982.

54. Idsoe O, Guthe T, Wilcox RR, DeWeck AL: Nature and extent of penicillin side-reactions, with particular reference to fatalities from anaphylactic shock. Bull WHO 38:159–188, 1968.

55. Shehadi WH: Adverse reactions to intravascularly administered contrast media: A comprehensive study based on a prospective survey. AJR 124:145–152, 1975.

56. Littner MR, Rosenfield AT, Ulreich S, Putman CE: Evaluation of bronchospasm during excretory urography. Radiology 124:17–21, 1977.

57. Fischer HW, Doust VL: An evaluation of pretesting in the problem of serious and fatal reactions to excretory urography. Radiology 103:497–503, 1972.

58. Yocum NW, Heller AM, Abels RI: Efficacy of intravenous pretesting and antihistamine prophylaxis in radiocontrast media-sensitive patients. J Allergy Clin Immunol 62:309–313, 1978.

59. Lasser EC: Adverse reactions to intravascular administration of contrast media. Allergy 36:369–373, 1981.

60. Lasser EC, Lang JH, Lyon SG, et al: Prekallikrein-kallikrein conversion: conversion rates as a predictor for contrast catastrophies. Radiology 140:11–15, 1981.

61. Brasch RC, Tsay YG, Xia ZL, et al: Isolation of specific IgE anti-radiocontrast medium antibodies from patients having radiocontrast sensitivity. Radiology 153:328, 1984.

62. Arroyave CM: An in vitro assay for radiographic contrast media idiosyncrasy. Invest radiol 15:S21–S25, 1980.

63. Cogen FC, Norman ME, Dunsky E, et al: Histamine release and complement changes following injection of contrast media in humans. J Allergy Clin Immunol 64:299–303, 1979.

64. Rockoff S, Brasch R, Kuhn C, Chraplevy N: Contrast media as histamine liberators. I. Mast cell histamine release in vitro by sodium salts of contrast media. Invest Radiol 5:503–509, 1970.

65. Rockoff S, Aker U: Contrast media as histamine liberators. VI. Arterial plasma histamine and hemodynamic response following angiocardiography in man with 75% Hypaque. Invest Radiol 7:403–406, 1972.

66. Ring J, Arroyave CM, Fritzler MJ, Tan EM: In vitro histamine and serotonin release by radiographic contrast media in man. J Allergy Clin Immunol 61:145, 1978.

67. Simon RA, Schatz N, Stevenson DD, et al: Radiographic contrast media infusions. Measurements of histamine, complement and fibrin split products in correlation with clinical parameters. J Allergy Clin Immunol 63:281–288, 1973.

68. Lang JH, Lasser EC, Kolb WP: Activation of serum complement by contrast media. Invest Radiol 11:303–308, 1976.

69. Arroyave CM, Bhat KN, Crown R: Activation of the alternative pathway of the complement system by radiographic contrast media. J Immunol 117:1866–1869, 1976.

70. Gonsette RE, Delmonte P: In vivo activation of serum complement by contrast media—a clinical study. Invest Radiol 15:52–55, 1980.

71. Siegle RL, Lieberman P, Jennings BR, Rice NC: Iodinated contrast material: studies relating to complement activation, atopy, cellular association and antigenicity. Invest Radiol 15:513–517, 1980.

72. Lasser EC, Lang JH, Lyon SG, Hamblin AE: Changes in complement and coagulation factors in a patient suffering a severe anaphylactoid reaction to injected contrast media: some considerations of pathogenesis. Invest Radiol 15:S6–S12, 1980.

73. Westaby S, Dawson P, Turner MW, Pridie RB: Angiography and complement activation. Evidence for generation of C3a anaphylatoxin by intravascular contrast agents. Cardiovasc Res 19:85–88, 1985.

74. Fareed J, Moncada R, Messmore Jr HL, et al: Molecular markers of contrast media-induced adverse reactions. Sem Thromb Haemost 10:306–328, 1984.

75. Paajanen H: The effect of ionic and nonionic contrast media on the metabolism of prostaglandin E_2 in rat lungs. Invest Radiol 19:216–220, 1984.

76. Lasser EC: Metabolic basis of contrast material toxicity. Status 1971. Am J Roentgenol Rad Ther Nucl Med 13:415–422, 1971.

77. Zeman RK: Disseminated intravascular coagulations following intravenous pyelography. Invest Radiol 12:203–204, 1977.

78. Lasser EC, Slivka J, Lang JH, et al: Complement and coagulation—causative considerations in contrast catastrophies. AJR 32:171–176, 1979.

79. Brasch RC: Allergic reactions to contrast media: Accumulated evidence. AJR 134:797–801, 1980.

80. May CD: The ancestry of allergy: Being an account of the original

81. experimental induction of hypersensitivity recognizing the contribution of Paul Portier. J Allergy Clin Immunol 75:485–495, 1985.

81. Sheffer AL: Anaphylaxis. J Allergy Clin Immunol 75:227–233, 1985.

82. Findlay SR, Dvorak AN, Kagey-Sobotka A, Lichtenstein LN: Hyperosmolar triggering of histamine release from human basophils. J Clin Invest 67:1604–1613, 1981.

83. Silber G, Naclerio R, Eggleston P, et al: In vivo release of histamine by hyperosmolar stimuli (abstr). J Allergy Clin Immunol 75:176, 1985.

84. Erffmeyer JE, Siegle RL, Lieberman P: Anaphylactoid reactions to radiocontrast material. J Allergy Clin Immunol 75:401–410, 1985.

85. Wasserman SI: Mediators of immediate hypersensitivity. J Allergy Clin Immunol 72:101–115, 1983.

86. Lasser EC, Walters AJ, Reuter SR, Lang JH: Histamine release by contrast media. Radiology 100:683–686, 1971.

87. Kaliner N, Dyer J, Merlin S, et al: Increased urine histamine and contrast media reactions. Invest Radiol 19:116–118, 1984.

88. Brown R, Igram RH, Wellman JJ, McFadden ER: Effects of intravenous histamine on pulmonary mechanics in non-asthmatic and asthmatic subjects. J Appl Physiol 42:221–227, 1977.

89. Littner MR, Ulreich S, Putman CE, et al: Bronchospasm during excretory urography: lack of specificity for the methylglucamine cation. AJR 137:477–481, 1981.

90. Austen KF: Diseases of immediate-type hypersensitivity. In Petersdorf RG, Adams RD, Braunwald E, et al (eds): Harrison's Principles of Internal Medicine, 10th Ed. pp. 372–373. New York, McGraw-Hill, 1983.

91. Kay J, Caldwell JL, Brasch RC: Inhibition studies of anticontrast medium antibodies. Invest Radiol 16:397, 1981.

92. Brasch RC, Caldwell JL: The allergic theory of radiocontrast agent toxicity: demonstration of antibody activity in sera of patients suffering major radiocontrast agent reactions. Invest Radiol 11:347–356, 1976.

93. Brasch RC, Caldwell JL, Fudenberg HH: Antibodies to radiographic contrast agents. Induction and characterization of rabbit antibodies. Invest Radiol 11:1–9, 1976.

94. Brasch RC, Kay J, Mark F, Nitecki D: Allergy to radiographic contrast media: Accumulated evidence for antibody-mediated human toxicity and a new animal model. In Amiel M (ed): Contrast Media in Radiology. New York, Springer-Verlag, 1982.

95. Kleinknecht D, Deloux J, Homberg JC: Acute renal failure after intravenous urography: Detection of antibodies against contrast media. Clin Nephrol 2:116–119, 1974.

96. Harboe N, Folling I, Haugen OA, Bauer K: Sudden death caused by interaction between a macroglobulin and a divalent drug. Lancet 2:285–288, 1976.

97. Wakkers-Garritsen BG, Houwerziji J, Nater JP, Wakkers PJM: IgE-mediated adverse reactivity to a radiographic contrast medium—a case report. Ann Allergy 36:122–126, 1976.

98. Miller WL, Doppman JL, Kaplan AP: Renal arteriography following systemic reaction to contrast material. J Allergy Clin Immunol 56:291–295, 1975.

99. Siegle RL, Lieberman P: Measurement of histamine, complement components and immune complexes during patient reaction to iodinated contrast material. Invest Radiol 11:98–101, 1976.

100. deWeck AL: Drug reactions. In Samter M (ed): Immunological Diseases, 3rd Ed. Little, Brown & Company, 1978, pp 418–421.

101. Lasser EC, Kolb WP, Lang JH: Contrast media activation of serum complement system (Letter to the Editor). Invest Radiol 9:6a, 1974.

102. Kolb WP, Lang JH, Lasser EC: Nonimmunologic complement activation in normal human serum induced by radiographic contrast media. J Immunol 121:1232–1238, 1978.

103. Lasser EC, Lang JH, Lyon SG, Hamblin AE: Complement and contrast material reactors. J Allergy Clin Immunol 64:105–112, 1979.

104. Lieberman P, Siegle RL: Complement activation following intravenous contrast material administration. J Allergy Clin Immunol 64:13–17, 1979.

105. Saito H: The contact system in health and disease. Adv Int Med 25:217–238, 1980.

106. Herxheimer H, Stresemann E: The effect of bradykinin aerosol in guinea pigs and in man. J Physiol 158:38–39, 1961.

107. Varonier HS, Panzani R: The effect of inhalations of bradykinin on healthy and atopic (asthmatic) children. Int Arch Allergy 34:293–296, 1968.

108. Lasser EC, Lang JH, Curd JG, et al: The plasma contact system in atopic asthma. J Allergy Clin Immunol 72:83–88, 1983.

109. Harpel PC, Lewin MF, Kaplan AP: Distribution of plasma kallikrein between C1̄ inactivator and α_2-macroglobulin in plasma

utilizing a new assay for α_2-macroglobulin-kallikrein complexes. J Biol Chem 260:4257–4263, 1985.

110. Wiggins RC, Loskutoff DJ, Cochrane CG, et al: Activation of rabbit Hageman factor by homogenates of cultured rabbit endothelial cells. J Clin Invet 65:197–206, 1980.

111. Shimada T, Kato H, Iwanaga S, et al: Activation of Factor XII and prekallikrein with cholesterol sulfate. Thromb Res 38:21–31, 1985.

112. Castellot JJ Jr, Favreau LV, Karnovsky MJ, Rosenberg RD: Inhibition of vascular smooth muscle cell growth by endothelial cell-derived heparin. J Biol Chem 257:11256–11260, 1982.

113. Lasser EC, Simon RA, Lyon SG, et al: Heparin-like anticoagulants in asthma. Submitted for publication.

114. Lasser EC: Unpublished data.

115. Hojima Y, Cochrane CG, Wiggins RC, et al: In vitro activation of the contact (Hageman Factor) system of plasma by heparin and chondroitin sulfate E. Blood 63:1453–1459, 1984.

116. Douglas WW: Polypeptides—angiotensin, plasma kinins, and other vasoactive agents: Prostaglandins. In Goodman LS, Gilman A (eds): The Pharmacologic Basis of Therapeutics. MacMillan, 1970, pp 663–676.

117. Kellermeyer RW, Graham RC Jr: Kinins—possible physiologic and pathologic roles in man. N Engl J Med 279:754–759, 1968.

118. Lalli AF: Reactions to contrast media: Testing the CNS hypothesis. Radiology 138:47–49, 1981.

119. Russell M, Dark KA, Cummins RW, et al: Learned histamine release. Science 225:733–734, 1984.

120. Zweiman B, Mishkin MM, Hildreth EA: An approach to the performance of contrast studies in contrast material-reactive persons. Ann Int Med 83:159–161, 1975.

121. Greenberger P, Patterson R, Kelly J, et al: Administration of radiographic contrast media in high-risk patients. Invest Radiol 15:S40–S43, 1980.

122. Small P, Satin R, Palayew MJ, Hyams B: Prophylactic antihistamines in the management of radiographic contrast reactions. Clin Allergy 12:289–294, 1982.

123. Greenberger P, Patterson R, Radin RC: Two pretreatment regimens for high-risk patients receiving radiographic contrast media. J Allergy Clin Immunol 74:540–543, 1984.

124. Ring J, Rothenberger K-H, Clauss W: Prevention of anaphylactoid reactions after radiographic contrast media infusion by combined histamine H$_1$- and H$_2$-receptor antagonists: Results of a prospective control trial. Int Arch Allergy Appl Immunol 78:9–14, 1985.

125. Agardh C-D, Arner P, Ekholm S, Boijsen E: Desensitisation as a means of preventing untoward reactions to ionic contrast media. Acta Radiol Diagn 24:235–239, 1983.

126. Barach EM, Nowak RM, Lee TG, Tomlanovich MC: Epinephrine for treatment of anaphylactic shock. JAMA 251:2118–2122, 1984.

127. Smith PL, Kagey-Sobotka A, Bleecker ER, et al: Physiologic manifestations of human anaphylaxis. J Clin Invest 66:1072–1080, 1980.

128. American College of Radiology Committee on Drugs: Prevention and Management of Adverse Reactions to Intravascular Contrast Media (monograph). July, 1977.

129. Goldberg M: Systemic reactions to intravascular contrast media—a guide for the anesthesiologist. Anesthesiology 60:46–56, 1984.

130. Hirata F, Schiffmann E, Venkatasubramanian K, et al: A phospholipase A$_2$ inhibitory protein in rabbit neutrophils induced by glucocorticoids. Proc Natl Acad Sci USA 77:2533–2536, 1980.

131. Blackwell GJ, Flower RJ, Nijkamp FP, Vane JR: Phospholipase A$_2$ activity of guinea-pig isolated perfused lungs: Stimulation, and inhibition by anti-inflammatory steroids. Br J Pharmacol 62:79–89, 1978.

132. DiRosa M, Flower RJ, Hirata F, et al: Nomenclature announcement: Anti-phospholipase proteins. Prostaglandins 28:441–442, 1984.

133. Dahlen S-E, Hedqvist P, Hammarstrom S, Samuelsson B: Leukotrienes are potent constrictors of human bronchi. Nature 288:484–486, 1980.

134. Hedqvist P, Dahlen S-E, Gustafsson L, et al: Biological profile of leukotrienes C$_4$ and D$_4$. Acta Physiol Scand 110:331–333, 1980.

135. Piper PJ: The evolution and future horizons of research on the metabolism of arachidonic acid by 5-lipooxygenase. J Allergy Clin Immunol 74:441–444, 1984.

136. Morris HG: Mechanisms of action and therapeutic role of corticosteroids in asthma. J Allergy Clin Immunol 75:1–13, 1985.

137. Zurier RB, Weissmann G, Hoffstein S, et al: Mechanisms of lysosomal enzyme release from human leukocytes. II. Effects of cAMP and cGMP, autonomic agonists, and agents which affect microtubule function. J Clin Invest 53:297–309, 1974.

138. Ignarro LJ, Colombo C: Enzyme release from polymorphonuclear leukocyte lysosomes: Regulation by autonomic drugs and cyclic nucleotides. Science 180:1181–1183, 1973.

139. Krzanowski JJ, Szentivanyi A: Refractions on some aspects of current research in asthma (editorial). J Allergy Clin Immunol 72:433–442, 1983.

140. Shelhamer JH, Marom Z, Kaliner M: Abnormal beta-adrenergic responsiveness in allergic subjects. II. The role of selective beta-2-adrenergic hyporeactivity. J Allergy Clin Immunol 71:57–61, 1983.

141. Kaliner M, Orange RP, Austen KF: Immunologic release of histamine and flow-reacting substance of anaphylaxis from human lung. IV. Enhancement by cholinergic and alpha-adrenergic stimulation. J Exp Med 136:556–567, 1972.

142. Ingall M, Goldman G, Page LB: β-blockade in stinging insect anaphylaxis (Letter to the Editor). JAMA 251:1432, 1984.

143. Stanley RJ, Pfister RC. Bradycardia and hypotension following use of intravenous contrast media. Radiology 121:5–7, 1976.

144. Fantozzi R, Masini E, Blandina P, et al: Nature 273:473–474, 1978.

145. Obeid AI, Johnson L, Potts J, et al: Fluid therapy in severe systemic reaction to radiopaque dye. Ann Int Med 83:317–321, 1975.

146. Rapaport SI, Bookstein JJ, Higgins CB, et al: Experience with metrizamide in patients with previous severe anaphylactoid reactions to ionic contrast agents. Radiology 143:321–325, 1982.

147. Bettman MA: Radiographic contrast agents—a perspective (editorial). N Engl J Med 317:891, 1987.

148. Wolf GL: Safer, more expensive iodinated contrast agents. How do we decide? Radiology 159:557, 1986.

149. White RI, Halden WJ Jr: Liquid gold: Low-osmolality contrast media. Radiology 159:559, 1986.

150. Cohan RH, Dunnick NR: Intravascular contrast media: adverse reactions. AJR 149:665, 1987.

151. Stacul F, Carraro M, Magnaldi S, et al: Contrast agent nephrotoxicity: Comparison of ionic and nonionic contrast agents. AJR 149:1287, 1987.

152. Lasser EC: A coherent biochemical basis for increased reactivity to contrast material in allergic patients: A novel concept. AJR 149:1281, 1987.

153. Miller DL, Chang R, Wells WT, et al: Intravascular contrast media: Effect of dose on renal function. Radiology 167:607, 1988.

154. Jacobsson BF, Jorulf H, Kalanter MS, Narasimham DL: Nonionic versus ionic contrast media in intravenous urography: Clinical trial in 1000 consecutive patients. Radiology 167:601, 1988.

155. Hattery RR, Williamson B Jr., Hartman GW, et al: Intravenous urographic technique. Radiology 167:593, 1988.

156. Cohan RH, Dunnick NR, Bashore TM: Treatment of reactions to radiographic contrast material. AJR 151:263, 1988.

157. Cochran ST, Ballard JW, Katzberg RW, et al: Evaluation of iopamidol and diatrizoate in excretory urography: A double-blind clinical study. AJR 151:523, 1988.

158. Gomes AS, Baker JD, Paredero M, et al: Acute renal dysfunction after major arteriography. AJR 145:1249, 1985.

159. Binz A, Rath C: Die chemie des uroselectans. Klin Woschr 9:2297, 1930.

160. Hoppe JO, Larsen A, Coulston F: Observations on the toxicity of a new urographic contrast medium sodium 3,5-diacetomido-2,4,6-triiodobenzoate (Hypaque sodium) and related compounds. J Pharmacol Expt Therap 116:394, 1956.

161. Evens RG: Low-osmolality contrast media: Good news or bad? Radiology 169:277, 1988.

162. Parfrey PS, Griffiths SM, Barrett BJ, et al: Contrast-induced renal failure in patients with diabetes mellitus, renal insufficiency, or both. N Engl J Med 320:143, 1989.

163. Schwab SJ, Hlatky MA, Pieper KS, et al: Contrast nephrotoxicity: A randomized controlled trial of a nonionic and an ionic radiographic contrast agent. N Engl J Med 320:149, 1989.

164. Kinnison ML, Powe NR, Steinberg EP: Results of randomized controlled trials of low- versus high-osmolality contrast media. Radiology 170:381, 1989.

165. Jacobson PD, Rosenquist CJ: The introduction of low-osmolar contrast agents in radiology: Medical, economic, legal and public policy issues. JAMA 260:1586, 1988.

166. Gold RP: The radiologist's role in treating reactions to contrast media. Radiology 169:875, 1988.

167. Gomes AS, Lois JF, Baker JD, et al: Acute renal dysfunction in high-risk patients after angiography: Comparison of ionic and nonionic contrast media. Radiology 170:65, 1989.

168. Benness GT, Fischer HW: Reactions to ionic and nonionic contrast media. Radiology 170:282, 1989.

5

Abdominal Plain Radiography

ZORAN L. BARBARIC ☐ HOWARD M. POLLACK

A radiograph of the abdomen has two major uses: as a means of primary examination of the abdomen and as an overture to a radiographic contrast examination of any anatomical structure in the abdomen, including the urinary tract. Synonyms that have been used over the years are KUB (short for kidneys, ureters, and bladder), scout film, plain film, and preliminary radiograph. The term "flat plate" is an anachronism and a throwback to the early days of radiology before the days of x-ray film. It has no place in current terminology. Only *preliminary radiograph of the abdomen, preliminary roentgenogram of the abdomen,* or, if the administration of a contrast medium is to follow, *preliminary roentgenogram of the pelvis,* are technically correct terms. The word *plain* frequently substitutes for the word *preliminary* and implies that no contrast has been administered. The term *abdominal plain radiography* seems a logical and acceptable compromise.

Four main reasons for obtaining a preliminary radiograph prior to a contrast examination are the following:

1. To check on the technical quality of the examina-

tion. It is improper to administer radiographic contrast material to the patient if the positioning is not correct, or if the radiograph is over- or under-exposed. The preliminary radiograph allows the necessary adjustments to be made before contrast material is given. A proper radiograph for the urinary tract examination must include the areas of both adrenal glands on the top and a point 2 cm below the inferior margin of the symphisis pubis on the bottom. Frequently, it is impossible to fit this large area on a single radiograph and two different film sizes have to be used (Fig. 5–1). The supine position is preferred for the plain radiograph. Prone and erect radiographs are reserved for special indications.

2. To detect calcific densities that could be urinary tract calculi. Contrast material in the collecting system may totally obliterate the image of some urinary calculi, especially if they are in the kidney. Without the preliminary radiograph, many renal calculi cannot be diagnosed. Frequently, it is impossible to determine from a single radiograph whether a calcific density is in the expected anatomical distribution of the urinary tract. An additional

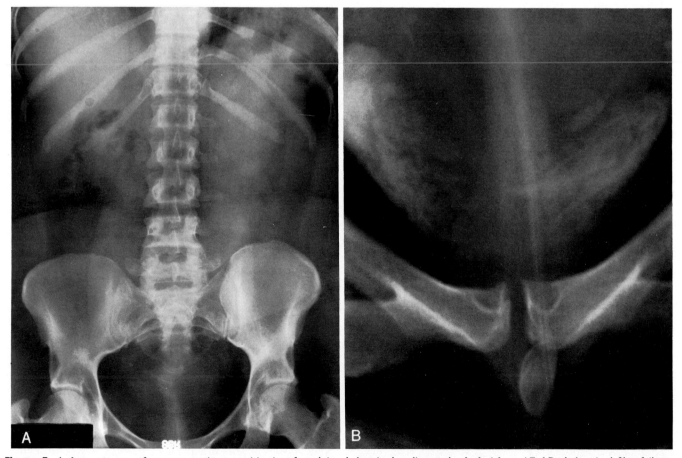

Figure 5–1. Importance of proper patient positioning for plain abdominal radiograph. *A,* A 14 × 17 AP abdominal film fails to include the inferior pubic angle. *B,* A subsequent film made to include only the pelvis reveals a large urethral calculus within a diverticulum in a 27-year-old woman.

oblique projection is often needed to take a second look at the calcification to see if it "moves" with the kidney (Fig. 5–2).

3. To determine whether a contraindication to abdominal compression exists. Compression is usually used in the course of obtaining an excretory urogram in order to distend the upper urinary tract system, thus better visualizing the collecting systems. Some contraindications to compression are (1) abdominal aortic or iliac artery aneurysm (Fig. 5–3), (2) abdominal distention (ileus, bowel obstruction, ascites), (3) acute abdomen (appendicitis, cholecystitis, abscesses, perforation), (4) recent abdominal surgery, (5) various types of urinary tract diversions and stomas, (6) abdominal trauma, (7) Greenfield filter (Fig. 5–4) or umbrella in the inferior vena cava, and (8) acute renal colic. Many of the radiographic signs contributing to diagnosis of the conditions enumerated above are present on the preliminary radiograph. This does not imply that other pathological entities are being ignored but merely that, if necessary, they can be detected on the other radiographs obtained in the course of the urographic contrast examination.

4. To determine if bowel preparation is adequate. Frequently the patient has residual contrast material, usually barium in his or her colon, from an earlier radiological examination or an inordinate amount of gas. A decision has to be made for each patient individually regarding whether or not to proceed with the contrast examination, depending on the indications, the amount of retained contrast material, and so forth. This may be one of the most trying decisions a radiologist is called upon to make. On one hand, cost constraints make it mandatory to perform studies without delay. On the other hand, a study that is technically inadequate owing to the obscuring effects of barium may be worse than no study at all, and may actually be a disservice to the patient.

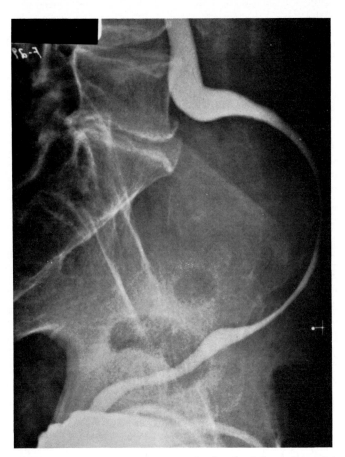

Figure 5–3. Lateral projection at the level of the pelvic inlet during a contrast examination of the urinary tract. The ureter is markedly displaced anteriorly by an iliac artery aneurysm. Faint calcification can be detected outlining the size of the aneurysm. External ureteral compression is definitely contraindicated in this case.

ANATOMICAL LANDMARKS

Organ Outlines. Larger parenchymal organs such as kidneys, liver, spleen, and urinary bladder are almost always identified on a plain abdominal radiograph. Their

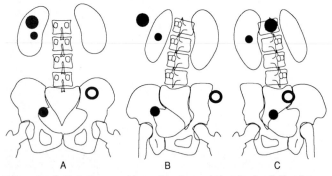

Figure 5–2. Relative position of various abdominal calcifications on different radiographic projections: A, AP; B, RPO; and C, LPO. The right upper-quadrant calcifications represent a gallstone and a renal calculus. The right lower-quadrant calcification is an appendicolith. The left lower-quadrant calcification is a granuloma in the gluteus maximus muscle. Note that with rotation the various types of calcification can usually be distinguished from each other by more or less typical changes in their relation to known structures.

outline is visible because of the contrasting radiolucent mesenteric or retroperitoneal fat that surrounds these organs. On careful inspection, even the right adrenal gland can sometimes be identified in the fat-filled triangular radiolucent suprarenal area. Numerous superimposed radiodensities and radiolucencies from the gas-filled bowel obscure much of the anatomical detail provided by the contrasting fat. The main function of tomographic techniques is to reduce unwanted bowel "noise."

Major Muscle Outlines. The psoas muscle is particularly well outlined by fat on plain radiographs. Disappearance of this outline may imply the presence of fluid in the compartment adjacent to the psoas muscle. One centimeter lateral and parallel to the psoas is the outline of the quadratus lumborum muscle. Although visualization of both psoas muscles is expected in the healthy patient, in fact, failure to clearly outline the psoas muscle on one side may be seen in up to 20% of abdominal radiographs in normal persons. In the pelvis, the outline of the internal obturator muscle forms the lateral wall of the pelvic fossa (obturator line).

Properitoneal Fat. Properitoneal fat is also known as the "flank fat stripe." It is the continuation of the posterior paranephric space and is sandwiched between transversalis fascia and the parietal peritoneum. The medial interface of this radiolucent stripe, therefore, identifies the lateral extent of the peritoneal cavity.

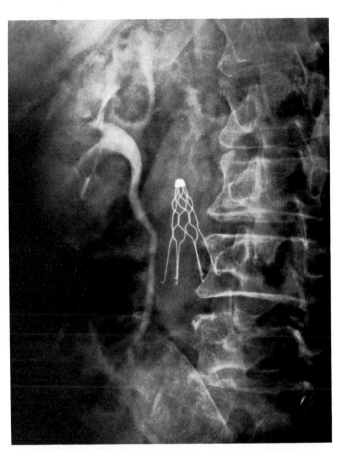

Figure 5—4. Greenfield filter in inferior vena cava. This is another contraindication to external ureteral compression.

Perivesical Fat Line. The top of the bladder, particularly when the bladder is empty, is outlined by a radiolucent strip of perivesical fat.

Stomach and Bowel Gas. Because the fundus is the most dependent part of the stomach when the patient is in the supine position, it is usually filled with fluid, whereas gas tends to accumulate in the antrum. On occasion a fluid-filled fundus may mimic a left upper-quadrant mass. (Fig. 5–5). The presence of a mass can be excluded by placing the patient in the prone position, in which the fluid and gas reverse their locations. The hepatic flexure of the colon is almost always in the subhepatic area. Occasionally, this part of the colon is interposed between the dome of the liver and the diaphragm (Chilaiditi's syndrome).

ACUTE ABDOMINAL DISORDERS

A plain radiographic examination of the abdomen should always be approached with seriousness. A referring clinician who requests an abdominal examination likely suspects an acute process to be excluded or confirmed. Many diseases outside the urinary tract mimic urinary tract symptoms, and vice versa. The patient probably exhibits nonspecific symptoms, usually pain or epigastric discomfort. All contrast examinations include a precontrast or a preliminary radiograph. A variety of abnormal findings and normal variants that could mimic a pathological process are likely to be encountered.

Renal Colic

A small renal or ureteral stone or poorly calcified stone may easily be missed on a plain radiograph. This frequently occurs in the presacral ureteral segment, where superimposed bony densities interfere with detection (Fig. 5–6). Presence of calcifications outside the urinary tract, particularly phleboliths and other vascular calcifications, may present difficulties and false-positive results.

Acute Appendicitis

A common need for an abdominal radiograph arises during triage in the emergency room for a patient with nonspecific right lower-quadrant pain. A specific radiographic sign for acute appendicitis is the presence of an appendicolith (Fig. 5–7). They are more common in children than in adults, and the overall incidence is 14%.[1] They are also more common in the retrocecal appendix.[2] Appendicoliths may be confused with ureteral calculi, and vice versa.

Other findings are a soft-tissue mass representing an abscess or edema that separates the cecum from the properitoneal fat line and, possibly, a slight curvature of the spine due to splinting. Perforation of the appendix may be suggested if no gas is seen in the ascending colon (spasm) while there is paralytic ileus of the transverse colon (dilated transverse colon sign).[3] Gas in the appendix must always be viewed as suspicious for appendicitis, although it is occasionally seen normally, especially in an incompletely rotated colon (Fig. 5–8).

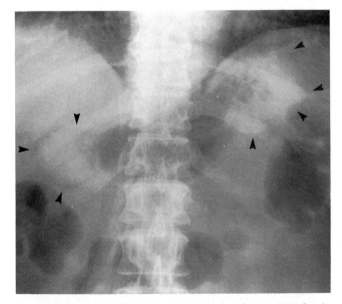

Figure 5—5. Pseudotumors produced by the gastric fundus and duodenal bulb. A plain abdominal radiograph demonstrates bilateral soft-tissue densities (*arrowheads*) superimposed over the upper portions of each kidney. On the left, the soft-tissue density is attributable to the gastic fundus; on the right, to the duodenal bulb. Care must be exercised in not misinterpreting these common artifacts as renal or adrenal masses.

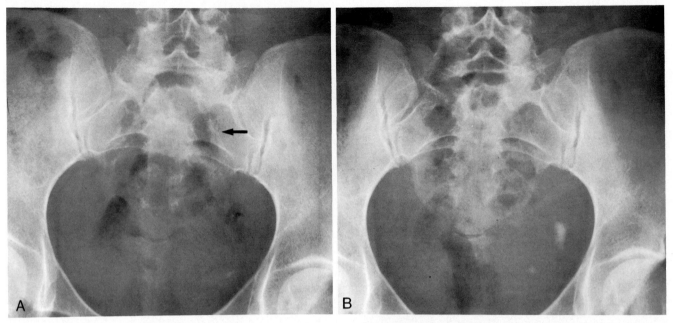

Figure 5–6. Inapparent ureteral calculus. *A*, Plain abdominal radiograph reveals a barely perceptible opacity superimposed over the sacrum (*arrow*). The patient was complaining of left flank pain and was told initially that there was "no evidence of a ureteral calculus." In retrospect, the calculus was identified. *B*, Film exposed 10 weeks later now reveals the calculus to be present in the distal left ureter. The opacity over the sacrum is no longer seen. In cases such as this, oblique films usually clarify the issue.

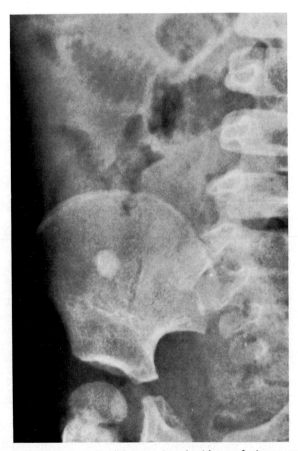

Figure 5–7. Appendicolith associated with a soft-tissue mass in the right lower quadrant is diagnostic of acute appendicitis. (Courtesy M.I. Boechat, M.D.)

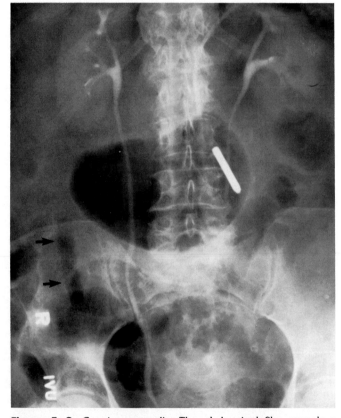

Figure 5–8. Gas in appendix. The abdominal film reveals a tubular gas-filled structure in the right lower abdomen (*arrows*) indicative of gas in the appendix. This 67-year-old woman complained of right lower-quadrant pain. Laparotomy revealed acute appendicitis. Although gas in the appendix is usually abnormal, it can occasionally be seen normally, especially in patients with retrocecal inverted appendices.

Intestinal Obstruction

Radiographic findings of intestinal obstruction depend on the level as well as on the completeness of the obstruction, and on the period of elapsed time between occurrence of the obstruction and performance of the examination. If enough time elapses, the intestine distal to the obstruction is nondistended and gas free. The intestine above the obstruction is dilated and contains gas, intestinal fluid, and perhaps food material. If the radiograph is obtained early after the obstruction has occurred, the distal intestine may still contain gas and fecal material, and the bowel proximal to the obstruction may not have had a chance to distend. Therefore, serial examinations may be necessary. A suspicion of bowel obstruction mandates the performance of the erect or possibly lateral decubitus radiograph, as well as the standard supine radiograph.

Gastric-outlet obstruction is caused by a hypertrophic pyloric stenosis and an antral web in neonates; it is caused by carcinoma, volvulus, scar due to gastric ulcer, or bezoar in adults.[4]

Duodenal obstruction has numerous developmental causes when seen in neonates.[5] In adults, duodenal obstruction is more likely due to tumor extension and invasion from pancreatic carcinoma, renal carcinoma, or metastatic lymph nodes. Other causes are duodenal ulcer, primary carcinoma of the duodenum or duodenal hematoma.[6] A peculiar type of duodenal obstruction may be caused by compression of the superior mesenteric artery and vein upon the third portion of the duodenum as it crosses the aorta. This tends to occur in patients in wholebody casts (cast syndrome) but interestingly is not associated with the "nutcracker" syndrome, in which similar superior mesenteric arterial compression is exerted upon the left renal vein.[7]

A classic radiographic finding is the "double bubble" sign (Fig. 5–9), in which two distinct air pockets, one in the stomach and the second in the duodenum, are seen. Jejunal obstruction may produce the "triple bubble" sign.[8]

Urologists in particular are concerned about small-bowel obstruction after dividing and reanastomosing the bowel during construction of various conduits and diversions. In the presence of small-bowel obstruction, dilatation of the bowel is proximal to the site of the obstruction. Air–fluid levels are seen particularly well on the upright or decubitus radiograph. The more distant the site of the obstruction, the more numerous are the air–fluid levels. No air or fecal material is identified in the large bowel some time after the acute event (Fig. 5–10).

Besides postsurgical adhesions, causes for small bowel obstruction are numerous and include intussusception, gallstone ileus, inflammatory bowel disease, periappendiceal abscess, small-bowel tumors, and hernias.[9] One should always look for inguinal hernias on the abdominal radiograph. They are seen as gas-containing soft-tissue masses in the groin area. One should also look for evidence of incisional hernia in patients known to have prior abdominal surgery. Bowel herniation through the foramina of Morgagni and Bochdalek may be seen.[10]

Common causes of large-bowel obstruction are colonic carcinoma, metastases, volvulus, diverticulitis, and fecal impaction in adults, and meconium plug syndrome, colonic atresia and anal atresia in neonates. Distention is again the diagnostic feature on a plain radiograph, while retained fecal material may be striking in quantity. Perforation is a hazard if the large bowel, usually the cecum, enlarges to 10 cm or more in diameter.

Ileus

A lack of peristaltic activity is also likely to cause bowel dilatation. Causes are numerous and include postoperative ileus, many systemic diseases, drugs, ischemic bowel

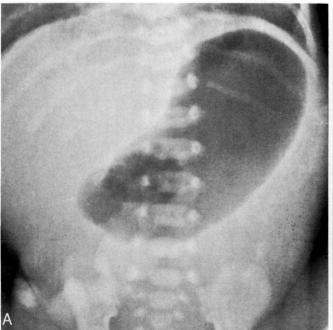 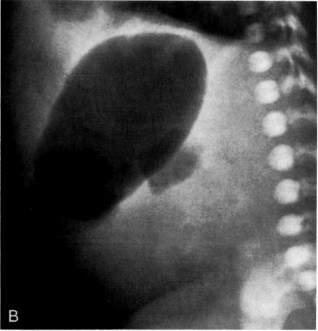

Figure 5–9. "Double bubble" sign in a neonate with congenital duodenal obstruction. *A,* Supine view. Only gas-filled stomach is seen. *B,* Same patient, lateral projection. The obstructed duodenum is now distended with gas. On occasion this sign may be better observed in a projection other than anteroposterior (AP). (Courtesy M.I. Boechat, M.D.)

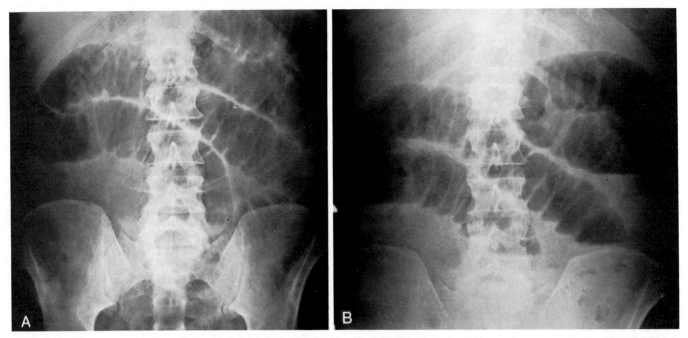

Figure 5–10. Proximal small bowel obstruction due to adhesions. *A,* In the supine position little or no gas is seen in the small or the large bowel distal to the obstruction site. *B,* Same patient in the upright position. Several air-fluid levels are now evident. (Courtesy Barbara M. Kadell, M.D.)

disease, neuromuscular disorders, uremia, hypokalemia, scleroderma, diabetes, and many more.[11–14]

Postoperative ileus is diffuse and usually appears after abdominal surgery. Characteristically, both the small and the large bowels are dilated. This is the important finding differentiating the disorder from acute small bowel obstruction.

Localized ileus is a reflection of a localized, isolated inflammatory process in the abdomen where there is inhibition of bowel motility adjacent to an inflammatory process. Prime examples are acute pancreatitis or acute cholecystitis (sentinel ileus) (Fig. 5–11).[15]

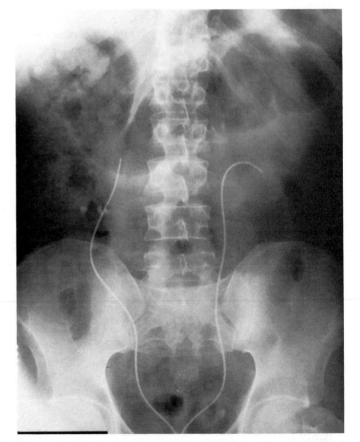

Figure 5–12. Colon "cutoff" sign. Following the passage of bilateral ureteral catheters in this patient with lymphoma, abdominal pain developed. The colon is dilated to the region of the splenic flexure, suggesting retroperitoneal irritation of the left side. The position of the tip of the left ureteral catheter suggests that it may have perforated the ureter at this point. The catheter was partially withdrawn and correctly repositioned, and the large-bowel ileus disappeared. Lateral deviation of right ureter is attributable to retroperitoneal adenopathy.

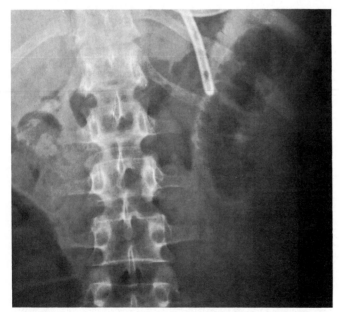

Figure 5–11. Sentinel ileus of a proximal loop of small bowel is shown in a patient with acute pancreatitis. (Courtesy Barbara M. Kadell, M.D.)

Ureteral colic is frequently accompanied by ileus. Renal inflammatory disease may be associated with a segmental type of large bowel ileus, the "colon cutoff" sign, in which the colon is dilated from the cecum to a point overlying the abnormal kidney and beyond which it is devoid of gas (Fig. 5–12).

Perforation

A perforated viscus allows gas to escape into the peritoneal cavity. The detection of this "free" gas is therefore mandatory. To facilitate detection of gas that might have collected in the lesser sac (e.g., posterior gastric wall perforation), the patient is placed in the left lateral decubitus position for at least 10 minutes. Gas thereby escapes from the lesser sac through the gastro-epiploic foramen and into the greater peritoneal cavity, where it is easily detected. Appropriate views should include (1) left lateral decubitus, (2) anterior-posterior (AP), and (3) chest (PA).[16] A cross-table lateral radiograph occasionally reveals free air just below the anterior abdominal wall, when the gas is equivocally demonstrated on other views.

Large amounts of intraperitoneal gas may contrast other intraperitoneal structures, such as the falciform ligament,[17] or may collect under the dome of the anterior abdominal wall (football sign),[18] and contrast any intra-peritoneal fluid (Fig. 5–13).[19] Both sides of the bowel wall, rather than the luminal side only (double-wall sign) (Fig. 5–14),[20] or gas trapped between several loops of bowel assuming triangular appearance (triangle sign)[21] may also be seen. Air can be found in the scrotum of children with pneumoperitoneum, retroperitoneal emphysema, or scrotal injury (Fig. 5–15).

Certain conditions may simulate gas in the peritoneal cavity, such as the intestine between diaphragm and liver (Chilaiditi's syndrome) or subdiaphragmatic fat.[22] Large amounts of free intraperitoneal air may be found normally up to a week after abdominal surgery.

Abdominal Fluid

Large amounts of peritoneal fluid can easily be detected on an abdominal radiograph, because the floating loops of bowel are localized in the central abdomen. An overall haze and increased density due to attenuation of x-rays by the fluid are also seen (Fig. 5–16A, B).

Smaller amounts of fluid (ascites, blood, intestinal contents) are more difficult to detect. The fluid tends to accumulate first in the most dependent parts of the

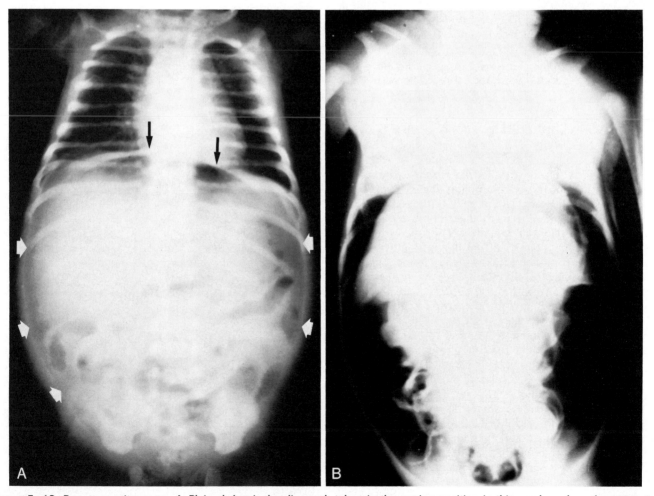

Figure 5–13. Pneumoperitoneum. *A,* Plain abdominal radiograph taken in the supine position in this newborn boy demonstrates free air distributed throughout the entire peritoneal space (*arrowheads*). The air is particularly well seen just below the diaphgram in the midline (*arrows*) ("football sign"). Diagnosis: perforated cecum. *B,* Abdominal film taken in the prone position results in redistribution of the intraperitoneal gas and a much clearer depiction of a massive pneumoperitoneum.

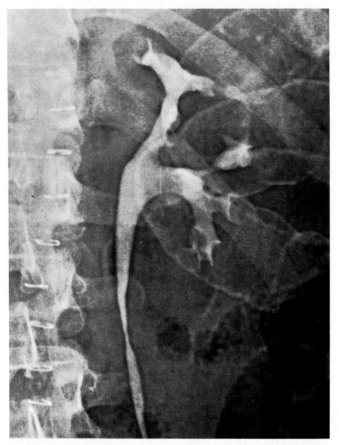

Figure 5–14. Double-wall sign pathognomonic for free intraperitoneal gas. Both the inside and outside of the bowel wall are outlined by gas. The visualized loops of bowel are distended.

The outline of this space may become visible on the plain radiograph, because it is contrasted from outside of Gerota's fascia by paranephric fat. The reverse is also true. A fluid-filled paranephric space contrasts the fat within the perinephric space (Fig. 5–19).[28–31]

Abscess

There is no doubt that the primary method for evaluating the abdomen for presence and distribution of intra-abdominal abscesses is computed tomography (CT). However, an abscess may frequently be seen on abdominal examination performed for other reasons, and it should not be overlooked. Intra-abdominal abscess is diagnosed with certainty only if gas is seen within a soft-tissue mass (Fig. 5–20). It is easy to confuse the gas within the abscess with that of bowel gas interspersed within fecal material, although multiple small gas bubbles are practically pathognomonic of abscess. Most intra-abdominal abscesses are complications of abdominal surgery (Fig. 5–21), diverticulitis,[32] and pancreatitis.[33]

Common locations for abscesses are as follows: anterior or posterior subphrenic space on the right, Morison's pouch, pelvis, lesser sac, anterior paranephric space, left subphrenic space, pericolic space, ischiorectal fossa (Fig. 5–22), and posterior paranephric space. Perivesical abscess is usually seen after bladder surgery.

Renal and perinephric abscesses are discussed elsewhere (see Chapter 22).

intraperitoneal cavity: (1) Douglas's pouch and peritoneal recesses in the pelvis, (2) the right paracolic gutter, and (3) Morison's pouch (hepatorenal angle). As the fluid accumulates in the pelvis, radiographic density increases. Characteristic appearance resembling dog ears can occur when the fluid fills the lateral pelvic recesses (Fig. 5–17).[23] Fluid in the right paracolic gutter is detected with greater ease than fluid in the pelvis. The fluid in the right paracolic gutter is contrasted from the outside by properitoneal fat and from the inside by the gas in the ascending colon.[24] If the measured distance between these two structures, which also includes the thickness of the colon wall, is greater than 4 mm, it is diagnostic of the presence of fluid.

As the fluid continues to accumulate, the tip of the liver becomes surrounded and obliterated, because mesenteric fat no longer provides contrast. The right lateral hepatic border may be displaced medially, if sufficient fluid is present (Hellmer's sign) (see Fig. 5–16B).[25]

Retroperitoneal fluid is somewhat more difficult to detect on plain radiographs. Obliteration of the psoas outline is a suggestive sign,[26] although the psoas is not well visualized in a number of patients even without fluid.[27] Also, large amounts of fluid are required to fill the retroperitoneal space along the psoas muscle, and the fluid must be interspaced between the muscle and retroperitoneal fat for this sign to become evident.

Fluid localized in the perinephric space obliterates the renal outline and the fat within that space (Fig. 5–18).

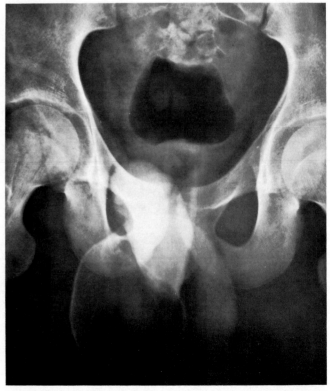

Figure 5–15. Right-sided pneumoscrotum associated with penetrating scrotal trauma.

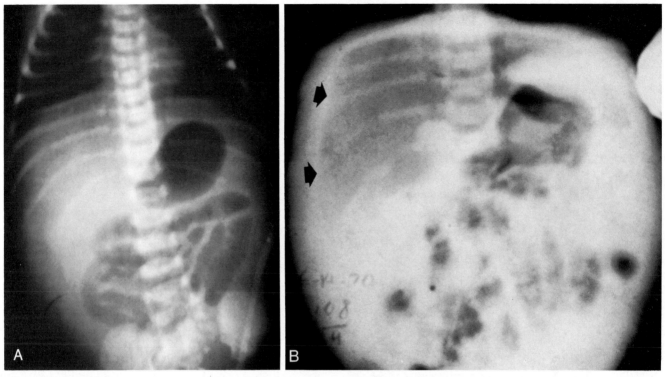

Figure 5–16. Ascites in the newborn. *A*, Plain abdominal radiograph in the supine position in this 2-day-old male infant reveals considerable fluid in the peritoneal space. The centralized or "floating" small-bowel loops are diagnostic. *B*, Abdominal radiograph taken after a cystogram demonstrates massive intraperitoneal accumulation of contrast material. The liver is particularly well outlined with contrast material, and the right hepatic border is displaced medially by the fluid (Hellmer's sign) (*arrowheads*). Diagnosis: intraperitoneal rupture of the urinary bladder secondary to catheterization.

Figure 5–17. Pelvic ascites. The plain abdominal radiograph demonstrates distention of the pelvic peritoneal cavity by fluid. The right and left peritoneal reflections (*asterisks*) overlap the lateral margins of the partially filled urinary bladder, indicating fluid in the pelvis. This sign is often the first—and sometimes the only—finding in patients with traumatic rupture of an abdominal organ. Note spina bifida occulta involving the upper sacrum.

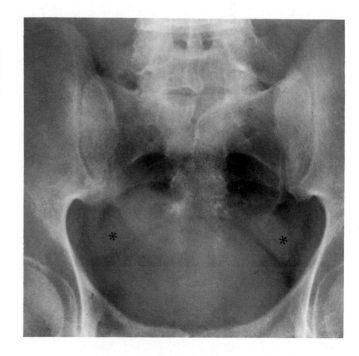

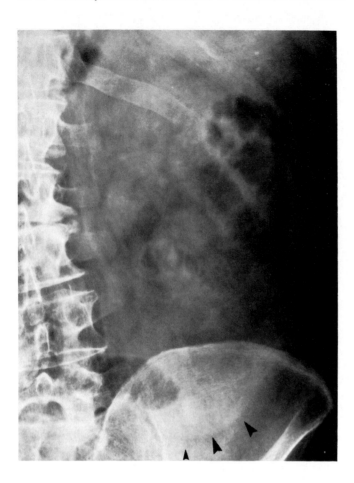

Figure 5–18. Patient with a ureteral obstruction and pyelosinus extravasation. Extravasated urine in this patient has accumulated in the perinephric space, obliterating the renal outline. The caudad extension of the fluid-filled perinephric space is outlined at the bottom of the illustration (*arrowheads*).

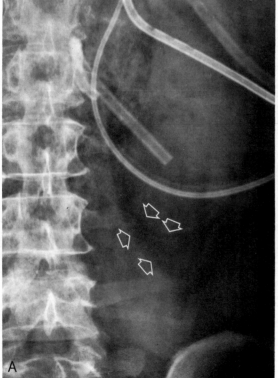

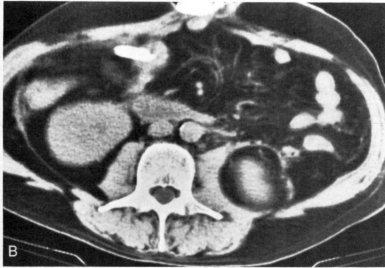

Figure 5–19. Renal "halo" sign. *A,* Fluid in the anterior paranephric space and outside of the renal fascia, outlines the perinephric fat. Kidney within the perinephric fat appears as if it is surrounded by a lucent halo (*arrowheads*). The sign is useful for diagnosing paranephric fluid. The patient had a pancreatic abscess. *B,* CT slice through the lower pole of the left kidney in the same patient demonstrates fluid in the anterior paranephric space and fat surrounding the lower pole of the left kidney.

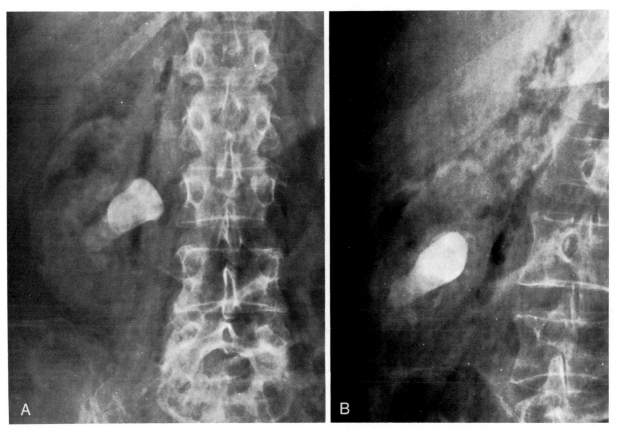

Figure 5–20. Right gas-forming perinephric abscess in a patient with pyohydronephrosis and a renal calculus. *A*, Except for the gas collection that parallels the psoas, one would have difficulty in differentiating the rest of the gas from bowel contents. *B*, RPO projection in the same patient clearly shows the gas to be anterior and posterior to the kidney.

Acute Cholecystitis

Gallstones are present in almost all patients with acute cholecystitis, but only 10% to 20% are visible on a radiograph. The most sensitive and pathognomonic sign is intramural and/or intraluminal gas (emphysematous cholecystitis),[34] an extreme form of acute cholecystitis

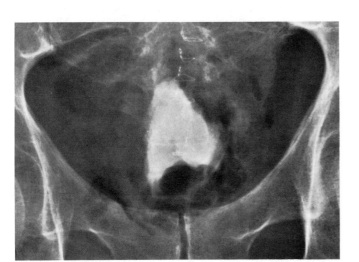

Figure 5–21. Gas-containing perivesical abscess after abdominoperineal resection. Contrast material in the bladder is from a cystogram.

(Fig. 5–23). An acutely inflamed gallbladder may perforate either into the peritoneal cavity or into the small bowel. The latter condition may result in acute bowel obstruction due to gallstone impaction as the stone travels down the intestinal tract (gallstone ileus). Gas may be evident in the biliary system of patients with gallstone ileus.[35]

Intramural Gas

Gas in the bowel wall is called *pneumatosis intestinalis*[36] and commonly involves the sigmoid and descending colons (pneumatosis coli),[37] although it may involve small bowel and stomach (emphysematous gastritis). Causes are numerous and include necrotizing enterocolitis in children,[38] intestinal obstruction, occlusion of the mesenteric vessels with bowel infarction, various types of bypass intestinal surgery, obstructive pulmonary disease, and pneumomediastinum. Many cases of pneumatosis coli, especially in adults, are completely asymptomatic and benign (Fig. 5–24).

Emphysematous cystitis (Fig. 5–25) is an acute bladder inflammation characterized by gas in the bladder wall.[39] Occasionally, gas may be found within the bladder lumen. Almost all patients have diabetes. Curiously, this disease causes only the minor symptoms of dysuria and frequency.

Emphysematous pyelonephritis is discussed elsewhere (see Chapter 21).

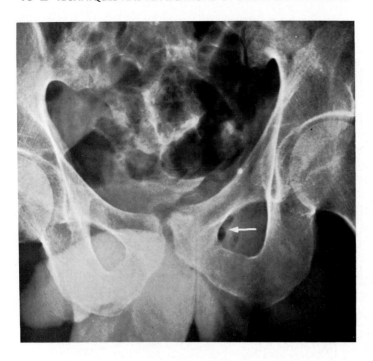

Figure 5–22. Ischiorectal fossa abscess. Gas projecting over the left obturator foramen (*arrow*) is too far lateral to be in the rectum. Differential diagnosis also includes an inguinal hernia, but the absence of the soft-tissue component militates against this diagnosis.

UNUSUAL GAS COLLECTIONS

Gaseous radiolucencies are frequently seen in the soft tissues of the abdominal wall (Fig. 5–26). This is most commonly the result of surgery in which some air is trapped in the subcutaneous tissues; or it may be due to chest tube placement or may even follow laryngostomy. On occasion, these collections become large. If the radiolucencies are tangential to the x-ray beam, for instance occurring in the flank, they are easily identified. On the other hand, if the air dissects through soft tissues of the anterior abdominal wall, it may cast confusing shadows.

During introduction of epidural anesthesia, small amounts of air are injected through the needle until a "give" signifies that epidural space has been reached. The injected air may dissect along the fascial planes of the dorsolumbar muscles in the form of streaky artifacts,[40] superficially mimicking retroperitoneal emphysema.

Gas may be seen in the biliary system after neocholedochoduodenostomy or after gallbladder perforation into the intestines. Gas in the portal system may occur with pneumatosis intestinalis and necrotizing enterocolitis. A benign form occurs in neonates with umbilical vein catheters that find their way into the portal system.[41]

Air is frequently found in the urinary tract in the presence of indwelling catheters or nephrostomy tubes, or after bladder and urethral instrumentation.

In patients with certain types of urinary tract diversion, gas reflux into the upper urinary tract system may occur. Prime examples are ureterosigmoidostomy (Figs. 5–27, 5–28) and ileal loop diversion. The presence of gas in the voided urine is called pneumaturia. Without a history of prior catheterization, it signifies either a gas-forming urinary tract infection or a fistula between the urinary and gastrointestinal tract. Few things are more frightening to the patient than a sudden, unexpected appearance of gas at the end of micturition.

Renal carcinoma, particularly if large, may show radiolucencies after complete embolization, even in the absence of acute infection.[42] This is similar to the subcutaneous or intravascular gas formation in a dead fetus.

A fresh vaginal tampon is seen as a radiolucent cylinder, usually pointing to the right or left lateral vaginal recess (see Fig. 5–62). Giant colonic diverticula may present as unusual abdominal gas collections.

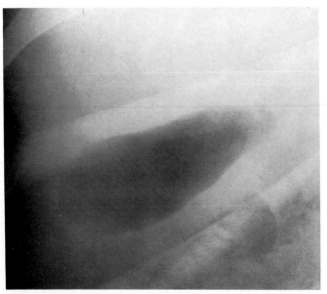

Figure 5–23. Emphysematous cholecystitis. A plain abdominal radiograph coned to the right upper quadrant reveals a gas-filled gallbladder. The patient was quite ill with right upper-quadrant pain, sepsis, and signs of peritoneal irritation. Emergency cholecystectomy revealed a gangrenous gallbladder.

CALCIFICATIONS

The number and types of calcifications encountered in the abdomen are many. McAfee and Donner have listed almost 200.[43] All abdominal calcifications consist of

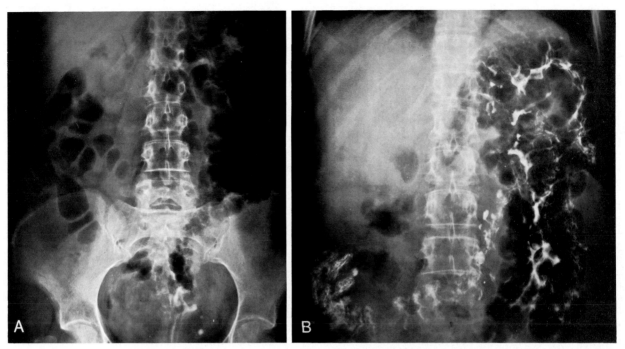

Figure 5–24. Pneumatosis coli. *A*, Plain radiograph shows normal-appearing right colon but an unusual appearance of the gas pattern in the splenic flexure and descending colon. *B*, Postevacuation radiograph after a barium enema shows the collapsed lumen of the left colon outlined by barium. Large blebs of intramural gas impress upon the barium. The patient was relatively asymptomatic and was followed with this problem over period of years. The pneumatosis eventually resolved spontaneously.

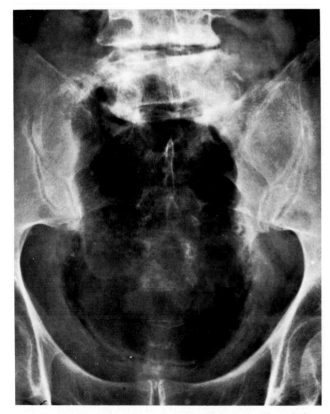

Figure 5–25. Emphysematous cystitis. This patient has diabetes and urinary tract infection with *Candida albicans*.

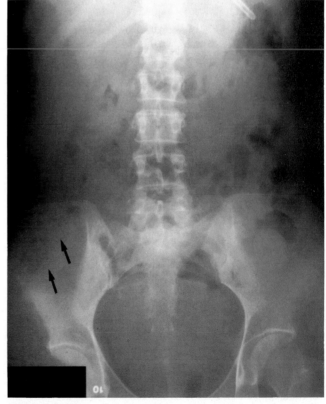

Figure 5–26. Abdominal-wall gas secondary to hypodermic injections. The patient is a 37-year-old female with deep vein thrombosis. She had been self-administering injections of heparin into the anterior abdominal wall, which accounts for the streaks of air (*arrows*). A nasogastric tube is seen superiorly, and a vaginal tampon inferiorly.

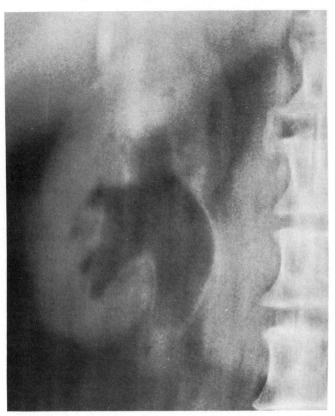

Figure 5–27. Gas reflux into the pyelocalyceal system from the sigmoid colon in a patient with ureterosigmoidostomy.

stones, dystrophic calcifications, vascular calcification, or heterotopic bone formation.[41]

Urinary tract calculi, nephrocalcinosis, and other calcifications of the urinary tract are addressed in detail elsewhere. Other common calcifications in the abdomen include vascular, biliary, prostatic, ligamentous, and soft tissue.

Vascular Calcifications

Arterial vascular calcifications are usually linear, and occasionally parallel. Their distribution matches the expected distribution of the vessels (Fig. 5–29), although very tortuous vessels may attain a different anatomical position. The splenic artery is likely to be the first to calcify (Fig. 5–30). Calcification in the abdominal aorta and iliac arteries may be best seen on left posterior oblique or lateral projections (see Fig. 5–52). In the presence of an abdominal aortic aneurysm (Fig. 5–31), ureteral compression by an external device is contraindicated. Therefore, care should be exercised in scrutinizing the preliminary radiograph for this disease. Vascular calcification is particularly pronounced in diabetics, in whom it may involve, for example, uterine or testicular vessels, or the branches of the renal artery, which is rarely encountered in nondiabetics (Fig. 5–32).

Renal and splenic-artery aneurysms (Fig. 5–33) are easily detected and should not be confused with cysts or neoplasms of these organs. Smaller than 2 cm in diameter, calcified aneurysms are benign, are not expected to rupture, and usually require no treatment. Aneurysms may grow to an extremely large size (Fig. 5–34).

Phleboliths (Fig. 5–35) are perhaps the most common intra-abdominal calcifications.[44] They may present difficulties when one is searching for a ureteral calculus. Characteristically, they are round and contain a radiolucent center (Fig. 5–36). Their distribution is usually below the ischial spines. Nonetheless, urography or pyelography is usually necessary for unequivocal differentiation of phlebolith from stones. By comparison with a prior examination, an unsuspected pelvic mass may be diagnosed by virtue of the fact that phleboliths have been displaced. Phleboliths may also appear in unusual locations, for instance in the periureteral plexus of veins (see Fig. 5–43) or in the plexus pampiniformis. A cluster of phleboliths in an unusual location (e.g., abdominal wall) may indicate a hemangioma (Fig. 5–37).

In infancy, an inferior vena cava thrombus may calcify, characteristically in the intrahepatic portion (Fig. 5–38). Pelvic veins may calcify following thrombophlebitis or radiotherapy (Fig. 5–39).

Intraluminal Calcifications

Gallstones are the most common visceral intraluminal calcifications (Fig. 5–40). In all sizes and shapes, they exhibit different radiodensities and may layer, showing a horizontal fluid–stone interface in the upright projection. Only 10% to 15% of all gallstones are sufficiently radiopaque to be seen on plain radiograph.[45] Gallstones are usually laminated or may exhibit radiolucent fissures (Mercedes Benz sign) (Fig. 5–41).[46–47] Another rare but most dramatic condition, "milk-of-calcium bile" exists in the presence of calcium carbonate suspension composed of microscopic calcifications in liquid forms. The milk-of-calcium layers can be seen in the erect or decubitus position.[48] One should always look for gallstones in the region of the common bile duct. Because of their characteristic location, gallstones are not often confused with

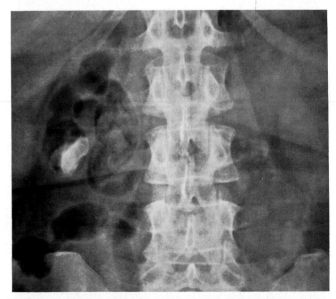

Figure 5–28. Gas, calculus, and an intraluminal filling defect are seen in the right renal pelvis in a patient with ureterosigmoidostomy. The filling defect proved to be a fungus ball. Note gas in the dilated right ureter.

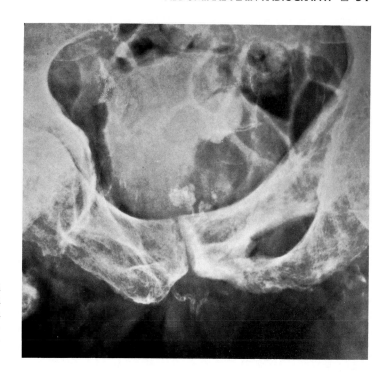

Figure 5–29. Calcification of the dorsal penile arteries in a patient with diabetes mellitus. Also present are prostatic calcification and Paget's disease involving the left pubic bone. Cortical thickening, coarse trabecula, and bone expansion are present and constitute the radiographic hallmarks of Paget's disease.

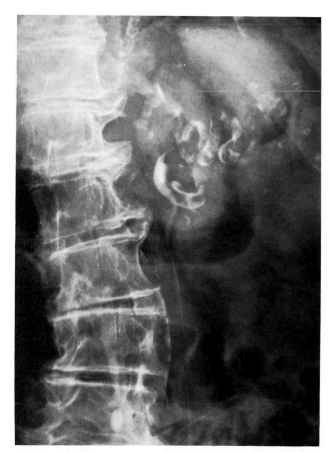

Figure 5–30. Heavy vascular atheromatous calcification involving aorta and splenic artery. The splenic artery tends to become tortuous. There is also pronounced degenerative disease of the lumbar spine.

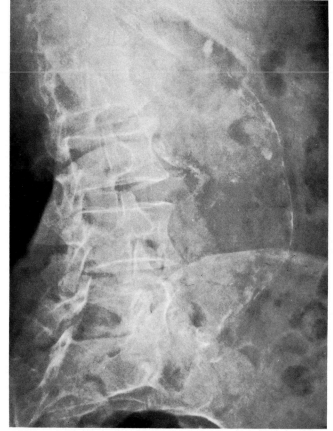

Figure 5–31. Calcified abdominal aortic aneurysm. The left posterior oblique projection is usually the optimal one for demonstrating these aneurysms.

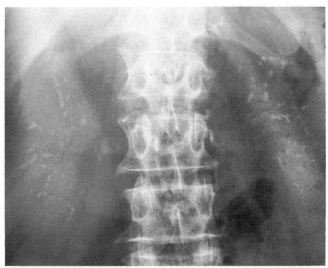

Figure 5–32. Calcification of the intrarenal branches of the renal artery. Plain abdominal radiograph demonstrates diffuse intrarenal vascular calcification in a 60-year-old diabetic woman. Such extensive intrarenal calcification is unusual and usually indicates diabetes mellitus.

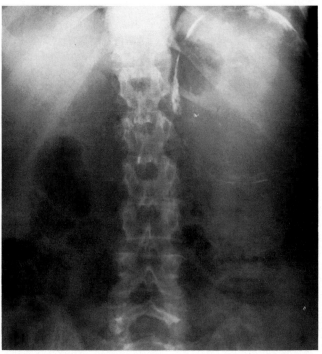

Figure 5–34. Abdominal calcification secondary to giant aneurysm of the splenic artery. This is a 74-year-old asymptomatic female.

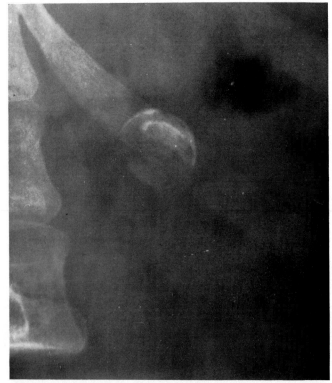

Figure 5–33. Calcified left renal artery aneurysm (atherosclerotic). The lesion is located in the renal hilus and involves the main renal artery.

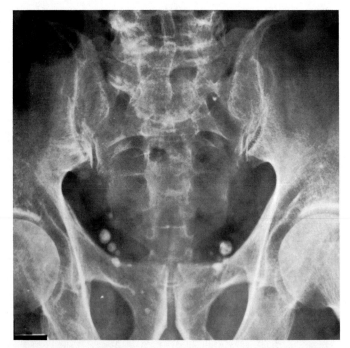

Figure 5–35. Phleboliths are calcified thrombi within the pelvic veins. They usually do not, but sometimes can present a diagnostic problem, because occasionally differentiation from distal ureteral calculus is impossible. The typical pelvic phlebolith lies below the level of the ischial spines and has a laminated or "bull's-eye" appearance. In fact, however, they can occur almost anywhere, and at times can only be differentiated from ureteral calculi by urography or retrograde studies.

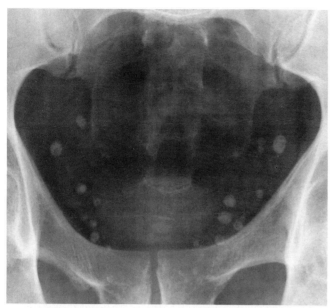

Figure 5–36. Phleboliths. Typical radiographic picture of multiple pelvic phleboliths. The phleboliths are clustered to either side of the pelvis and arranged in the distribution of the pelvic veins. The phleboliths tend to be round and fairly opaque, and they commonly measure 2 to 6 mm in diameter, although there are numerous exceptions.

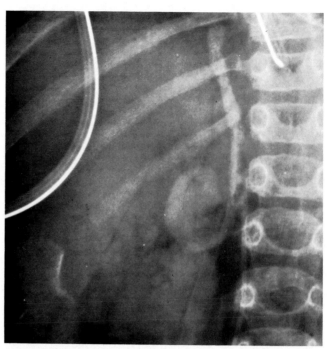

Figure 5–38. Calcified thrombus in the intrahepatic part of the inferior vena cava in an infant. (Courtesy M. I. Boechat, M.D.)

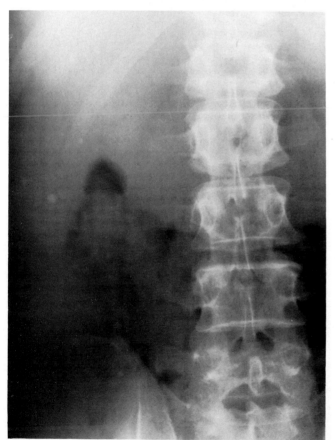

Figure 5–37. Cavernous hemangioma of abdominal wall. Plain abdominal radiograph demonstrates numerous small, round radiolucencies in the right midabdomen. These represented phleboliths within blood vessels of a giant cavernous hemangioma of the anterior abdominal wall. (Courtesy E. Darracot Vaughan, Jr., M.D.)

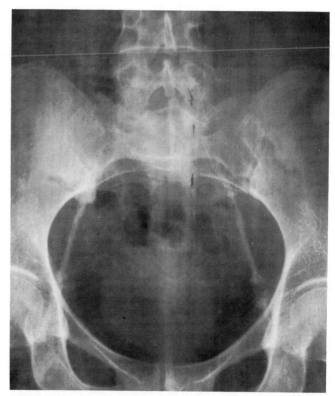

Figure 5–39. Calcified iliac veins. Years earlier, this middle-aged female had undergone radiotherapy to the pelvis for uterine carcinoma. A plain abdominal radiograph demonstrates dense calcification of the iliac and femoral veins bilaterally. The location of the calcification was proved by means of phlebography.

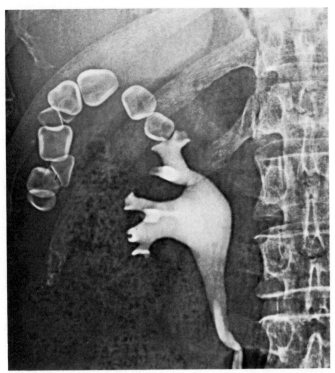

Figure 5—40. Gallstones. The multiple, faceted, similar-appearing calcifications are typical. Deposition of calcium bilirubinate around a cholesterol nucleus gives the gallstones a lucent center and a ring shape.

urinary stones, but on occasion this distinction may prove challenging.

Pancreatic calcifications are almost always associated with chronic pancreatitis (Fig. 5–42). These have a characteristic distribution starting from the C-shaped loop of the duodenum and extending toward the splenic hilus (Fig. 5–43). They are almost always intraductal (calcium carbonate) and less commonly occur in areas of fat necrosis (calcium hydroxyapatite). A pancreatic pseudocyst presents as a mass, frequently showing rim calcification, and usually originates in the pancreatic tail. A similar appearance may occur with pancreatic cystadenocarcinoma. Pancreatic calcifications in children are associated with hereditary pancreatitis and cystic fibrosis.[49]

An appendicolith is a fecolith (coprolith) found in the lumen of the appendix (Fig. 5–44).[2] This finding is almost always associated with acute appendicitis. Other fecoliths may be found in a Meckel's diverticulum (meckolith) or in other parts of the gastrointestinal tract (Figs. 5–45 and 5–46).

Renal, ureteral, and bladder calculus diseases are discussed elsewhere. Suffice it to say, urinary-tract calculi have a variety of radiographic appearances (Figs. 5–47, 5–48). The presacral area must always be scrutinized for their presence, as this is a site where they are commonly missed (Fig. 5–49).

Occasionally, a closed-off calyceal diverticulum contains crystals of calcium phosphate and, occasionally, calcium carbonate. The condition is known as milk-of-calcium urine, and the crystals layer so that a fluid–fluid interface is seen on an upright or cross-table lateral projection (Fig. 5–50).

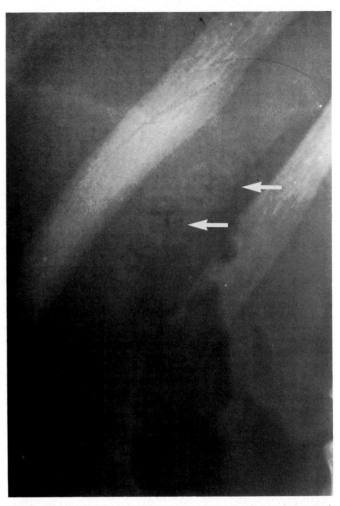

Figure 5—41. Gas-containing gallstones. A plain abdominal radiograph coned to the right upper quadrant reveals several gallstones with radiolucent centers (*arrows*). The triradiate appearance of the gas within the gallstones has given rise to the term "Mercedes Benz" sign. (Courtesy Thomas C. Beneventano, M.D.)

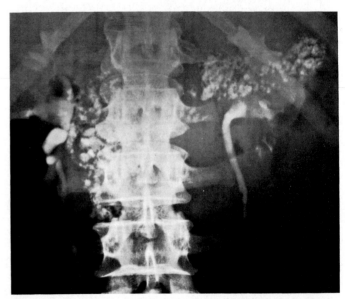

Figure 5—42. Pancreatic calcifications in a patient with chronic pancreatitis. Most of the pancreatic calcification is intraductal.

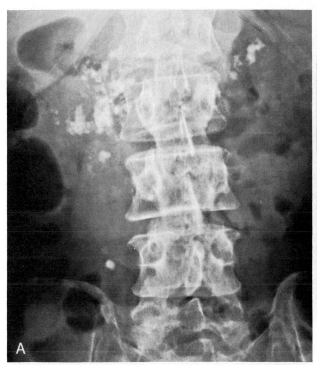

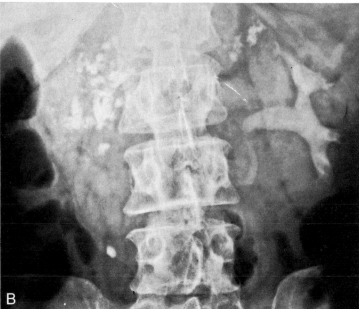

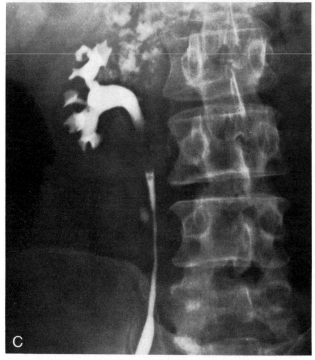

Figure 5–43. Coexistent pancreatic and venous calcification. *A,* Heavy pancreatic calcification is present. Calcific density to the right of L5 vertebral body could be a ureteral calculus. *B,* Excretory urogram on the same patient demonstrates no excretion by right kidney and ureteral calculus has not been excluded. *C,* Retrograde pyelogram excludes obstruction. Calcific density is probably a phlebolith in periureteral venous plexus or gonadal vein and not a ureteral calculus. Renal function is absent because of renal artery occlusion demonstrated on a subsequent angiogram.

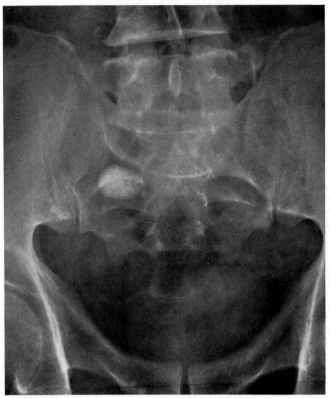

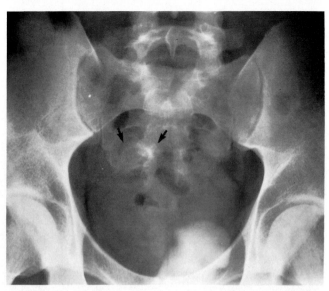

Figure 5—46. Calculi in Meckel's diverticulum. A plain abdominal radiograph of the pelvis demonstrates several laminated calculi overlying the sacrum (*arrows*). Originally these calculi were thought to be within the lower urinary tract, but they eventually proved to reside within a Meckel's diverticulum. (Courtesy John Rawlings, M.D.)

Figure 5—44. A very rare occurrence of a pelvic kidney harboring a calculus mimicking an appendicolith.

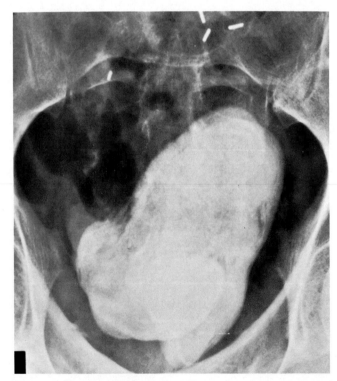

Figure 5—45. Large rectal fecolith forming around an exposed nonabsorbable suture in a patient with ureterosigmoidostomy.

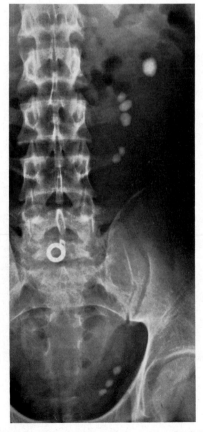

Figure 5—47. An array of nine urinary-tract calculi in left kidney and ureter. A surgical gown snap overlays the sacrum.

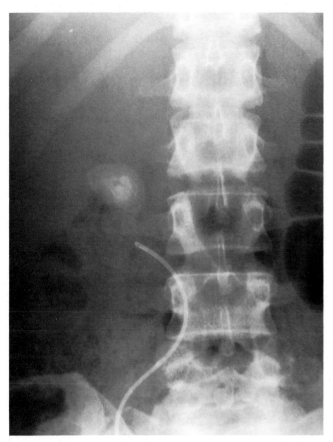

Figure 5–48. Laminated kidney stone simulating gallstone. The laminated appearance of this right upper-quadrant calculus is suggestive of a gallstone. However, the stone was impacted in the ureteropelvic junction. It is not always possible to judge the origin of a calculus based on its location or appearance.

Prostatic calcifications are very common (see Fig. 5–29). These are small intratubular calcific concrements that are usually asymptomatic, but which at times may be associated with an inflammatory process. Most prostatic calcifications occur between areas of adenomatous hyperplasia and the surgical capsule of the prostate.

Parenchymal and Intramural Calcifications

Extraurinary

Mesenteric lymph-node calcification is the most common type of parenchymal calcification in the abdomen. Calcified nodes have a "popcorn" appearance and a characteristic distribution along the expected propagation of the mesenteric root. Calcification of the retroperitoneal, porta hepatis, retrocrural, and pelvic lymph nodes is rare. As is the case with other abdominal calcifications, calcified lymph nodes may be confused with renal or ureteral calculi. Tuberculous mesenteric lymphadenitis may have a striking appearance (Fig. 5–51).

Gallbladder-wall calcification has a very characteristic appearance, and is called "porcelain gallbladder" (Fig. 5–52).[50]

The liver is a common site for metastases (Fig. 5–53). Mucin-producing adenocarcinoma, particularly from the gastrointestinal tract, generates a psammomatous type of calcification. Curvilinear calcifications are seen in echi-

nococcal cysts (Fig. 5–54).[51, 52] Other causes of liver calcifications include tuberculosis, portal vein thrombosis, granulomatous disease of childhood,[53] hepatoblastoma, abscess, aneurysm, and giant hemangioma.[54, 55]

Splenic parenchymal calcifications are common, usually a result of the healing of small histoplasmosis granulomas. Rare causes of splenic calcifications are splenic cyst, splenic infarct (Fig. 5–55), brucellosis, hydatid disease (Fig. 5–56), and old splenic hematoma. Splenic cyst may be confused with a splenic artery aneurysm (see Fig. 5–34).

Adrenal gland calcifications are due to a variety of causes and may or may not be associated with an adrenal mass.[56] Both neoplastic and benign diseases exhibit calcification, so this finding alone does not provide a definitive diagnosis. Differential diagnosis includes hemorrhage, tuberculosis, metastases, cysts (Fig. 5–57), neuroblastoma, Wolman's disease, adenocarcinoma (Fig. 5–58), and, rarely, pheochromocytoma.

Uterine calcifications, particularly heavy and dense ones, are seen in uterine leiomyomas and are quite characteristic (Figs. 5–59 to 5–61; see Fig. 5–59). Cystadenoma and cystadenocarcinoma of the ovary show amorphous calcification in half of all cases. Dermoid cysts usually have calcified elements (Figs. 5–62, 5–63) although they may also be suspected in the presence of radiolucent fat (Fig. 5–64). Fat within and outside of the

Text continued on page 63

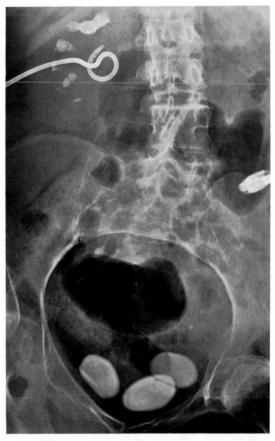

Figure 5–49. Multiple calculi in the bladder and the kidney in a patient with multiple sclerosis. Right ureteral calculus is present just below the pelvic inlet. The ureteral calculus is causing obstruction, requiring a percutaneous nephrostomy tube. Tip of a gastrostomy tube is seen on the left.

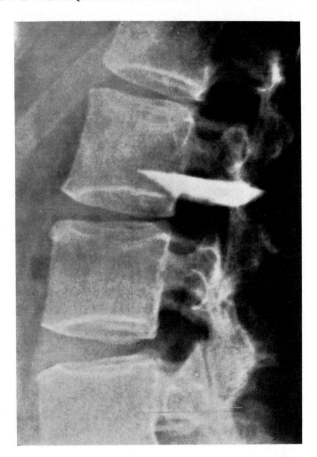

Figure 5–50. "Milk-of-calcium urine" in an obstructed calyceal diverticulum. Fluid–fluid interface is present on an upright lateral projection.

Figure 5–51. Calcified mesenteric lymph nodes secondary to tuberculosis. The abdominal plain radiograph reveals densely calcified mesenteric lymph nodes. Some of the nodes are unusually large and demonstrate an amorphous type of calcification, which suggests underlying caseation necrosis. Calcified mesenteric nodes are a very common finding in abdominal radiographs. They usually have a fairly characteristic appearance and location. Large irregularly calcified nodes such as this, however, are uncommon.

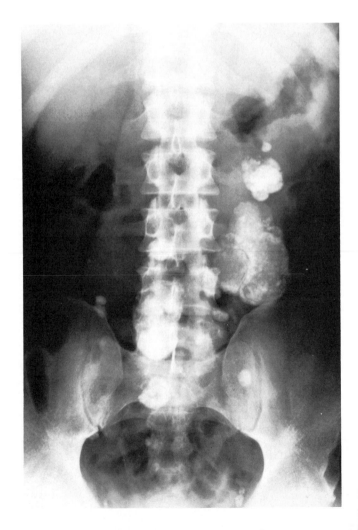

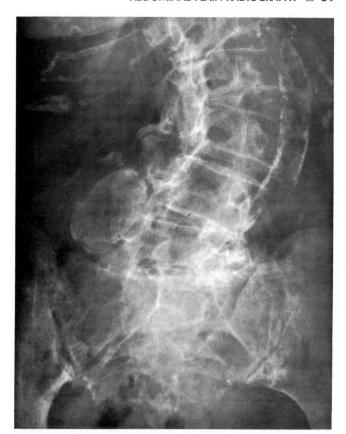

Figure 5–52. Porcelain gallbladder. Oval, egg-shaped calcification is seen to the right of the spine. The gallbladder is low because of marked scoliosis. There is dense calcification of the abdominal aorta.

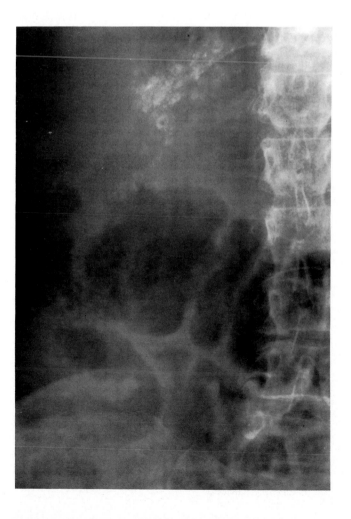

Figure 5–53. Calcified liver metastases. The right upper-quadrant calcification represents diffuse hepatic metastases from primary carcinoma of the breast. Calcified liver metastases are usually associated with primary mucus-secreting tumors of the gastrointestinal tract.

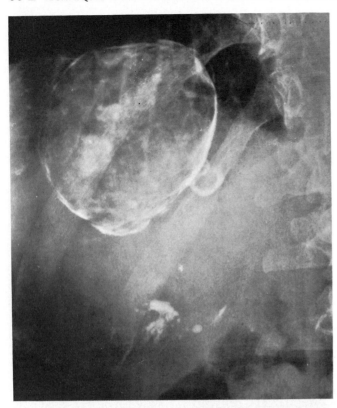

Figure 5–54. Calcified echinococcal cyst of the liver. (Courtesy Barbara M. Kadell, M.D.)

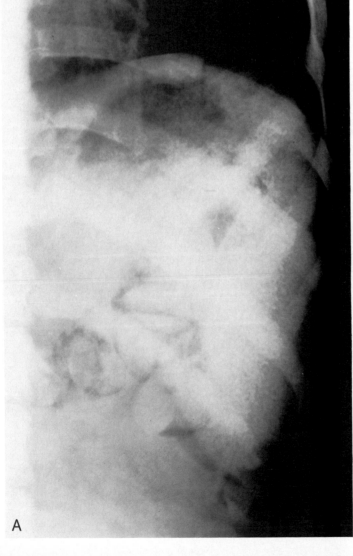

Figure 5–55. Splenic calcification secondary to sickle cell anemia. *A*, A 21-year-old male with diffuse splenic calcification secondary to multiple splenic infarcts. The appearance in this case simulates that seen in thorium dioxide (Thorotrast) deposition, but the opacities are much denser with the contrast material. *B*, In another patient with the same disease, the spleen has atrophied and now is only a fraction of its normal volume. Again, it is diffusely calcified.

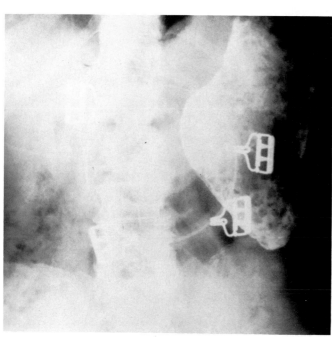

Figure 5–56. Calcification of the spleen secondary to echinococcus disease.

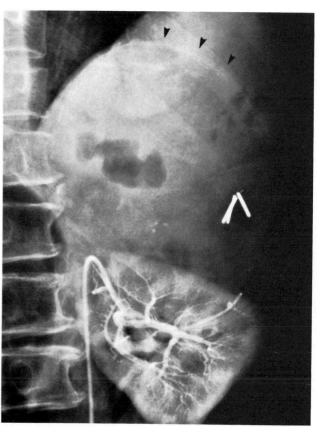

Figure 5–58. Rim calcification (*arrowheads*) in left adrenal adenocarcinoma. Large left adrenal mass is displacing left kidney.

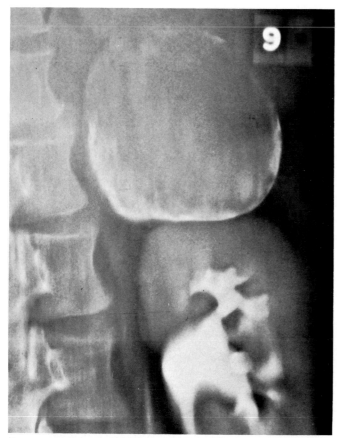

Figure 5–57. Large calcified benign adrenal cyst. There is inferior displacement and flattening of the top of the kidney, as well as flattening of the inferior surface of the cyst.

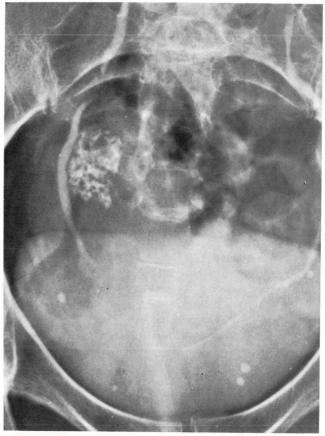

Figure 5–59. Calcification in a small uterine leiomyoma. These can be among the most dense calcifications in the body. Several phleboliths are also present. Myomatous calcifications may also be ring shaped.

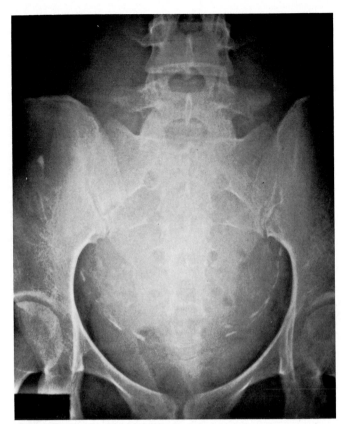

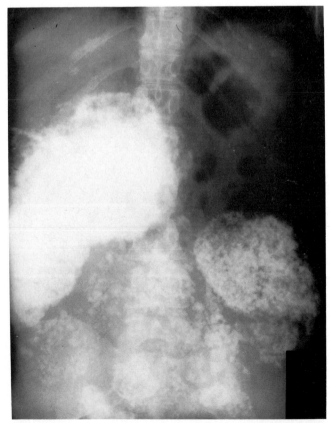

Figure 5—60. Calcified uterine fibroids. Plain abdominal radiograph of the pelvis demonstrates extensive calcification within large uterine fibroids. This appearance is considered to be typical for that associated with calcification in uterine fibroids.

Figure 5—62. Ovarian teratoma. Rim calcification is present in the pelvic mass. A vaginal tampon is seen as a radiolucency pointing toward the right vaginal fornix.

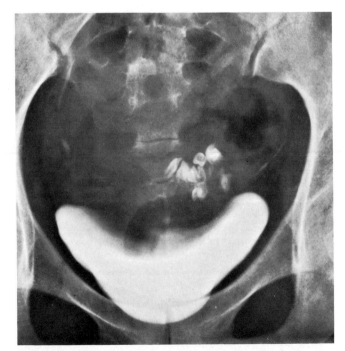

Figure 5—61. Calcified uterine fibroids. The plain abdominal radiograph demonstrates multiple huge calcified leiomyofibromata originating in the uterus. The densely and diffusely calcified masses have a characteristic appearance. Giant fibroids of this type sometimes undergo malignant degeneration.

Figure 5—63. Teeth in a dermoid tumor. Usually, fat is more abundant in these tumors.

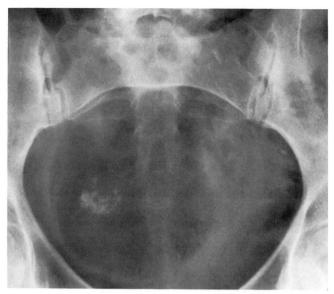

Figure 5–64. Dermoid cyst of the ovary. This 36-year-old female has a palpable pelvic mass. The abdominal radiograph demonstrates a rounded radiolucency in the pelvis attributable to a fat-filled dermoid tumor, in the center of which calcification is seen. Calcification in a dermoid cyst may have an amorphous appearance, such as this, or may resemble teeth. The fat, however, is characteristic of the cyst.

cyst contrast, respectively, the inside and outside of the fibrous capsule encapsulating the tumor.[57] Rare causes of calcifications in the female pelvis include lithopedion (Fig. 5–65), endometriosis, pelvic inflammatory disease, and calcification in the ovary.

Urinary

Calcifications involving the kidneys are numerous and are discussed in detail in the sections addressing specific diseases elsewhere in this book. Here, suffice it to say that the presence of calcification within a renal mass on a plain radiograph makes the diagnosis of a renal carcinoma very likely (Fig. 5–66). Other renal lesions that may exhibit focal areas of calcifications are renal cyst, polycystic renal disease, echinococcal cyst, renal infarct, pyelonephritic scar, renal tuberculosis (Fig. 5–67), bilharziasis (schistosomiasis), renal adenoma, metastases from mucinous adenocarcinoma or osteosarcoma, subcapsular and intraparenchymal hematoma, abscesses, amyloidosis of the renal pelvis,[58] aneurysms, and failed renal transplant (Fig. 5–68). Nephrocalcinosis is diffuse parenchymal calcification most often involving the renal medulla, and occasionally cortex. This topic is discussed in detail elsewhere (see Section 7).

Calcification of the vas deferens occurs mainly in patients with diabetes mellitus and has a characteristic parallel track appearance (Fig. 5–69).[59] Calcifications may also be seen in conjunction with tuberculosis or bilharziasis. However, as many as 50% of all cases have no identifiable cause.

Intramural bladder and, occasionally, distal ureteral calcifications are seen in patients with schistosomiasis (Fig. 5–70).[60] Bladder tumors also may calcify.[61, 62]

Calcifications in Muscles, Ligaments, and Cartilage

Injection granulomas are the most common type of intramuscular calcifications (Fig. 5–71). They may result from almost any type of medication, including quinine and penicillin. These also have a popcorn appearance and characteristic distribution over the gluteal areas. Occasionally, the residua of heavy metals such as mercury and arsenic, which were used to treat syphilis in the preantibiotic era, may be seen in the buttocks (Fig. 5–72). Calcified intramuscular hematomas (myositis ossificans), retroperitoneal hematomas, and calcified tuberculous psoas abscesses (Fig. 5–73) are occasionally seen. Calcification or ossification in the anterior rectus sheath following laparotomy can be confused, on occasion, with renal calculi (Fig. 5–74).

Ligamentous calcifications are seen in Cooper's ligament (Fig. 5–75) and may resemble periosteal elevation over the upper margin of the superior ramus of the symphysis pubis. The sacrotuberous and sacrospinous ligaments may also calcify (Figs. 5–76, 5–77).

Soft-tissue calcifications are commonly seen around the hip joints of paralytic patients and may become very prominent. Polymyositis is associated with soft-tissue calcification (Fig. 5–78).

Calcifications of the rib cartilage can be seen early in

Text continued on page 68

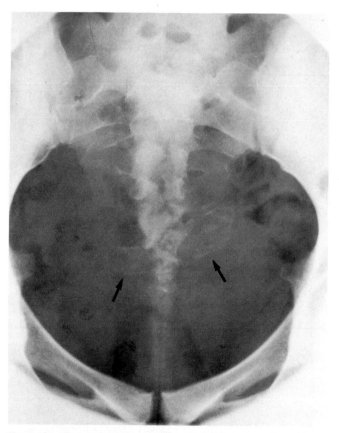

Figure 5–65. Lithopedion. A 21-year-old female with a missed abortion. The fetus was never expelled. Plain pelvic radiograph demonstrates calcification and mummified fetus *(arrows)*. At surgery the fetus was found to be lying free in the pelvic portion of the peritoneal cavity.

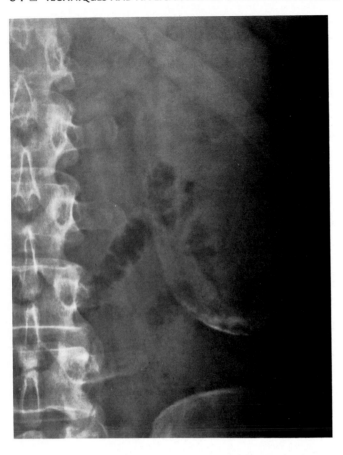

Figure 5–66. Curvilinear calcification in a renal cell carcinoma. More often the calcification is flocculent and centrally located but a ring-shaped calcification in a renal mass represents malignancy in a significant percentage of cases. (Courtesy Thomas S. Mitchell, M.D.)

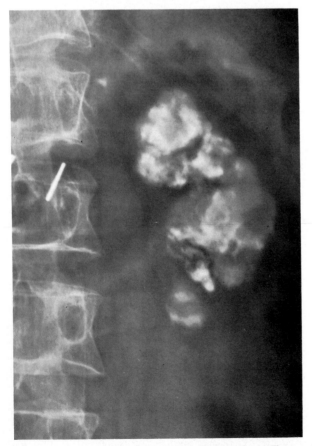

Figure 5–67. Autonephrectomy in renal tuberculosis. The small scarred kidney is heavily calcified ("putty kidney").

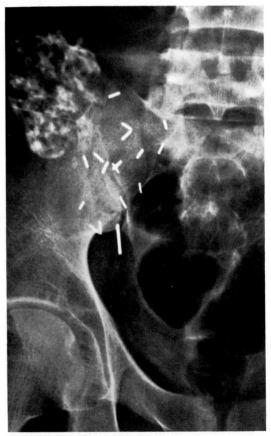

Figure 5–68. Autonephrectomy of a transplanted kidney. The diffusely calcified, shrunken allograft suggests that the kidney had become infarcted.

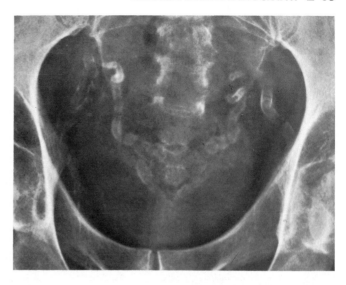

Figure 5–69. Heavy calcification of vas deferens and seminal vesicles in a patient with diabetes mellitus. While diabetes mellitus is the most common cause of vasal calcification, it may also occur in tuberculosis, schistosomiasis, and in many cases without demonstrable cause.

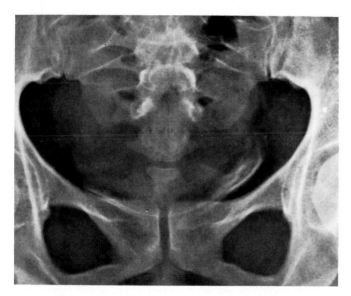

Figure 5–70. Bladder wall calcification in a patient with schistosomiasis. Bladder calcification may be seen in a variety of conditions, including tuberculosis, amyloidosis, and carcinoma.

Figure 5–71. Injection granulomas and abdominal aorta aneurysm. Injection granulomas are seen overlying left iliac bone. A huge calcified abdominal aortic aneurysm is also present. (Courtesy Barbara M. Kadell, M.D.)

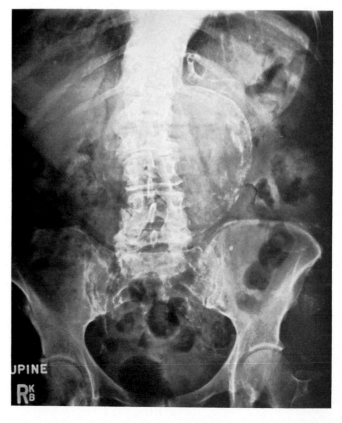

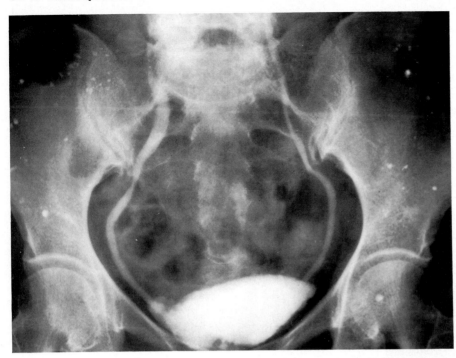

Figure 5–72. Heavy metal injection. Multiple small metallic densities are scattered over the pelvis and hips. These represent the residua of heavy metal injections administered for the treatment of lues 35 years earlier.

Figure 5–73. Calcified tuberculous abscesses ("cold" abscess). Plain abdominal radiograph reveals bilateral paravertebral calcification representing tuberculous abscesses in this 42-year-old man with tuberculous spondylitis (Pott's disease) involving vertebral bodies T9 to T12.

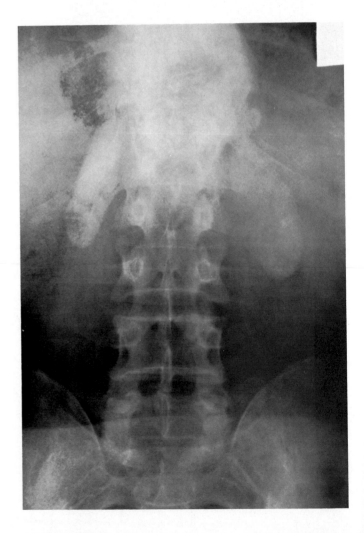

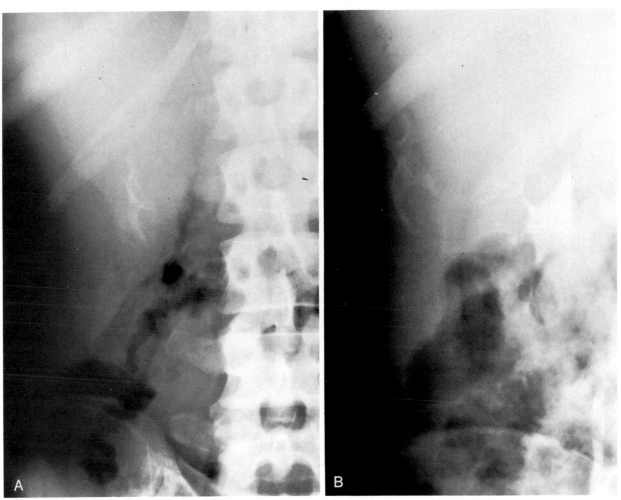

Figure 5–74. Ossified abdominal scar simulating renal calculus. *A,* An AP view of the abdomen demonstrates a hook-shaped opacification overlying the upper pole of the right kidney. *B,* A right posterior oblique view from an excretory urogram demonstrates the structure, which now has a stalactite configuration, lying anterior to the kidney. This density represented an ossified hematoma in the rectus sheath secondary to a previous laparotomy through a right paramedian incision. (Courtesy Matthew S. Pollack, M.D.)

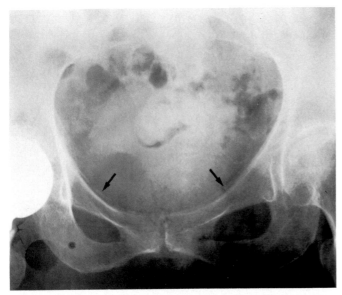

Figure 5–75. Bilateral calcification in Cooper's ligaments (*arrows*). This is easily confused with calcification in the bladder or in the peritoneal reflection. Note the right femoral head prosthesis.

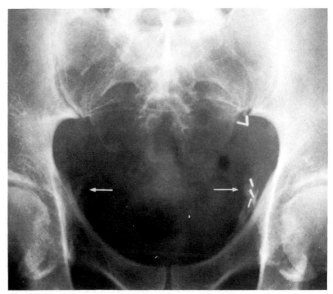

Figure 5–76. Bilateral sacrospinous ligament calcification. This was secondary to diffuse idiopathic skeletal hyperostosis (DISH) (*arrows*).

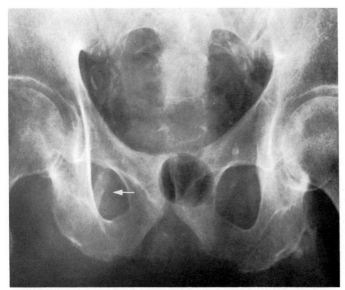

Figure 5–77. Calcified sacrotuberous ligament. The right sacrotuberous ligament is extensively calcified and, in fact, may actually be ossified (*arrow*). Extensive arterial calcification and several phleboliths can be seen. Early calcification in the ligamentous tissues about the left ischial tuberosity is also apparent.

life, even in the third and occasionally as early as the second decade of life. They are a nuisance, making the exclusion of urinary tract calcification, for example, that much more difficult (Fig. 5–79).

Intraperitoneal Calcifications

Epiploical appendices may twist, lose their blood supply, detach from the omentum, and become loose in the peritoneal cavity. On occasion, these fatty globules calcify and can be seen in different locations at different time periods. Similar to these, but smaller, are ring-like calcifications precipitating around globules formed from min-

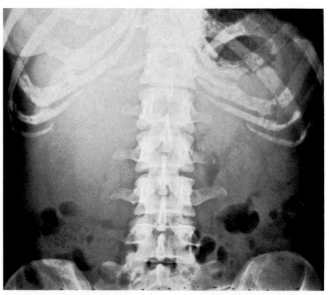

Figure 5–79. Heavy calcification of costochondral cartilages. Such calcification may interfere with visualization and detection of other calcifications within the abdomen.

eral oil, which half a century ago used to be instilled into the peritoneal cavity to prevent postsurgical adhesions.

A penduculated fibroid, or even an ovary, may twist on its pedicle, infarct, calcify and detach from its point of origin, free to meander through the peritoneal cavity as a calcified mass of puzzling origin (Fig. 5–80).

A few conditions produce widespread calcification throughout the peritoneal cavity. Tuberculous peritonitis of long duration is a cause (Fig. 5–81), as is infestation with the tongue worm *Armillifer armillatus*, a parasite found in African pythons and other snakes (Fig. 5–82).[63]

Peritoneal metastases, especially from ovarian carcinoma, may calcify extensively. The lesions may involve the liver, the entire peritoneal cavity, and the omentum.

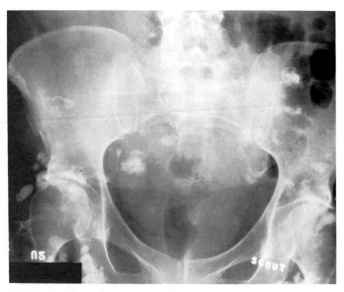

Figure 5–78. Polymyositis with soft-tissue calcification (calcinosis cutis). The multiple abdominal calcifications represent dystrophic soft-tissue calcification sometimes seen in this disease.

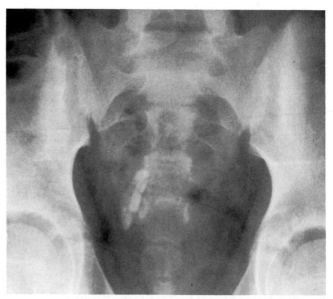

Figure 5–80. "Wandering ovary." A 13-year-old female with an elliptical calcification in the pelvis is shown. The calcification was noted on many occasions and rarely was in the same location. At surgery the right tube and ovary were absent; the left was normal. The calcification represented an infarcted ovary, probably secondary to torsion.

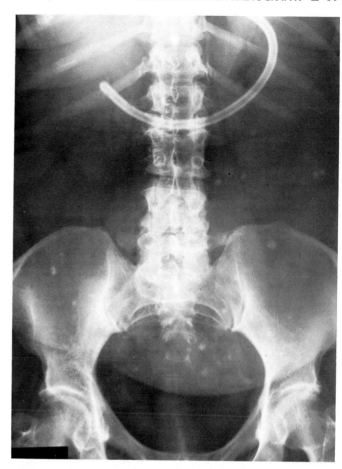

Figure 5–81. Tuberculous peritonitis. The numerous small calcifications are attributable to small tuberculous granulomas studded on the peritoneal surfaces.

Figure 5–82. Calcified larvae of *Armillifer armillatus*. The plain abdominal radiograph demonstrates multiple abdominal calcifications especially prominent over the liver. These C-shaped or comma-shaped calcifications, especially in the right upper quadrant, are typical of the calcified larvae of the African tongue worm *A. armillatus*.

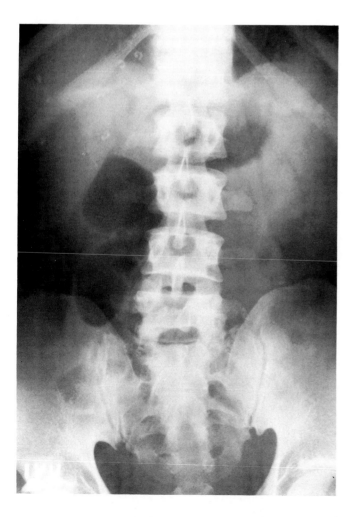

Serous cystadenocarcinomas are most likely to do this, producing either the small psammomatous (Fig. 5–83) or larger flocculent and diffuse types of calcifications (Fig. 5–84). Multiple intraperitoneal phleboliths can be seen with visceral hemangiomatosis and/or Klippel-Trenaunay-Weber syndrome.

Calcified Hematomas and Abscesses

Hematomas anywhere in the abdomen may occasionally undergo calcification (Fig. 5–85). Psoas abscesses, particularly cold abscesses due to tuberculosis may calcify (Fig. 5–86). Calcifications may be found in the soft tissues following a variety of surgical procedures, some of which represent calcified hematomas (Fig. 5–87).

FOREIGN MATERIAL

The abdomen is a mecca for a great variety of foreign material. Surgical clips, bowel staples, and wire sutures lead the way. Various metallic fragments, bullets, shrapnel, shotgun pellets (Fig. 5–88), a variety of ingested metallic artifacts including coins and droplets of mercury, and bobby pins in the urethra and bladder are examples

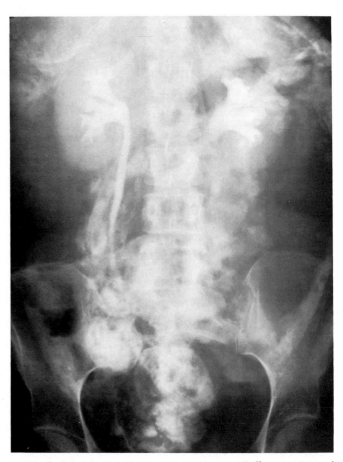

Figure 5–84. Metastatic ovarian carcinoma. Diffuse peritoneal calcifications are present in this 39-year-old female with serous cystadenocarcinoma of the ovary. The pattern of calcification from ovarian peritoneal metastases varies widely from small psammomatous lesions (Fig. 5–83) to diffuse peritoneal calcification, as in this patient. Note how the calcifications extend over the peritoneal surfaces of the liver and spleen.

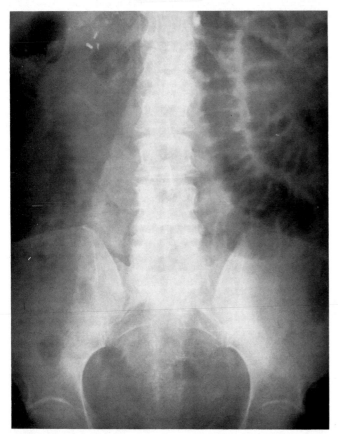

Figure 5–83. Psammomatous calcification. This 60-year-old female has small bowel obstruction secondary to diffuse peritoneal metastases from serous cystadenocarcinoma of the ovary. Multiple small opacities scattered throughout the abdomen and most prominently displayed to the right of the psoas muscle are attributable to small foci of lightly calcified tumor, which studded the peritoneal cavity. (Compare with Fig. 5–84.)

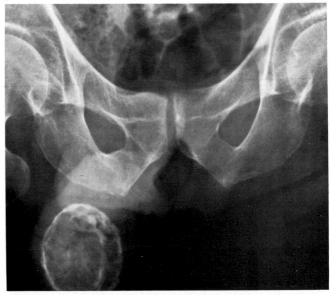

Figure 5–85. Calcified scrotal hematoma several years after trauma.

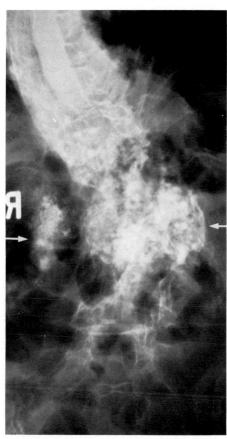

Figure 5–86. Bilateral calcified cold psoas abscess in tuberculosis of the spine (*arrows*). Marked deformity of the spine, including gibbus, is present. Myelographic contrast material is seen in the thoracic spine. (Courtesy R. H. Gold, M.D.)

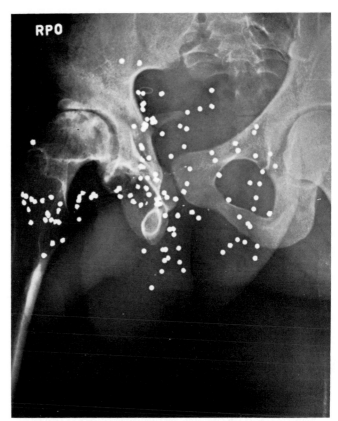

Figure 5–88. Shotgun pellets in the lower abdomen.

of some objects that, because of their marked x-ray attenuation, are usually apparent.

Residual radiographic contrast material may be present after an examination. Barium may be retained in large bowel diverticula, the rectum (Fig. 5–89) or the appendix

(Fig. 5–90) for a long period of time, rarely precipitating acute appendicitis. Extravasated barium from rectal perforation during barium examinations persists indefinitely and may be quite confusing (see Fig. 5–104). Old, oily myelographic contrast material is retained for years in the subarachnoidal space. Since ablation of renal cysts can be accomplished by percutaneous instillation of oily myelographic agents, residual contrast material from that procedure may occasionally be seen (Fig. 5–91).

Lymphangiographic oily contrast material is also retained in the lymph nodes and gradually disappears. However, traces may even be detected 5 or 6 years after obtaining the lymphangiogram. Oily contrast medium, if

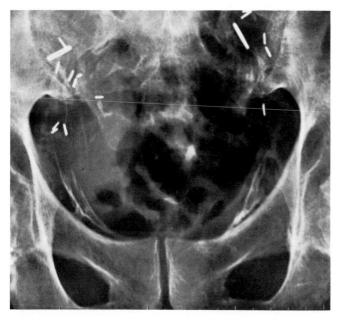

Figure 5–87. Calcifications in the pelvis following radical cystectomy.

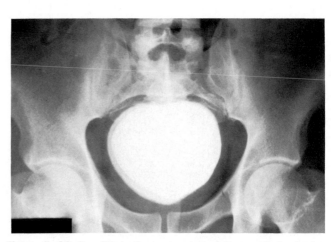

Figure 5–89. Barolith in the rectum simulating vesical calculus. This 28-year-old man had an anal stricture and, following a barium enema, was unable to completely evacuate the barium. This abdominal film was taken 3 weeks after the barium study.

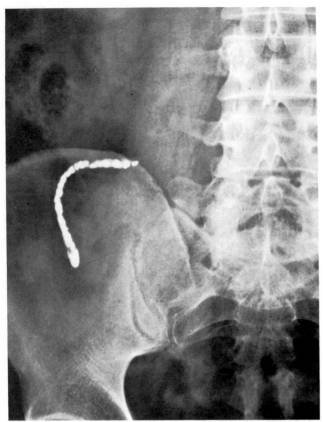

Figure 5–90. Retained barium in the appendix several weeks after an upper gastrointestinal barium study. Patient is asymptomatic.

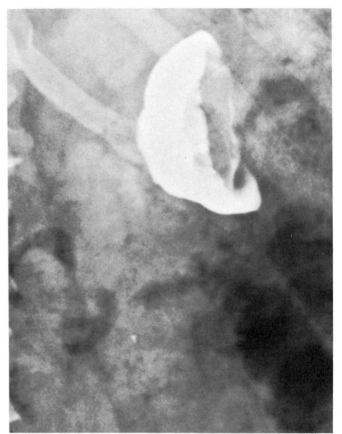

Figure 5–91. Contrast medium (Pantopaque) in a partially collapsed renal cyst. Once instilled in the cyst, the contrast remains unchanged for years. Renal cyst ablation using this particular agent has largely been abandoned in favor of alcohol or other sclerosing agents.

used for hysterosalpingography, may also be seen in the pelvis for many years (Fig. 5–92). Thorotrast, an early colloidal intravascular contrast agent, which is no longer in use because of its sarcogenic potential, is taken up by the reticuloendothelial cells in the liver and spleen, where it may be seen for years (Fig. 5–93).

Vaginal tampons (see Fig. 5–62), pessaries (Fig. 5–94), diaphragms and a diminishing variety of intrauterine contraceptive devices are found (Fig. 5–95). Small symmetrical rounded rings on each side of the uterus are sometimes seen after tubal ligation (Fig. 5–96). Similar clips are occasionally seen in the scrotum after vasectomy.

A variety of anti-incontinence and anti-impotence prosthetic devices are encountered in male patients (Fig. 5–97). Even hollow metallic testicular prostheses have been used at one time or another (Fig. 5–98). Battery-operated vibrators are among the more common of a large list of foreign bodies and implements that have been lost in the rectum (Fig. 5–99).

Condoms filled with illegal drugs are occasionally seen within the intestine. Usually, the patient presents with acute small- or large-bowel obstruction or is treated for

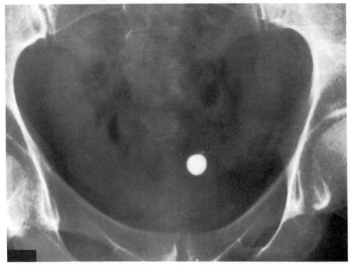

Figure 5–92. Residual contrast material (Lipiodol) in the pelvis from previous hysterosalpingography. This patient had undergone a hysterosalpingogram 8 years previously, with Lipiodol used as the contrast agent. Now, many years later, the retained contrast material is still visible as a small collection, either in a hydrosalpinx or possibly in a loculated intraperitoneal compartment.

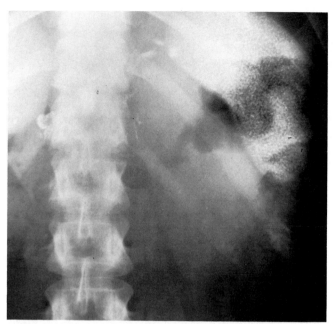

Figure 5–93. Contrast material (Thorotrast) retained in the spleen. The plain abdominal radiograph demonstrates a diffuse stippled opacification throughout the entire spleen. The opacities are extremely dense, consistent with the presence of metal. Note similar opacification involving several regional lymph nodes. This composite picture is particularly pathognomonic for retained Thorotrast and, indeed, 20 years earlier at the age of 6 the patient had undergone cerebral angiography with Thorotrast as the contrast agent.

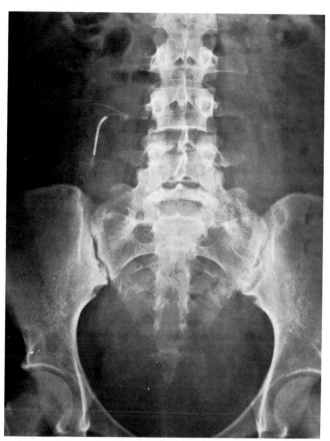

Figure 5–95. Lost intrauterine device. The device (copper-7) is clearly outside of the normal-size uterus (established by physical examination).

drug overdose subsequent to a condom rupture.[64, 65] Broken acupuncture needles are occasionally seen especially in those immigrating from the Far East (Fig. 5–100).

Most of the foreign material described above is easily detected and needs no further elaboration. However, there are two categories that need further analysis.

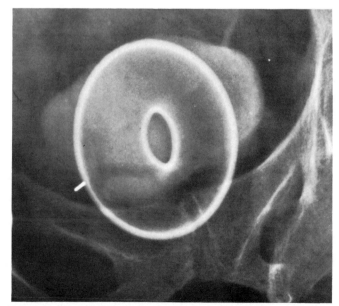

Figure 5–94. Vaginal pessary used to prevent bladder prolapse.

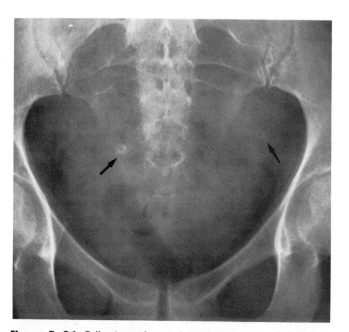

Figure 5–96. Fallopian tube occlusion rings and vaginal tampon. The two small, donut-shaped structures in the pelvis are attributable to fallopian tube occlusion devices (*arrows*), which were placed laparoscopically. The rectangular, oblique radiolucency above the symphysis pubis represents gas in the vagina secondary to a tampon.

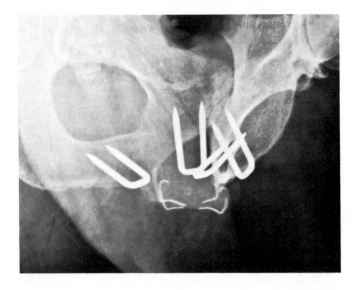

Figure 5–97. Kaufman II anti-incontinence prosthesis. Two staples in each inferior pubic ramus suspend a metallic cage with a silicon cushion on top. Extrinsic compression upon the bulbous urethra helps to maintain urinary continence.

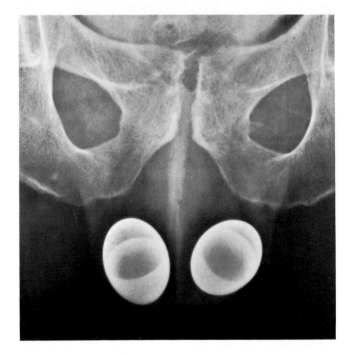

Figure 5–98. An older version of a testicular prosthesis is shown.

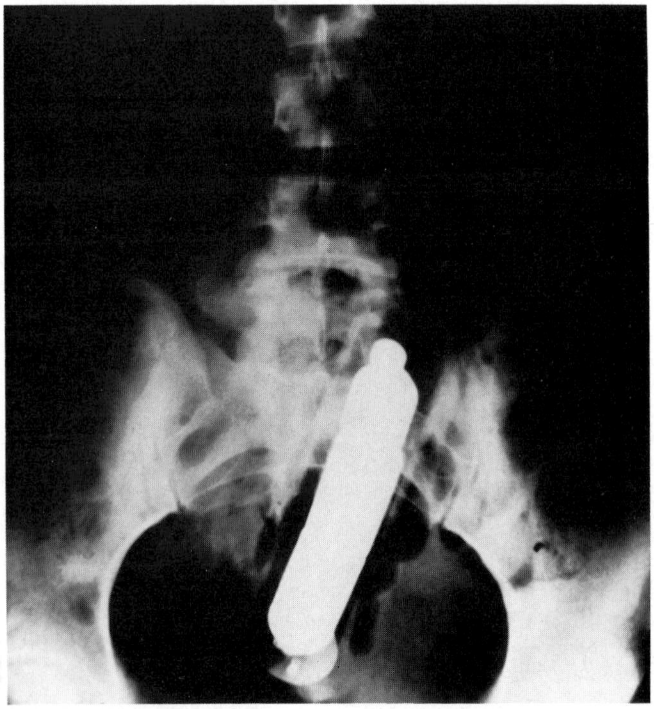

Figure 5–99. Foreign body in the rectum. An abdominal plain radiograph demonstrated the unexpected finding of a vibrator in the rectum of this 17-year-old female.

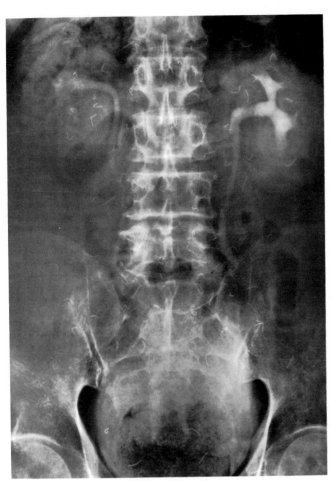

Figure 5–100. Acupuncture needles. This 56-year-old man lived most of his life in Vietnam. Numerous metallic foreign bodies are visible on this abdominal film exposed during an intravenous urogram. Their metallic densities, short lengths, and curvilinear configurations suggest that these are broken acupuncture needles located in the subcutaneous tissues.

Foreign Bodies Related to Surgery or Interventional Procedures

Surgical sponges usually have a radiodense marker for easy identification. Battery Packs and other hardware related to pacemakers and automatic defibrillators are obvious in their abdominal wall locations (see Fig. 5–102). Curvilinear metallic densities are most likely lost or broken surgical needles (Fig. 5–101). Over a period of time, these may migrate considerable distances in the body. Lost surgical clamps or needle holders are occasionally seen. Even draining tubes, which look innocent enough in their expected positions, may be lost in other parts of the body (Fig. 5–103). Ureteral double-pigtail stents may migrate from the bladder into the ureter and require ureteroscopic or cystoscopic retrieval (Fig. 5–104), may form a nidus for calcific deposits (Fig. 5–105), or may fracture spontaneously (Fig. 5–106). Gianturco occlusive steel coils, used for vascular embolization, are sometimes found in a part of the vascular system for which they were not intended. An inferior vena cava umbrella may be found in the intrahepatic portion of the inferior vena cava, well above the take-off of the renal veins, a position that is obviously undesirable (Fig. 5–

107). During total hip replacement, orthopedic cement may leak into the pelvis through a defect created in the medial acetabular wall (Fig. 5–108). Radioactive seeds (Fig. 5–109) or brachytherapy sources (Fig. 5–110) are easily recognized, as is the characteristic appearance of ventriculoperitoneal shunts (Fig. 5–111).

"What Is That Density?"

Frequently, radiopaque materials of varying densities, sizes, shapes, and numbers are seen in the abdomen and are difficult to place in an appropriate anatomical location. These may be due to ingested food such as caraway seeds and chicken bones or medications such as tablets and vitamin caplets. Examples of pills and other medications that are radiopaque include iron, potassium iodide, Pepto-Bismol, and other bismuth-containing compounds. Enteric coated pills are frequently covered by a layer of titanium oxide to delay absorption (Fig. 5–112).

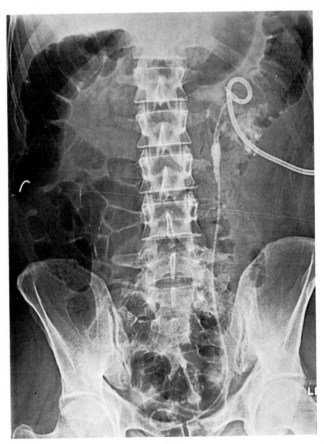

Figure 5–101. Lost surgical needle demonstrated on digital radiograph. Metallic curved radiodensity in the right flank is difficult to mistake for anything else. Percutaneous nephrostomy is in the left kidney to relieve obstruction caused by impacted calculus debris in the proximal left ureter, subsequent to extracorporeal lithotripsy. A double-pigtail stent is also obstructed and therefore afunctional. This radiograph is obtained with the patient in a prone position. Pointed iliac wings, foreshortened pelvic inlet, and a magnified sacrum are the telltale signs that the film was taken in prone position. This image was acquired, processed, and edge-enhanced by digital technology, without the use of a film screen combination.

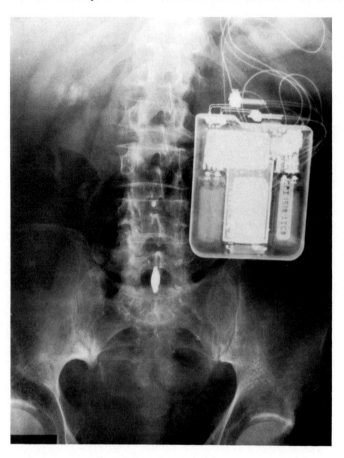

Figure 5–102. Defibrillator. Plain abdominal radiograph demonstrates the presence of an automatic self-regulated ventricular defibrillator located subcutaneously in the left anterior abdominal wall. There are stones in the right kidney and residual contrast material (Pantopaque) in the subarachnoid space.

Figure 5–103. A drainage tube *(arrow)* was unintentionally left in the left abdomen during an abdominal operation. Percutaneous nephrostomy tube is in place because of postoperative distal right ureteral obstruction. There is a drain in the pelvis and air in the bladder.

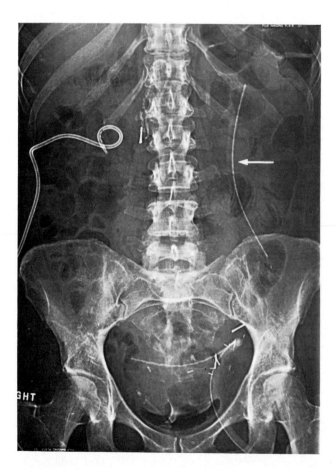

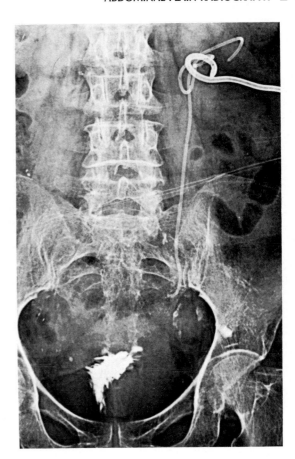

Figure 5–104. Retracted left ureteral stent. Distal end of the ureteral stent cannot be retrieved by simple cystoscopy. Either ureteroscopy or percutaneous extraction are necessary. Contrast material seen in the pelvis is barium in the soft tissues from a rectal perforation during a barium enema study several years earlier. Vascular calcification is present, as well as a bone island above the left acetabulum.

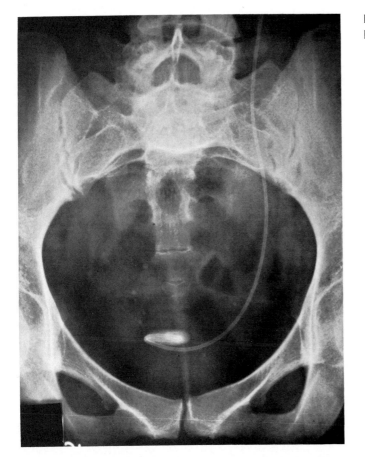

Figure 5–105. Stone forming at the distal end of a double-pigtail ureteral stent.

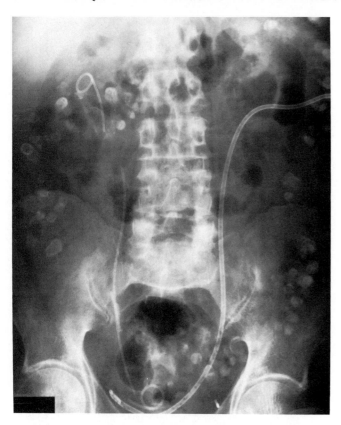

Figure 5–106. Spontaneous fracture of ureteral stent. This patient had retroperitoneal fibrosis and was treated with permanent indwelling stents. A double-pigtail stent in the right ureter has undergone spontaneous fracture at multiple sites. This stent had been in place and unchanged for approximately 18 months. A combined nephrostomy–single-pigtail ureteral stent is seen traversing the left renal pelvis and left ureter. This stent is intact. Multiple abdominal opacities are attributable to retained barium and colonic diverticulae.

Figure 5–107. Inferior vena cava umbrella. Plain abdominal radiograph demonstrates an umbrella in the inferior vena cava (*curved arrow*). Note the unusually oblique angle of the umbrella, suggesting that it may be protruding into the right renal vein. Also seen on this film are bilateral renal calculi (*arrows*) and a bone graft (*arrowheads*) between the transverse processes of L3 and L4.

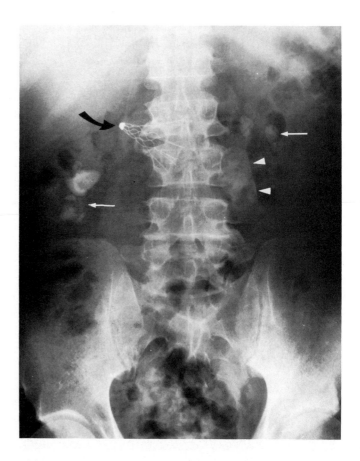

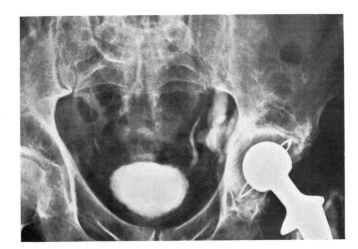

Figure 5–108. Foreign material (cement) in the pelvic cavity from a total hip replacement operation.

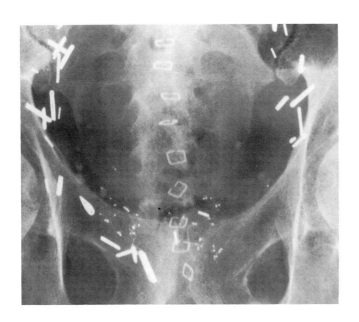

Figure 5–109. Radioactive seeds in the prostate. This patient underwent staging lymphadenectomy for carcinoma of the prostate. Stage-D disease was demonstrated, and palliative treatment of the prostatic carcinoma by means of the implantation of iodine-125 seeds was undertaken. The seeds are visualized as tiny, small opacities superimposed over the symphysis pubis. The large metallic clips overlying the lateral borders of the pelvic inlet are from the lymphadenectomy; the midline row of clips are in the skin.

Figure 5–110. Brachytherapy radiation source applicator. Plain radiograph of the pelvis reveals in situ applicators for radium or cesium-137 sources commonly employed in the treatment of carcinoma of the uterus. Two Fletcher ovoids are seen on either side of a slender intrauterine tandem source. An opacified Foley balloon is in the urinary bladder. (Courtesy Beatriz Amendola, M.D.)

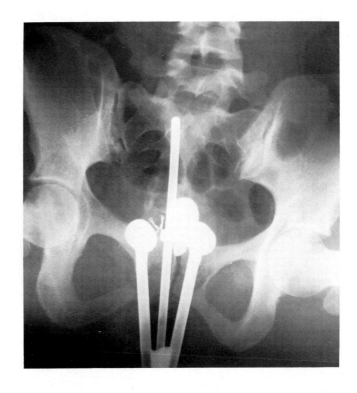

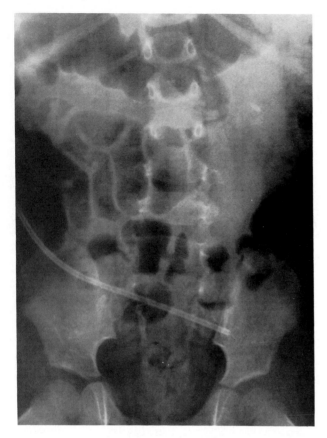

Figure 5–111. Ventriculoperitoneal shunt in child with meningomyelocele: left renal calculus. Plain abdominal radiograph demonstrates a tube (originating in the cerebral ventricles) in the peritoneal cavity of a child with hydrocephalus secondary to a meningomyelocele. The spinal defects attending meningomyelocele are evident in all of the vertebral bodies caudal to L2. Note also the small left renal calculus secondary to chronic urinary tract infections and a neuropathic bladder.

Iodine-impregnated suppositories—vaginal, urethral, and various rectal suppositories—may be seen (Fig. 5–113). External or intracavitary iodiform gauze packing and tantalum mesh (Fig. 5–114) may also be seen on plain radiographs.

Extraneous shadows, such as a skin fold (Fig. 5–115), a stoma bag, a smudge of contrast material on the skin, clothing, print on T-shirts, or items in pockets, may cast peculiar shadows on the radiograph.

Finally, peculiar radiopacities may be traced to spilled contrast residua on the top of the radiographic table, cassette, and grid or to improper film handling in the dark room, for example, handling film with greasy or lotion-treated hands.

The main inconvenience is that these densities may interfere with the proper recognition of urinary tract calculi and contribute to either false-positive or false-negative diagnoses in all organ systems. Additional views, repeated examinations, or an alternate imaging examination may be required.

SOFT-TISSUE DENSITIES

Radiodense Organs

Radiodense Kidneys. The kidneys, which are normally of soft-tissue density, may be more opaque than usual on a plain radiograph. Although various causes have been suggested for this appearance, including the presence of iron pigment (renal siderosis), the more likely explanation is that the patient has recently received intravascular contrast material. Under these circumstances, the appearance of radiodense kidneys on the plain radiograph should alert the physician to impending renal failure. A prolonged nephrogram, which may linger for 48 hours, is a harbinger of contrast nephropathy. Oliguria and renal failure may follow.[66] No more contrast material should

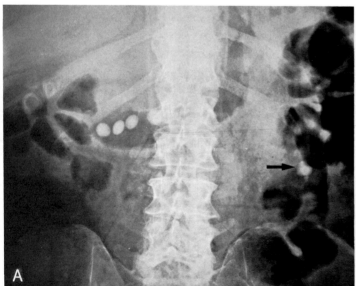
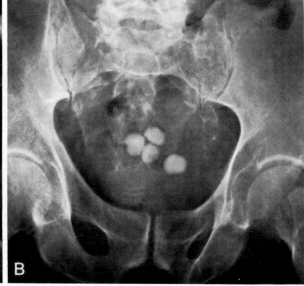

Figure 5–112. Pills, urinary calculi, and gallstones. *A,* Four tablets are seen in the gas-filled antrum of the stomach. Several gallstones are in the right upper quadrant. There is also left renal calculus of 1 cm in diameter (*arrow*), which is difficult to recognize immediately because of superimposed bowel gas. *B,* Same patient as in *A.* Four bladder calculi are clearly seen. There is also vascular calcification in the left pelvis. A multitude of different radiopacities may present diagnostic difficulties, particularly in patients with urolithiasis. (Courtesy Barbara M. Kadell, M.D.)

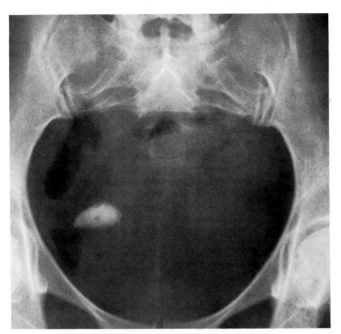

Figure 5–113. Confusing abdominal opacification produced by iodine-containing rectal suppository (povidone).

be administered until the patient's renal status has been normalized.

Radiodense Liver. Rarely, the radiodensity of the liver may be increased in patients with hemosiderosis or hemochromatosis.[43]

Bowel Wall

Occasionally, abnormal thickness of the bowel wall can be observed on the plain radiograph, because the thickened valvulae conniventes or haustrae are contrasted by

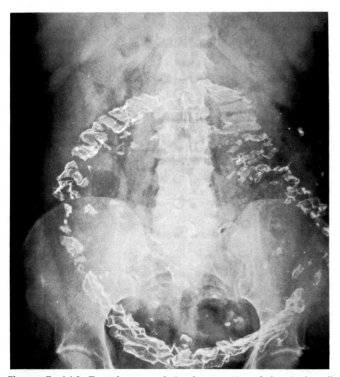

Figure 5–114. Tantalum mesh in the anterior abdominal wall following closure of surgical wound dehiscence. (Courtesy Barbara M. Kadell, M.D.)

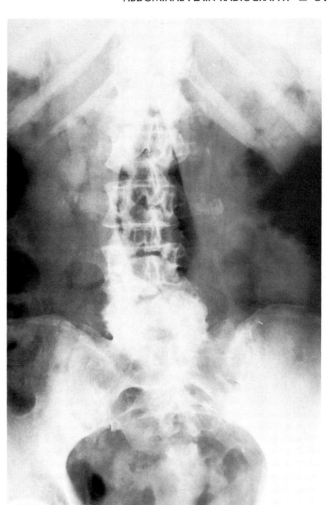

Figure 5–115. Air entrapment by dorsal skin folds. A plain abdominal radiograph performed with the patient in the supine position reveals a teardrop-shaped radiolucency superimposed over the spine. This is attributable to air that is trapped between redundant skin folds protruding from the patient's back.

intestinal gas. The presence of Crohn's disease or ulcerative colitis may be suspected on this basis. Similarly, the classic "apple-core" appearance of colon carcinoma may be an unexpected finding on the plain radiograph (Fig. 5–116).

Organomegaly

Hepatomegaly. Liver enlargement is difficult to determine from plain radiographs unless the enlargement is gross, because anatomical variations, relative position of the diaphragm, and the patient's habitus render any measurements impractical. Riedel's lobe is a normal anatomical variant of the right liver lobe, which extends inferiorly along the right flank as low as the pelvis.

Splenomegaly. Measurements to determine spleen size on a plain radiograph are not commonly used and are not even mentioned in standard textbooks on gastrointestinal radiology. It seems that a more precise estimation of the size is obtainable by the use of ultrasound, nuclear medicine, or CT. Nevertheless, a spleen measuring more than 14 cm in the longest axis is abnormal. A grossly enlarged spleen may displace the fundus of the stomach medially and the left kidney anteromedially (Fig. 5–117), despite the fact that the spleen is an intraperitoneal organ

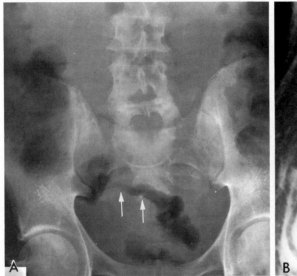
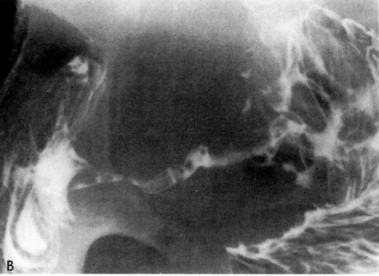

Figure 5–116. Carcinoma of the colon detected on plain abdominal radiograph. *A,* A plain abdominal film reveals abnormal narrowing of the rectosigmoid (*arrows*). *B,* A barium enema examination confirms a long "apple-core" lesion of the sigmoid colon that proved to be adenocarcinoma.

and the kidney is a retroperitoneal organ. Occasionally, the left kidney may be displaced, at least partially, across the midline by an enormous spleen.

Uterine Enlargement. A diamond-shaped soft-tissue density of the normal uterus is seen on 15% of plain abdominal radiographs. Inferiorly, it is contrasted by the perivesical fat stripe, and superiorly by the mesenteric fat. An enlarged uterus may be suggested on the plain radiographic examination, but fluid-filled loops of bowel may have a similar appearance.

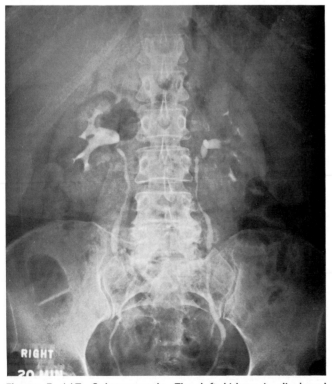

Figure 5–117. Splenomegaly. The left kidney is displaced anteromedially.

Soft-Tissue Masses

Most soft-tissue masses in the abdomen are of "water density," which means that x-ray attenuation differences between the mass and water (urine, cyst fluid, bile, spinal fluid) and parenchymal organs are so small (i.e., less than 3%) that they cannot be recorded on a plain radiograph. Therefore, a mass can only be detected if it is contrasted by surrounding fat or air.

On rare occasions, a very large fluid-containing structure, such as a large renal cyst or a giant hydronephrosis, when in immediate proximity to a homogeneous soft-tissue structure such as the liver, may be detectably radiolucent under optimal conditions of radiographic exposure.[67]

Fat-containing masses, if large enough, may also be detected on a properly exposed radiograph. Fatty masses, which are recognized by their characteristic radiolucency, have already been mentioned in conjunction with dermoids of the ovary. Further examples of special interest to urologists include angiomyolipomas and lipomas of the kidney, and myelolipomas of the adrenal gland (Fig. 5–118).

Abdominal wall masses protruding from the skin are easy to recognize because they are surrounded and contrasted by atmospheric air and are therefore rendered visible. Examples include neurofibromas (Fig. 5–119), moles, stoma sites (Fig. 5–120), anterior wall hernias (Fig. 5–121), and supernumerary nipples (Fig. 5–122).

Internal soft-tissue masses may arise from within any abdominal organs, fascial layers, muscles, lymph nodes, and so forth. Usually, they must grow to a rather large size before their presence can be detected. On the plain radiograph a soft-tissue mass may be detected as an abnormality in organ contour. For example, a bulge of the renal outline suggests a renal mass, whereas a bulge of the psoas muscle suggests a psoas tumor.

The anatomical origin of the mass may also be judged by the direction of displacement of adjacent organs. An

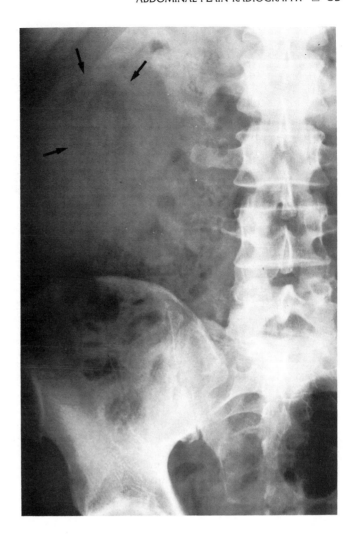

Figure 5—118. Radiolucency secondary to an angiomyolipoma. Plain abdominal radiograph on this 47-year-old male demonstrates a large right upper-quadrant mass. A radiolucent component (*arrows*) in this mass identifies it as containing fat and suggests the diagnosis of a renal angiomyolipoma. This was confirmed by CT.

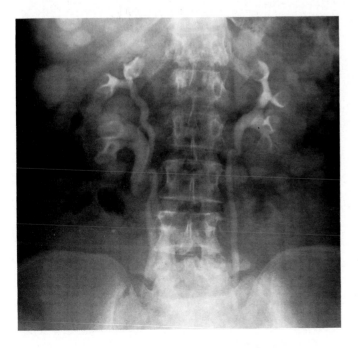

Figure 5—119. Neurofibromatosis. Abdominal film from excretory urogram demonstrates numerous round soft-tissue densities superimposed over the upper abdomen. These are attributable to multiple neurofibromata on the anterior and posterior abdominal wall.

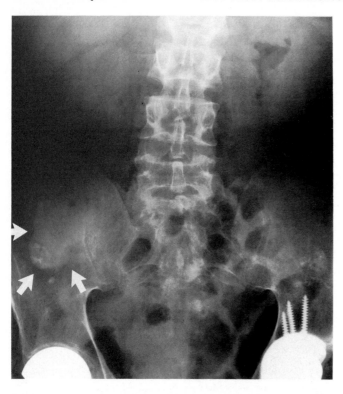

Figure 5–120. Prolapsed ileostomy stoma. Plain abdominal radiograph reveals an unusual soft-tissue density projected over the right iliac bone (*arrows*). This was attributable to a prolapsed ileostomy stoma. Note also the bilateral hip replacements and opacities attributable to the injection of medication into each buttock.

adrenal mass, for example, may displace the kidney in the caudad direction, whereas a primary retroperitoneal tumor may displace the kidney anteriorly and cephalad (Fig. 5–123). Sufficiently large masses may displace gas-filled loops of bowel, further pinpointing the likely site of origin. A mass originating in the right lobe of the liver should displace the hepatic flexure caudad, whereas a retrocecal appendiceal mucocele usually displaces the cecum in the anterior direction.

Finally, a pelvic mass is differentiated from a full bladder if the perivesical fat stripe can be identified (Figs. 5–124, 5–125).

Poor discrimination of x-ray attenuation differences between various soft tissues on plain radiographs and the need to maximize radiographic recording of these differences led to the development of modern radiographic contrast materials and, ultimately, to the development of CT.

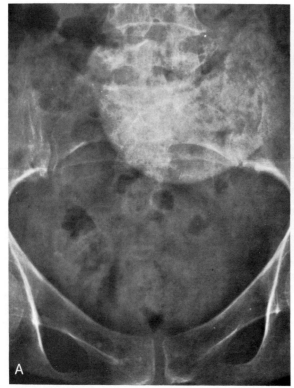

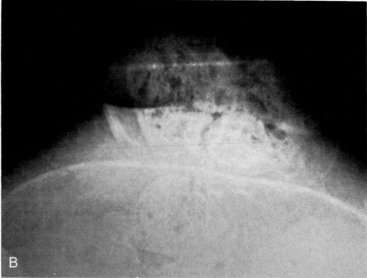

Figure 5–121. Hernia of the anterior abdominal wall. *A*, Soft-tissue mass projecting over the lower abdomen. The inferior part of the mass is well outlined by atmospheric air, but the superior portion is not ("incomplete wall sign"). *B*, Cross-table lateral view of the mass demonstrates the mass to be hernia of the anterior abdominal wall. The incomplete wall sign is explained by the hernia merging superiorly with the abdominal soft tissues.

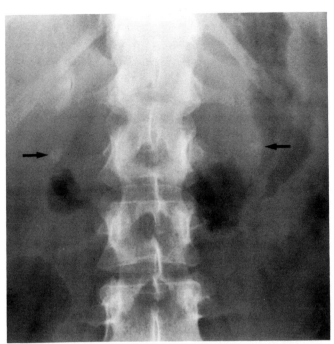

Figure 5–122. Supernumerary nipples in a 35-year-old female simulating intra-abdominal calcification. A plain film of the abdomen demonstrates bilaterally symmetrical densities overlying the areas of the renal collecting systems (*arrows*). These were found to be produced by supernumerary nipples on the anterior abdominal wall.

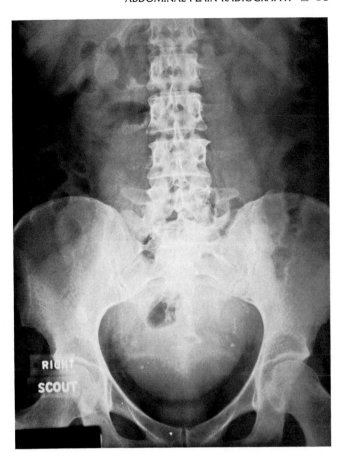

Figure 5–124. Perivesical fat outlines the empty bladder just below the large noncalcified pelvic mass. The mass is a large ovarian cyst. It is usually not possible to differentiate a soft-tissue parenchymal mass from a fluid-filled structure on the plain radiograph.

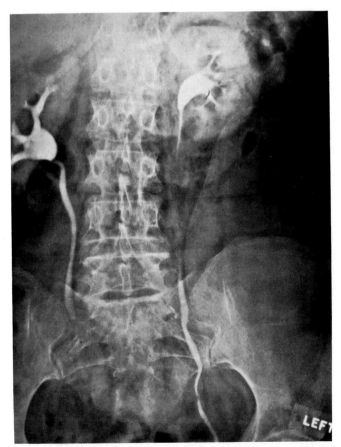

Figure 5–123. A large retroperitoneal mass is in the left abdomen. The kidney is displaced in the anterior and superior direction. The mass is a large lymphocele resulting from pelvic surgery. If on ultrasound a mass of this size proves to be solid, primary retroperitoneal sarcoma would be the diagnosis of choice.

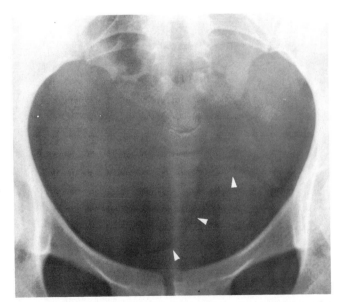

Figure 5–125. Perivesical fat stripe. Note the presence of a radiolucent fat stripe (*arrowheads*) surrounding the bladder and separating it from a large uterine myoma that asymmetrically indents the bladder. The perivesical fat stripe is an important landmark that often makes possible the separation of abdominal masses and ascites from a distended urinary bladder on a plain abdominal radiograph.

SKELETAL DISEASES

Degenerative Changes

Degenerative changes of the lumbar spine are common, and they increase with age.[68] Narrowing of the intervertebral disc space, formation of osteophytic spurs, osteosclerosis, and narrowing of the facetal joints and occasional "vacuum phenomena" in the disc space are the usual radiographic findings associated with the disease (Fig. 5–126). Sacroiliitis may be seen in short-bowel syndrome (Fig. 5–127) and rheumatoid spondylitis. Intercostal and the facetal joints may also be involved. The earliest changes consist of irregularity of the sacroiliac joints attributable to patchy deossification. Later, sclerosis on both sides of the joint ensues. In advanced cases, complete obliteration and ankylosis of the joints can be seen. Ossification of the longitudinal spinous ligaments may result in a radiographic appearance called "bamboo spine" (Fig. 5–128).

Spondylolisthesis and Spondylolysis

Spondylolisthesis is anterior slippage of one vertebral body over the other. It is usually associated with degenerative disc disease and degenerative disease of the facetal joints.[69] Spondylolisthesis of L5 may be suspected if, on the frontal radiograph, the slipped vertebral body is superimposed on the sacrum, giving it a characteristic appearance (inverted "Napoleon's hat" sign).[70] Otherwise, lateral and oblique projections are necessary. There is also frequent association with disruption of the pars interarticularis of the posterior vertebral elements, a condition known as spondylolysis.

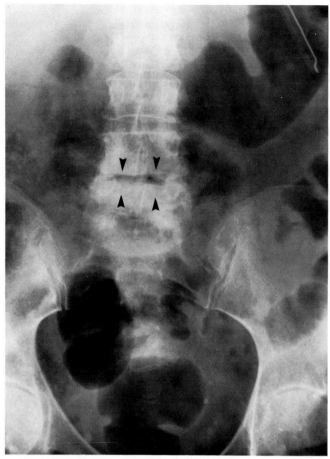

Figure 5–126. Vacuum disc. A plain abdominal radiograph demonstrates radiolucency within the L4–L5 interspace, representing the "vacuum disc" (*arrowheads*) indicative of intervertebral disc disease. Note the abundant dense reactive new bone about the superior surface of L5.

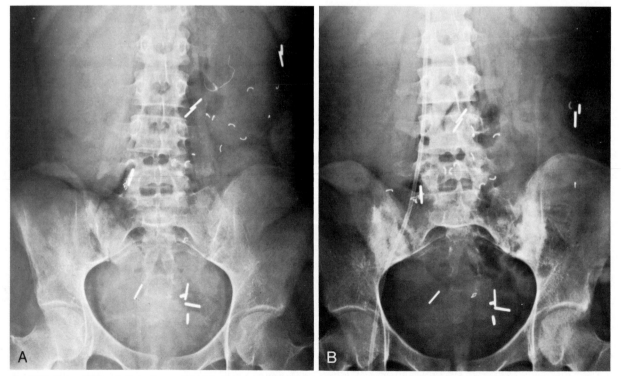

Figure 5–127. Sacroiliitis. *A,* Baseline radiograph in a patient with short-bowel syndrome. Note mild bone reabsorption around right sacroiliac joint. There is also moderate liver enlargement. *B,* Several years later, dense sclerotic changes are present at both sacroiliac joints, predominantly on the iliac side.

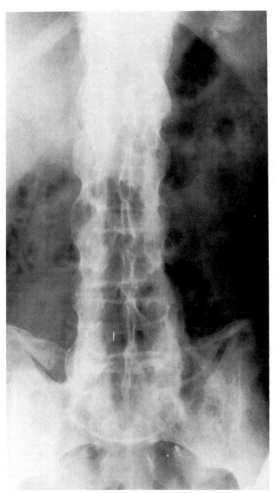

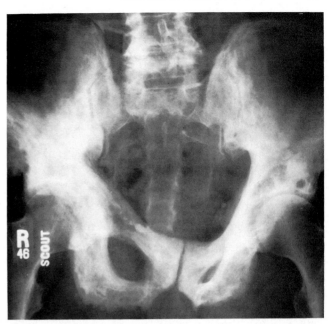

Figure 5–129. Paget's disease. A plain pelvic radiograph demonstrates diffuse involvement of the pelvis by Paget's disease. Note the increased bone density throughout the pelvis accompanied by pronounced cortical thickening and accentuation of trabecular markings throughout the involved bones. The involvement ends abruptly at the acetabula, the femurs being uninvolved. The asymmetry of the pelvis is probably attributable to bone softening—a frequent accompaniment of Paget's disease—with resulting early protrusion of the right femoral head into the acetabulum.

Figure 5–128. Ankylosing spondylitis. The abdominal radiograph of this middle-aged man reveals diffuse calcification involving the longitudinal ligaments of the lumbar spine with partial obliteration of the sacroiliac joints. This is the classic appearance of the "bamboo spine." (Courtesy Murray K. Dalinka, M.D.)

Paget's Disease

Paget's disease is a destructive bone process undergoing a concurrent reparative process. Several radiographic phases (destructive, combined, sclerotic, and malignant) are recognized. The phase of the disease most commonly seen in the dorsolumbar spine and pelvis is the combined phase, where bone destruction and reparation occur concomitantly. Classic radiographic findings in this phase are (1) coarsening of the bony trabeculae, which also become fewer in number, (2) thickening of the bony cortex, (3) bone expansion, and (4) bone deformity (Fig. 5–129).

The earliest involvement of the pelvis is often at the iliopectineal line. In more pronounced cases, the pubis, ischium, or ilium is enlarged, and its cortices thickened (see Fig. 5–129).[71] Few coarse trabeculae are present. Deformation of the bone may occur in the form of acetabular protrusion (Fig. 5–130). Similar changes are seen in the proximal femur. The remodeling changes in this bone have a distinct appearance called "shepherd's-crook" deformity.

The vertebral body also enlarges and the thickened cortex causes it to have a "picture-frame" appearance (Fig. 5–131). Pedicles and spinous processes may also be involved. Coarse trabeculae are also present in heman-

gioma of the vertebral body, but in this pathological condition there is no expansion, nor is there cortical thickening.

In the sclerotic phase, the trabeculae are obliterated and differentiating this disease from osteoblastic bone metastases becomes difficult. Occasionally osteoblastic metastasis may occur in bone already involved with Paget's disease, which makes the diagnosis of malignancy exceedingly difficult. Malignant transformation to osteogenic sarcoma and fibrosarcoma is an uncommon but well-known complication of Paget's disease.[72]

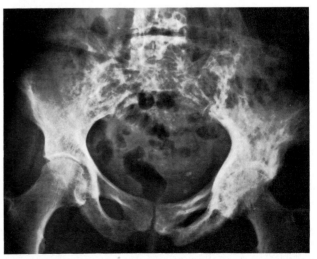

Figure 5–130. Paget's disease involving left hemipelvis. In addition to cortical thickening, coarse trabecular pattern, and bone expansion, there is acetabular protrusion involving the left hip.

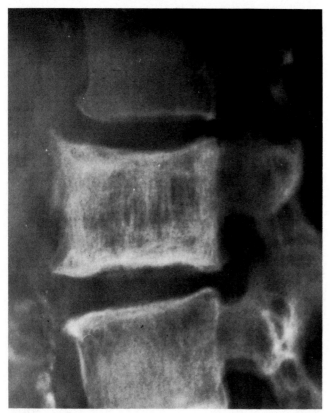

Figure 5–131. Paget's disease. Lateral projection of the lumbar spine. Bone expansion, cortical thickening, and coarse trabecular pattern are diagnostic of this disease.

Osteoblastic Metastases

The most common osteoblastic metastases are from carcinoma of the prostate (Figs. 5–132 and 5–133) in males and carcinoma of the breast in females. Prostatic cancer produces pure osteoblastic change in 80% (Fig. 5–134), mixed osteoblastic and lytic change in 15% (Fig. 5–135), and pure lytic disease in 5% of cases.[73] Many other carcinomas and lymphomas are capable of producing various degrees of osteoblastic reaction (Fig. 5–136). Metastases may be solitary, multiple, or diffuse (Fig. 5–137). Obliteration of the trabecular pattern occurs gradually and the inner cortical margin becomes unidentifiable once the contrasting marrow fat is totally replaced. A solitary metastasis may be seen in the pedicle of the vertebral body or in the vertebral body itself (ivory vertebra). Diffuse metastases may involve every bone visible on the radiograph. Differentiation from other benign or malignant osteosclerotic diseases may occasionally be difficult. Renal carcinoma is almost always osteolytic, only exceptionally producing other varieties of metastasis.[74]

Osteosclerotic Bone Diseases

Many benign and malignant osteosclerotic bone disorders may mimic osteoblastic bone metastases and must be considered when, for example, a patient with a prostatic carcinoma undergoes staging.

Bone Island. A bone island is compact cortical bone within the cancellous bone (Fig. 5–138).[75] It usually has

margins sharper than those of metastases (Fig. 5–139). The best way to differentiate a bone island from a metastasis is to consult a past radiographic examination to see if the lesion was present at that time. Skeletal scintigraphy reveals no abnormal uptake in bone islands, although usually enhanced uptake is seen in patients with osteoblastic skeletal metastases.

Myelofibrosis. This progressive fibrosis of the bone marrow is associated with osteosclerosis, anemia, leukemoid disorder, and splenomegaly and is usually seen in patients over 50 years of age.[76] The pelvis and spine are commonly involved (Fig. 5–140), and splenomegaly is usually very pronounced. Normochromic normocytic anemia, immature leukocytes, and red blood cells are present on the smear.

Tuberous Sclerosis. Patients who have this familial disease present with epilepsy, adenoma sebaceum, and, frequently, mental retardation. Renal angiomyolipoma is one of many types of benign hamartomas involving several organs that may be seen in this condition. Solitary or multiple osteosclerotic focal areas are detected mostly in the spine and pelvis.[77] Calcifications may be found in the brain, next to the lateral ventricles.

Hemangioma of the Vertebra. This may be confused with an ivory vertebra due to osteoblastic metastatic disease (prostate, lymphoma) or Paget's disease. Coarse trabeculae may resemble those seen in Paget's disease, but they usually have a vertical orientation ("corduroy"). Unlike Paget's disease there is no bone expansion and no cortical thickening.[78]

Mastocytosis. An abnormal proliferation of the tissue mast cells occurs in this disorder, which may involve a number of organs, including the bone marrow. Its cutaneous manifestation is known as urticaria pigmentosa. The spectrum of osteosclerotic bone changes ranges from mild trabecular thickening to diffuse bone involvement.[79]

Fluorosis. This is a response of bone to overfluorinated drinking water.[80] The symptoms are mild, compared with the extensive and pronounced osteosclerosis. Large osteophytes and ligamentous calcifications may develop.

Osteoid Osteoma. A painful benign bone tumor, osteoid osteoma is radiographically characterized by a central radiolucent nidus surrounded by a varying amount of

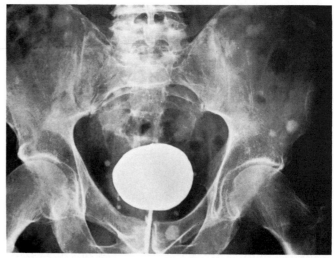

Figure 5–132. Diffuse osteoblastic metastases in a patient with a prostatic carcinoma. A cystogram has been performed.

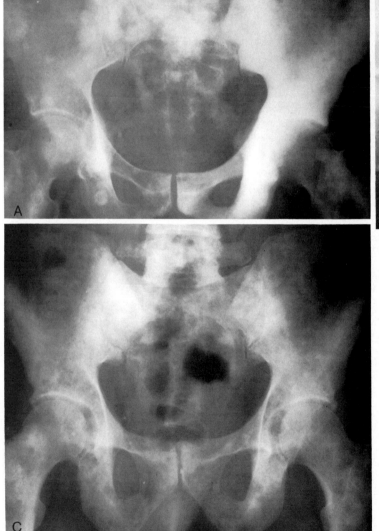

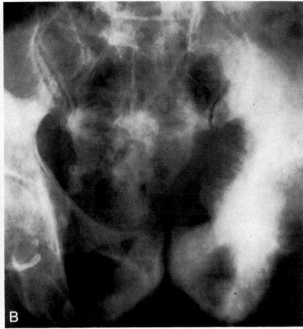

Figure 5–133. Metastatic prostate carcinoma: various examples. *A,* Diffuse blastic involvement of the left hemipelvis with focal blastic nodules on the right and in the last two lumbar vertebrae. There is also involvement of the sacrum and both femurs. Note that, in contrast to Paget's disease, there is no evidence of cortical thickening or accentuation of the trabecular pattern. The bones are not enlarged. *B,* Unusually severe involvement of the left ilium and ischium. The tumor extends beyond the bone and begins to encroach upon the left sacral foramen. There is extensive involvement elsewhere. *C,* Mixed lytic and blastic metastases are present. In addition to areas of increased bone density, small punched-out radiolucencies are in both femurs and in the pubic bones.

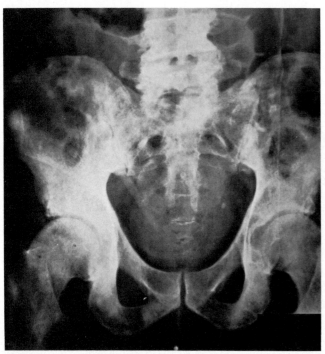

Figure 5–134. Another patient has diffuse osteoblastic metastases from carcinoma of the prostate.

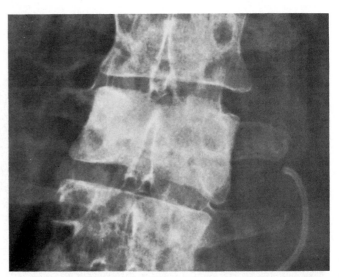

Figure 5–136. Osteoblastic bone metastases in a patient with a malignant pheochromocytoma. Individual trabeculae are not discernible, there is no bone expansion, and the cortex is not thickened.

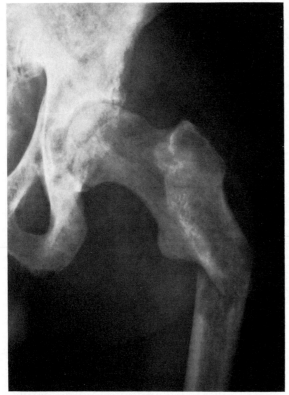

Figure 5–135. Mixed osteoblastic and osteolytic metastases from carcinoma of the prostate. Pathological fracture has occurred in the proximal femoral shaft where a predominantly lytic lesion is present.

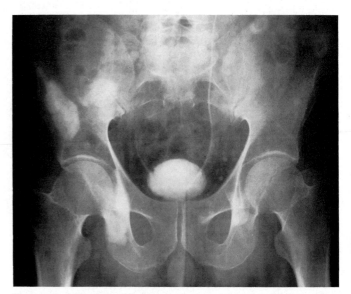

Figure 5–137. Osteoblastic prostatic metastases. A plain radiograph of the pelvis demonstrates an unusual configuration to the metastatic lesions. They are sharply demarcated, very dense, variegated in size, and separated by large areas of relatively normal-appearing bone.

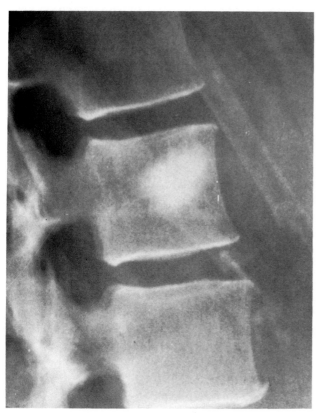

Figure 5–138. Bone island in a lumbar vertebral body. This was also found on a 10-year-old radiographic study, which helped to exclude osteoblastic metastasis.

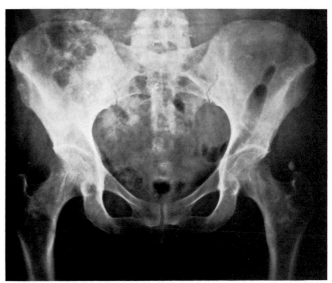

Figure 5–140. Myelofibrosis. Osteosclerotic bone densities are scattered throughout the pelvis making difficult the differential diagnosis from metastatic carcinoma of the prostate based on radiographic findings alone. (Courtesy R. H. Gold, M.D.)

reactive osteosclerosis.[81] Osteosclerosis may be the dominant part of a tumor and may obscure the nidus and mimic osteoblastic metastasis.

Osteitis Condensans Ilii. A triangular area of osteosclerosis involves bone on the ileal side of the sacroiliac joint in this disorder.[82] This is found in the female population, is thought to represent an aftermath of childbirth, and has no clinical significance.

Other Diseases. Numerous additional diseases may cause localized or diffuse increase in bone density, including osteopetrosis,[83] osteopoikilosis,[84] hypervitaminosis D, idiopathic hypercalcemia, and Ewing's sarcoma (Fig. 5–141).

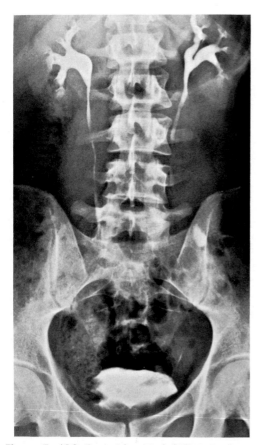

Figure 5–139. Bone island in left ilium is shown.

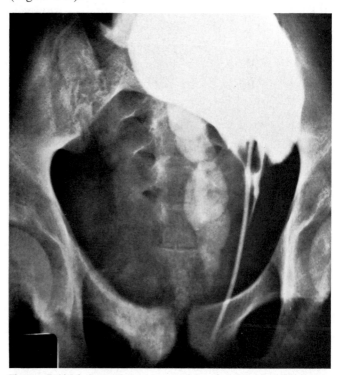

Figure 5–141. Ewing's sarcoma arising from right pubic bone, which shows inhomogeneous osteoblastic response. A large noncalcified soft-tissue component displaces contrast-filled rectum and bladder.

Osteolytic Metastases

Osteolytic metastases are relatively radiolucent compared with bone because the normal bony matrix is replaced by tumor growth (Fig. 5–142). Axial skeleton, ribs, and pelvis are all common sites for metastases. Overlapping gas radiolucencies from the bowel may render detection difficult. Discontinuity, cortical loss, scalloping of the inner cortx, loss of bony trabecula, and an absent pedicle (Fig. 5–143),[85] or spinous process are the radiographic findings. Renal carcinoma (Fig. 5–144), transitional cell carcinoma (Fig. 5–145), carcinoma of the urethra, renal and retroperitoneal sarcomas, and, occasionally, carcinoma of the prostate and carcinoma of the seminal vesicle are the urinary-tract sources of osteolytic bone metastases. Renal carcinoma metastases have an occasional tendency to expand bone outwardly and are occasionally found in the cortex (Fig. 5–146). Pathological fractures are possible and usually involve the proximal femur or pelvis. Diffuse osteoporosis or the presence of multiple lucencies in the pelvis are seen in multiple myeloma (Fig. 5–147).

Osteitis Pubis

In the acute stage this disease is characterized by intense and incapacitating pain over the symphysis pubis.[86] Osteitis pubis usually follows pelvic surgery or transurethral prostatectomy and is thought to be ischemic in origin. Treatment is bed rest and empiric antibiotics. During the acute stage, there is rarefaction of the pubic bone on each side of the symphysis (Fig. 5–148A). After healing has taken place, the radiolucent appearance of

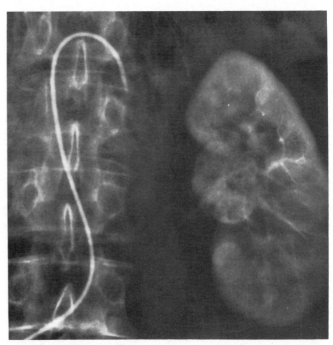

Figure 5–143. Renal cell carcinoma in the hilar region of the left kidney with a solitary metastasis to the right pedicle of the L2 vertebral body. Each vertebral pedicle must be compared with the adjacent pedicles.

bone rarefaction is replaced with varying degrees of osteosclerosis (Fig. 5–148B).

Avascular Necrosis of the Femoral Head

This entity is associated with a number of diseases (Fig. 5–149), but in uroradiological practice it is likely seen in

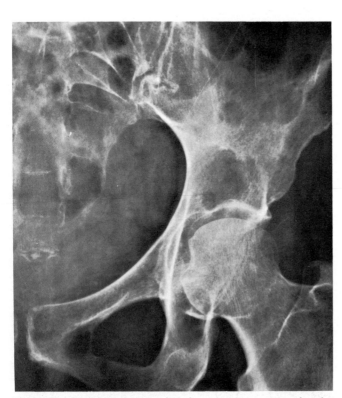

Figure 5–142. Multiple osteolytic bone metastases involve the left hemipelvis and proximal femur.

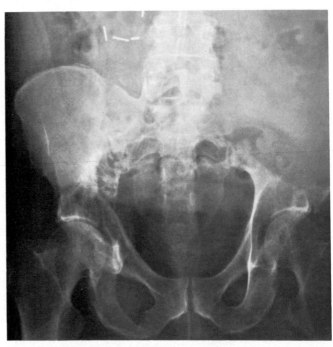

Figure 5–144. Large osteolytic metastasis from renal cell carcinoma. Most of the left ilium and part of the sacrum are involved. Metastases from renal cell carcinoma are usually hypervascular.

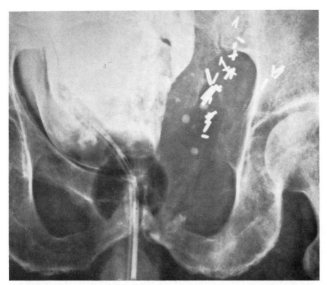

Figure 5–145. Osteolytic bone metastasis from transitional cell carcinoma destroying left pubic bone. The bone destruction is attributable to direct extension of tumor.

the renal transplant patient population on corticosteroid therapy. The process is thought to represent vascular infarct, possibly venous, resulting in osseous necrosis. The earliest findings are osteosclerosis and a radiolucent subcortical band (rim sign)[87] under the weight-bearing area of the femoral head. Collapse of the cortex, fragmentation, and sclerosis are late findings. MRI promises to be the examination of choice for early detection.[88]

Bladder Exstrophy—Epispadias Complex

In this condition, a wide separation exists at the symphysis pubis and there is "squaring" of the iliac notch (Fig. 5–150). Lesser degrees of exstrophy, or epispadias,

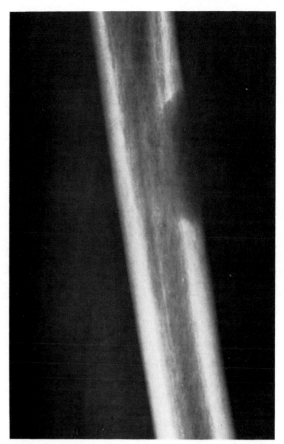

Figure 5–146. Renal cell carcinoma. Osteolytic metastasis is seen in the femoral cortex.

are associated with less pubic separation (Fig. 5–151). An interpubic distance of greater than 1 cm is considered abnormal. Cleidocranial dysostosis must be considered in the differential diagnosis (Fig. 5–152). Rarely, symphysial diastasis may be a normal finding or may be associated with other anomalies.[92]

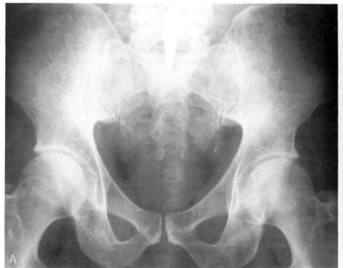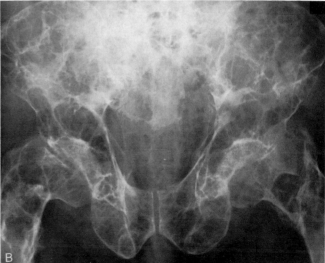

Figure 5–147. Multiple myeloma. *A,* The pelvic radiograph demonstrates multiple small radiolucencies throughout the iliac bones, the sacrum, the pubic rami, and ischia in this 41-year-old male with multiple myeloma. The findings are extremely suggestive of the diagnosis. Residual contrast medium (Pantopaque) is seen in the subarachnoid space. *B,* In this far-advanced myeloma, the entire pelvis is involved by plasma cell infiltration resulting in total loss of trabeculae and innumerable large lytic defects, producing a "bubbly" appearance. This is a very unusual picture. (*B,* Courtesy Alan J. Davidson, M.D.)

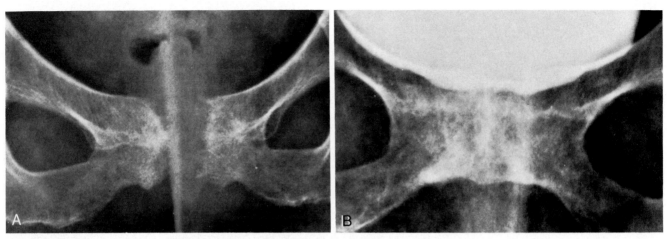

Figure 5–148. Osteitis pubis. *A*, Osteitis pubis is characterized initially by bone reabsorbtion at the symphysis. *B*, Same patient as in *A*. Osteosclerosis of varying degrees is seen after healing has taken place.

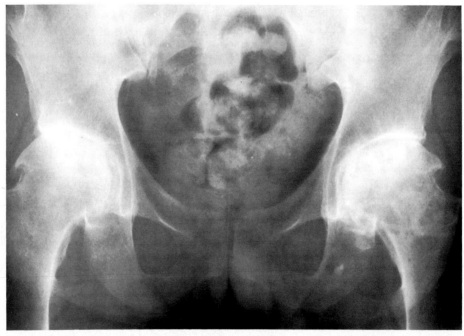

Figure 5–149. Aseptic necrosis of the hips. This 42-year-old male with Crohn's disesase had been on steroids for several years. Plain radiograph of the pelvis demonstrates narrowing of both hip joints, irregularity of the bone in each femoral head, and increased bone density, all indicative of aseptic necrosis, probably as a result of steroids.

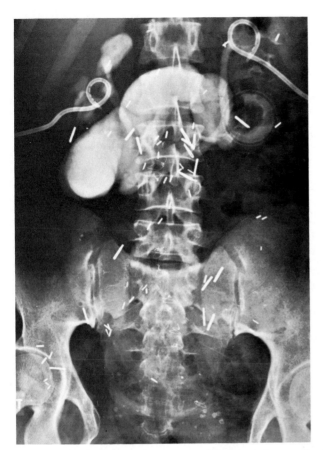

Figure 5–150. Wide gap between pubic bones in a patient with bladder exstrophy. The entire pelvis has a somewhat "squared" appearance. Bilateral ureteral diversion has been performed. In epispadias, the interpubic space is also widened, but usually less than in exstrophy.

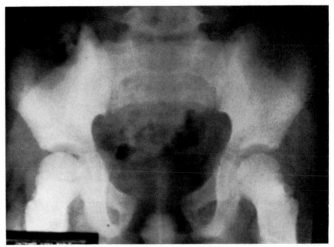

Figure 5–151. Epispadias. Note the wide separation of the symphysis pubis in this 5-year-old boy with epispadias. Epispadias and exstrophy are associated with this defect, although it tends to be less severe in the former. The upper limit of normal for the intersymphysial distance is 1 cm.

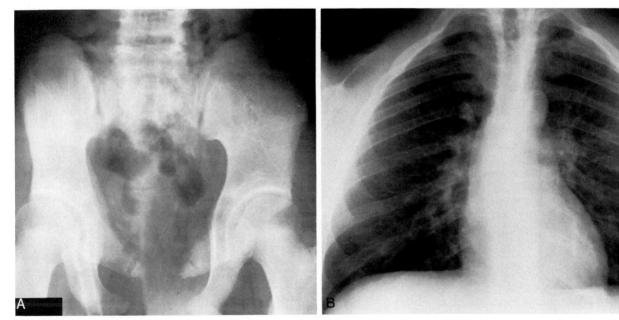

Figure 5–152. Cleidocranial dysostosis. A 17-year-old male. *A*, AP radiograph of the pelvis demonstrates separation of the pubes. Although this condition is sometimes confused with exstrophy on pelvic radiographs, the two conditions are unrelated. Cleidocranial dysostosis is an autosomal dominant disorder associated with multiple bone abnormalities, including failure of normal ossification of the cartilages forming the os pubis. Note in this case the lack of normal flaring of the iliac crests. The sacral iliac joints are not widened. *B*, A PA radiograph of the chest in the same patient reveals bilateral absence of the clavicles. The clavicles may be totally or partially absent in this condition.

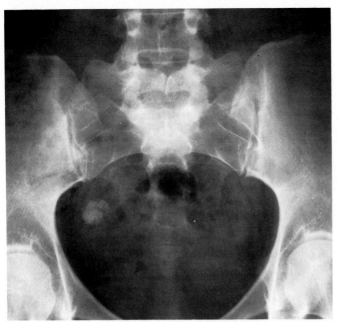

Figure 5–153. Spina bifida occulta. This 31-year-old woman has a spina bifida occulta at L5–S1. There is a partial segmentation anomaly of the distal lumbosacral spine, making it difficult to identify the bifid vertebrae as being either L5 or S1. An incidental calcified fibroid is seen in the pelvis.

Spina Bifida

Incomplete fusion of the posterior neural arches, usually involving lower lumbar vertebrae, is called spina bifida. If the fusion defect is small and asymptomatic, the entity is known as spina bifida occulta (Fig. 5–153; see Fig. 5–17).[89] Large defects may be associated with meningomyelocele and tethered cord (Fig. 5–154). The meningomyelocele may be seen as a soft-tissue mass.

Diseases of the Sacrum

The sacrum is almost always seen on a plain radiograph, although it may be partly obscured by the overlapping bowel. The common primary neoplasm involving the sacrum is chordoma, which presents as an osteolytic destructive process (Fig. 5–155).[90, 91] Other tumors of the sacrum are rare (Fig. 5–156). Sacral agenesis has a characteristic appearance in which the iliac bones fill the void. Associated deformities of other bones may be present. Sacral agenesis may be total or partial. In either case, neuropathic disease of the bladder may be associated (Fig. 5–157).

Postoperative Changes

Skeletal changes resulting from surgery are of some importance to both urologist and radiologist. Prior surgery on the kidney can be suspected if the 12th rib has been resected (Fig. 5–158). Some periosteum is almost always left behind, and almost linear new bone formation ensues.

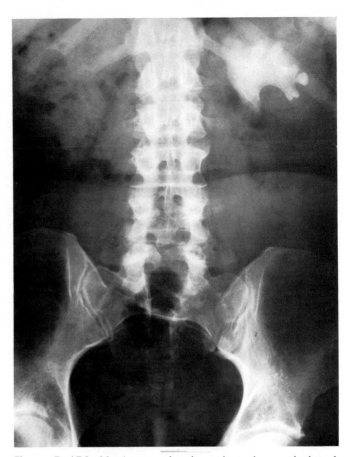

Figure 5–154. Meningomyelocele and staghorn calculus. A plain abdominal radiograph demonstrates the typical spinal deformity seen with meningomyelocele. The interpediculate distances are widened in the lumbosacral spine, and some of the posterior elements of the vertebral bodies are missing and/or incompletely formed. Also noted is a large left-sided staghorn calculus. The patient had a neuropathic bladder.

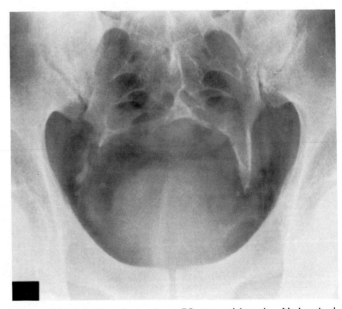

Figure 5–155. Chordoma in a 52-year-old male. Abdominal plain film demonstrates a large bony defect in the sacrum secondary to a chordoma. The appearance is extremely suggestive, if not typical, of this lesion.

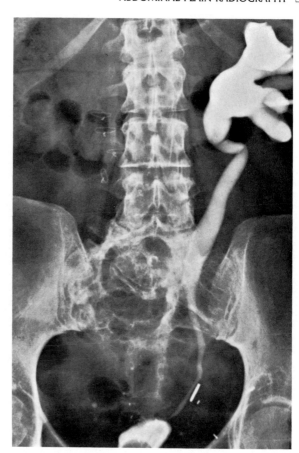

Figure 5–156. Epithelioid tumor involving the sacrum. Sacral tumors are somewhat difficult to detect because of the overlying bowel contents.

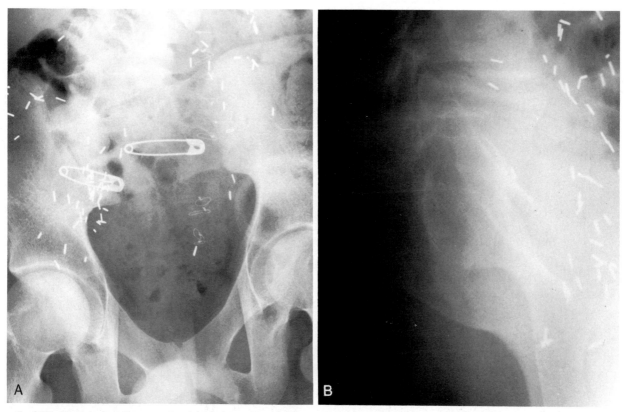

Figure 5–157. Partial sacral agenesis. *A*, A plain pelvic radiograph reveals absence of the distal sacral segments. The upper sacrum is present, and the spacing between the iliac bones is relatively normal. The multiple surgical clips are attributable to urinary diversion to a sigmoid conduit. Although the entire sacrum is not absent in this condition, clinically significant bladder neuropathy may exist. *B*, Lateral film of the sacrum demonstrates absence of the distal segments.

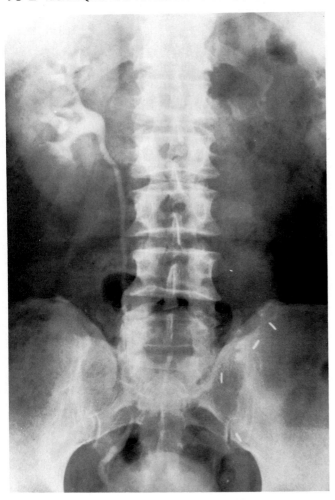

Figure 5–158. Previous left nephrectomy. Note the resection of the left 12th rib. When this finding is encountered on a plain radiograph, it usually suggests that renal surgery has occurred, as in this patient who had undergone left nephrectomy for calculus disease.

Figure 5–159. Laminectomy defect. The plain abdominal radiograph demonstrates surgical loss of the posterior vertebral elements of L4–L5. Bone grafts have been inserted bilaterally, bridging L3–L4 and L4–L5. Residual contrast medium (Pantopaque) droplets are seen in the caudal sac. Large laminectomy defects such as these are no longer frequently encountered since the development of new surgical techniques that do not require removal of the vertebral laminae.

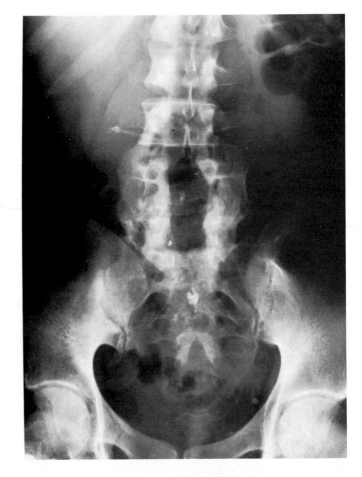

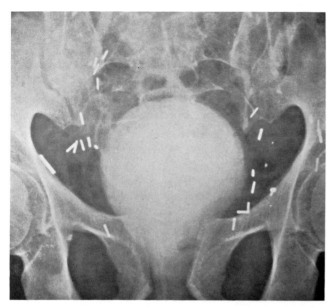

Figure 5–160. Resection of the symphysis pubis during radical prostatectomy. There is also an osteoblastic metastasis in the right ischium.

A spectrum of changes is seen after laminectomy. Either only several chips are taken from the inferior margin of the lamina (usually unilaterally), or the lamina is missing (hemilaminectomy or laminectomy), or the lamina and the spinous processes are absent. These findings may involve only one or several posterior arches (Fig. 5–159).

Posterior spinal fusion has a very characteristic appearance. Masses of trabecular bone are seen along the posterior arches. The spinous processes are no longer visualized since they have blended into the added bony mass. The ilium will have gaps and deformities from the areas where the bone chips were harvested. Fusion may also be performed along the Transverse processes (see Fig. 5–107).

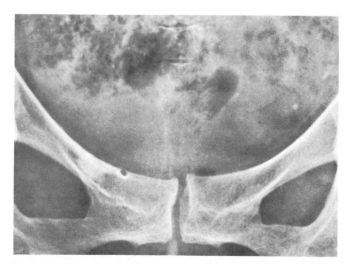

Figure 5–161. Peculiar bone defect following Pereyra urethral suspension for urinary incontinence. The defect is caused either by the needle, which is used to deliver the suspension suture from the anterior abdominal wall to vagina, or by the suture itself.

The symphysis pubis may be resected during prostatectomy or urethral reconstruction, leaving a wedge defect that can be seen on radiographs (Fig. 5–160). A peculiar defect is occasionally seen at the superior margin of the pubic bones following the Pereyra urethral suspension operation for urinary incontinence (Fig. 5–161).

References

1. Shimkin PM: Radiology of acute appendicitis—commentary. AJR 130:1001–1004, 1978.
2. Vaudagna JS, McCort JJ: Plain film diagnosis of retrocecal appendicitis. Radiology 117:533–536, 1975.
3. Swischuk LE, Hyden CK Jr: Appendicitis with perforation: the dilated transverse colon sign. AJR 135:687–689, 1980.
4. Szemes GC, Amberg JR: Gastric bezoars after partial gastrectomy. Report of five cases. Radiology 90:765–768, 1968.
5. Salomen IS. Study of 66 patients including a histopathological study of annular pancreas and a follow-up of 36 survivors. Acta Pediatr Scand (Suppl)272:1–12, 1978.
6. Fullen WD, Selle JG, Whitely DH, et al: Intramural duodenal hematoma. Ann Surg 179:549–556, 1974.
7. Bisla RS, Louis HJ: Acute vascular compression of the duodenum following cast application. Surg Gynecol Obstet 140:563–570, 1975.
8. Swischuk LE: Radiology of the Newborn and Young Infant. Baltimore, Williams & Wilkins, 1980.
9. Currarino G: Incarcerated inguinal hernias in infants: Plain film and barium enemas. Pediatr Radiol 2:247–253, 1974.
10. Blatt ES: Roentgen findings in obstructed diaphragmatic hernia. Radiology 79:648–657, 1962.
11. Hyson EA, Burrell M, Toffler R, et al: Drug-induced gastrointestinal diseases. Gastrointest Radiol 2:183–186, 1977.
12. Weiner MJ: Myotonic megacolon in myotonic dystrophy. AJR 130:177–179, 1978.
13. Kelvin FM, Rice RP: Radiologic evaluation of acute abdominal pain arising from the alimentary tract. Radiol Clin North Am 16:25–39, 1978.
14. Meyers MA: Colonic ileus. Gastrointest Radiol 2:37–45, 1977.
15. Weens HS, Walker LA: The radiologic diagnosis of acute cholecystitis and pancreatitis. Radiol Clin North Am 2:89–103, 1964.
16. Johnson CD, Rice RP: Acute abdomen: Plain radiographic evaluation. Radiographics 5:259–271, 1985.
17. Schultz EH: An aid to the diagnosis of pneumoperitoneum from supine abdominal films. Radiology 70:728–731, 1958.
18. Miller RE: Perforated viscus in infants: A new roentgen sign. Radiology 74:65–67, 1960.
19. Han SY, Shin MS, Tishler JM: Plain film findings of hydropneumoperitoneum. AJR 136:1195–1197, 1981.
20. Rigler LG: Spontaneous pneumoperitoneum. A roentgenologic sign found in the supine position. Radiology 37:604–607, 1941.
21. Miller RE, Nelson SW: The roentgenologic demonstration of tiny amounts of free intraperitoneal gas: Experimental and clinical studies. AJR 112:574–585, 1971.
22. Miller RE: The radiologic evaluation of intraperitoneal gas (pneumoperitoneum). CRC Crit Rev Radiol Sci 4:61–85, 1973.
23. McCort JJ: Radiological examination in blunt abdominal trauma. Radiol Clin North Am 2:121–143, 1964.
24. Laurell A: A contribution to the differential diagnosis in the presence of free fluid in the abdomen. Acta Radiol 16:424–427, 1935.
25. Jorulf H: Roentgen diagnosis of intraperitoneal fluid. A physical, anatomic and clinical investigation. Acta Radiol (Suppl)344:1975.
26. Moskowitz M: The psoas sign, hepatic angle, normal patients, and everyday practice. Gut 14:308–310, 1973.
27. Williams SM, Harned RK, Hultman SA, Quaife MA: Psoas sign: Reevaluation. Radiographics 5:525, 1985.
28. Meyers MA: Dynamic Radiology of the Abdomen: Normal and Pathologic Anatomy. New York, Springer-Verlag, 1976.
29. Meyers MA, Oliphant M, Berna AS, Feldberg MAM: The peritoneal ligaments and mesenteries: Pathways of intraabdominal spread of disease. Radiology 163:593–604, 1987.
30. Fritzsche P, Toomey FB, Ta HN: Alteration of perirenal fat secondary to diffuse retroperitoneal infiltration. Radiology 131:27–29, 1979.
31. Susman N, Hammerman AM, Cohen E: The renal halo sign in pancreatitis. Radiology 142:323–327, 1982.

32. Fleishner FG, Ming SC: Revised concepts of the colon, II. So-called diverticulitis, diverticular sigmoiditis and perisigmoiditis, diverticular abscess, fistula and frank peritonitis. Radiology 84:599–609, 1965.

33. Aquos JW, Holmes RB: Gas in the pancreas as a sign of abscess. AJR 80:60–66, 1958.

34. Campbell EW, Rogers CL: Submucosal gallbladder emphysema. JAMA 227:790–792, 1974.

35. Rigler LG, Borman CW, Nobel JF: Gallstone obstruction pathogenesis and roentgen manifestations. JAMA 117:1753–1754, 1941.

36. Meyers MA, Ghahremani GG, Clements JL, Goodman K: Pneumatosis intestinalis. Gastrointest Radiol 2:91–98, 1977.

37. Bloch C: Natural history of pneumatosis coli. Radiology 123:311–314, 1977.

38. Kogutt MS: Necrotizing enterocolitis of infancy. Radiology 130:367–370, 1979.

39. Carson CC, Malek RS, Remine WH: Urologic aspects of vesicoenteric fistulas. J Urol 119:744–746, 1978.

40. Roberts MC, Pollack HM, Banner MP, et al: Interstitial emphysema associated with epidural anesthesia for extracorporeal shock-wave lithotripsy. AJR 148:301–302, 1987.

41. McCort JJ: Abdominal Radiology. Baltimore, Williams & Wilkins, 1981.

42. Rankin RN: Gas formation after renal tumor embolization without abscess; a benign occurrence. Radiology 130:317–320, 1979.

43. McAfee JG, Donner MW: Differential diagnosis of calcifications encountered in abdominal radiographs. Am J Med Sci 243:609, 1962.

44. Dovey P: Pelvic phleboliths. Clin Radiol 17:121–125, 1966.

45. Berk RN: Radiology of the gallbladder and bile ducts. Surg Clin North Am 53:973–978, 1973.

46. Meyers MA, O'Donohue N: The Mercedes-Benz sign: Insight into the dynamics of formation and disappearance of gallstones. AJR 119:63–70, 1973.

47. Strijik SP: Calcified gallstone fissures: reversed Mercedes-Benz sign. Gastrointest Radiol 12:152–154, 1987.

48. Holden WS, Turner MJ: Disappearing limy bile. Clin Radiol 23:500–502, 1972.

49. Brenner RW, Stewart CF: Cholecystitis in children. Rev Surg 21:327–333, 1964.

50. Cornel CM, Clarke R: Vicarious calcifications involving the gallbladder. Ann Surg 149:267–270, 1959.

51. Rossi P, Gould HR: Angiography and scanning in liver disease. Radiology 96:553–562, 1970.

52. Beggs I: Radiology of the hydatid disease. AJR 145:639–648, 1985.

53. Shackelford GD, Kirks DR: Neonatal hepatic calcification secondary to transplacental infection. Radiology 122:753–757, 1977.

54. Gelfand DW: The liver: Plain film diagnosis. Semin Roentgenol 10:177–207, 1975.

55. Adam YG, Huvos AG, Fortner JG: Giant hemangiomas of the liver. Ann Surg 172:239–246, 1970.

56. Kenny PJ, Stanley RJ: Calcified adrenal masses. Urol Radiol 9:9–12, 1987.

57. Pantoja E, San Pedro CA, Jittivanich U: The radiographic wall-sign of ovarian dermoids. Rev Interam Radiol 2:33–35, 1977.

58. Gardner KD, Castellino RA, Kempson R, et al: Primary amyloidosis of the renal pelvis. N Engl J Med 284:1196–1198, 1971.

59. Camiel MR: Calcification of vas deferens associated with diabetes. J Urol 86:634–636, 1961.

60. Jorulf H, Lindstedt E: Urogenital shistosomiasis: CT evaluation. Radiology 157:745–747, 1985.

61. Sumers EH, Gittes RF: Calcified tumor of the urinary bladder: Sonographic diagnosis and distinction from a bladder calculus. J Ultrasound Med 4:681–682, 1985.

62. Pollack HM, Banner MP, Hodson CJ, Martinez LO: Diagnostic considerations in bladder wall calcifications. AJR 136:791, 1981.

63. Mapp EM, Pollack HM, Goldman LH: *Armillifer armillatus* infestation in man. J Nat Med Assoc 68:198, 1976.

64. Beerman R, Nunez D Jr, Wetli CV: Radiographic evaluation of the cocaine smuggler. Gastrointest Radiol 11:351–354, 1986.

65. Pinsky MF, Ducas J, Ruggere MD: Narcotic smuggling: the double condom sign. J Can Assoc Radiol 29:79–81, 1978.

66. Older RA, Korobkin M, Cleeve DM, et al: Contrast-induced acute renal failure: Persistent nephrogram as clue to early detection. AJR 134:339–342, 1980.

67. Fisher MS: Case of the summer season. Semin Roentgenol 12:161, 1977.

68. Resnik D: Annual oration: Degenerative diseases of the vertebral column. Radiology 156:3–14, 1985.

69. Rosa M, Capellini C, Canevari MA, et al: CT in low back pain due to lumbar canal osseous changes. Neuroradiol 28:237–242, 1986.

70. Gehweiler JA, Osborne RL, Becker RF: The Radiology of Vertebral Trauma. Philadelphia, WB Saunders, 1980.

71. Goldman AB, Bullough P, Kammerman S, Ambos M: Osteitis deformans of the hip joint. AJR 128:601–606, 1977.

72. Price CHG, Goldie W: Paget's sarcoma of bone. J Bone Joint Surg 51B:205–224, 1969.

73. Whitmore WF: The natural history of prostatic cancer. Cancer 32:1104, 1973.

74. Reidy JF: Osteoblastic metastases from a hypernephroma. Br J Radiol 48:225–227, 1975.

75. Blank N, Lieber A: The significance of growing bone island. Radiology 85:508–511, 1965.

76. Meszaros WT, Sisson M: Myelofibrosis. Radiology 77:958–967, 1961.

77. Komar NN, Gabrielsen TO, Holt JF: Roentgenographic appearance of lumbosacral spine and pelvis in tuberous sclerosis. Radiology 89:701–705, 1967.

78. Laredo JD, Reizine D, Bard M, Merland JJ: Vertebral hemangiomas: Radiologic evaluation. Radiology 161:183–187, 1986.

79. Barer M, Peterson LF, Dahlin DC, et al: Mastocytosis with osseous lesions resembling metastatic malignant lesions in bone. J Bone Joint Surg 50A:142–152, 1968.

80. Morris JW: Skeletal fluorosis among Indians of the American Southwest 94:608–615, 1965.

81. Swee RG, McLeod RA, Beabout JW: Osteoid osteoma. Radiology 130:117–123, 1979.

82. Isley JK, Baylin GJ. Prognosis in osteitis condensans ilii. Radiology 72:234–237, 1959.

83. Pincus JB, Gittleman IF, Kramer B: Juvenile osteopetrosis. Am Dis Child 73:458–472, 1947.

84. Green AE, Ellswood WH, Collins JR: Melorheostosis and osteopoikilosis. AJR 87:1096–1111, 1962.

85. Patel NP, Kumar R, Kinkhabwala M, Wengrover S: Radiology of lumbar vertebral pedicles: Variants, anomalies and pathologic conditions. Radiographics 7:101–137, 1987.

86. Warwick RTT: The pathogensis and treatment of osteitis pubis. Br J Urol 32:464–472, 1960.

87. Mitchell DG, Rao VM, Dalinka MK, et al: Femoral head avascular necrosis: Correlation of MR imaging, radiographic staging, radionuclide imaging and clinical findings. Radiology 162:709–715, 1987.

88. Thickman D, Axel L, Kressel HY, et al: Magnetic resonance imaging of avascular necrosis of the femoral head. Skeletal Radiol 15:133, 1986.

89. Boone D, Parsons D, Lachmann SM, Sherwood T: Spina bifida occulta: Lesion or anomaly. Clin Radiol 36:159–161, 1985.

90. Amorosa JK, Weintraub S, Amorosa LF, et al: Sacral destruction: Foraminal lines revisited. AJR 145:773–775, 1985.

91. Smith J, Ludwig RL, Marcove RC: Sacrococcygeal chordoma: Clinicoradiological study of 60 patients. Skeletal Radiol 16:37–43, 1987.

92. Steidle CP, Kennedy HA, Mitchell ME, Rink RC: Symphysial diastasis in the absence of the exstrophy—epispadias complex. J Urol 140:349, 1988.

6

Excretory Urography

RICHARD M. FRIEDENBERG □ J. S. DUNBAR

EXCRETORY UROGRAPHY IN THE ADULT

RICHARD M. FRIEDENBERG

The number of excretory (intravenous) urograms performed nationally has decreased sharply over the past 10 years.[58] This trend has paralleled the increased use of computed tomography (CT) and ultrasound as new methods of triage before considering the intravenous urogram. Ultrasonography is generally used as the initial study for determining the presence or absence of a kidney, identifying hydronephrosis, and localizing masses as well as determining their nature (cystic or solid). More recently, it has been used for the follow-up of transplanted kidneys, and even for evaluating interstitial diseases. CT is frequently used as the first study in patients with significant renal trauma and in evaluating the extent of renal masses, a function previously performed by renal angiography.

More recently, magnetic resonance imaging (MRI) has had an impact on abdominal imaging, particularly of the liver, gynecological organs, and bladder. MRI has less spatial resolution than CT, and motion artifacts are frequent because of the long imaging times. However, MR scans provide excellent contrast, which can be altered by varying the amount of T1 and T2 weighting inherent in a given set of images. MRI also presents the potential for metabolic assessment of organs that is not available with other modalities. The advent of fast scanning, our current ability to measure flow, and our future ability to measure perfusion, diffusion and other parameters, will increase the importance of MRI in abdominal imaging. Table 6–1 is a personal assessment of CT, MRI, and ultrasonography in the evaluation of renal pathology at the time of this writing.

Although fewer urograms are performed currently than in the past, they remain the primary modality for visualization of the pyelocalyceal system and the ureter, and for assessment of calculi and renal infection.

Table 6–1. Evaluation of Renal Lesions

Type or Location of Lesion	CT	Ultrasound	MRI	Urogram
Masses	1	2*	3	4
Calculi	1	2	3	1
C-M junction	2	3	1	4
Calyces and pelvis	1	3	2	1
Abscess, central	1	2*	2	4
Abscess, perinephric	1	2	2	4
Hydronephrosis	2	1	3	1
Ureter	2	3	2	1

1 represents the most information, 4 the least.
C-M = corticomedullary.
*Simplest method, frequently used first, although it may provide less detail.

EXCRETORY UROGRAPHY

Within this section we use the term urogram to refer to the visualization of kidney parenchyma, calyces, and pelvis resulting from the intravenous injection of contrast media. The term pyelogram is reserved for retrograde studies visualizing only the collecting system. The commonly used colloquial term intravenous pyelogram (IVP) is really a misnomer; it implies visualization of the pelvis and calyceal system alone without visualization of the parenchyma and is actually synonymous with the retrograde pyelogram. The term cystography is used to describe visualization of the bladder, whereas urethrography refers to visualization of the urethra, and cystourethrography to the combined study. Additional terms include antegrade pyelogram for percutaneous puncture of the collecting system and injection of opaque contrast material, percutaneous nephrostomy for the insertion of a tube into the renal pelvis, and antegrade or retrograde seminal vesiculography for visualization of the seminal vesicles and vas deferens. (The discussion of these specialized examinations can be located using the index.)

Preparation of Patient

It is never necessary to postpone an urgent examination to prepare a patient for a urogram. Differences of opinion are considerable concerning the value of catharsis and dehydration in preparing patients for excretory urography.[242]

Catharsis

Conventional enemas are not desirable, because they are inadequate for colon cleansing and frequently leave residual fluid and air that detract from the examination. In scheduled cases, catharsis is recommended to eliminate fecal material from the colon and to reduce the amount of gas in the bowel. Castor oil is an effective catharsis administered in a dose of 1 to 2 ounces. Many satisfactory proprietary medications (e.g., X-prep, Dulcolax) can be substituted for castor oil. In older or sedentary patients, it is frequently advisable to utilize a suppository in addition to oral catharsis. Some proprietary distal colon enema preparations are quite effective in cleaning the distal bowel and can be utilized in place of the suppository.

Dehydration

With modern contrast media, most uroradiologists believe that, although overhydration must be avoided, dehydration is unnecessary. Infants and young children should never be dehydrated before the examination. Dehydrated patients are more prone to protein precipitation (Tamm-Horsfall, Bence Jones) in the renal tubules producing intrarenal obstruction leading to oliguria or anuria. Dehydration increases the risk of renal shutdown in renal failure, particularly in diabetics with mild to moderate azotemia. Dehydration in infancy may lead to renal vein thrombosis. The rationale for the use of dehydration is that it stimulates production of antidiuretic hormone, which in turn increases water reabsorption in the distal nephron, increasing the contrast density in the collecting system. This is rarely accomplished by overnight abstinence from fluids, and in practice, dehydration has not proved to be of significant value.[234]

In some instances, evaluation of the early contrast films suggest variations in the examination. Some patients may show normal volume within the calyces with poor contrast density. This appearance may be related to overhydration or osmotic diuresis due to the hyperosmotic effect of a large dose of contrast material. Later films may show improved contrast as the diuresis decreases, or an injection of less contrast medium may provide better contrast detail (Fig. 6–1). If, on the other hand, the initial contrast film shows thin, poorly filled, spidery calyces resulting from low volume and insufficient contrast medium, then larger doses of the medium are suggested to increase diuresis (Fig. 6–2). A usual compromise for patients scheduled in the early morning is to omit fluids after 11:00 PM and to omit breakfast, which decreases the chance of vomiting as well as producing slight dehydration. For patients examined later in the day, a light breakfast is usually advisable.

Overhydration interferes with the quality of the examination. A patient arriving in the radiology department with an infusion running frequently shows poor or no visualization of the collecting system, although renal function is normal. In such patients, shutting off the infusion and waiting 30 minutes frequently solves the problem (Fig. 6–3). Collecting system opacification may be further enhanced by reinjection of contrast material (Fig. 6–2).

Technique

Plain Abdominal Radiograph (Scout Film)

The previous chapters have described the value of the scout film and have discussed contrast media. It is impossible to place too much emphasis on the importance of obtaining a scout film of the abdomen prior to the injection of contrast media. Careful analysis of this film often provides considerable information and frequently indicates the probable diagnosis. In many cases, the urogram may be misleading without a scout film. Some of the primary uses of the scout film are described in the following list (for detailed discussion and illustrations, see Chapter 5):

1. *Calculus.* A suspicious calculus seen on the scout film may not be seen in any of the postexcretion films. Calculi do not always obstruct. If a suspicious calcification is suggestive of calculus, it may be worthwhile to take an oblique film to check whether its localization is within the area of the kidney or ureter (Fig. 6–4).

2. *Skeletal abnormality.* Congenital abnormalities, such as exstrophy, absence of the abdominal muscles, and spinal abnormalities provide clues to abnormalities that may be present in the urinary tract (Fig. 6–5). Metabolic changes in bone such as rickets assist in the diagnosis of renal abnormalities.

3. *Intestinal gas pattern.* Ileus or obstruction may explain symptoms. Ileus is frequently present with renal pain (Fig. 6–6).

4. *Calcifications.* The location and nature of the calcifications may provide strong indications as to whether

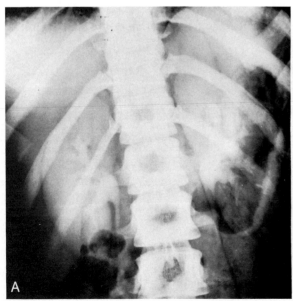 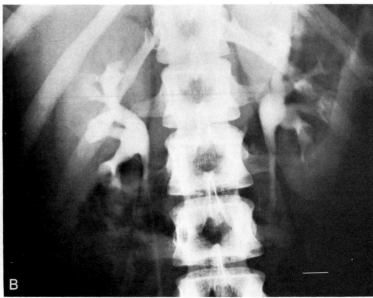

Figure 6–1. *A,* A 3-minute film of a urogram following 100 cc of contrast medium. Pelvis and calyces are distended, but contrast is poor. *B,* A 25-minute film. Osmotic diuresis has decreased. Contrast is now excellent.

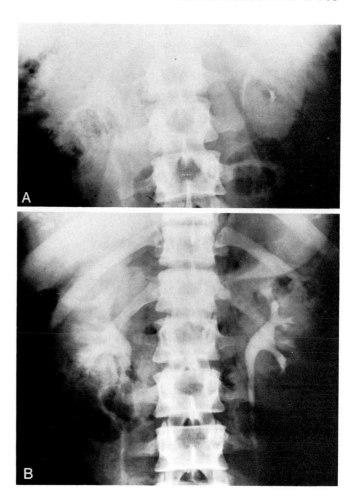

Figure 6–2. *A*, Thin spidery calyces with poor density and filling of collecting system, following the initial injection of a contrast bolus. *B*, A second bolus of 50 cc of contrast medium was injected, producing sufficient diuresis to distend the collecting system and to increase contrast density.

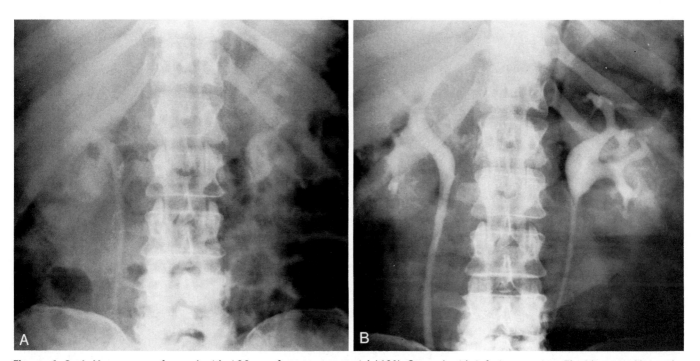

Figure 6–3. *A*, Urogram performed with 100 cc of contrast material (60% Conray) with infusion running. The diuresis dilutes the contrast medium, and visualization of the pyelocalyceal system is poor. *B*, Reinjection 1 hour after infusion stopped with 50 cc of 60% Conray provides excellent visualization of the pyelocalyceal system.

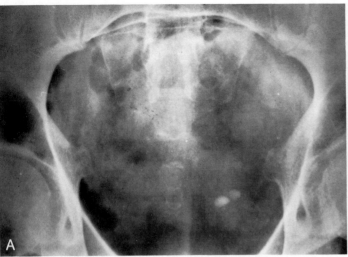
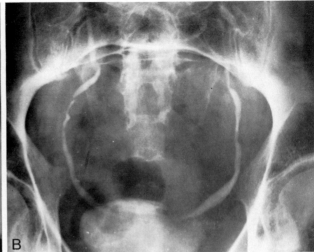

Figure 6–4. *A,* Plain radiograph reveals two calculi in the distal left ureter. *B,* Contrast material in urogram completely obscures the calculi. There is no evidence of obstruction.

infection, vascular abnormalities, tumor, or metabolic diseases are present (Fig. 6–7).

5. *Abdominal masses.* A mass may be seen more clearly on the scout film and may suggest special views to elucidate its nature in the urogram.

6. *Foreign bodies.* Opaque foreign bodies noted in the scout films may influence the type of examinations performed.

Contrast Media

The amount of contrast medium administered varies with the method of administration. Table 6–2 illustrates the common ionic contrast media available today, the usual dose administered for a bolus injection, and the

grams of iodine per 100 cc injected. The newer (dimers and ratio-3) contrast media that are becoming available are discussed in Chapter 4. Nonionic contrast media are described in Table 6–3. Many reports suggest a lesser incidence of reactions with these newer media partly because of their lower osmolarity.[172] Contrast density may

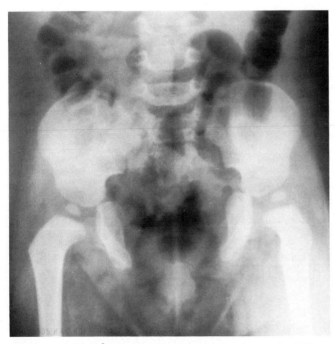

Figure 6–5. Exstrophy of the bladder in an 18-month-old boy. The bony pelvis is incomplete anteriorly, and the symphysis pubis is widely separated.

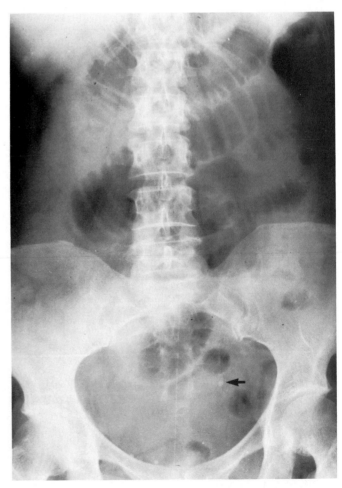

Figure 6–6. Opaque calculus in the distal left ureter (*arrow*). Secondary ileus involving primarily the small intestine.

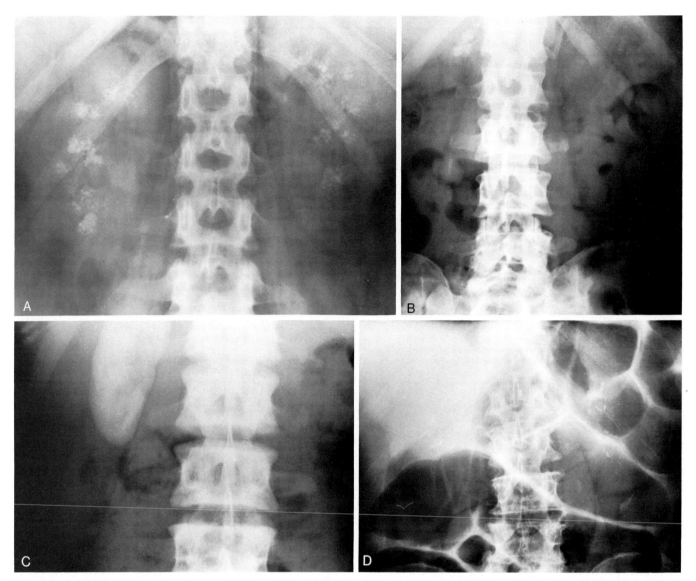

Figure 6–7. Findings encountered on preliminary abdominal radiograph. *A*, Nephrocalcinosis secondary to lupus erythematosus. *B*, Calcification of the right adrenal gland, post-trauma. *C*, Scout film showing a densely calcified right kidney in a patient with renal failure and oxalosis. The entire renal parenchyma is calcified. The opposite kidney is absent. *D*, Fine calcifications bilaterally in the vascular structures of both kidneys with minimal calcification of the aorta in a patient with hypertension. Intrarenal arterial calcification is most commonly seen in hyperparathyroidism, diabetes mellitus, and hypertension.

be slightly improved as well.[72, 78a] The high cost of nonionic contrast media has inhibited their general use for urography.[63, 78b] Within the next few years, however, current ionic media will probably be largely replaced by the new contrast media. Pretesting does not provide reliable information regarding sensitivity to contrast media and therefore is not performed prior to the injection, as described in Chapter 4.

The dose of contrast is variable, depending on patient size and the radiologist's preference. A dose of 200 mg iodine/pound body weight is an average adult dose. For most patients, this means a dose of between 20 and 30 gm. It is usually not necessary to exceed a dose of 30 gm of iodine, except for very large patients. Most injections of contrast medium are performed by rapidly injecting the contrast as a bolus, using either one or two 50-cc syringes. In most cases, a butterfly 18-gauge needle is inserted into the antecubital vein and the syringe connected to the tubing. In some cases, smaller needles may

be used for other veins that seem accessible. Injection is usually completed within 30 to 60 seconds. The density of the nephrogram relates directly to the plasma level of contrast media.[157] More injected iodine increases the density of the nephrogram (Figs. 6–8 and 6–9). Large doses of contrast medium increase diuresis, which distends the collecting system and, by increasing volume, usually increases the diagnostic usefulness of the urogram, if contrast density is sufficient. Although the bolus injection, as described above, is the most commonly used method, certain variations may be helpful. Occasionally, on the early films in a patient not in renal failure the collecting system may appear spidery and poorly filled, or in patients who have poor concentrating ability or who are overhydrated the diuresis may dilute the contrast. In the former situation, a higher dose of contrast medium increases contrast, whereas in the latter, a smaller dose of contrast improves visualization of the pyelocalyceal system (see Figs. 6–1 to 6–3).

Table 6–2. Ionic Contrast Media

Generic Name	Cation	Percentage in Solution	Trade Name	Iodine (mg/ml)	Osmolality (mOsm/kg)	Viscosity 25°C	Viscosity 37°C	Size and Availability
Iodamide	Meglumine	24*	Renovue-Dip	111	433	1.8	1.4	300 ml B
Iothalamate	Meglumine	30*	Conray-30	141	600	2.0	1.5	50 ml V
								100 ml V
								150 ml B
								200 ml B
								300 ml B
Diatrizoate	Meglumine	30*	Hypaque 30%	141	633	1.92	1.43	100 ml B
								300 ml B
Diatrizoate	Meglumine	30*	Reno-M-Dip	141	566	1.9	1.4	300 ml B
Diatrizoate	Meglumine	30*	Urovist Meglumine DIU/CT	141	640	1.9	1.4	300 ml B
Diatrizoate	Meglumine	25*	Hypaque 25%	150	696	1.55	1.17	300 ml B
Iothalamate	Meglumine	43*	Conray-43	202	1000	3.0	2.0	50 ml V
								100 ml V
								150 ml B
								100 ml B
Diatrizoate	Meglumine	60	Angiovist 282	282	1400	6.1	4.1	50 ml V
								100 ml V
								150 ml V
Iothalamate	Meglumine	60	Conray	282	1400	6.0	4.0	20 ml V
								30 ml V
								50 ml V
								100 ml V
								100 ml B
								150 ml B
								200 ml B
Diatrizoate	Meglumine	60	Hypaque 60%	282	1415	6.16	4.10	20 ml V
								30 ml V
								50 ml V
								100 ml V
								100 ml in 200 ml B
								150 ml in 200 ml B
								200 ml in 200 ml B
Diatrizoate	Meglumine	60	Reno-M-60	282	1500	4.6	4.0	10 ml V
								30 ml V
								50 ml V
								100 ml V
								100 ml B
								150 ml B
Diatrizoate	Sodium 8% Meglumine 52%	60	Angiovist 292	292	1500	5.9	4.0	30 ml V
								50 ml V
								100 ml V
Diatrizoate	Sodium 8% Meglumine 52%	60	MD-60	292	1539	6.2	5.0	30 ml V
								50 ml V
Diatrizoate	Sodium 8% Meglumine 52%	60	Renografin-60	292	1420	5.9	4.0	10 ml V
								30 ml V
								50 ml V
								100 ml V
								100 ml B
Diatrizoate	Sodium	50	Hypaque 50%	300	1550	3.43	2.43	20 ml V
								30 ml V
								50 ml V
								150 ml in 200 ml B
								200 ml in 200 ml B
Diatrizoate	Sodium	50	MD-50	300	1522	3.2	2.4	30 ml V
								50 ml V
Iodamide	Meglumine	65	Renovue-65	300	1558	8.7	5.7	50 ml V
								300 ml B
Diatrizoate	Sodium	50	Urovist Sodium 300	300	1550	3.3	2.4	50 ml V
Diatrizoate	Sodium 29.1% Meglumine 28.5%	57.6	Renovist II	309	1517	5.6	3.8	30 ml V
								50 ml V
Iothalamate	Sodium	54.3	Conray-325	325	1700	4.0	3.0	30 ml V
								50 ml V
Diatrizoate	Meglumine	76	Diatrizoate Meglumine USP 76%	358	1980	15	9.2	50 ml V
Diatrizoate	Sodium 10% Meglumine 66%	76	Angiovist 370	370	2100	13.8	8.4	50 ml V
								100 ml V
								150 ml B
								200 ml B

Table 6–2. Ionic Contrast Media *Continued*

Generic Name	Cation	Percentage in Solution	Trade Name	Iodine (mg/ml)	Osmolality (mOsm/kg)	Viscosity 25°C	Viscosity 37°C	Size and Availability
Diatrizoate	Sodium 10% Meglumine 66%	76	Hypaque-76	370	2016	13.34	8.32	30 ml V 50 ml V 100 ml V 100 ml in 200 ml B 150 ml in 200 ml B 200 ml in 200 ml B
Diatrizoate	Sodium 10% Meglumine 66%	76	MD-76	370	2140	14.7	9.1	50 ml V 100 ml B 150 ml B 200 ml B
Diatrizoate	Sodium 10% Meglumine 66%	76	Renografin-76	370	1940	13.8	8.4	20 ml V 50 ml V 100 ml B 200 ml B
Diatrizoate	Sodium 35% Meglumine 34.3%	69.3	Renovist	371	1900	9.1	5.7	50 ml V
Diatrizoate	Sodium 25% Meglumine 50%	75	Hypaque-M, 75%	385	2108	12.69	7.99	20 ml V 50 ml V
Iothalamate	Sodium	66.8	Conray-400	400	2300	7.0	4.5	25 ml V 50 ml V
Iothalamate	Sodium 26% Meglumine 52%	78	Vascoray	400	2400	17.0	9.0	25 ml V 50 ml V 100 ml B 150 ml B 200 ml B
Diatrizoate	Sodium 30% Meglumine 60%	90	Hypaque-M, 90%	462	2938	34.7	19.50	50 ml V
Iothalamate	Sodium	80	Angio-Conray	480	2400	14.0	9.0	50 ml V

*Contrast medium used for infusions.
Note: B = bottle; V = vial.
From Fischer HW: Catalog of intravascular contrast media. Radiology 159:561–563, 1986.

Table 6–3. Nonionic Contrast Media

Generic Name	Dimer	Percentage in Solution	Trade Name	Iodine (mg/ml)	Osmolality (mOsm/kg)	Viscosity 25°C	Viscosity 37°C	Size and Availability
Iohexol		38.8	Ominpaque	180	411	2.81	2.05	10 ml V 20 ml V
Iopamidol		40.8	Isovue-M 200	200	413	3.3	2.0	20 ml V 50 ml V
Iohexol		51.8	Omnipaque	240	504	4.43	3.08	10 ml V 100 ml V 200 ml B
Iopamidol		61	Isovue 300	300	616	8.8	4.7	20 ml V 50 ml V 100 ml B 200 ml B
Iohexol		64.7	Omnipaque	300	709	10.35	6.77	10 ml V 30 ml V 50 ml V 100 ml V
Ioxaglate	Sodium 19.6% Meglumine 39.3%	58.9	Hexabrix	320	600	15.7	7.5	20 ml V 30 ml V 50 ml V 100 ml in 150 ml B 150 ml in 150 ml B 200 ml in 250 ml B
Iohexol		75.5	Omnipaque	350	862	18.50	11.15	50 ml V 100 ml V 200 ml B
Iopamidol		76	Isovue 370	370	796	20.9	9.4	20 ml V 50 ml V 100 ml B 200 ml B

Note: B = bottle; V = vial.
From Fischer HW: Catalog of intravascular contrast media. Radiology 159:561–563, 1986.

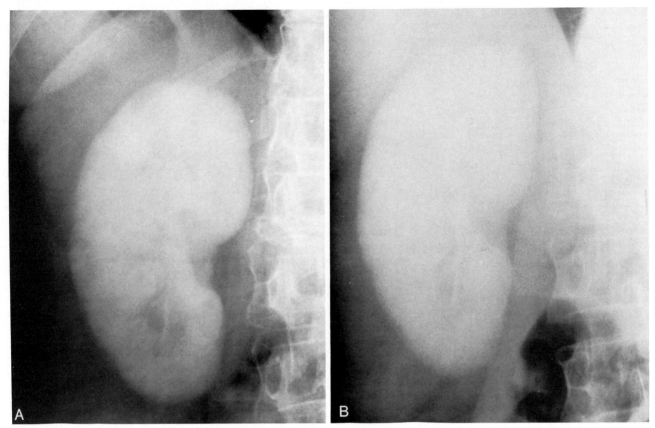

Figure 6–8. Nephrogram obtained during a cardiac angiogram. The intensity of the nephrogram is directly proportional to the iodine level in the plasma. *A,* Nephrogram obtained soon after an injection of a large bolus of contrast material into the heart. *B,* Nephrogram obtained after the injection of a second bolus a few minutes later. Note that both nephrograms are very intense with the second nephrogram more intense because of the added bolus of contrast material.

A method of examination that was popular some 15 years ago and is still used in some institutions today is the drip infusion technique. This method is a convenient way of delivering large doses of contrast material over a prolonged time. Infusion kits may be purchased contain-

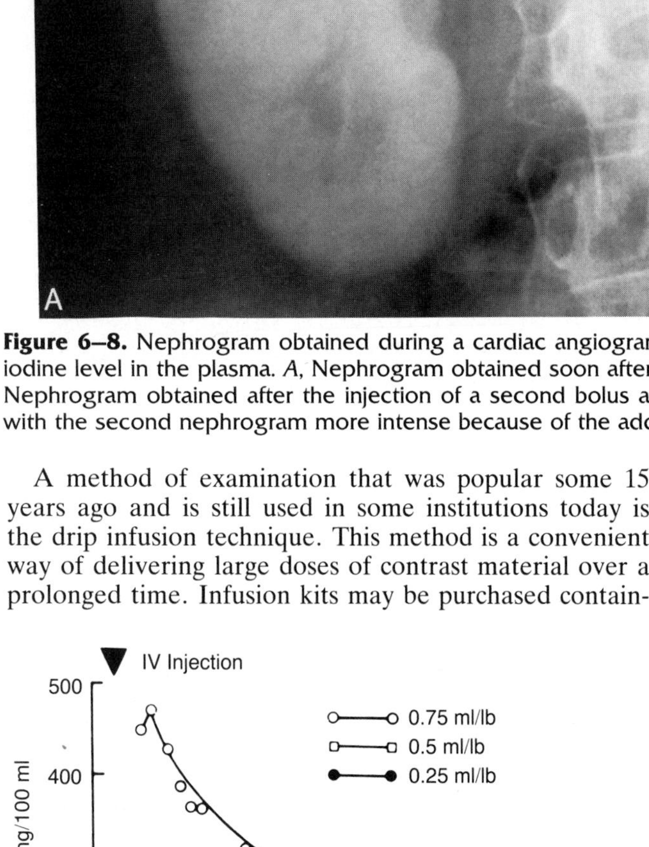

Figure 6–9. Plasma concentrations of sodium diatrizoate following single injections of increasing doses. The larger the dose, the higher the plasma level of contrast medium and the better the nephrogram. (From Catell WR, Fry IK, Spencer AG, Purkiss P: Excretory urography; factors determining excretion of Hypaque. Br J Radiol 40:561, 1967.)

ing 40 to 45 gm of iodine, which is delivered in 250 to 400 cc of fluid. The advantages of the drip infusion as compared with bolus injection are as follows:

1. There is a markedly prolonged (not more intense) nephrogram (Fig. 6–10).

2. Enhanced diuresis from the additional contrast material and water volume more fully distends the collecting system and ureters (Fig. 6–11). Relatively rapid distention of the urinary bladder may also contribute to this increased fullness of the ureters, renal pelvis, and calyces.

3. The collecting system is visualized for a longer time, providing more flexibility in filming.

4. No significant increase in reactions occurs, and, in fact, nausea and vomiting may be less frequent than with bolus injections.

5. Ureteral compression need not be used because excellent ureteral visualization is usually obtained (Fig. 6–11).

6. Administration is easy.

The disadvantages of drip infusion include the following:

1. It overloads the normal patient with more iodine than necessary.

2. Calyceal blunting may be produced, suggesting abnormal dilatation.

3. It may lead to pyelosinus extravasation and significant pain in patients with partial obstruction.

4. The increased diuresis produced may decrease visualization, if there is a low fixed specific gravity (Fig. 6–12).

5. Drip infusion may occasionally produce congestive

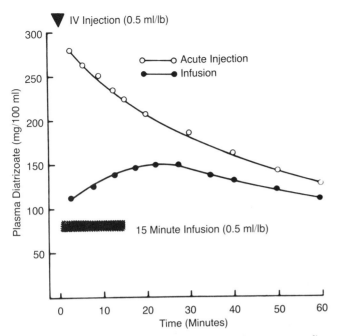

Figure 6–10. Comparison of plasma levels of contrast medium following bolus and infusion injections. Rapid injections produce higher peak plasma levels. (From Catell WR, Fry IK, Spencer AG, Purkiss P: Excretory urography; factors determining excretion of Hypaque. Br J Radiol 40:561, 1967.)

heart failure in patients with borderline cardiac compensation.

6. An initial vascular nephrogram is not obtained.

Filming Technique

This subject has recently been reviewed in detail by Hattery and associates at the Mayo Clinic.[237a] The object is to obtain satisfactory contrast and spatial resolution. This is accomplished by using relatively low kV and high mA. The kilovoltage range is usually 65 to 75 kV, and the milliamperage 600 to 1000 mA, which allows an exposure of less than 0.1 sec (approximately 50 mA) (Fig. 6–13). In children, exposures should not exceed 50 msec. Tomographic technique should also utilize low kV (60 to 75) to emphasize contrast. A tube arc of 25 to 30 degrees will provide a relatively thick section of 0.3 to 0.4 cm, which is more desirable than thinner cuts for general use. In uncooperative patients, exposure time must be decreased and kV therefore increased. Screen-film combinations are used at the discretion of the radiologist and usually reflect personal preferences regarding contrast and latitude, as well as cost considerations. All modern film systems for abdominal radiology should incorporate the advantages of rare-earth screens, which permit more rapid exposures (and, thus, lower radiation doses) without significant loss of detail in comparison with older systems.

Filming Sequences

There are many acceptable variations in filming sequences. Normally, contrast material is excreted rapidly and the calyces are visualized within 2 minutes. The sequence of filming should allow for visualization of the nephrogram, early and late visualization of the collecting system, visualization of the ureters, and "tailoring" the examination according to the clinical history and findings in the early images. In our institution, a usual schedule for adults is the following: The patient is placed supine and a 14 × 17 scout film is obtained with the symphysis pubis positioned 2 or 3 inches above the bottom of the film. In large patients, two scout films may be required to cover the entire abdomen. After viewing the scout film, a compression device is placed over the ureters and

Figure 6–11. Diuresis secondary to drip infusion of contrast. *A,* Shows the distention of the collecting system and ureter obtained in a patient 15 minutes following drip infusion. *B,* Same patient at a different time with urography performed by bolus technique. Note the poorer visualization of the ureters and relative lack of filling of the collecting system.

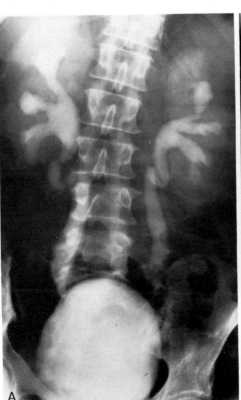

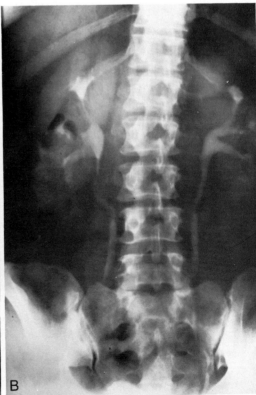

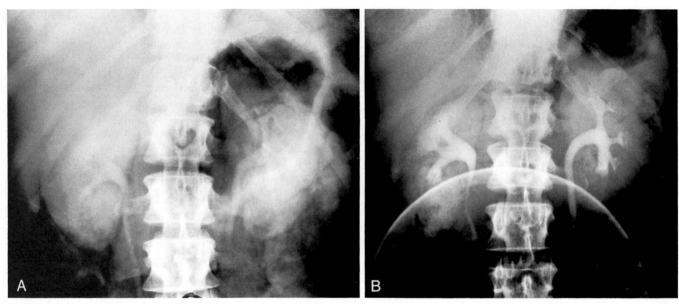

Figure 6–12. *A,* Drip infusion of contrast in a patient with a low fixed specific gravity reveals inability to concentrate the contrast medium resulting in poor visualization of the collecting systems. *B,* Same patient at a subsequent date after administration of a bolus of 50 cc of contrast medium with compression, showing excellent visualization of the collecting systems.

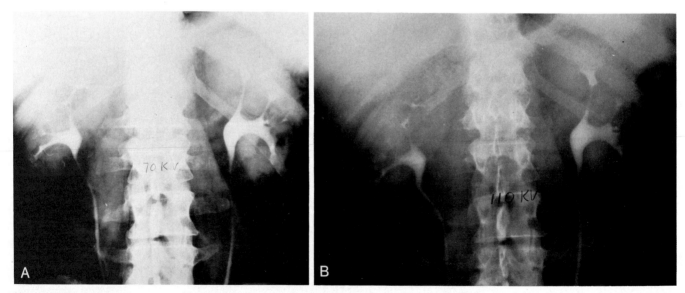

Figure 6–13. The disadvantage of high kV. *A,* Exposure at 70 kV and, *B,* exposure at 110 kV. The 70 kV film provides much better contrast of the renal parenchyma, collecting systems and ureters, improving definition of these anatomical structures.

the contrast medium is injected rapidly (Figs. 6–14 and 6–16). *Compression should not be used* if there is a strong suspicion of *ureteral calculi, obstruction, recent surgery, nephrostomy, severe hypertension, or abdominal aneurysm.* Compression applied too tightly may result in forniceal rupture and contrast extravasation, but this is usually of no consequence. Following injection and compression of the ureters, our sequence is as follows (Figs. 6–15 to 6–17):

1. 1-minute film—10 × 12, renal area
2. 3-minute film—14 × 17, abdomen
3. 4-minute film—Three tomographic sections of the renal area (10 × 12) taken immediately after the 3-minute film, usually at 8 cm to 10 cm from posterior abdominal wall
4. 10-minute film—14 × 17, supine immediately after release of compression
5. 20-minute film—14 × 17, supine
6. 20-minute film—14 × 17, prone

The examination should always be tailored to answer specific questions suggested by the patient's symptoms or the referring physician's clinical examination. On this basis, the number of films can frequently be reduced, particularly when the problem has been identified following the tomographic films, or perhaps by a single properly timed delayed film. Tomograms of 25 degrees to 30 degrees are used routinely in all patients over 40 years of age, selectively in patients between 20 and 40, and rarely in those under 20. In the average patient, the tomograms are obtained at 8, 9, and 10 cm from the table top. In heavier patients, the sections may be 9 through 11 cm and in thin patients, 7 through 10 cm. These levels may vary with individual tomographic units. A nomogram has been developed, based on AP abdominal thickness.[233] In practice, tomography significantly increases the recognition of renal masses, fine renal calcifications, and para-

nephric structures (Figs. 6–18 to 6–20). For the obliteration of overlying bowel gas, a 10-degree tube arc (zonogram) is adequate. The tomograms should be obtained just before or just after the 3-minute films to ensure a satisfactory nephrogram and early calyceal filling. At this point, all of the films obtained should be reviewed to determine whether any special views are required. If the examination is a repeat study performed for a specific purpose, it should be tailored to answer the questions at issue, rather than to repeat the entire routine study. If the information can be obtained with fewer films, the examination should be terminated early. In females, except for the scout film and the 10- and 20-minute 14 × 17 films, *the ovarian area should be shielded. In male patients, gonadal shields should be used routinely throughout the examination.* Although it is desirable to limit the number of films to that required for the diagnosis, nothing is more frustrating than completing the study and finding that another view is necessary to clarify the diagnosis. Therefore, careful monitoring of the films at the time they are taken is required to prevent repeating the examination.

In children, the minimum number of films that are needed to answer the questions posed must be utilized. This requires constant supervision of the examination. Urography is of limited value in the first week of life because of the decreased glomerular filtration and concentrating ability of the kidney. The technique for children is discussed in the second part of this chapter. Special views may be required in certain instances. Often, a film coned to a specific area of interest, such as a renal calyx, will provide enough improvement in detail to establish a diagnosis such as renal papillary necrosis and dispel the need for additional studies. An extension cone (i.e., paranasal sinus cone) works very well for this purpose.

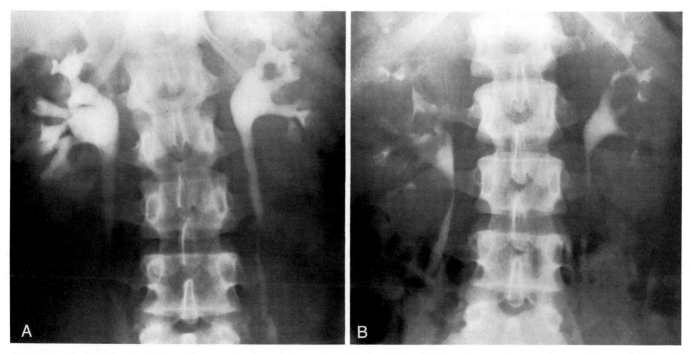

Figure 6–14. *A*, A 3-minute film with compression of the ureters. Compression distends the proximal ureters and the pyelocalyceal system, rendering them fully visible. *B*, A film taken after the release of compression shows incomplete filling of the calyceal systems.

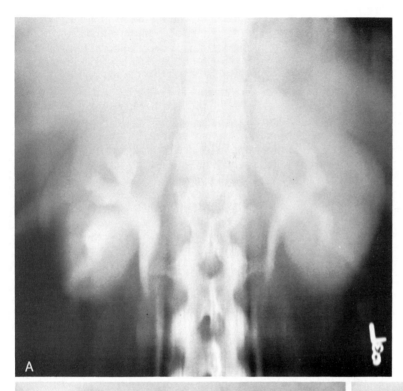

Figure 6–15. Normal excretory urogram. *A*, Tomogram at 3 minutes shows distention of the collecting systems from the ureteral compression. There is good visualization of the nephrograms. *B*, A 10-minute film with compression maintained shows excellent visualization of the collecting systems and proximal two-thirds of the ureters above the area of compression. Note the symmetrically placed, fully inflated compression balloons overlying the pelvic portions of the ureters. *C*, A 30-minute supine film. After release of compression, the calyces are slightly less dilated and the ureters not as well filled, indicating satisfactory drainage. The bladder is fully distended.

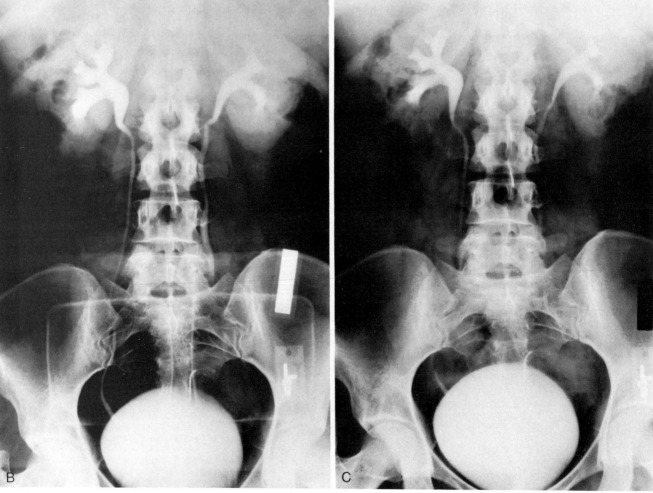

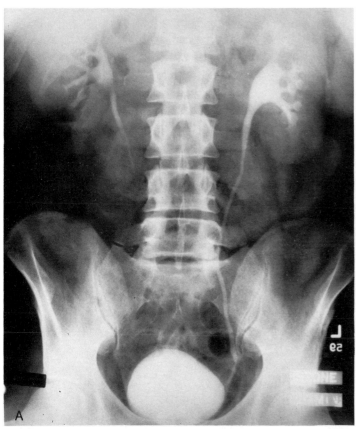
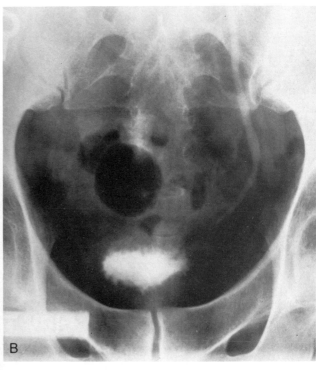

Figure 6–16. Normal excretory urogram. *A*, Prone film taken at 20 minutes reveals good visualization of the left ureter and partial visualization of the right ureter. The prone film is excellent for ureteral filling, noting changes in position of the kidney, visualizing bladder hernias, and demonstrating filling defects on the anterior bladder wall. Normally, the collecting systems should empty rapidly in the prone position. *B*, Postvoiding film (taken in all men over the age of 60) shows a normal amount of residual urine. The postvoiding film must be taken immediately after the patient has returned from the bathroom. Any delay will result in the mimicked presence of residual urine.

Oblique Views. Routine use of oblique views has largely given way to tomography. Oblique films are still of value for questionable ureteral lesions, differentiation of extrinsic and intrinsic renal or ureteral masses, and visualization of the posterolateral aspects of the bladder (Fig. 6–21).

Delayed Views. These may be obtained from 1 hour to 48 hours after injection. They are of value in cases of obstruction in which an early nephrogram is seen but the collecting system is not visualized (Fig. 6–22), in long-standing hydronephrosis in which rim signs (thinned renal parenchyma) are seen but the collecting system is not visualized until many hours later (Figs. 6–23 and 6–24), and in certain congenital lesions such as a nonvisualized upper-calyceal system with an ectopic or otherwise obstructed ureter. Delayed views are generally unrewarding in the total absence of an early nephrogram.

Prone Film. This is useful for viewing filling of ureteral areas that are not seen in the supine position (Fig. 6–17). It is also a good view for renal ptosis and for demonstrating bladder hernias (Figs. 6–25 and 6–26).

Erect Film. The erect film is the optimal view for demonstrating renal ptosis, bladder hernias, and cystocele. It best provokes emptying of the urinary tract. This view demonstrates layering of calculi in cysts or abscesses (milk of calcium) and occasionally demarcates areas of obstruction in the ureter better than does the prone film (Fig. 6–27). It also demonstrates small amounts of urinary tract gas not appreciated on other views.

Postvoiding Film. In many institutions, this is routinely taken in older male patients (over 60 years) to determine residual urine. The film *must* be obtained immediately after voiding; otherwise the residual urine cannot be estimated. An empty bladder rules out residual urine, the presence of which may signify obstruction but may also signify the inability of the patient to void in a busy impersonal x-ray department, or a delay in taking the film after voiding. This view is occasionally helpful in improving demarcation of the bladder wall and visualization of bladder mucosal lesions and diverticula (Fig. 6–28). Vesicoureteral reflux may be demonstrated in the postvoiding film.

Even the most thorough "routine" urogram, regardless of the number of films exposed, occasionally is unsatisfactory or inadequate for the purposes for which it is intended. Such unfortunate results can only be prevented by careful attention to the radiographs as they are being processed and not after the patient has left the radiology department. The importance of careful in-progress monitoring of every urogram cannot be overemphasized.

Text continued on page 125

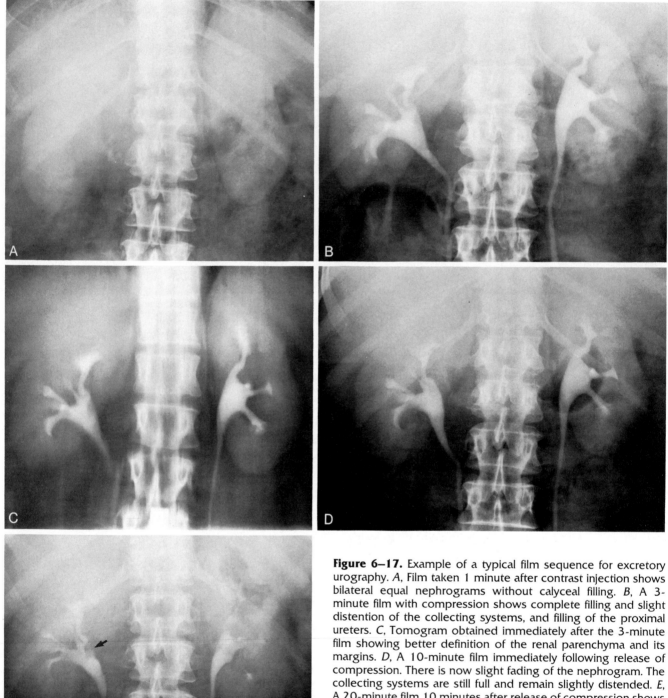

Figure 6–17. Example of a typical film sequence for excretory urography. *A,* Film taken 1 minute after contrast injection shows bilateral equal nephrograms without calyceal filling. *B,* A 3-minute film with compression shows complete filling and slight distention of the collecting systems, and filling of the proximal ureters. *C,* Tomogram obtained immediately after the 3-minute film showing better definition of the renal parenchyma and its margins. *D,* A 10-minute film immediately following release of compression. There is now slight fading of the nephrogram. The collecting systems are still full and remain slightly distended. *E,* A 20-minute film 10 minutes after release of compression shows normal calyceal structure without distention. The calyces are not as well filled, and not all calyces are equally well visualized. A vascular impression on the right renal pelvis (*arrow*) is now apparent. On the compression films, this area was distended and less apparent.

Figure 6–18. Tomography during urography. *A*, Urographic film shows slight bulge on the lateral contour of the right kidney (*arrow*). *B*, Tomogram shows detail of intrarenal mass (cyst) interrupting normal lateral contour. *C*, Another patient with a renal cyst whose urogram shows a mass in the lower pole of the right kidney. *D*, Tomogram reveals the detail of the mass and more clearly defines the cyst walls (*arrows*).

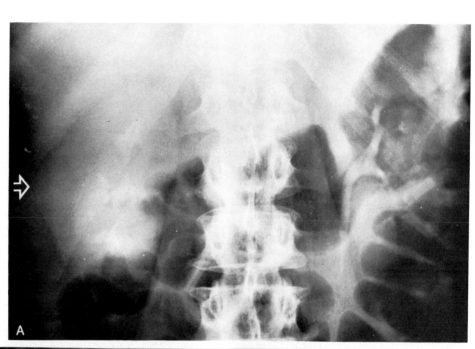

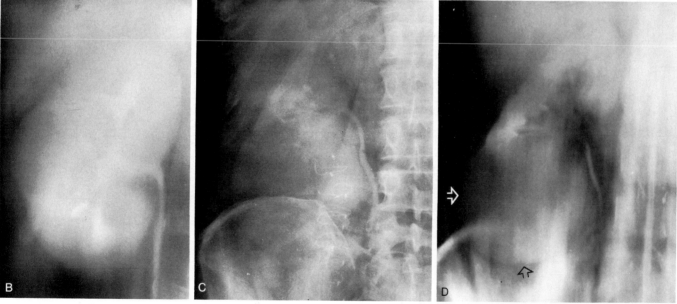

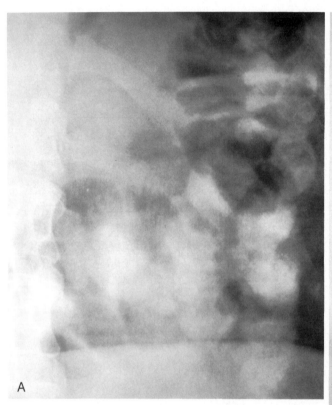

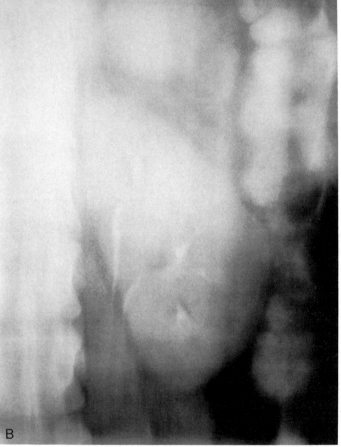

Figure 6–19. Value of tomography. *A*, Scout film with barium in the descending and transverse colon overlying the left kidney. *B*, A 4-minute tomogram with excellent nephrogram and good pyelocalyceal visualization. The barium in the anteriorly placed transverse colon is not visualized in the tomogram.

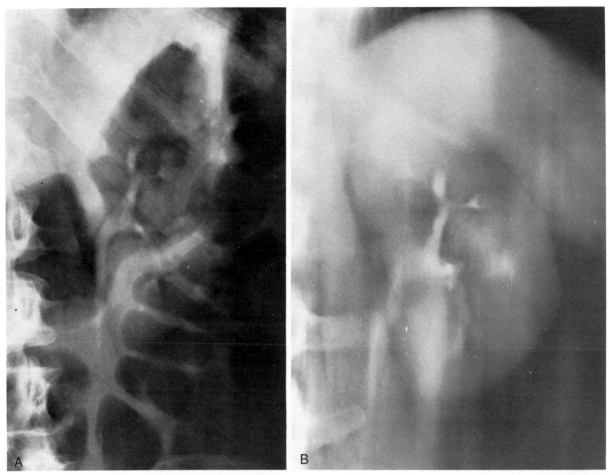

Figure 6–20. Further advantages of tomography. *A*, Film from an excretory urogram reveals that most of the renal contour is obscured by overlying colonic gas. *B*, Tomogram delineating the renal outline and showing the nephrogram in good detail.

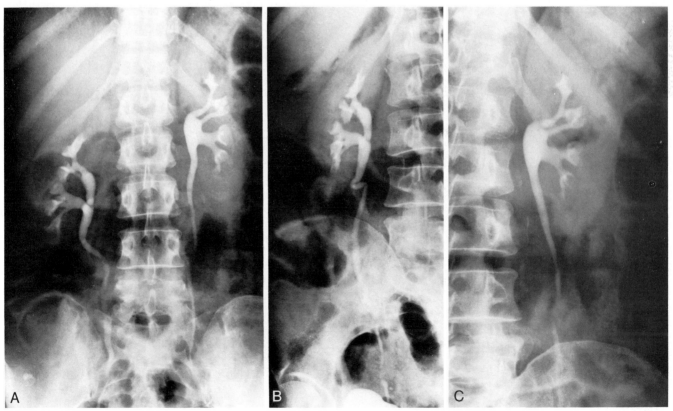

Figure 6–21. Usefulness of oblique views. *A*, Supine film of a urogram with good visualization of the collecting systems and ureters. *B*, *C*, Right and left posterior oblique views project the ureters away from the spine. Oblique views are useful for questionable ureteral lesions in the frontal projection and for projecting renal masses outside of the renal contour.

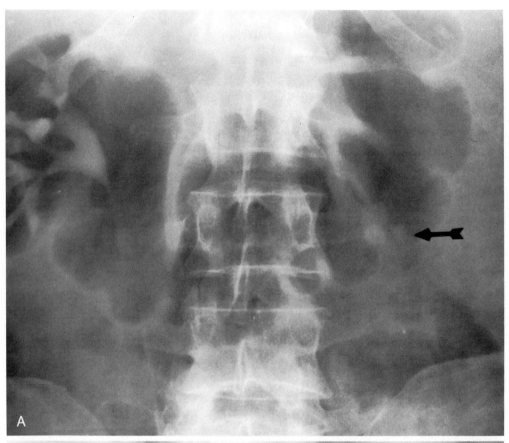

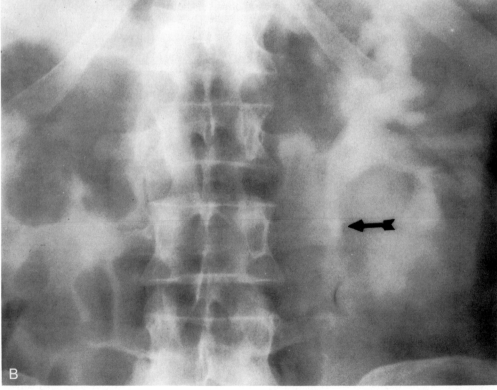

Figure 6–22. Value of delayed urographic films. *A*, A 10-minute film of an excretory urogram shows a calculus (*arrow*) in the proximal left ureter with a faint nephrogram. The right kidney functions normally. *B*, An 8-hour film again shows the calculus (*arrow*) with a moderately dilated collecting system filled proximally to the stone. Contrast material has long since cleared from the right kidney.

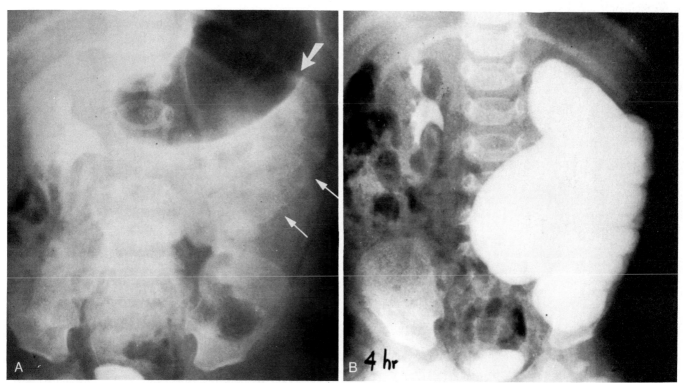

Figure 6–23. Use of delayed films. *A*, A 10-minute film from an intravenous urogram reveals the right kidney to be functioning normally. The left kidney is markedly enlarged owing to a ureteropelvic junction obstruction. There is a peripheral nephrogram, evidenced by rims of opacified parenchyma, outlining the margin of the kidney (*arrows*) and some of the columns of Bertin. *B*, A 4-hour film reveals the severe hydronephrosis now filled with contrast material. There is no opacification distal to the ureteropelvic junction, suggesting obstruction at this point.

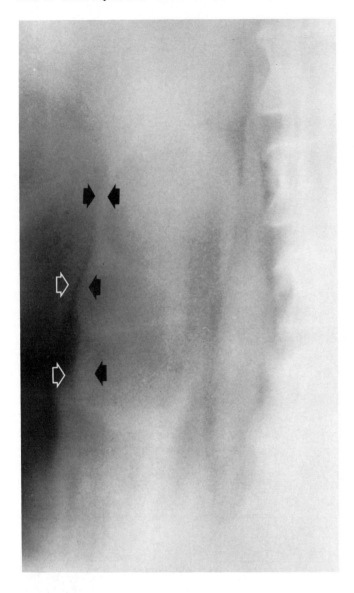

Figure 6–24. Severe hydronephrosis with rim sign of thinned renal parenchyma (*arrowheads*).

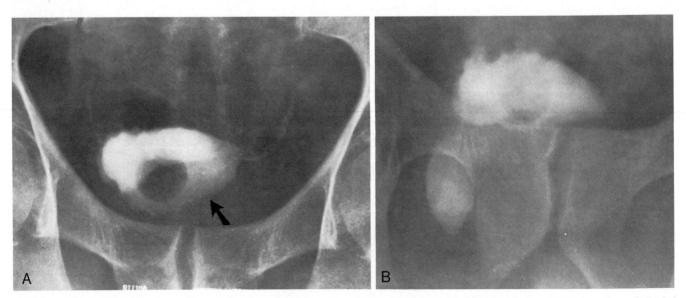

Figure 6–25. Value of the prone film. *A*, On the supine film, the bladder appears normal, aside from slight elevation of the left half of the bladder above the symphysis pubis (*arrow*). *B*, Prone film at the same time now reveals a right-sided hernia of the bladder into the inguinal canal. The prone position demonstrated the hernia, whereas the supine position did not. (Courtesy Milton Elkin, M.D.)

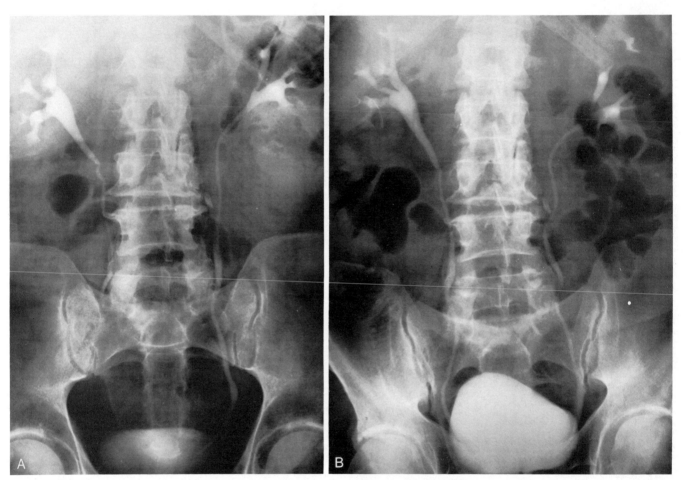

Figure 6–26. Value of prone film. *A*, Supine 10-minute film from a urogram with poor visualization of distal right ureter. *B*, Prone film shows complete visualization of both ureters.

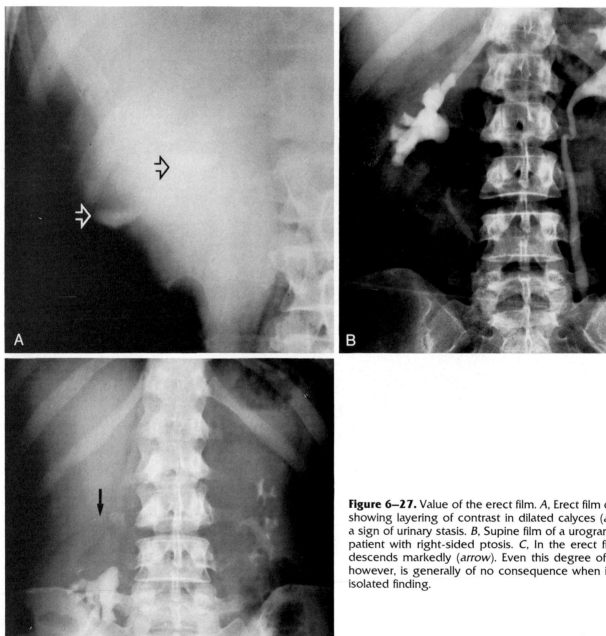

Figure 6–27. Value of the erect film. *A,* Erect film of the urogram showing layering of contrast in dilated calyces (*arrows*). This is a sign of urinary stasis. *B,* Supine film of a urogram in a different patient with right-sided ptosis. *C,* In the erect film the kidney descends markedly (*arrow*). Even this degree of nephroptosis, however, is generally of no consequence when it occurs as an isolated finding.

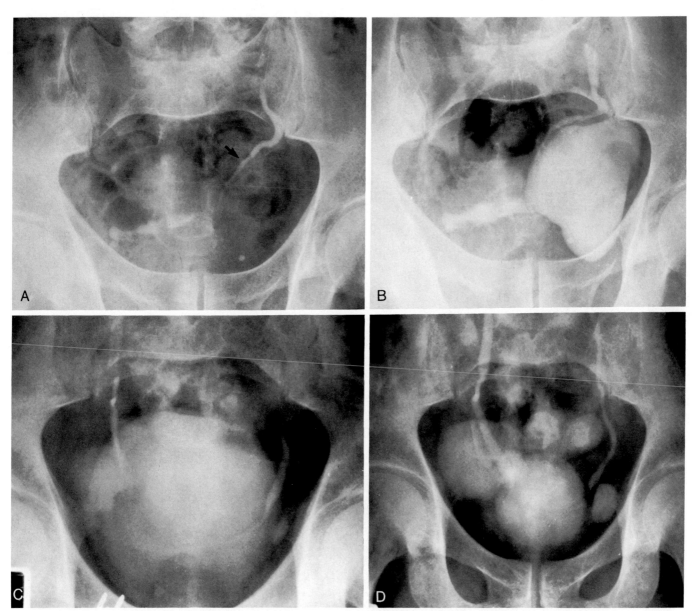

Figure 6–28. Value of the postvoid film—several examples: *A,* Urogram demonstrating typical medial deviation of the distal end of the left ureter (*arrow*) suggestive of vesical diverticulum. However, no diverticulum was demonstrated on the urogram. *B,* Postvoiding film now shows filling of the diverticulum. *C,* A second case with multiple diverticula obscured by the contrast-filled urinary bladder. *D,* A postvoiding film clearly demonstrates the diverticula.

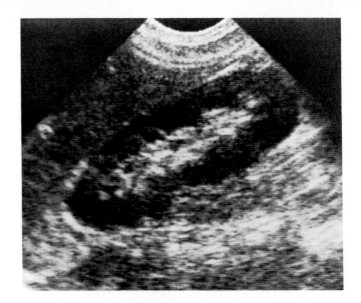

Figure 6–29. Normal renal sonogram. The kidney is well visualized in the sagittal plane showing the highly echogenic sinus fat and central pyelocalyceal structures and the clear demarcation of the less echogenic cortex.

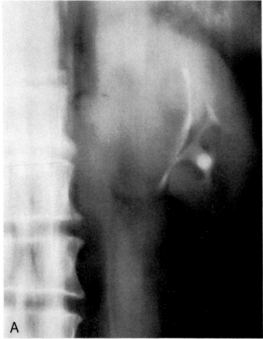

Figure 6–30. Correlation of urography and sonography. *A,* Tomogram from a urogram revealing a large mass in the upper pole of the left kidney displacing the calyceal system laterally. *B,* Transverse sonogram reveals a well-defined mass with lack of echogenicity within it typical of a renal cyst. Note the enhanced through transmission. *C,* A different case showing increased echogenicity within the kidney (*arrows*) typical of gas or fat. However, the poorly defined acoustical shadowing is more in keeping with gas.

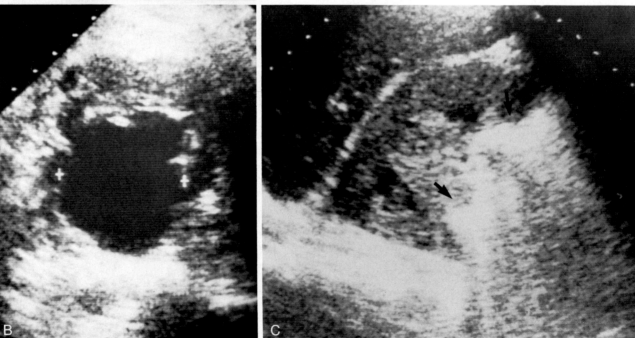

Complementary Studies; Other Technological Choices in Imaging the Urinary Tract and Their Relationship to the Urogram

The greatest value of the urogram is its ability to demonstrate and localize calculi and calcifications, to visualize the ureter, and to reveal changes in the collecting system resulting from infection or tumor. It is of less value in determining the nature of masses (unless characteristic calcification or fat is present) or in delineating contour lesions of the kidney and lesions of the perinephric space.

Today, with the increasing number and variety of technological approaches available for the work-up of genitourinary tract problems, it is appropriate to define the place of these techniques and their complementary or supplementary effects on each other.

Ultrasonography (See Chapter 12.)

Ultrasonography has become a triage technique for many conditions affecting the kidney. As far as is known, there is no significant adverse biological effect from diagnostic ultrasound, and, of course, no radiation is produced. The technique is excellent for the following purposes (Figs. 6–29 to 6–31):

1. To determine the presence or absence of a kidney
2. To evaluate the size of the kidney (Fig. 6–29)
3. To assess for the presence of significant hydronephrosis (Fig. 6–31)
4. To evaluate masses disturbing the contour of the kidney (i.e., to determine cyst or tumor) (Fig. 6–30)
5. In the detection of fat (Fig. 6–30)
6. In the detection of an end-stage kidney

Ultrasonography is useful but less reliable for the following purposes:

1. Solid lesions not disrupting renal contour
2. Moderate degrees of interstitial nephritis
3. Renal calculi over 4 or 5 mm in size
4. Minimal degrees of hydronephrosis

Ultrasonography has little or no value for these purposes:

1. Determining function of the kidney
2. Observing details of pelvic and calyceal structures
3. Observing ureteral abnormalities

More recently, attempts have been made to use ultrasonography for tissue characterization, which may yield further information on the nature of lesions within the kidney and may possibly detect microcalcifications within the kidney that cannot be visualized on x-ray film. Because ultrasonography does not involve radiation, it has become a frequent first-stage evaluation of renal abnormalities.

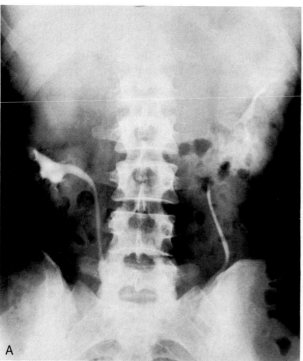

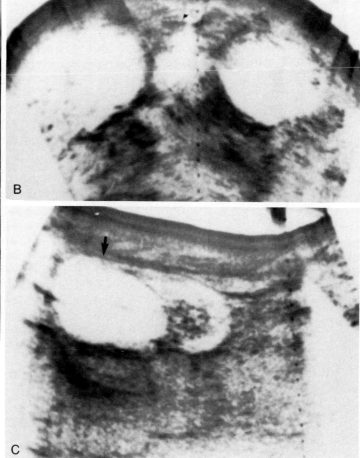

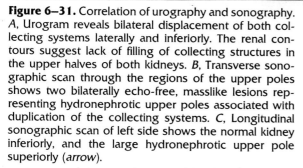

Figure 6–31. Correlation of urography and sonography. *A,* Urogram reveals bilateral displacement of both collecting systems laterally and inferiorly. The renal contours suggest lack of filling of collecting structures in the upper halves of both kidneys. *B,* Transverse sonographic scan through the regions of the upper poles shows two bilaterally echo-free, masslike lesions representing hydronephrotic upper poles associated with duplication of the collecting systems. *C,* Longitudinal sonographic scan of left side shows the normal kidney inferiorly, and the large hydronephrotic upper pole superiorly (*arrow*).

Computed Tomography (See Chapter 13.)

CT, because of its ability to visualize multiple organs in the renal examination and to clearly demonstrate renal contours and the circumrenal spaces, has become the procedure of choice for significant abdominal trauma. It is frequently the initial work-up for patients suspected of having renal masses, although it is more logical to first define the lesion by ultrasonography, and, if the mass is not a typical cyst, then proceed to CT. CT is of value in evaluating abscesses, neoplasms, or other lesions that produce subcapsular or perinephric extensions (Figs. 6–32 to 6–34). Although it is not the first choice in diffuse renal infection, it has very suggestive patterns that support the clinical diagnosis of lobar nephronia (Figs. 6–35 and 6–36), abscesses, or xanthogranulomatous pyelonephritis. CT does not show calyceal detail (Fig. 6–37) and is not of significant use for evaluation of ureteral lesions. It is excellent for differentiation of nonopaque stones from luminal masses in the renal pelvis.

Aside from its use in trauma, CT should probably not be the initial procedure of choice, because it produces significant radiation and is costly.

Nuclear Medicine (See Chapter 18.)

The principal studies in nuclear medicine include renal imaging, radionuclide phlebography, radionuclide angiography, radionuclide cystography, and renography.

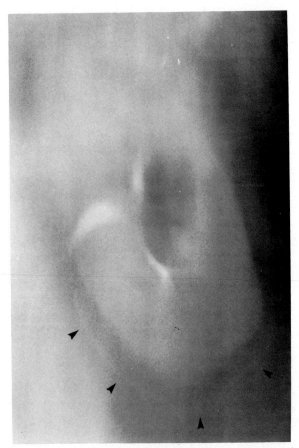

Figure 6–32. Visualization of Gerota's fascia in normal patient. A 30-year-old obese male with no known history of renal or other abdominal disease. Urinalysis is normal. Tomogram from excretory urogram reveals clear visualization of Gerota's fascia (*arrowheads*), which does not appear abnormally thick.

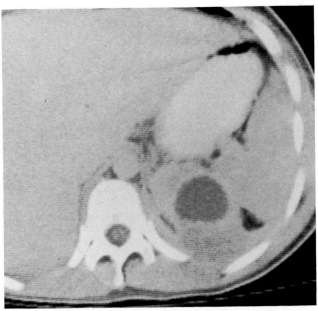

Figure 6–33. Value of CT in renal masses. A 22-year-old woman presented with fever. CT scan shows a large renal abscess in the upper pole of the left kidney (*arrow*) with extension into the perinephric and posterior paranephric spaces. CT provides better definition of such lesions than does urography. Note the dense rim surrounding the abscess.

Studies in nuclear medicine provide more functional information than do x-ray studies, but less anatomical detail. Nuclear medicine has the advantage of utilizing different agents, which may be excreted purely by glomerular filtration or may be actively secreted by the renal tubules. Renography is of value in comparative studies between both kidneys, depicting radionuclide uptake and excretion by the kidney. Patterns have been established that are suggestive of obstruction to the excretory system or to the vascular system. Radionuclide scintigrams can help to differentiate mechanical obstruction from physiological hydronephrosis (Fig. 6–38). Nuclear medicine studies are useful to determine whether masses represent normal-functioning renal tissue (pseudotumors) (Fig. 6–39 and 6–40) or represent bona fide pathological entities such as tumors or abscesses (Fig. 6–41). Radionuclides may also be utilized to identify residual urine within the bladder and to detect vesicoureteral reflux. The resolution with nuclear medicine techniques is poor; consequently, studies for reflux are more effectively utilized as follow-up studies than for detecting the presence and degree of reflux in the initial study. Because of their extreme functional sensitivity, radionuclide studies are advantageous when renal insufficiency precludes urography.

Therefore, nuclear medicine is particularly valuable for providing functional information in comparative studies between the two kidneys.

Vascular Procedures (See Chapter 15.)

Vascular catheter procedures, which were used to detect tumors in the 1960s and 1970s, have given way to CT, which is preferred for this purpose. Today, most catheter procedures may be classified as interventional radiologic, relating to dilatation of renal arteries, embolic procedures, stenting of ureters, nephrostomies, and so forth, and to visualization of the renal arteries or veins

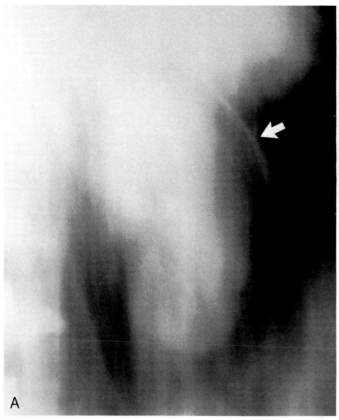

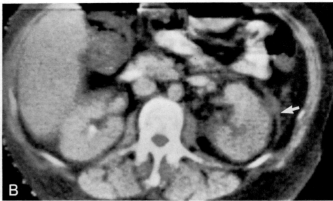

Figure 6–34. *A,* Tomogram from a urogram in a patient with chronic urinary tract infection demonstrating thickening of Gerota's fascia (*arrow*). *B,* CT shows the irregularly thickened fascia (*arrow*) and its relationship to the kidney and perinephric space in greater detail.

in patients with hypertension or obstruction. The use of diagnostic angiography of the kidneys has decreased markedly, as use of CT has increased.[227]

Digital Radiography (See Chapter 16.)

Digital subtraction angiography is a useful method of visualizing the vascular anatomy of the proximal renal arteries. It may be used as a screening examination to detect renal arterial stenosis, renal artery aneurysm, anatomy of the renal arteries, and comparative hemodynamics in the early phases of the vascular filling of both kidneys.

Digital subtraction angiography has the potential of providing quantitative information on renal blood flow.

Digital subtraction urography is of limited value because of its poor spatial resolution and because of the difficulty in obtaining satisfactory masks for use with the contrast-filled kidneys. As the technique for digital radiography of all parts of the body is perfected, digital renal radiography (digital urography) will become available. With the ability to use computer manipulation on each image, enhancing low-contrast objects, as well as immediate digital storage and recall and the ability to obtain sequential examinations with lower dosage to the

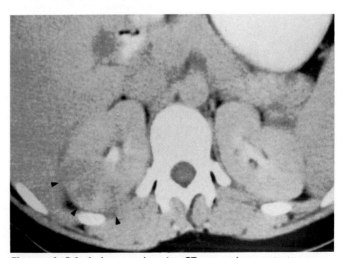

Figure 6–35. Young woman with fever and right flank pain. CT scan shows three discrete areas of lobar nephronia (inhomogeneous nephrogram) involving the right kidney, separated by the columns of Bertin. This represents a segmental pattern of pyelonephritis involving individual lobes of the kidney. CT provides greater detail of the anatomy of the lesion than does urography.

Figure 6–36. Lobar nephronia. CT scan demonstrates poor opacification of three individual renal lobes (*arrowheads*) in a patient with clinical pyelonephritis. The septa of Bertin between the lobes are opacified. Poor opacification is the result of the infection producing either vascular spasm, preventing contrast from entering the nephrons, or nephrons filled with pus.

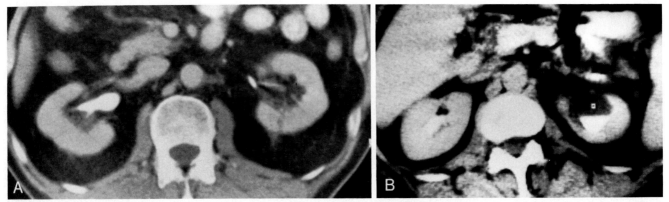

Figure 6–37. *A,* Normal CT scan of the kidneys with contrast enhancement. Definition of calyces with CT is poor compared with conventional urography. However, the definition of the renal outlines and perinephric spaces is far superior to that achieved with urography. *B,* CT scan of patient with left ureteral obstruction. The dilated renal pelvis is clearly shown with layering of contrast in the dependent portion of the pelvis. Back pressure atrophy has decreased the size of the kidney. The individual calyces are not well seen in this projection.

abdomen, digital urography may eventually replace routine film radiography.[229, 240]

Antegrade Percutaneous Pyelography (See Chapter 113.)

If obstruction of the ureteropelvic junction (UPJ) or ureter is sufficient to prevent visualization of the urinary tract and, if retrograde pyelography is not successful or feasible, an 18-gauge needle or Teflon-sheath needle may be inserted into the renal pelvis under local anesthesia. After a small quantity of urine is removed, contrast medium may be injected. This provides excellent antegrade visualization of the distended excretory system and supplies urine for culture or cell block (Fig. 6–42). Assuming transparenchymal needle placement, it may also be utilized for renal drainage by substituting a catheter for the needle and provide a percutaneous nephrostomy or other types of drainage (Fig. 6–43). It is often useful to drain an infected/obstructed system by catheter or percutaneous nephrostomy prior to corrective surgery. The antegrade approach may be also used for catheter stenting of the ureter. The antegrade approach should be avoided, if possible, in the face of known or strongly suspected transitional cell carcinoma, because of the propensity for urothelial tumors to seed onto new surfaces. (See Chapter 7.)

Retrograde Pyelogram

Between 1910 and 1930, retrograde pyelography was the only means of visualizing the urinary tract. In the

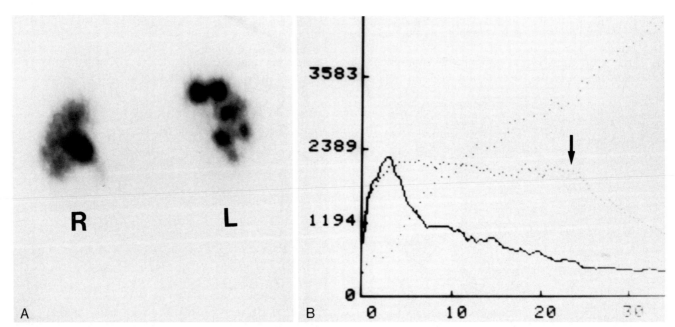

Figure 6–38. Use of radionuclide renography, in lieu of urography, to view obstruction. Differentiation of mechanical obstruction from nonmechanical hydronephrosis. *A,* Young adult with ureteropelvic-junction (UPJ) obstruction. Because of sensitivity to contrast material, the initial study was a technetium-99m DTPA scintiscan, which reveals a hydronephrotic pattern on the left with clear demarcation of the dilated calyces by the radioisotope. The pelvis is not yet filled. *B,* Iodine-131 iodohippurate study. The right kidney (*solid line*) is normal. The left kidney (*arrow*) shows a prolonged excretion phase. Furosemide (Lasix) was administered at 20 minutes. Response was adequate (no mechanical obstruction) with over a 60% drop within 10 minutes of injection. The third broken line is the curve of bladder activity.

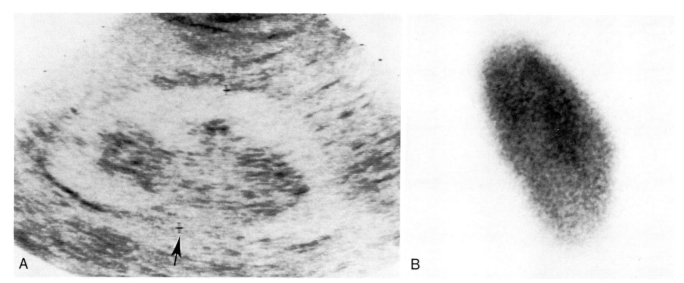

Figure 6–39. Radionuclide scintiscan complementing urography and ultrasonography. Renal pseudotumor. A 45-year-old woman admitted for microscopic hematuria. Ultrasonography was performed because of her sensitivity to contrast material. *A,* Sagittal plane sonogram of the left kidney suggests a mass (*arrow*) along the lateral border of the kidney. *B,* A nuclear medicine study with technetium-99m DMSA reveals no cold area in the kidney and in fact suggests slightly more activity in the region of the proposed mass. This was considered to be a column of Bertin. No surgical confirmation was appropriate.

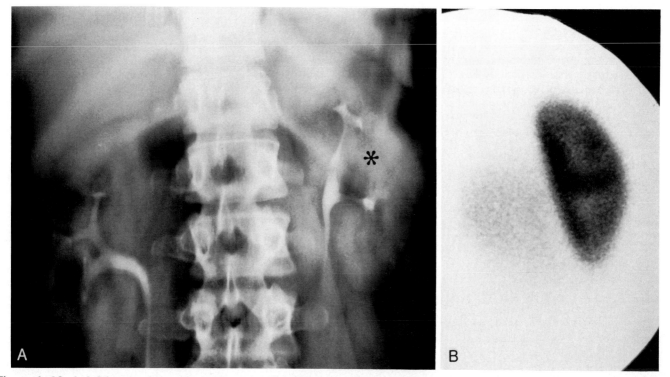

Figure 6–40. *A,* A 39-year-old woman with uterine fibroid tumors. The urogram suggested a mass (*asterisk*) in the left kidney. *B,* Technetium-99m glucoheptonate renal scintiscan shows only normal corticomedullary differential excretion, with no evidence of a pathological mass. The columns of Bertin are well demonstrated. (Courtesy A.J. DeRogatis, M.D.)

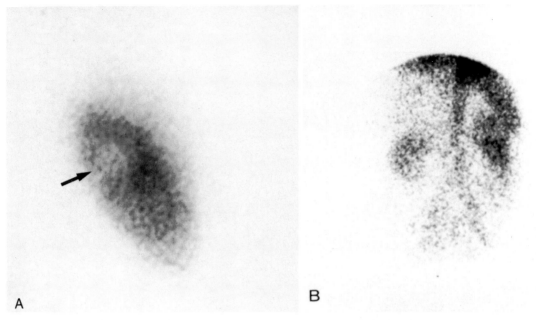

Figure 6—41. Renal tumor. Middle-aged woman with hematuria. *A,* Technetium-99m glucoheptonate image shows a clear-cut defect in the upper portion of the left kidney (*arrow*). *B,* Selected frame from a flow study shows that this area in the left kidney becomes hypervascular. The lack of uptake in the glucoheptonate image indicates that this is not renal parenchyma, whereas the increased flow suggests that it is a hypervascular lesion. At surgery, this represented a renal cell carcinoma.

1930s Uroselectan became the first practical contrast medium for urography. By the late 1950s pyelograms were largely replaced by intravenous studies to visualize the urinary tract. However, the retrograde pyelogram still has a very specific place in diagnosis. Indications for retrograde pyelography include the following:

1. Nonvisualization in the urogram. The retrograde pyelogram may delineate an area of obstruction in the ureter or may demonstrate a normal collecting system, suggesting occlusion of the vascular pedicle.

2. In patients with unexplained recurrent gross hematuria in which other modalities have not revealed the cause of the hematuria, the retrograde pyelogram may show an intraluminal lesion of the ureter, pelvis or calyces (Fig. 6–44).

3. Whenever a questionable area in the collecting system is not well visualized by other modalities, the retrograde study may show it to better advantage.

4. It may be used for selective separate collection of urine from each kidney.

In almost all instances, the retrograde pyelogram should not be the first study but instead should be preceded by the urogram, ultrasound, or CT examination. The incidence of contrast reactions appears to be much lower with the retrograde study than with urography. However, because extravasation of contrast material into the lymphatic and venous structures is extremely common, the decreased incidence is thought to be primarily due to the sedation or anesthesia of the patient.

Catheters are almost routinely opaque so that they can be seen on the x-ray film. The catheter must be manipulated carefully to avoid traumatizing the ureterovesical

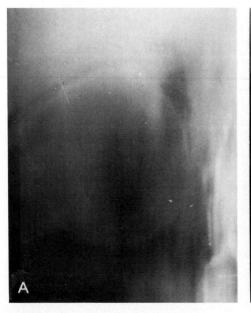

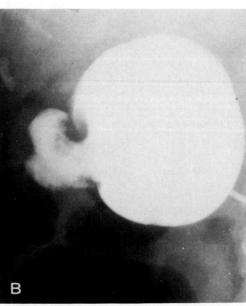

Figure 6—42. Antegrade percutaneous pyelogram. Woman with longstanding UPJ obstruction. *A,* Tomogram from urogram shows hydronephrosis with no contrast filling of the dilated pelvis. *B,* Percutaneous puncture with injection of contrast medium shows in greater detail the hydronephrosis and the level of the obstruction. The calyceal filling defect proved to be a transitional cell carcinoma. The risk of tumor seeding from needling urothelial neoplasms is much greater than from renal cell carcinoma.

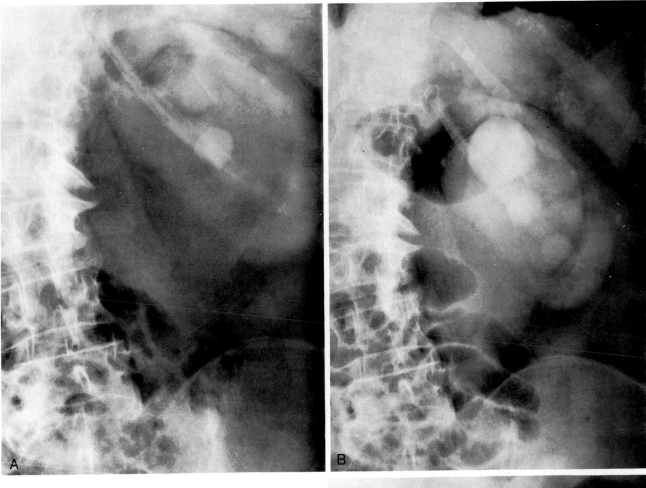

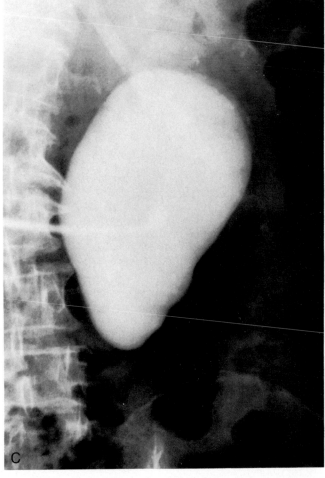

Figure 6—43. A 74-year-old man with chronic urinary tract obstruction. *A*, Early film from the urogram reveals displacement of the middle and lower portion of the left kidney laterally by a vague central mass. Dilated hydronephrotic calyces show early filling. *B*, A 20-minute film of the urogram reveals increasing density within the central mass medial to the kidney. Further filling and distention of the dilated calyces are noted. *C*, The mass was percutaneously punctured, and contrast medium was injected. There is excellent definition of the mass, which represented a urinoma. A catheter was left in situ for drainage.

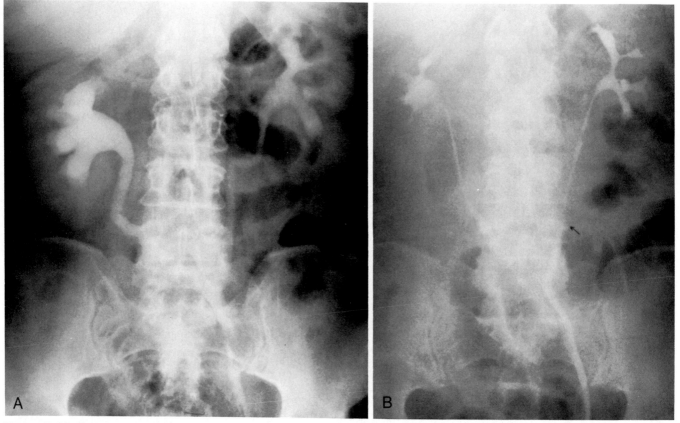

Figure 6–44. Patient postcystectomy with transureteroureterostomy. Patient at this point presented with hematuria. *A,* Urogram did not reveal a lesion in either kidney or ureter. *B,* Retrograde pyelogram revealed a transitional cell carcinoma (*arrow*), which was not obstructing and was not visualized on the urogram.

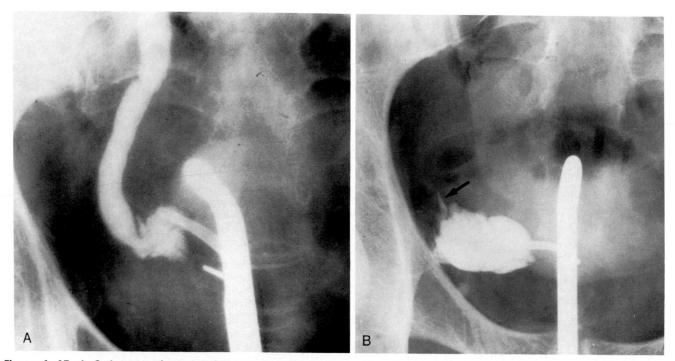

Figure 6–45. *A,* Catheter perforation submucosally at the ureteral orifice. Contrast material has extravasated submucosally and extends in a typical fan-shaped appearance around the ureteral orifice. The material does not enter the bladder lumen. *B,* Intramural perforation of the distal ureter. Contrast material has extended around the ureter, limited by the bladder musculature, and is just beginning to extend into the retroperitoneal area (*arrow*).

junction or the ureters. The most common area for failure of catheterization is at the ureterovesical orifice. Rarely, the catheter perforates the wall of the ureter, usually near the ureterovesical junction, and the injection of contrast material reveals submucosal, intramural, or most commonly retroperitoneal contrast (Fig. 6–45).

Variations in retrograde examinations include the following (for details, see Chapter 7):

1. Bulb tip catheter—This produces distention of the entire ureter and renal pelvis because of the obstruction produced by the bulb distally.

2. Instrumental catheters—Numerous types of instrumental catheters can be used for brushing, performing biopsy, and removing stones.

Two variations that may be utilized with retrograde studies include the following:

1. *Air pyelogram or double-contrast pyelogram*—This technique, which is frequently underutilized, can provide exquisite visualization of the mucosa of the ureter and renal pelvis (Fig. 6–46), as well as demonstrate poorly visualized filling defects. It may take from 10 to 20 cc of air to fill the normal renal pelvis. If one wishes to see primarily the renal pelvis and upper ureter, it is wise to elevate the head of the table so that the air will stay within the upper portion of the collecting system. The air

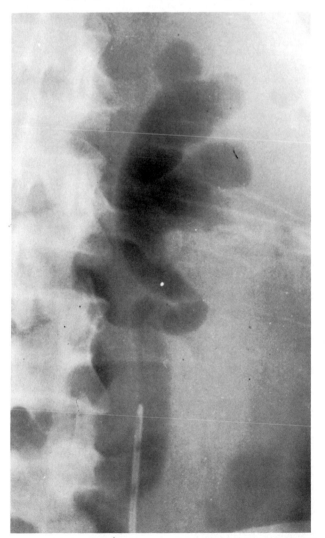

Figure 6–46. Pneumopyelogram. Injection of air via the catheter into the proximal ureter and renal pelvis. Visualization of the mucosa of the ureter and pelvis is excellent.

pyelogram can be performed immediately after routine contrast pyelography for a "double contrast" effect (Fig. 6–47).

2. *Delayed pyelogram*—The delayed pyelogram is used to demonstrate the presence of stasis or obstruction in the pelvis or ureter. After obtaining the pyelogram, the catheter is removed and the patient is allowed to sit or stand for 10 minutes. Any residual contrast on the subsequent film indicates a delay in emptying (Fig. 6–48). If the delay seems to be due to ureteropelvic obstruction, the possibility of spasm or edema from the procedure must be considered.

Modifications of the Urogram

The following are modified versions of the urogram:

1. *Hypertensive urogram*—The hypertensive urogram, in vogue in the 1960s, produced too many false positives and false negatives to be of practical value. The major findings in the urogram of a hypertensive individual that suggest renovascular hypertension are (1) a small kidney (smaller than the opposite side by more than 1.5 cm), (2) delayed appearance of the nephrogram and contrast material in the calyces, and (3) hyperconcentration in the late film as a result of the increased water reabsorption from the decreased urine volume leading to a more concentrated mixture of contrast material and urine (Fig. 6–49). Although these specific findings are of value, the urogram is not considered the screening procedure for hypertension. In patients under the age of 50 with a short history of significant hypertension or in patients who cannot be controlled by antihypertensive therapy, the work-up for renal hypertension must consist of visualization of the renal arteries and an assessment of the renin output from each kidney. This may be accomplished by digital subtraction angiography, or by direct arteriography, together with measurement of the levels of renin from each renal vein. A renin ratio greater than 1.5 to 1 is suggestive of renovascular hypertension when coupled with the presence of a stenotic lesion.

With the advent of angioplasty, many authorities believe that, in patients under the age of 50 who have significant hypertension being controlled by medical therapy, angiography should be performed, if the hypertension is of relatively recent origin. Although there is no indication, as yet, that long-term antihypertensive therapy is harmful, it remains a possibility to consider in the individual patient. In addition, a stenotic lesion producing hypertension controlled by medical therapy may nevertheless progress to occlusion of the artery, radically reducing renal reserve. Therefore, in young patients with controlled renovascular hypertension of recent onset, it is logical to evaluate the renal arteries and to perform an angioplasty to attempt to correct significant stenotic lesions rather than to use long-term medical therapy.

2. *Hydration urogram*—Hydration urography is useful when intermittent obstruction is suspected but cannot be confirmed on the standard study. Here, the use of diuretics such as furosemide, 40 mg, administered during the study will demonstrate an acutely developing hydronephrosis if true intermittent hydronephrosis is present (see Chapter 55, Obstructive Uropathy).

3. *Tailored urogram*—This expression, coined by Lalli,[230] emphasizes the importance of modifying the urogram to provide the information needed to include or

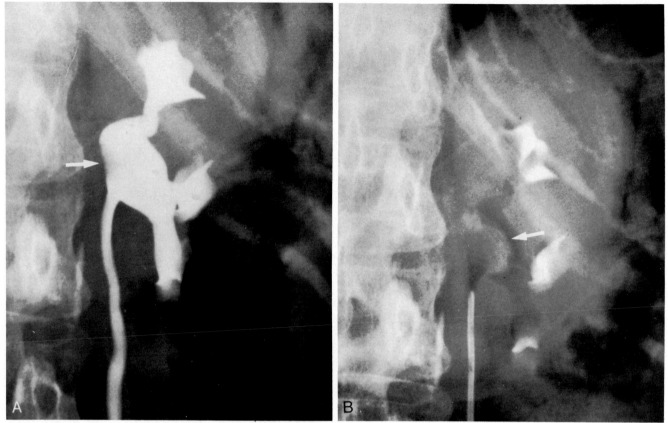

Figure 6—47. Transitional-cell carcinoma of the renal pelvis. Double-contrast pyelogram. *A,* Retrograde study suggesting marginal defect on the medial aspect of the renal pelvis (*arrow*). *B,* Following drainage of the contrast, air was injected. The air pyelogram reveals a well-defined lobulated mass in the renal pelvis (*arrow*). The margins of the mass are better seen with air contrast.

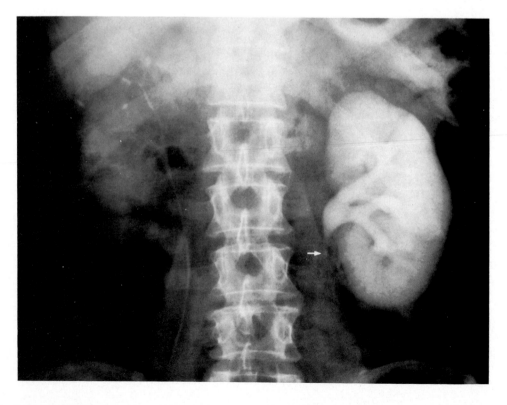

Figure 6—48. Value of the delayed film. The initial 5-minute film (not shown) showed a dense nephrogram without calyceal visualization. The 45-minute film of the urogram now shows a dilated collecting system proximal to a small calculus in the ureter (*arrow*). The nephrogram remains very dense.

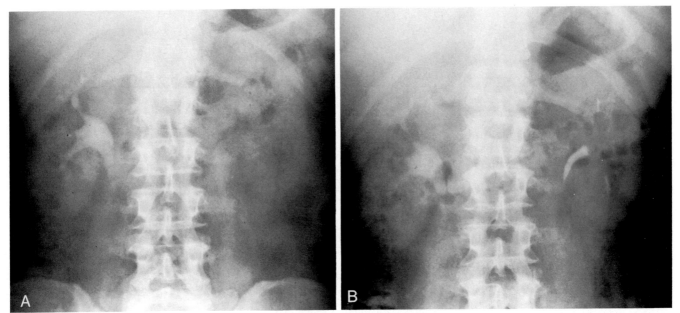

Figure 6–49. Hypertensive urogram. A 52-year-old woman with renovascular hypertension. *A,* The 3-minute film from an excretory urogram reveals no calyceal opacification in the left kidney. *B,* The 20-minute film shows thin calyces and infundibula, with increased density of the late-appearing contrast.

exclude the clinical problem. When performing the urogram, it is of the utmost importance to answer the question posed by the clinician and to tailor the urogram to that purpose. Repeat urograms should be modified to the specific purpose of the repeat examination. Urograms in children should be limited to include or exclude the nature of the clinical problem. A corollary to this is that it is always worthwhile to take an additional film to prove or disprove the findings on the urogram, rather than to provide the clinician with an incomplete diagnosis that requires further work-up.

Although it is difficult to provide algorithms for a particular patient, Table 6–4 shows the uses of the preceding procedures in patients who present with definitive findings. With significant trauma to the abdomen, CT is the triage examination of choice. The urogram is still the study of choice for calculi. It can readily be performed on an emergency basis, and the images can, if necessary, be transmitted in digitized form over long distances for consultation.[228] If pseudotumor is suspected, nuclear medicine is the triage of choice. In infection, CT is the preferred choice if a mass is revealed; the urogram is best for visualizing calyceal distortion. CT is the most sensitive detector of renal masses. Although urography is very sensitive with masses greater than 3 cm in diameter (85%), it is very unreliable in detecting smaller lesions.[241]

RENAL DEVELOPMENT AND ANATOMY

Embryology

The human kidney is demarcated during the fourth week of gestation and arises from the paraxial mesoderm. The classical concept originally presented by Felix in 1912[3] delineated three separate stages: (1) the early appearance of a vestigial pronephros, (2) the later appearance of the mesonephros, and (3) the ultimate development of the metanephros. Fraser in 1920[4] and Torrey

in 1954[13] believed that kidney development occurs in a continuous manner with the formation of glomeruli and tubules, proceeding caudally in the nephrogenic mesoderm. Resorption follows formation, and only the most caudal and latest-formed units remain as the definitive kidney of the adult. This concept considers kidney formation as a continuum, in contrast to the classical concept (Felix) that delineates three separate stages. The formation of the adult kidney (metanephros) depends on the existence of the embryonic kidney and mesonephric duct. The mesonephric or wolffian duct forms the ureter, renal pelvis, calyces, and collecting tubules. When the ureteral bud and the metanephros join, the kidney begins its ascent and rotation. It is presumed by Gruenwald[6] that the ascent of the kidney is produced by the straightening of the embryo, which occurs at this time. When the kidney is at the level of the S2 and S3 vertebrae it is approximately 7 mm in size, and when it reaches its final position it is approximately 25 mm in size. During the seventh and eighth weeks, the kidneys rotate 90 degrees with the renal pelvis, changing from a ventral to a medial position.

Failure of the ureteral bud to form or to join with the nephrogenic blastema leads to absence, aplasia, or dysgenesis of the kidney. Duplication of the ureteral bud as it grows into the kidney results in various duplications of the kidney and ureter. Problems associated with the ascent of the kidney during the sixth and seventh weeks relate to ectopia of the kidney or various types of renal fusion.

Renal Fascia

An understanding of the fascial relationships in the retroperitoneal area around the kidney is essential to understanding the localization and spread of fluid and infection around the kidney. The retroperitoneal space and its subdivisions, from the region anterior to the

Table 6–4. Examples of Procedures Applied to Patients with Definitive Urographic Findings

A. Persistent gross hematuria

B. Renal mass detected on urography

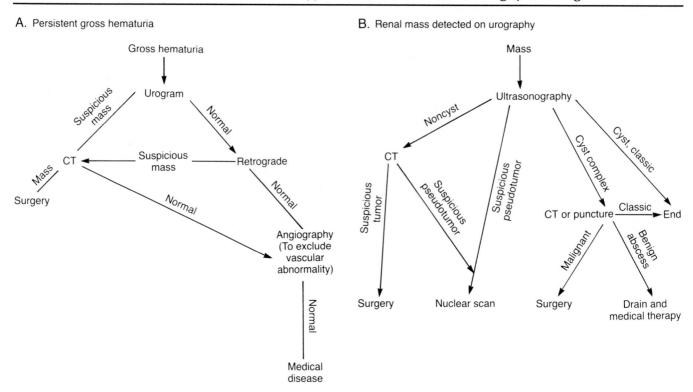

Note: Retrograde pyelograms are not necessary if *all* parts of the collecting system and ureter are well visualized.

C. Renal Infection

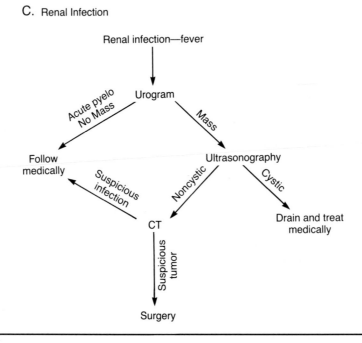

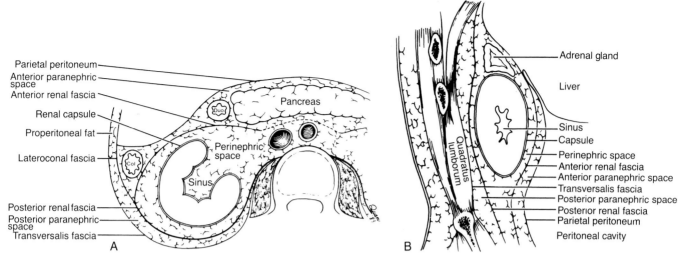

Figure 6–50. *A*, Diagram of the cross-sectional anatomy of the right side of the retroperitoneum at the level of the renal sinus and the subdivisions created by the renal fascial planes. *B*, Diagram of the parasagittal anatomy of the right side of the retroperitoneum at the level of the renal sinus. (From Davidson AJ: Radiology of the Kidney, Philadelphia, WB Saunders Company, 1985, p 630.)

kidney to the transversalis fascia posteriorly, consists of the posterior parietal peritoneum, the anterior paranephric space, the anterior renal fascia, the perinephric space (space of Gerota) containing the kidney, the posterior renal fascia, the posterior paranephric space, and the transversalis fascia. These fascial relationships form fairly well demarcated spaces (Fig. 6–50). The renal fascia, which is clearly visible by CT, is occasionally visualized by urography in the normal patient (see Fig. 6–32). This observation is made much more frequently in the presence of perinephric disease, when the fascia becomes thickened (see Figs. 6–33 and 6–34).[118]

Anterior Paranephric Space

The anterior paranephric space is delineated by the posterior parietal peritoneum in front, and by the anterior renal fascia behind. This space is only partially closed, medially by the fusion of the fascial planes along the course of the aorta and inferior vena cava, and laterally by the lateroconal fascia. It opens inferiorly into the iliac fossa and there communicates with the posterior paranephric space. The anterior paranephric space contains paranephric fat, the duodenal loop, and pancreas; on the right is the ascending, and left the descending, colon. Infections of the colon, pancreas, duodenum, or retrocecal appendix may produce abscesses in the anterior paranephric space (Fig. 6–51). If this space enlarges with fluid collections, pressure effects may be seen on the colon and on the proximal ureter, which runs through the paranephric space. Infections in this space may communicate with the posterior paranephric space in the pelvis.

Perinephric Space

The perinephric space lies between the anterior and posterior renal fascia. It is closed superiorly, medially, and laterally but may open into the iliac fossa inferiorly, communicating with the anterior and posterior paranephric spaces. The normal perinephric space contains

kidney, fat, and adrenal gland. Almost all lesions occurring here are secondary to renal disease. Renal abscesses may rupture into the perinephric space. Renal trauma may produce hemorrhages into the space, and renal neoplasms may extend into it (Fig. 6–52). Urinomas, either spontaneous or traumatic, frequently occupy the inferior medial aspect of the perinephric space (Fig. 6–53).

Posterior Paranephric Space

The posterior paranephric space lies between the posterior renal fascia in front and the transversalis fascia in back. Along the lateral aspect of this compartment, the posterior renal fascia joins the anterior renal fascia to

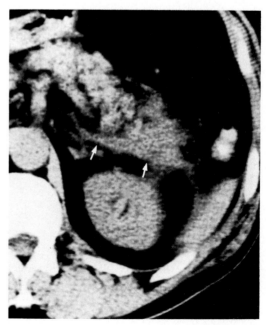

Figure 6–51. Pancreatic abscess in the anterior paranephric space (*arrows*) clearly demarcated from the perinephric space.

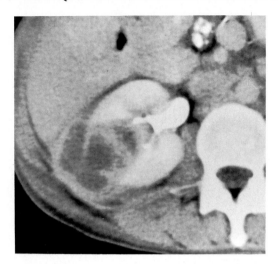

Figure 6–52. Abscess in the right perinephric space. A large renal abscess has ruptured into the perinephric space. The anterior and posterior paranephric spaces are essentially uninvolved.

and hematomas may occur there, and fluid collections from the anterior paranephric or perinephric spaces may freely communicate with it (Fig. 6–54).

Renal Capsule

The renal capsule is a fibrous envelope covering the kidney that is firmly adherent to the renal substance. A potential space exists between the kidney and its capsule, which in abnormal situations may contain blood, pus, or urine (Fig. 6–55). Medially, the capsule extends into the renal sinus and is loosely attached to the renal pelvis. It can usually be separated from the pelvis by increasing intrarenal pressure, allowing extravasation of urine into the perinephric space and, less commonly, the anterior paranephric space. Presumably, capsular attachments vary widely and in a given kidney may allow subcapsular and/or intrarenal collections, if the attachments cannot be separated.

form the lateroconal fascia. The medial aspect of the posterior paranephric space is closed by the fusion of the posterior renal fascia with the psoas fascia. This space continues behind the lateroconal fascia to join the properitoneal fat. Inferiorly, it communicates with the anterior paranephric space and contains no organs. Abscesses

Renal Sinus

The renal sinus contains fat and areolar tissue, as well as the renal arteries, nerves, and lymphatics. The sinus extends around the pelvis, infundibula, and calyces and may be continuous with the perinephric fat (Fig. 6–56).

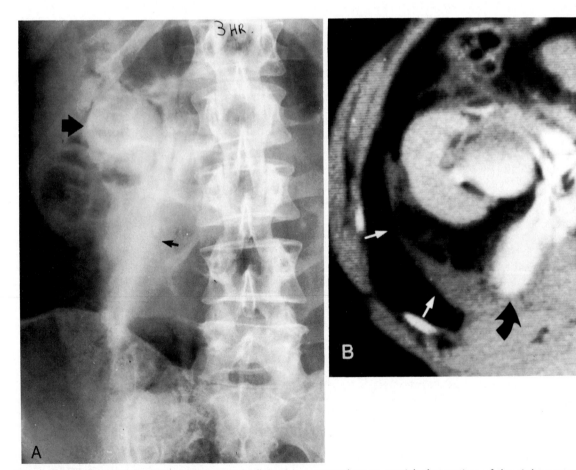

Figure 6–53. Spontaneous urinoma in perinephric space secondary to partial obstruction of the right ureter. *A,* A 3-hour film of the urogram with typical extravasation of contrast containing urine into the perinephric space. The contrast parallels the psoas margin and primarily lies lateral to the psoas (*arrow*). The renal pelvis is dilated (*large arrow*). *B,* CT scan with fluid sharply demarcated in the perinephric space on the right (*arrows*). Contrast-containing urine is entering the compartment (*curved arrow*).

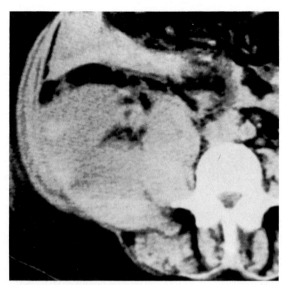

Figure 6—54. Massive hemorrhage in the right posterior paranephric space extends subhepatically.

Renal Vascular Anatomy

The renal arteries usually arise from the anterolateral aspect of the aorta between the lower two-thirds of the body of L1 and the upper one-third of the body of L2. Approximately 20% to 30% of individuals have multiple renal arteries and 10% have multiple renal veins, the latter occurring primarily on the right side. Multiplicity of arteries is approximately equal bilaterally. The right renal artery usually arises more cephalad and more anteriorly than the left, and the right renal vein usually enters the vena cava more posteriorly than the left. Sykes described the main renal artery as dividing near the hilus into anterior (ventral) and posterior (dorsal) branches, from which several (three to six) segmental branches arise.[144] In the absence of multiple arteries, the anterior

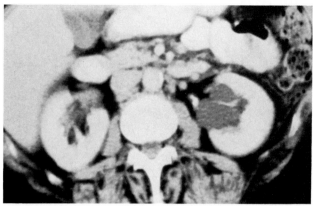

Figure 6—56. CT scan through the region of the renal hilus. The left kidney has an increased amount of renal sinus fat compressing the contrast-filled pelvis and extending medially from the kidney to the contrast-filled ureter. The density of the fat in the renal sinus is frequently greater than that of the fat in the perinephric space, probably due to the presence of increased fibrous tissue within the fat, which may be secondary to infection or repeated small urinary extravasations. The fat in the renal sinus may be continuous with the perinephric fat. Parapelvic cysts may have a similar appearance but are of water density and are differentiable by ultrasonography, as well.

division supplies the anterior parenchyma and usually the lower pole of the kidney. The posterior division supplies the upper pole of the kidney (Fig. 6–57). Occasionally, the renal artery divides into multiple branches in the renal hilus, without the demarcated anterior and posterior divisions. The segmental branches divide into interlobar arteries, which parallel the sides of the pyramids and then branch into the arcuate arteries along the corticomedullary junction. The arcuate arteries give off numerous small perpendicular branches, called the interlobular arteries. The arcuate arteries occasionally communicate

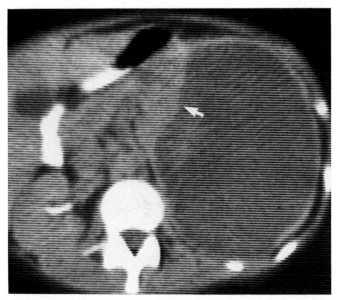

Figure 6—55. Large subcapsular hematoma with a thick capsule displacing the kidney anteromedially (*arrow*). The kidney and hematoma are in the perinephric space, which now occupies most of the left abdomen at this level.

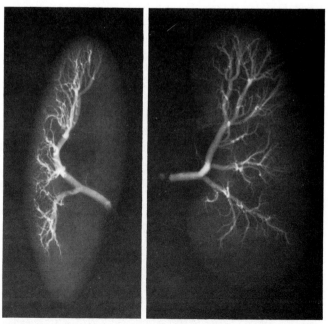

Figure 6—57. Specimen radiograph following injection of the posterior division of the renal artery, lateral and frontal views. The posterior division supplies the upper pole and the posterior parenchyma.

with perforating capsular arteries and with arcuate arteries in adjacent lobes, but the arcuate arteries essentially are end arteries (Fig. 6–58). The following are important concepts regarding renal vascular supply:

1. The posterior (dorsal) artery is usually the first branch of the renal artery.

2. Discrete polar arteries arise directly from the aorta in approximately 10% of people.

3. The inferior adrenal and capsular arteries arise from the renal artery.

4. When multiple branches arise from the aorta, they usually do not communicate with other branches in the kidney.

Anatomical Relationships of the Kidney

The kidneys lie behind the peritoneum, surrounded by the perinephric fat between the anterior and posterior renal fascia (see Fig. 6–50). They lie lateral to and roughly parallel to the lateral border of the psoas. The renal fossa is bounded medially by the psoas muscle, posteriorly by the quadratus lumborum muscle, laterally by the broad abdominis muscles, and superiorly by the diaphragm (Fig. 6–59). Anterolaterally, the kidneys are covered by peritoneum; posteriorly the twelfth rib crosses the left kidney at a 45-degree angle, with approximately one-third or more of the left kidney above the inferior margin of the thoracic cage. On the right side, however, the position of the kidney is lower. Organs intimately associated with the kidney include the adrenal glands, which tend to be directly superior to the kidney on the right side and anteromedial to the kidney on the left. The upper portion of both kidneys rests against the diaphragm, and the posterior aspect of the remaining portions, from medial to lateral borders, are in contact with the psoas, quadratus lumborum, and the tendons of the transversus abdominis muscle. The anterior surface of the right kidney, above and downward, is in contact with the right adrenal gland, the right lobe of the liver, the second portion of the duodenum, and the hepatic flexure of the colon. The organs in apposition to the anterior surface of the left kidney are (above and downward) the left adrenal gland, the stomach, the pancreas, and (on the extreme lateral margin) the spleen and splenic flexure of the colon.

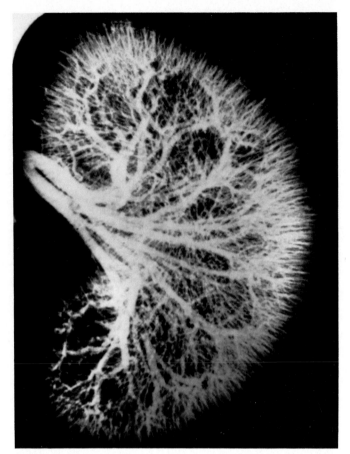

Figure 6–58. Injected specimen of a dog kidney shows the fine interlobular arteries extending into the cortex of the kidney from the arcuate arteries.

Renal Anatomy

Although the kidneys are paired retroperitoneal organs and one might expect symmetrical architecture in a given individual, the lobar distribution and calyceal systems in the two sides are often different in number and distribution.

As previously described, the renal cortex surrounds the medullary pyramids. The cortex is thickest in the polar

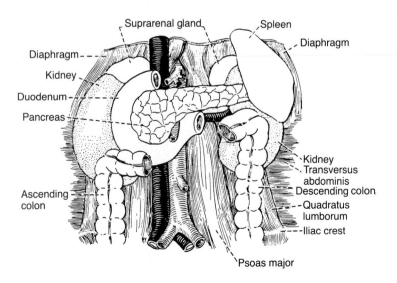

Figure 6–59. Diagram shows the anatomical relations of the kidney to the spleen, pancreas, duodenum, colon, and diaphragm.

areas and along the lateral contour of the kidney. The cortical columns in the midportion of the kidney separate the renal pyramids forming the lobar architecture of the kidney (Fig. 6–60).

Lobar Development

An understanding of the lobar development of the kidney provides insight into several anomalies and diseases of the kidney such as fetal lobations, pseudotumors, compound calyces and intrarenal reflux, and various types of lobar dysmorphism. The rat kidney consists of a single renal lobe containing a medullary pyramid surrounded by cortex and draining through a single papilla into a single calyx. A whale kidney consists of numerous such lobes connected by a network of infundibula to the pelves and ureter. Its appearance is much like a bunch of grapes on a stalk (Fig. 6–61). The pig kidney shows renal lobes grouped like those of the human kidney, but frequently nonfused (Fig. 6–62). The human kidney during embryonic development consists of a large number of separate renal lobes (renunculi) similar to those present in lower mammals, each made up of a medullary pyramid surrounded by cortex, drained by a single calyx and one artery and vein. The renal lobes fuse together, and the areas of fusion are marked by indentations or grooves over the cortical surface of the kidney. When the separate

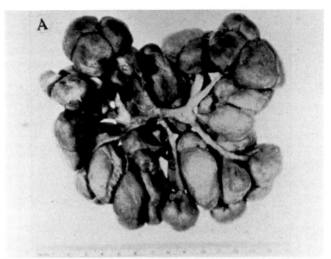

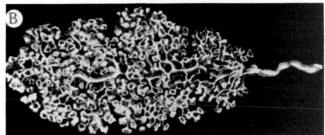

Figure 6–61. Kidney of large mammal (whale). *A*, The kidney consists of numerous renunculi, each representing a renal lobe containing a medullary pyramid, capped by a calyx, and surrounded by cortex. *B*, Calyces, infundibula, and ureter following dissolution of parenchyma. (From Nickel R: Viscera of Domestic Mammals. New York, Springer-Verlag, 1977.)

renal lobes fuse, the outer areas of two adjacent lobes are incorporated within the kidney, representing the cortical renal columns or septae of Bertin (Fig. 6–64; see also Fig. 6–60). The interlobar vessels are located in the septae, branching at the corticomedullary junctions into the arcuate vessels, which then give off the interlobular vessels from their outer aspects radiating into the peripheral cortex (Fig. 6–63; see also Fig. 6–58). The surface grooves or lobulations of the neonate kidney usually disappear during childhood so that the teenage kidney has a smooth-appearing cortical surface. Persistence of surface grooves in the adult kidney is referred to as fetal lobation (Fig. 6–64). Occasionally, fusion does not occur in segments of the kidney (Fig. 6–65), or a kidney may present with abnormality in fusion. It has been stated that approximately half of all adult kidneys show some evidence of persistent lobation, with 4% or 5% showing the complete delineation of the fused lobes. Lobation is usually more prominent on the anterior surface of the kidney. This process of fusion of individual lobes explains why cortex is present in the center of the kidney abutting the renal sinus (cortical columns).

The cortex of the kidney contains both glomeruli and uriniferous tubules, whereas the medulla contains only tubules. Near the apex of the pyramid (papilla) the tubules coalesce, forming larger collecting tubules, known as the collecting ducts of Bellini, which pierce the tip of the papilla and open into a calyx. The average papilla contains from 10 to 24 papillary collecting ducts. Each papilla projects into a calyx, which in turn drains into the

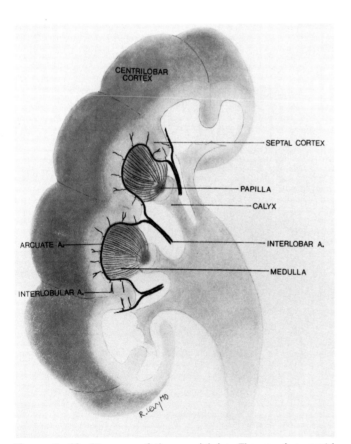

Figure 6–60. Diagram of the renal lobe. The renal pyramid (medulla) is covered by cortex laterally and on its sides (septal cortex; columns of Bertin). The interlobar artery divides into arcuate arteries that traverse the corticomedullary junction, giving off the interlobular arteries. The lobe is the anatomical unit of the kidney.

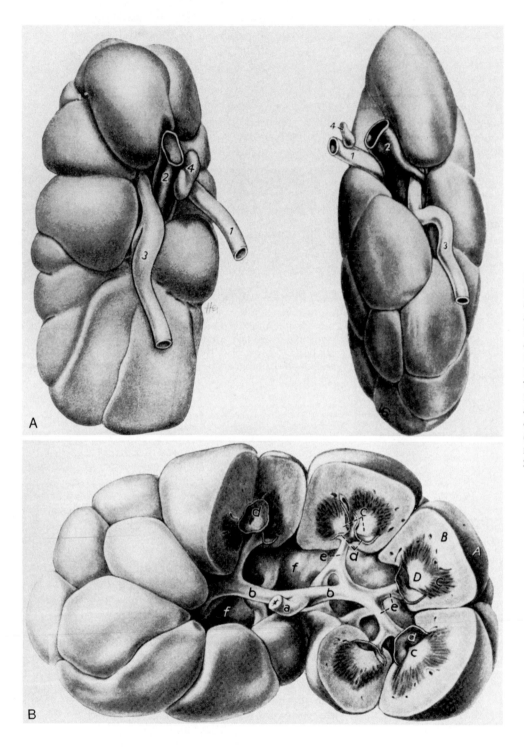

Figure 6–62. Lobar structure of pig kidney. *A*, The renal lobes, although still clearly defined, are partially fused. *B*, Most lobes contain a single pyramid and calyx, although some totally fused areas show multiple pyramids. (1 = artery, 2 = vein, 3 = ureter, 4 = lymph nodes, A and B = cortex, C and D = medulla, a to e = collecting system, f = sinus.) (From Nickel R: Viscera of Domestic Mammals. New York, Springer-Verlag, 1977.)

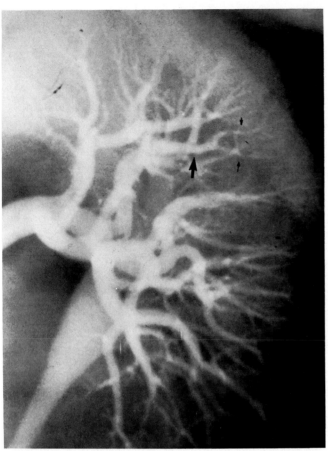

Figure 6–63. Magnified angiogram reveals the segmental renal arteries dividing into the interlobar arteries (*large arrow*) and then into the interlobular arteries (*small arrows*), which give off radiating branches into the cortex. The interlobar arteries course around the medullary pyramids.

renal pelvis and ureter, thus forming a closed system from glomeruli to bladder. The tip of each papilla is convex, and the openings of the collecting ducts are oval shaped (Figs. 6–66 and 6–67). This combination resists reflux of urine from the calyx into the papilla. The opening of the papillary ducts in some of the upper-pole calyces and, to a lesser extent, the lower pole calyces may be round rather than oval shaped. This is thought to explain the propensity for intrarenal reflux to occur in these locations. The tips of the papilla and calyces are surrounded by renal sinus fat of varying amounts.

The anatomical unit of the kidney is the renal lobe, which consists of the renal medulla surrounded by cortex. The collecting ducts drain through the papilla of the pyramid into the calyx. The renal lobe receives its blood supply from two intralobar arteries, which run on each side of the renal lobe (see Figs. 6–60 and 6–63). The usual number of lobes reported in the human kidney varies considerably but averages at about 14 to 16. The lobes are distributed in anterior and posterior groups, with the posterior group of lobes more medially placed and the anterior group found more laterally. This is partially due to the position of the renal hilus, which is anteromedially placed, rather than being directly medial (Fig. 6–68). Because of the position of the anterior and posterior lobes, the anterior calyces usually extend to within 1.5 to 2 cm of the lateral cortical margin, and the posterior calyces are closer to the renal pelvis (Fig. 6–68;

see also Fig. 6–105). With simple calyces, each minor calyx caps one papilla; therefore, the number of calyces relates directly to the number of lobes. Where the cortical columns are deficient, most commonly in the polar areas, multiple renal pyramids fuse forming compound calyces. In compound calyces, multiple papillae may enter into a single multiheaded calyx (Figs. 6–69 and 6–70; see also Fig. 6–66). Compound calyces are more common in the upper lobe, less common in the lower lobe, and least common in the central portion of the kidney. It is estimated that 70% of persons have one or more compound calyces.[8] The compound calyx is the result of a tendency for renal columns to be absent or very thin in the polar areas, allowing multiple pyramids to coalesce and drain into a single lobulated calyx. Compound calyces have also been referred to in the literature as T-shaped or hammerhead calyces, and they have assumed new importance because of their association with intrarenal reflux and an increased probability of pyelonephritis. The tendency of atrophic pyelonephritis (reflux nephropathy) to occur in the polar area of the kidney approximately relates to the frequency of compound calyces with their associated round, rather than oval, ductal openings in these areas. Individuals without compound calyces are more resistant to intrarenal reflux and, therefore, are less likely to develop atrophic pyelonephritis.

Renal Size

Kidney size is directly related to the body surface area of the individual. In the average adult at autopsy, the kidney measures approximately 11.25 cm in length, 5.0 to 7.5 cm in breadth, and 2.5 to 3.5 cm in thickness, and it weighs from 115 to 170 gm. The radiographic size of the kidneys is considerably larger as a result of normal distention associated with blood and fluids and the magnification obtained on the x-ray film (approximately 18%). The average normal mean lengths and widths observed on roentgenograms are listed in Table 6–5.

In Moell's survey of 100 males and 100 females 20 to 49 years of age,[206, 208] he measured the roentgenographic length of the kidney as the maximum distance between the upper and lower poles, and the width at right angles to the length at the widest lateral-to-medial aspect of the kidney, including the hilar area. Studies by Griffiths,[238] Ludis (1967),[239] and others have attempted to establish more sophisticated means of estimating kidney size, but the simple measurement of renal length appears to be adequate for daily use.

The usual length in the normal adult ranges between 11 and 14 cm, but the kidneys can be expected to be larger in individuals with large body surface areas and smaller in diminutive individuals. Women tend to have smaller kidneys than do men, simply because they generally have a smaller body surface area. The normal renal length approximates the height of three to four lumbar

Table 6–5. Normal Mean Length and Width of Kidneys[206, 208]

	Males		Females	
	RIGHT	LEFT	RIGHT	LEFT
Length	12.9	13.2	12.3	12.6
Width	6.2	6.3	5.7	5.9

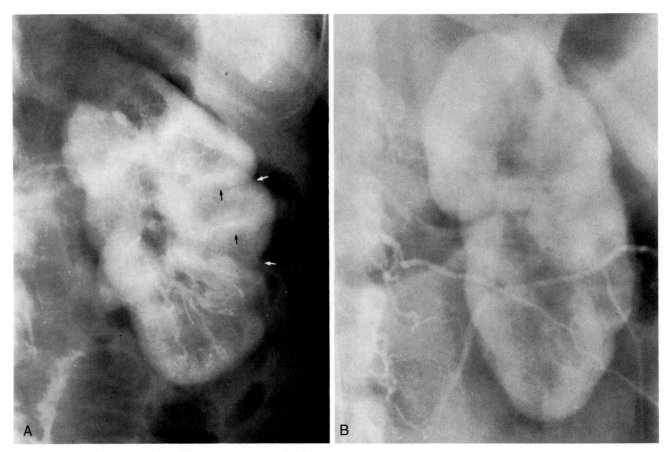

Figure 6–64. Examples of fetal lobation. *A,* The nephrographic phase of the renal arteriogram clearly demarcates the more densely staining cortex from the medullary pyramids. When the renal lobes fuse during development, the outer margins of the lobes become incorporated into the kidney at the columns of Bertin (*black arrows*). If fusion is incomplete, areas of fetal lobation may persist, presenting as indentations of the cortex at the points of fusion of two adjacent lobes opposite the column of Bertin (*white arrows*). *B,* Nephrographic phase of an angiogram reveals multiple areas of fetal lobation along the lateral aspect of the kidney.

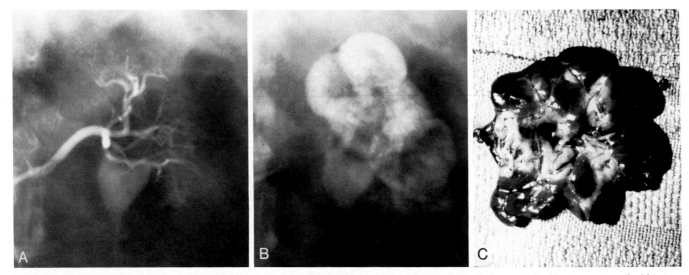

Figure 6–65. Incomplete fusion of renal lobes. A 4-year-old child presents with microscopic hematuria. Urogram revealed bizarre contours and poor function of the left kidney. *A,* Renal angiogram reveals the renal artery to divide into segmental vessels without the usual major divisions. *B,* Late film of the angiogram shows the two superior lobes to be almost nonfused. Fusion is incomplete in other areas of the kidney as well. *C,* The incomplete fusion is better seen in the nephrectomy specimen.

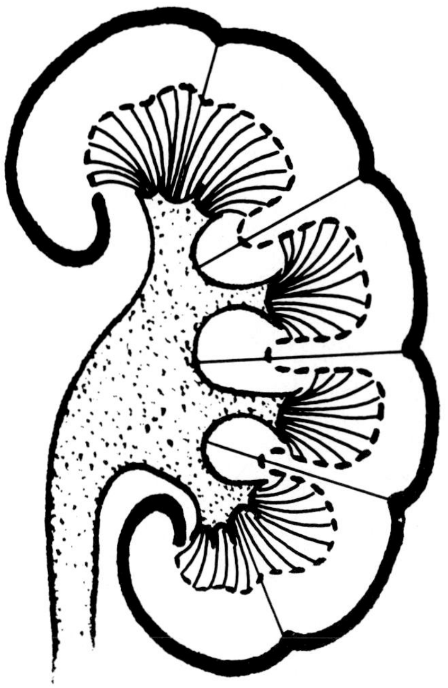

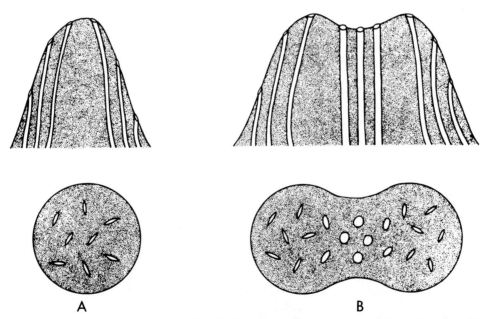

Figure 6–66. The renal lobes are well defined along the lateral margin of the kidney. There is usually a one-to-one ratio of medullary pyramid to calyx. In the upper pole, and less commonly in the lower pole, the column of Bertin is frequently incomplete, allowing adjacent medullary pyramids to fuse. In such cases, multiple pyramids may enter into a single calyceal stem, forming a compound calyx. (From Davidson AJ: Radiology of the Kidney. Philadelphia, WB Saunders Company, 1985, p 80.)

A

B

Figure 6–67. Diagram of simple and compound papillae. *A*, Simple papilla seen tangentially and en face. The papilla is convex with collecting ducts running to its surface, which is covered by the cribriform plate. In the en face view, note that the openings of the collecting ducts are slitlike. When pressure increases within the calyx, the openings of the collecting ducts close, preventing intrarenal reflux. *B*, Compound papilla with more than one papilla entering into a compound calyx. Over the convex portions of the papilla, the anatomy is similar to that of the simple papilla. However, in the region where the two papillae fuse, concavity stretches the orifice of the collecting ducts so that they become round or widely oval in appearance. These collecting ducts frequently allow free intrarenal reflux. (From Davidson AJ: Radiology of the Kidney. Philadelphia, WB Saunders Company, 1985, p 80.)

X-RAY BEAM

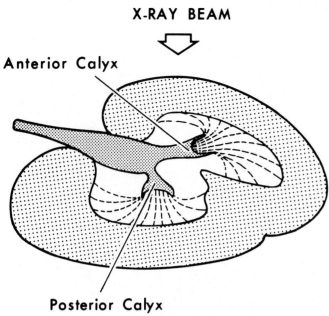

Anterior Calyx

Posterior Calyx

Figure 6–68. Diagram of the kidney in situ. The x-ray beam is entering on the anteroposterior axis of the body. Note that the renal hilus is placed anteromedially, which places the anterior calyces more lateral than the posterior calyces. (From Hodson CJ: The lobar structure of the kidney. Br J Urol 44:246, 1972.)

vertebral bodies. During excretory urography, the size of kidneys may increase by as much as 1 cm owing to the diuretic effect of the contrast medium, and during episodes of shock the kidneys may decrease by 1 cm or more in size owing to blood loss (Fig. 6–71). The right kidney is usually 0.5 cm smaller than the left. The rule of thumb is that a left kidney should be at least 1.5 cm larger than the right to be considered abnormally large, whereas the right should be at least 0.5 cm larger than the left. This rule should be approached with caution, because variability is common. Numerous charts are available relating

kidney size to height, weight, and body surface area (Fig. 6–72). The right kidney is 1 to 2 cm lower than the left, with the right renal pelvis usually opposite the L2 vertebra. In 10% of patients, the right kidney may be higher than the left when the patient is in the supine position, and in about 30% of patients, when in the prone position, the right kidney is higher than the left. A normal range of mobility during respiration varies from 1 to 4 cm. During inspiration the ureters may become kinked, mimicking adhesions or obstructions (Fig. 6–73). Urograms are best obtained in the expiratory phase. Studies correlating renal size measurements obtained at urography with those obtained sonographically have shown a 10% to 15% discrepancy. The smaller values determined by ultrasonography are probably attributable to both the elimination of magnification in sonography and diuresis-induced nephromegaly in urography.[236]

The kidney grows rapidly in the first few years of life, reaching maximum size in the early twenties, and stabilizes until the fifth decade, decreasing in the sixth and seventh decades. Renal mass in old age may decrease over 20%, while renal length decreases about 10%. The more significant decrease in renal mass is related to the replacement of parenchyma by fat. In the healthy adult, renal cortex contributes approximately 50%, medulla 35%, and sinus fat 15% to the overall volume of the kidney. The cortex, in turn, volumetrically consists of 80% tubules, 10% glomeruli, and 10% interstitial tissue.[235]

In summary, renal size is related to body surface area. Tall heavy-set individuals may have a "normal" length of 15 cm or more (Fig. 6–74). Practically, renal size is measured as renal length. Difference in renal size of over 2 cm is usually significant (Fig. 6–75). Additional significant aspects affecting renal size and calyceal position include the following:

1. Always measure both kidneys in the same film and in supine position.

2. Duplex systems are larger than expected for that individual by as much as 10%. A duplex system is the

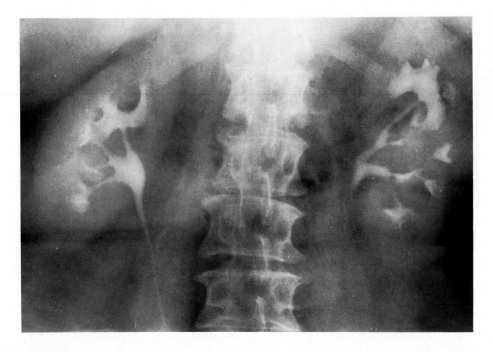

Figure 6–69. Compound calyces. Bilateral upper- and lower-pole compound calyces. The compound calyces in the upper pole are more numerous and present an appearance that has often been referred to as T-shaped or hammerhead.

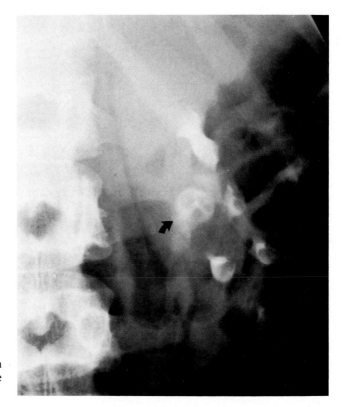

Figure 6–70. Compound calyx in the center of the kidney seen en face (*arrow*). The free papillae entering the calyx produce negative defects. (Courtesy A.J. Palubinskas, M.D.)

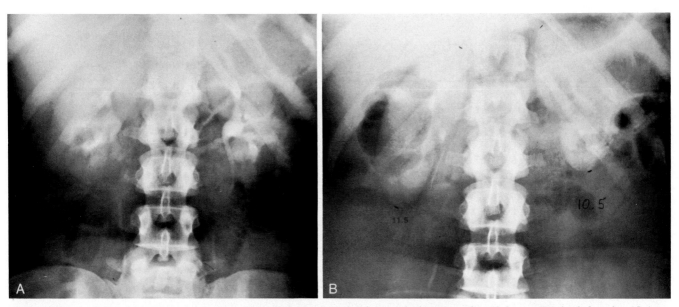

Figure 6–71. *A*, A 3-minute film of the urogram reveals the length of the right kidney to be 13.2 cm and the left to be 12.1 cm. The patient had a reaction to the contrast medium and became hypotensive. *B*, A film taken at 10 minutes reveals a persistent nephrogram with the collecting system almost empty. Renal size has decreased with the right kidney now measuring 11.5 cm and the left 10.5 cm. The decrease in size is due to decreased blood flow through the kidneys.

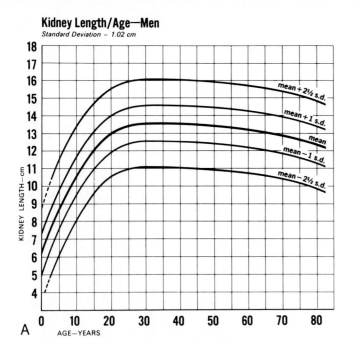

Kidney Length/Age—Men
Standard Deviation = 1.02 cm

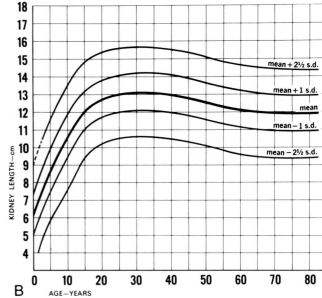

Kidney Length/Age—Women
Standard Deviation = 1.02 cm

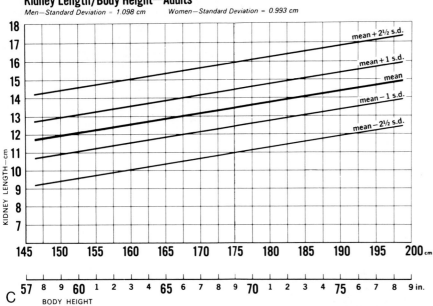

Kidney Length/Body Height—Adults
Men—Standard Deviation = 1.098 cm   Women—Standard Deviation = 0.993 cm

Figure 6–72. *A,* Kidney length by age in males. *B,* Kidney length by age in females. *C,* Kidney length by body height in adults. *D,* Kidney length by body height in children. (Modified from Hodson CJ, Drewe JA, Karn MN, King A: Renal size in normal children: A radiographic study during life. Arch Dis Child 35:616, 1962.)

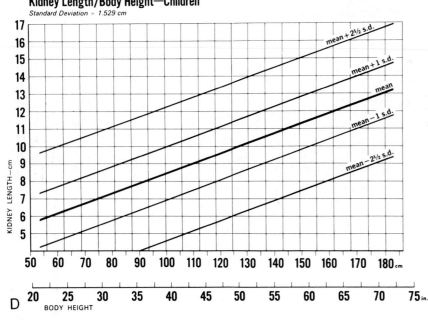

Kidney Length/Body Height—Children
Standard Deviation = 1.529 cm

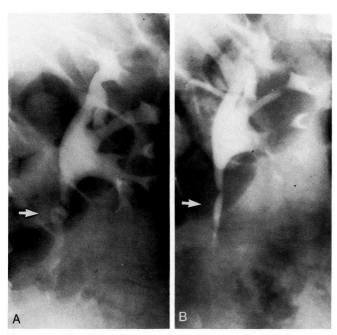

Figure 6–73. Kink of ureter during inspiration. *A,* Patient in deep inspiration with a kink of the ureter just below the ureteropelvic junction *(arrow)*. *B,* Patient in partial expiration. The ureteral kink is no longer present.

single most common cause of an enlarged unilateral kidney (Fig. 6–76).

3. A solitary kidney at birth often approximates the mass of two kidneys by the age of 1 year.

4. In the lateral projection, the anterior and posterior calyces can be seen separately (Fig. 6–77).

5. In the lateral projection, the kidney on the side closest to the film normally lies posterior to the anterior border of the spine. A few of the anterior calyces may project beyond the anterior border of the spine. The kidney farthest from the film usually is more forward and lies anterior to the vertebral bodies (Fig. 6–78).

Anatomical Relationships of the Ureters

The ureters are conduits approximately 25 to 29 cm in length, with lumens of 2 to 4 mm in size. The ureter is conveniently divided into two parts, an abdominal ureter and a pelvic ureter (Fig. 6–79). The abdominal portion begins at the junction with the renal pelvis and runs over the anterior surface of the psoas muscle in the anterior paranephric space. It is usually described as coursing over the lateral portion of the transverse processes. A ureter that lies more than 1.5 cm lateral to the transverse process is suspected of being laterally deviated; a ureter that crosses over the pedicle is suspected of being medially deviated; and a ureter that is medial to the pedicle is usually abnormal. In prone or inspiratory films, kinking of the proximal ureter occurs commonly (Fig. 6–73). The abdominal ureter crosses the brim of the pelvis at the bifurcation of the common iliac artery and becomes the pelvic ureter. The pelvic ureter runs abruptly backward and laterally, following the contour of the pelvis. In the region of the ischial spine, the ureter turns medially and forward to enter the bladder. The pelvic ureter, therefore, has a convex lateral appearance. There are three normal areas of narrowing in the ureter (Fig. 6–80): (1) at the ureteropelvic junction, (2) where the ureter crosses the iliac vessels at the pelvic brim, and (3) at its entrance into the bladder.

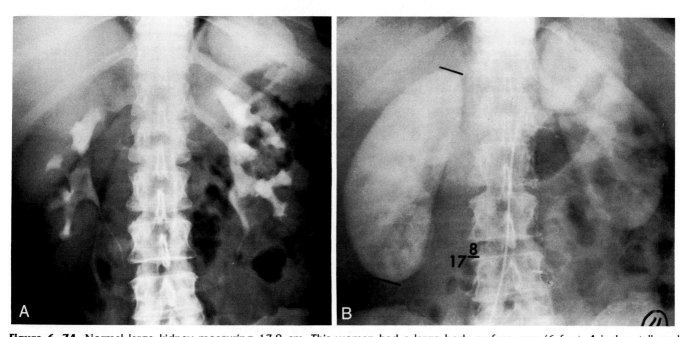

Figure 6–74. Normal large kidney measuring 17.8 cm. This woman had a large body surface area (6 foot, 4 inches tall, and weighed over 200 pounds). *A,* A 10-minute film from urogram. *B,* Nephrographic phase from aortogram. (Courtesy A.J. Palubinskas, M.D.)

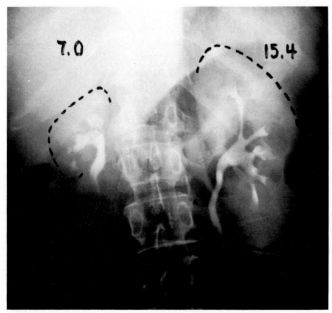

Figure 6–75. A 64-year-old female with hypertension secondary to renal artery stenosis. The right kidney measures 7 cm, the left 15.4 cm. Marked difference in renal size is due to decreased perfusion of right kidney.

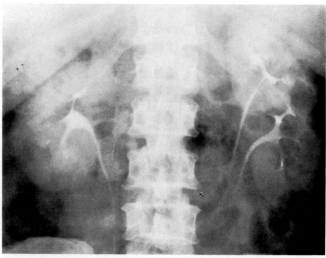

Figure 6–76. Duplex system, left. A complete double collecting system and double ureter are present on the left side. The left kidney measures 17.5 cm, and the right kidney measures 14 cm. A duplex system is usually 0.5 to 2 cm larger than its mate, partly owing to the increased size of the hilus of the kidney. In this instance, the left double kidney is almost 20% larger than the right kidney.

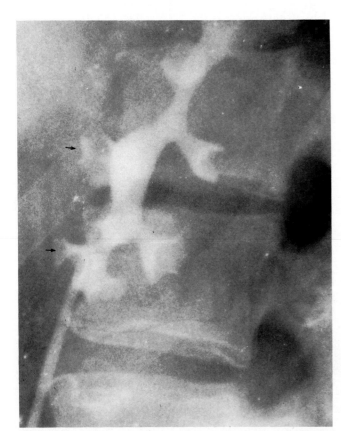

Figure 6–77. Lateral projection of kidney. The anterior and posterior calyces are separated, the anterior calyces extending just anterior to the spine (*arrows*).

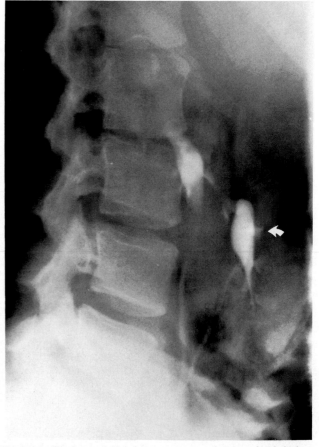

Figure 6–78. Lateral film from urogram showing both kidneys. The kidney on the side farthest from the table is more anterior (*arrow*). Left kidney is down; right kidney is up. Right kidney is more anterior.

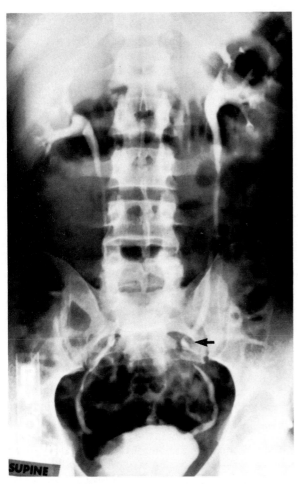

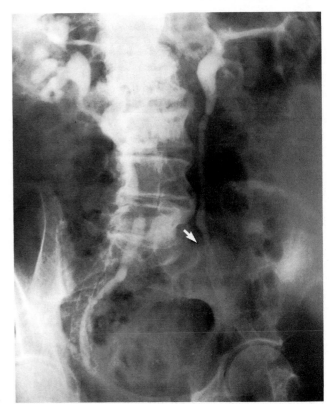

Figure 6–80. Oblique film of the urogram shows the left ureter crossing the calcified iliac artery (*arrow*), where it becomes the pelvic ureter. This is one of the areas of normal narrowing in the course of the ureter.

Figure 6–79. Normal ureters. The left ureter overlies the lateral aspects of the transverse processes of the vertebral bodies down to the pelvic brim, where it curves medially as it crosses the iliac vessels (*arrow*). The ureter above the arrow is the abdominal ureter; below it is the pelvic ureter. The right ureter is normal but more medially placed than the left. It remains lateral to the pedicles of the vertebral bodies. Note the normal lateral convexity of the pelvic ureters down to the ureterovesical junctions.

THE NORMAL INTRAVENOUS UROGRAM

Anatomy and Physiology of Excretion

The kidney is responsible for the stability of the internal environment of the body. It regulates the water content and the maintenance of a proper electrolyte balance, and it has the responsibility for the excretion of wastes such as urea, uric acid, creatinine, and creatine. At the glomerulus, the kidney filters all substances of the plasma, except for the cellular constituents and the plasma protein. In addition, the kidney selectively reabsorbs the necessary valuable substances required by the body.

The function of the kidney is the sum of the functions of the individual nephrons. Each normal adult kidney contains approximately 1,250,000 nephrons. Many variables affect the function of the nephrons, including the circulation through the glomerular capillary, changes in blood flow or redistribution of blood flow in the kidney or systemic circulation, and diseases that affect varying amounts of renal parenchyma. In the normal adult, about 120 to 140 ml of filtrate is formed each minute. This represents approximately 180 L per day of filtrate, which has approximately the same composition as plasma, except for protein. The average daily urine excretion is approximately 1000 ml (1 L); therefore, approximately 179 L of filtrate are reabsorbed. It has been suggested that 80% of this reabsorption occurs in the proximal tubule, and 20% in the distal tubular structures. In the collecting tubule, the absorption of water is in excess of solute, and this relationship determines the final concentration of urine that reaches the bladder. Tubular reabsorption may be characterized as active or passive. In the active form, the reabsorption of substances occurs against a concentration gradient. Movement of the substance from an area of low concentration to an area of high concentration requires energy. Passive reabsorption occurs from areas of high concentration to low concentration. The few plasma proteins that are filtered are usually reabsorbed, probably by an active process. Glucose is an example of a substance that is actively reabsorbed.

The functional microscopic unit of the kidney is the nephron (Fig. 6–81). The nephron consists of the glomerulus and proximal convoluted tubules in the cortex. It also includes Henle's loop, with a descending limb entering the medullary tissue and an ascending limb going back toward the cortex, where the distal convoluted tubule is located; finally, it empties into the collecting ducts, which again enter the medullary tissue and open into the calyx. Approximately 20% of the total glomeruli are juxtamedullary, located in the cortical columns or borders of the medullary pyramid. The gross anatomical functioning unit of the kidney is the renal lobule. It

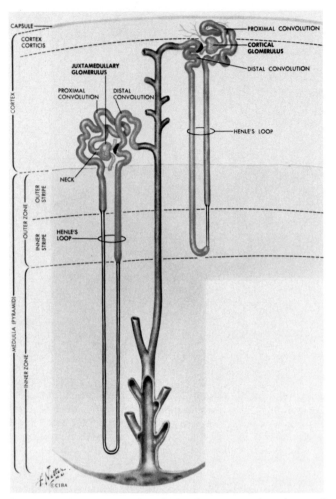

Figure 6–81. Diagram of nephron. Cortex contains glomeruli, proximal and distal convoluted tubules, and part of Henle's loop. The medullary pyramid contains Henle's loop and the collecting tubules. (Copyright 1973. CIBA-GEIGY Corporation. Reproduced with permission from the CIBA COLLECTION OF MEDICAL ILLUSTRATIONS by Frank H. Netter, MD. All rights reserved.)

consists of the medullary pyramid, with its apex in the calyx in the region of the renal sinus, its base covered by peripheral cortex, and its sides enclosed between the renal cortical columns. The collecting ducts that drain the nephron perforate a thin cribriform plate over the tip of the papilla, in order to gain access to the renal calyx. Thin pericalyceal muscles extend from the calyces to the tips of the pyramids and aid in squeezing urine from the collecting ducts into the calyx.

Urogram

The urogram is a physiological study that permits a rough assessment of renal function. As opposed to retrograde pyelography, it provides an undistorted view of pyelocalyceal and ureteral anatomy.

Following administration of contrast medium, which for all practical purposes is excreted solely by glomerular filtration with currently used agents, significant fluid and ionic shifts occur.[71] Serum osmolality rapidly increases, causing influx of water from the interstitial space into the blood stream, and blood volume increases as much as 16%. Concurrently, cardiac output increases. Simultaneously, there is rapid diffusion of the contrast agent into

the extravascular space, 70% disappearing within 2 minutes, and gradually being rereleased into the circulation. Hemodynamic changes consist of transient hypotension, peripheral vasodilatation, increased pulmonary artery pressure, and tachycardia. Electrocardiographic abnormalities are also known to occur. These cardiovascular effects are much less pronounced with nonionic contrast agents than with the ionic ones. There may be a slight lowering of the serum calcium as a result of chelating agents in the contrast preparation. On rare occasions, this may lead to clinical tetany. Owing to rapid excretion and equilibration of the contrast agent, the plasma half-life is relatively short, about 30 minutes for bolus injections, to several hours for drip infusions.[77]

After glomerular filtration, within 20 seconds of a bolus injection of contrast agent, a cortical nephrogram normally appears. Its density depends on the amount and rate of injection of contrast material. This represents contrast in the proximal nephron. The nephrogram provides excellent visualization of the renal parenchyma and frequently provides diagnostic clues. The passage of the opaque medium along the nephron is rapid, with the contrast material in the calyces usually visible approximately 2 minutes after injection. During its transit, it may be concentrated as much as 50 times, producing a relatively dense pyelogram.

Although the plasma contrast concentrations are identical for equal doses of sodium or methylglucamine salts of ionic contrast media, the urinary concentration is significantly greater with the sodium salts. The basis of this effect is the fact that methylglucamine is not reabsorbed from the renal tubule, whereas sodium is reabsorbed. The net effect is an osmotic diuresis with the methylglucamine agents, which effectively lowers urinary iodine concentration. A further increase in urinary iodine concentration is provided by the nonionic media, by virtue of their relatively low osmolality and decreased osmotic diuresis, while maintaining a high molecular iodine content.

A kidney that fails to excrete radiographically detectable amounts of contrast agent into its collecting system is termed *nonvisualizing.* Although the terms "nonfunctioning" or "nonexcreting" kidney have been applied to this failure in the past, they wrongly imply information that cannot be inferred from urography alone and are, therefore, not recommended.

Urography is the procedure of choice when anatomical details of the calyces, pelvis, or ureter are desired. If function is sufficient, the urogram localizes the obstruction. Its primary uses today appear to be in the areas of known or suspected calculi, ureteral obstruction, congenital anomalies, infection, and intraluminal tumors. All other things being equal, it is the study of first choice in patients with unexplained gross hematuria or pyuria, and in those requiring thorough screening of the entire urinary tract.

Retrograde Pyelography

The retrograde pyelogram is not a physiological study. Distortion of anatomy occurs following pressure injections and distention of the collecting system (Fig. 6–82). No nephrogram is obtained, and a retrograde study

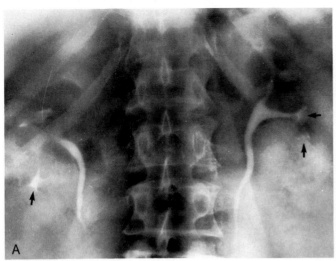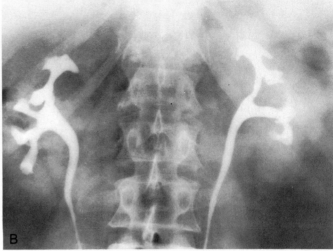

Figure 6–82. Retrograde distention. *A,* Urogram in this adult male with incomplete visualization of the collecting system. The calyces (*arrows*) are cupped and normal in appearance. *B,* Retrograde pyelogram, same patient, reveals the typical overdistention of the calyces due to the force of injection. These should not be interpreted as overdistended or hydronephrotic calyces.

always introduces the possibility of infection and trauma through manipulation. It is primarily valuable when visualization in the urogram is inadequate or when more detail in a specific area of the kidney or ureter is desired. In general, retrograde pyelography is not performed without a prior urogram.

Variations in the excretory system are protean, and both radiologists and urologists often have difficulty in differentiating normal variations from early pathological changes. The renal pelvis receives urine from the two rows of anterior and posterior minor calyces, which point anteriorly or posteriorly, respectively (see Fig. 6–77). Each calyx drains by means of an infundibulum into the renal pelvis. There is considerable variation in the kidneys of different individuals, and, unfortunately, the two kidneys in a given individual may or may not be symmetrical. Therefore, direct comparisons between the two kidneys may not be helpful.

As previously stated, the right renal pelvis is usually located opposite the L2 vertebra, and the left renal pelvis is usually 0.5 to 1 cm higher. Variations in position of the kidney in the transverse, longitudinal, and anteroposterior axes of the body are not uncommon. When these occur as dominant findings, they are considered congenital anomalies. However, minor degrees of changes in position are frequent and are considered normal variations. The following guidelines help to assess these variations:

1. An excursion of up to two lumbar vertebral bodies from the mean position of the kidney is considered to be within normal limits. Every normal kidney has a moderate degree of mobility, which usually falls within this limit. Displacement of a greater degree is referred to as nephroptosis if it is positional, and ectopia if it is permanent (Figs. 6–83 and 6–84). Ectopic kidneys have short ureters, whereas ptotic kidneys have a ureter of normal length. Even severely ptotic kidneys rarely produce symptoms, although ptosis rarely may be associated with obstructions. When acute intermittent hydronephrosis of a ptotic kidney is associated with colicky-type pain, it is referred to as *Dietl's crisis.*

2. Occasionally, a laterally placed kidney is seen; the entire kidney is 2 or 3 cm more distant from the spine than is usual. In such cases the upper pole of the kidney may lie lateral to the transverse process of T12 to L1. Occasionally, the upper pole of the kidney is in normal position but the lower pole of the kidney is laterally rotated so that the oblique axis of the kidney increases to over 45 degrees (Fig. 6–85). It is important to recognize that these may be normal variations, but one must always exclude the presence of a mass displacing the kidney.

3. The kidney may be slightly rotated along its transverse axis, in which case the upper pole of the kidney is posterior and the lower pole of the kidney tends to fall more anteriorly. The calyces tend to overlie each other, and the contour of the kidney becomes somewhat circular, a "tennis-ball" kidney (Fig. 6–86). This kidney can be easily distinguished by obtaining a lateral film that will show the kidney placed in the anteroposterior direction. When obtaining lateral films of the kidney, as mentioned previously, the side in question should always be closest to the film.

In the anatomical description of the kidney, it was stated that the renal pelvis may be completely intrarenal, completely extrarenal, or a combination of both. Pelves are obviously extrarenal when they project beyond the medial border of the kidney in the urogram (Figs. 6–87 and 6–88). Nevertheless, pelvis may still be extrarenal and present anterior to the kidney without projecting medially. Large extrarenal pelves may impinge upon the psoas muscle in the supine position but fall anterior to the psoas in the prone position (Fig. 6–89). Occasionally, the entire renal pelvis is outside of the renal hilus. In such cases the infundibula arise from the pelvis outside of the kidney and penetrate the renal mass individually ("extrarenal calyces") (Fig. 6–90). It is important not to confuse a large extrarenal pelvis that has normal calyces with a partially obstructed system that has dilated calyces. Approximately 10% of renal pelves may be bifid, and less than 0.1% trifid.

Numerous variations affect the anatomical arrangements at the ureteropelvic junction. The renal pelves may be thin and long, or broad and flat. They are frequently classified into two types: a "funnel" pelvis, which merges

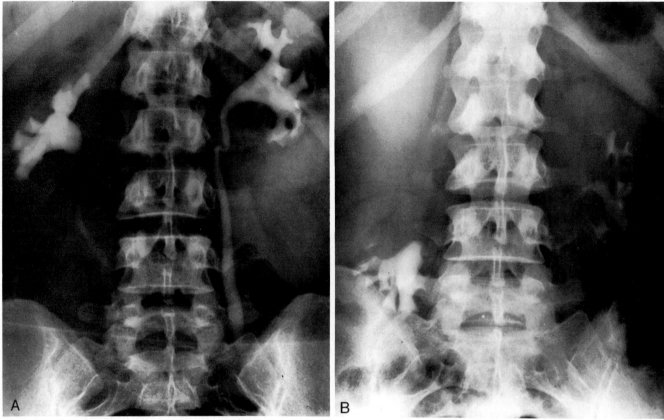

Figure 6–83. Excessive renal mobility (ptosis). *A*, Patient in supine position with the left kidney opposite the interspace between L1 and 2, the right kidney opposite the second lumbar vertebral body. *B*, Same patient, erect position. The left renal pelvis is now opposite the interspace between L3–L4. The right kidney has descended and rotated with the calyces pointing inferiorly. The right renal pelvis is now opposite the interspace between L4–L5.

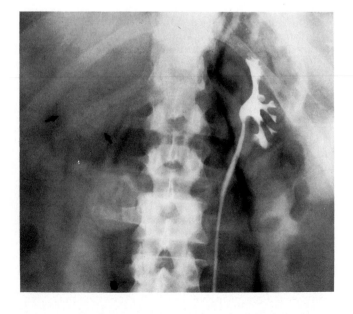

Figure 6–84. High position of the kidneys. Retrograde study shows the left kidney and pelvis to be at the interspace between T12 and L1. The lower pole of the right kidney (*arrows*) is opposite the first lumbar vertebral body, with the renal hilus either at T12 or above.

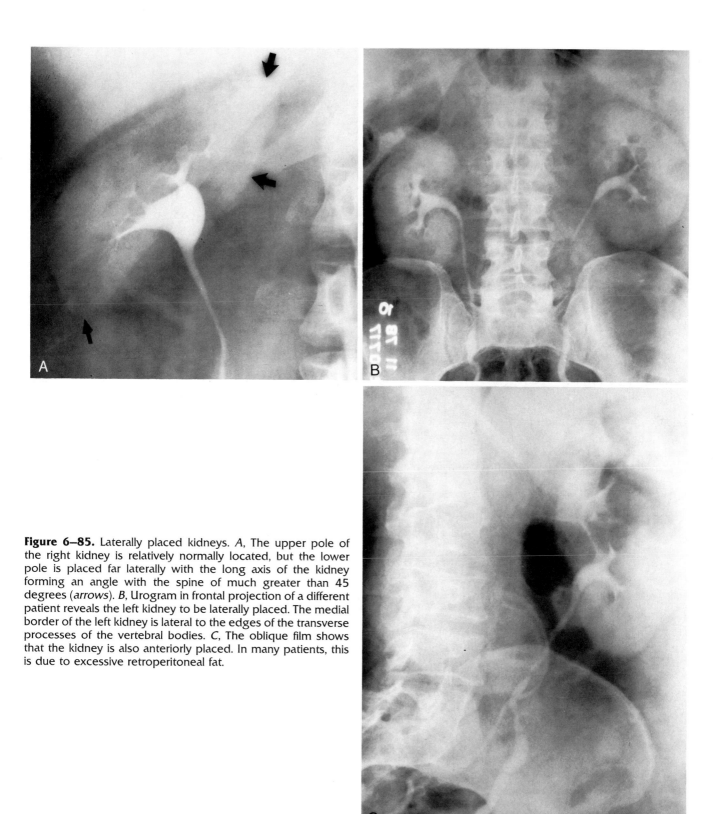

Figure 6—85. Laterally placed kidneys. *A*, The upper pole of the right kidney is relatively normally located, but the lower pole is placed far laterally with the long axis of the kidney forming an angle with the spine of much greater than 45 degrees (*arrows*). *B*, Urogram in frontal projection of a different patient reveals the left kidney to be laterally placed. The medial border of the left kidney is lateral to the edges of the transverse processes of the vertebral bodies. *C*, The oblique film shows that the kidney is also anteriorly placed. In many patients, this is due to excessive retroperitoneal fat.

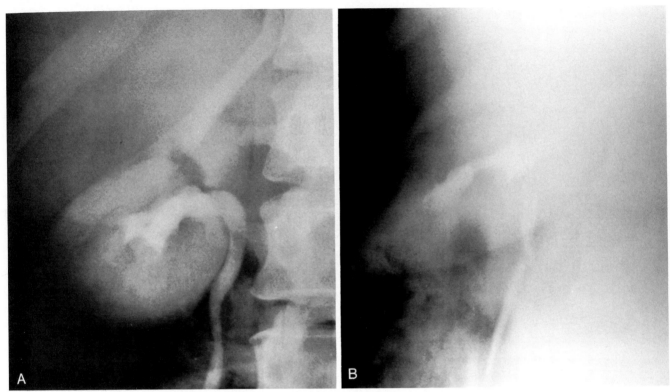

Figure 6–86. Rotation of kidney on transverse axis. *A*, In the nephrogram, the kidney appears round in the frontal projection, with the calyces superimposed on each other. *B*, The lateral film shows the kidney to be rotated on its transverse axis. The upper pole is posterior, and the lower pole is anterior.

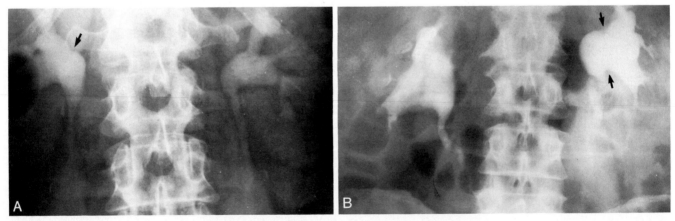

Figure 6–87. Partial extrarenal pelves. The normal renal pelvis projects anteromedially from the kidney and therefore may be partially extrarenal without extending beyond the medial outline of the kidney. Occasionally, a notch within the renal outline is seen, where the pelvis projects anteromedially through the hilar lip. *A*, Bilateral partial extrarenal pelves projecting beyond the medial contour of the kidney. Note the notch (*arrow*) in the right kidney. *B*, Somewhat larger, bilateral, partially extrarenal pelves. Again, note the notch (*arrows*) on the superior and inferior surface of the renal pelvis of the left kidney, where it protrudes through the hilar lip.

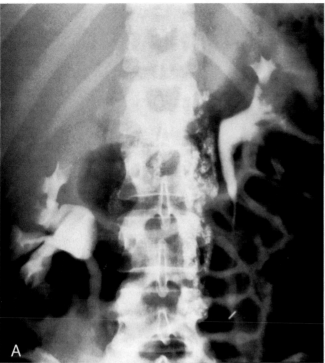

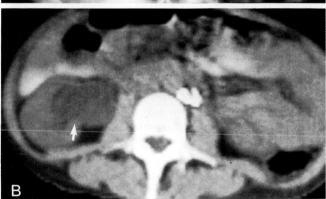

Figure 6–88. Partially extrarenal pelvis. *A,* Excretory urography reveals that the right renal pelvis is partially extrarenal. The paravertebral densities are from a previous lymphogram. *B,* CT reveals the pelvis extending through the hilar lip, which is indenting the pelvis in this projection (*arrow*) and dividing the intrarenal from the extrarenal pelvic segment. A large extrarenal pelvis should not be confused with an obstructed pelvis.

imperceptibly into the proximal ureter, and a "box" pelvis, displaying a more definite division between ureter and pelvis. Most pelves fall between these categories. In the usual funnel-type pelvis (Fig. 6–91), it is sometimes difficult to determine where the ureter anatomically begins. Radiologists frequently describe this area as the ureteral cone, implying a segment that is functionally a ureter but where the anatomical demarcation is not clear. In the boxlike pelvis, drainage is less efficient and some degree of pelvic distention may occur. In addition, many variations of ureteropelvic attachments are inefficient for function, such as ureters that insert rather high into the renal pelvis (high insertion of the ureter) and ureters that insert more anteriorly or posteriorly into the renal pelvis and not in the most dependent position (Fig. 6–92). Such anomalous arrangements tend to lead to some degree of stasis and occasionally obstruction and infection.

The pelvis exits from the kidney anteromedially. As a pelvis becomes more extrarenal, there is a tendency for the infundibula to insert directly into the renal pelvis and, of course, for the pelvis to dilate (Figs. 6–87 to 6–90). This should not be confused with obstruction. The dilatation is due to the decreased pressure around the extrarenal pelvis and is not accompanied by any calyceal blunting. Entirely intrarenal pelves tend to be small, whereas completely extrarenal pelves tend to be large.

Peristaltic activity may change the size and shape of the calyces, pelvis, and ureter from film to film (Figs. 6–93 and 6–94). Peristalsis is active. The calyces "milk" the papillae by contraction of the small pericalyceal muscles. The calyces fill, contract, and fill the renal pelvis. The pelvis contracts with a continuous peristaltic wave moving down the ureter, pushing the urine into the bladder. The complete emptying of the kidney several times an hour is an important protective mechanism, removing bacteria that may be present in the upper tract. Absence of active peristalsis (i.e., stasis) frequently leads to infection. Although the capacity of the renal pelves varies widely, it averages from 3 to 12 cc. The more unusual variations of the pelves and calyces, including malrotation, fusion, abnormal insertions of the ureter, rotations, and displacements are discussed in the section Congenital Anomalies.

Segmentations and duplications of the pelvis and/or ureters are secondary to segmentation of the wolffian duct, which forms the collecting system. Renal pelves, as previously mentioned, are bifid in approximately 10% of individuals (Fig. 6–95). Unusual appearances of segmentation are occasionally seen that should not be interpreted as abnormalities (Fig. 6–96). The bifid collecting system usually has a single upper calyceal segment and multiple lower calyceal segments (Figs. 6–97 and 6–98). With complete ureteral duplication, the ureter draining the upper renal segment enters the bladder ectopically, below the ureter draining the lower segment. The upper-seg-

Text continued on page 162

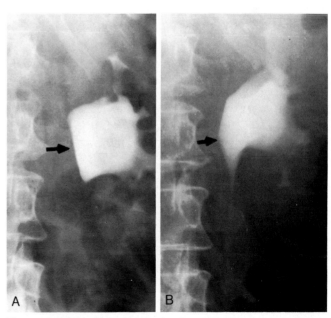

Figure 6–89. *A,* The extrarenal pelvis extends to and impinges upon the psoas muscle (*arrow*), producing a sharp lateral edge to the pelvis. *B,* Same patient in the prone position in which the pelvis falls anterior to the psoas and therefore does not show the impression.

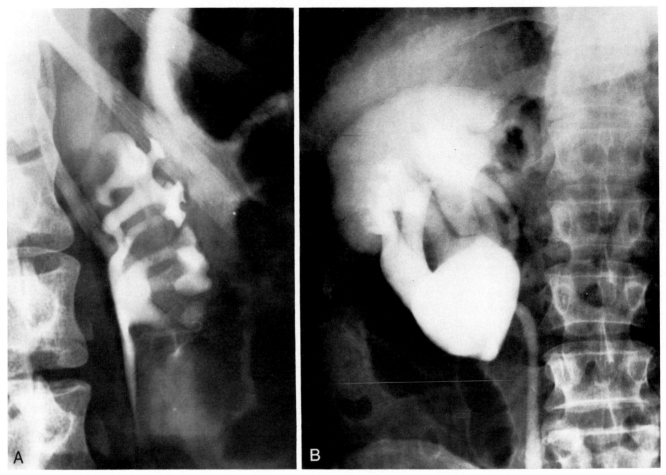

Figure 6–90. Completely extrarenal pelves and infundibula. *A*, The entire pelvis is extrarenal, with the infundibula penetrating the kidney substance individually. *B*, Another example of a completely extrarenal pelvis with the infundibula extending from the pelvis outside of the kidney into the renal substance. Completely extrarenal pelves may be associated with some degree of renal dysplasia.

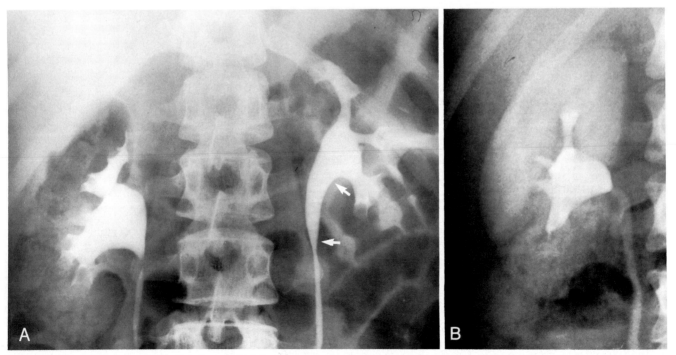

Figure 6–91. *A*, The left renal pelvis is a typical funnel pelvis, lacking clear demarcation of the ureteropelvic junction. The area between the pelvis (*upper arrow*) and abdominal ureter (*lower arrow*) has been termed the *ureteral cone*. The right renal pelvis is a box-type pelvis with a clear demarcation of where the ureter begins. *B*, The right renal pelvis is a box-type pelvis. The box pelvis is a less efficient drainage configuration than the funnel pelvis.

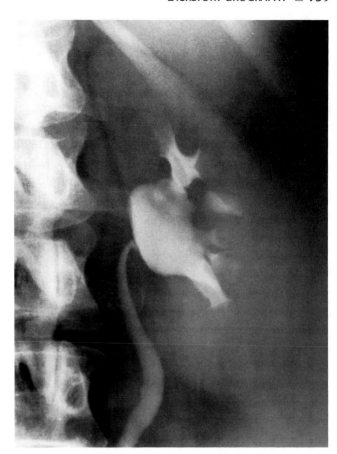

Figure 6–92. High insertion of the ureter into the renal pelvis. This leads to inefficient drainage and pelvic dilatation. It may be secondary to obstruction when the pelvis dilates significantly and the ureteropelvic junction is no longer dependent.

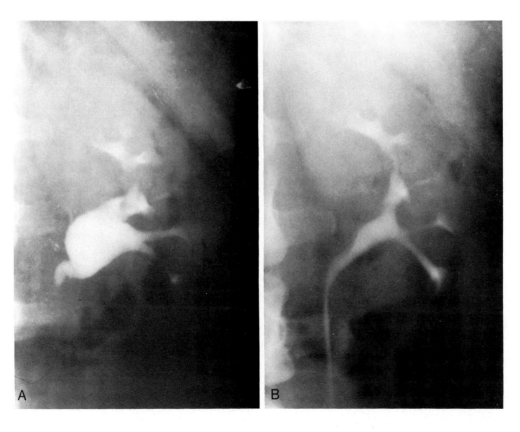

Figure 6–93. Peristalsis in the kidney. *A,* The calyces have contracted and the pelvis is relaxed. *B,* The pelvis has now contracted, and contrast material is in the ureter. The calyces are beginning to dilate as they fill with urine from the nephrons and, in a retrograde fashion, with urine from the renal pelvis.

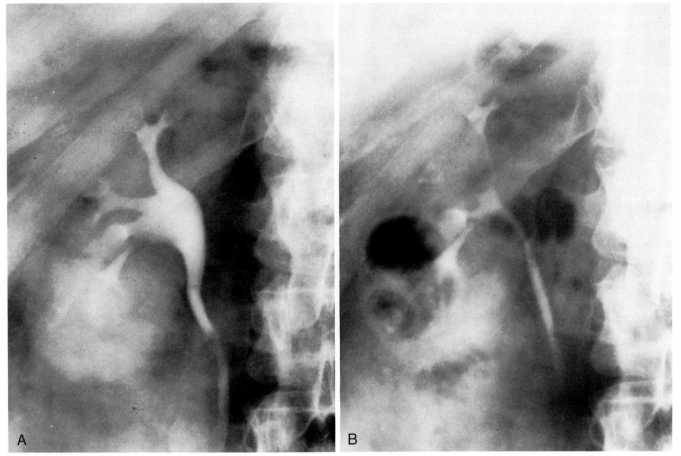

Figure 6–94. *A*, The calyces and renal pelvis are dilated, with the pelvis beginning to empty into the ureter. *B*, Less than 1 minute later, the calyces and pelvis have completely contracted and will now refill with urine.

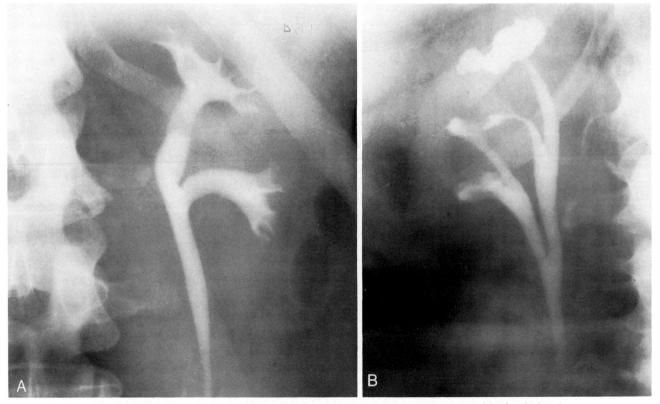

Figure 6–95. *A, B,* Two examples of bifid renal pelves with a single ureter (duplex kidney).

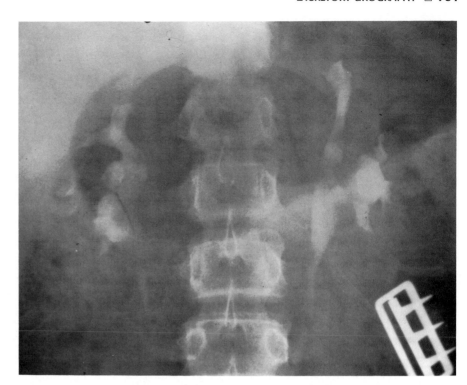

Figure 6–96. An unusual example of segmentation of the right renal pelvis with a bifid left renal pelvis. The renal pelvis on the right is divided by a thin band of tissue, seen as a lucent line on the contrast-filled pelvis.

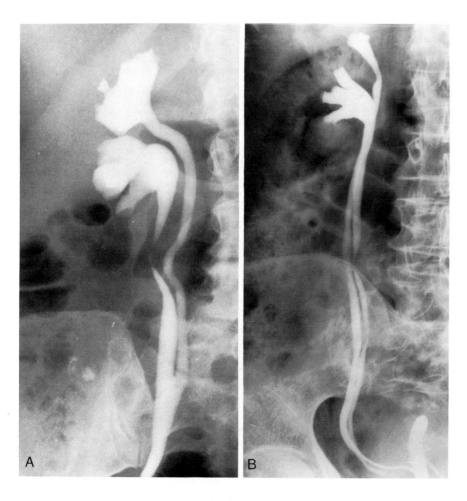

Figure 6–97. *A*, Double renal pelvis and double proximal ureter joining in the middle third of the ureter. *B*, Double renal pelvis and complete duplication of the ureter. In such cases the ureter draining the upper moiety enters the bladder below the ureter draining the lower moiety. The upper moiety contains fewer calyces than does the lower.

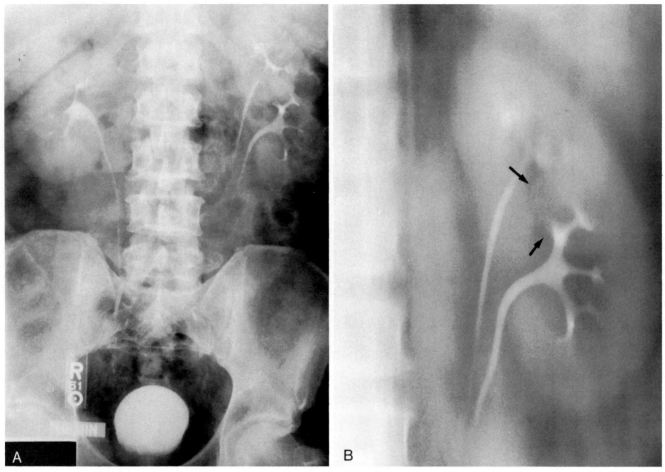

Figure 6–98. *A*, Complete duplication of the collecting system of the left kidney. Two ureters entered the bladder separately. *B*, Tomogram of the left kidney reveals two separate renal hila as shown by the areas of lucency around each renal pelvis, separated by a large column of Bertin (*arrows*) protruding into the sinus fat. The left kidney measured 17 cm, approximately 3 cm larger than the right kidney. Duplication of the collecting system is one of the most common causes of an enlarged kidney.

ment ureter is prone to obstruction at its orifice (stenosis), whereas the lower-segment ureter is prone to reflux (Fig. 6–99). Far more unusual are the rare trifid pelves and ureters (Figs. 6–100 and 6–101). Up to six ureters have been reported to drain one kidney. Various types of pelvic segmentation have been reported to produce bizarre appearances referred to as compartmentalization (Fig. 6–102). These unusual appearances are often associated with vascular impressions that appear in underfilled pelves in the supine patient and disappear when the pelves are totally filled or the patient is in the prone position.

Anatomy textbooks frequently divide calyces into major and minor components. The usual description states that three major calyceal systems arise from the renal pelvis, subdividing into three to five minor calyces. The minor calyx is then divided into the branching infundibula, the calyx proper, and the fornix, which surrounds the sides of the renal papilla. This definition leads to confusion when applied to clinical cases, because of numerous variations. Not infrequently, two or four or more infundibula (major calyceal systems), each leading to single or multiple calyces, arise separately from the pelvis (Fig. 6–103*B*). Infundibula leading to the pelvis may be long (Fig. 6–103*A*) or short, and in some instances calyces appear to arise directly from the pelvis because of very short, stubby infundibula (Figs. 6–103*B* and 6–

104). At times, these are very confusing (see Aberrant Papilla, pages 192, 235).

For practical purposes, we speak of the renal pelvis. All branches from the pelvis, whether single or multiple, are termed infundibula. The calyx is the cup receiving the tip of the papilla, and the fornices represent the side projections of the calyx surrounding the papilla. The variations in the outline of the renal pelvis and calyces are shown in Figures 6–95 to 6–121. Although the two kidneys are frequently not symmetrical, any unusual appearance of bilateral pelves or calyces can usually be assumed to be a normal variation (Fig. 6–105).

The average number of calyces is seven to nine per kidney, but it may be as low as four or five, or as high as 18 or 19, or more ("polycalycosis") (Fig. 6–106). With simple papillae, there is a one-to-one ratio of calyx to pyramid. Multiple papillae (two or more) draining into a single calyx are referred to as a compound calyx (see Fig. 6–70).

The calyx is a physiologically active unit connected to the papilla by thin pericalyceal muscles, which contract and help to drain the collecting ducts into the calyx. The calyx, in effect, passes through systolic and diastolic phases, where urine is collected into the calyx and propelled forward to the renal pelvis (see Figs. 6–93 and 6–94). The fornices of the calyx are usually thin and pointed,

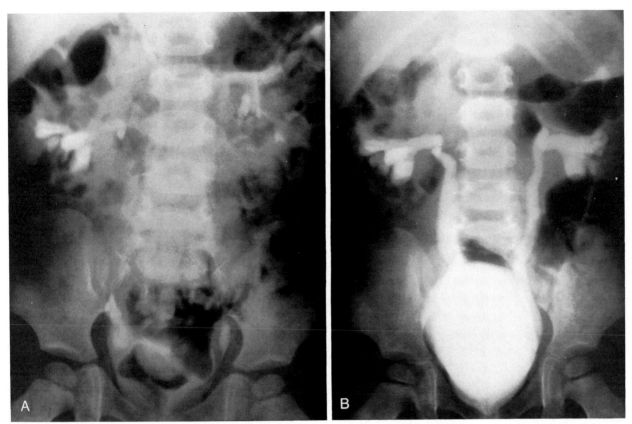

Figure 6–99. Bilateral double collecting systems with stenosis of the ureteral orifices of both upper poles producing obstruction. There is gross reflux in both lower poles. *A,* Urogram showing partial filling of the lower-pole segments of both kidneys without visualization of the upper poles. *B,* Cystogram showing gross reflux into both lower poles. With duplicated systems, the upper poles tend to be become obstructed; the lower poles tend to display reflux.

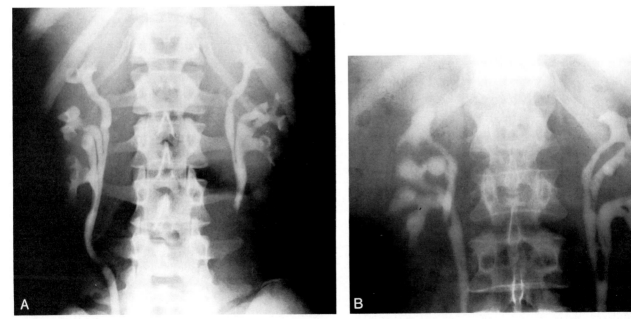

Figure 6–100. *A,* Triplication of the renal pelvis. There is a trifid pelvis on the right and a bifid pelvis on the left. *B,* In a different patient, trifid pelvis on the left is associated with three ureters joining in the proximal third of the ureter. There is a bifid pelvis on the right joining in the proximal portion of the ureter.

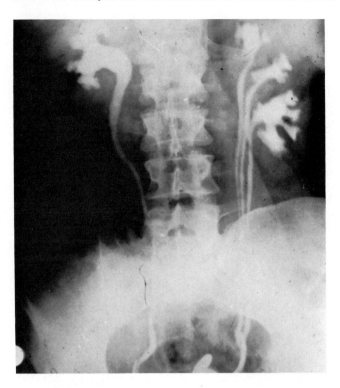

Figure 6–101. Triplication of the renal pelves on the left and triplication of the ureter. The three ureters join just proximal to the ureterovesical junction.

when seen tangentially (Fig. 6–107). The size of the calyx correlates to the size of the papilla that projects into it. The calyces may be shallow or deep, narrow or wide. Occasionally, unusually large calyces are seen (Fig. 6–108). These may suggest edema of the papilla, such as might occur in early medullary necrosis, but they usually represent a normal variant. Very shallow or small calyces, again, are usually a normal variant suggesting small or hypoplastic pyramids (Figs. 6–109 and 6–110). When calyces are seen end-on, they have a distinctive en face appearance (see Fig. 6–105). Because the anterior and posterior rows of calyces project anteriorly and posteriorly, respectively, end-on calyces are not uncommon. The renal hilus points anteromedially; therefore, the anterior calyces are more lateral, and the posterior calyces more medial (see Figs. 6–104 and 6–105). Calyces may occasionally be superimposed, presenting a bilobed appearance (Figs. 6–108 and 6–111). The upper-pole calyces fill best in the supine position, because the upper pole is more posterior than the lower pole. Turning the patient into the prone position fills the lower calyceal system and ureter, and tends to empty the upper calyceal system (Fig. 6–112). The pyelocalyceal appearance in children is similar to that in adults, although the ureteropelvic angle in children tends to be more acute (Fig. 6–113).

Because calyces cap pyramids, the displacement of lobes (referred to as dysmorphism) places calyces in unusual positions (see Fig. 6–115). These dysmorphic appearances may also produce peculiar lobulations or angulations of renal contour (see Pseudotumors, pages 191, 228).

Unusual Variations in Calyces

Many unusual appearances of calyces bridge the area between normal variations and congenital abnormalities.

These result from deviations in the collecting system, which is formed by racemose branching of the wolffian duct within the metanephros. More detailed discussion will be found in the section Congenital Lesions of the Kidney in Chapter 19.

Microcalyces and Macrocalyces. A microcalyx usually occurs between two branching infundibula. If visualized, it is seen as a slender infundibulum approximately 1 mm in size with a very small tapered calyx at its end (Fig. 6–114). The calyx diameter frequently measures only 3 or 4 mm. The microcalyx often does not function and is filled by retrograde flow. It has no particular clinical significance, aside from the fact that it might be mistaken for a finding of more consequence, such as a small cavity.

Macrocalyces are large in diameter and depth; presumably the enlargement is secondary to an enlargement of the underlying medullary papilla. The calyx itself is tapered and normal in appearance, although the fornices are spread and encircle a large piece of the papilla (see Fig. 6–108). In most instances this is a normal variation, although anything that enlarges the papilla such as interstitial edema might produce such a finding.

Dysmorphism. Occasionally, the renal lobes may be displaced during their formation and may present in unusual positions within the kidney. The calyces that cap these pyramids will also appear in unusual positions and occasionally in unusual structures. Unless a problem of drainage exists, leading to stasis and its complications, there is no particular significance to this variation (Fig. 6–115; see also Figs. 6–157 and 6–158).

Absent Calyces or Diminished Number of Calyces. Variations in the formation of the collecting system may lead to bizarre appearances both in the contour of calyces and in the number of calyces. If an insufficient number of calyces is present, reflecting a deficient number of renunculi, renal function may be affected (Figs. 6–116 and 6–117).

Text continued on page 173

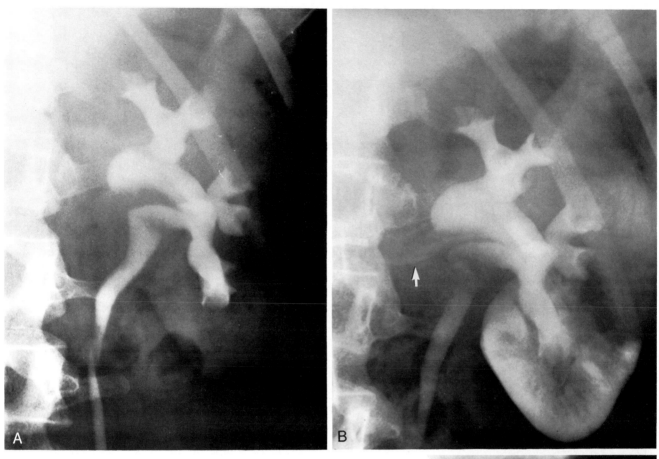

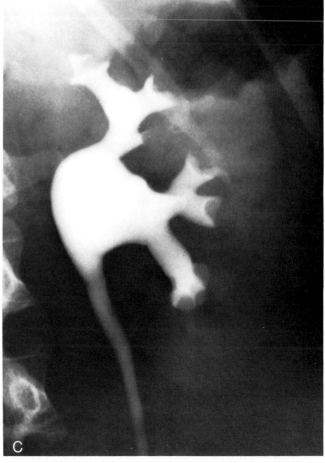

Figure 6–102. Compartmentalization of the renal pelvis. This usually results from a vascular impression, attributable to either a major artery or vein. *A*, The pelvis appears to be segmented in the urogram. *B*, A late film of the arteriogram reveals faint filling of the renal vein (*arrow*), which is producing the segmentation defect. *C*, Retrograde pyelogram with distention of the pelvis does not show the defect. The renal vein is displaced by the distended pelvis.

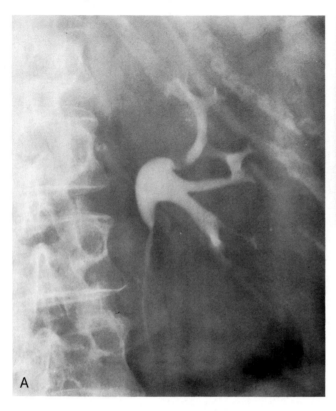

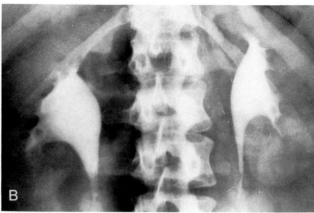

Figure 6–103. Examples of the differences in infundibula in normal kidneys. *A*, Long tapered infundibula leading to the peripheral calyces. *B*, Calyces appear to arise directly from the renal pelvis on short infundibula.

Figure 6–104. Aberrant calyx. A calyx arises directly from a main infundibulum without an identifiable stalk (*arrows*). (Courtesy A. J. Palubinskas, M.D.)

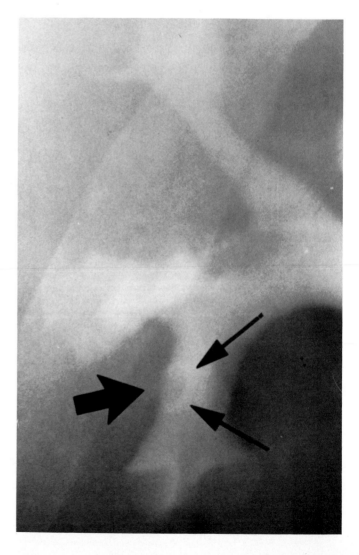

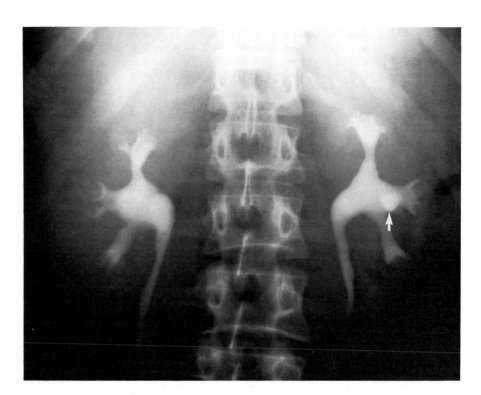

Figure 6–105. Symmetry of infundibular and calyceal structure bilaterally. Even in this instance, differences in the position of minor calyces are observed. Total symmetry is rarely present. The arrow points to a calyx seen end-on. This medially placed calyx is a posterior calyx (*arrow*).

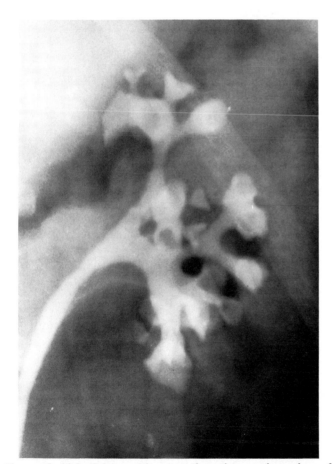

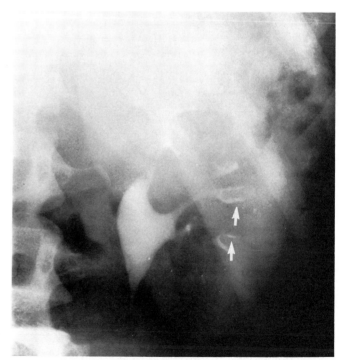

Figure 6–106. Kidney with more than the usual number of calyces ("polycalycosis"). The lateral calyces are anterior, and the medial ones are posterior. The number of calyces usually relates directly to the number of pyramids within the kidney. Compound calyces are present in the midportion of the kidney. It is uncommon to see an adult kidney with more than 14 calyces.

Figure 6–107. The lower two calyces are visualized tangentially. They appear elongated. Note the thin walls representing the fornices of the calyces (*arrows*).

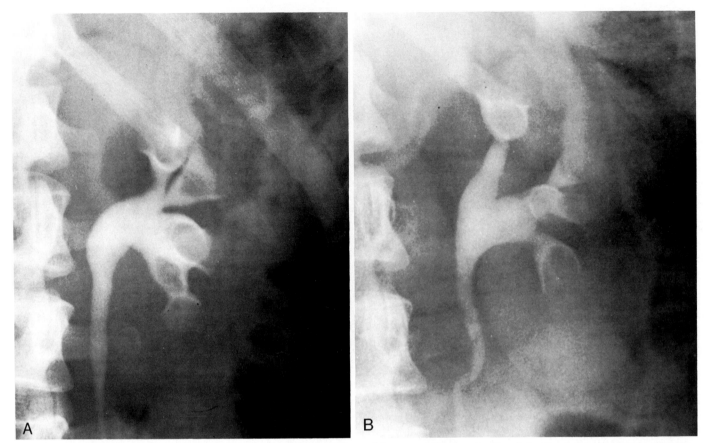

Figure 6–108. Examples of large calyces, presumably the effect of large papillae protruding into the calyx. These are usually normal variants, although they may be seen in diseases that produce edema of the pyramids, such as sickle cell disease. *A,* Two interpolar calyces are superimposed, one on the other, producing a bilobed appearance. Note the thin fornices of each calyx. *B,* A bilobed or cleft calyx receiving two pyramids perpendicular to each other is seen in the lower pole of the left kidney. A thin calyceal fornix seperates the two.

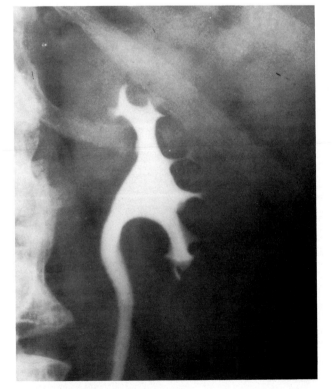

Figure 6–109. The calyces visualized in the midportion of the left kidney appear small and finely tapered. Presumably, this relates to the size of the papillae of the pyramids in this region.

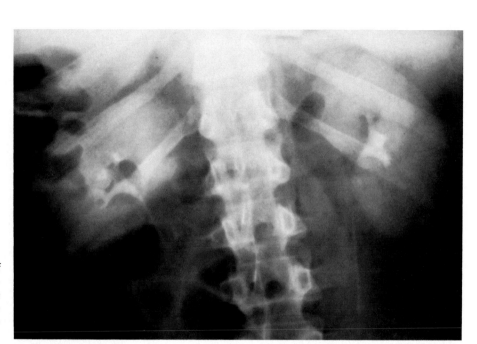

Figure 6–110. Variation in the size of the collecting system in a normal individual. Small pelves and calyces relative to the size of the kidney. A similar appearance may be seen in infiltrative diseases that increase cortical thickness.

Figure 6–111. Bilobed or cleft lower-pole calyx (*arrow*).

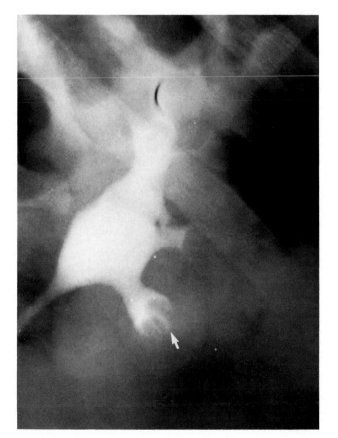

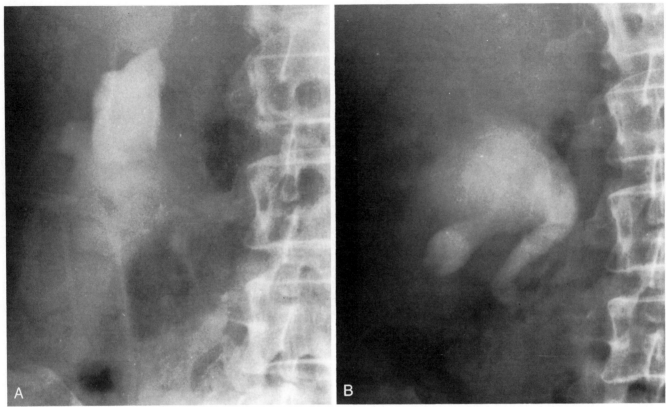

Figure 6–112. Partially obstructed kidney demonstrating the differences in filling in the prone and supine positions. *A,* Supine view shows that contrast, which is heavier than urine, has pooled in the superior calyceal system, which is the most dependent. *B,* Prone view shows that the contrast material has moved into the lower calyceal system and proximal ureter. The lower pole of the kidney and the proximal ureter are placed more anteriorly than the upper pole of the kidney. Consequently, they fill more readily in the prone position.

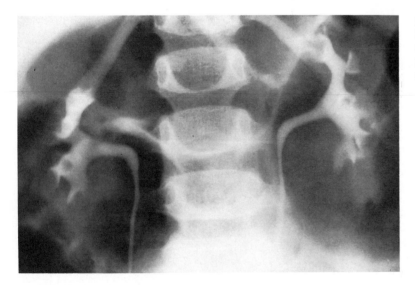

Figure 6–113. Urogram in an 8-year-old child. Pyelocalyceal anatomy is similar to that of the adult. The ureteropelvic angle approaches 90 degrees on the right. In young children the angle tends to be more acute than in adults.

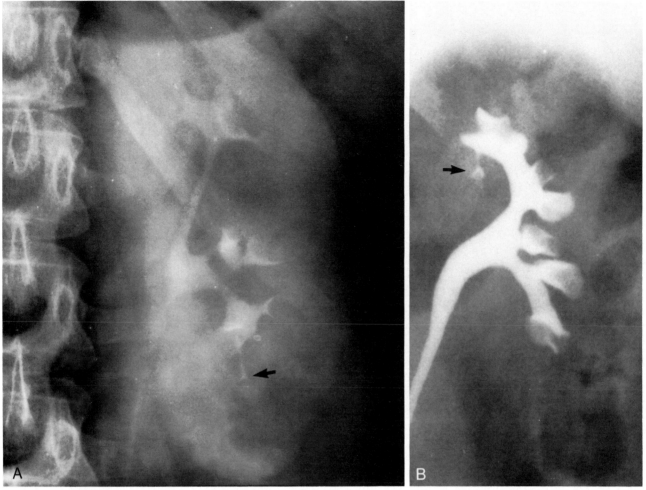

Figure 6–114. Microcalyces are related to abnormalities in the branching of the wolffian duct, which forms the collecting system. *A,* Microcalyx extending from the fornix of a lower-pole calyx *(arrow)* into the renal parenchyma. The tiny calyx does not cap a functioning pyramid. It fills by retrograde flow. *B,* Another example of a microcalyx extending from the fornix of an upper calyx.

Figure 6–115. Dysmorphism. Occasionally, the orderly placement of the anterior and posterior lobes does not occur during renal development, and lobes appear in unusual sites. The urogram illustrates abnormal placement of lower-pole lobes, which are capped by partially dysplastic calyces.

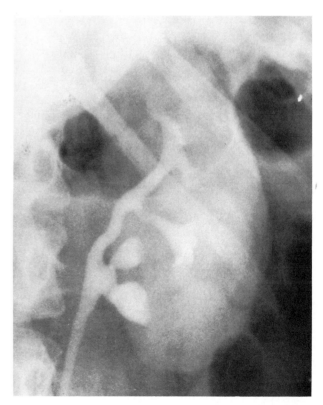

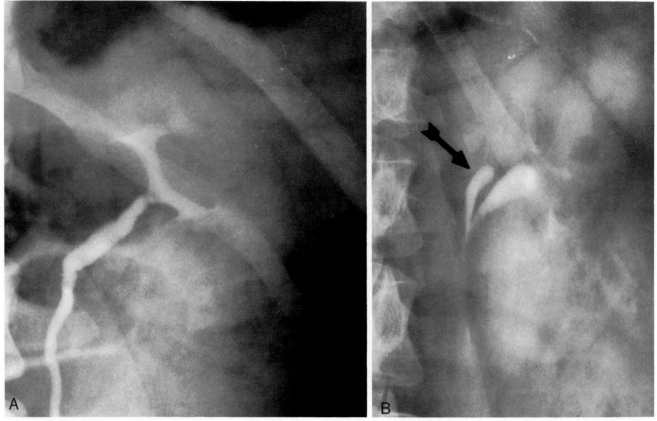

Figure 6–116. Calyceal dysplasia. *A,* Deficiency of renal lobes manifested by the presence of only two functioning calyces. The opposite kidney also had a calyceal abnormality. The patient did not develop elevated blood urea nitrogen (BUN) until 48 years of age. This variant may also be viewed as a form of renal hypoplasia. *B,* Bifid pelvis without any calyces developing from the upper branch (*arrow*), which is blind ended.

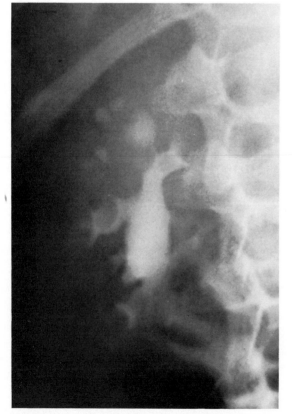

Figure 6–117. Abnormal formation of calyces and collecting tubules in the upper pole of the right kidney. The upper-pole calyx is abnormal, and numerous collections of contrast material are seen in dilated dysplastic tubules. This represents a focal dysplasia of the collecting system in the upper pole.

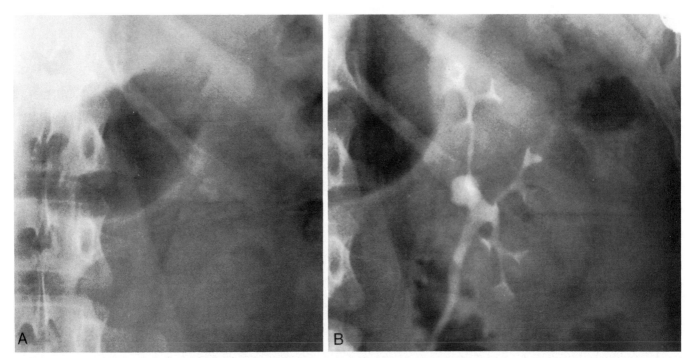

Figure 6–118. Diverticulum of renal pelvis. *A,* Scout film shows three small calculi overlying the silhouette of the left kidney. *B,* Urogram shows the calculi to be within a diverticulum of the renal pelvis. This may represent a dilated rudimentary infundibulum.

Infundibular Variations. Numerous variations may occur affecting both the size and distribution of infundibula within the kidney. Occasionally, diverticular pouches are seen in association with what appears to be blind-ending infundibular buds (Figs. 6–118, 6–119, and 6–121).

Miscellaneous Variations. Any combination of lobes may occur, producing peculiar configurations of calyces.

A right-angled kidney may occur as a form of lobar dysmorphism (Fig. 6–120). In such cases the upper and lower lobes meet at right angles. The kidney may appear incomplete, unless viewed in the lateral projection. Compound calyces, which have been previously discussed, occur when the renal column between pyramids is absent.

In evaluating the normal urogram, in addition to care-

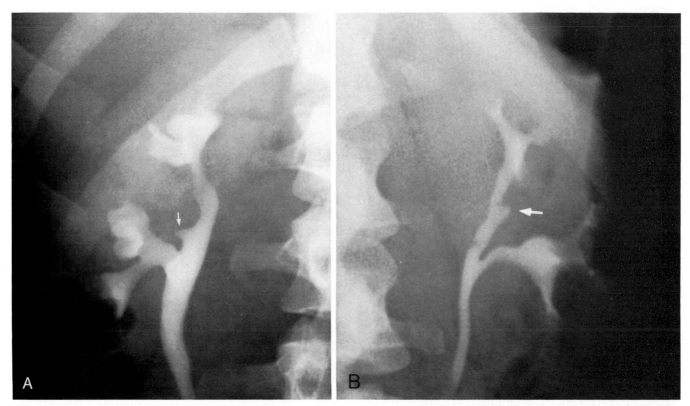

Figure 6–119. Infundibular variations. *A,* Blind-ending infundibulum (*arrow*) arises in the midportion of the kidney. *B,* Blind-ending diverticulum is seen in the upper segment of the bifid pelvis in the left kidney (*arrow*).

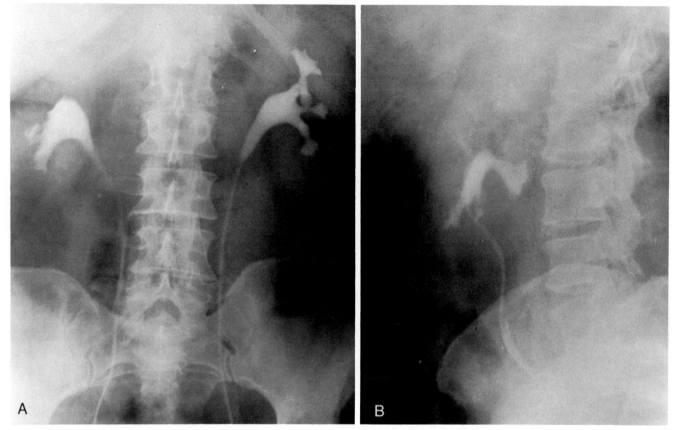

Figure 6–120. "Right-angled" kidney. *A,* Retrograde pyelogram with good filling of the collecting system fails to define the upper pole of the right kidney. *B,* Lateral film shows that the right upper pole extends directly posteriorly, and therefore is invisible in the frontal view. This is a form of lobar dysmorphism producing a right-angled kidney.

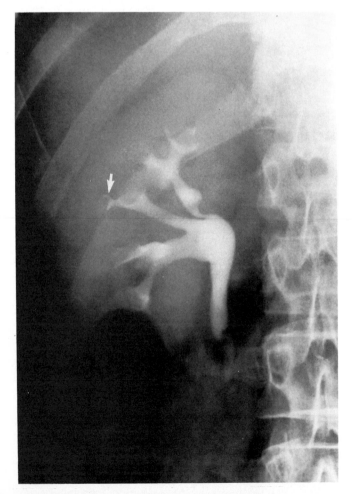

Figure 6–121. A calyx is seen arising from the fornix of an adjacent calyx (*arrow*). This, again, is a developmental anomaly related to the wolffian duct.

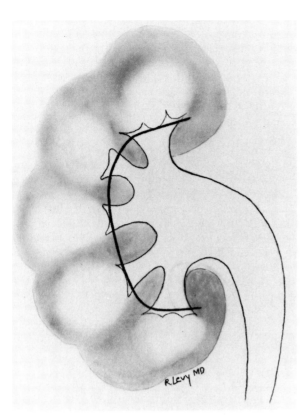

Figure 6–122. Interpapillary line. Diagram illustrates the inter-papillary line drawn through the bases of all calyces. The distance from the nonpolar calyces to the lateral surface of the kidney is fairly constant. Polar distances are greater, but in a particular kidney they are usually equal (see text). The inter-papillary line is useful as a guide for judging normal renal corticomedullary thickness.

fully evaluating renal contour, measuring the length of the kidney, and analyzing calyceal structure, the observer should also pay careful attention to the thickness of the renal parenchyma. A line drawn through the tips of the papilla (base of the calyces), known as the interpapillary line, is a useful landmark for evaluating loss of normal parenchyma (Hodson)[198] (Fig. 6–122). The distance from the interpapillary line to the lateral cortex of the kidney averages 2.5 to 3 cm; this is the thickness of the renal lobe. Distances less than 2 cm are suggestive of paren-chymal loss, and distances greater than 3.5 cm are sugges-tive of mass lesions or interstitial infiltration. Parenchyma is thicker in the area of the polar regions of the kidney. The distance from the interpapillary line at the upper pole of the kidney to the outer edge of the upper pole, and from the interpapillary line of the lower calyx of the kidney to the outer edge of the kidney, should be between 3 and 3.5 cm. Most importantly, the distances in both polar areas should be within 1 or 2 mm of each other (Figs. 6–122 and 6–123).

The following is a summary of some of the more useful guidelines for evaluation of possible abnormalities of the collecting system or cortex:

1. Measurement of cortical thickness, discussed earlier.

2. Bizarre calyceal appearances may occur in the upper and lower poles from compound calyces. Vascular impres-sions, mimicking true filling defects, may cross the infun-dibula (see later discussion).

3. Calyceal and pelvic contours change with peristaltic activity. On any single film, such change may simulate abnormality.

4. There may be considerable variation in the degree of obliquity of the renal pelvis. The renal pelvis tends to be more right-angled in young children (see Fig. 6–113). Any ureteropelvic junction in adults with an angle 90 degrees or greater should be suspected for possible mass displacement.

5. The long axis of the kidney usually runs in the same inclination as the psoas muscle, with the upper pole of the kidney closer to the spine, the lower pole farther away. Abnormality should be suspected if the long axis of a kidney runs either vertically or more than 45 degrees from the vertical. This may occur normally in laterally placed kidneys (see Fig. 6–85). (In the section Congenital Anomalies, malrotations of the kidney on its long axis, transverse axis, and AP axis are considered in detail.)

6. Approximately 10% of young children and 4% of older children and adults have single or multiple inden-tations of the lateral cortex of the kidney, representing persistent fetal lobations. The indentations (valleys) occur at the renal columns (columns of Bertin) at the sites of fusion of the renal lobules (see Fig. 6–64). This is usually easily distinguished from the scarring from infection that occurs between the columns of Bertin overlying the calyx.

7. A common variation in contour on the left side is the splenic impression and dromedary hump. The impres-sion represents contact of the splenic border along the lateral upper half of the renal contour. The dromedary hump represents a bulge at the end of the splenic impres-sion, where the kidney reverts to its normal convexity (Fig. 6–124).

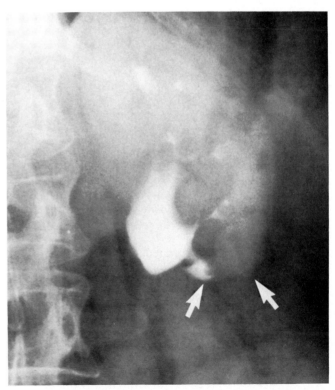

Figure 6–123. Patient with atrial fibrillation and embolic renal infarction. Loss of parenchyma is marked in the region of the lower pole of the left kidney (*arrows*), with the lower-pole calyx extending to the outer margin of the kidney.

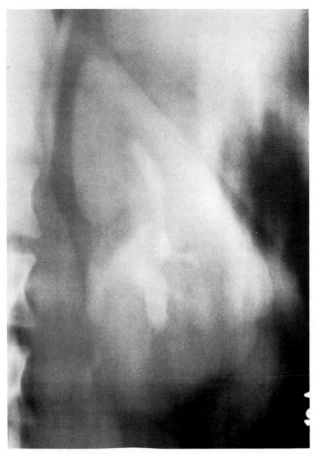

Figure 6–124. Dromedary hump. There is flattening of the upper two-thirds of the lateral border of the left kidney, most likely from splenic pressure, producing a dromedary hump. This pseudotumor is associated with multiple fetal lobations in the lower third of the lateral renal contour.

URETER

The course and relations of the normal ureter have been described previously (Fig. 6–125; see also Figs. 6–79 and 6–129). Variations in the appearance of the ureter may mimic abnormalities. The following are useful diagnostic aids in evaluating the ureter:

1. The ureter is normally compressed as it crosses the iliac vessels (see Fig. 6–80). In some individuals the proximal dilatation may mimic an obstruction. In such instances, it will be noted that there are changes from film to film, that the pelvis and calyces are not dilated, and that there is no delay in emptying on the prone or erect film.

2. Peristaltic activity, redundancy, or crossing vessels may simulate areas of narrowing or stricture (Figs. 6–126 to 6–128).

3. Marked respiratory movement or moderate renal ptosis may produce kinks or angulations of the ureter (see Fig. 6–73). The ureter may be bowed laterally by the psoas muscle (Fig. 6–129).

4. Contrast media may produce diuresis sufficient to simulate dilatation of the entire ureter (see Fig. 6–11).

5. A "jet sign" may be seen through the mixture of urine and contrast in the bladder. This represents concentrated contrast material ejected from the ureteral orifice by peristalsis and seen passing obliquely through the less dense contrast material in the urinary bladder (Fig. 6–

130). This can easily be distinguished from ureteral ectopia, since the jet crosses the midline, whereas ectopic ureters do not.

6. Because of x-ray beam divergence, the distal ureters may appear to insert abnormally low in the prone position and should not be mistaken for ectopic ureters.

7. A ureter that crosses medial to a pedicle is usually abnormally displaced (Fig. 6–131). A ureter crossing over a pedicle is suspect.

8. A ureter that is concave laterally in the pelvic area is usually abnormal. A straight ureter with a convex mate is also suspected of abnormality. If both pelvic ureters are straight (i.e., no convexity or concavity) and are not medially displaced, they may be normal. The usual causes of concavity and medial displacement of a single ureter in the pelvis include bladder diverticulum (see Fig. 6–28A), enlarged hypogastric nodes, or aneurysmal dilatation of the hypogastric artery (Fig. 6–132). The usual causes of medial placement of both pelvic ureters include retroperitoneal fibrosis, pelvic lipomatosis, and postabdominoperineal surgery (Fig. 6–133).

9. The ureter usually is within 1 cm of the outer edge of the transverse process (see Fig. 6–125). Although this is variable, a ureter over 1.5 cm lateral to the margin of the transverse process is suspected of abnormality.

10. A ureter that remains completely filled in all films, even though it is not significantly dilated, is suspected of minimal ureterovesical obstruction, possibly a small calculus.

11. A distended urinary bladder may cause abnormal ureteral fullness.

THE NEPHROGRAM

A nephrogram is the opacification of the renal parenchyma following the administration of contrast medium. The contrast medium causing opacification is primarily

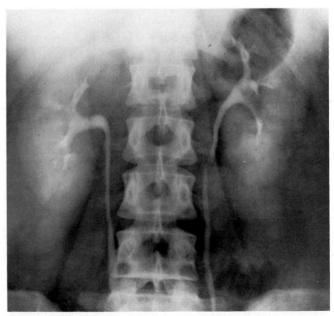

Figure 6–125. Normal proximal half of the left ureter crosses over the transverse processes of the vertebral bodies and lies lateral to the pedicles. Normal right ureter is slightly more medially placed (L4) than usual.

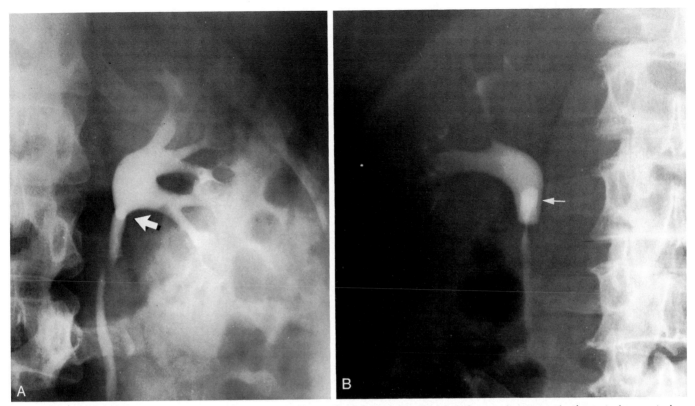

Figure 6–126. Examples of ureteral redundancy ("kinks"). *A,* The ureter is visualized end-on as it courses in the anterior-posterior direction, producing increased density simulating a dense calculus. *B,* Kinking of the ureter with redundancy without obstruction. In the AP projection two segments of proximal ureter are superimposed by the redundancy (*arrow*).

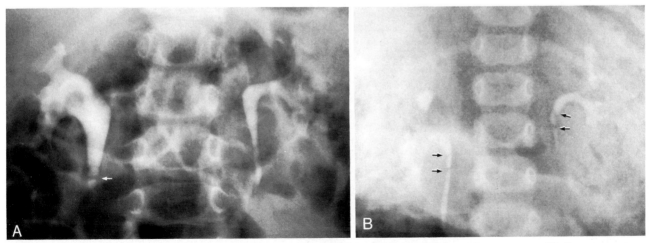

Figure 6–127. Folds or webs in ureter. In the infant and young child mucosal redundancy is common with the appearance of folds or webs within the ureter. They do not behave as valves and do not produce obstruction. *A,* A linear bandlike lucency across the proximal ureter of this 3-year-old child probably represents a mucosal fold. *B,* Multiple mucosal folds are visualized in the ureter of an infant.

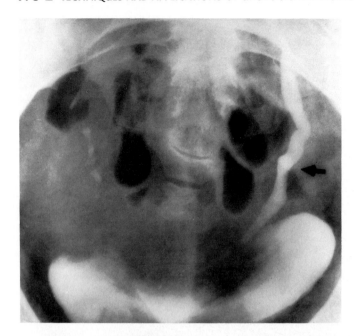

Figure 6–128. Redundancy of the pelvic ureter is shown (*arrow*).

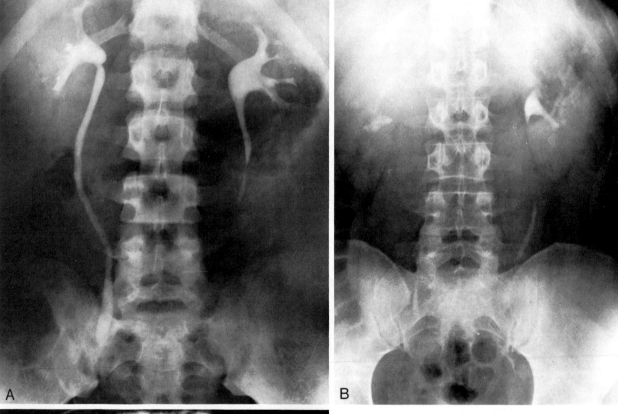

Figure 6–129. *A,* Bowing of the proximal ureters laterally. This appearance suggests that the ureter is caught upon the outer margin of a prominent psoas muscle. The ureter crosses over the psoas in the region of the L4 vertebral body. *B, C,* Another example of bowing of the left ureter on the edge of a prominent psoas. *B,* The distal segment of the bowing is visualized on the urogram. *C,* CT scan shows the right ureter to be in normal position with the left ureter (*arrow*) resting on the outer edge of the psoas muscle.

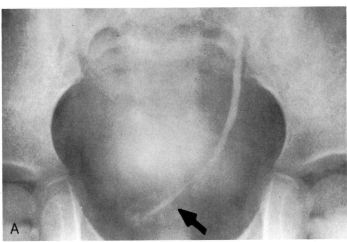
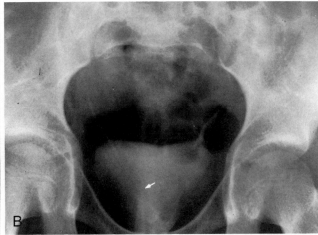

Figure 6–130. *A,* Ureteral jet (*arrow*) traversing obliquely through the bladder, impinging on the opposite wall. This is a manifestation of ureteral peristalsis. *B,* Another example of a ureteral jet (*arrow*) visualized because of the higher density of contrast in the ureteral urine at this stage of bladder filling.

within the lumen of the nephron. Therefore, the density of the nephrogram will depend upon the plasma concentration (amount of contrast given and the length of time over which it is given), the glomerular filtration rate, the number of functioning nephrons, the volume of the individual nephron, and the ability of the kidney to concentrate the contrast medium within the tubule by water reabsorption.[157, 232] In a given injection, the concentration of contrast medium in the filtrate depends primarily on the plasma concentration of the contrast medium, the only variable in the above factors. Therefore, the nephrogram is dose dependent. Sixty to eighty per cent of water reabsorption occurs in the proximal tubule and is closely related to the reabsorption of sodium. It is to some extent time dependent; the longer the filtrate is in contact with the proximal tubule wall, the more water will be reabsorbed. The remaining amount of water reabsorption occurs in the distal tubule controlled mainly by antidiuretic hormone. Obviously, in the context of renal den-

sity, the proximal reabsorption is much more significant in regard to the intensity of the nephrogram.

The normal nephrogram can be divided into two major phases that blend with each other in vivo in an imperceptible manner.

Vascular Nephrogram

A pure vascular nephrogram can be obtained by the injection of a material such as thorium dioxide (Thorotrast), which fills the vascular structures but is not excreted by the kidney. A pure vascular nephrogram may be seen, then, by the injection of thorium dioxide; the vascular nephrogram appears within about 1 second of the initial injection and disappears within several seconds depending on the amount of the contrast medium used, the speed of delivery, and the state of renal blood flow (Fig. 6–134). The vascular nephrogram, therefore, refers to the radiodensity of the kidney caused by opacified

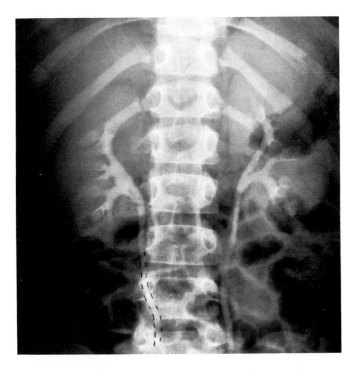

Figure 6–131. Deviation of ureter medial to vertebral pedicle. Urogram shows deviation of the right ureter (dotted lines) medial to the pedicle of L5 secondary to a retroiliac ureter.

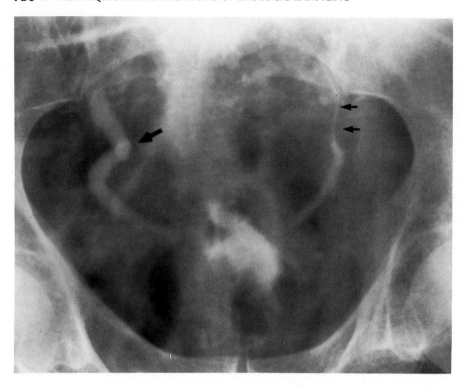

Figure 6–132. Aneurysmal dilatation of the right hypogastric artery displacing the right ureter medially (*large arrow*). There is a similar but less dramatic impression of the left hypogastric artery upon the left ureter (*small arrows*). Faint calcifications of the hypogastric artery are seen at those sites.

blood within the renal circulation. It is best seen during selective renal artery injection during angiography. Utilizing the usual contrast medium for urography and angiography, the vascular nephrogram is a transient and minor part of the total nephrogram and rapidly gives way to the excretory nephrogram as the contrast medium is collected in the renal tubules.

Excretory ("Tubular") Nephrogram

The nephrogram observed during urography is almost entirely caused by the accumulation of contrast medium within the tubules as a result of glomerular filtration and tubular concentration (see Fig. 60–8). Contrast may be visualized in the nephron within 30 seconds after injection. Depending on the volume and the length of time over which it is delivered, the nephrogram may last 30 minutes or longer. This excretory nephrogram is caused by opacified urine in the lumina of the nephron, the density increasing as the contrast is concentrated by water reabsorption.[157] In most instances, the excretory nephrogram is most intense during the first few minutes after injection. The excretory nephrogram may be prolonged by drip-infusion technique or by using multiple large doses of contrast medium (Fig. 6–134; see also Figs. 6–8, 6–15, and 6–20).

Abnormal Nephrograms

There are many causes of abnormal nephrograms, a few of which will be described here.[91] The characteristic of a nephrogram is frequently helpful during the diagnostic study. *Nephrograms of increased density* may be subclassified into those increased immediately after injection and those slowly producing an increased nephrogram over a prolonged period of time. *Nephrograms of decreased density* usually result from impaired renal function or blood flow. The following is a list of some of the more important causes of increased and decreased nephrograms:

A. Increased nephrogram
    1. Obstructive nephrogram
        a. Extrarenal obstruction (see Figs. 6–48, 6–137, and 6–138)
        b. Intrarenal obstruction (see Figs. 6–139 and 6–140)
    2. Hypotensive nephrogram (shock) (see Figs. 6–141 and 6–142)
    3. Renal vein thrombosis (see Fig. 6–143)
    4. Acute tubular necrosis (Fig. 6–135)
B. Decreased nephrogram
    1. Chronic renal failure (see Fig. 6–144)

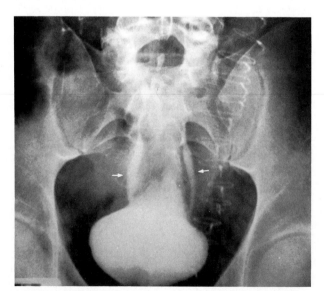

Figure 6–133. Medial position of both ureters (*arrows*) following abdominal perineal surgery for carcinoma of the rectosigmoid. The ureters tend to fall medially following dissection and reperitonealization of the posterior peritoneum.

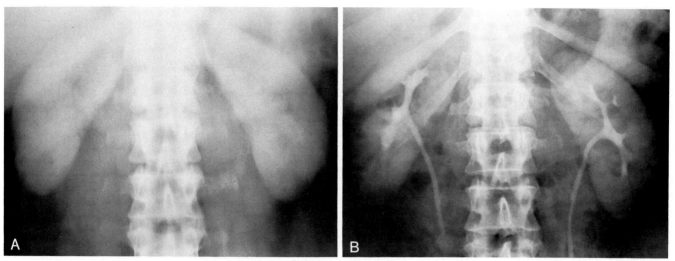

Figure 6–134. Bolus nephrogram. *A,* Tomogram exposed 1 minute after bolus injection of contrast shows bilateral dense nephrograms. *B,* Film 5 minutes after injection shows rapid disappearance of the nephrogram.

2. Renal artery occlusion
3. Renal transplant rejection
4. Renal infection (Fig. 6–136; see also Fig. 6–35)

The following classification is adapted from that of Fry and Cattell:[86]

A. **Immediate, dense, persistent nephrogram**

1. *Acute tubular necrosis.* The density of the nephrogram is maximal at the end of injection, similar to that seen in normal subjects, but may persist unchanged for hours or even days (Fig. 6–122). This is presumed to be due to the disruption of the tubular structures secondary to the acute tubular necrosis with contrast extravasating into the parenchyma. Although there is little or no urine production, circulation of urine occurs via the lymphatics and renal veins. There have been a few reports of an immediate, dense, persistent nephrogram in *acute suppurative pyelonephritis,* which

again is believed to be due to the disruption of the tubular structures and perhaps tubular blockage by pus and casts. This nephrogram is frequently patchy and irregular in appearance (see Figs. 6–35 and 6–136). In most cases of acute infection, a faint nephrogram is seen.

B. **Increasingly dense nephrogram**

1. *Acute extrarenal obstruction.* This is the common type of obstructive nephrogram usually secondary to a calculus in the ureter with progressive increase in parenchymal opacification over minutes or hours (see Fig. 6–48). The nephrogram may be most intense from 2 to 24 hours after urography (Fig. 6–137). Nephrograms that become intense relatively early usually signify that calyceal filling will occur if delayed films are obtained. In acute obstruction the nephrogram may be intense enough to visualize clumps of nephrons within the kidney.

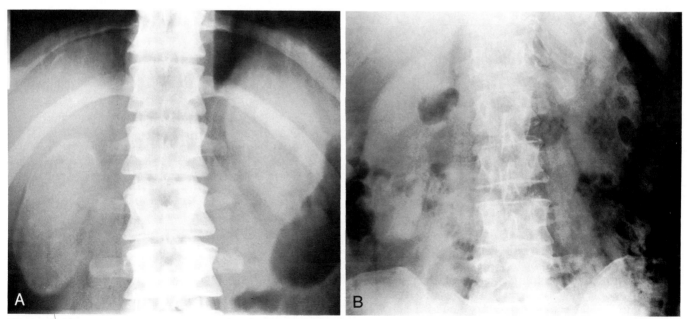

Figure 6–135. Nephrogram of acute tubular necrosis (ATN). *A,* Immediately following injection, patchy irregular nephrograms are present bilaterally with slightly increased density in the peripheral cortices. The nephrograms persisted for 4 hours before fading. *B,* A second case of ATN with persistent nephrogram at 15 minutes. The nephrogram was still visible at 24 hours.

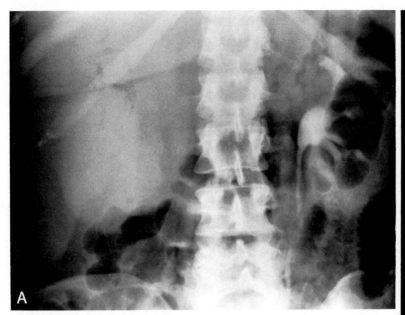

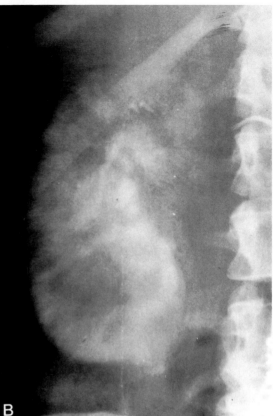

Figure 6–136. Striated nephrogram in acute bacterial pyelonephritis. *A,* Intravenous urogram in a 33-year-old diabetic woman, with acute sepsis. The left kidney is normal. The right kidney is large with a faint nephrogram. Calyces were not visualized. *B,* The nephrogram following renal arteriography shows patchy striated areas of contrast in the renal parenchyma. The lucent areas represent nonvisualized nephrons obstructed either by pus or by vascular spasm.

This striated pattern has been termed "medullary rays" (Fig. 6–138). Although the intensity of the nephrogram is greatest in incomplete obstruction, there will be some increase in density even in complete obstruction, probably secondary to continued reabsorption of water and salt, and lymphatic transport of urine.

2. *Intrarenal obstruction.* Intrarenal obstruction is usually bilateral. The nephrogram gradually becomes increasingly dense over a period of minutes to hours. The most common causes are the precipitation in the tubular lumina of either Tamm-Horsfall protein or crystals (uric acid, sulphite) (Figs. 6–139 and 6–140). Tamm-Horsfall proteinuria with precipitation of protein in the nephron is seen in dehydrated children and in dehydrated patients with myeloma or debilitating diseases. Uric acid precipitation occurs most commonly in lymphoproliferative diseases but also in gout, or after administration of potent uricosurics. Crystallization or protein precipitation in contrast-containing urine occurs more frequently in dehydrated patients. As the tubular blockage develops, a progressively denser nephrogram is seen. It is presumed that the increasingly dense nephrogram is produced by continuing minimal glomerular filtration with stasis of fluid within the nephron. The prolonged contact with the nephron allows increased reabsorption of water from the filtrate, concentrating the contrast medium as well as causing slight dilatation of the tubules; both factors increase the intensity of the nephrogram. The collecting structures are not commonly visualized. The process is usually reversible, but occasionally permanent dialysis is required.

Intratubular obstruction rarely occurs in hydrated patients, which is another reason for not dehydrating patients prior to urography.

Azotemic patients, especially diabetics, may develop acute renal failure following the administration of contrast medium. The exact mechanism is not known, and adequate hydration does not always prevent the renal shutdown. These patients may present with an increasingly dense nephrogram. In all patients whose renal failure is due to intratubular obstruction, the kidney tends to enlarge during the examination. When compared with the scout film, there may be an increase in renal length of as much as 1 to 2 cm, presumably due to the dilatation of the individual tubules and edema within the kidney itself. In the absence of alternative explanations, a bilateral nephrogram that persists beyond 30 minutes in any patient should be taken as a warning of a possible developing renal insufficiency.

3. *Hypotension.* This may present with increasingly dense bilateral nephrograms without visualization of the collecting structures during the hypotensive episode (Figs. 6–141 and 6–142). As soon as blood pressure returns to normal, the nephrogram rapidly fades and a urogram appears. Hypotension is usually caused by either a reaction to the contrast medium or shock from some other cause (i.e., trauma). The sudden drop in blood pressure results in a severe reduction in glomerular filtration and leads to stasis within the tubules. Salt and water reabsorption continues, concentrating the contrast medium in the tubules. In the previously described prolonged nephrogram seen with protein or crystal precipitation, the kidney was enlarged. In hypo-

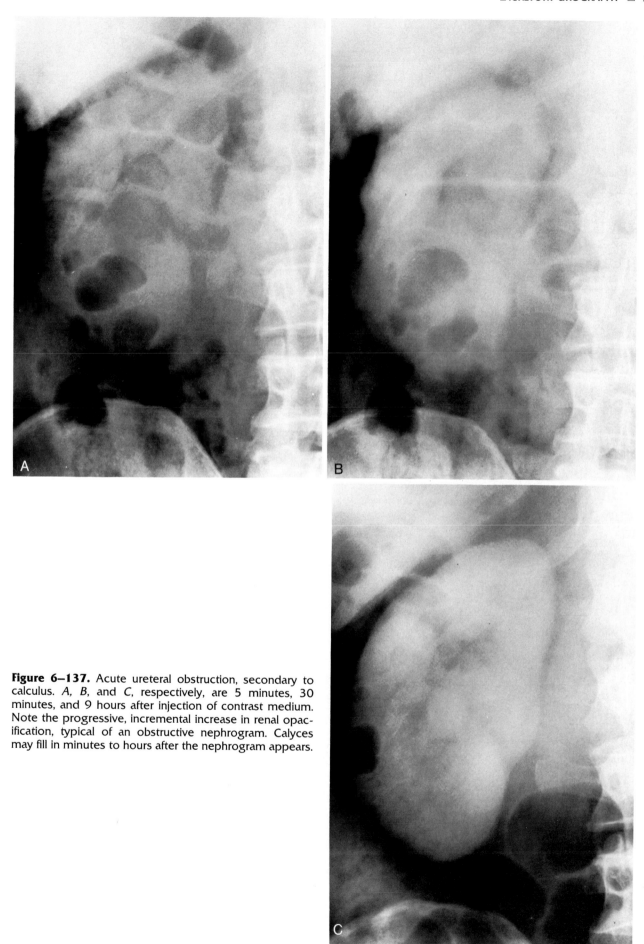

Figure 6–137. Acute ureteral obstruction, secondary to calculus. *A, B,* and *C,* respectively, are 5 minutes, 30 minutes, and 9 hours after injection of contrast medium. Note the progressive, incremental increase in renal opacification, typical of an obstructive nephrogram. Calyces may fill in minutes to hours after the nephrogram appears.

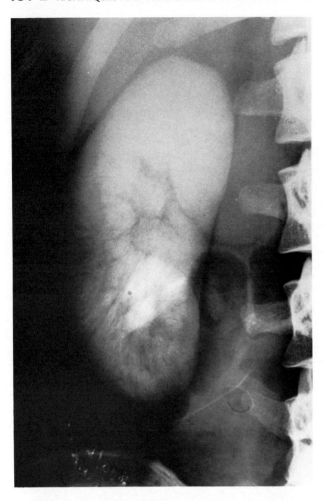

Figure 6–138. Acute obstructive nephrogram; calculus in the ureter. Marked intensity of obstructive nephrogram is obtained at 20 minutes after contrast medium injection. Note the fine linear striations (medullary rays) best seen along the lateral and inferior aspects of the kidney. These represent groups of nephrons containing high concentrations of contrast medium that are separated by areas of interstitial edema.

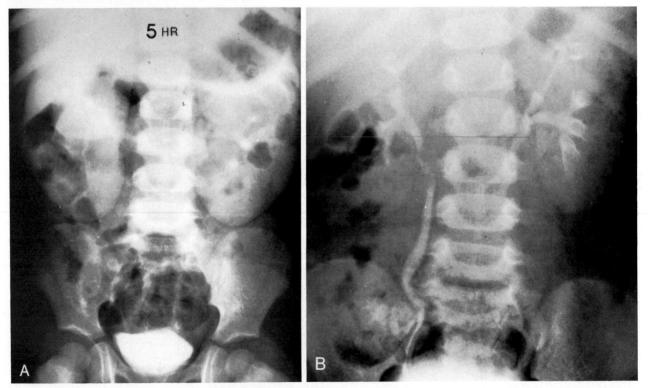

Figure 6–139. *A,* A dehydrated 6-month-old boy received an injection of contrast medium for a urogram. A 5-hour film reveals a persistent nephrogram with huge kidneys, markedly enlarged in the scout film. The obstruction is not complete, as revealed by contrast medium in the bladder. The obstruction, probably attributable to Tamm-Horsfall proteinuria, lasted for 24 hours and was followed by a brisk diuresis. *B,* A repeat urogram, obtained when the patient was well hydrated 2 months later, reveals normal kidneys, about 35% smaller than in the obstructed state.

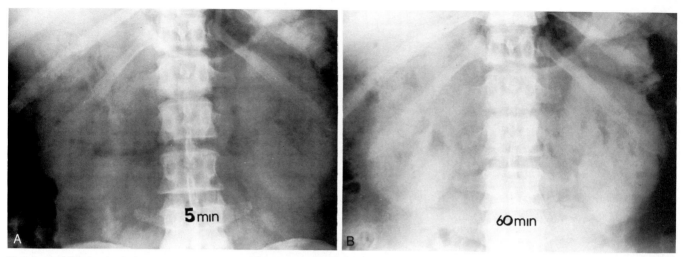

Figure 6–140. Intratubular uric acid precipitation. A 35-year-old man with lymphoma received an injection of contrast medium. The patient had hyperuricemia. Uric acid crystals precipitated within the nephron, producing a complete renal block. Five-minute urogram film (A) and the 60-minute film (B) reveal increasingly dense nephrograms with swollen and enlarged kidneys. The calyces are not visualized. The patient diuresed 48 hours later.

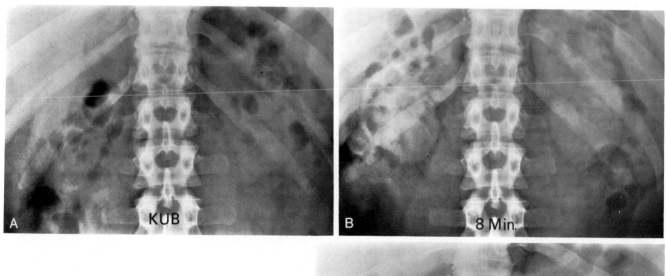

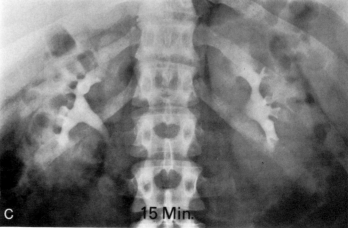

Figure 6–141. Hypotensive nephrogram. Hypotension following injection of contrast medium. The patient received 50 cc of contrast after the scout film (A). A hypotensive episode followed and lasted approximately 10 minutes. A film taken at 8 minutes (B) shows bilateral persistent nephrograms without evidence of calyceal filling. The kidneys are now slightly smaller. Following restoration of blood pressure, a 15-minute film (C) shows good calyceal filling. Both kidneys have increased in size by about 1.5 cm.

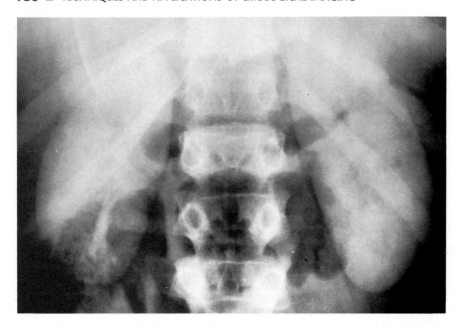

Figure 6–142. A 5-year-old boy who was admitted following an automobile accident. Although conscious, he was markedly hypotensive. The 10-minute film after contrast medium injection shows a bilaterally persistent nephrogram related to his hypotensive episode.

tension, the kidneys are usually smaller during the episode of hypotension because of the reduction in blood flow. If hypotension occurs during the study (reaction to contrast material), the first film may show normal excretion, and later a bilateral hypotensive nephrogram will appear. Similar nephrograms have been reported to develop on a unilateral basis in ischemia. These are usually in patients with hypertension, in whom a unilaterally increased nephrogram occurs due to marked reduction in glomerular filtration on the side of severe ischemia.

4. *Acute renal vein thrombosis.* Acute renal vein thrombosis may result in a unilateral or bilateral nephrogram increasing in density over several hours (Fig. 6–143). It has been suggested that a reduction in renal perfusion may be secondary to increased intrarenal venous pressure, which may produce the dense nephrogram similar to that found in patients with ischemia; or that edema of the kidney may cause intrarenal obstruction due to compression of the tubules by interstitial edema. The mechanism has not been accurately defined.

5. *Acute renal failure.* Occasionally, acute renal failure and acute glomerular disease may initially produce an increasingly dense bilateral nephrogram. In this group the mechanisms are not well understood, and the type of nephrogram that may occur is not predictable.

C. **Faint or decreased nephrogram.** Many conditions may produce a decreased or absent nephrogram (Fig. 6–144). Among these are chronic renal failure, renal

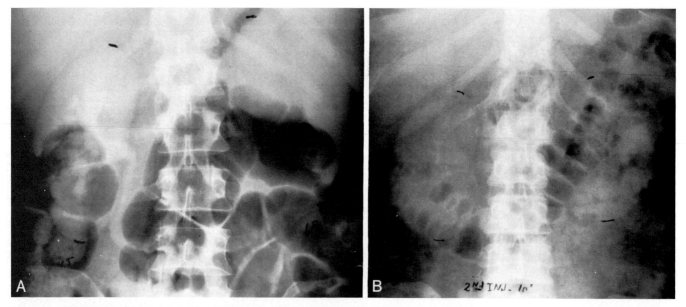

Figure 6–143. Nephrogram in renal vein thrombosis. *A,* A 15-minute film from an excretory urogram in a patient with bilateral renal vein thrombosis shows slight enlargement of both kidneys, bilateral faint nephrograms, and moderate calyceal filling on the right. *B,* A 10-minute film from a urogram in a second patient with renal vein thrombosis shows a mottled faint nephrogram with minimal calyceal filling.

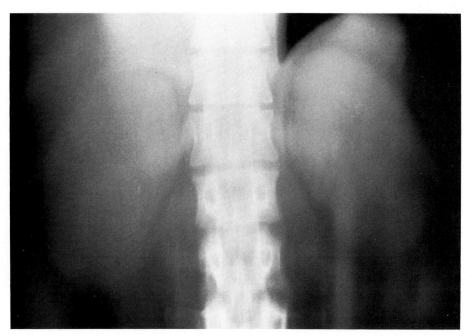

Figure 6–144. Chronic renal failure. Middle-aged man with chronic glomerulonephritis. Following administration of a large bolus of contrast medium, the nephrogram is faint bilaterally without definition of cortex or medullary tissue. The kidneys are slightly smaller than normal. There is no evidence of calyceal opacification.

artery occlusion, renal transplant rejection, acute bacterial pyelonephritis, and longstanding renal obstruction.

Pyramidal Blush

In normal and abnormal conditions, contrast may be seen in the collecting ducts of the pyramid producing a blush or fan effect, particularly when large doses of nonionic contrast medium are utilized[244] (Fig. 6–145). This can be simply classified as follows:

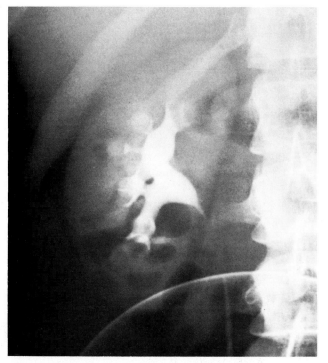

Figure 6–145. Pyramidal blush. It is not uncommon to see contrast within the papilla and pyramid of the normal kidney as an area of increased density or "blush." This is especially notable with tight ureteral compression.

1. Normal: pyramidal blush (caused by large doses of contrast media and/or compression of ureters)
2. Abnormal: obstruction (pyramidal blush, medullary rays); medullary sponge kidney (tubular ectasia)

The pyramidal blush has no clinical significance and, in fact, frequently signifies a well-functioning kidney with good concentrating ability. It does *not* represent pyelotubular "backflow," which in fact cannot be recognized on excretory urography. The normal tubular blush is increased by ureteral compression, which in effect is "normal" partial obstruction (Fig. 6–145). Medullary sponge kidney, which is discussed under Renal Cystic Disease, produces a somewhat similar appearance, owing to ectasia of the collecting ducts, and may be present with or without associated intraductal calculi. The severe cases of medullary sponge kidney are easily defined (Fig. 6–146). In the more minimal cases it may be difficult to differentiate a medullary sponge kidney from a pyramidal blush. A good rule of thumb is to report medullary sponge kidney only when the observer can distinguish individual, defined, linear, radiating, contrast-filled ducts ("brush" appearance) greater than 0.3 mm in diameter.[243] In obstructive lesions, particularly in acute obstruction, groups of nephrons become dilated and produce long, linear, radiating, contrast-filled ducts in the pyramid and through the thickness of the cortex. These have been defined as medullary rays, simply representing dilated nephrons after acute obstruction (see Fig. 6–138). They are not usually confused with pyramidal blush or sponge kidney.

Sinus Lipomatosis

A varying amount of fat and fibrous tissue is always present within the renal sinus extending around the hilum and around the infundibuli to the calyces. It is more prominent in patients with duplicated renal pelves and extrarenal pelves (see Fig. 6–98). The fatty/fibrous tissue usually is bilaterally symmetrical (Fig. 6–147). It is best visualized in tomograms of the urogram and in CT. When the fatty/fibrous tissue increases, the renal pelvis may

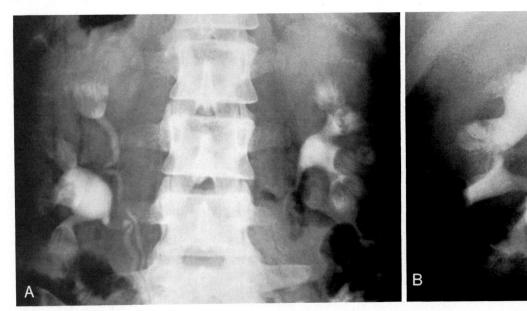

Figure 6–146. Medullary sponge kidney (tubular ectasia). *A*, Ectasia of the collecting ducts produces a linear ("brush") pattern in the papilla and proximal pyramid, in which groups of collecting ducts can be individually distinguished. *B*, The process is more advanced. Small cystic areas can be distinguished in the regions of the collecting ducts containing contrast medium.

appear slightly compressed, and the infundibula appear elongated, stretched, and spread apart. The calyces are thin and frequently "trumpet-like" in appearance. At times the deformity is sufficient to suggest the presence

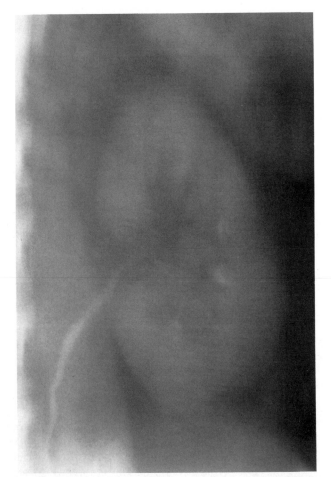

Figure 6–147. Sinus lipomatosis. The tomogram of the urogram demonstrates the extensive sinus fat around the renal pelvis. The fat infiltrates around the infundibula and peripheral calyces.

of one or more parapelvic cysts, a distinction that can readily be made by means of ultrasonography. In fact, many cases previously thought to represent sinus lipomatosis may actually represent parapelvic cysts or localized urinomas. The following is a simple classification of increased renal sinus fat:

A. Symmetrical
  1. Obesity. This is the most common cause of increased sinus fat and may show increases or decreases with changes in weight of the individual. Bilateral increases in sinus fat may also be seen in patients on steroids.
  2. Renal senility. Aging produces gradual atrophy of renal parenchyma, which is replaced by fat in the inner aspects of the kidney. Like obesity, this replacement is relatively symmetrical bilaterally.

B. Asymmetrical sinus lipomatosis
  1. Infection. Chronic infection, particularly when associated with calculi, tends to produce asymmetrical increases in sinus fat and fibrous tissue following destruction of parenchyma (Fig. 6–148). The process, which is also termed "replacement fibrolipomatosis," is usually unilateral and may occur in younger individuals. Occasionally, increased fat and fibrous tissue may simulate a renal mass (Fig. 6–149).

Renal Hyperplasia and Hypertrophy

Compensatory renal growth usually occurs as a response to renal loss. Growth may occur either by hyperplasia (the growth of new cellular elements) or hypertrophy (the enlargement of existing elements). In the newborn, compensatory renal growth consists of both hyperplasia and hypertrophy. In the child and adult, compensatory growth is basically hypertrophy with dilatation occurring primarily in the proximal convoluted tubules. Duplication of the renal pelvis and compensatory renal hypertrophy are the common causes of a unilaterally

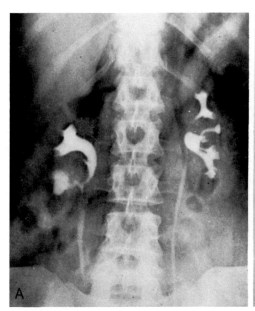
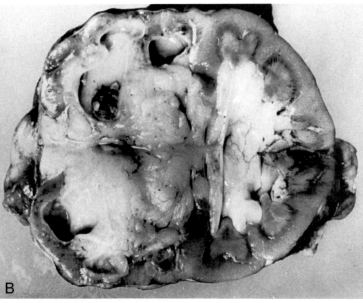

Figure 6–148. Replacement fibrolipomatosis; history of chronic right pyelonephritis with calculi. *A,* Excretory urography demonstrates central mass impression and partial obliteration of right calyceal structures. *B,* Nephrectomy specimen showing massive lipomatosis replacing renal parenchyma centrally. This degree of fatty infiltration is beyond that seen with ordinary sinus lipomatosis. When associated with loss of renal parenchyma, this entity has been termed replacement fibrolipomatosis. (Courtesy Morton Bosniak, M.D.)

enlarged kidney. In children born with unilateral renal agenesis or multicystic dysplastic kidney, compensatory growth of the contralateral kidney will usually produce a unilateral renal mass approximately equal to the total renal mass expected in that infant by the age of 12 to 18 months (Fig. 6–150). Children who have nephrectomies for Wilms' tumor show rapid compensatory growth for approximately 2 years after the tumor is removed. Compensatory renal growth, therefore, is most marked in the

infant, is less in the child, and is minimal in the middle-aged adult (Fig. 6–151). If total renal function is threatened (i.e., loss of 75% of the functioning renal parenchyma), hypertrophy will occur at any age (obligatory hypertrophy), although it is not necessarily radiographically detectable.

Compensatory growth in the contralateral kidney is probably hormone mediated, possibly resulting from renotropin secretion, and represents an attempt to maintain

Figure 6–149. Sinus lipomatosis presenting as a renal mass. *A,* Urogram in a woman with a history of repeated urinary tract infections. Calyces are dilated and there was clinical and radiographic evidence of pyelonephritis. *B,* Repeat urogram 1 year later reveals a mass impinging on the pelvis and upper infundibulum (*arrow*). At surgery this represented asymmetrical proliferating sinus fat secondary to the chronic low-grade infection.

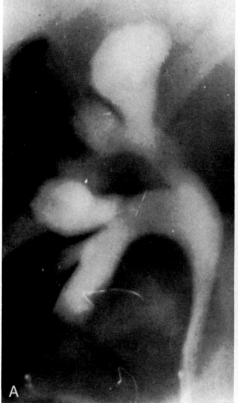
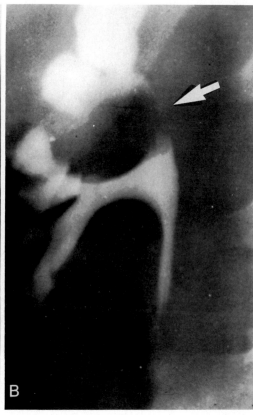

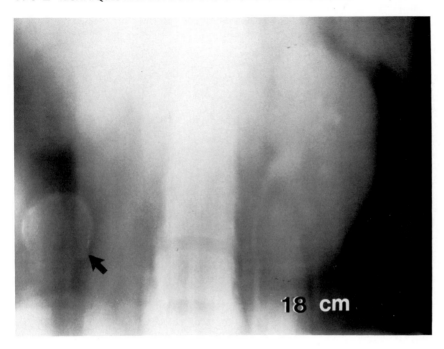

Figure 6–150. Compensatory hypertrophy in patient with contralateral renal dysplasia. This is a right multicystic kidney with calcification (*arrow*). The left kidney measured 18 cm. The kidney is approximately 50% longer than would be expected, and the renal mass is probably close to twice that of the average normal kidney. Compensatory hypertrophy is greater, the earlier in life it occurs.

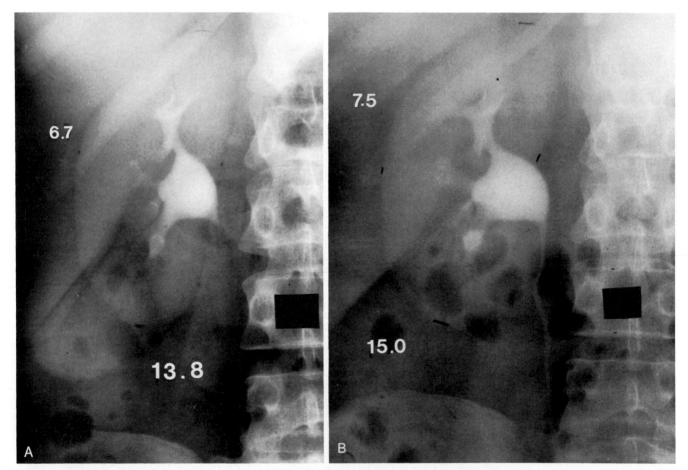

Figure 6–151. Compensatory hypertrophy. *A,* A 55-year-old male with left renal cell carcinoma. The right kidney measures 13.8 cm in length and 6 to 7 cm in width. *B,* Nine years postnephrectomy the length of the right kidney measures 15 cm. Note the increase in transverse diameter, as well, to 7.5 cm. Compensatory hypertrophy is minimal if overall renal function is not threatened in the middle-aged or older adult.

renal mass and function.[34] Renotropin is a serum factor, capable of undergoing dialysis, that stimulates functional and structural elements within proximal convoluted tubules.

Factors reported to stimulate renal growth include renal agenesis, multicystic kidney, nephrectomy, ureteral ligation, acidosis, thyroxine, testosterone, growth hormone, and mineralocorticoids.

In severe focal renal disease (i.e., bilateral pyelonephritis), islands of remaining normal tissue may hypertrophy and simulate mass lesions of the kidney. This is discussed under Pseudotumor (see Figs. 6–161 and 6–162).

Pseudotumor

Pseudotumor refers to normal renal tissue that may mimic an abnormal mass. The term is not usually applied to cysts, hemorrhage, abscess, hydronephrosis, or other specific abnormal lesions of the kidney. Pseudotumors have been reviewed thoroughly by Feldman and colleagues.[112]

Congenital Pseudotumors

Column of Bertin. A prominent, thick column ("cloison") of Bertin projecting into the renal sinus can produce deformities of adjacent calyces and infundibula and an intense "stain" in the angiogram and nephrogram (Figs. 6–152 to 6–154). This is the most common form of pseudotumor, occurring most commonly in patients with bifid or duplicated renal pelves, and it is characteristically located at the junction of the upper and middle thirds of the kidney (Figs. 6–152 and 6–153). It does not produce any bulge on the outer cortex. The radiographic appearance includes the following:

1. Urogram. Usually a double or bifid renal pelvis is seen, with displacement and compression of one or more calyces at the junction of the middle and upper thirds of the kidney.

2. Nephrogram. A dense blush in a masslike nodule of cortical tissue appears and fades at the same time as the cortical nephrogram. Since it projects into the renal sinus, it is usually surrounded on its medial, superior, and inferior aspects by a radiolucent halo of sinus fat (Fig. 6–152).

3. Angiogram. Displacement of normal vessels is seen, without any neovasculature.

When a patient presents with microscopic hematuria and a suggestive mass at the junction of the upper and middle thirds of the kidney, the simplest method for diagnosing pseudotumor is to perform a radionuclide renal scan. If the lesion is over 2 cm in size, the scan will show that it is composed of normal functioning tissue (see

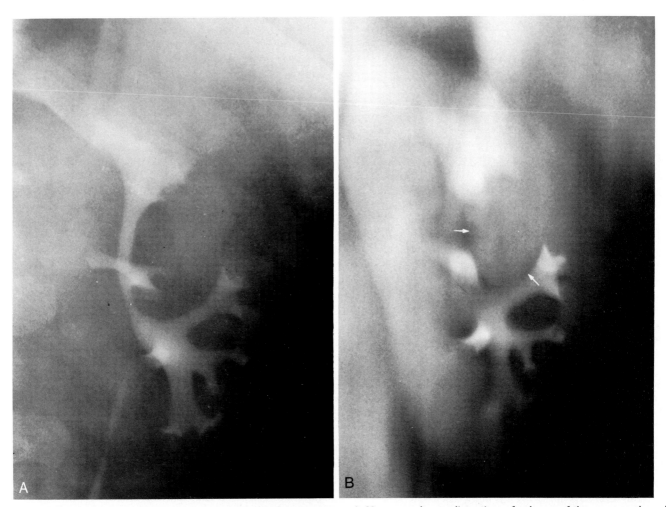

Figure 6–152. Column of Bertin pseudotumor, typical appearance. *A*, Urogram shows distortion of calyces of the upper calyceal system. *B*, Tomogram shows a large column of Bertin projecting between the upper and middle calyceal system, displacing calyces medially. A halo can be seen around the central two-thirds of the column where it presses into the sinus fat (*arrows*).

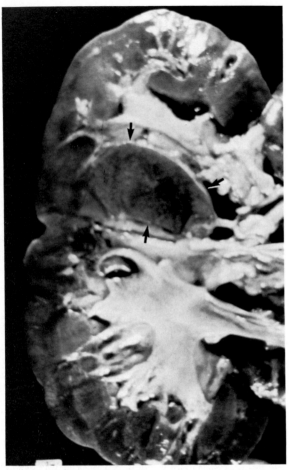

Figure 6–153. Renal specimen showing a typical large column of Bertin projecting into the renal sinus fat in a double collecting system and compressing adjacent calyces (*arrows*). The column typically occurs at the junction of the upper and middle third of the kidney, most often in bifid or double renal pelves.

Figs. 6–39 and 6–154). If the lesion represents tumor, the area will be identified as a photopenic defect in the scan (see Fig. 6–41). CT and MRI are more expensive but equally reliable methods of confirming the diagnosis. They are best employed only in equivocal cases.

Suprahilar or Infrahilar Bulges. The suprahilar and infrahilar areas frequently present with an overgrowth of normal parenchyma that may mimic a mass just above or below the hilus (Figs. 6–155 and 6–156). Infrahilar bulges appear to be more common than suprahilar ones. Large hilar pseudotumors may occasionally be associated with an accessory artery (Fig. 6–157). Hilar pseudotumors are identified at presentation as normal renal tissue, in a manner similar to that of the column of Bertin.

Cortical Dysmorphism. Variation in renal lobe formation may simulate an abnormal mass, most commonly on the lateral aspect of the kidney. Misplaced pyramids surrounded by cortex may produce bizarre configurations (Figs. 6–157 to 6–159).

Fetal Lobation. Asymmetrical fetal lobation that occurs at the demarcation of only one or two lobes of the kidney may occasionally mimic a pseudotumor (see Figs. 6–64, 6–65, and 6–124).

Dromedary Hump. This has been discussed previously. Like other pseudotumors, it can usually be confirmed by scintigraphy.

Aberrant Papilla. An ectopic papilla may project into the renal pelvis or an infundibulum, mimicking a filling defect in the collecting system (see Fig. 6–104). If tangential films are obtained, the papilla may be visualized as an extraluminal pyramid-shaped mass impinging upon the collecting system (Fig. 6–160). It is usually surrounded by an opaque halo, corresponding to the circular calyceal fornix.

Acquired Pseudotumor

Kidneys affected by severe focal disease such as reflux nephropathy frequently have islands of unaffected parenchyma adjacent to the renal lesions. The residual normal parenchyma may mimic a mass lesion producing displacement or impression on neighboring calyces (Figs. 6–161 and 6–162). If the lesions are bilateral or the opposite kidney is diseased, overall renal function may be threatened and hypertrophy of the remaining parenchyma may result. In both cases, a radionuclide renal scan can define the masslike lesion as normal tissue.

Vascular Impressions

Intrarenal and extrarenal vascular impressions are quite common and fortunately are usually readily recognized. Intrarenal vascular impressions are commonly seen on the upper infundibulum and renal pelvis (Figs. 6–163 and 6–164). Baum and Gillenwater[159] reported 42 patients with such defects resulting from pressure from normal renal arteries. They listed the most common defects as follows:

1. Crossing defect on the superior infundibulum—42%
2. Extrinsic impression on the infundibulum simulating mass—26%
3. Filling defect in the renal pelvis—12%
4. Crossing defect of the renal pelvis—14%
5. Arterial impression at the ureteropelvic junction—6%

Larger defects upon the superior infundibulum and pelvis may be produced by crossing veins (Fig. 6–165). Vascular impressions on the renal pelvis may mimic an intraluminal lesion, particularly when the artery presses on the posterior aspect of the renal pelvis (Figs. 6–165 and 6–166; see also Fig. 6–159). Hematuria may be associated with vascular impressions presumably resulting from congestion of the local mucosa from pressure. Occasionally, crossing defects and the collecting system may be so intimate that partial obstruction may result. In these instances, pain is produced, particularly during times of diuresis with distention of the collecting system distal to the impression. Fraley described such a sequence in the upper infundibulum in 1966.[184] The upper infundibulum appears to be the most common site of both impressions and the occasional case of partial obstruction.

Extrarenal vascular impressions are common in anomalies and in the presence of multiple renal arteries. Multiple renal arteries occur in 20% to 30% of kidneys. The great majority supply the lower-pole segment. This may produce an impression near the ureteropelvic junction. Accessory or multiple extrarenal arteries usually do not cause obstruction unless other factors such as fixation of the ureter, nephroptosis, or associated bands are

Text continued on page 201

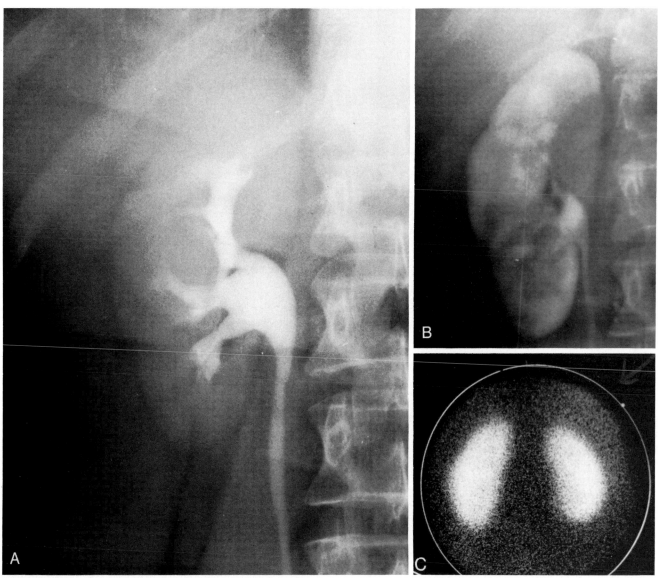

Figure 6–154. Middle-aged man presenting with microscopic hematuria. *A*, The urogram shows displacement of upper and middle calyces in the middle third of the right kidney. *B*, An arteriogram was performed showing a very large intense "stain" equaling the density of the cortical nephrogram projecting into the junction of the middle and upper thirds of the kidney. This was believed to be a pseudotumor. *C*, A technetium-99m DMSA scan shows excellent visualization of the right kidney without evidence of a photopenic area, confirming the diagnosis of pseudotumor.

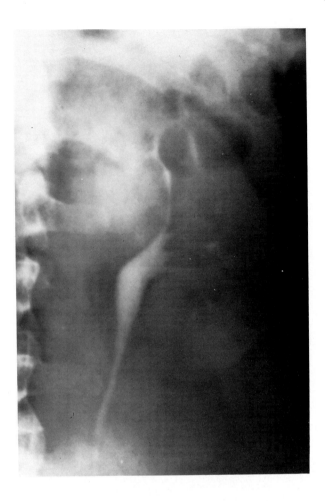

Figure 6–155. Suprahilar pseudotumor. An overgrowth of the renal parenchyma in the suprahilar area impresses the upper infundibulum laterally. The density of this area is similar to that of the remainder of the cortical nephrogram. Cortical overgrowth in the suprahilar and infrahilar areas ("uncus") is common.

Figure 6–156. Infrahilar pseudotumor. Lobular mass projecting from the kidney in the region of the infrahilar area represents a cortical pseudotumor.

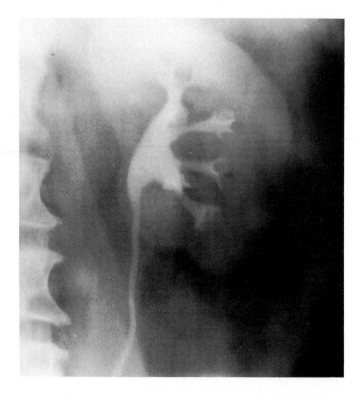

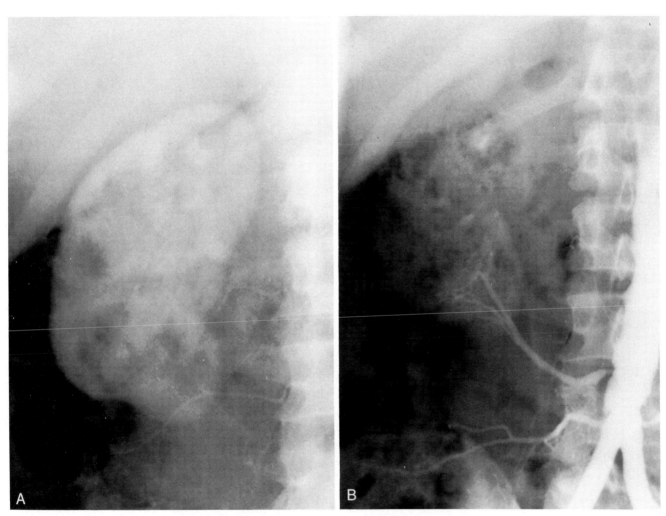

Figure 6–157. Cortical dysmorphism. *A*, Bizarre projection from the region of the infrahilar area of the right kidney suggests a renal lobe (a pyramid surrounded by cortex). *B*, Aortogram reveals this area to be supplied by an accessory vessel.

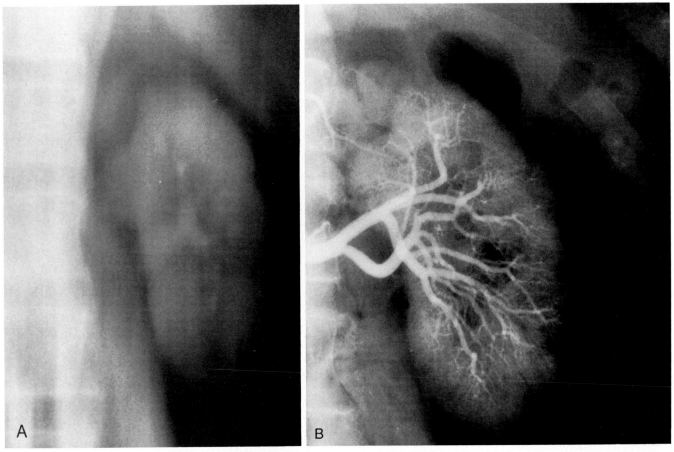

Figure 6–158. Cortical dysmorphism pseudotumor. *A,* Lobular projection of renal parenchyma extending medial to the upper pole of the left kidney is seen in the tomogram. *B,* Renal arteriogram shows the projection of renal parenchyma from the medial aspect of the upper pole. The vascular structures supplying it are normal vessels similar to those of the rest of the cortex.

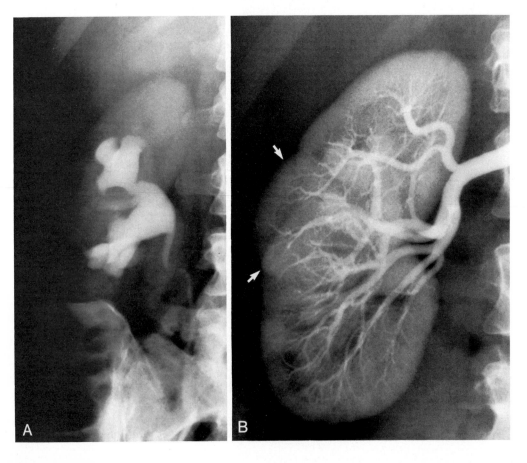

Figure 6–159. Cortical dysmorphism pseudotumor. Middle-aged patient presenting with microscopic hematuria. *A,* Urogram shows poor filling of a middle calyx. *B,* Renal arteriogram shows a dysmorphic lobe (*arrows*), which is pressing on the calyx and projecting as a hump from the kidney.

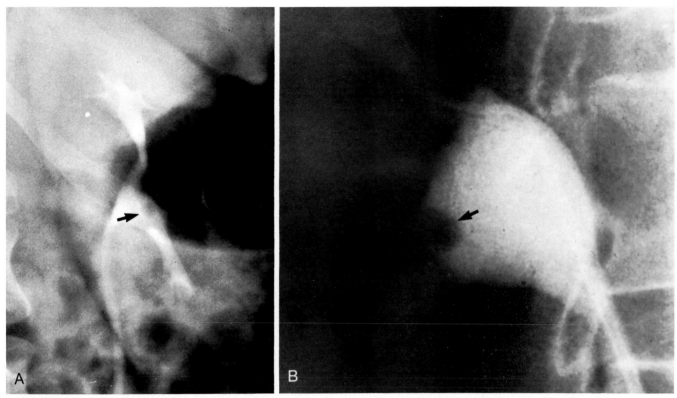

Figure 6–160. *A, B,* Two examples of ectopic papillae projecting into the renal pelvis (*arrows*). An ectopic papilla may mimic a filling defect in the collecting system. This is another form of pseudotumor that represents normal renal tissue presenting as a defect in the collecting system.

Figure 6–161. Acquired pseudotumor (nodular hypertrophy). Late film from the angiogram in a patient with longstanding chronic atrophic pyelonephritis reveals the right kidney to be small with thin cortical margins. A residual area of normal cortical tissue is not affected by the focal infection, which presents as a mass lesion—a pseudotumor (*arrow*).

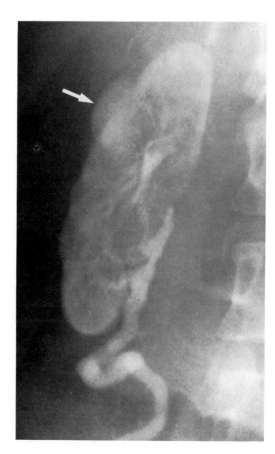

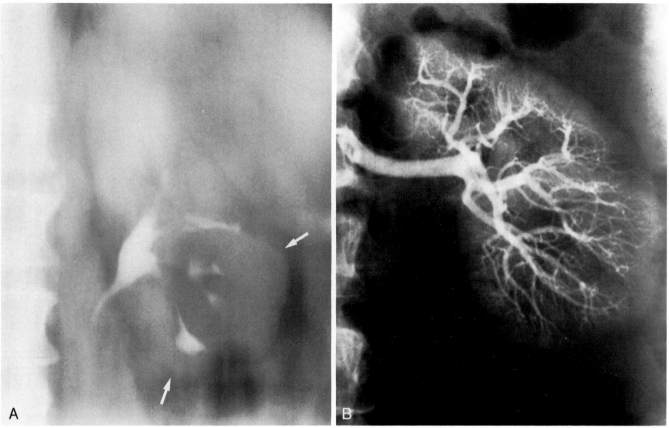

Figure 6–162. Acquired pseudotumor. The patient has a longstanding history of chronic pyelonephritis that has affected both poles and the upper middle portion of the left kidney. *A,* The tomogram reveals a masslike lesion in the lower pole (*arrows*), displacing the middle and lower calyceal systems. *B,* The renal arteriogram shows normal vascularity in this region. This represents residual normal parenchymal tissue that is unaffected by the chronic pyelonephritis, which has attenuated the remainder of the kidney.

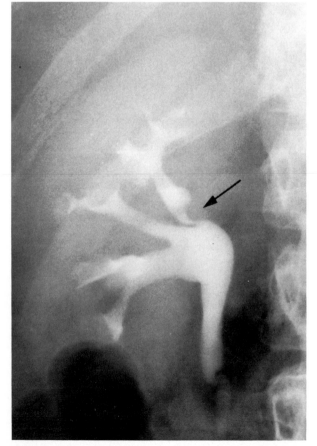

Figure 6–163. Vascular impression. Urogram demonstrates a notchlike defect on the base of the superior infundibulum (*arrow*), typical of the defects produced by crossing vessels.

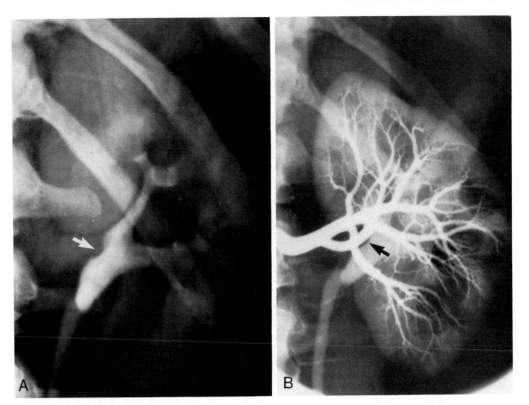

Figure 6–164. Patient presenting with microscopic hematuria. *A*, Urogram reveals a defect on the medial aspect of the renal pelvis (*arrow*) suspicious of a tumor of the renal pelvis. *B*, Angiogram shows that the wall of the renal pelvis is impressed by a branch of the renal artery (*arrow*), which is responsible for the defect seen in the urogram.

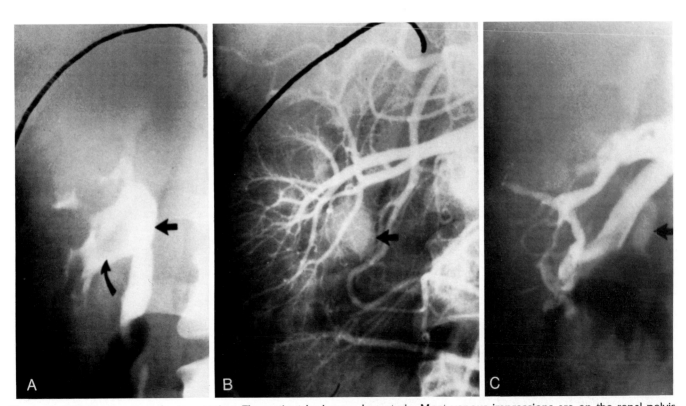

Figure 6–165. Venous vascular impression. The patient had gross hematuria. Most venous impressions are on the renal pelvis. *A*, A defect in the renal pelvis simulates a pelvic tumor (*arrows*). *B*, Angiogram shows that the arterial vessels do not contribute to the vascular defect. The arrow points to the partially filled renal pelvis. *C*, Phlebogram. A branch of the renal vein crosses directly over the renal pelvis, impressing it at that point. Arrow points to the medial margin of the renal pelvis with the vein producing the defect seen originally. (Courtesy A. J. Palubinskas, M.D.)

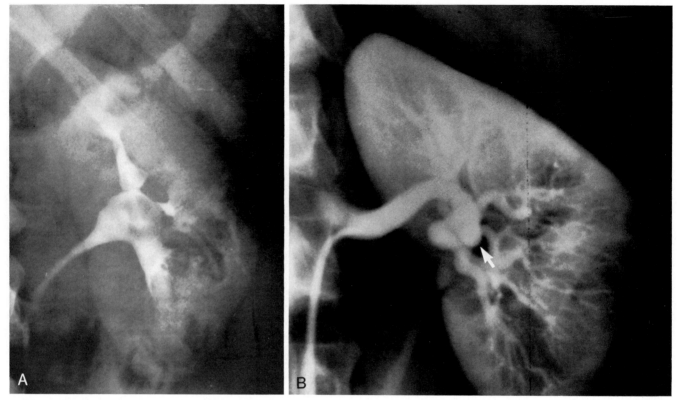

Figure 6–166. Vascular defect mimicking intraluminal lesion in a patient presenting with microscopic hematuria. *A,* Urogram reveals a large irregular filling defect occupying the central area of the renal pelvis. *B,* Arteriogram demonstrates a knuckle of the tortuous renal artery (*arrow*) protruding into the posterior aspect of the renal pelvis, producing the radiolucent defect originally seen.

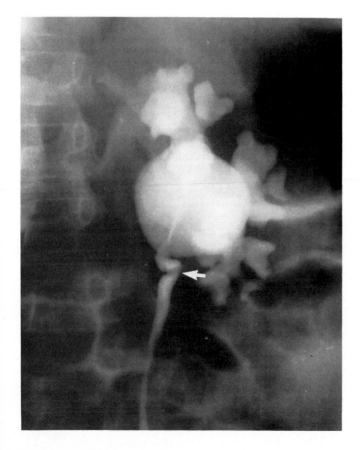

Figure 6–167. Vascular impression on proximal ureter. A linear transverse crossing defect is produced by an accessory artery (*arrow*), in this instance associated with partial proximal obstruction. At surgery, a congenital band was found fixing the ureter. The band, rather than the crossing vessel, was responsible for the obstruction.

present (Fig. 6–167). Veins as well as arteries may produce extrinsic defects on the ureter or outer margins of the pelvis. It is usually not difficult to distinguish vascular impressions from intraluminal filling defects. Usually, oblique views clearly demonstrate the extrinsic nature of vascular crossings, whereas abdominal compression or retrograde pyelography shows the extrinsic defects to be effaced with collecting system distention.

Pyelosinus Backflow

The different types of backflow were described in the 1930s, in connection with retrograde studies. Of the various types (pyelosinus, pyelotubular, pyelovenous, and pyelolymphatic), pyelosinus is the most common. Pyelosinus backflow, which results from fornix rupture, is occasionally encountered during urography and probably represents a physiological release mechanism to reduce the intrapelvic pressure in the acutely obstructed renal collecting system (Figs. 6–168 and 6–169). Fornix rupture may result from the use of ureteral compression as well as from pathological obstruction. Rarely, pyelolymphatic backflow can be recognized during urography (Fig. 6–170).

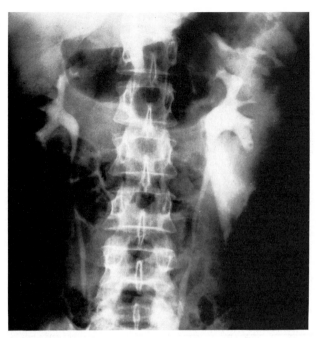

Figure 6–169. Pyelosinus extravasation from the fornices of the calyces extends out through the renal pelvis into the perinephric space. Note that the contrast remains lateral to the psoas margin and does not extend down to the iliac crest. It is confined within the perinephric space.

Bladder and Urethra

A question frequently asked is whether the bladder and urethra can be evaluated following the urogram.[231] A routine postvoid film (10 × 12) of the bladder area is frequently obtained in men over 60 years old to estimate residual urine. This study is valuable, providing that (1) the patient has totally voided as much as possible and (2) the film is obtained within 3 minutes after the patient has voided. Frequently, patients are kept waiting 20 or 30 minutes for their postvoiding film, which allows significant accumulation of urine in the bladder. There is no reason for routine postvoiding films in women who have no specific voiding problems.

In a small but significant number of children and a lesser number of adults, a good cystourethrogram can be obtained posturography. If the density of contrast medium in the bladder is sufficient, the procedure may be attempted. In our experience, in cooperative children with voiding problems who have a urogram for other reasons, a cystourethrogram should be attempted to avoid the need for catheterization. If the patient is going to be catheterized or if the examination is specifically for the bladder and urethra, a routine voiding cystourethrogram (VCU) should be performed. One of the disadvantages of the posturographic VCU is the uncertainty of determining vesicoureteral reflux.

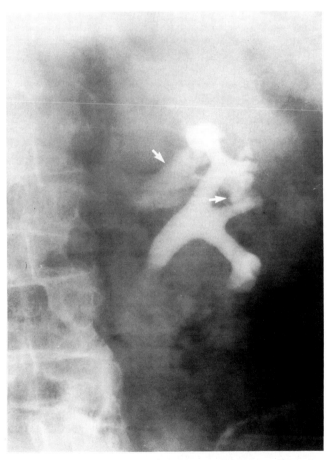

Figure 6–168. Patient with partially obstructing nonopaque calculus in the upper ureter. Marked diuresis follows the intravenous injection of contrast medium, dilating the collecting system and increasing the intrapelvic pressure. Pyelosinus extravasation (*arrows*) occurs at multiple sites, relieving the high intrapelvic pressure.

RISK FACTORS IN UROGRAPHY

The adverse effects of contrast media have been described in detail in the section on Contrast Media. The following is a brief analysis of the major risk factors, which, if present in a given individual, may increase the

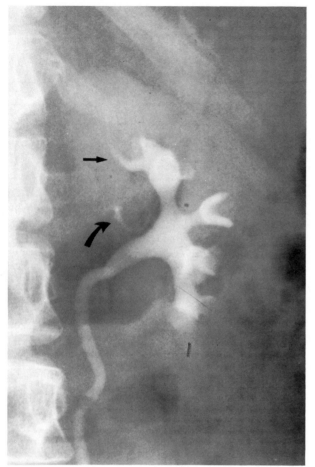

Figure 6–170. Pyelolymphatic backflow during excretory urography. A 10-minute film reveals fornix rupture adjacent to upper-pole calyx (*arrow*) with opacification of hilar lymphatics (*curved arrow*). This was believed to be attributable to excessively tight ureteral compression.

reactions associated with the intravenous injection of contrast media in common use today. The new contrast media (dimers and nonionic) produce fewer reactions than do our current ionic agents.

Dehydration

Dehydrated patients have a far greater tendency toward renal shutdown, secondary to intratubular obstruction by precipitation of proteins or crystals. Children, particularly, are affected. Renal shutdown is associated with the increasingly intense nephrogram described previously. In most instances, the precipitating protein is Tamm-Horsfall, the only protein produced by the kidney. Patients with multiple myeloma and hyperuricemia, as well as those receiving poorly soluble sulfa drugs, are also prone to intratubular block when dehydrated.

Diabetics with Azotemia

Diabetic patients with mild to moderate azotemia are particularly prone to nephrotoxic contrast media effects. It has been stated that approximately 1 in 2000 patients with diabetes and azotemia will develop renal shutdown

following contrast medium administration. The mechanism of the renal failure is not clearly understood. It does not appear to be significantly influenced by hydration.

Cardiac Decompensation

Patients with cardiac decompensation should not be examined when in cardiac failure. The hyperosmotic contrast medium will intensify the congestive failure, and in addition there is a greater likelihood of azotemia.[78] Patients with compensated heart failure requiring urography are probably best studied with the meglumine rather than with the sodium-containing agents.

Allergic History

Patients with an allergic history have approximately a twofold increase in reactions. It is not clear, however, whether this increased risk applies to life-threatening reactions.

Previous Reactions to Contrast Media

Patients with a history of previous reactions to similar contrast media have a three-times-greater chance for reaction following subsequent injection. The reaction is usually not more severe than the original reaction. Patients who have had a previous life-threatening reaction should be re-examined with caution. The indications for the examination should be very clear, anesthesia should be available, and a physician should be with the patient throughout the examination. Patients with such previous reactions often have no reaction on re-examination. Pretreatment with steroids and the use of nonionic agents should be considered. This topic is discussed in more detail in Chapter 4.

Renal Failure

Ordinarily, the triage examination for renal failure should be ultrasonography. The usual reason for examination is to exclude hydronephrosis. If contrast medium is used, it is frequently necessary to increase the dose to obtain a useful degree of visualization. In such cases there is usually at least a temporary increase in BUN and creatinine. If the urogram is believed to be clinically necessary, tomograms obtained 2 or 3 minutes after an injection of 1.5 to 2 cc/kg of contrast medium and a subsequent 5-minute film may visualize the collecting system. No arbitrary level of serum creatinine is established, above which the urogram has no diagnostic value. In general, the higher the creatinine level, the less likely is the urogram to be helpful. This will vary with the cause of the azotemia to some extent. For example, in obstructive uropathy delayed visualization with eventual pooling of the contrast to the level of obstruction is seen often, even with relatively high levels of creatinine. However, this is not so with renal parenchymal disease. The serum creatinine is not always a reliable barometer of urographic quality, because it varies greatly with muscle mass, state of hydration, and so forth. As a rule of thumb, urography is probably wasteful in patients with medicorenal disease whose creatinine level is above 4.0 mg/dl.

Recent Contrast Studies

Patients who have undergone multiple contrast studies, such as CT, angiography, and oral cholecystography, on consecutive days immediately before urography may be at risk for contrast nephropathy if the study is done without an intervening rest period of 1 or 2 days. During this time, suitable hydration should be carried out.

Acknowledgment

The author thanks the J. B. Lippincott Company for permission to use many illustrations from Ney C, Friedenberg RM: Radiographic Atlas of the Genitourinary System, 2 Ed., 1981.

References

Embryology

1. Baum S, Gillenwater JY: Renal artery impressions on the renal pelvis. J Urol 95:139–145, 1986.
2. Cook IK, Keats TE, Seale DL: Determination of the normal position of the upper urinary tract on the lateral abdominal urogram. Radiology 99:499–502, 1971.
3. Felix W: The development of the urogenital organs. In Keibel F, Mall FP (eds): Manual of Human Embryology, Vol II. Philadelphia, JB Lippincott Co, 1912.
4. Fraser EA: The pronephros and early development of the mesonephros in the cat. J Anat 54:287–304, 1920.
5. Frimann-Dahl J: Normal variations of the left kidney: An anatomical and radiologic study. Acta Radiol 55:207–216, 1961.
6. Gruenwald, P: The normal changes in the position of the embryonic kidney. Anat Res 85:163, 1943.
7. Gruenwald P: The relation of the growing mullerian duct to the wolffian duct and its importance for the genesis of malformations. Anat Rec 81:1, 1941.
8. Hodson CJ: The lobar structure of the kidney. Br J Urol 44:246–261, 1972.
9. Hodson CJ, Drewe JA, Karn MN, King A: Renal size in normal children. Arch Dis Child 37:616–622, 1962.
10. Meyers, MA: The reno-alimentary relationship: Anatomic roentgen study of their clinical significance. Am J Nephrol 123:386–400, 1975.
11. Sykes D: The arterial supply of the human kidney with special reference to accessory renal arteries. Br J Surg 50:368–374, 1963.
12. Sykes D: The correlation between renal vascularization and lobulation of the kidneys. Br J Urol 36:549, 1964.
13. Torrey TW: The early development of the human nephros. Contrib Embryol Carnegie Inst Wash 35:175–197, 1954.

Compensatory and Obligatory Hypertrophy

14. Boner G, Sherry J, Rieselback RE: Hypertrophy of the human kidney following contralateral nephrectomy. Nephron 9:364–370, 1972.
15. Eklof O, Lax I, Lundell G, et al: Renoprival growth following treatment of unilateral Wilms' tumor. Acta Radiol [Diagn] (Stockh) 25:231–236, 1984.
16. Eklof O, Ringertz H: Kidney size and growth in unilateral renal agenesis in the remaining kidney following nephrectomy for Wilms' tumor. Acta Radiol [Diagn] (Stockh) 17:601–605, 1976.
17. Fine L: The biology of renal hypertrophy. Kidney Int 29:619–634, 1986.
18. Fleck C, Braunlich H: Kidney function after unilateral nephrectomy. Exp Pathol 25:3–18, 1984.
19. Galla JH, Klein-Robenhaar T, Hayslett JP: Influence of age on the compensatory response in growth and function to unilateral nephrectomy. Yale J Biol Med 47:218–226, 1974.
20. Lafortune M, Constantin A, Breton G, Vallee C: Sonography of the hypertrophic column of Bertin. AJR 146:53–56, 1986.
21. Laufer I, Griscom NT: Compensatory renal hypertrophy. Absence in utero and development in early life. AJR 113:464–467, 1971.
22. Lytton B, Schiff M, Bloom N: Compensatory renal growth: Evidence for a tissue-specific factor of renal origin. J Urol 101:648–652, 1969.
23. Lapson JS, Owen JP, Robson RA, et al: Compensatory renal hypertrophy after donor nephrectomy. Clin Radiol 36:307–310, 1985.
24. Laufer I, Griscom NT: Compensatory renal hypertrophy. Absence in utero and development in early life. AJR 113:464–467, 1971.
25. Leekam RN, Matzinger MA, Brunelle M, et al: The sonography of renal columnar hypertrophy. J Clin Ultrasound 11:491–491, 1983.
26. Lytton B, Schiff M, Bloom N: Compensatory renal growth: Evidence for a tissue-specific factor of renal origin. J Urol 101:648–652, 1969.
27. Martinez LO, Frances DA, Schilling KJ, Cohen BM: Diagnosis of polar hypertrophy of the kidney revisited. Mt Sinai J Med (NY) 51:697–701, 1984.
28. Monn E, Nordshus T: Hereditary renal dysplasia. Acta Paediatr Scand 73:278–80, 1984.
29. Morag B, Rubinstein ZJ, Itzchak Y: Computerized tomography in the evaluation of localized renal cortical hypertrophy. J Urol 130:438–439, 1983.
30. Orecklin JR, Craven JD, Lecky JW: Compensatory renal hypertrophy: A morphologic study in transplant donors. J Urol 109:952–954, 1973.
31. Prando A, Pereira RM, Marins JL: Sonographic evaluation of hypertrophy of septum of Bertin. Urology 24:505–510, 1984.
32. Segel MC, Lecky JW, Slosky BS: Diabetes mellitus: The predominant cause of bilateral renal enlargement. Radiology 153:341–342, 1984.
33. Shames D, Murphy JJ, Berkowitz H: Evidence for a humoral factor in unilaterally nephrectomized dogs stimulating renal growth in isolated canine kidneys. Surgery 79:573–576, 1976.
34. Silber SJ: Compensatory and obligatory renal growth in babies and adults. Aust NZ J Surg 44:421–423, 1974.
35. Silber SJ, Malvin RL: Compensatory and obligatory renal growth in rats. Am J Physiol 226:114–117, 1974.
36. Wikstad I, Pettersson B, Elinder G, Aperia A: A comparative study of size and function of the remnant kidney in patients nephrectomized in childhood for Wilms' tumor and hydronephrosis. Acta Paediatr Scand 75:408–414, 1986.

Contrast Media

37. Ansell G: Adverse reactions to contrast agents. Scope of problems. Invest Radiol 5:374–391, 1970.
38. Ansell G, Tweedie MCK, West CR, et al: The current status of reactions to intravenous contrast media. Invest Radiol (suppl)15:S32, 1980.
39. Assen ESK, Bray K: The release of histamine from human basophils by radiological contrast agents. Br J Radiol 56:647, 1983.
40. Baltzer G, Kuni H, Dombrowski H, et al: Investigations on renal function during and after intravenous administration of contrast media. Urol Nephrol 1:127, 1969.
41. Bartley O, Bengtsson U, Cederbom G: Renal function before and after urography and angiography with large doses of contrast media. Acta Radiol [Diagn] (Stockh) 8:9, 1969.
42. Benness GT: Urographic contrast agents. A comparison of sodium and methylglucamine salts. Clin Radiol 21:150–156, 1970.
43. Bettmann MA, Morris TW: Recent advances in contrast agents. Radiol Clin North Am 24:347–357, 1986.
44. Brasch RC: Allergic reactions to contrast media: Accumulated evidence. AJR 134:797, 1980.
45. Cattell WR: Excretory pathways for contrast media. Invest Radiol 5:473, 1970.
46. Cattell WR, Fry IK, Spencer AG, et al: Excretion urography. I. Factors determining excretion of Hypaque. Br J Radiol 40:561–571, 1967.
47. Fry IK, Cattell WR, Spencer AG, et al: Excretion urography. II. The relation between Hypaque excretion and the intravenous urogram. Br J Radiol 40:572, 1967.
48. Davidson AJ, Becker J, Rothfield NM: An evaluation of the effect of high dosage urography in previously impaired renal and hepatic function in man. Radiology 97:249–254, 1970.
49. Davies P, Roberts MB, Roylance J: Acute reactions to urographic contrast media. Br J Med 2:434, 1975.
50. Diaz-Buxo JA, Wagoner RD, Hattery RR, et al: Acute renal failure after excretory urography in diabetic patients. Ann Intern Med 83:155–158, 1975.
51. Dure-Smith P: The dose of contrast medium in intravenous urography: A physiologic assessment. AJR 108:691–697, 1970.
52. Fischer HW: Catalog of intravascular contrast media. Special report. Radiology 159:561–563, 1986.

53. Fischer HW, Doust VL: An evaluation of pretesting in the problem of serious and fatal reactions to excretory urography. Radiology 103:497–501, 1972.

54. Fortune JB, Brahme J, Mulligan M, Wachtel TL: Emergency intravenous pyelography in the trauma patient. A reexamination of the indications. Arch Surg 120:1056–1059, 1985.

55. Gooding CA, Berdon WE, Brodeur AE, et al: Adverse reactions to intravenous pyelography in children. AJR Rad Ther Nucl Med 123:802–804, 1975.

56. Greganti MA, Flowers WM Jr: Acute pulmonary edema after the intravenous administration of contrast media. Radiology 132:583, 1979.

57. Kawada TK: Iohexol and iopamidol: Second-generation nonionic radiographic contrast media. Drug Intell Clin Pharm 19:525–529, 1985.

58. Kelly M, Golman K: Metabolism of urographic contrast media. Invest Radiol 16:159, 1981.

59. Kleinknecht D, Deloux J, Homberg JC: Acute renal failure after intravenous urography: Detection of antibodies against contrast media. Clin Nephrol 2:116–119, 1974.

60. Lalli AF: Urographic contrast media reactions and anxiety. Radiology 112:267–271, 1974.

61. Lang EK, Foreman J, Schlegel JU, et al: The incidence of contrast medium induced acute tubular necrosis following arteriography. A preliminary report. Radiology 138:203, 1981.

62. Lieberman P, Siegle RL, Treadwell G: Radiocontrast reactions. Clin Rev Allergy 4:229–245, 1986.

63. McClennan BL, Becker JA: Excretory urography: Choice of contrast material. Clin Radiol 100:591–595, 1971.

64. Morris TW, Fischer HW: The pharmacology of intravascular radiocontrast media. Annu Rev Pharmacol Toxicol 26:143–60, 1986.

65. Olin T: Adverse reactions to intravascularly administered contrast media. Acta Radiol [Diagn] (Stockh) 27:257–263, 1986.

66. Owen JP, Keir MJ, Lambolle AK, et al: Comparative study of the sodium salts of iodamide and iothalamate in clinical urography. Clin Radiol 34:353–357, 1983.

67. Pfister RC, Yoder IC, Hutter AM, et al: The effect of intravenous urography on cardiac rhythm and ischaemia. The 60th Scientific Assembly & Annual Meeting, the Radiological Society of North America, Chicago, December 5, 1974.

68. Shehadi WH: Adverse reactions to intravascularly administered contrast media. AJR 124:145–152, 1975.

69. Shehadi WH: Contrast media adverse reactions: Occurrence, recurrence and distribution patterns. Radiology 143:11, 1982.

70. Siegle RL: Current problems of contrast materials. Invest Radiol 21:779–81, 1986.

71. Spataro RF: Newer contrast agents for urography. Radiol Clin North Am 22:365, 1984.

72. Spataro RF, Katzenberg RW, Fischer HW, McMannis MJ: High-dose clinical urography with the low osmolality contrast agent Hexabrix: Comparison with a conventional contrast agent. Radiology 162(Pt1):9–14, 1987.

73. Stanley RJ, Pfister RC: Bradycardia and hypotension following use of intravenous contrast media. Radiology 121:5, 1976.

74. Velchik MG: Radionuclide imaging of the urinary tract. Urol Clin North Am 12:603–631, 1985.

75. Witten DM, Hirsch FD, Hartman GW: Acute reactions to urographic contrast medium. AJR Rad Ther Nucl Med 119:832–840, 1973.

76. McClennan BL: Low osmolality contrast media: Premises and promises. Radiology 162:1, 1987.

77. Sovak M: Radiocontrast Agents. New York, Springer-Verlag, 1984, p 136.

78. Talierico CP, Vlietstra RE, Fisher LD, Burnett JC: Risks for renal dysfunction with cardiac angiography. Ann Intern Med 104:501, 1986.

78a. Jacobsson BF, Jorulf H, Kalantar MS, Narasimham DL: Nonionic vs ionic contrast media in intravenous urography: Clinical trial in 1,000 consecutive patients. Radiology 167:601, 1988.

78b. Evens RG: Low-osmolality contrast media: Good news or bad? Radiology 169:277, 1988.

Nephrogram

79. Anigstein IR, Elkin M, Roland P, et al: The obstructive nephrogram—microradiologic studies. Invest Radiol 72:24–32, 1972.

80. Berdon WE, Schwartz RH, Becker J, et al: Tamm-Horsfall proteinuria—its relationship to prolonged nephrogram in infants and children and to renal failure following intravenous urography in adults with multiple myeloma. Radiology 92:714–722, 1969.

81. Bosniak MA: Nephrotomography: A relatively unappreciated but extremely valuable diagnostic tool. Radiology 113:313–321, 1970.

82. Coel MV, Talner LB: Obstructive nephrogram due to renal vein thrombosis. Radiology 101:573–574, 1971.

83. Dyer R, Miller S, Anderson BL, et al: The segmental nephrogram. AJR 145:321–322, 1985.

84. Elkin M: Radiology of urinary tract. Some physiologic considerations. Radiology 116:259–270, 1975.

85. Elkin M, Meng CH, Mendez L: Angiographic appearance of the canine kidney in acute hemorrhagic shock. Modification by saline infusion, Tham infusion, and reinfusion of blood. AJR 111:716–728, 1971.

86. Fry IK, Cattell WR: The nephrographic patterns during excretory urography. Br Med Bull 28:227–232, 1972.

87. Hamilton G: The vascular nephrographic phase of excretory urography and its implications. Radiology 102:37–40, 1972.

88. Hunnani GR, Sherwood T: Striated nephrogram in rhabdomyolisis. Br J Radiol 58:682–683, 1985.

89. Korobin M: The nephrogram of hemorrhagic hypotension. AJR 114:673–683, 1972.

90. Rosenberg HK, Gefter WB, Lebowitz RL, et al: Prolonged dense nephrograms in battered children. Suspect rhabdomyolisis and myoglobinuria. Urology 21:325–330, 1983.

91. Newhouse JH, Pfister RC: The nephrogram. Radiol Clin North Am 17:213, 1979.

92. Binder R, Korobin M, Clark RE, et al: Aberrant papillae and other filling defects of the renal pelvis. AJR Rad Ther Nucl Med 114:746–752, 1972.

93. Braunstein P, Hernberg SG, Bosniak MA, et al: Scintiscan evaluation of prominent renal columns. Radiology 104:103–106, 1972.

94. Charghi A, Dessureault P, Drouin G, et al: Malposition of renal lobe (lobar dysmorphism); condition simulating renal tumor. J Urol 105:326–329, 1971.

95. Cooperman LR, Lowman RN: Fetal lobulations of the kidneys. AJR 92:273–280, 1964.

96. Elgazzar AH, Fernandez-Ulloa M, Powers GT: Pseudovascular tumor in a renal flow study. Clin Nucl Med 10:201–202, 1985.

97. Felson B, Moskowitz M: Renal pseudotumors: The regenerated nodule and other lumps, bumps, and dromedary humps. AJR 107:720–729, 1969.

98. Gain DL, Parfrey NA: Unusual renal pseudotumor (cloison) in a young woman with chronic rejection of a transplanted kidney. Urol Radiol 7:112–115, 1985.

99. Goldstein HM, Reuter SR, Wallace S: Pseudotumor of the renal pelvis caused by arterial impression. J Urol 111:735–737, 1974.

100. Green WM, Pressman BD, McClennan BL, et al: "Columns of Bertin:" Diagnosis by nephrotomography. AJR Rad Ther Nucl Med 116:714–723, 1972.

101. Hartman GW, Hodson LJ: Duplex kidney and other abnormalities. Clin Radiol 20:387–400, 1969.

102. King M, Friedenberg RM, Tena LB: Normal renal parenchyma simulating tumor. Radiology 91:217–222, 1968.

103. Kyaw MM: Renal pseudotumor due to infolding column of Bertin. JAMA 219:1634, 1972.

104. Leekam RN, Matzinger MA, Brunelle M, et al: The sonography of renal columnar hypertrophy. J Clin Ultrasound 11:491–494, 1983.

105. Mahony BS, Jeffrey RB, Laing FC: Septa of Bertin: A sonographic tumor. J Clin Ultrasound 11:317–319, 1983.

106. Moss GD, Malvar TC: CT demonstration of an ectopic pancreatic tail causing a renal pseudotumor. J Comput Assist Tomogr 7:724–726, 1983.

107. Murasawa M, Kizu N, Mouta T: [Two cases of renal pseudotumor in pyelonephritis]. Rinsho Hoshasen 30:141–144, 1985.

108. Schwartz DB, Mindelzun R: Ectopic (retropelvic) renal papilla. J Urol 108:28–29, 1972.

109. Simpson EL, Mintz MC, Pollack HM, et al: Computed tomography in the diagnosis of renal pseudotumor. J Comput Tomogr 10:341–348, 1986.

110. Vitti RA, Maurer AH: Single photon emission computed tomography and renal pseudotumor. Clin Nucl Med 10:501–503, 1985.

111. Wolfson JJ, Stowell DW: Aberrant renal papilla simulating an intrarenal mass. Report of two cases. Radiology 93:812–814, 1969.

112. Feldman AE, Pollack HM, Perri AJ Jr, et al: Renal pseudotumors: An anatomic-radiologic classification. J Urol 120:133, 1978.

Renal Fascia

113. Congdon ED, Edson JN: The cone of renal fascia in the adult white male. Anat Rec 80:289–313, 1941.

114. Meyers MA, Whalen JP, Evans JA: Diagnosis of perirenal and

subcapsular masses: Anatomic-radiologic correlations. AJR 121:523–538, 1974.

115. Meyers MA: The reno-alimentary relationship: Anatomic roentgen study of their clinical significance. Am J Nephrol 123:386–400, 1975.

116. Meyers MA, Whalen JP, Peelee K, et al: Radiologic features of extraperitoneal effusions. An anatomic approach. Radiology 104:249–258, 1972.

117. Raptopoulos V, Kleinman PK, Marks S Jr, et al: Renal fascial pathway: Posterior extensions of pancreatic effusions within the anterior pararenal space. Radiology 158:367–374, 1986.

118. Kochkodan EJ, Haggar AM: Visualization of the renal fascia: A normal finding in urography. AJR 140:1243, 1983.

Renal Insufficiency

119. Becker JA: Before and after dialysis urography. Radiology 109:271–275, 1973.

120. Becker JA, Berdon WE: Blood clearances of contrast material in patients with impaired renal function. Radiology 93:1301–1304, 1969.

121. Becker JA, Gregoire A, Berdon W, et al: Vicarious excretion of urographic media. Radiology 90:243–248, 1968.

122. Fulton RF, Witten DM, Wagoner RD: Intravenous urography in renal insufficiency. AJR 106:623, 1969.

123. Keeton GR, Pillay GP: Diagnostic role of intravenous urography in acute and chronic renal failure. Urol Radiol 8:72–76, 1986.

124. Knapp MS: Renal failure after contrast radiography. Br Med J 287:3, 1983.

125. MacEwen DW, Dunbar JS, Nogrady MB: Intravenous pyelography in children with renal insufficiency. Radiology 78:893–903, 1962.

126. Nelson CMK, Brown RC, Culp DA: The extrarenal excretion of urographic contrast material. J Urol 110:104–110, 1973.

127. Rao SR, Mieza MA, Leiter E: Renal failure in diabetes after intravenous urography. Urology 15:577, 1980.

128. Talner LB: Urographic contrast media in uremia. Physiology and pharmacology. Radiol Clin North Am 10:421–432, 1972.

129. van Waes PFGM: High dose urography in oliguric and anuric patients. Amsterdam, Excerpta Medica, 1972.

130. Webb JAW, Reznek RH, Cattell WR, Fry IK: Renal function after high dose urography in patients with renal failure. Br J Radiol 54:479, 1981.

Renal Sinus Lipomatosis

131. Dana A, Musset D, Ody B, et al: Abnormal renal sinus: Sonography patterns of multilocular parapelvic cysts. Urol Radiol 5:227–231, 1983.

132. Faegenburg D, Bosniak M, Evans JA: Renal sinus lipomatosis: Its demonstration by nephrotomography. Radiology 83:987–998, 1964.

133. Olsson O, Weiland P: Renal fibrolipomatosis. Acta Radiol 1:1061–1070, 1963.

134. Roth LJ, Davidson HB: Fibrous and fatty replacement of renal parenchyma. JAMA 111:233–239, 1938.

135. Simril WA, Rose DK: Replacement lipomatosis and its simulation of renal tumors: A report of two cases. J Urol 63:588–592, 1951.

136. Subramanian BR, Bosniak MA, Horu SC, et al: Replacement lipomatosis of the kidney: Diagnosis by computed tomography and sonography. Radiology 148:791–792, 1983.

137. Suramo I, Paivansalo M, Myllyla V: Echo-free and relatively "echo-free" renal sinus findings. ROFO 138:558–560, 1983.

138. Tizzani A, Cocimano V, Fea B, Botto A: [Lipomatosis of the renal sinus]. Minerva Urol Nefrol 36:311–313, 1984.

Ureter

139. Benness GT: Urographic excretion study—dehydration and dose. Australas Radiol 11:261, 1967.

140. Davidson AJ: Radiology of the Kidney. Philadelphia, WB Saunders Company, 1985.

141. Harath P: The hydromechanics of the calyx renalis. J Urol 43:145, 1940.

142. Moell H: Kidney size and its deviation from normal in acute renal failure. Acta Radiol [Diagn] (Stockh) 56(Suppl):5, 1961.

143. Seldino RM, Palubinskas AJ: Medial placement of ureter: A normal variant which may simulate retroperitoneal fibrosis. J Urol 107:582, 1972.

144. Sykes D: The correlation between renal vascularization and lobulation of the kidneys. Br J Urol 36:549, 1964.

Urinomas

145. Adzick NS, Harrison MR, Flake AW, deLormier AA: Urinary extravasation in the fetus with obstructive uropathy. J Pediatr Surg 20:608–615, 1985.

146. Allison MC, McLean L, Robinson LQ, Locrance CJ: Spontaneous urinoma due to retroperitoneal fibrosis and aortic aneurysm. Br Med J (Clin Res) 291:176, 1985.

147. Bernardino ME, McClennan BL: High dose urography: Incidence and relationship to spontaneous peripelvic extravasation. AJR 127:373, 1976.

148. Eklof O, Elle B, Thonell S: Pseudotumor of the kidney secondary to posterior urethral valves: The role of renal backflow and perirenal extravasation. Pediatr Radiol 14:215–219, 1984.

149. Friedenberg RM, Moorehouse H, Gade M: Urinomas secondary to pyelosinus backflow. Urol Radiol 5:23–29, 1983.

150. Kinoshita N, Yamasaki Y, Kato M, et al: [Six cases of spontaneous peripelvic extravasation from the renal pelvis]. Hinyokita Kiyo 31:1171–1182, 1985.

151. Kramer RL: Urinoma in pregnancy. Obstet Gynecol 62(3 Suppl):265–285, 1983.

152. Lang EK, Glorioso L 3d: Management of urinomas by percutaneous drainage procedure. Radiol Clin North Am 24:551–559, 1986.

153. Macpherson RI, Gordon L, Bradford BF: Neonatal urinomas: Imaging considerations. Pediatr Radiol 14:396–399, 1984.

154. Patel MR, Mooppan MM, Kim H: Subcapsular urinoma: Unusual form of "page kidney" in newborn. Urology 23:585–587, 1984.

155. Urbain D, Vanderauwera J, Dewit S, Vandendris M: Perirenal urinoma secondary to prostatic obstruction. J Urol 134:967–968, 1985.

Urography

156. Anto HR, Shyan-Yih C, Porush JG, Shapiro WB: Infusion intravenous pyelography and renal function. Effects of hypertonic mannitol in patients with chronic renal insufficiency. Arch Intern Med 141:1652, 1981.

157. Banner MP, Pollack HM: Evaluation of renal function by excretory urography. J Urol 124:437, 1980.

158. Batson PG, Keats TE: The roentgenographic determination of normal adult kidney size as related to vertebral height. AJR 116:737–739, 1972.

159. Baum S, Gillenwater JY: Renal artery impressions on the renal pelvis. J Urol 95:139–145, 1986.

160. Becker JA: Drip infusion pyelography. Its evaluation as a routine examination. AJR 98:96–101, 1966.

161. Becker JA: Before and after dialysis urography. Radiology 109:271, 1973.

162. Benness GT: Double dose urography. J Coll Radiol Australas 9:78–82, 1965.

163. Benness GT: Urographic excretion study—dehydration and dose. Australas Radiol 11:261, 1967.

164. Benness GT, Evill CA: Urographic physiology and contrast materials. In Friedland GW, et al (eds): Uroradiology. An Integrated Approach. London, Churchill Livingstone, 1983, pp 155–166.

165. Berdon WE: Techniques and application of urography in infants and children. Syllabus for Categorical Course in Genitourinary Radiology, RSNA, 1975, pp 137–150.

166. Berdon WE, Baker DH, Becker HA: Danger of dehydration in pyelography. N Engl J Med 281–167, 1969.

167. Berg GR, Hutter AM, Pfister RC: Electrocardiographic abnormalities associated with intravenous urography. N Engl J Med 289:87, 1973.

167a. Riggs W Jr, et al: Anatomic changes in the normal urinary tract between supine and prone urograms. Radiology 94:107–113, 1970.

168. Danford RO, Davidson AL, Goldman RL: Drip infusion pyelography. N Engl J Med 280:1022, 1964.

169. Daniel WW, Hartman GW, Witten DM, et al: Calcified renal masses. A review of ten years experience at the Mayo Clinic. Radiology 103:503–506, 1972.

170. Davidson AJ: Radiology of the Kidney. Philadelphia, WB Saunders Company, 1985.

171. Davidson AJ, Becker J, Rothfield N, et al: An evaluation of the effects of high-dose urography on previously impaired renal and hepatic function in man. Radiology 97:249, 1970.

172. Dawson P, Heron C, Marshall J: Intravenous urography with low-osmolality contrast agents: Theoretical considerations and clinical findings. Clin Radiol 35:173–175, 1984.

173. Diaz-Buxo J, Wagoner RD, Hattery RR, Palumbo PJ: Acute renal

failure after excretory urography in diabetic patients. Ann Intern Med 83:155, 1975.

174. Dure-Smith P: Fluid restriction before excretory urography: Is it obsolete? *In* Proceedings of the National Uroradiological Conference, New Orleans, American College of Radiology, 1974, p 24.

175. Dure-Smith P: Opacification of the urinary tract during excretory urography. Concentration vs. amount of contrast medium. Invest Radiol 7:407–410, 1972.

176. Dure-Smith P, Rose NR, Stern A, et al: Physiology of the excretory urogram. 3. A densitometric and subjective assessment of change in contrast medium concentration. Invest Radiol 9:104–108, 1974.

177. Edling NPG, Melander CG, Renck L: Correlation between contrast excretion and arterial and intrapelvic pressures in urography: Experimental study in rabbits. Acta Radiol 42:442–450, 1954.

178. Elkin M: The prone position in intravenous urography for study of the upper urinary tract. Radiology 76:961–967, 1961.

179. Elkin M: Supine and prone positions in intravenous urography for diagnosis of bladder lesions. Radiology 78:904–913, 1962.

180. Elkin M, Cohen G: Diagnostic value of psoas shadow. Clin Radiol 13:210–217, 1962.

181. Ettinger A, Fainsinger MH: Zonography in daily radiological practice. Radiology 87:82, 1966.

182. Filly R: Ultrasonography. *In* Friedland GW, et al (eds): Uroradiology. An Integrated Approach. London, Churchill Livingstone, 1983, pp 311–322.

183. Finberg H: Renal ultrasound: Anatomy and technique. Semin Ultrasound 2:7, 1981.

184. Fraley EE: Vascular obstruction of superior infundibulum causing nephralgia: A new syndrome. N Engl J Med 275:1403–1409, 1966.

185. Fred HL, Eiband JM, Collins LC: Calcification in intra-abdominal and retroperitoneal metastases: Review of the roentgenographic features. AJR 91:138–148, 1964.

186. Brenner BN, Rector FC: The Kidney. Philadelphia, WB Saunders Company, 1976.

187. Fry IK, Cattell WR: Radiology in the diagnosis of renal failure. Br Med Bull 27:148, 1971.

188. Gondos B: Roentgenographic evaluation of the size and shape of the kidneys. Med Ann DC 31:158–161, 1962.

189. Griffiths GJ: Loss of renal tone in the elderly. Br J Radiol 49:111–117, 1976.

190. Griscom NT: The roentgenology of neonatal abdominal masses. AJR 93:447–463, 1965.

191. Gup AK, Schlegel JU: Physiological effects of high dosage excretory urography. J Urol 100:85–87, 1968.

192. Handel J, Schwartz S: Value of the prone position for filling the obstructed ureter in the presence of hydronephrosis. Radiology 71:102–103, 1958.

193. Harkonen S, Kjellstrand CM: Exacerbation of diabetic renal failure following intravenous pyelography. Am J Med 63:939, 1977.

194. Harkonen S, Kjellstrand CM: Intravenous pyelography in nonuremic diabetic patients. Nephron 24:268, 1979.

195. Hartman GW, Hattery RR, Witten DM, Williamson B Jr: Mortality during excretory urography: Mayo Clinic experience. AJR 139:919, 1982.

196. Havey RJ, Krumlovsky F, delGreco F, Martin HG: Screening for renovascular hypertension: Is renal digital-subtraction angiography the preferred noninvasive test? Special Communications. JAMA 254:388–393, 1985.

197. Hodson CJ: The effect of disturbance of flow in the kidney. J Infect Dis 120:56–60, 1969.

198. Hodson CJ, Drewe JA, Karn MN, et al: Renal size in normal children: A radiographic study during life. Arch Dis Child 37:616–622, 1962.

199. Johnson JL, Abernathy DL: Diagnostic imaging procedure volume in the United States. Special Report. Radiology 146:851–853, 1983.

200. Jorulf H, Nordmark J, Jonsson A: Kidney size in infants and children as assessed by area measurement. Acta Radiol (Diagn) 19:154–162, 1978.

201. Kelley WM: Uricosuria and x-ray contrast agents. N Engl J Med 284:975, 1971.

202. Kumar R, Schreiber MH: The changing indications for excretory urography. *In* Jacobson HG, Edeiken J (eds): Topics in radiology/diagnostic radiology. JAMA 254:403–405, 1985.

203. Liberson M, Coleman JW: Kidney size variation during arteriography in hypertensive patients. J Urol 97:798–803, 1967.

204. Mandell GA, Swacus JR, Rosenstock J, Buck BE: Danger of urography in hyperuricemic children with Burkitt's lymphoma. J Can Assoc Radiol 34:53–55, 1983.

205. Mitty HA, Schapira HE: Total body opacification in the adult. AJR 115:630–635, 1972.

206. Moell H: Kidney size and its deviation from normal in acute renal failure. Acta Radiol [Diagn] (Stockh) 56(Suppl 206):5, 1961.

207. Moell H: The position of the kidneys. Acta Radiol [Diagn] (Stockh) 1:22–28, 1963.

208. Moell H: Size of normal kidneys. Acta Radiol [Diagn] (Stockh) 46:640–645, 1956.

209. Narath P: The hydromechanics of the calyx renalis. J Urol 43:145, 1940.

210. O'Connor JF, Neuhauser EB: Total body opacification in conventional and high dose intravenous urography in infancy. AJR 90:63–71, 1963.

211. Pfister RC, Hutter AM: Cardiac alterations during intravenous urography. Invest Radiol 15(Suppl):S239, 1980.

212. Pollack HM: Some limitations and pitfalls in excretory urography. J Urol 116:537–543, 1971.

213. Pollack HM, Banner MP: Current status of excretory urography. A premature epitaph? Urol Clin North Am 12:585–601, 1985.

214. Riggs WJ Jr, Hagood JH, Andrews JE: Anatomic changes in normal urinary tract between supine and prone urograms. Radiology 94:107–113, 1970.

215. Rosenfield AT, Littner MR, Ulreich S, et al: Respiratory effects of excretory urography: A preliminary report. Invest Radiol 12:295, 1977.

216. Rosenfield AT, Taylor KJW, Jaffe CC: Clinical applications of ultrasound tissue characterization. Radiol Clin North Am 18:31, 1980.

217. Saldino RM, Palubinskas AJ: Medial placement of ureter: A normal variant which may simulate retroperitoneal fibrosis. J Urol 107:582–585, 1972.

218. Schenker B: Drip infusion pyelography: Indications and applications in urologic diagnosis. Radiology 83:12, 1964.

219. Schencker B, Marcuie RW, Moody DL: Simplified nephrotomography: The drip infusion technique. AJR 95:283–280, 1965.

220. Sherwood T, Breckenridge A, Dollery CT, Doyle FH: Intravenous urography and renal function. Clin Radiol 19:296, 1968.

221. Swanson DP, Dick TJ, Simms SM, Thrall JH: Product selection criteria for intravascular ionic contrast media. Clin Pharmacol 4:527–538, 1985.

222. Talner LB: Urographic contrast media in uremia. Physiology and pharmacology. Radiol Clin North Am 10:421, 1972.

223. Tenti L, Belli I: Uretero-pyelo-pneumotography. Ann Radiol 5:879–884, 1962.

224. Webb JAW, Fry IK, Charlton CAC: An anomalous calyx in the mid-kidney: An anatomical variant. Br J Radiol 48:674–677, 1975.

225. Whitaker RH, Edwards D: Congenital hypertrophy of a renal papilla. Br J Urol 38:287–289, 1966.

226. Wolpert SM: Variations in kidney length during intravenous pyelogram. Br J Radiol 38:100–103, 1965.

227. Chait A: Current status of renal angiography. Urol Clin North Am 12:687, 1985.

228. DiSantis DJ, Cramer MS, Scatarige JC: Excretory urography in the emergency department: Utility of teleradiology. Radiology 164:363, 1987.

229. Fajardo LL, Hillman BJ, Hunter TB, et al: Excretory urography using computed radiography. Radiology 162:345, 1987.

230. Lalli AF: Tailored Urologic Imaging. Chicago, Year Book Medical Publishers, 1980.

231. Morewood DJW, Scally JK: Evaluation of the post-micturition radiograph following intravenous urography. Clin Radiol 37:499, 1986.

232. Pfister RC, Shea TE: Nephrotomography: Performance and interpretation. Radiol Clin North Am 9:41, 1971.

233. Rhodes RA, Fried AM, Lorman JG, Kryscio RJ: Tomographic levels for intravenous urography: CT-determined guidelines. Radiology 163:673, 1987.

234. Trewhella M, Forsling M, Richards D, Dawson P: Dehydration, antidiuretic hormone and the intravenous urogram. Br J Radiol 60:445, 1987.

235. Dunnill MS, Halley W: Some observations on the quantitative anatomy of the kidney. J Pathol 110:113, 1973.

236. Brandt TD, Neiman HL, Dragowski MJ, et al: Ultrasound assessment of normal renal dimensions. J Ultrasound Med 1:49, 1982.

237. Saxton HM: Urography. Br J Radiol 42:321, 1969.

237a. Hattery RR, Williamson B Jr, Hartman GW, et al: Intravenous urographic technique. Radiology 167:593, 1988.

238. Griffiths GJ, Cartwright G, McLachlan MSF: Estimation of renal size from radiographs: Is the effort worthwhile? Clin Radiol 26:249, 1975.
239. Ludin H: Radiologic estimation of kidney weight. Acta Radiol (Diagn) 6:561, 1967.
240. Fajardo LL, Hillman BJ: Image quality, diagnostic certainty, and accuracy: Comparison of conventional and digital urograms. Urol Radiol 10:72, 1988.
241. Warshauer DM, McCarthy SM, Street L, et al: Detection of renal masses: Sensitivities and specificities of excretory urography/linear tomography, US and CT. Radiology 169:363, 1988.
242. Roberge-Wade AP, Hosking DH, MacEwan DW, Ramsey EW: The excretory urogram bowel preparation: Is it necessary? J Urol 140:1473, 1988.
243. Saxton HM: Opacification of collecting ducts at urography. Radiology 170:16, 1989.
244. Ohlson L: Normal collecting ducts: Visualization at urography. Radiology 170:33, 1989.

EXCRETORY UROGRAPHY IN INFANTS AND CHILDREN

J. S. DUNBAR

The primacy once enjoyed by excretory urography in imaging of the urinary tracts of infants and children is now shared by ultrasonography and to some extent by radionuclide imaging.[94] Nonetheless, it remains a vital tool in evaluating the pediatric urinary system and is likely to retain this role in the foreseeable future. Urography and ultrasonography are frequently required in evaluating the infant and child, since 15% of all births involve a genitourinary variant or anomaly. Anomalies of the genitourinary tract are commonly associated with anomalies of other systems, particularly the cardiac and vertebral systems.

Although the principles of excretory urography in children are not basically different from the principles underlying urography in adults, some modifications are necessary to address the unique clinical and physiological problems encountered in young patients.

DIFFERENCES FROM ADULTS

Indications for excretory urography in pediatric work differ from those in adult work as follows:

1. In pediatrics, much emphasis is placed on detection of vesicoureteral reflux and renal scarring in the assessment and management of recurrent urinary tract infection.

2. The discovery of an abdominal mass in the loin or flank in the neonate (or its discovery in utero by ultrasonography) is a common problem in pediatrics, and prompt and urgent investigation and management are important. However, ultrasonography is replacing excretory urography for most such cases.

3. Malformations of the urinary tract and general malformation syndromes usually present in early life. Examples are renal hypoplasia/dysplasia, and renal cystic disease (except for the solitary cyst of the kidney, which is rare in infants and children).

4. Renal trauma is common in children (although less common than liver and spleen trauma), but bladder and urethral trauma are comparatively rare. Thus, cystograms and (retrograde) urethrograms for bladder rupture or urethral tear are infrequently needed. When they are needed, however, the technique used is similar to that used in assessing lower tract trauma in the adult, except for the use of small catheters and Foley-type balloons.

Any discussion of the indications for urography in children should be coupled with an admonition about nonindications. For example, urography is not recommended for the evaluation of urinary tract infection unless preliminary VCU reveals reflux or some other compelling indication (e.g., ureterocele).[87] Enuresis and congenital anomalies such as penile hypospadias and cryptorchism coexist with significant urinary tract disorders so infrequently as to make urography unrewarding in these settings.[88] The study by Pedersen and coworkers suggests that excretory urography is overutilized in children.[89]

INDICATIONS FOR PEDIATRIC EXCRETORY UROGRAPHY

The indications for excretory urography in infants and children include the following clinical situations:

1. An overview of the urinary tract is needed, and cannot readily be provided by an alternative method; for example, abdominal pain compatible with urinary colic, or a congenital anomaly of another system such as cardiac or vertebral.

2. Other methods, such as ultrasonography, CT, or nuclear medicine, are not available, or are not available under conditions suitable for infants and children.

3. A comparison with previous studies is needed, such as postoperative study after surgical relief of urinary obstruction.

4. A condition exists, or is suspected, that involves the upper and lower urinary system, such as the Eagle-Barrett syndrome (prune-belly syndrome) or neurogenic bladder.

5. Renal scarring is present or suspected because of recurrent urinary tract infections and/or significant vesicoureteral reflux, and other methods of showing or confirming the scarring are not sufficient or have produced equivocal results.

6. Operation on the urinary tract is contemplated or planned, and the surgeon needs the complete demonstration of the urinary system that excretory urography provides.

7. Abdominal trauma has occurred and involvement of the urinary tract is deemed unlikely, but some reassurance short of CT is needed.

8. Urinary tract obstruction is present or suspected, and its severity and location need assessment; the combination of anatomy and function provided by the excretory urogram is very valuable.

9. A malformation of the genitalia or a systemic

malformation syndrome requires investigation and/or assessment. An example is Turner's syndrome (ovarian agenesis).

10. Confirmation of an abnormality detected during intrauterine ultrasonography is required. One example is hydronephrosis.

RADIOGRAPHIC TECHNIQUE

Pediatric urography should be done with equipment that permits rapid (millisecond) exposures, low patient dosage, and high-resolution images. Such results can be achieved only when well-trained technologists work with excellent facilities.

Filters

Filters should have a half-value layer of not less than 3.7-mm aluminum, including inherent filtration. Rare earth filters have been shown to reduce exposure substantially, and should probably be used for patients of all ages—but particularly for children, because radiation protection is so important for the pediatric patient.[36, 79]

Film-Screen Combinations

Rare earth intensifying screens have proved their worth in reducing exposure levels and exposure times and should be used for all pediatric urography. In addition, the quality of fast films is now sufficient to justify wide acceptance. We use rare earth screens, and our film-screen combination is rated at an ASA speed of 400. With the development of low-attenuation cassettes and faster film-screen combinations, ASA speeds of 2000 are now available and are said to have good gray-scale and resolution characteristics.[80]

Radiographic Equipment

Equipment should be capable of very short exposures, not to exceed 5 msec, with a moving grid (Bucky) or a fine-line stationary grid. Longer exposures lead to motion blurring, which should not be accepted.

In small infants in the few weeks of life, a nongrid urographic technique can be used. This reduces radiation, and permits fast exposures of approximately 1 to 2 msec. A rule of thumb that we have found helpful is to use a grid (stationary or moving) when the AP diameter of the abdomen, or the longest dimension of the beam, exceeds 10 cm.

Fast exposures require high-capacity radiographic equipment. A seeming contradiction results: heavy-duty equipment for radiography of small patients. However, the extra cost of the high-capacity equipment is well justified by the improvement in image quality made possible by eliminating motion blur and by reducing the need for repeat exposures. The apparatus permits the use of small focus tubes (1.2 mm—very fine focus is not necessary). Adequate source-to-image distance (SID) is needed, of at least 40 inches (1 m).

Preparation

No pediatric patient should ever be purposely dehydrated for urography. Dehydration does not substantially improve urographic quality[21] and is dangerous to young and/or sick patients. It is important that the colon be empty for satisfactory urography. In principle, this can be achieved by laxatives; however, the results of laxatives are unpredictable, and compliance in their administration by parents is erratic. Cleansing enemas are also effective, but here again one cannot depend on their being given properly at home. We issue instructions to parents at home, and to personnel in the hospital for bowel preparation for urography but find that very frequently the results are unsatisfactory. Therefore, we have a program of administering cleansing enemas in the radiology department, as necessary. The preliminary film is first made, and if it shows undue gas and/or feces in the colon, our technologists or nurses administer a cleansing enema, using soap suds. This is necessary in approximately 75% of cases, and is usually effective (Fig. 6–171; see also Fig. 6–214). Although many uroradiologists believe that cleansing enemas tend to leave too much gas in the bowel, we have not found any other method of preparation as satisfactory as this.

In children under the age of 2, cleansing enemas are more difficult to administer, and perhaps harder on the patient, so are infrequently used.

The patient who is to have urography must not have a full stomach, because of the risk of vomiting. So, the pediatric patient is given nothing by mouth for 3 to 4 hours before the contrast material is injected (Figs. 6–172 and 6–173).

Restraint

In pediatric urography, as in pediatric radiography generally, infants and young children frequently need restraint. We have found the Octostop* to be very effective. This is a board of low radiographic attenuation, with an octagonal aluminum handle at each end. It is furnished with Velcro belts, and makes immobilization relatively easy without impairing access to the patient, and with maximum flexibility in use of radiographic facilities and positioning of the patient (Fig. 6–174).

For children who are too large for the Octostop, sandbags and/or human restraint, best accomplished by accompanying parents or guardians, is needed. When necessary, technologists, radiologists, nurses, or aides of the hospital (radiology) staff are able to soothe and at the same time hold or restrain the patient. Strict attention must always be paid to the use of lead aprons and gloves for protection of personnel and to the need for tight collimation. Exposure of personnel in the room, and of the patient, is greatly reduced when the x-ray beam is carefully limited to the area being examined.[57]

Contrast Medium

We have used and recommended sodium meglumine diatrizoate for many years. The tri-iodinated contrast

---

*Octostop Entreprises, C.P. 1476 St Laurent, Montreal, Canada, H4L 4Z1.

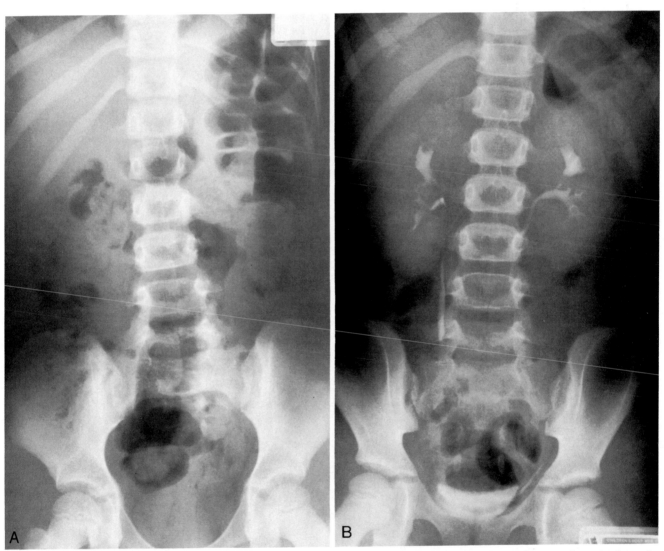

Figure 6–171. Preparation for intravenous urogram by cleansing enema. *A*, Preliminary film shows feces and gas in the colon. *B*, Prone (PA) urographic film was obtained after cleansing enema and 15 minutes after contrast medium injection. The urinary tract is almost completely unobscured by gut content. This is because of the cleansing enema and the prone position, which displaces gas-containing bowel away from the kidneys.

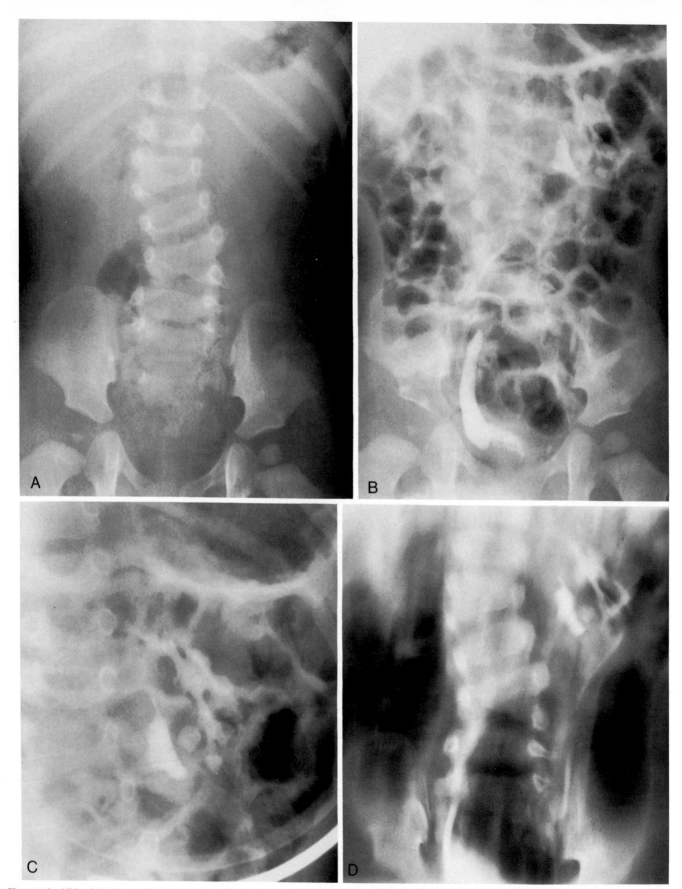

Figure 6–172. Gas in gut from crying. *A*, Preliminary film for intravenous urogram (IVU) of 18-month-old boy. The gut is almost completely free of gas and feces. There are malformations of the vertebral column and the right hip. *B*, Postinjection supine radiograph at 7 minutes. The child had cried a lot during the contrast injection, and there is now gas throughout the entire bowel, partially obscuring triplication of the kidneys. One is at and just to the right of the midline, and two fused and malformed kidneys are on the left. *C*, "Paddle" compression confirming the fused left kidneys. *D*, Linear tomography shows the right lower ureter and portions of the left lateral ureter. Voiding cystourethrography (VCU) (not shown) demonstrated reflux into the two left ureters, but not into the right ureter.

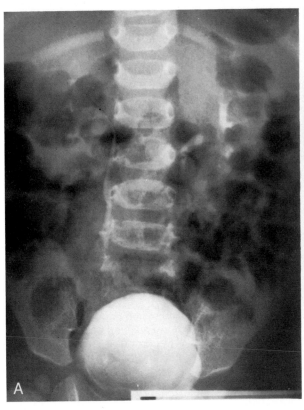

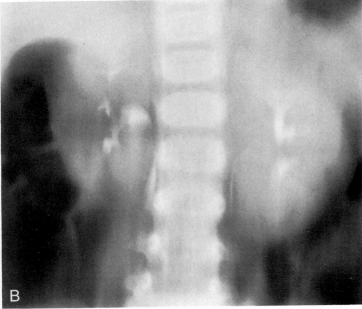

Figure 6–173. Value of tomography in urography. *A*, An 11-month-old boy has intestinal gas that partially obscures the urinary tract. *B*, Linear tomogram made with a 40-degree sweep, with 1-second exposure. The kidney parenchyma is adequately visualized.

media are well tolerated by pediatric patients, and urographic results are good. The dose is 1 to 2 ml/kg body weight, up to a maximum of 100 ml of 60% contrast. The dose is injected as rapidly as can be done without causing discomfort to the patient; the "drip infusion" method[72] is not used.

In the neonate (usually defined as a newborn in the first month of life, but with particular emphasis on the first few days of life) the dose is the same: 1 to 2 ml/kg body weight. The concentrating ability of the kidney is not fully developed at birth,[93] so the radiopacity is less than in the older child or adult. In addition, the maximum

opacity is developed more slowly in the neonatal urogram;[59] thus the nephrogram and pyelogram are less dense, and are later in appearing, than in older subjects. Therefore, films should be exposed relatively late, in comparison to the practice in children and adults. The first film should be made at 15 to 20 minutes after injection, and further films correspondingly delayed to 30 minutes; other films may be exposed even later, as necessary.

It must be re-emphasized that the very young patient is particularly susceptible to dehydration, and to disruption of acid-base balance. Therefore, excretory urography

Figure 6–174. Immobilization device for young infants—the Octo-stop.

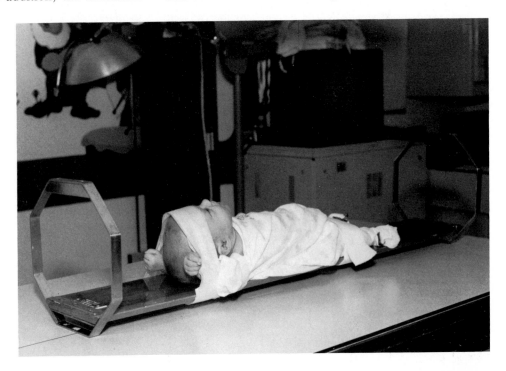

must not be undertaken without skilled pediatric personnel and equipment at hand.

When there is any reason to be concerned about clinical stability or renal insufficiency, when large doses must be introduced, or when the patient is a newborn, we use low-osmolality contrast agents.[84] They are used at the same dose rates as the diatrizoates, and with the same method of injection. In particular, we have used ioxaglate (Hexabrix,* a low-osmolality dimer) and iohexol (Omnipaque,† a nonionizing monomer). Both have been shown to be about equally effective in producing a low incidence of discomfort and reaction and in providing highly satisfactory urographic images. Iohexol, being a monomer, appears to be slightly superior. Given the high cost of these low-osmolality agents, and the very low incidence of reactions in pediatric patients, we continue to use the diatrizoates for routine purposes,[15, 17, 81] although others use nonionics routinely in pediatric practice.[90] The vial from which the contrast medium is taken should, of course, be carefully checked before the syringe is loaded. Furthermore, the vial should be kept, whether partly empty or empty, until the examination is complete and the patient is well. If an adverse reaction occurs, the vial and any remaining contrast medium must be impounded.

Injection Technique and Sites

A needle connected to a syringe by a soft tube is used. "Butterfly" scalp sets of 21 and 23 F are suitable for this purpose. A needle connected directly to a syringe should not be used, because if the child moves the needle can easily be displaced.

Venipuncture is not always easy in a tiny infant, or a struggling child, but with patience, experience, and adequate help, a vein can almost always be found; subcutaneous or intramuscular injections should not be used.

In older children, injection sites are the same as those used for adults. In young children and infants, antecubital veins and posterior hand and wrist veins are usually acceptable. We frequently inject into posterior wrist veins, with good results (Fig. 6–175). We recommend using anterior wrist veins, but only with particular caution because extravasation into the relatively tight tissues of the anterior wrist can cause swelling in the unyielding carpal tunnel; severe pain and even hand and/or wrist ischemia can occur. Femoral veins should not be used because of the danger of septic arthritis of the hip.[12]

Other available sites include the foot (dorsal aspect), the scalp veins, and the external jugular vein.

The external jugular vein is often prominent and easily visible in infants—even fat infants, and when the child cries the vein becomes still more prominent. It is thus a good site for intravenous injection, but only in skilled hands. A danger of pneumothorax is said to exist because of the proximity of the lung apex; however, we have not found this to be a problem. A more important danger is in positioning the patient, when damage to the neck or the cervical vertebral column might possibly occur because the head must be extended and at the same time turned to the side to expose the vein. Caution and gentleness should therefore be used. If blood extravasates

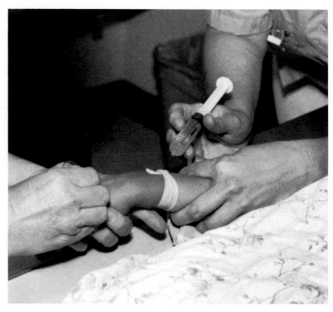

Figure 6–175. A needle being inserted into the posterior wrist vein of a pediatric patient. The needle is fused to a soft tube, which will be connected to the contrast-containing syringe after spontaneous backflow is obtained.

in the neck, an ugly hematoma results, but usually nothing more serious. Finally, the procedure is frightening for the child. Therefore, external jugular vein injection should be reserved for infants and children in whom no other vein can be found and should be performed only by skilled personnel.

When kidney function is surprisingly poor on the initial radiograph, and/or when the child complains to an unusual degree of pain in or around the injection site, extravasation must be suspected and confirmed or excluded by fluoroscopy or radiography (Fig. 6–176). Extravasation can be surprisingly extensive without producing obvious signs or symptoms.

Occasionally, extensive extravasation causes pain, temperature changes (cold or hot), and swelling of part or all of the extremity. Treatment usually consists of elevation of the extremity and observation (the child should not leave the department until the reaction has subsided). Occasionally, we have considered more aggressive treatment such as steroids or even surgical decompressive measures, but they have never been necessary.

Reactions

Reactions to contrast media are much less frequent and much less severe in infants and young children than in adults.[27] The most common reactions are nausea and vomiting; uritcaria is the next most common, and only infrequently is severe. Treatment is usually necessary for urticaria only when the swelling or itching is distressing to the child; otherwise, the child is observed until the reaction has subsided. In more severe or troublesome cases, diphenhydramine hydrochloride (Benadryl*) is used intravenously if the intravenous needle has been left in place after the contrast injection, otherwise by intramuscular injection. The dose is 10 to 50 mg. The urticaria

*Mallinckrodt, Inc., P.O. Box 5840, St. Louis, Missouri 63134

†Winthrop-Breon Laboratories, 90 Park Avenue, New York, New York 10016

*Parke-Davis, Division of Warner-Lambert Company, 201 Tabor Road, Morris Plains, New Jersey 07950

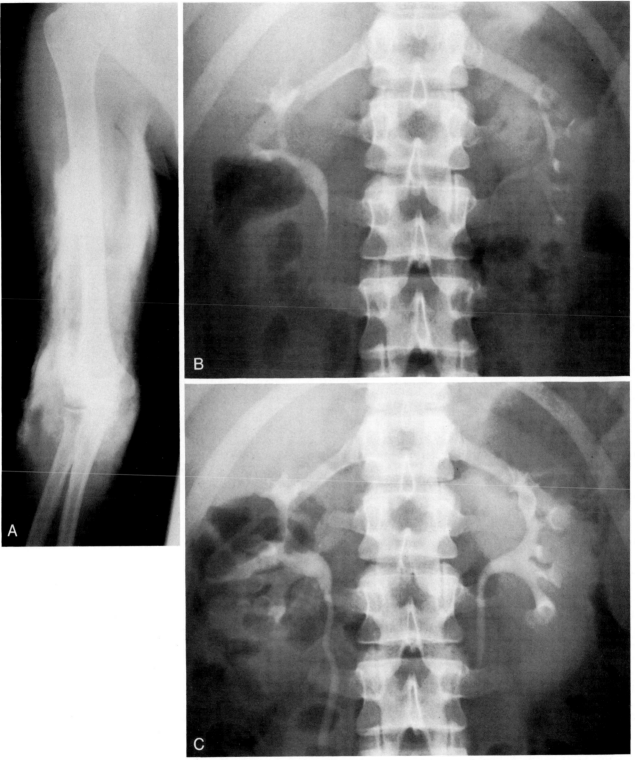

Figure 6–176. Contrast extravasation during injection. *A*, Needle had been inserted into the antecubital vein without difficulty, and satisfactory blood return was obtained during the injection, with no soft-tissue swelling adjacent to the needle. Immediately after the injection, the child complained of swelling of the extremity, which progressed for almost 2 hours, becoming brawny edema from the proximal third of the forearm to the axilla. The reaction gradually subsided over the next 1 to 2 hours, and recovery was complete. One clue of such asymptomatic massive extravasations is decreased and/or delayed urographic visualization. *B*, A 2-minute renal film. Nephrogram and pyelogram densities are less than anticipated. *C*, Ureteral compression film. Nephrogram and pyelogram are adequate.

can occasionally recur or persist for 24 hours or more, so repeated treatment with diphenhydramine hydrochloride may be necessary at home.

Wheezing is much less frequent, and although usually mild is occasionally severe. It too is usually treated by observation, but if severe or persistent, by subcutaneous epinephrine, 1:1000 aqueous solution, in a dose of 0.01 ml/kg body weight, to a maximum dose of 0.50 ml. This dosage can be repeated at 20-minute intervals for two additional doses.

A steroid, hydrocortisone sodium succinate (Solu-Cortef*) is kept available in case needed for very severe hypersensitivity or allergic reactions, but we have almost never used it. The adult dose is 100 to 500 mg intravenously over 30 seconds to 10 minutes. The maximum dose, either intravenous or intramuscular, is 100 to 200 mg/m^2 body surface/day. When treating contrast reactions, the intravenous route is preferred, and the amount and speed of injection must be related to the severity of the reaction and the patient's response to the drug. The minimum effective dosage is 25 mg.

There is no way of predicting which pediatric patient will have a reaction to intravenously injected contrast medium, just as there is no way to do so in adults. Pretesting is unreliable. A history of a previous reaction is not a dependable indicator of another reaction. Nonetheless, it is wise, when there is such a history, to leave the needle in the vein at the end of the injection, so medication can be administered easily and promptly if necessary.

Therefore, in spite of the low incidence of reactions, and the even lower incidence of serious reactions, a "crash cart" (Fig. 6–177) must be immediately available, as must oxygen, suction, face masks in a selection of sizes, sphygmomanometer, and emergency medication (Fig. 6–177).

Hypotension occasionally occurs, manifested by faintness and/or dizziness. It can usually be treated expectantly.

In a patient of any age who is paraplegic due to a spinal cord lesion at or above T6, the possibility of autonomic hyperreflexia[73] caused by distention of a viscus, such as the bladder, must be anticipated, even though it is very rare. It is heralded by headaches, heat, perspiration and flushing of the head and neck, and severe hypertension; it is a reflex response to distention of a hollow viscus. The treatment is to relieve the viscus distention immediately and, if this does not promptly control the hypertensive reaction, to use a hypotensive drug such as diazoxide. Diazoxide is given intravenously in a dose of 3 to 5 mg/kg and may have to be repeated.

Rarely, a "shock nephrogram" occurs (Fig. 6–178) because of hypotension and transient renal ischemia. Precipitation of Tamm-Horsfall proteins as a cause or contributing cause has been suggested[6] but is not universally accepted.[18] Usually, prolonged observation and late films show recovery of kidney function within 30 minutes to 1 or 2 hours. The child should be kept recumbent during such a hypotensive or shock reaction. Avner and colleagues reported severe oliguria, renal enlargement, and sonographic findings, indistinguishable from infantile polycystic disease of the kidneys, in an asymptomatic premature infant given 5 ml of diatrizoate (Renografin).

---

*The Upjohn Company, Kalamazoo, Michigan 49001

Spontaneous diuresis finally began at age 3.5 days, with full recovery.[2]

Mandell and colleagues[52] have drawn attention to the importance of monitoring uric acid levels in children with lymphoma, particularly if Burkitt's lymphoma is diagnosed or suspected, because of the possibility of uric acid nephropathy complicating excretory urography.

McAlister and colleagues[55] reported severe pulmonary edema, with complete recovery, in an 18-day-old girl given 4.7 ml diatrizoate (Hypaque 60). They suggested a dose of no greater than 3 mg/kg in early infancy. Wood and Smith[84] reported six infants under 1 week of age in whom pulmonary edema complicated excretory urography; their experience indicated that this complication is impossible to predict in the newborn.

Angioneurotic edema, with severe spasm and/or swelling of the larynx, appearing clinically as dyspnea and stridor, is fortunately only rarely observed in infancy and childhood. It can cause supraglottic swelling that closely mimics acute epiglottitis. The treatment is as outlined above for allergic reactions, with diphenhyramine hydrochloride being the mainstay.

Radiation Protection

The following measures are necessary to assure maximum protection to infants and children undergoing excretory urography.

1. Adequate filtration ($\geq$ 3.7 mm Al equivalent)
2. A kVp as high as practicable. This means about 65 to 75 kVp in pediatric urography; kilovoltages higher than this diminish the radiographic density of the iodinated contrast medium.
3. Adequate focal film distance (SID): 40 inches (1 m). Shorter distances increase the radiation absorbed by the patient and decrease the quality of the radiographs.
4. Adequate collimation. The region exposed radiographically should be only the area of urographic interest. A wider area greatly increases the total absorbed dose and decreases film quality because of increased scattered radiation.
5. Fast film-screen combinations. An ASA rating of at least 400 is appropriate, and film-screen combinations with a rating of 2000 are now available and radiographically satisfactory.[80]
6. Minimum number of films. For routine radiography, we use three films: an AP preliminary, a small (kidney area) AP 2-minute film, and a PA 7-minute film. This suffices in a large majority of patients.
7. Gonadal protection. Although lead masking of the ovaries is not practicable during excretory urography,[57] the male gonads should always be lead shielded and should, by the use of strict collimation, be outside the main beam.

Film Sequence

An anteroposterior preliminary film is first made in order to assess preparation and to identify abnormalities such as calculi, renal calcification, a mass, or important extraurinary disease.

As noted earlier, if preparation is inadequate in patients

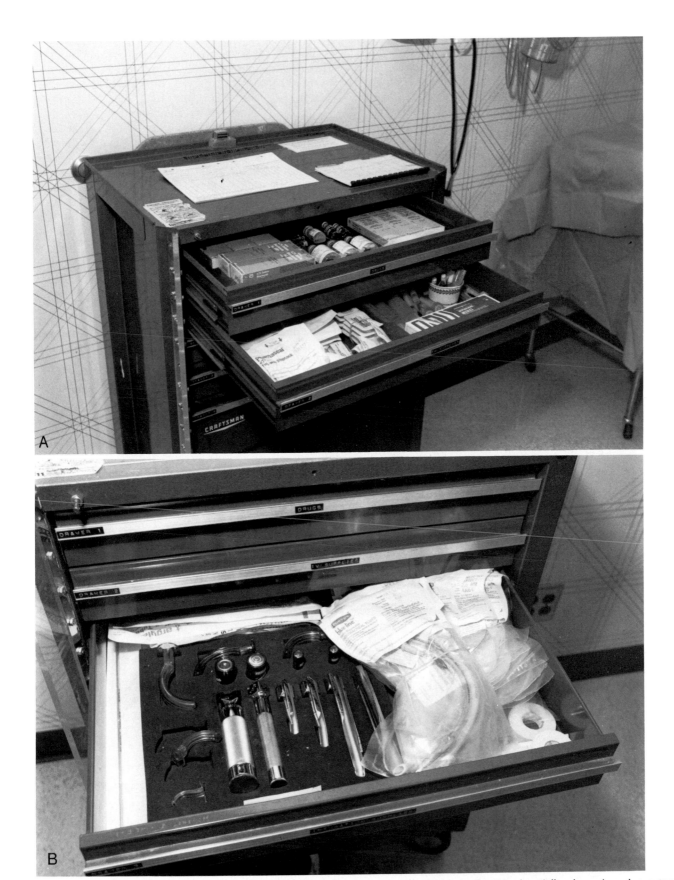

Figure 6–177. *A, B,* "Crash cart" containing emergency medications and instruments. Suction (partially shown) and oxygen outlets are available in each radiographic room. (See Chapter 4 for full list of medications and supplies that should be available.)

over the age of 2, a cleansing enema is given (see Fig. 6–171). The preliminary film is *not* repeated after this enema; the additional radiation would not be justified.

It bears repeating that the number of films in pediatric urography should be kept to a minimum. Most excretory urograms can be accomplished with one preliminary film and two postinjection films. In more difficult or complicated cases, however, further filming is necessary and justifiable.

Urographic films should consistently be made in *expiration*, and each film should be carefully monitored by the attending radiologist.

The first postinjection film is made at 2 minutes and is restricted to the kidneys. The patient is supine (Fig. 6–179A).

The second film is made at 7 minutes, with the patient prone (Fig. 6–179B).[7] The prone film is valuable because it tends to disperse laterally gas-containing gut and causes the kidneys to assume a position closer to the coronal plane, thus improving their visualization (Fig. 6–179). In addition, it provides a second look and thus demonstrates whether a questionable finding is constant and therefore likely to be significant.

If the kidney outline is not completely visualized, a posterior oblique film, with a sharply collimated beam, is useful (see Fig. 6–196).

Lateral projections are sometimes helpful, usually to clarify anteroposterior relationships. For example, when a ureterocele is suspected, or when it is recognized but requires further anatomical definition, a lateral film may be used. It is also useful in abdominal masses.

If gas-containing bowel obscures the kidney, particularly in young children, we use the "paddle-compression" technique (Figs. 6–172, 6–180, and 6–181). A pneumatic paddle, the same as those familiar in gastrointestinal spot filming, is used to gently compress the abdomen over the kidney with the patient in the supine position. This successfully disperses the gas-containing bowel and improves visualization of the kidney. In young infants, a single paddle-compression exposure can be used to show both kidneys, but generally one kidney at a time is shown by this technique (see Figs. 6–172C and 6–181). The paddle-compression radiograph can be made in oblique projection, if desired.

When distention of the pelvis and calyceal system is insufficient, the lower ureters can be compressed and

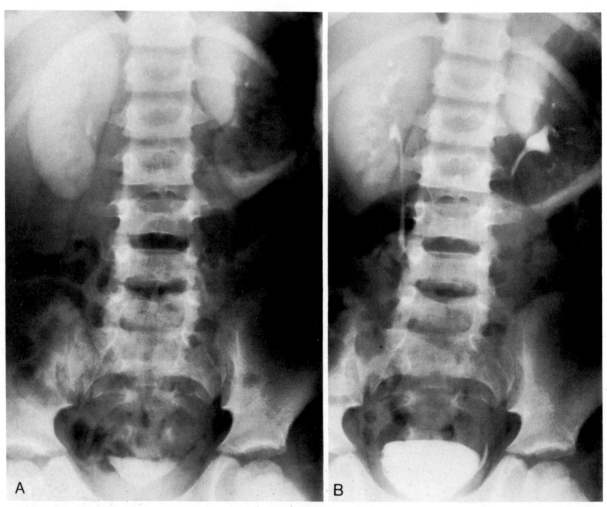

Figure 6–178. "Shock" nephrogram in a 5.5-year-old boy who vomited and developed hives, conjunctival edema, nasal mucosal edema, and mild laryngeal spasm, after contrast was injected. He became hypotensive, without tachycardia or bradycardia. He was treated with intramuscular diphenhydramine hydrochloride, subcutaneous epinephrine, and intravenous fluids, and was placed in Trendelenburg position. He recovered fully in a few hours. *A,* A film at 25 minutes shows an enhanced and delayed bilateral nephrogram, with an almost empty bladder. *B,* A film was made at 60 minutes when urinary function had almost fully recovered. A right upper-pole calyceal diverticulum is an incidental finding.

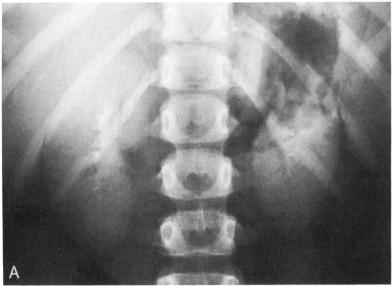

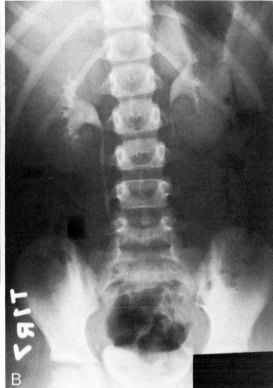

Figure 6–179. Advantages of prone radiography. *A,* A 2-minute postinjection radiograph was obtained with beam confined to the kidneys. *B,* A 7-minute prone radiograph shows the abdomen. The kidneys are slightly broader because in the prone position they are closer to the coronal plane than in the supine position. Gas-containing gut is largely displaced laterally and therefore does not obscure the urinary system.

Figure 6–180. "Paddle" compression is applied. This is useful in dispelling gas from selected areas of the child's abdomen.

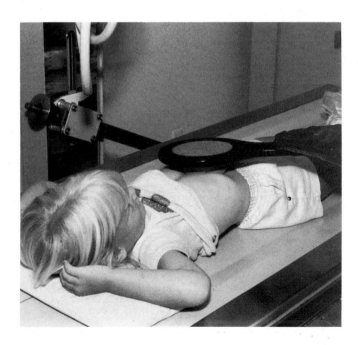

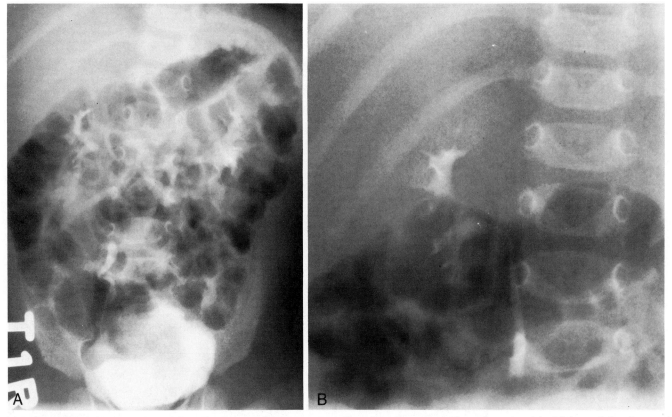

Figure 6–181. *A*, Prone radiograph at 7 minutes after contrast medium injection shows the urinary tract, but it is partially obscured by gas-containing gut in a 2-month-old child. *B*, Paddle compression used immediately after *A*. Visualization, particularly of the renal parenchyma, is improved.

partially obstructed, thereby distending the upper collecting systems in a fashion similar to the technique used in adults. The technique is not used in very small infants but is highly effective in pediatric patients of all other ages. Indeed, if the resulting radiograph does not show distention of the upper collecting system, it is likely that the method has not been properly applied. Commercial devices are available for this purpose, but we prefer the following: a folded blood-pressure cuff (sphygmomanometer) (Fig. 6–182*A*) is placed under a Velcro belt at the level of the anterior-superior iliac spines, with the patient supine (Fig. 6–182*B*). The blood-pressure cuff is then gently and carefully inflated until the patient begins to feel discomfort. The compression is maintained for 5 minutes, and a radiograph of the upper collecting system is obtained (Fig. 6–183). Occasionally, the ureteral obstruction produced by the lower adominal compression causes mild caliectasis (Fig. 6–184).

It is *very* important, before an upper abdominal paddle or lower ureteral compression is applied, that the condition of the patient be known and the preliminary film carefully inspected for any evidence of a contraindication to compression—such as a mass, evidence of appendicitis, or perforation.

If opacification of the ureters is important but is inadequate on the standard prone projection at 7 minutes, we use the "postcompression release technique." This is accomplished by compressing the distal ureters, as described earlier, for 5 minutes, and then obtaining a full abdominal radiograph immediately after the compression is released. Usually, the ureters promptly fill and are radiographically visible (Fig. 6–185).

When urinary obstruction, as by a calculus, is suspected or identified on the early films, delayed films must be made. The delayed films are made at increasing intervals until opacification is sufficient and/or again begins to diminish. This is not predictable, and the film timing must be judged on a patient-by-patient basis. Sometimes it must be carried on for 24 hours; usually, however, a shorter time, such as 3 to 6 hours, suffices.

Delayed filming is also used for nonobstructive renal insufficiency and for nonobstructive hydronephrosis.

Distention of the stomach by administration of a carbonated beverage has been recommended to improve visualization of the kidneys and the collecting systems when they are obscured by gut content.[35] In our experience this has rarely been a useful method. The distended stomach does improve visualization of much of the left kidney, but seldom in its entirety, and only part of the right kidney is better shown, because the distal portion of the stomach is smaller than the proximal part (Fig. 6–191). In addition, the gas that has been introduced passes to the small bowel and may obscure, rather than clarify, urinary anatomy on subsequent films. Distention of the stomach with water has also been recommended;[50] this too improves visualization, but not of the whole kidney or kidneys.

A second injection of contrast medium is occasionally justified, when the density achieved during the excretory urogram is insufficient. We have used the second injection to improve visualization, for example, when hydronephrosis or cystic disease is present.

When bilateral hydronephrosis and hydroureter are present, the examination should not be considered com-

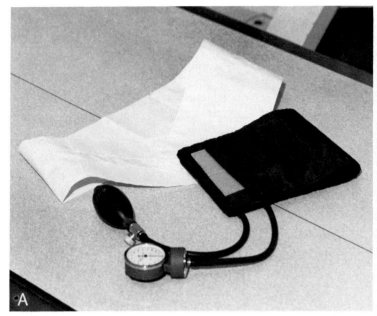

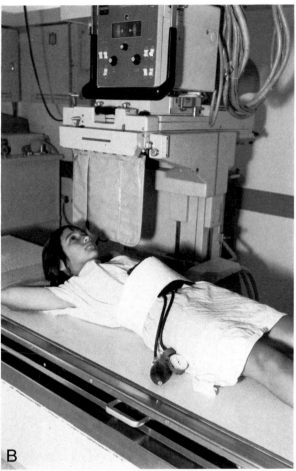

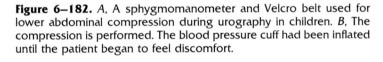

Figure 6–182. *A,* A sphygmomanometer and Velcro belt used for lower abdominal compression during urography in children. *B,* The compression is performed. The blood pressure cuff had been inflated until the patient began to feel discomfort.

plete until a final film has been made with the bladder empty.[5, 45] If the child cannot empty the bladder, it must be accomplished by catheterization.

In young infants, excretion of contrast medium is not as prompt as in the child or adult; delayed films are therefore more frequently needed in young patients, especially for those in the first month of life.[59]

When pediatric patients cry they tend to swallow air, which may introduce enough gas into the gut to spoil the excellent preparation that had been achieved (Fig. 6–172). To displace gas, which obscures the kidneys, we use "paddle compression" or lower abdominal (ureteral) compression. If that is unsuccessful, we occasionally must resort to tomography. Linear tomography usually suffices; it is simple to operate and achieves the fastest exposures of any tomographic method. Three linear cuts are made, the center cut at one-third of the AP diameter from the back, and the other at 1 cm anterior and 1 cm posterior, respectively, to this level.

Since the minimum duration of exposure for linear tomography is about 0.5 seconds, movement of the child may ruin the examination.

Excretory Micturition Cystourethrography (EMCU)

The common, and usually the best, method of visualizing the bladder and urethra in pediatric uroradiology is the voiding cystourethrogram (VCU). This is performed by catheterizing the bladder, filling it with contrast medium until the child is ready to void or begins to void, and recording the micturition sequence on television tape, with spot films of important events observed during voiding. Sometimes it is difficult or inopportune to catheterize the bladder, for example, when a child cannot tolerate catheterization, when parents refuse to have it performed, or when a referring physician or radiologist believes it to be contraindicated. In these circumstances, an adequate study may often be obtained by using the contrast medium in the urinary bladder at the end of the excretory urogram.

The problem is how to produce adequate density (concentration) of the contrast medium in the bladder. The solution is to be sure that the bladder is empty when excretion of the intravenously injected contrast begins, so that undiluted contrast reaches the bladder and can be imaged during micturition. This is accomplished by making the intravenous injection immediately before or immediately after urination, so that the contrast-containing urine reaching the bladder is not diluted.

Figure 6–186 illustrates a patient in whom this method was used. The child had urgency; he was catheterized without difficulty, and filling the bladder with contrast material (drip method) was almost complete, when he suddenly urinated. The single image that was obtained (Fig. 6–186*A*) was believed to be inadequate, yet we hesitated to recatheterize him. We obtained an excretory urogram after the VCU, making sure that he had emptied his bladder just before the intravenous injection of con-

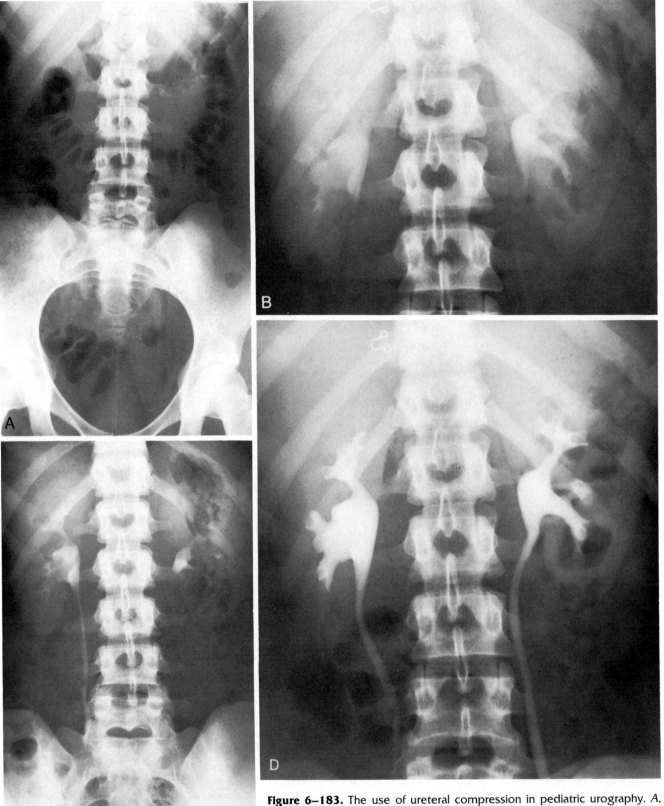

Figure 6–183. The use of ureteral compression in pediatric urography. *A*, Supine preliminary radiograph shows moderate fecal and gas content in the colon. *B,C*, Supine kidney and prone abdominal radiographs incompletely show the kidneys and their collecting systems. *D*, Upper abdominal radiograph after 5 minutes of lower ureteral compression. The entire upper ureter and upper collecting system on each side are now distended and clearly shown.

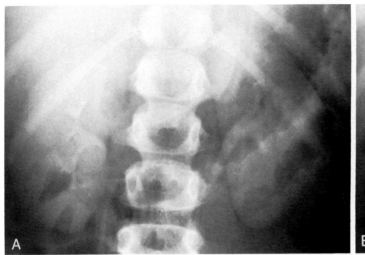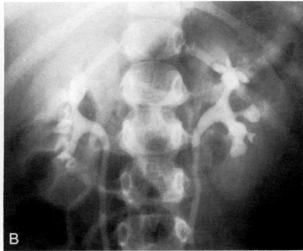

Figure 6–184. Mild caliectasis caused by lower ureteral compression. *A,* Visualization of the upper collecting system is incomplete. *B,* Similar exposure after 5 minutes of lower ureteral compression. Visualization is improved, and the compression has produced mild caliectasis.

trast material. Without the irritation of a catheter in his bladder, he was able to void on command, and a satisfactory cystourethrogram was obtained (Fig. 6–186*B*).

This method is not recommended for routine use (i.e., to replace the standard VCU). It requires intravenous injection of contrast, which is not needed for lower-tract study. There is difficulty in controlling the density and volume of bladder urine, and the urge to urinate is less predictable when the bladder is filling slowly (and more physiologically) by excretion, than when it is filled directly and more rapidly by catheter.

Vesicoureteral reflux, at least of a minor degree, is much more difficult to detect and record by EMCU. However, minor reflux is arguably of such slight significance that overlooking it may not be very important.

THE NORMAL PEDIATRIC KIDNEY

Shape

The shape of the kidney of the infant or child does not differ substantially from that of the adult, with the exception of fetal lobation.

Size

Much attention has been given to the size of the kidney in pediatric work, mostly because of scarring and impaired growth caused by urinary tract infection and/or vesicoureteral reflux. A number of systems of measurement of the kidneys have been devised. All the radiographic methods use supine films, which must therefore be used if any of them is to be applicable. It has been said that the apparent renal size is magnified on prone films; this is only partially true. The kidneys appear larger on the prone radiograph, primarily because in this position they rotate forward into the coronal plane, seeming to be broader; that is, their full breadth is visualized in the prone position. This observation is easily confirmed by ultrasonography in supine and prone positions.

Almost all the systems that have been proposed use kidney length; no practical radiographic system that measures volume has been devised; ultrasonography is superior for volume measurements. For radiographic measurement, correlations with age, body height, body surface area, and lumbar vertebral heights have been made. Klare and colleagues[95] thoroughly reviewed most proposed methods. The simplest method, and a good one, is to compare the kidney height with the combined heights of the first four vertebral bodies and their interspaces; the correlation is close and direct, ± 1 cm, after the first 18 months of life.

We have found the system suggested by Eklöf and Ringertz[92] to be useful and convenient. It compares kidney length with vertebral height and offers a nomogram that is readily used to obtain means and standard deviations. As with other biological measurements, however, the range of normal is sufficiently broad that no method of measurement is entirely satisfactory. It is useful to make measurements when comparing serial and follow-up urograms.

Radiographic factors can alter kidney measurement, particularly when examinations have been in different radiographic rooms, and/or using different focus-film distances. When comparison with vertebral length is used, these changes are unlikely to be of clinical significance; however, every effort should be made to standardize radiographic factors. This is particularly important when follow-up studies are performed, and growth of the kidney is an important consideration.

Normal Variants

Total Body Opacification

The phenomenon of increased radiographic density of all organs in the body following administration of contrast material is particularly evident in young infants, and it has been shown to have diagnostic value in the presence of a nonvascularized, space-occupying mass or collection of fluid.[30, 61] This effect is sometimes striking in an infant with a full bladder that is visualized as a negative density

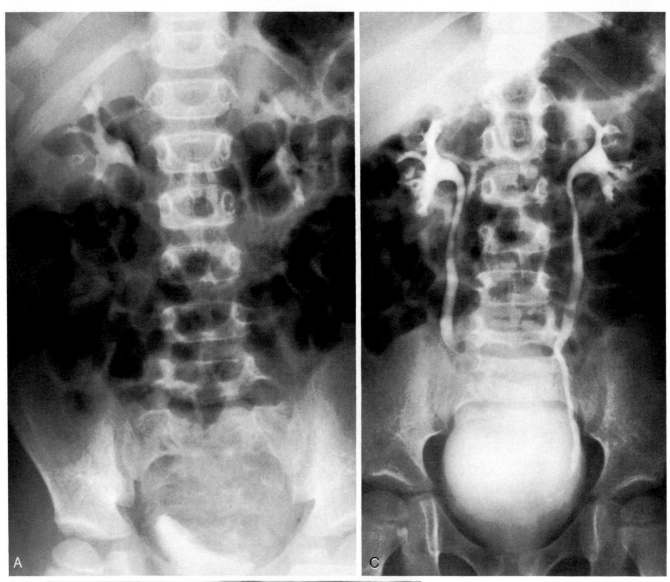

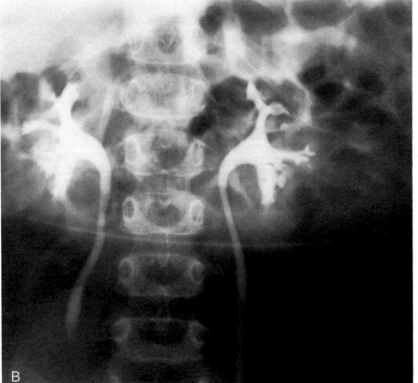

Figure 6–185. Compression and release technique. *A*, A 7-minute prone radiograph incompletely visualizes the urinary system and the ureters, in particular. *B*, Upper abdominal film was taken after 5 minutes of lower ureteral compression. The upper collecting systems and upper ureters are distended and well visualized. *C*, Supine abdominal radiograph exposed immediately after release of compression. Ureteral visualization is much improved.

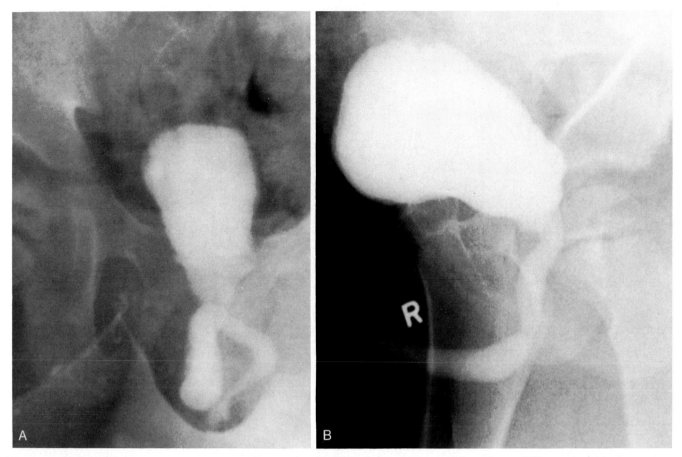

Figure 6–186. Excretory micturition cystourethrography (EMCU). *A,* Precipitous voiding during VCU occurred before proper positioning and filming could be obtained in this 5-year-old boy. This single AP film was believed to be inadequate. *B,* Rather than recatheterize the child, an EMCU study was attempted at the conclusion of an intravenous urogram. The film clearly demonstrates a normal bladder neck and posterior urethra.

shortly after contrast injection. Another example is, in adrenal hemorrhage of the newborn, the appearance of the hemorrhagic suprarenal mass as a negative density because of surrounding organ enhancement. The displacement of the ipsilateral kidney and flattening of the upper pole of the kidney make the diagnosis possible (Fig. 6–187). (With CT scanning, the phenomenon of total body opacification is much easier to recognize, and is referred to as contrast enhancement.)

Bowel Wall Opacification

The bowel wall may become slightly to moderately opacified after contrast medium injection, even if renal function is normal (Fig. 6–188). This is most striking in the newborn and is accentuated in renal insufficiency.[3]

Gallbladder Opacification

Rarely, the gallbladder opacifies following standard contrast medium injection. With the use of low-osmolality contrast media, opacification of the gallbladder, presumably representing excretion through the liver and concentration in the gallbladder, is common. It is most often reported following administration of ioxaglate.[68] Figure 6–189 is a plain film of the abdomen made approximately 1 day after intravenous ioxaglate administration. It clearly

shows gallbladder opacification, which lasted at least 48 hours.

The heterotopic excretion of ioxaglate through the liver does not indicate impaired renal function; nor, as far as we are aware, does it influence the incidence of adverse reactions to the contrast medium.

Adrenal Calcification

Adrenal calcification is occasionally visualized (Fig. 6–190), usually bilaterally. It is generally presumed to be the result of neonatal adrenal atrophy and hemorrhage. When discovered as an incidental finding and when small and triangular, it is almost always insignificant. In the past, it has been attributed to tuberculosis or has been thought to be associated with Addison's disease. Although cases of such findings are on record, they are now rare indeed. In the healthy child, adrenal calcification is an incidental finding of no clinical significance.[54]

Prone versus Supine Radiographs

During prone radiography, the kidneys assume a more coronal position, and thus appear broader in transverse diameter than during supine radiography (see Fig. 6–177). Furthermore, in the prone position the left kidney may appear depressed in comparison with the right, and

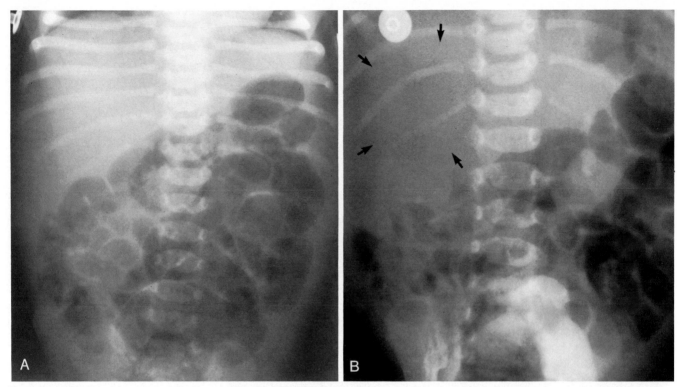

Figure 6–187. Total body opacification. In this 3-day-old infant, a right upper abdominal mass was palpated. *A,* The preliminary radiograph shows no abnormality, but the gut contains much gas. *B,* Prone radiograph during total body opacification. A nonvascularized right suprarenal mass (*arrows*) is shown by its (relative) decrease in density and by inferior displacement of the kidney, with flattening of its upper pole. The diagnosis of neonatal hemorrhage was confirmed by ultrasound and by clinical and sonographic follow-up, showing resolution of the hematoma.

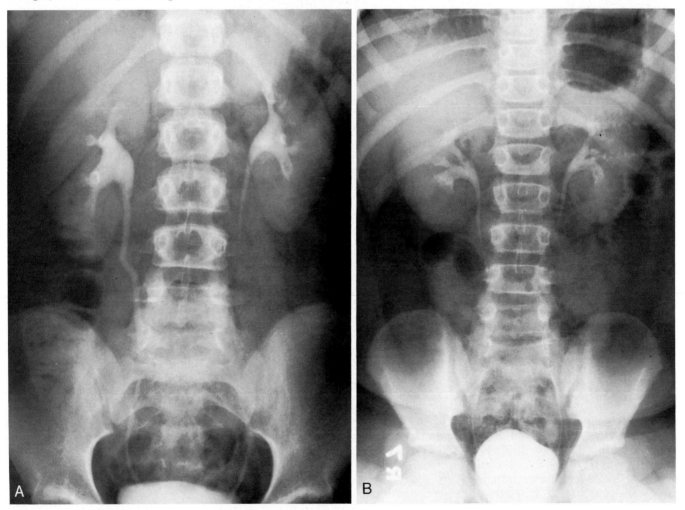

Figure 6–188 *See legend on opposite page*

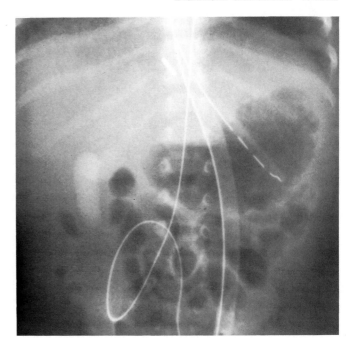

Figure 6–189. Gallbladder opacification after ioxoglate injection in a 13-day-old baby who had an angiocardiogram because of congenital heart disease. A follow-up film made 1 day later shows persistent opacification of the gallbladder.

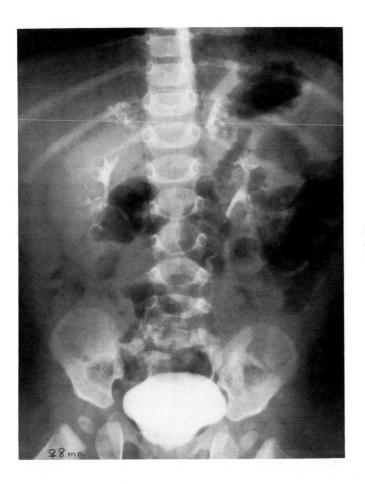

Figure 6–190. Adrenal calcification incidentally discovered in an 8-month-old girl. The adrenals are calcified, but normal both in size and in their approximately triangular configuration.

Figure 6–188. Gut wall opacification during urography. *A,* The patient is a 7-year-old girl. On a standard PA (prone) postinjection radiograph at 7 minutes, the wall of the right colon is partially opacified; it was not opacified on the preliminary film. Urinary function was normal, as was this IVU. *B,* In an 8-year-old boy, opacification of the wall of the stomach and some segments of small bowel after contrast injection are shown.

in comparison with its appearance in the supine position (Fig. 6–191). This normal phenomenon must not be confused with kidney displacement or abnormal position.

Fetal Lobation

The fetal kidney is frequently lobular, a configuration that tends to smooth out or disappear by birth. However, in early postnatal life the lobation may persist and must be distinguished from scars. The lobes are usually well defined, with sharp indentations between them (Fig. 6–192), rather than the flattened or irregular indentations produced by scars. In addition, the indentations are between—not opposite—the calyces and are not associated with calyceal blunting or deformity. The lobation may be unilateral or bilateral.[14]

Duplication

Duplication of the upper collecting system is common and usually is clinically insignificant. It is associated with increased length of the kidney (Fig. 6–193A,B). The duplication may involve part or all of the ureter. Some attempt should be made to determine the extent of the duplication, since there is evidence that the more complete the duplication, the more likely is reflux and/or infection.[33, 34] To demonstrate the ureter (or ureters)

completely, the compression and release technique is valuable (see page 218).

Campbell[11] showed that when incomplete ureteral duplication is present, peristalsis is frequently unusual or abnormal, with peristaltic waves descending one loop of the Y and ascending the other. This he thought was insignificant, except in the event of infection when the incoordinated peristalsis would predispose to complications.

Size Asymmetry

Some minor variation in the size of the two kidneys may occur normally (Fig. 6–194). Any measurement of over 1-cm difference between the two kidneys is probably abnormal. Careful search should be made for scarring or deformity of the smaller of the two kidneys, and for compensatory hypertrophy of the opposite kidney. When the small kidney is closer to the vertebral column than usual (or than normal), it is more likely to represent hypoplasia than normal asymmetry of size. When the smaller kidney is on the same side as vesicoureteral reflux, it is more likely to be scarred and contracted than to be a normal variant. If there is a history of urinary tract infection, voiding cystourethrography (VCU) should be done to look for ipsilateral reflux.

Templeton and Thompson[76] reported on and recom-

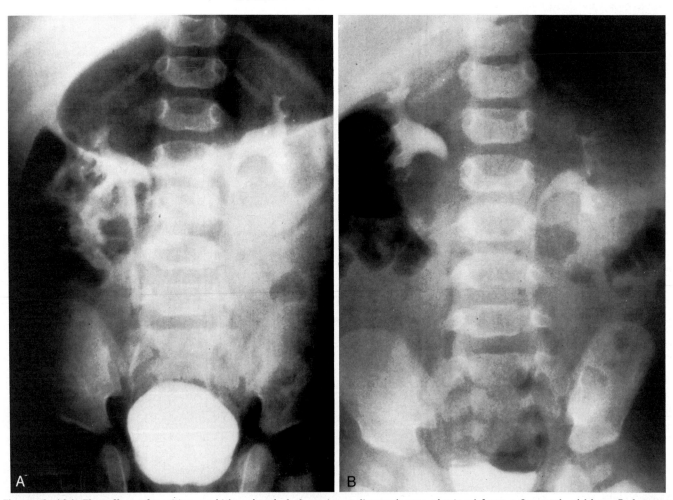

Figure 6–191. The effect of position on kidney level. A, A supine radiograph was obtained from a 9-month-old boy. B, A prone radiograph was made immediately after A. The left kidney is now lower. Note that the stomach is distended with gas, but that this does not help much in visualizing the kidneys.

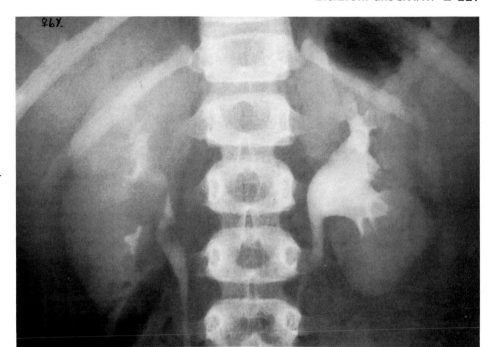

Figure 6–192. Mild bilateral fetal lobation is more marked on the right.

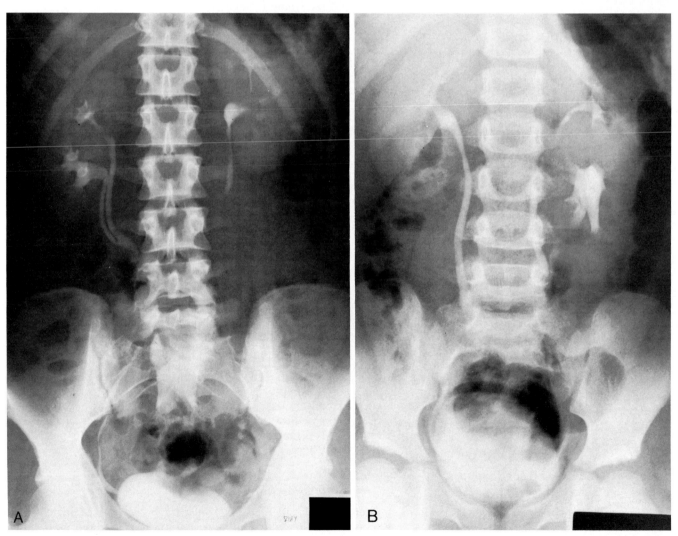

A

B

Figure 6–193. Duplication of collecting system and part of the ureter. *A,* Prone radiograph shows duplication of the right upper collecting system and upper ureter. The right kidney is longer than the left. This is a Y-shaped duplication. *B,* Shown is duplication of the left upper collecting system and partial duplication of the kidney and of the left upper ureter. The left kidney is much longer than the right.

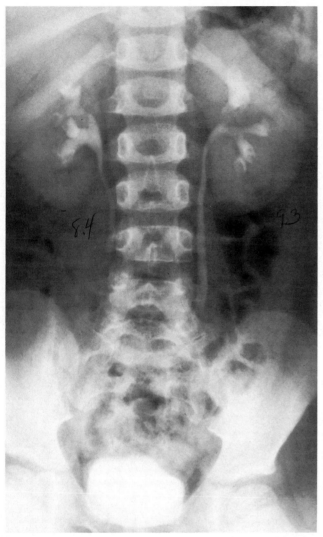

Figure 6–194. Unilateral small kidney. The right kidney (8.4 cm) is smaller than the left (9.3 cm), slightly more vertical in orientation, and slightly closer to the midline. Vesicoureteral reflux was shown bilaterally, but was more severe on the left. It resolved spontaneously with further growth and development. It was therefore inferred that the small right kidney was a normal variant (mild hypoplasia), rather than a scarred kidney.

mended aortography to differentiate between congenital and acquired small kidneys. If the origin of the ipsilateral renal artery was narrow, the kidney was congenitally small. If the origin was normal, the diminutive kidney was acquired. Such studies are not indicated today. In the presence of urinary tract infection, ipsilateral reflux, or hypertension, ultrasonography can be performed to help determine whether a unilateral small kidney is structurally normal.

Renal Pseudomasses (Pseudotumors)

Just as in adults, splenic indentation can produce or be associated with thinning of the renal cortex in children. This occurs at and immediately adjacent to the point where the spleen indents the left kidney. The contiguous cortex bulges prominently enough to simulate, occasionally, a mass in the kidney (Fig. 6–195).

A normal but prominent inferior hilar lip may indent

the ureteropelvic junction so strikingly as to suggest a mass (Fig. 6–196).

A hump may be present on either kidney because of thick parenchyma, but without any other deformity and with an intact pyelocalyceal system (Fig. 6–197). This "dromedary hump" is common and usually is properly overlooked. It is more often seen on the left side.

Papillary Blush

A papillary blush is seen when contrast material in the collecting ducts (ducts of Bellini) is radiopaque. Since these ducts are the site of the last stage of absorption of water to produce normally concentrated urine, it is not surprising that their opacity occasionally approaches that achieved in the calyx. Their appearance on excretory urography was first described by Fleischner and colleagues,[24] who refuted the notion that the appearance was due to pyelotubular backflow.

The normal papillary blush is a fan-shaped density occupying the distal papilla. For reasons that are not understood, we believe it is more common on the right side than on the left (Fig. 6–198). It may be restricted to only a few calyces, and if the urogram is repeated at a later date these calyces will again show the phenomenon with no change and no progression.

When the opacification of the collecting ducts is unusually dense, it may resemble renal tubular ectasia (medullary sponge kidney).

The papillary blush may be increased when films are made after compressing the lower ureters (Fig. 6–199), presumably because the resulting obstruction slows excretion through the ducts, leading to a higher concentration of urine.

Calyceal Diverticulum

A calyceal diverticulum is usually an incidental finding on excretory urography. Timmons and associates reported its incidence as 3.3/1000 pediatric excretory urograms.[77] It is most frequent in the upper pole of one kidney, intimately related to a calyx, which is usually normal, as is the remainder of the kidney (Fig. 6–200; see also Fig. 6–177). In children, calculi rarely form in such a diverticulum, but in adults the incidence of this complication rises to 40%.[48, 77] Infection and hematuria are reported in association with diverticula. However, it is difficult to determine, if there is no calculus and if the related calyx is anatomically normal, what role (if any) the diverticulum plays in the hematuria or infection. Because of the possibility of calculus, it is important to have adequate preliminary films, since the calculus is obscured after injection by the excreted contrast medium (Fig. 6–201). (Further discussion of calyceal diverticula is provided in Chapter 19).

Solitary Calyx

A single calyx, presumably serving a single papilla (unipapillary kidney), may be encountered as a variant in a patient with no urinary disease when the opposite kidney is normal. However, Peterson and colleagues[65] have pointed out that it is usually associated with other, serious, malformations.

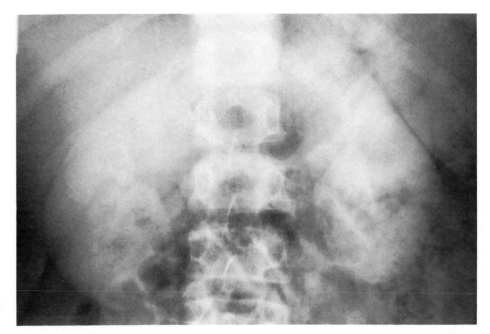

Figure 6–195. Mild deformity of the left kidney caused by the spleen. The renal parenchyma is thin where the splenic indentation occurs superiorly, and thick just beyond the area of contact with the spleen.

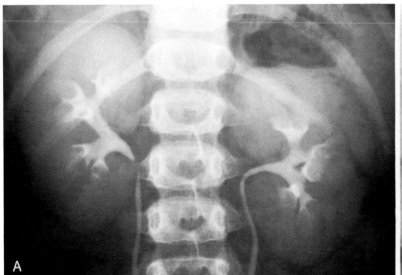

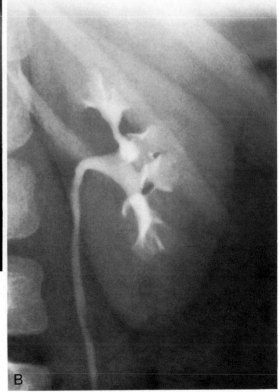

Figure 6–196. Large normal renal hilar lips, IVU. *A*, On the 2-minute AP radiograph, both inferior hilar lips appear large, deforming the pelves and displacing the upper ureters at the ureteropelvic junctions. This is more marked on the left side. *B*, Left posterior oblique projection confirms the normal nephrogram and absence of any invasion, destruction, or obstruction of the collecting system or ureter by the pseudomass.

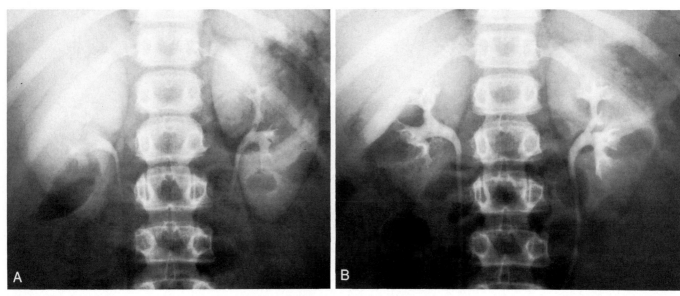

Figure 6–197. "Dromedary hump" seen on IVU. *A*, On the 2-minute radiograph, localized thickening of the renal parenchyma causes protrusion of the right lateral border of the kidney just below its midpoint. The collecting system appears to be normal. *B*, This is confirmed by a film made after ureteral compression, which shows the collecting system to be entirely normal.

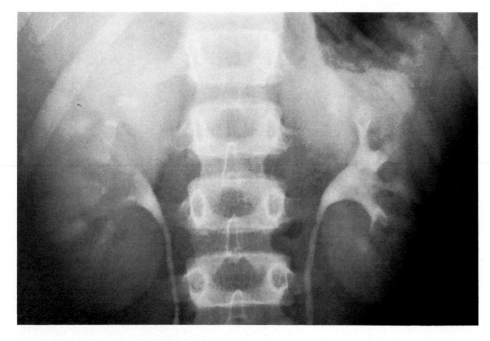

Figure 6–198. IVU shows papillary blush which is much more marked on the right than on the left side in normal kidneys.

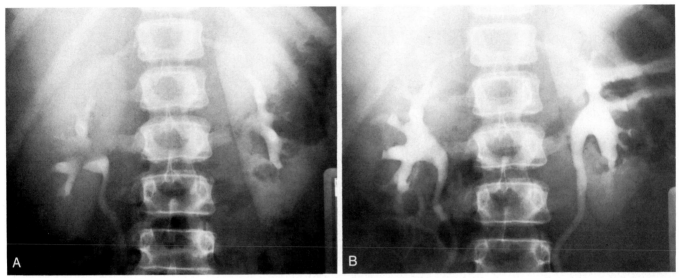

Figure 6–199. Papillary blush produced by lower ureteral compression during IVU. *A*, Standard 2-minute postinjection AP kidney radiograph shows little or no papillary blush. *B*, With ureteral compression a moderate papillary blush is produced, which is greater on the right than on the left.

Figure 6–200. Calyceal diverticulum. An approximately spherical collection of contrast medium appears in relation to a left upper-pole calyx on this IVU. There was no calcification on the preliminary film. The kidney parenchyma is normal.

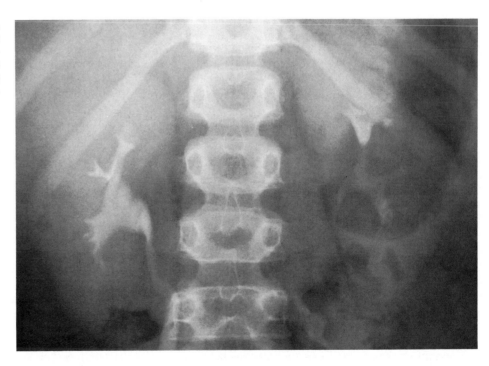

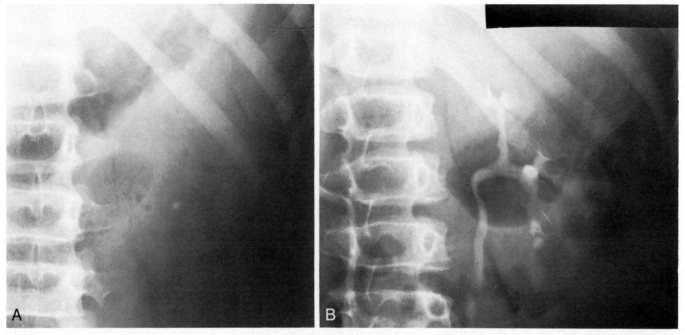

Figure 6–201. Calyceal diverticulum containing a calculus. *A,* A close-up from the preliminary film of an IVU shows a calcification overlying the left lower pole. *B,* Left posterior oblique urographic film shows that the calcification is in a calyceal diverticulum. The calculus would have been missed had the preliminary film not been made, or had gas or feces obscured the lower pole of the kidney.

Long Calyceal Infundibulum

Usually, long infundibula are confined to the upper poles of the kidney. Occasionally, as in Figure 6–202, one or more nonpolar infundibula may be exceptionally long, extending into what appears to be cortical renal tissue. If the calyx is otherwise structurally intact, and there is no evidence of contiguous cortical scarring, we believe this to be a normal finding, as are the much-more-frequent short infundibula.

Large Papillae

Occasionally, excretory urography reveals unusually broad, deep calyces, presumably indicating large papillae. However, in the absence of deformity of the calyces or other urographic abnormality, this represents a normal variant (Fig. 6–203). Large papillae are often seen in medullary sponge kidney, but the disorder is infrequent in children.

Multiple Calyces (Polycalycosis)

Most normal kidneys have from six to 12 minor calyces. However, the number varies and the number of calyces is often difficult to count accurately, especially when compound calyces exist. Figure 6–204 illustrates normal kidneys with approximately 16 calyces on the right side, and approximately 13 on the left.

The great variability in number is worth keeping in mind when the possibility of congenital megacalyces is considered, since one criterion for that diagnosis is an increased number of calyces (Fig. 6–205).

Compound Calyces

Each kidney may have simple or compound calyces, or both. The compound varieties are most frequent in the upper pole, next most frequent in the lower pole, and least frequent in the interpolar part of the kidney.

Some evidence shows that intrarenal reflux occurs most easily in compound calyces, because their orifices are more patulous than those of simple calyces. This may explain the tendency for reflux nephropathy to be most frequent and most severe in the upper pole of the kidney.[67] Simple and compound calyces are illustrated in Figure 6–204. The radiographic distinction of simple from compound calyces is often difficult and necessarily arbitrary.

Fraley's Syndrome

In both children and adults, the upper calyceal group, comprising one major and several minor calyces, is occasionally dilated, and the distal portion of the major calyx constricted or compressed (Fig. 6–206*A*). This led Fraley[25] to explain renal pain by associating it with obstruction of a major calyx. Since his report, some observers[4, 70] have concluded, as have we, that the radiological findings of Fraley's syndrome usually represent a normal variant. The entity is seen more frequently on the right than on the left side, is virtually always in the upper pole, and does not change or progress. It is likely due to an intrarenal vessel (or vessels) crossing the superior major calyx and compressing it.[19] The impression producing the apparent constriction of the major calyx can be eliminated radiographically by the distention following lower ureteral compression (Fig. 6–206*B*).

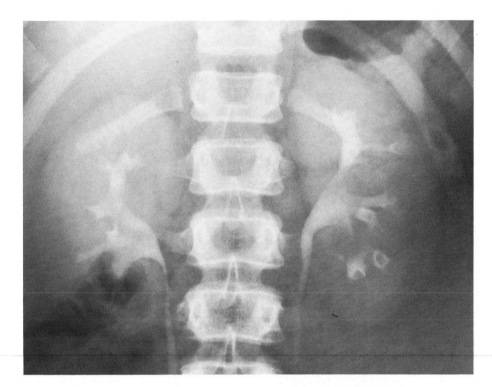

Figure 6–202. Normal variant on IVU: long, normal calyceal infundibula. There is some inconsistency of the lengths of the calyceal infundibula on both sides. In the upper pole of the left kidney and the lower pole of the right kidney are single long calyces, which are structurally normal, even though they protrude beyond the interpapillary line. The renal parenchyma is also normal.

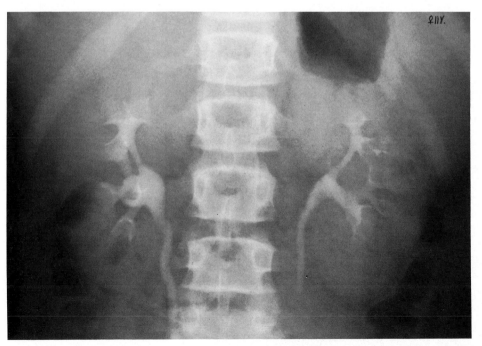

Figure 6–203. Normal variant on IVU: Broad, deep calyces representing large papillae are seen bilaterally in normal kidneys.

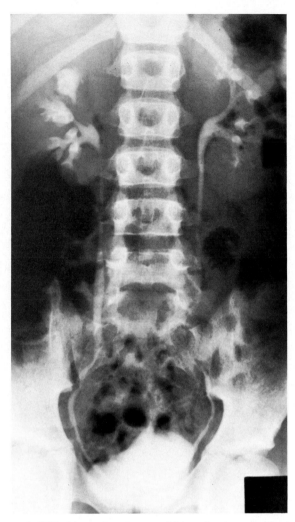

Figure 6–204. Normal variant on IVU: polycalycosis. On both sides, the calyces are more numerous than usual, particularly on the right where compound middle and upper-pole calyces drain multiple minor calyces.

Column of Bertin

The column of Bertin, originally described by Bertin[8] as a septum ("cloison"), is a thickened aggregate of cortical tissue, in place of the usual thin cortical septum that separates two pyramids. Since it forms a mass that displaces contiguous structures, it may simulate a neoplasm. It usually occurs near the junction of the middle and upper thirds of the kidney, frequently associated with a collecting system that is bifid or shows a tendency toward being bifid. The enlarged column of Bertin is often drained by a dwarfed and seemingly misdirected calyx (Fig. 6–207). Hodson and Mariani[34] showed that the enlarged column of Bertin often contains medullary tissue in its center, thereby explaining the paradox of a calyx seeming to drain cortical tissue.

The calyces surrounding the cloison, although usually displaced and deformed, are not invaded, obstructed, or destroyed.

On angiography, the enlarged column of Bertin shows normal or increased vasculature, but no evidence of tumor vascularity. On radionuclide study, there is increased uptake of the technetium-99m–labeled radionuclide by the renal cortical tissue constituting the mass.[62] Likewise, on excretory urography, the mass is either equal in opacity to the rest of the renal parenchyma during the nephrogram phase of the urogram, or it shows a slight increase corresponding to the increased vasculature and increased radionuclide uptake. These findings are well shown by nephrotomography.[29]

Given the criteria of typical site, tendency toward collecting system bifidness, displacement but not destruction of contiguous structures, and normal or increased density during the nephrogram, the diagnosis can usually be made with confidence from excretory urography alone. If not, a radionuclide scan clarifies the diagnosis. Angiography is almost never needed. Lafortune and colleagues have stated that sonographic findings are characteristic and obviate further investigation;[44] Simpson and associ-

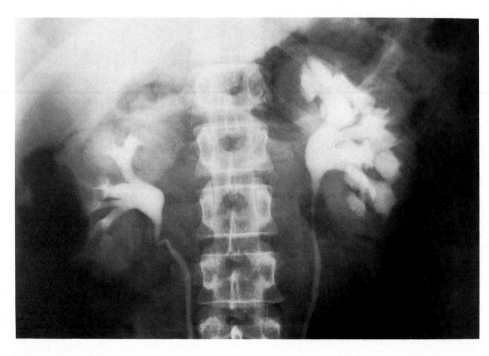

Figure 6–205. Unilateral congenital megacalyces. The left kidney is enlarged and its renal parenchyma is thin. There are numerous (multiple) calyces, all of which are dilated, the calyces are flattened (faceted) on contiguous surfaces, and there is no obstruction. No calculi were demonstrated, and the process was unchanged over a number of years.

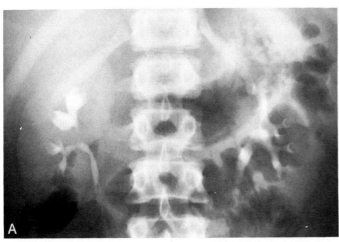
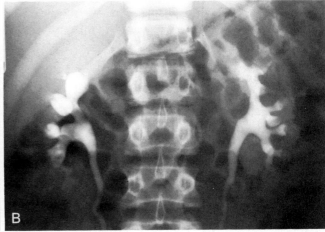

Figure 6–206. Fraley's syndrome. The right superior major calyx is compressed, and its minor calyces are dilated, as revealed by IVU. The remainder of both upper collecting systems is normal. AP radiographs, *A*, without compression, and *B*, with compression. The narrowing of the major calyx is no longer apparent. All calyces on both sides show mild dilatation with compression.

ates have shown that the same distinction can be clearly drawn using CT.[91]

Aberrant Papillae

Rarely, a renal papilla is ectopic or aberrant, and protrudes into a normal calyx in an unusual position.[83] It appears as a rounded, sharply circumscribed mass outlined by a "halo" of contrast in the calyx or pelvis (Fig. 6–208). The diagnosis is by exclusion, since a polyp, a neoplasm, or a blood clot can produce a similar appearance radiographically. An anteriorly or posteriorly directed calyx ("on end") can produce the same appearance but can be easily excluded or confirmed by an oblique radiograph.

The diagnosis is rarely confirmed histologically, since finding an aberrant papilla is only occasionally sufficient reason for any interventional procedure,[9, 23] in either adults or children.

Psoas Hypertrophy

In a heavily muscled subject, the psoas muscles may be strikingly larger than usual, indeed large enough to displace the kidneys anterolaterally, and increase their supramedial to inferolateral orientation (Fig. 6–209). Psoas hypertrophy is usually easy to recognize radiographically, but when in doubt one can confirm the condition by oblique films or ultrasonography. The ureters may be displaced anterolaterally by large psoas muscles.[31]

Ureteral Valves (Fetal Valves)

Although valves in the ureter are known to be a rare cause of obstruction, they are occasionally seen as folds or valves in a ureter that is otherwise normal and, in particular, not obstructed.

These valves or valvelike protrusions are known as "fetal valves," particularly because of the work of Os-

Figure 6–207. Column of Bertin. On this IVU, both collecting systems show a tendency toward being bifid. On the right, a mass just above the middle of the kidney slightly displaces contiguous calyces and shows slight enhancement of density. Similar but less marked changes appear on the left. On both sides, dwarfed and slightly misdirected calyces appear to be related to and presumably drain the mass, which, as shown by Hodson,[34] is likely to contain medullary tissue.

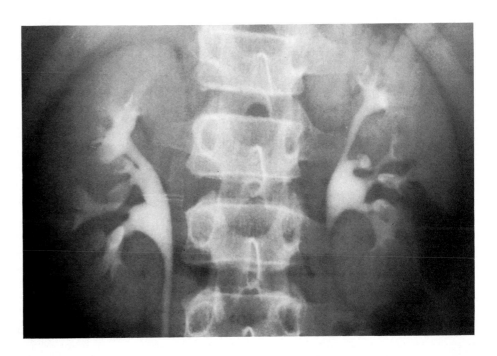

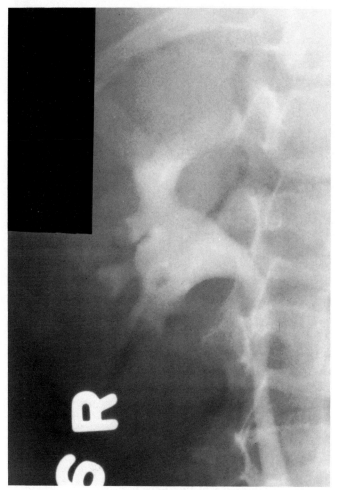

Figure 6–208. Aberrant papilla. Excretory urogram, right anterior oblique projection, shows a filling defect within the renal pelvis. The lucency is round and smooth, and it is ringed by contrast medium, of a slightly increased density ("halo"). No further investigation was undertaken.

tling,[63] who studied autopsy material from 250 fetuses in various stages of development. He found that, although the ureter in small embryos has an open lumen with no folds, by 4 to 5 months most fetal ureters show kinks in the upper portion of the ureter, occasionally extending as far as the pelvic brim. These were nonobstructive, and most disappeared with further maturation, prenatally and postnatally. Accordingly, they are occasionally seen in young infants at urography but are rarely seen in children. They are usually multiple and striking, even "corkscrew" in appearance (Fig. 6–210), but clinically insignificant—or at least not requiring surgical treatment.[46]

Medial Position of Ureters

The usual position of ureters as shown in Figures 6–184 and 6–185 is approximately vertical with slight undulations, crossing most of the transverse processes and/or the lateral portion of the pedicles from the ureteropelvic junction to the pelvic cavity, where lateral deviation is common.

However, considerable medial displacement of the ureters is not unusual and not necessarily abnormal.[71] Figure 6–211 shows mild, abrupt medial deviation or "hooking" that is likely over the normal psoas muscle. It simulates circumcaval ureter, but the medial displacement of the midureter is less than in that condition. Furthermore, obstruction is absent, whereas it characteristically is present in circumcaval ureter.

Medial displacement of the ureters inferiorly, as shown in Figure 6–212, may be marked, yet normal. We have no quantitative criteria on which to base the diagnosis of normal as opposed to abnormal medial displacement of the middle and distal ureters, but two qualitative criteria seem to suffice: absence of obstruction and absence of progression.

Figure 6–213 is an example of undulating medial displacement of the middle and lower ureters and no evidence of abdominal abnormality or urinary obstruction; it is thus acceptable as a normal variant. The same appearance, with low kidneys, occurs when the exposure is made during inspiration.

Ureteral Dilatation Proximal to Common Iliac Vessels

At the level of the upper sacral alae, the normal ureters undergo slight medial displacement and compression, with associated minimal proximal dilatation. This may be so slight as to be barely detectable (Fig. 6–214) or so marked as to simulate or suggest clinically significant obstruction (Fig. 6–215). Apparently, it is due to fixation at the point where the ureter crosses the iliac vessels. It was seen in about one-third of normal pediatric patients: on the right side in 55%, on the left side in 15%, and on both sides in 30% of patients in a review by Kaufman and coworkers.[38] No gender difference exists, but the incidence is low in young children, reaching peak incidence at age 12 in the pediatric population.

It would be expected that true ureteral obstruction, such as by stenosis or nonopaque calculus, could cause the same radiographic appearance, but generally the urographic findings reliably indicate that this is a normal variant.

Urinary Jet

During excretory urography, the spurt or jet of urine emerging from the ureteral orifice may be observed radiographically (Fig. 6–216).[37, 85] This phenomenon is also observed endoscopically; the flow from each ureter into the bladder is seen to be intermittent and forceful, and is called *efflux* by the endoscopist. It will be shown on IVU only when the bladder is partially opacified, because it must be seen through the contrast medium (Fig. 6–216).

Kuhns and associates[43] reported not only that the jet phenomenon is a normal finding in excretory urography, but also that the presence of such a jet is a good sign that vesicoureteral reflux is not present. Of 19 ureters with a jet sign, only one had minimal transient ureteral reflux, whereas in 39 ureters without a jet sign, 15 had reflux. We agree that the jet phenomenon usually means that no vesicoureteral reflux is present. In the prone radiograph, the jet may simulate an ectopic ureteral orifice (Fig. 6–217). This is because the heavy contrast medium accumulates in the bladder fundus, which is dependent in this position. The bladder is dependent in this position, and the urine in the base of the bladder may be nonopacified.

Text continued on page 242

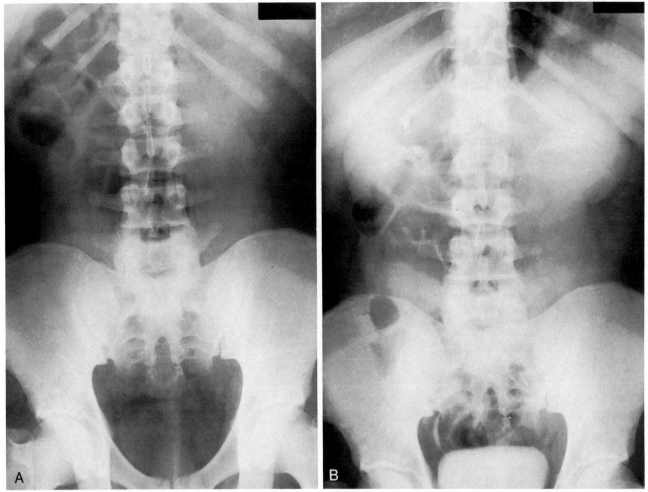

Figure 6–209. Psoas hypertrophy. *A*, Preliminary film shows unusually large psoas muscles in a well-developed 17-year-old boy. *B*, IVU demonstrates lateral displacement of the kidneys by the large psoas muscles.

Figure 6–210. Ureteral valves. Boy 7 months old has multiple ureteral valves bilaterally, particularly striking on the right, where there is a tendency to a "corkscrew" configuration. There is no obstruction.

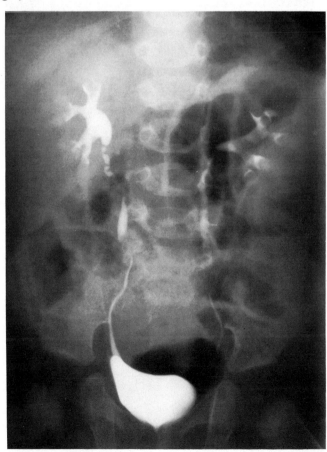

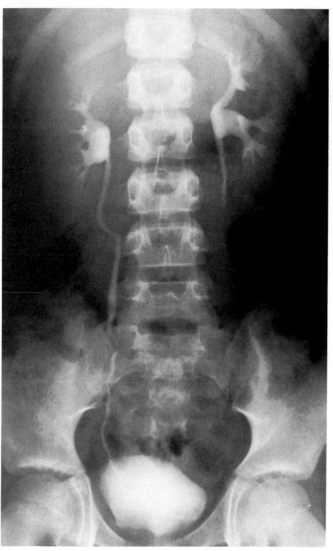

Figure 6–211. Normal localized medial deviation of the ureters. The right ureter abruptly courses medially, probably over the psoas, at the level of the inferior pole of the right kidney. The deviation is less than that of a circumcaval ureter, and there is no obstruction.

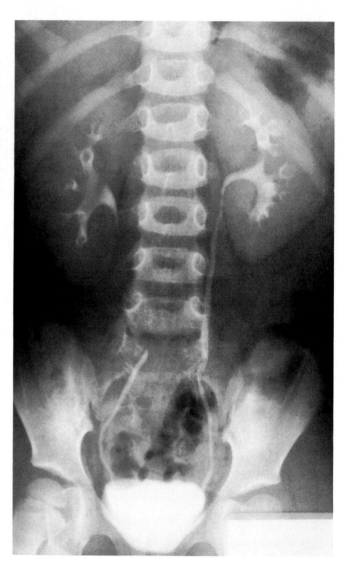

Figure 6–212. Normal medial deviation of the ureters. Each ureter deviates medially at approximately the point where it crosses the common iliac vessels. There is no obstruction.

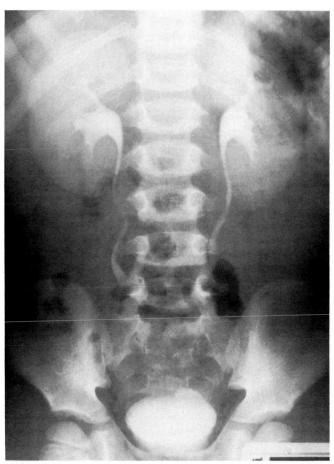

Figure 6–213. Normal medial deviation of the ureters. Undulating medial displacement of both ureters, maximum at the level of the L5 vertebra. There is no obstruction.

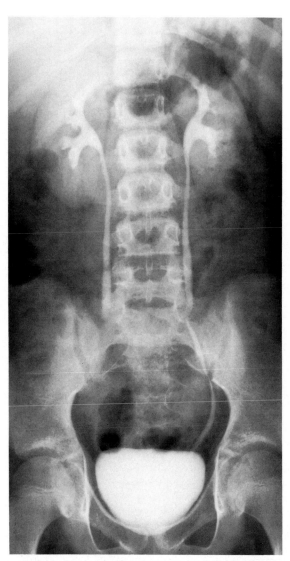

Figure 6–214. Ureteral dilatation proximal to the iliac vessel crossing point. There is mild and continuous dilatation of both middle and upper ureters proximal to this point.

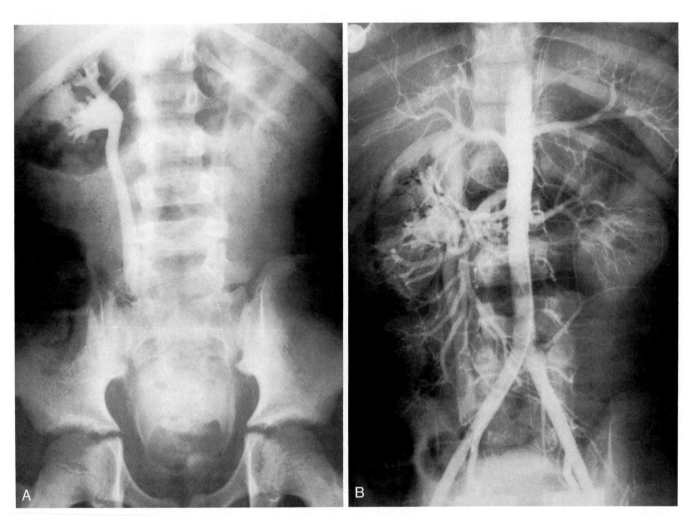

Figure 6–215. Marked dilatation of the right ureter proximal to the iliac vessel crossing point, on the right side only. *A*, Excretory urogram shows the dilatation involving the pelvis and, minimally, the calyces. *B*, Aortogram for abdominal trauma. The vessels are normal, and the crossing of ureter over right iliac vessels as well as dilatation proximal to this point is clearly shown.

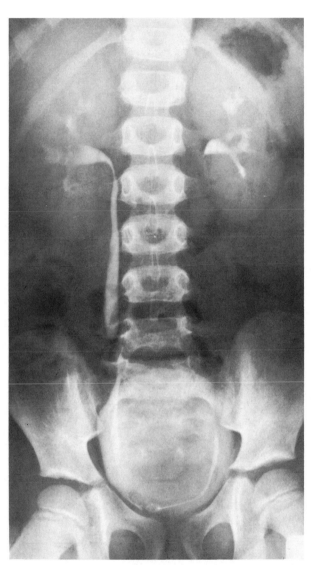

Figure 6–216. Bilateral ureteral urinary jets. They are asymmetrical, but almost synchronous, and are well shown because the bladder is only partially opacified by excreted contrast medium.

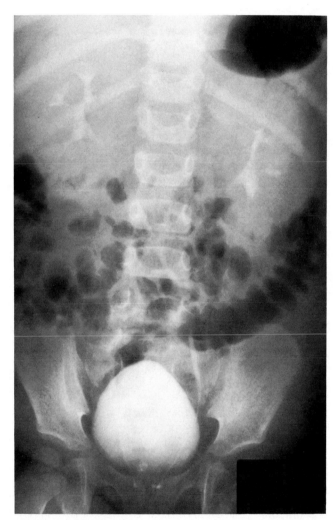

Figure 6–217. Bilateral synchronous ureteral urinary jets simulating ectopic ureters. The contrast medium in this prone radiograph is collected in the most dependent portion of the bladder, which is the fundus, and the jets pass through nonopacified urine in the bladder base, mimicking ectopic ureters.

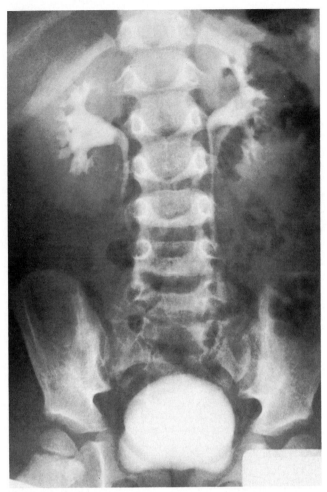

Figure 6–218. Bladder "ears." The bladder protrudes inferolaterally just lateral to its base, as shown in this prone radiograph during excretory urography of a 4-year-old boy. The "ears" are more common in young infants.

The urinary jet then looks like a ureter outside the bladder lumen. Occasionally, this may be observed bilaterally (Fig. 6–217).

"Bladder Ears"

In young infants, usually less than 6 months of age, inferomedial protrusions of the bladder lumen may be present; these are usually called "bladder ears." They are demonstrated in 9% of urograms of infants under the age of 1 year (Fig. 6–218). The protrusions are most often seen when the bladder is partially filled, and they are transitory. Their occurrence is probably related to the size and position of the bladder in infants and to the persistence of a large inguinal ring. This suggestion is reinforced by the higher incidence of bladder ears in infants having inguinal hernias.

References

1. Athanasoulis CA, Brown B, Baum S: Selective renal venography in differentiation between congenitally absent and small contracted kidney. Radiology 108:301–305, 1973.
2. Avner ED, Ellis D, Jaffe R, Bowen D: Neonatal radiocontrast nephropathy simulating infantile polycystic kidney disease. J Pediatr 100:85–87, 1982.
3. Becker JA, Gregoire A, Berdon W, Schwartz D: Vicarious excretion of urographic media. Radiology 90:243–248, 1968.
4. Benz G, Willich E: Upper calyx reno-vascular obstruction in children: Fraley's syndrome. Pediatr Radiol 5:213–218, 1977.
5. Berdon WE, Baker DH: The significance of a distended bladder in the interpretation of intravenous pyelograms obtained on patients with "hydronephrosis." AJR 120:402–409, 1974.
6. Berdon WE, Schwartz RH, Becker J, Baker DH: Tamm-Horsfall proteinuria. Its relationship to prolonged nephrogram in infants and children and to renal failure following intravenous urography in adults with multiple myeloma. Radiology 92:714–722, 1969.
7. Berdon WE, Baker DH, Leonidas J: Advantages of prone positioning in gastrointestinal and genitourinary roentgenologic studies in infants and children. AJR 103:444–455, 1968.
8. Bertin M: Memoire pour servir a l'histoire des reins. In Histoire de l'Acadamie Royale des Sciences. Paris, Academie Royale des Sciences, 1744, pp 77–111.
9. Binder R, Korobkin M, Clark RE, Palubinskas AJ: Aberrant papillae and other filling defects of the renal pelvis. AJR 114:746–752, 1972.
10. Bree RL, Green B, Keiller DL, Genet EF: Medial deviation of the ureters secondary to psoas muscle hypertrophy. Radiology 118:691–695, 1976.
11. Campbell JE: Ureteral peristalsis in duplex renal collecting systems. AJR 99:577–584, 1967.
12. Chacha PB: Suppurative arthritis of the hip joint in infancy: A persistent diagnostic problem and possible complication of femoral venipuncture. J Bone Joint Surg 53A:538–544, 1971.
13. Chang SF: Pear-shaped bladder caused by large iliopsoas muscles. Radiology 128:349–350, 1978.
14. Cooperman LR, Lowman RM: Fetal lobulation of the kidneys. AJR 92:273–280, 1964.
15. Cremin BJ, Rhodes AH: Letter to the Editor: Contrast media in paediatric radiology. Br J Radiol 56:779, 1983.
16. Curtis JA, Sadhu V, Steiner RM: Malposition of the colon in right renal agenesis, ectopia, and anterior nephrectomy. AJR 129:845–850, 1977.
17. Davies P, Panto PN, Buckley J, Richardson RE: The old and the new: A study of five contrast media for urography. Br J Radiol 58:593–597, 1985.
18. Dawson P, Freedman DB, Howell MJ, Hine AL: Contrast-medium–induced acute renal failure and Tamm-Horsfall proteinuria. Br J Radiol 57:577–579, 1984.
19. Doppman JL, Fraley EE: Arteriography in the syndrome of superior infundibular obstruction. A simplified technic for identifying the obstructing vessel. Radiology 91:1039–1041, 1968.
20. Dretler SP, Olsson C, Pfister RC: The anatomic, radiologic and clinical characteristics of the pelvic kidney: An analysis of 86 cases. J Urol 105:623–627, 1971.
21. Dunbar JS, MacEwan DW, Hebert F: The value of dehydration in intravenous pyelography—an experimental study. AJR 84:813–836, 1960.
22. Emanuel B, Nachman R, Aronson N, et al: Congenital solitary kidney: A review of 74 cases. Am J Dis Child 127:17–19, 1974.
23. Feldman AE, Rosenthal RS, Shaw JL: Aberrant renal papilla: A diagnostic dilemma. J Urol 114:144–146, 1975.
24. Fleischner FG, Bellman S, Henken EM: Papillary opacification in excretory urography, so-called pyelotubular reflux. Radiology 74:567–572, 1960.
25. Fraley EE: Vascular obstruction of superior infundibulum causing nephralgia. A new syndrome. N Engl J Med 275:1403–1409, 1966.
26. Gay BB, Dawes RK, Atkinson GO, Ball TI: Wilms tumor in horseshoe kidneys: Radiologic diagnosis. Radiology 146:693–697, 1983.
27. Gooding CA, Berdon WE, Brodeur AE, Rowen M: Adverse reactions to intravenous pyelography in children. AJR 123:802–804, 1975.
28. Grandone CH, Haller JO, Berdon WE, Friedman AP: Asymmetric horseshoe kidney in the infant: Value of renal nuclear scanning. Radiology 154:366, 1985.
29. Green WM, Pressman BD, McClennan BL, Casarella WJ: "Column of Bertin:" Diagnosis by nephrotomography. AJR 116:714–723, 1972.
30. Griscom NT, Neuhauser EBD: Total body opacification. J Pediatr Surg 1:76–79, 1966.
31. Haines JO, Kyaw MM: Anterolateral deviation of ureters by psoas muscle hypertrophy. J Urol 106:831–832, 1971.
32. Harrison RB, Wood JL, Gillenwater JY: A solitary calyx in a human kidney. Radiology 121:310, 1976.

33. Hartman GE, Hodson CJ: The duplex kidney and related anomalies. Clin Radiol 20:387–400, 1969.
34. Hodson CJ, Mariani S: Large cloisons. AJR 139:327–332, 1982.
35. Hope JW, Campoy F: Use of carbonated beverages in pediatric excretory urography. Radiology 64:66–71, 1955.
36. Johnson MA, Burgess AE: Clinical use of a gadolinium filter in pediatric radiology. Pediatr Radiol 10:229–232, 1981.
37. Kalman EH, Albers DD, Dunn JH: Ureteral jet phenomenon. Stream of opaque medium simulating an anomalous configuration of the ureter. Radiology 65:933–934, 1955.
38. Kaufman RA, Dunbar JS, Gole DE: Normal dilatation of the proximal ureter in children. AJR 137:945–949, 1981.
39. Kelalis PP, Malek RS, Segura JW: Observations on renal ectopia and fusion in children. J Urol 110:588–592, 1973.
40. Kirks DR, Currarino G, Weinberg AG: Transverse folds in the proximal ureter: A normal variant in infants. AJR 130:463–464, 1978.
41. Kozakewich HPW, Lebowitz RL: Congenital megacalyces. Pediatr Radiol 2:251–258, 1974.
42. Kuchta SG, Manco LG, Evans JA: Prominent iliopsoas muscles producing a gourd-shaped deformity of the bladder. J Urol 127:1188–1189, 1982.
43. Kuhns LR, Hernandez R, Koff S, et al: Absence of vesico-ureteral reflux in children with ureteral jets. Radiology 124:185–187, 1977.
44. Lafortune M, Constantin A, Breton G, Vallee C: Sonography of the hypertrophied column of Bertin. AJR 146:53–56, 1986.
45. Lebowitz RL, Avni FE: Misleading appearances in pediatric uroradiology. Pediatr Radiol 10:15–31, 1980.
46. Leiter E: Persistent fetal ureter. J Urol 122:251–254, 1979.
47. Levine RB, Forrester D, Halpern M: Ureteral deviation due to iliopsoas hypertrophy. AJR 107:756–759, 1969.
48. Lister J, Singh H: Pelvicalyceal cysts in children. J Pediatr Surg 8:901–905, 1973.
49. Lundius B: Intrathoracic kidney. AJR 125:678–681, 1975.
50. Lutzker LG, Goldman HS: A method for improved urographic visualization in children. Radiology 111:217–218, 1974.
51. Majd M: Nuclear medicine. In Kelalis, King, Belman (eds): Clinical Pediatric Urology, 2nd Ed. Philadelphia, WB Saunders Company, 1985, pp 145–146.
52. Mandell GA, Swacus JR, Rosenstock J, Buck BE: Danger of urography in hyperuricemic children with Burkitt's lymphoma. J Can Assoc Radiol 34:274–277, 1983.
53. Mascatello V, Lebowitz RL: Malposition of the colon in left renal agenesis and ectopia. Radiology 120:371–376, 1976.
54. McAlister WH, Lester PD: Diseases of the adrenal. Med Radiogr Photogr 47:62–81, 1971.
55. McAlister WH, Siegel MJ, Shackelford GD: Pulmonary oedema following intravenous urography in a neonate. Br J Radiol 52:410–411, 1979.
56. Mindell HJ, Kupic EA: Horseshoe kidney: Ultrasonic demonstration. AJR 129:526–527, 1977.
57. NCRP Report No 68: Radiation Protection in Pediatric Radiology. Washington, DC, National Council on Radiation Protection and Measurements, 1981, p 19.
58. Nogrady MB, Dunbar JS: The technique of roentgen investigation of the urinary tract in infants and children. Progr Pediatr Radiol 3:3–50, 1970.
59. Nogrady MB, Dunbar JS: Delayed concentration and prolonged excretion of urographic contrast medium in the first month of life. AJR 104:289–295, 1968.
60. Nogrady MB, Dunbar JS: On the use of the pneumatic compression paddle for improved visualization of the upper urinary tract in pediatric patients. AJR 103:218–222, 1968.
61. O'Connor JF, Neuhauser EBD: Total body opacification in conventional and high-dose intravenous urography in infancy. AJR 90:63–71, 1963.
62. Older RA, Korobkin M, Workman J, et al: Accuracy of radionuclide imaging in distinguishing renal masses from normal variants. Radiology 136:443–448, 1980.
63. Ostling K: The genesis of hydronephrosis. Acta Chir Scand (Suppl)86:72, 1942.
64. Persky L, Owens GH: Genitourinary tract abnormalities in Turner's syndrome (gonadal dysgenesis). J Urol 105:309–313, 1971.
65. Peterson JE, Pinckney LE, Rutledge JC, Currarino G: The solitary renal calyx and papilla in human kidneys. Radiology 144:525–527, 1982.
66. Pfister-Goedeke L, Brunier E: Intrathoracic kidney in childhood (with particular emphasis on a case secondarily displaced through a Bochdalek hernia). Helv Paediatr Acta 34:345–357, 1979.
67. Ransley PG: Opacification of the renal parenchyma in obstruction and reflux. Pediatr Radiol 4:226–232, 1976.
68. Rickards D, Dawson P: Letter to the Editor: Hexabrix and gallbladder visualization. Br J Radiol 59:79, 1986.
69. Rivard DJ, Milner WA, Garlick WB: Solitary crossed renal ectopia and its associated congenital anomalies. J Urol 120:241–242, 1979.
70. Rusiewicz E, Reilly BJ: The significance of isolated upper pole calyceal dilatation. J Can Assoc Radiol 19:179–182, 1968.
71. Saldino RM, Palubinskas AJ: Medial placement of the ureter: A normal variant which may simulate retroperitoneal fibrosis. J Urol 107:582–585, 1972.
72. Schencker B, Marcure WR, Moody DL: Simplified nephrotomography. The drip infusion technique. AJR 95:283–290, 1965.
73. Scher AT: Autonomic hyperreflexia: A serious complication of radiological procedures in patients with cervical or upper thoracic spinal cord lesions. S Afr Med J 53:208–210, 1978.
74. Smith DW: Chromosomal abnormality syndromes. In Recognizable Patterns of Human Malformation, 3rd Ed. Philadelphia, WB Saunders Company, 1982, p 72.
75. Talner LB, Gittes RF: Megacalyces. Clin Radiol 23:355–361, 1972.
76. Templeton AW, Thompson IM: Aortographic differentiation of congenital and acquired small kidneys. Arch Surg 97:114–117, 1968.
77. Timmons JW, Malek RS, Hattery RR, Deweerd JH: Caliceal diverticulum. J Urol 114:6–9, 1975.
78. Tregut H, Schulze K, Schulze H-J, Meiisel P: Malignant tumors in horseshoe kidneys. RoFo 130:287–290, 1979.
79. Wang Y, McArdle GH, Feig SA, et al: Clinical applications of yttrium filters for exposure reduction. RadioGraphics 4:479–505, 1984.
80. Wesenberg RL, Amundson GM, Mueller DL: Kevlar cassettes: Further reduction in radiation exposure during routine pediatric radiography. Paper No 39, Washington, DC, Society for Pediatric Radiology Annual Meeting, 1986.
81. White RI, Halden WJ: Liquid gold: Low-osmolality contrast media. Radiology 159:559–560, 1986.
82. Whitehouse GH: Some urographic aspects of the horseshoe kidney anomaly: A review of 59 cases. Clin Radiol 25:107–114, 1975.
83. Wolfson JJ, Stowell DW: Aberrant renal papilla simulating an intrarenal mass. Radiology 93:812–814, 1969.
84. Wood BP, Smith WL: Pulmonary edema in infants following injection of contrast media for urography. Radiology 139:377–379, 1981.
85. Zanca P, Barker KG, Pye TH, et al: Ureteral jet stream phenomenon in adults. AJR 92:341–345, 1964.
86. Zondek LH, Zondek T: Horseshoe kidney and associated congenital malformations. Urol Int 18:347, 1964.
87. Lebowitz RL, Mandell J: Urinary tract infection in children: Putting radiology in its place. Radiology 165:1, 1987.
88. Pollack HM, Banner MP: Current status of excretory urography: Premature epitaph? Urol Clin North Am 12:585, 1985.
89. Pedersen HK, Gudmundsen TE, Ostensen H, Pape JF: Intravenous urography in children and youth. Pediatr Radiol 17:463, 1987.
90. Fjelldal Å, Nordhus T, Eriksson J: Experiences with iohexol (Omnipaque) at urography. Pediatr Radiol 17:491, 1987.
91. Simpson EL, Mintz MC, Pollack HM, et al: Computed tomography in the diagnosis of renal pseudotumors. Comput Tomogr 10:341, 1986.
92. Eklöff O, Ringhertz H: Kidney size in children. A method of assessment. Acta Radiol (Diagn) 17:617, 1976.
93. Guinard JP: Renal function in the newborn infant. Pediatr Clin North AM 29:777, 1982.
94. Haller JO, Cohen HL: Pediatric urosonography: An update. Urol Radiol 9:99, 1987.
95. Klare B, Geiselhardy B, Welsh H, et al: Radiological kidney size in childhood. Pediatr Radiol 9:153, 1080.
96. General Reference: Aaronson IA, Cremin BJ: Clinical Pediatric Uroradiology. Edinburg, Churchill-Livingstone, 1984.

7

Retrograde Pyelography

THOMAS J. IMRAY □ ROBERT P. LIEBERMAN

Retrograde pyelography is the roentgenographic demonstration of the renal pelvis and ureter by the retrograde injection of radiopaque contrast material through the ureter. Prior to the development of intravenous urography, this was the only radiographic method of examining the urinary tract. Although still a valuable technique, retrograde pyelography is performed less frequently today. This trend is primarily due to technical improvements in intravenous urography and, to a lesser extent, to the development of ultrasonography and computed tomography (CT).

EARLY HISTORY OF RETROGRADE PYELOGRAPHY

The development of retrograde techniques followed advances in cystoscopy. Although primitive cystoscopes were first devised in 1806, it was not until 1877 that Nitze developed a practical instrument with an electric light source and lens system.[34] The first attempt to opacify the urinary tract for roentgenography was by Tuffier in 1897, only 2 years after Roentgen's initial discovery of x-rays. He suggested the combination of a radiopaque ureteral catheter and abdominal x-ray examination. Schmidt and Kolischer, in 1901, independently published roentgenograms demonstrating the course of the ureter by means of a ureteral catheter containing a radiopaque wire.

Klose, in 1904, suggested the injection of a bismuth emulsion into the renal pelvis and ureter to opacify the collecting system during roentgenography. He did not perform retrograde pyelography using bismuth because he feared that the renal pelvis might be irritated by this emulsion.[5]

In 1906 Voelcker and von Lichtenberg were the first to successfully demonstrate the renal pelvis and ureter utilizing colloidal suspension of silver (Collargol). While obtaining a cystogram with this solution, they found that the colloidal silver had refluxed into the ureter and renal pelvis. This finding inspired them to inject colloidal silver through a ureteral catheter to obtain a successful retrograde pyelogram. Within 4 years, this method became widely utilized.

In 1909 Uhle and Pfahler suggested the use of silver iodide solution for retrograde pyelography. Higher concentrations of the solution produced clearer delineations of the collecting system, but also caused more irritation to the urothelium.

In 1911 von Lichtenberg and Dietlen reported a series of retrograde pyelograms performed with oxygen as a contrast agent. This method, however, was not widely accepted because of the problem of differentiating gas in the ureter and kidney from that in bowel.

Cameron in 1918 was the first to employ a solution of sodium and potassium iodide. Potassium iodide proved to be toxic, but sodium iodide was widely utilized in retrograde pyelography.

Bluhbaum, Frick, and Kalkbrenner in 1928 advocated

a new colloid, thorium dioxide (Thorotrast), which gained rapid acceptance because of its excellent radiopacity and patient tolerance. This early enthusiasm was short-lived. The thorium precipitated and adhered to the urothelium for prolonged periods. It also was found to induce malignant change in tissues due to its radioactivity.

Subsequent improvements in the procedure have come about with the development of less toxic contrast agents, improvement in fluoroscopic equipment, and newer, less traumatic catheter materials. (For a detailed history of the early years of retrograde pyelography, see Braasch[5] or Narath.[24])

TECHNIQUE OF RETROGRADE PYELOGRAPHY

Bowel preparation with cathartics is not routinely performed. However, if the bowel is opacified from previous contrast examinations, cathartics are indicated. A preliminary radiograph of the abdomen is mandatory. This and all subsequent films should be numbered to avoid confusion during interpretation.

Failure to use cathartics to clear a contrast-filled colon may result in an inadequate study (Fig. 7–1).

The retrograde opacification of the undiverted, nonrefluxing urinary tract requires cystoscopic manipulation.

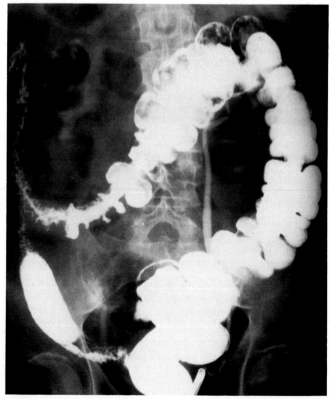

Figure 7–1. Inadequate bowel preparation and failure to obtain a preliminary film may result in a worthless examination.

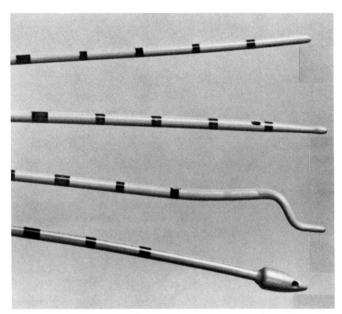

Figure 7–2. Commonly used ureteral catheters, from top to bottom, have round, olive, spiral, and cone or "bulb" tips.

The ureteral orifices must be identified and catheterized. The procedure may be performed under local anesthesia utilizing intraurethral lidocaine jelly, although general anesthesia is often required, especially in males. Sterile technique is mandatory.

Many kinds of ureteral catheters are commercially available. The most commonly used sizes range from 4 to 7 F. The whistle, round, and olive-tipped catheters are general-purpose instruments used for retrograde pyelography, urine collection, and drainage. The spiral-tipped catheter is useful in negotiating curves and kinks in the ureter. The acorn-, bulb-, and cone-tipped catheters have enlarged ends designed to obstruct the ureteral orifice (Fig. 7–2). These catheters have closed ends that assist their penetration of the ureteral orifice. Open-end catheters have recently gained popularity because they allow not only retrograde pyelography, but also the passage of a guide wire, thereby facilitating the introduction of curved catheters and stents.

Most ureteral catheters used today are radiopaque. This feature permits not only fluoroscopic visualization during manipulation, but also documentation of catheter position on subsequent abdominal roentgenograms. The opaque catheter can be used to identify the course of the ureter and to determine if a pelvic calcification is within the ureter. The catheter may obscure a small calcification, but this problem can usually be solved with oblique films.

One technique of retrograde pyelography involves wedging an acorn-, bulb-, or cone-tipped catheter in the ureteral orifice and injecting contrast material with a syringe or by gravity flow. This type of study often facilitates an excellent evaluation of the ureters and upper collecting system before the passage of ureteral catheters.[29] Three to five milliliters of contrast medium is injected, slowly to avoid extravasation. If suboptimal opacification of the ureter or renal pelvis is obtained, the injection may be repeated with a larger volume. This type of study can rule out obstruction, demonstrate the course of the ureter, and, if the delineation of the collecting system is adequate, may obviate the need for subsequent

passage of ureteral catheters (Fig. 7–3). Occlusive-tip or "bulb" pyeloureterography is useful when difficulty is experienced in passing a ureteral catheter. Its major disadvantage is the need to constantly observe the catheter tip through the cystoscope to insure that it remains wedged in the ureteral orifice. This can be awkward when the patient must be rotated into the oblique position.

Another technique of retrograde pyelography involves passing a catheter to the upper ureter or renal pelvis (Fig. 7–4). The catheter is advanced to a distance that varies among patients. The distance from the ureteral orifice to the ureteropelvic junction is approximately 25 cm in most adults. Correct assessment of this distance in the individual patient is important. If the catheter is advanced too far or if too much force is employed, the catheter may perforate a calyx and penetrate the renal parenchyma (Fig. 7–5). Ureteral catheters occasionally break, leaving a portion of the catheter in the renal pelvis or ureter (Fig. 7–6). Coiling of the catheter presents another risk of overzealous advancement, because twisting or withdrawal of a coiled catheter may form a knot within the renal pelvis or ureter (Fig. 7–7). Several measures can be undertaken to avoid these complications. Because most patients undergo intravenous urography before retrograde catheterization, the position of the kidneys should be noted and this information should be used to determine the distance catheters are passed. The preliminary film of

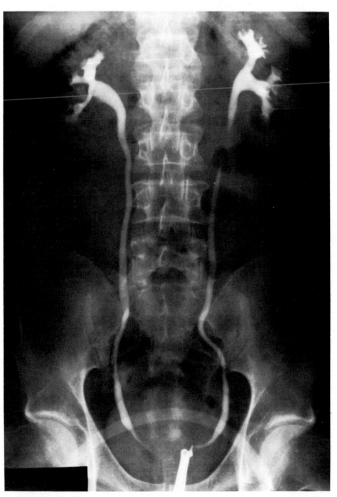

Figure 7–3. Normal bulb pyelogram shows the entire collecting system outlined from a single injection.

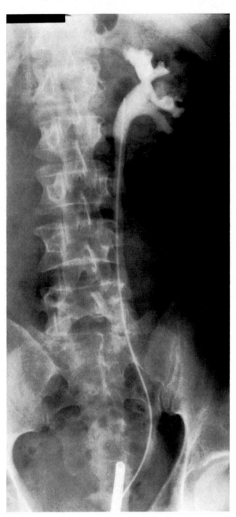

Figure 7–4. Normal retrograde pyelogram is shown, utilizing ureteral "whistle-tip" catheter.

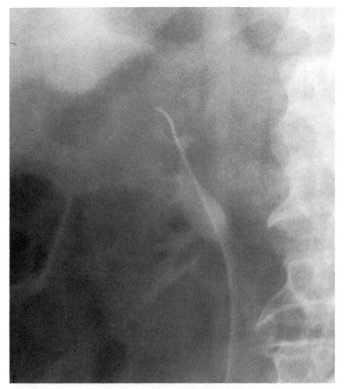

Figure 7–5. Ureteral catheter has perforated an upper-pole calyx and entered the renal parenchyma.

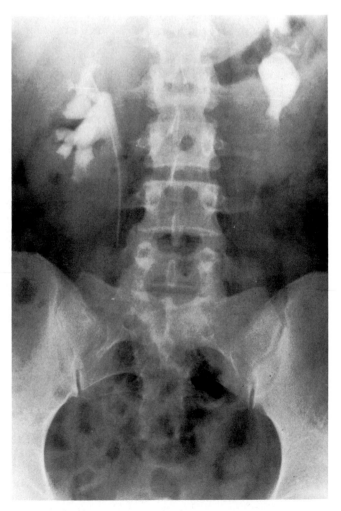

Figure 7–6. Intravenous urogram demonstrates a ureteral catheter fragment retained in the right renal pelvis and ureter. The catheter broke when it was being withdrawn. The catheter fragment was successfully removed 4 months later by means of a retrogradely passed stone basket.

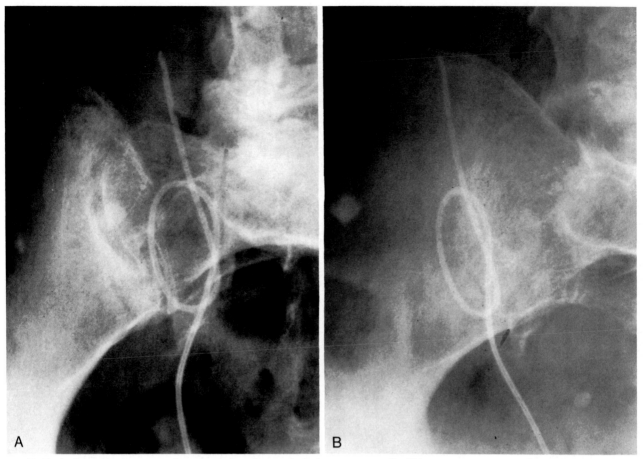

Figure 7–7. A, Retrograde ureteral catheter has knotted during passage. B, Oblique projection confirms that the catheter is knotted.

the retrograde study may also assist in localizing the approximate level of the ureteropelvic junction. If fluoroscopy is available, the passage of the catheter can be monitored.

Contrast material may be injected by syringe or instilled by means of gravity. The syringe method, which is less time consuming, is the method generally employed. If the gravity method is used, the container should be elevated no more than 50 cm above the level of the kidney to prevent extravasation and to minimize the risk of backflow.[33] If a syringe is used, the injection should be made slowly and carefully, and the injection should be terminated if the patient complains of fullness or pain in the flank. Three to five milliliters is usually adequate in a nondilated upper collecting system. If fluoroscopy is available, monitoring can reduce the risk of overdistention.

Any of the contrast agents currently used for intravenous urography may be employed for retrograde pyelography. A 15% to 45% concentration of the contrast medium will give adequate opacification of the collecting system, but care must be taken when using the more concentrated solutions not to obscure small or poorly opacified filling defects, especially in a voluminous renal pelvis.

Filming technique is similar to the plain film. Low kilovoltage technique (65 to 75 kVp) should be employed to enhance visualization of calculi and the contrast medium. After 3 to 5 ml of contrast medium has been injected, an exposure is taken immediately, with the patient supine, to obtain maximum opacification. Oblique or lateral films, although difficult to obtain in this setting, may provide significant additional information.

If the films obtained are not adequate, it is important to leave a catheter in the upper ureter and to repeat the examination. The patient can be transferred to a fluoroscopic suite in the radiology department for further filming under fluoroscopic control. The patient can be moved and positioned to obtain optimal visualization of any area in question.

Delayed films after retrograde pyelography can be helpful to determine the presence of significant ureteral obstruction. These films should be obtained after the patient has been standing or sitting for 5 to 15 minutes. The films may be taken with the patient supine or erect. Retention of contrast material in the renal pelvis or ureter on delayed films is abnormal and implies obstruction (Fig. 7–8). The possibility of catheter-induced ureteral spasm must also be considered.

AIR PYELOGRAPHY AND DOUBLE-CONTRAST PYELOGRAPHY

Calculi are sometimes difficult to delineate on positive contrast retrograde pyelography, because the density of the contrast can obscure the calculus. In this instance, an air pyelogram can be helpful. Fifteen to twenty milliliters of air is introduced into the renal pelvis. The head of the table should be elevated to retain the air and displace the

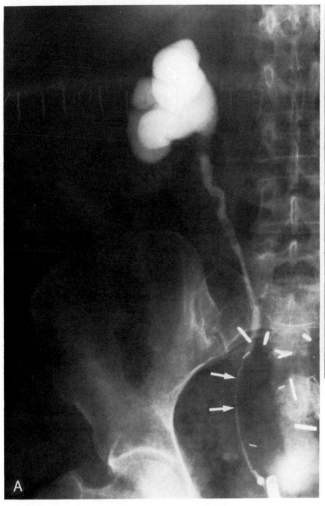

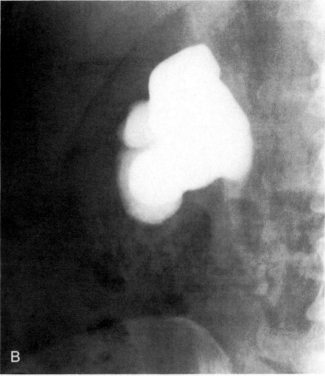

Figure 7–8. *A,* Retrograde pyelogram shows moderate hydronephrosis and narrowing of the lower ureter (*arrows*). *B,* Thirty minutes later, film shows retention of contrast material, indicating significant obstruction.

urine from the upper collecting system.[6] If a double-contrast study is desired, 3 to 5 ml of contrast media is injected immediately prior to instillation of air (Fig. 7–9).[6] Air embolism has been reported with air pyelography, so the injection should be slow and the study preferably monitored by fluoroscopy.[25] If larger volumes of gas are required, CO_2 may be used to reduce the risk of air embolism. Because of the need to maneuver the patient during the injection, this technique is most efficiently performed on a tilting fluoroscopic table. Gas pyelography is now rarely performed, and CT and/or ultrasonography is utilized in the evaluation of most renal pelvic defects. However, double-contrast pyelography has the potential for yielding a great deal of information about intraluminal renal pelvic and ureteral lesions. One problem is that current contrast media, which are extremely water-soluble, lack the mucosal coating properties necessary to produce ideal double-contrast studies.

INDICATIONS, CAUTIONS AND COMPLICATIONS

Retrograde pyelography allows controlled opacification of the renal pelvis and ureter. Situations in which retrograde pyelography is indicated include the following:

1. Absent or unsatisfactory visualization of the collecting system on the intravenous urogram. (If a diagnosis can be made with another study, such as CT or ultrasonography, the retrograde pyelogram may not be necessary.)
2. Unexplained hematuria, when the ureters have not been completely visualized by intravenous urography.
3. Evaluating persistent intraureteral or intrapelvic filling defects seen on intravenous urography.
4. Quantifying the emptying of the upper urinary tract.
5. Performing air pyelography or double-contrast pyelography.
6. Demonstrating the exact site of a ureteral fistula.
7. Brushing and/or biopsy of suspected lesions.
8. Evaluating the collecting system in patients who cannot receive intravenous contrast medium. (Contrast reactions are possible but rare with retrograde studies.)

It should be emphasized that unless contraindicated, intravenous urography should be performed prior to retrograde pyelography.[20] Intravenous urography is a more physiological study and provides much more information regarding the renal parenchyma than retrograde pyelography.[3] Retrograde catheterization must be performed with caution if there is a small calculus in the distal ureter. Injection could force the calculus into the proximal ureter or renal pelvis and make removal more difficult or impossible.[29]

The retrograde pyelogram is an invasive procedure that requires cystoscopy and catheter manipulation of the ureters. Complications include perforation of the ureter

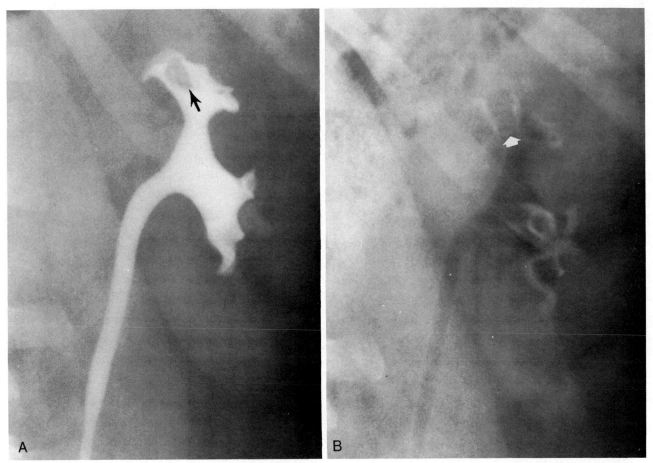

Figure 7–9. *A,* Retrograde pyelogram shows a filling defect in the upper-pole calyx *(arrow).* Plain film showed no calcification in this area. *B,* Double-contrast pyelogram indicates that the lesion is attached to the wall of the calyx *(arrow).* This lesion was a benign fibrourothelial polyp. (Courtesy Hal Mardis, M.D.)

or renal pelvis (Figs. 7–10 and 7–11). This complication is more likely to occur with larger, stiffer catheters and rough handling. Although withdrawal of the ureteral catheter and conservative therapy often result in healing, urinomas or abscesses may form, especially in the presence of distal obstruction or infected urine.

Introduction of infection is also a risk. Breach of sterile technique is common during retrograde catheterization. Bacteria can be introduced into the upper collecting system or into the blood stream, resulting in sepsis. Injection of contrast medium above a point of obstruction can lead to fulminant sepsis requiring prompt intervention. Retrograde pyelography should be undertaken cautiously in the presence of an active urinary tract infection or obstruction.

Although it has often been erroneously assumed that contrast material is not absorbed during retrograde pyelography, life-threatening and even fatal reactions have occurred during these procedures.[8, 17, 21] Because of potential absorption, only contrast agents safe for intravenous use should be employed.[27] Lipid contrast medium carries the risk of pulmonary emboli. In patients with a history of serious contrast reactions, these studies should be approached with caution. Consideration should be given to using nonionic contrast media. The physician performing retrograde pyelography should be competent in the treatment of contrast reactions.

Over the years, there has been debate regarding the advisability of bilateral retrograde pyelograms performed on the same day.[10, 18, 28] Hydronephrosis and acute renal failure have been reported to follow bilateral retrograde catheterization.[1, 14–16, 26] These complications appear to result from edema and obstruction secondary to trauma of the intramural ureter. Considering the large number of uneventful bilateral retrograde catheterizations and pyelograms performed daily, this type of complication must be unusual. It is probably still advisable to restrict retrograde pyelography to the side of interest and to utilize the smallest-size catheter consistent with a successful study. Retrograde pyelography should not be performed merely because the patient is undergoing cystoscopy.

BACKFLOW

During retrograde pyelography, contrast material sometimes extravasates from the collecting system into surrounding tissues even in the absence of prior catheter trauma. This phenomenon, called *backflow,* results from excessive injection pressure.[13] Several radiographically distinct types of backflow have been recognized.[24]

Intrarenal backflow is characterized by wedge-shaped areas of fine striations or a blush of contrast radiating from a calyx, often reaching the outer surface of the kidney (Fig. 7–12).[31] The phenomenon may involve only

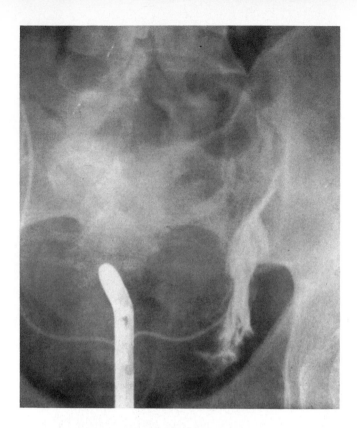

Figure 7–10. Perforation of the distal left ureter during retrograde catheterization is shown. Injected contrast material documents the perforation.

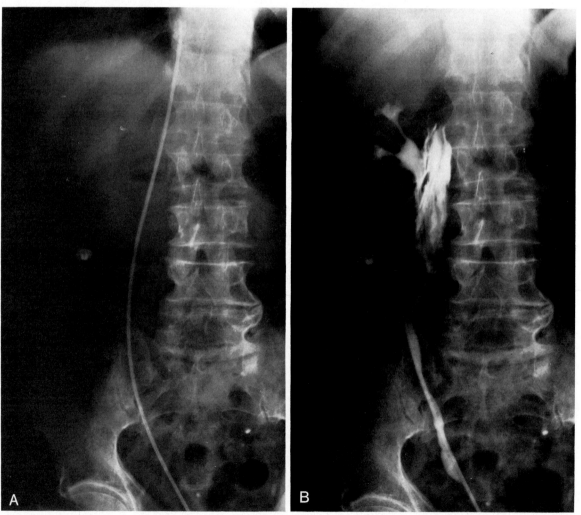

Figure 7–11. Perforation of the renal pelvis during retrograde catheterization is shown. *A,* Catheter has been passed retrograde well beyond the right kidney. *B,* The catheter has been withdrawn to the L5 level. Injected contrast material extravasates from the renal pelvis.

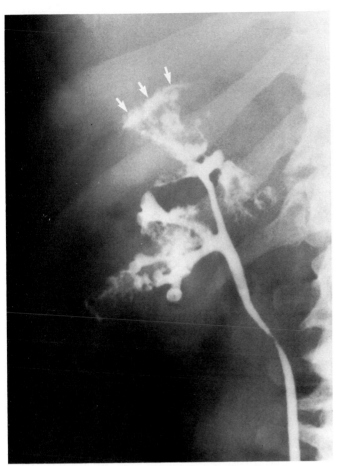

Figure 7–12. Intrarenal backflow during right retrograde pyelogram. Contrast extravasates into the renal parenchyma and extends to the capsule of the kidney *(arrows).*

one calyx or all calyces and is more common at the upper and lower renal poles. The contrast material enters the collecting ducts and may extend as far as the glomeruli. Under increased pressure, it enters the interstitium through tubular leakage.[32] Usually, however, it is not radiographically possible to differentiate pyelotubular from pyelointerstitial backflow (Fig. 7–13). It should be noted that the term *intrarenal reflux* is to be reserved for the phenomenon occurring during voiding cystourethrography, even though intrarenal reflux may have the same pathophysiology as intrarenal backflow.

Pyelosinus backflow is caused by microscopic tears in the mucosa of the calyces at the fornices, secondary to overdistention of the renal pelvis and calyces during retrograde pyelography. The extravasated medium enters the renal sinus and may obscure the collecting system (Fig. 7–14).[30]

Intrarenal extravasation of contrast material or its absorption from the renal sinus may lead to opacification of lymphatics (pyelolymphatic backflow).[24] This is easily recognized by the opacification of multiple fine vascular channels in the hilum of the kidney directed toward the para-aortic lymph nodes (Figs. 7–15 and 7–16). These channels generally follow the course of the renal veins. Occasionally, the extravasated contrast medium may enter venous channels (pyelovenous backflow).[4] This occurrence is rarely documented on radiographs, probably because the amount of medium entering the veins is

small, and the flow in renal veins is rapid, leading to dilution (Fig. 7–17).

Intrarenal backflow should be avoided because it decreases the overall diagnostic quality of the examination and increases the risk of sepsis. Intrapelvic pressure should be kept within a range of 0 to 30 mmHg during retrograde pyelography, using slow injection or gravity to instill contrast material. Small nonocclusive catheters also reduce the risk of backflow, because they allow flow around the catheter and down the ureter. Backflow occurring at normal pressures should raise the possibility of decreased viability of renal parenchyma, such as may occur in renal artery occlusion or renal vein thrombosis.

RETROGRADE URINE COLLECTION, BRUSHING, AND FORCEPS BIOPSY

Retrograde catheterization is often performed to evaluate a persistent filling defect within the renal pelvis or ureter. If urine is to be collected for cytological examination, urine specimens are best collected before the injection of any contrast material.[2] Hypertonic contrast solution causes dehydration and distortion of the urothelial cells, making cytological evaluation more difficult.[23]

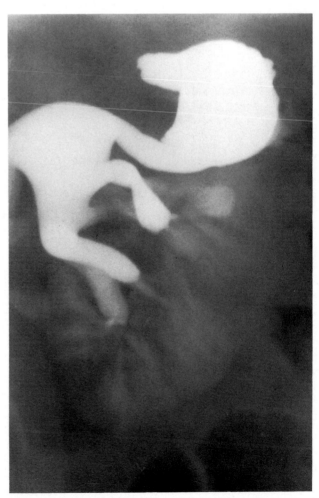

Figure 7–13. Intrarenal backflow during retrograde pyelography. This may represent pyelotubular backflow or a combination of pyelotubular and pyelointerstitial backflow.

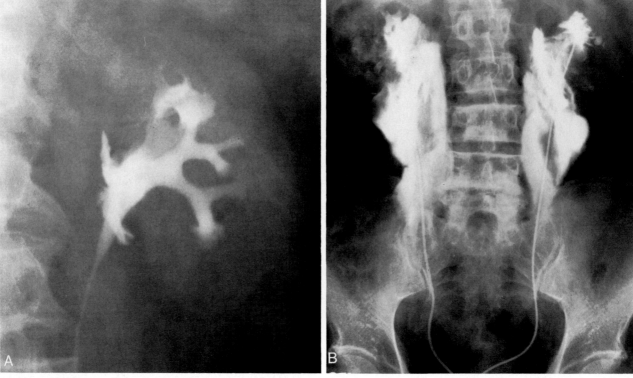

Figure 7–14. Pyelosinus backflow during retrograde pyelography is shown in two different patients. *A,* Contrast leaks from upper-pole calyces into renal sinus, obscuring detail of the renal pelvis. *B,* Following bilateral retrograde injection, there is massive pyelosinus backflow leading to extensive bilateral extravasation throughout the retroperitoneum.

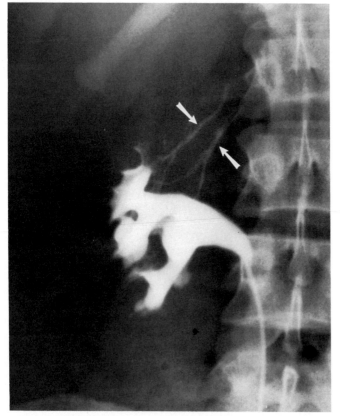

Figure 7–15. Pyelolymphatic backflow is shown. Right retrograde pyelogram shows slight overdistention of the renal pelvis and filling of renal hilar lymphatics (*arrows*).

If contrast medium must be used before urine collection, one of lower concentration or one of the newer low-osmolality agents should be employed. The literature also suggests irrigating out contrast material with a saline solution before the collection of urine for cytological examination. Because diagnostic cells may be flushed out during irrigation, the urologist should not discard the contrast-containing irrigant solution.

Unfortunately, cytological study of urine has a relatively high rate of false-negative results (22% to 67%), in part owing to the well-differentiated appearance of many urothelial tumors.[11] To increase the yield of positive cytological examinations, nylon or steel bristle brushes can be introduced through open-ended catheters to obtain cells.[12] This is best performed under fluoroscopic guidance. If a forceps biopsy is contemplated, a sheathed (coaxial) catheter should be inserted into the ureter. The inner catheter is then removed, leaving a semiflexible sheath as a conduit for the biopsy forceps. The sheath also facilitates brushing, lavage, and contrast pyelography.[19] Cystoscopy is needed to insert the coaxial catheter but not to pass instruments through it. Therefore, the biopsy can be performed in a standard fluoroscopic suite with much more mobility of the patient (Fig. 7–18).

Retrograde pyelography has also been used to localize the level of obstruction as a guide to a fine-needle percutaneous biopsy.[9, 22]

In summary, retrograde pyelography is a time-honored diagnostic tool that can yield important information in certain settings. However, whenever retrograde pyelography is contemplated, the following questions should be

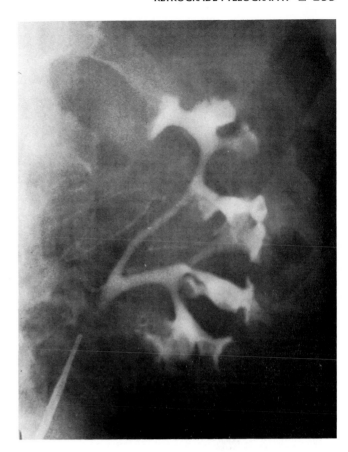

Figure 7–16. Pyelolymphatic backflow is shown in a left retrograde pyelogram.

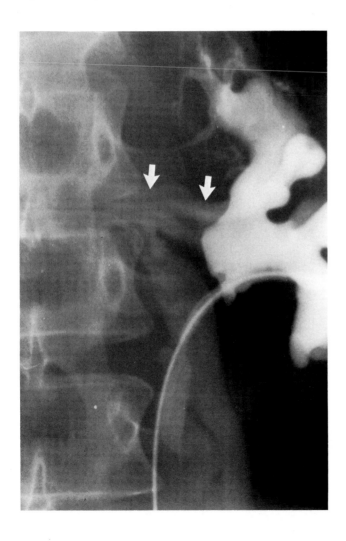

Figure 7–17. Retrograde pyelogram shows overdistention and pyelovenous backflow. Note filling of left renal vein (*arrows*).

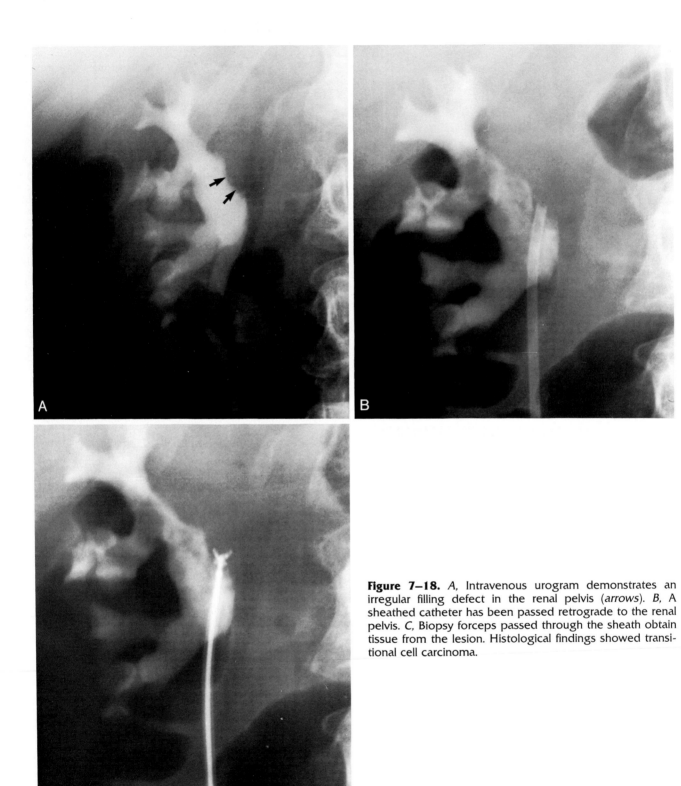

Figure 7–18. *A*, Intravenous urogram demonstrates an irregular filling defect in the renal pelvis (*arrows*). *B*, A sheathed catheter has been passed retrograde to the renal pelvis. *C*, Biopsy forceps passed through the sheath obtain tissue from the lesion. Histological findings showed transitional cell carcinoma.

asked: (1) Will retrograde pyelography provide important information in the diagnostic evaluation of this patient? (2) Would the information be more easily and effectively obtained by using less invasive techniques, such as intravenous urography with tomography, ultrasonography, or CT? The performance of retrograde pyelography because the patient is undergoing cystoscopic examination is hardly justified. The performance of retrograde pyelography as a result of a technically inadequate intravenous urogram is only to be condemned.

References

1. Alfrey AC, Rottschafter OW, Hutt MP: Acute parenchymal dysfunction with acute anuria induced by retrograde pyelography. Arch Intern Med 119:214–217, 1967.
2. Barry JM, Murphy JB, Nassir E, et al: The influence of retrograde contrast medium on urinary cytodiagnosis: A preliminary report. J Urol 119:633–634, 1978.
3. Bell EG, McAfee JG, Makhuli ZN: Medical imaging of renal diseases—suggested indications for different modalities. Semin Nucl Med 11:105–127, 1981.
4. Bidgood WD, Cuttino JT, Clark RL, Volberg FM: Pyelovenous and pyelolymphatic backflow during retrograde pyelography in renal vein thrombosis. Invest Radiol 16:13–19, 1981.
5. Braasch WF: Pyelography (Pyelo-Ureterography). Philadelphia, WB Saunders Company, 1915.
6. Christiansen J: Retrograde pyelography with double contrast: A preliminary report. Acta Chir Scand 136:435–439, 1970.
7. Christiansen J: Retrograde pyelography with gas (carbon dioxide) as contrast medium. Acta Chir Scand 136:441–445, 1970.
8. Currarino G, Weinberg A, Putnam R: Resorption of contrast material from the bladder during cystourethrography causing an excretory urogram. Radiology 123:149–150, 1977.
9. Ekelund L, Gothlin J: Fine needle biopsy of metastases at retrograde pyelography, directed by fluoroscopy. Scand J Urol Nephrol 10:261–262, 1976.
9a. Elkin M: Radiology of the Urinary System. Boston, Little, Brown & Company, 1980.
10. Epstein M, Shelp WD, Weinstein AB: Acute renal failure following retrograde pyelography. Invest Urol 2:355–364, 1965.
11. Gibod LB, Chice R, Dalian D, Steg A: Upper tract urothelial tumors—diagnostic efficiency of radiology and urinary cytology. Eur Urol 8:145–147, 1982.
12. Gill WB, Lu CT, Thomsen S: Retrograde brushing: A new technique for obtaining histologic and cytologic material from ureteral, renal pelvic and renal caliceal lesions. J Urol 109:573–578, 1973.
13. Green N, Fingerhut AG, French S: Mechanism of renovascular backflow. Radiology 92:531–536, 1969.
14. Harrow BR, Sloane JA: Anuria and hydronephrosis following ureteral catheterization. JAMA 180:415–417, 1962.
15. Hope JW, Michie AJ: Hydronephrosis following retrograde pyelography. Radiology 72:844–849, 1959.
16. Hurley RM: Acute renal failure secondary to bilateral retrograde pyelography. Case reports. Clin Pediatr 18:754–756, 1979.
17. Johenning PW: Reactions to contrast material during retrograde pyelography. Urology 16:442–443, 1980.
18. Levant B, Yardumian K: Reflex anuria following retrograde and excretory investigation: The urologic and cutaneous review. 48:554–556, 1944.
19. Lieberman RP, Cummings KB, Leslie SW: Sheathed catheter system for fluoroscopically guided retrograde catheterization, and brush and forceps biopsy of the upper urinary tract. J Urol 131:450–453, 1984.
20. Lowe PP, Roylance J: Transitional cell carcinoma of the kidney. Clin Radiol 27:503–512, 1976.
21. Marshall WH, Castellino RA: The urinary mucosal barrier in retrograde pyelography: The role of the ureteric mucosa. Radiology 97:5–7, 1970.
22. McCanse L, Whittier F, Cross D, Mebust W: Percutaneous renal biopsy with localization by retrograde pyelography. J Urol 114:521–523, 1975.
23. McClennan BL, Oreterl YC, Malmgren RA, Mendoza M: The effect of water-soluble contrast material on urine cytology. Acta Cytol 22:230–233, 1978.
24. Narath PA: Renal Pelvis & Ureter. New York. Grune & Stratton, 1951.
24a. Ney C, Friedenberg RM: Radiographic Atlas of the Genitourinary System, 2nd Ed. Philadelphia, JB Lippincott, 1981.
25. Pyron CL, Segal AJ: Air embolism: A potential complication of retrograde pyelography. Case reports. J Urol 130:125–126, 1983.
26. Quinby WC, Austen G: Suppression of urine complicating pyelography. N Engl J Med 221:814–816, 1939.
27. Siegle RL, Lieberman P: A review of untoward reactions to iodinated contrast material. J Urol 119:581–587, 1978.
28. Sirota JH, Narins L: Acute urinary suppression after ureteral catheterization—the pathogenesis of "reflux anuria." N Engl J Med 257:1111–1113, 1957.
29. Taylor RJ, Bennett AH, Schwentker FN, Friedman HW, Geller RA: Use and abuse of retrograde pyelography. Urology 14:536–539, 1979.
30. Thomsen HS, Dorph S: Pyelorenal backflow during retrograde pyelography after renal transplantation. Scand J Urol Nephrol 12:175–179, 1978.
31. Thomsen HS, Dorph S: Pyelorenal backflow during retrograde pyelography in adult patients. Scand J Urol Nephrol 15:65–68, 1981.
32. Thomsen HS, Larsen S: Intrarenal backflow during retrograde pyelography with graded intrapelvic pressure. Acta Path Microbiol Immunol Scand 91A:245–252, 1983.
33. Thomsen HS: Pressures during retrograde pyelography. Acta Radiol (Diagn) (Stockh) 24:171–175, 1983.
33a. Walsh PC, Gittes RF, Perlmutter AD, Stamey TA: Campbell's Urology, 5th Ed. Philadelphia, WB Saunders Company, 1986.
34. Wershub LP: Urology from Antiquity to the Twentieth Century. St. Louis, Warren H. Green, 1970.
35. Witten DM, Myers GH, Utz DC: Emmett's Clinical Urography, An Atlas and Textbook of Roentgenologic Diagnosis, 4th Ed. Philadelphia, WB Saunders Company, 1977.

8

Cystourethrography

MARJORIE HERTZ

HISTORY OF THE RADIOLOGICAL EVALUATION OF THE LOWER URINARY TRACT

The human bladder and urethra have been studied with x-ray techniques ever since the early days of radiology. In 1905, Wulf wrote the first description of cystographic techniques using retrograde filling.[84] Other researchers focused on the urethra and demonstrated strictures and prostatic cancers by means of retrograde urethrography.[1–3] In the early 1930s, intravenous urography made it possible to visualize the bladder, which accumulated contrast material after excretion by the kidneys. Today, excretory urography remains the primary radiological study in most adults with symptoms deriving from the upper urinary tract.

Adequate visualization of the entire bladder is most reliably achieved by a retrograde cystogram. This examination has been largely replaced by voiding cystourethrography (VCU), performed under fluoroscopic control. Edling,[3] in a study on male urethrocystography, emphasized that in order to adequately visualize the bladder and urethra in the adult male, the micturition method should be used. Kjellberg and coworkers[4] wrote the first comprehensive account of the child's lower urinary tract based on their experience with 1461 children. Burrows' monograph on urethral lesions in children, published in 1965, was based on findings obtained by micturition studies.[5] Shopfner popularized micturating cystourethrography in the 1960s and wrote extensively on the methodology and physiology of the bladder and urethra.[6–9] He exposed many fallacies in previous concepts of bladder pathology. His observations refuted an earlier belief that congenital bladder neck obstruction and female meatal stenosis were frequent causes of urinary disorders. His ideas are now universally accepted. These new concepts completely changed the urological approach to the lower urinary tract in children.

Cinecystourethrography in children was very popular in the late fifties and early sixties, but the cine film image was not as sharp as spot films, and the dose to the gonads was much higher. The 70-mm and the later 105-mm camera have replaced the spot film technique and greatly reduced the radiation dose to the gonads, while preserving excellent visualization of bladder and urethra (Table 8–1).[10,11]

In adults, VCU is also recognized as a useful examination for the demonstration of the bladder and urethra.

Originally, retrograde urethrography had been performed using penile clamps and other devices. McCallum and Colapinto[12] popularized the use of a Foley catheter in the distal urethra to help retain contrast material in the urethra after filling. They called their method of exposing a film during injection *dynamic retrograde urethrography*, as distinct from static urethrography, which consisted of retrograde injection, clamping the urethra and then filming. Davis and Cian[13] advocated the use of a special catheter for retrograde demonstration of the much shorter urethra in women.

Contrast Material

Over the years, a variety of substances have been employed for the radiological demonstration of the bladder and urethra. Cunningham first published a paper on the roentgenographic examination of the urethra using a 50% argyrol injection.[1] Uray injected a bismuth suspension into the urethra, whereas Pfister used a barium sulphate suspension.[14,15] In 1924, Sicard and Forestier introduced lipiodol as a contrast medium for retrograde urethrography, while Kohnstam and Cave report its use in 26 patients.[16,17]

However, there were serious drawbacks to all these materials. The silver reagents used early in this century produced artifacts during leaking and were insufficiently radiopaque. The high viscosity of oily contrast material makes injection into the urethra more difficult. Furthermore, oily media will not mix with urine, and embolism may occur in patients with mucosal lesions through urethrocavernous reflux.[18] Four fatal cases resulting from oil embolism following urethrography with lipiodol were reported by Crabtree.[19] With barium suspension, barium impaction may occur in the upper collecting system following reflux. This medium may also induce a foreign body reaction in the kidney in the event of intrarenal reflux.[20] Solutions of sodium iodide and bromide induce severe local irritation.[5]

Even the more modern urographic contrast media can be irritating to the bladder. Shopfner found sodium acetrizoate to be irritating to the bladder, whereas meglumine diatrizoate was not.[88] McAlister and coworkers examined the histological effect of 30% acetrizoate and 25% meglumine diatrizoate and Renografin-30 in the bladder of rats. There was marked inflammatory response to all three contrast media, but inflammation was less

Table 8–1. Gonadal Doses for Different Techniques of VCU (Children Four Years of Age)

Male	Female	Technique	Reference Number
55 to 62 mrad	33 to 35 mrad	Single overhead film	Aspin[82]
105 mrad	269 mrad	70 mm without fluoroscopy	Kaude and Reed[77]
140 mrad	260 mrad	70 mm with fluoroscopy	Hertz and Werner[78]
±450 mrad	±1305 mrad	Spot film technique	Hertz and Werner[78]
±1.100 R	±1.100 R	Cine	Gross and Sanderson[83]

when medium was administered by gravity drip rather than by hand injection. Dilution of the media by 10% also reduced the inflammation.[21, 72]

Contrast media for cystourethrography must be adequately radiopaque and sufficiently viscous to demonstrate the urethra as well as the bladder, inexpensive, nonirritating to the mucosa, miscible with urine, and sterile and harmless if introduced into the circulation or into the kidney by reflux.[86] The meglumine salts of diatrizoate and iothalamate are now almost universally employed for this examination. Solutions of 15% are generally adequate for cystography, while 30% solutions usually render adequate opacification of the urethra, although 50 to 60 cc of 60% opaque medium may be added to improve visualization in adult men.

RADIOLOGICAL ANATOMY AND PHYSIOLOGY OF BLADDER AND URETHRA

Children

Bladder

In the newborn infant the bladder lies above the symphysis pubis (Fig. 8–1), but as the child grows the bladder descends, until at about 5 years of age the bladder floor lies at, or somewhat below, the level of the symphysis pubis (Fig. 8–2). During filling with contrast material, the bladder distends and assumes a round (Fig. 8–3) or oval shape (Fig. 8–4); it can adopt a horizontal position (Fig. 8–4) or a vertical position (Fig. 8–5), which

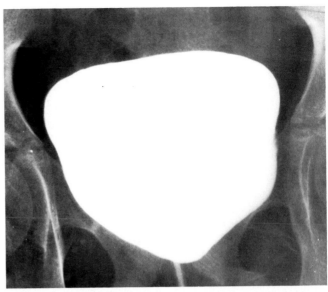

Figure 8–2. Cystogram of a 12-year-old child. The bladder base reaches the lower border of the symphysis.

is seen more frequently in small children. These variants may be seen in the same child on different examinations.

The wall of a fully distended normal bladder is smooth. As the bladder fills it may show an irregular border due to mucosal folds (Fig. 8–6), which will disappear on further filling. It is important, therefore, to ensure adequate distention to prevent mistaking an incompletely filled bladder for cystitis.

Shopfner and Hutch divide the bladder into two units: the vault—the upper part—and the bladder floor.[7] When the patient is in either the supine or upright position, the top of the bladder appears round. Often, air enters the bladder along with contrast material. A fluid level is visualized just beneath the bladder roof when the film is

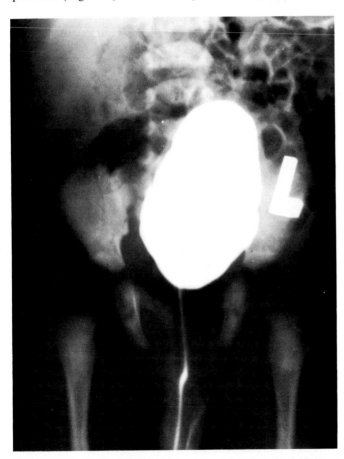

Figure 8–1. Cystogram of a 1-week-old infant. The bladder lies above the symphysis pubis.

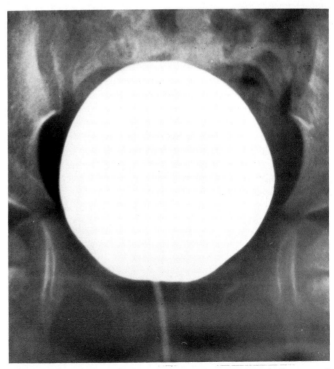

Figure 8–3. Filled bladder in this child has a round shape and flat base.

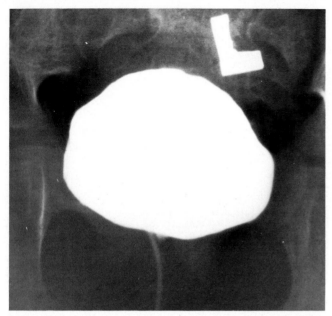

Figure 8–4. Cystogram shows a somewhat oval-shaped bladder, with the largest diameter in the transverse plane.

taken with the patient standing upright (Fig. 8–7). Sometimes an indentation is seen at both sides of the distended bladder giving the effect of a "waist"[4] (Fig. 8–7). The waist, which disappears on urination, is a normal phenomenon but is more pronounced in cases of urinary tract infection with cystitis (Fig. 8–8).

In infants under the age of 1 year, transitory herniation

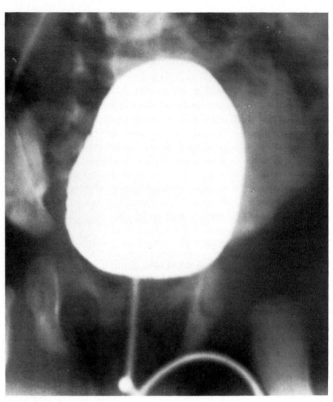

Figure 8–6. Cystogram reveals slight irregularity of the lateral bladder wall, attributable to incomplete filling. This represents mucosal folds.

of the bladder may occur because of still-incompetent inguinal rings. This is seen on an excretory urogram as a pouch lateral to the bladder. It is not visible on a cystogram. The pouches, which have been termed "blad-

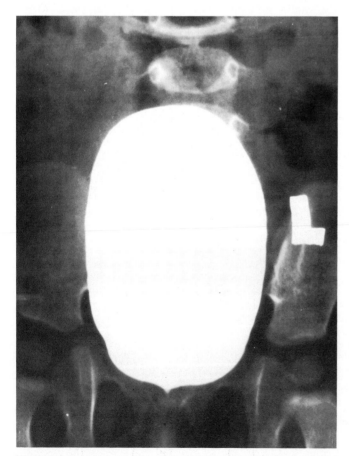

Figure 8–5. Bladder in this child is oriented vertically. A vertical position is often seen in the very young.

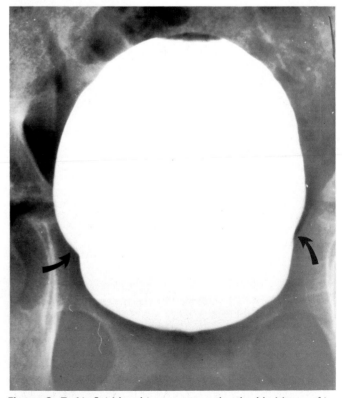

Figure 8–7. Air-fluid level is present under the bladder roof in this upright patient. Arrows show "waist," which is normal.

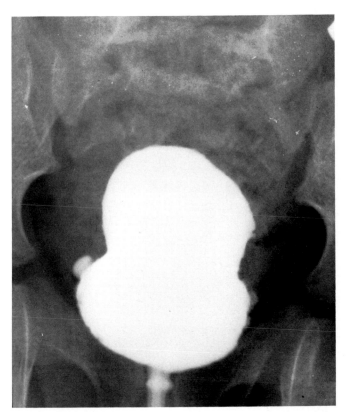

Figure 8–8. Bladder waist becomes more pronounced in severe cystitis. Note irregular bladder wall and bilateral small diverticula.

der ears" by Allen and Condon, can be unilateral or bilateral[22] (Figs. 8–9A,B and 8–10).

The base of the bladder is flat in the supine position (Figs. 8–3 and 8–4) and becomes cone shaped when the patient stands upright (Fig. 8–11). Its lowest point is anterior to the internal urethral orifice. Therefore, in the

anteroposterior view the bladder is superimposed on both the bladder outlet and proximal urethra. As a result, voiding studies must always be filmed in the steep oblique to lateral projection.

Most of the bladder floor is occupied by the base plate, which is circular when the bladder is full and at rest.[7, 23] It consists of an anterior and posterior trigonal plate with the vesicourethral junction slightly anterior to its center. It is best identified on a lateral cystogram as the postero-inferior wall of the bladder, extending from its most dependent point to a small indentation representing the interureteric ridge, which is part of the trigone (Fig. 8–12).

Voiding takes place when the smooth muscles of the vault (detrusor) contract and the pelvic floor muscles, chiefly the levator ani, relax. As the bladder descends, it changes form. The detrusor contraction elevates both halves of the base plate, while the progressive narrowing of the angle between them results in a cone formation. At the end of voiding, the two halves are vertical and parallel, creating the trigonal canal.

The bladder wall musculature is composed of three layers: outer and inner, longitudinal, and middle circular, the latter terminating at the internal urethral orifice. Both the inner and outer longitudinal layers continue into the urethral wall. The trigonal canal is therefore continuous with the posterior urethra. The final configuration of the trigonal canal, first cone-shaped and then tubular, can be observed only at the end of voiding when the bladder is nearly empty. When voiding stops, the canal reverts to its normal flat position. While voiding takes place, the contraction of the detrusor muscle can be seen on the cystogram in the lateral projection as an irregular posterior bladder wall (Fig. 8–13). This image should not be considered indicative of an obstructive lesion. In obstruction, the entire bladder wall, not just the posterior wall, is irregular (Fig. 8–14).

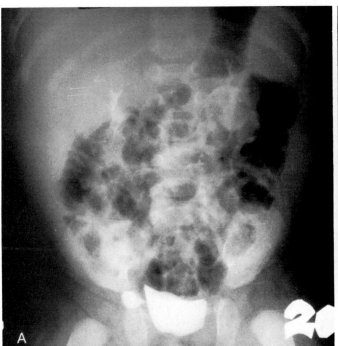

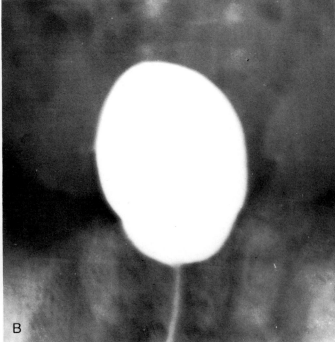

Figure 8–9. *A,* "Bladder ear." Urogram of a 2.5-month-old infant. Small collection to the right of the bladder represents protrusion into an as yet incompetent inguinal ring. *B,* Cystogram of same infant. Bladder ears are not now visualized.

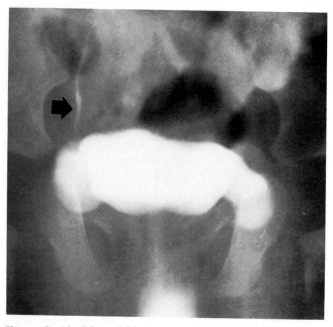

Figure 8–10. Bilateral bladder ears are seen on intravenous urogram of an infant. Arrow indicates right ureter.

The shape of the bladder may be altered by pressure from adjacent organs such as a gas-distended sigmoid colon (Fig. 8–15), a dilated ureter (Fig. 8–16), or an ectopic kidney (Fig. 8–17).

The Urethra

MALE CHILD

The male urethra has three sections: the prostatic and membranous (diaphragmatic) parts, together referred to as the posterior urethra, and the cavernous part (anterior urethra), which consists of the bulbar and pendulous

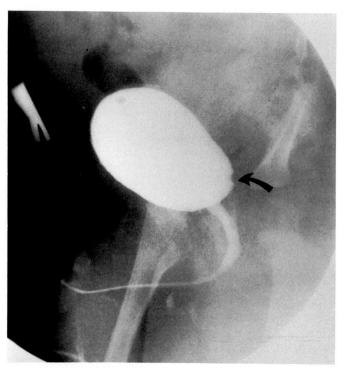

Figure 8–12. Cystourethrogram in a near-lateral projection. The small indentation in the posterior inferior bladder wall defines the interureteral ridge (arrow).

penile urethra. The prostatic urethra originates in the bladder base and ends distal to the verumontanum, a narrow longitudinal ridge on the posterior wall. The ejaculatory ducts enter the verumontanum on either side, the prostatic utricle passes through its center, and multiple prostatic ducts open on its surface. On the lateral urethrogram, the verumontanum is indicated as an oval filling

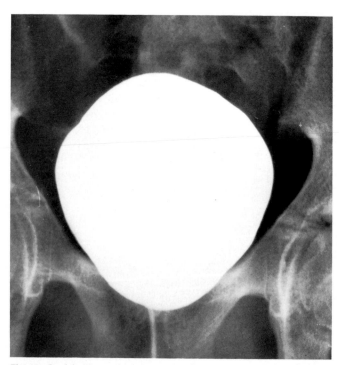

Figure 8–11. Normal cystogram of patient in upright position. Bladder base becomes cone shaped.

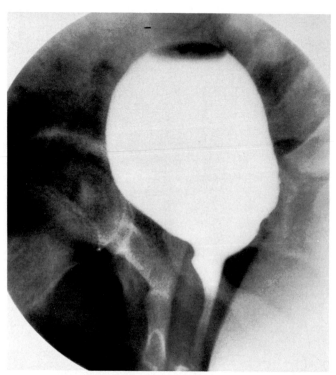

Figure 8–13. Cystourethrogram in steep oblique projection. Irregular posterior bladder wall caused by muscular contraction during voiding is a normal phenomenon.

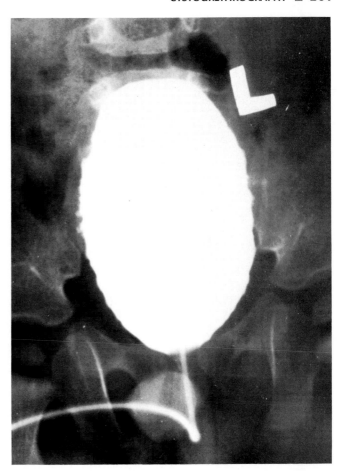

Figure 8–14. Cystogram of 6-year-old boy with obstructing polyp in the posterior urethra (not shown). Note trabeculated bladder wall caused by the obstruction.

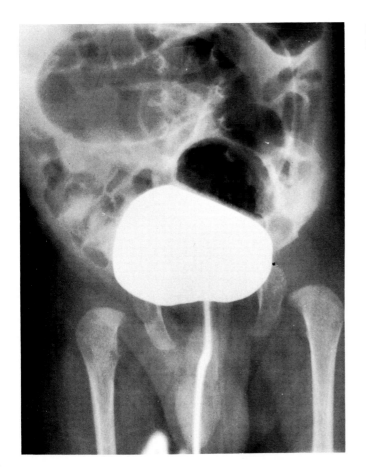

Figure 8–15. Impression on left side of bladder dome is produced by a distended sigmoid colon.

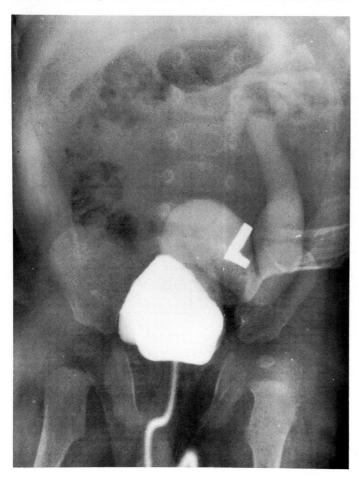

Figure 8–16. Impression on bladder by a very dilated and tortuous left ureter. Cystogram with residual contrast material diluted by urine from reflux into the left kidney and ureter.

Figure 8–17. Intravenous urogram reveals flattening of bladder roof attributable to left pelvic kidney.

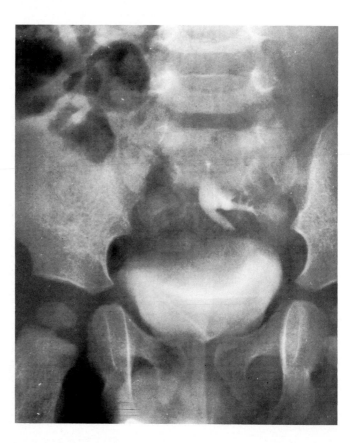

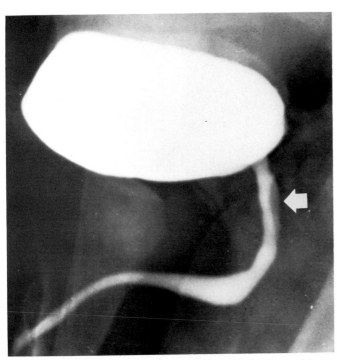

Figure 8–18. Voiding cystourethrogram (VCU), steep oblique projection. Shallow filling defect in posterior wall of prostatic urethra delineates the verumontanum *(arrow).*

defect in the posterior urethra (Fig. 8–18). Immediately below it lies the external sphincter. The verumontanum is the only constant landmark in the male urethra.

During voiding of contrast material the urethra has the appearance of a long tube, broad at its base and tapering off toward the meatus (Fig. 8–19). Sometimes an indentation can be seen in the proximal penile urethra (Fig. 8–20), representing the point where the smooth muscle running from the upper half of the urethra joins the

striated muscle of the distal urethra. The indentation is usually not concentric and does not cause disturbance to the urinary flow. It should not be interpreted as posterior urethral valves (Fig. 8–21). Occasionally, a slight narrowing is seen where the urethra passes the urogenital diaphragm, formed by the transversus perinei profundus muscle and its fasciae.[24] Contraction of this muscle may produce a constriction of the urethra. The distal or anterior part of the urethra has no normal indentations or constrictions. In the uncircumcised child, contrast material may collect under the prepuce (Fig. 8–22). The most distal portion of the urethra can show local widening: this is the navicular fossa (Figs. 8–22 and 8–23).

The following points about VCU in the male child should be emphasized:

1. The vesicourethral junction is wide open during voiding; congenital bladder neck obstruction is rare, if it does, in fact, exist.[25]

2. The exact location of the external sphincter cannot be determined on a micturition cystourethrogram.

3. Anterior indentations are caused by pressure from the urogenital diaphragm and by the incisura intermuscularis. Additional defects in the contrast-filled male urethra may occasionally be produced by other normal structures including the constrictor nudae muscle (extensions of the bulbocavernosus) and the plicae semilunares (vestigial müllerian structures extending distally from the verumontanum).

4. The verumontanum is the only consistent landmark and is situated in the posterior wall of the prostatic urethra.

FEMALE CHILD

The female urethra is much shorter than that of the male. As in the male, the smooth muscular layers of the

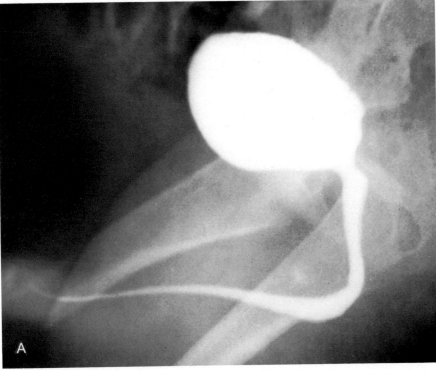

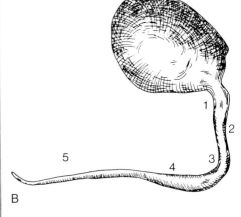

Figure 8–19. *A,* Normal VCU of a male child. Lateral projection. *B,* Diagram of *A:* (1) prostatic urethra, (2) verumontanum, (3) membranous urethra, (4) bulbar urethra, and (5) pendulous urethra.

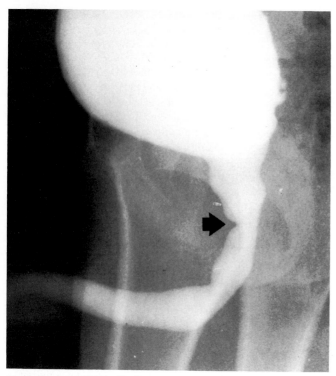

Figure 8–20. VCU. Shallow anterior indentation in proximal urethra represents incisura intermuscularis *(arrow)*. Note normal width of entire urethra. Compare with Figure 8–21.

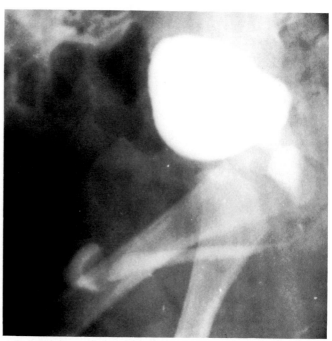

Figure 8–22. Contrast material collecting under prepuce in VCU of an uncircumcised child.

bladder continue into the urethra up to the urogenital diaphragm. From this point on, the urethral wall of the distal segment is almost entirely collagenous and, unlike the proximal part, is not distensible. The urethra passes obliquely downward, horizontally, or vertically, depending on the descent of the bladder base during straining. The vesicourethral junction is often somewhat superior and posterior to the lowest point of the bladder (Fig. 8–24). The diameter at the vesicourethral junction is variable and usually as wide or wider than the urethra itself. The width of the urethra is also variable and depends on the amount and velocity of the urine streaming through it (Fig. 8–25). It is slightly wider in older girls.

Two places in the female urethra do not expand: the incisura intermuscularis and the meatus with its collage-

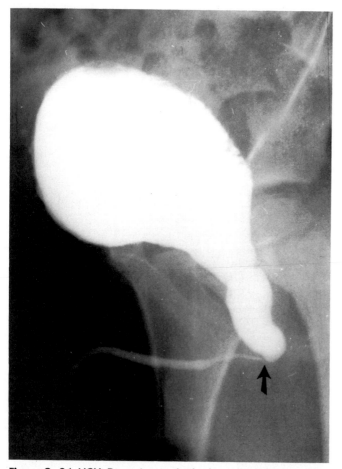

Figure 8–21. VCU. Posterior urethral valves are present *(arrow)*. Note marked dilatation of urethra proximal to valve, with distal narrowing. This is unlike the appearance in Figure 8–20, in which the entire urethra is normally distensible.

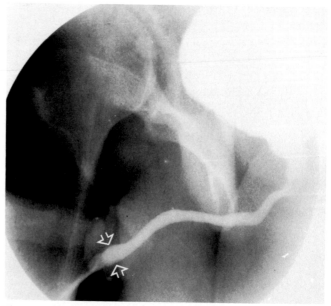

Figure 8–23. VCU. The fossa navicularis is seen as widening of most distal part of urethra *(arrows)*.

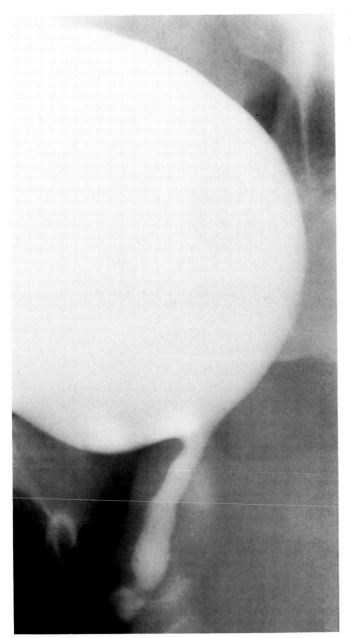

Figure 8–24. VCU in a girl, oblique projection. Note that bladder base is located somewhat anteriorly and inferiorly from vesicourethral junction.

nous structure. The space between them is named the fossa navicularis.

Contraction of the transverse fibers of the sphincter compressae urethrae muscle, located in the distal segment of the urethra, may give rise to an apparent narrowing on the urethrogram. The urethrographic image produced has been likened to an onion, a turnip, or a spinning top (Fig. 8–26). At one time this appearance was thought to indicate the presence of meatal stenosis, but it is now appreciated as being well within normal limits. The spinning top appearance is, however, sometimes seen in children with detrusor instability or the so-called congenital wide bladder-neck anomaly (CWBNA).[106] Shopfner in 1967 proved that there is no relationship between the shape of the urethra, intravesical pressure, and the width of the external urethral meatus.[26]

When voiding takes place, some of the contrast material

may reflux into the vagina. This occurs to some extent in 75% of all female children, regardless of whether they are in the supine or the upright position[23, 27] (Figs. 8–27 and 8–28). The phenomenon is demonstrated in the lateral view as the filling of an elongated cavity posterior to the urethra, reaching upward to the posteroinferior part of the bladder (Fig. 8–27). A sharp horizontal filling defect in the distal part of the vagina represents the hymen (Fig. 8–28).

During voiding, the bladder empties and the vagina progressively fills, remaining full until after voiding has stopped (Fig. 8–29). The horizontal rugae, characteristic of the vagina, seen on the anteroposterior film should not be mistaken for irregular urethral folds. (A lateral film separates and distinguishes between urethra and vagina (Fig. 8–29B), whereas in the anteroposterior projection one structure is superimposed on the other.)

In summary, the urethra in the female child is short with an obliquely downward course. Its width is variable and depends on the amount and velocity of the urine flowing through it. The distal segment is not distensible owing to the collagen content of its wall. Sometimes it produces a spinning top appearance simulating meatal stenosis. However, meatal stenosis in girls exists rarely, if at all. Reflux into the vagina is a physiological phenomenon and should not be interpreted as evidence of a fistula connecting urethra and vagina. Vaginal reflux may be accentuated in hypospadias and labial fusion, and occasionally may account for postmicturitional dribbling. After separation of the labia, the dribbling usually subsides.[28]

Adults

Bladder

The adult bladder is not much different from the child bladder. It has a smooth wall and is usually oval-shaped with its greatest diameter in the vertical (Fig. 8–30) or, especially in women, the horizontal position (Fig. 8–31). In the upright position, the bladder descends to a level lower than in children (Fig. 8–32). This is more pronounced in older women who have slackening of the perineal muscles as a result of child bearing and at times may interfere with complete emptying of the bladder. Normally, urine is held at the bladder neck. If the posterior urethra fills before voiding begins (Fig. 8–33), a neurogenic bladder should be suspected, unless the patient has undergone a recent prostatectomy. In the former case the finding would be due to incompetence, and in the latter would result from ablation of the internal sphincter.

Male Urethra

The urethra in the adult male has the same characteristics as in the child, except for its greater length. The posterior urethra extends from the bladder neck to the external sphincter. Its proximal or prostatic part passes through the prostate, and during micturition it is normally the widest section of the entire urethra, measuring approximately 3.5 cm at the vesicourethral junction. The verumontanum, or urethral crest, in the posterior wall of the prostatic urethra is usually well defined in the adult

Text continued on page 271

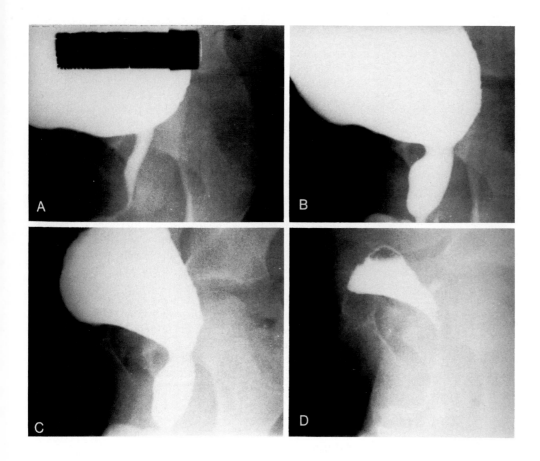

Figure 8–25. VCU in a young girl. Normal voiding sequence *(A–D)* shows variable width of urethra during micturition.

Figure 8–26. VCU in a female. "Spinning top" configuration represents a normal variant.

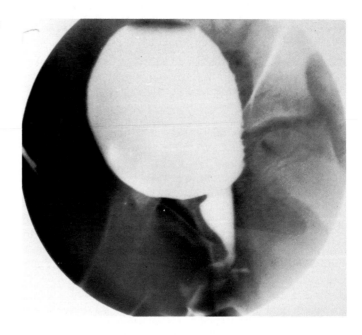

Figure 8–27. VCU voiding sequence in an infant girl. *A,* Cystogram, frontal projection. Catheter is still in urethra. *B,* Cystogram lateral projection. *C,* Catheter withdrawn; voiding starts. Trigonal canal formed. Vagina starts to fill. *D–G,* Vagina continues to fill as bladder empties. *H,* Film in frontal projection. Bladder is empty; vagina remains filled.

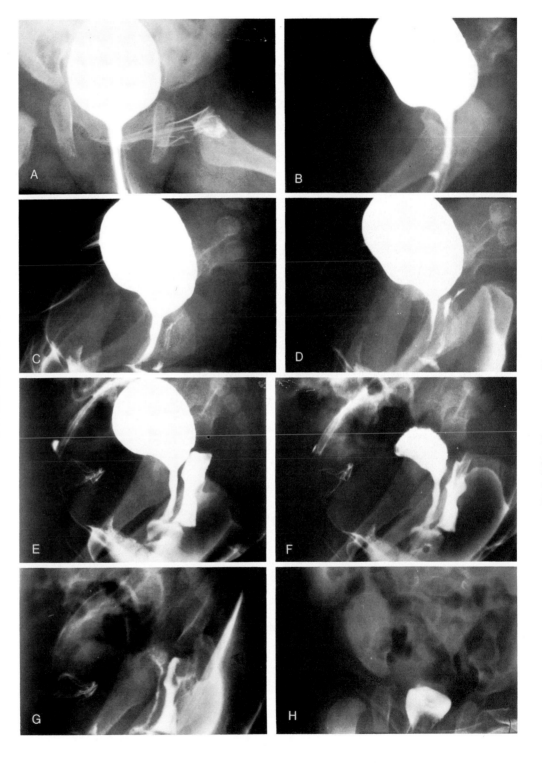

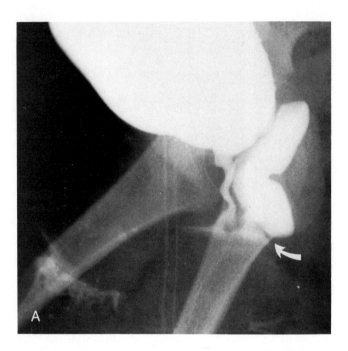

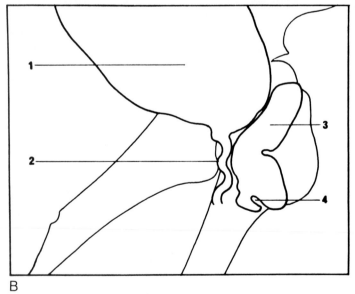

Figure 8–28. *A,* VCU. Marked filling of vagina during voiding. Horizontal filling defect in distal part of vagina represents the hymen *(arrow). B,* Drawing shows (1) bladder, (2) urethra, (3) vagina, and (4) hymen.

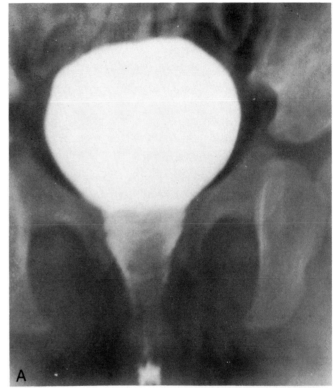

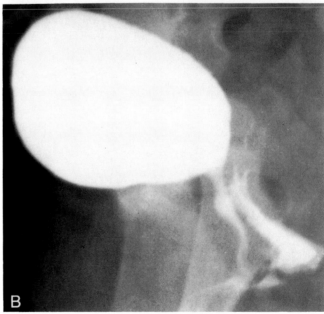

Figure 8–29. Simultaneous filling of vagina and urethra seen in *A*, frontal projection (horizontal rugae indicate vagina), and in *B*, lateral projection.

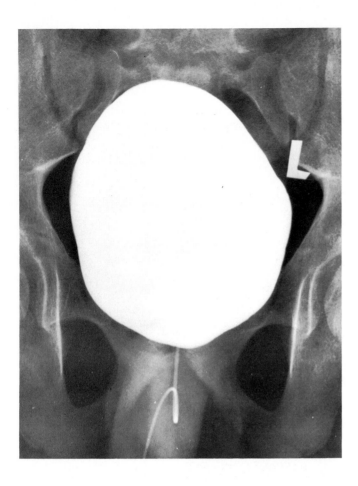

Figure 8–30. Cystogram of normal adult male bladder, which is oriented vertically.

Figure 8–31. Adult female. Bladder has a horizontal orientation.

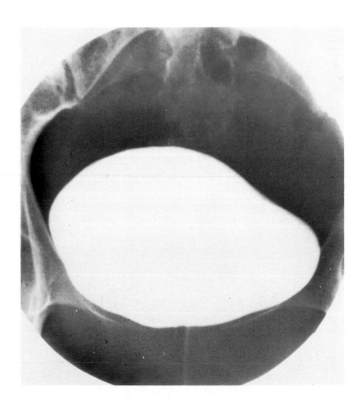

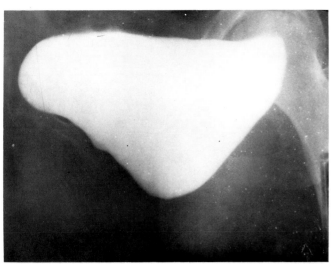

Figure 8–32. Cystogram of a 50-year-old female. Bladder descends markedly in erect position.

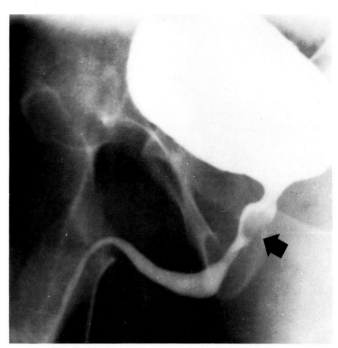

Figure 8–34. VCU of normal male adult urethra. Verumontanum is clearly demonstrated *(arrow).*

urethrogram (Fig. 8–34). The prostatic utricle, a vestige of the müllerian duct, opens in its center.[12] The membranous portion is short (1 cm) and narrow and is surrounded by the fibers of the external sphincter. The anterior urethra can be subdivided into the bulbous and pendulous parts. The bulbous portion reaches from the external sphincter to the penoscrotal junction. Here, the pendulous urethra is suspended by the suspensory ligament and continues to the external meatus. The most distal portion, known as the fossa navicularis, is somewhat wider (Fig. 8–35). The entire urethra forms a reverse "S" bend in the lateral projection: the first bend appears in the bulbous urethra, and the second at the penoscrotal junction (Fig. 8–36). During voiding, the air that entered the bladder along with contrast material is expelled, and a double-contrast "air urethrogram" may be demonstrated (Fig. 8–37). Filling of the prostatic ducts may occur normally (although it is much more commonly seen in patients with urethral strictures). Occasionally, the seminal vesicles and even the ductus deferens are demonstrated (Fig. 8–38). Two small ducts (Cowper's ducts) occasionally fill with contrast material. These ducts are situated posteriorly and lateral to the membranous urethra and extend from Cowper's glands to enter the floor of the cavernous portion of the urethra (Fig. 8–39). While the periurethral Littre's glands may sometimes opacify normally, they are more commonly seen in acute or chronic urethritis (Fig. 8–40). In recent years, prostheses have been implanted in the penis (Fig. 8–41). Barring complications, such as fistula formation, the urethrogram in these patients is normal (Fig. 8–42).

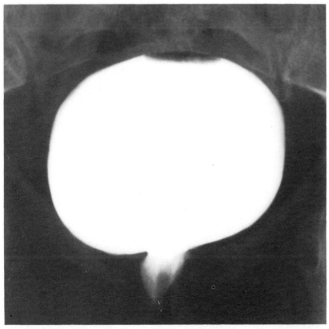

Figure 8–33. Cystogram before voiding in a 59-year-old patient with spinal cord injury. Note involuntary filling of posterior urethra to level of external sphincter.

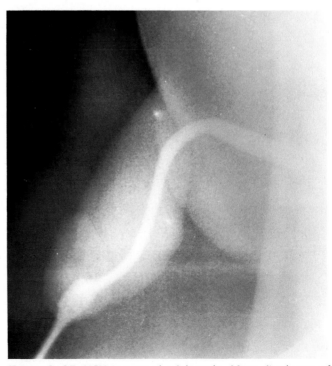

Figure 8–35. VCU in normal adult male. Most distal part of urethra shows typical widening of fossa navicularis.

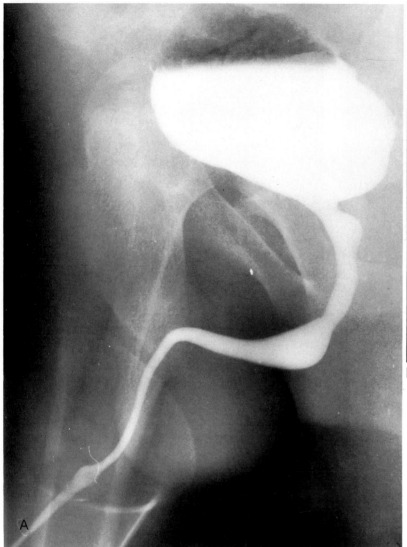

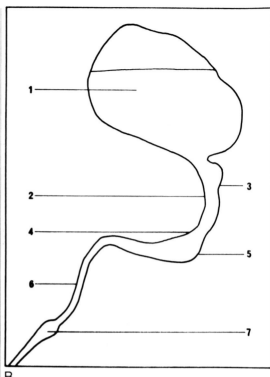

Figure 8–36. *A*, VCU showing normal course of male urethra with reverse S bend. *B*, Diagram of *A* showing (1) bladder, (2) prostatic urethra, (3) verumontanum, (4) membranous urethra, (5) bulbar urethra, (6) pendulous urethra, and (7) fossa navicularis.

Figure 8–37. Terminal phase of a VCU sometimes produces a double-contrast urethrogram, with air and contrast material outlining the lumen.

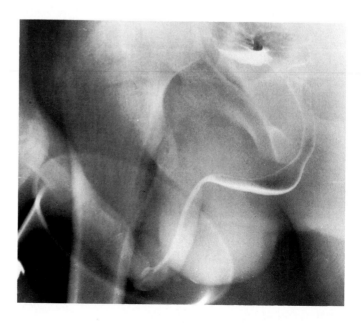

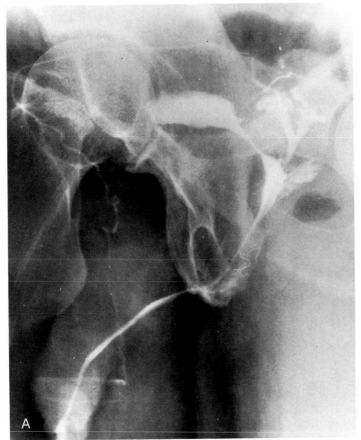

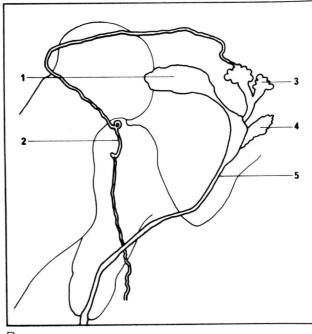

B

Figure 8–38. *A,* Filling of seminal vesicles, prostatic ducts, and vas deferens during VCU in a 65-year-old patient 7 years after prostatectomy. The patient is suffering from recurrent bilateral epididymo-orchitis. *B,* Drawing of *A* shows (1) bladder, (2) ductus deferens, (3) seminal vesicles, (4) prostatic ducts, (5) urethra.

Figure 8–39. Cowper's ducts demonstrated on VCU. Small channel is visualized posterior to the membranous urethra where stricture *(arrow)* causes both proximal urethral dilatation and filling of duct. Visualization of Cowper's ducts may also be seen normally.

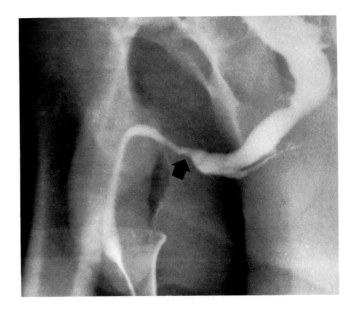

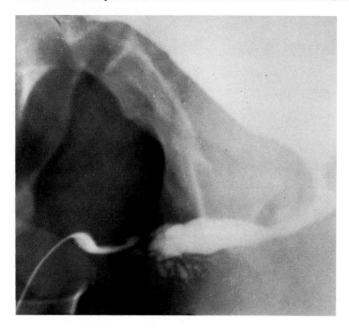

Figure 8–40. VCU demonstrating Littre's glands. Many small ducts are opacified around the bulbar urethra. A stricture accounts for the dilated urethra.

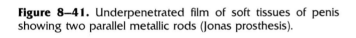

Figure 8–41. Underpenetrated film of soft tissues of penis showing two parallel metallic rods (Jonas prosthesis).

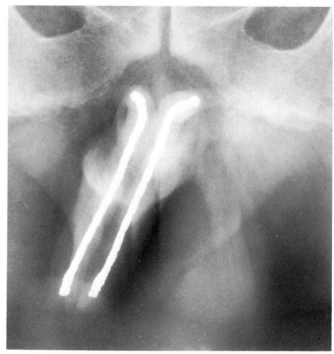

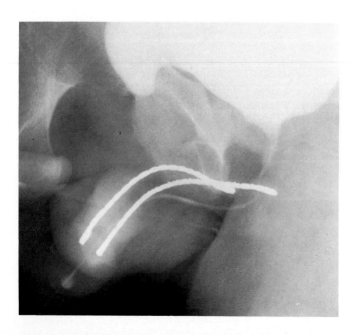

Figure 8–42. Normal cystourethrogram in patient with Jonas penile prosthesis.

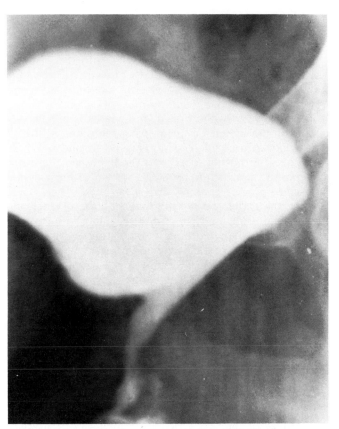

Figure 8–43. VCU of a normal adult female. Urethra courses obliquely forward and downward.

Female Urethra

The urethra in the adult woman is about 4 cm long and extends from the internal to the external urethral orifice. Its course is obliquely downward and slightly curved (Fig. 8–43), and there are many variations of its contour (Fig. 8–44). The urethral meatus is anterior to the vaginal opening, but in women (unlike girls) the contrast material usually does not enter the vagina during voiding.

TECHNIQUES OF EXAMINATION

Voiding Cystourethrography (VCU)

VCU is the most widely used examination for the radiological evaluation of the bladder and urethra in both children and adults. It is a specific roentgenological procedure that should be performed with fluoroscopic control. Its purpose is to demonstrate the bladder and urethra by retrograde filling of the bladder with contrast material and visualize the urethra during voiding.

Children

No preparation is needed for the child; no cleansing enema, fasting, or anesthesia is required. In fact, it is preferable that the child be awake. It is often helpful to have a parent or other familiar adult accompany and remain with the child throughout the examination, which is performed by a radiologist under fluoroscopic control. The older child should receive a simple explanation of the procedure and is asked to empty his or her bladder before the procedure commences. When completely undressed, the child lies on the x-ray table covered by a sheet. Using sterile technique, a catheter is introduced into the bladder. A No. 5 feeding tube with side holes is used for babies, and in older children No. 8 or No. 10 polyethylene or soft rubber catheters with end holes are quite suitable.

The meatus in girls, situated anteriorly to the vagina, is a slitlike opening that is usually not difficult to identify. After an initial inspection of the perineum to identify an obvious abnormality such as urethral prolapse,[18] or labial fusion, the urethral catheter is inserted. When it enters the bladder, a varying amount of urine will flow through it. If there is no flow, the catheter is advanced somewhat until urine is obtained. Suprapubic pressure is sometimes helpful in expressing a small amount of urine in the near empty bladder. The urine may be retained for microbio-

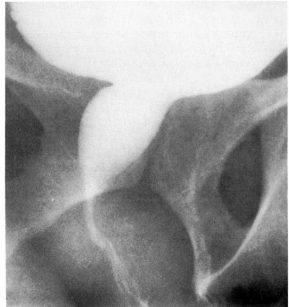

Figure 8–44. VCU of spinning top variety of urethra in an adult woman. This is a normal appearance.

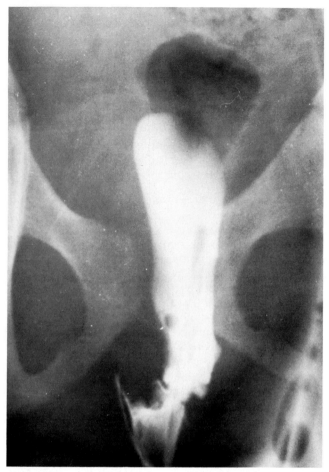

Figure 8–45. Inadvertent catheterization and filling of vagina, which is pear-like in shape. Note contrast material flowing out of cavity.

the bladder. In the older child, gentle pressing often produces the same result. Alternatively, some contrast material can be injected through the catheter into the posterior urethra to facilitate passage into the bladder. Rarely is obstruction sufficient to prevent passage of a small catheter, even when posterior urethral valves are present.

In a boy with hypospadias, the meatus is abnormally placed on the underside of the penis, causing the stream to flow backward or downward (Figs. 8–46 and 8–47). In about one-third of these patients the hypospadiac meatus is stenosed, and a catheter of very small caliber should be used.

Once the catheter has safely reached the bladder and the residual urine has been removed, filling with contrast material can begin. Although some radiologists fill the bladder by means of hand-injected contrast we prefer the gravity method, which is usually less uncomfortable for the child. An infusion set is connected to the catheter, and the contrast-filled bottle is suspended above the table to a height of 35 to 40 cm. A 30% solution of meglumine diatrizoate or iothalamate is satisfactory. The amount necessary to fill the bladder well and induce voiding is variable and depends on the age and sex of the child. Berger and coworkers[89] and Koff[93] estimate bladder capacity in children in order to standardize urodynamic studies. They claim that normal bladder capacity can be estimated as follows: ounces = age (in years) + 2. In the bladder of the newborn, 30 to 50 cc can be instilled with ease. From about 3 years of age, girls can hold 200 to 250 cc, and from 12 years of age, even more. The capacity in boys is less: 100 to 150 cc up to 5 to 6 years of age, and 250 cc in older boys. This is a rough estimate, and the amount must be adjusted individually.

logical studies, if clinically indicated. If no urine is obtained, it is advisable to learn whether the catheter has inadvertently been inserted into the vagina. If this is the case, then the catheter is left in the vagina and another sterile catheter is introduced into the urethral meatus. The vaginal catheter is removed only when it is certain that the second catheter is inside the bladder. An inexperienced radiologist may not observe a faulty position of the catheter and start filling the vagina. This error can be observed on the screen as a pear-shaped image (Fig. 8–45) and by the fact that the contrast material immediately empties around the catheter, wetting the sheet. When in doubt, the radiologist can check by turning the child onto her side. An anterior cavity filled with contrast medium represents the bladder, and a more posterior one, the vagina.

The meatus in boys is located at the tip of the glans and is easy to see in the circumcised child. In the uncircumcised boy, the foreskin should be retracted to facilitate a sterile preparation. After catheterization, the foreskin should be replaced to prevent paraphimosis.

The catheter should be copiously lubricated with an anesthetic jelly and inserted slowly and gently into the urethra holding the penis in an almost vertical position. The catheter can be easily advanced up to the external sphincter, which resists further passage. If, in the infant, there is crying at this stage, the radiologist waits for a deep breath. At this moment the sphincter usually relaxes, and the catheter can be advanced until it enters

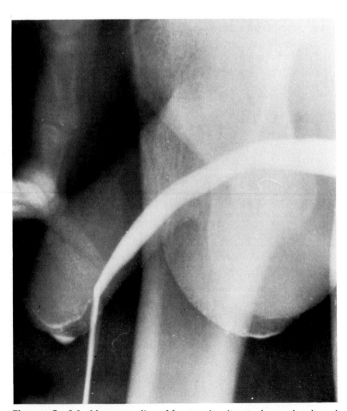

Figure 8–46. Hypospadias. Meatus is situated proximal and ventral to the glans and is clearly indicated during voiding. Downward voiding is shown.

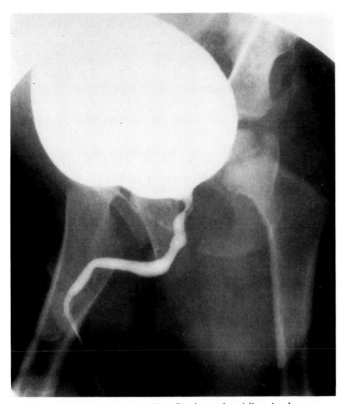

Figure 8–47. Hypospadias. Backward voiding is shown.

Capacity is reached when the child becomes uncomfortable and restless or begins voiding around the catheter, or when bladder and infusion pressure become equal and flow ceases or reverses. Forceful flexion of the toes sometimes signifies that bladder capacity has been reached. The volume of contrast material instilled in the bladder should be recorded.

During filling, fluoroscopic screening takes place at short intervals to see if vesicoureteral reflux or diverticula or other abnormalities are present. The child is turned slightly to the left and to the right to ensure that minimal reflux is not overlooked. If reflux appears, films are taken in the oblique projection (Fig. 8–48). If the bladder appears normal, one film is taken in the posteroanterior position at the end of filling. The infant under 2 years of age is then turned in the steep oblique position; the examination table is elevated slightly in the reverse Trendelenburg direction and the 105-mm camera or the spot film device is prepared for exposures. The catheter is not removed until all this is done.

Voiding often starts in infants at the moment the catheter is removed. Well-coned films of the urethra filled with contrast material should now be made with fluoroscopic monitoring and in the steep oblique projection. At the end of voiding, a frontal film is again made of the entire abdomen, including the kidney region, in order to prevent overlooking vesicoureteral reflux, which is sometimes apparent only on termination of voiding and may reach the upper collecting system without being easily discerned on the screen.

If the infant does not start to void, patience is required. One can try spraying cold water on the lower abdomen and perineum, keeping one's hand near the urethral meatus to glimpse the first spurt, without the need for screening. Another way to induce voiding is to give the infant a bottle. Otherwise, another catheter can again be introduced into the urethra and a small amount of additional contrast injected. When the catheter is withdrawn, the child usually starts urinating.

In the older child, the catheter is removed after one film of the full bladder has been taken. The table and the child on it are together placed upright, and another film of the bladder is obtained. The child is then turned to the steep oblique position, a receptacle is put into place (in front of the boy, or between the legs of a girl), and the child is asked to void.

Boys generally have no difficulty in urinating while upright. For girls this is not so easy. It is helpful to give the child something to drink or to turn on the tap. Some patients are sent to the lavatory to start voiding and are then usually able to complete voiding in the examination room.

The upright position is physiological for voiding and less untidy. Moreover, we have seen cases when reflux appeared in the upright and not in the supine position (Fig. 8–49). Nonetheless, in most instances, satisfactory films can be obtained in the supine position, if desired. It should be stressed that no study is complete without visualization of the urethra during voiding. To adequately assess the presence and degree of reflux, visualization must be obtained during and after urination. Reflux that was not present during filling may suddenly appear during, or even after, voiding. If reflux is present, additional

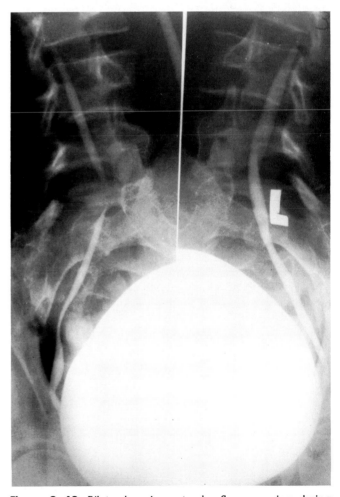

Figure 8–48. Bilateral vesicoureteral reflux occurring during bladder filling in a young boy. Films made in both oblique projections with spot film technique, dividing cassette into two vertical halves.

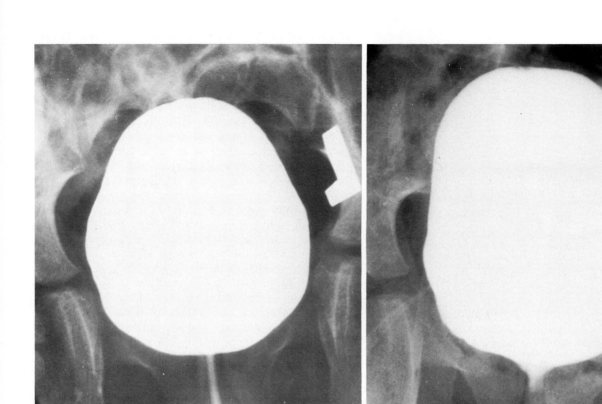

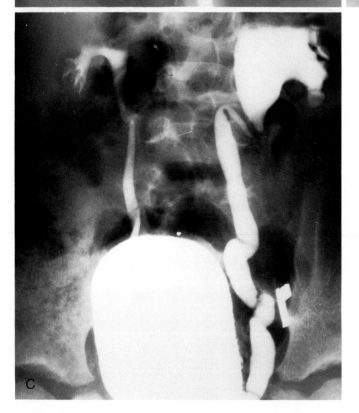

Figure 8–49. Vesicoureteral reflux appearing only in upright position during attempt at voiding. A 9-year-old boy with urinary tract infection. *A,* Cystogram, patient in supine position; catheter still in bladder. *B,* Patient upright. Catheter withdrawn. *C,* Sudden marked reflux into both kidneys before voiding has started.

films of the ureter and bladder are taken in the oblique projection. It is then possible to demonstrate whether a paraureteral Hutch's diverticulum is present (Fig. 8–50) and if the ureter ends in the trigone or ends ectopically.

The kidney area should be filmed in the frontal view in order to evaluate the grade of reflux. When premicturitional reflux is marked, the bladder is not filled to its maximal capacity. However, films are made during and after voiding to see whether the bladder empties completely before it refills from the kidney, and to exclude an obstructive lesion in the urethra.

Adults

Male. Straight rubber 14- to 18-F or Foley catheters are usually employed for cystourethrography in the adult male.

The bladder is filled in the usual way and, as in the older child, voiding takes place in the upright position. If possible, voiding studies are made in the steep oblique projection. The patient is able to urinate physiologically and has no difficulty initiating voiding. He voids into a receptacle that is radiolucent and should be careful not to press the penis against its edge, so as to prevent artificial obstruction with hold-up of the contrast material at the level of the penoscrotal junction[29] (see Fig. 8–75). Both thighs should be positioned to avoid superimposing either femur over the urethra. The voiding study in male adults can be modified by getting the patient to void against resistance; either he himself can close off the meatus by pinching the distal part of the penis, or a penile clamp such as Zipser's clamp is utilized. This is known as "choke" cystourethrography, and often enhances the visualization of the urethra by the artificial distention so produced.[30]

Patients with neurogenic dysfunction of the lower urinary tract, in the course of their follow-up examinations, often require a routine micturating cystourethrogram. Although the paraplegic or tetraplegic patient does not

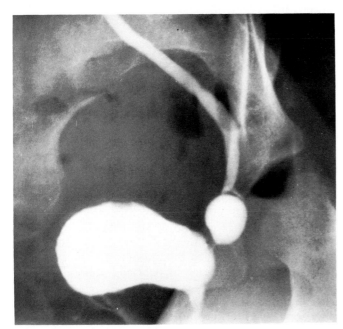

Figure 8–50. VCU of a child. Film taken in oblique projection at end of voiding shows vesicoureteral reflux and large "Hutch's" diverticulum.

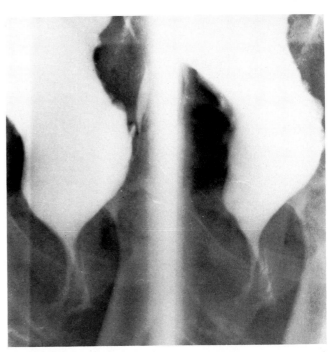

Figure 8–51. Voiding by Credé's method in a child with neuropathic bladder. Seven-year-old girl compressing her lower abdomen in order to achieve voiding. Note indentation on anterior bladder wall produced by abdominal wall pressure.

usually have satisfactory bladder control, the examination can be "tailored" to the habits acquired by the individual during his illness. A Foley catheter can be used to prevent involuntary expulsion of fluid. The patient can manually compress the meatus to improve visualization of the urethra. Voiding can be induced by a patient's self-established trigger mechanism, involving the lower abdomen or anal stimulation, for example. Abdominal compression by the Credé method (Fig. 8–51) can also help to empty the bladder at least partially. By these means, the entire urethra can be visualized (Fig. 8–52). Bladder trabeculation, vesicoureteral reflux, and narrowing of bladder neck or urethra, if present, will be successfully demonstrated.

The interpretation of the VCU in conjunction with urodynamic data determines the type of treatment the patient requires.

Female. The VCU procedure in women is essentially the same as in girls. However, it is worth filling the bladder with a large amount of contrast material, as young women often experience great difficulty in initiating voiding and are often "infrequent voiders."[95] In addition to the standard exposures, a doubly exposed film taken both at rest and during straining demonstrates the degree of bladder descensus, if any (Fig. 8–53).

Other Techniques

Excretion Micturition Cystourethrography (EMCU)

This is a method of demonstrating the bladder and urethra by making use of contrast material accumulated in the bladder during an excretory urographic examination. In 1965 Nogrady and Dunbar reported their experience with EMCU.[31] They observed successful visuali-

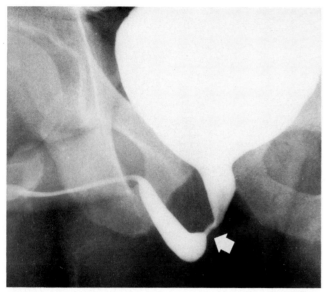

Figure 8–52. Neuropathic bladder in a 20-year-old patient. Voiding by abdominal tapping produces good demonstration of entire urethra. External sphincter dyssynergia is present *(arrow)*.

zation of the lower urinary tract in 75% of their patients and listed the following advantages of the method: (1) avoidance of the physical and psychic trauma of catheterization, (2) avoidance of possible infection by urethral catheterization, and (3) a more physiological and thus more reliable examination.

The method has several disadvantages, however: In children older than approximately 2 years of age, visualization is not usually adequate; the examination takes longer than VCU, and, most importantly, vesicoureteral reflux cannot be reliably detected. However, in children in whom it is difficult or impossible to catheterize the bladder, the EMCU is certainly an alternative for demonstrating the urethra.

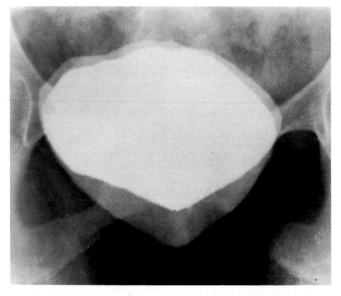

Figure 8–53. Double exposure on single film of bladder, both at rest and during straining. Demonstrates degree of bladder descensus, if any.

Double-Contrast Cystography (Pneumocystography)

This technique consists of instilling into the urinary bladder both gas and contrast material, usually for the purpose of evaluating neoplasms. With the advent of cross-sectional imaging, there is currently little need for double-contrast cystography. The study is sometimes helpful in evaluating suspected neoplasms within bladder diverticula, especially when the lesion is thought to involve the neck of the diverticulum. Double-contrast cystography, used in conjunction with computed tomography (CT), has been reported to facilitate the assessment of bladder neoplasms[32] (Fig. 8–54).

Bartley and Helander used double-contrast cystography in 75 patients, 20 of whom had bladder tumors.[33] They correctly diagnosed the neoplasm in all 20. Bartley and Eckerbom combined perivesical and intravesical instillation of gas to outline the thickness of the involved bladder wall, and by estimate, the degree of infiltration of the tumor.[34] When performing double-contrast studies, prone and supine films are necessary to move urinary collections away from the dependent part of the bladder. Films in the oblique projection and with a horizontal beam may also be used. Johannessen also listed the advantages of pneumocystography in patients with tumors.[35] He stated that in a series of 429 patients, 17 tumors were found that were not seen on cystoscopy. This might be due to the location of the tumor, such as near the bladder neck or in a diverticulum, or because active bleeding occurred. The author used barium sulphate in an aqueous suspension and a carbon dioxide mixture in 22 cases, allowing excellent visualization of the bladder tumor. These methods are now considered to be of historical interest only.

Suprapubic Micturition Cystourethrography

This study utilizes the technique of percutaneous needle puncture and filling of the bladder. The examination was developed after 1959, when Pryles and coworkers[36] introduced into pediatric practice suprapubic bladder puncture to aspirate sterile urine.

The bladder should be full prior to puncture; this can be achieved by means of an IV injection of furosemide (Lasix) and confirmed, if necessary, by ultrasonography. After 10 to 15 minutes, the bladder can be punctured at a site 1 to 2 cm above the symphysis. After aspiration of the urine, the bladder is filled by a concentrated contrast agent to ensure adequate visualization. The needle is withdrawn when the patient has an urge to void. X-ray films of bladder and urethra are taken in the same way as conventional VCU. Its reported advantages are the avoidance of catheterization and simplicity of technique. Complications include paravesical accumulations, bleeding, and intestinal perforation (see Fig. 8–64).[37]

A variant of this method is the technique of bladder filling through a cystostomy tube, which is inserted, for example, after trauma to the urethra. This is a noninvasive way of visualizing the bladder and urethra following its rupture and repair (Fig. 8–55).

Retrograde Urethrography

Although in most cases the micturating cystourethrogram satisfactorily visualizes the urethra, in some patients

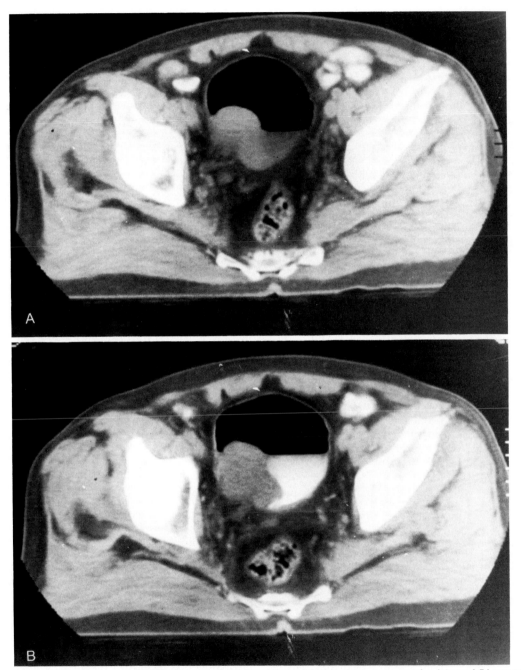

Figure 8–54. CT scans of transitional cell tumor of the bladder with double-contrast cystography (air and IV contrast) before *(A)* and after *(B)* intravenous contrast material injection. Tumor is clearly visible in right posterior part of bladder while anterior wall is well shown by air introduced into bladder.

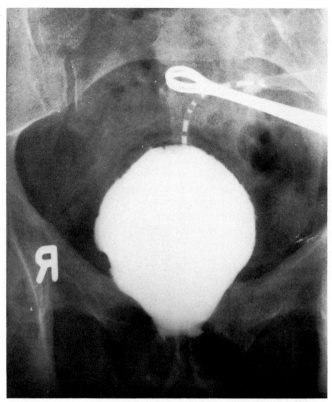

Figure 8–55. Filling of bladder through a cystostomy tube in a 63-year-old man with voiding difficulties following suprapubic prostatectomy. Bladder has an irregular wall. Subsequent urethrogram (not shown) demonstrated stricture of urethra.

a retrograde urethrogram is necessary for the adequate demonstration of strictures or anterior urethral disease. The contrast material used is sodium or meglumine diatrizoate, 30% in children and 50% to 60% in adults. McCallum and Colapinto in their experience with over 1000 studies using retrograde urethrography did not encounter local or systemic complications with this medium, even in patients with extravasation.[12]

The examination, which is mainly carried out on men, uses essentially the same technique in adults and children. In older boys and adults, perhaps the best method is to use a small Foley catheter, taking care that the balloon is placed in the fossa navicularis, which is the most distal part of the urethra (Fig. 8–56). The balloon, distended with 1 to 2 ml of saline, should effectively close off the urethral meatus. We do not use a local anesthetic, as it may cause mucosal edema, increased permeability, and vascular stasis,[12] as well as poor retention of the balloon, which may slip out of the urethra, or leakage of the contrast material.[38] Contrast material can now be injected and will visualize the anterior urethra facilitated by the resistance of the external sphincter. The presence of air bubbles in the urethra is prevented by inserting the catheter and simultaneously injecting contrast medium into the urethra until the catheter balloon is inflated.[39] The exposures are made with the patient in a 45° oblique position lying on either side, with the dependent thigh acutely flexed. The examination is fluoroscopically controlled throughout (Fig. 8–57A). If there is sufficient contrast material in the bladder, a VCU can be added at the conclusion of the retrograde study to outline the proximal and distal extents of a lesion (Fig. 8–57B).

The retrograde urethrogram is not a physiological ex-

amination. Contrast material is often injected under pressure to overcome the resistance of a stricture. The increased pressure in the urethra may lead the contrast material to avenues other than the urethral lumen, and various channels that are usually not demonstrated on micturating cystourethrography may become opacified. Inflammation, which accompanies most strictures, enhances venous and lymphatic filling. Mukerjee and coworkers reported on two patients with marked urethrovascular reflux.[40] In one patient, visualization of the entire collecting system was demonstrated through absorption of the contrast material and subsequent excretion by the kidneys. They recommend ascertaining whether the patient is allergic to drugs and contrast solutions before commencing the retrograde study. They also advise antibiotic coverage to protect the patient from possible gram-negative sepsis.

Filling of the corpora cavernosum and spongiosum, and venous and lymphatic intravasation may occur when the contrast medium accumulates and is obstructed by a urethral stricture (Fig. 8–58).

The balloon catheter as an aid in retrograde urethrography has largely replaced the older clamps to compress the penile urethra. Knutsson in 1929 described an instrument consisting of an adjustable clamp with limbs to hold the penis behind the corona and a cannula for fastening to the clamp.[41] In 1941, Brodny introduced a somewhat similar device that enjoyed widespread popularity in the United States for many years (Fig. 8–59).[103]

Henriet in 1969 devised a spring clip for urethrographic use.[43] The instrument consists of a straight clip and an injection cannula joined with an elastic band. The set is autostatic, and the injection can be carried out from a distance.

Lapides and Stone in 1968 stated that they avoid instrumentation as much as possible and instill contrast material directly from the syringe into the urethra.[44] Although such a technique has the virtue of simplicity, its routine use should be discouraged because of the radiation dosage to the operator's hands. A simple technique for retrograde urethrography in male infants was

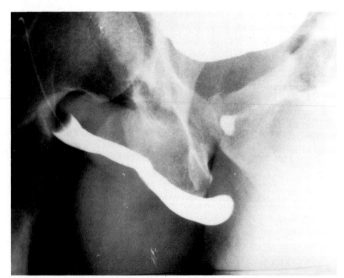

Figure 8–56. Retrograde urethrogram of a 34-year-old patient after a motor vehicle accident, with trauma to the pelvis. Inflated balloon of Foley catheter is in fossa navicularis and contrast material fills penile and bulbar urethra. Contrast will not fill proximal bulbar urethra because of strictures.

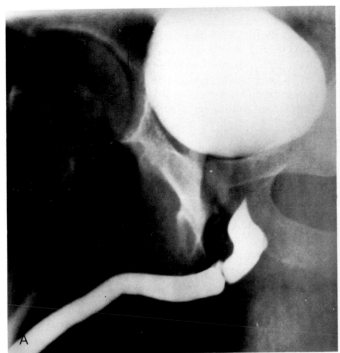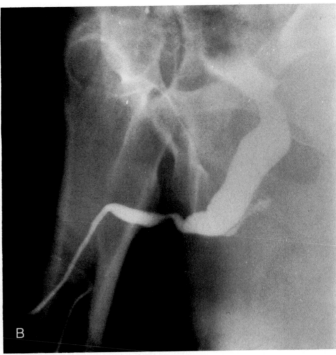

Figure 8–57. Residual stricture in 20-year-old man, after repair of urethral rupture. *A,* Retrograde urethrogram shows stricture in the bulbous part of the urethra. Contrast material has passed stricture and fills urethra to the external sphincter. *B,* VCU shows same stricture with proximal dilatation of urethra and filling of Cowper's duct.

reported by Lucaya.[45] After introducing the catheter into the urethra, he used collodion USP to bind it firmly to the meatus. After the examination, the collodion and the catheter are easily removed by peeling off the border of the film; the rest of the film lifts off in one piece. Double-contrast studies with this method have been used by Yokoyama and coworkers. They were able to clearly visualize small anterior urethral lesions with this technique.[46]

Retrograde urethrograms in females are rarely necessary. They are less readily performed than in males, because it is technically difficult to completely close the external urethral orifice. The examination is performed primarily when a urethral diverticulum is suspected but cannot be confirmed by VCU.

Davis and Cian were perhaps the first to use a double-

balloon catheter in the female, one balloon occluding the vesical neck and the other the urethral meatus.[13] A first injection is made, occluding the bladder neck only to clear the urethra of air, urine, and pus. The second balloon is then pressed against the external meatus followed by a further injection of viscous contrast material. The pressure in the urethra effects filling of a urethral diverticulum, if one is present. Lang and Davis reported satisfactory experience with this method in 108 examinations.[46a]

Andersen in 1964 devised an instrument consisting of eight cannulae with end-plates of different diameters (4 to 18 mm).[47] A suitable cannula is introduced into the urethra. No fluid will escape when an aqueous contrast material is injected. The author tested the instrument in 100 patients with carcinoma of the genital tract. He found

Figure 8–58. Retrograde urethrogram in a patient with stricture shows filling of corpus cavernosum and spongiosum, as well as extensive intravasation into blood vessels, which resulted from excessively high injection pressures.

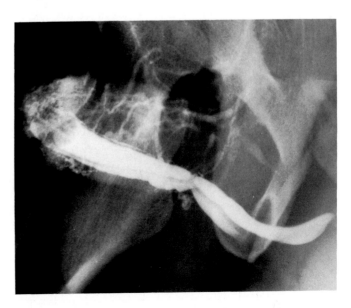

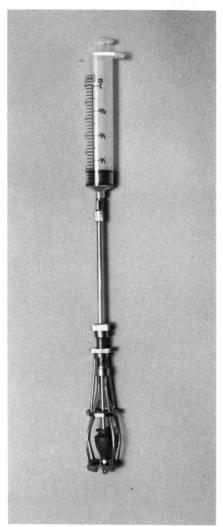

Figure 8–59. Brodny's clamp simultaneously obturates urethral meatus and compresses glans behind corona. It is sometimes cumbersome to fit clamp properly, or difficult to maintain a watertight seal, but once clamp is appropriately positioned, it produces satisfactory studies.

the method effective and did not encounter complications, except dysuria, which subsided within 24 hours after the investigation.

Greenberg and coworkers used a Trattner catheter to evaluate the female urethra.[48] This catheter has both a proximal and a distal balloon, each with its own tube for inflation. A third conduit runs between the two and into the urethra. The authors demonstrated the normal urethra, small outpouchings, true diverticula, and filling of periurethral glands (Fig. 8–60A–C).

INDICATIONS FOR CYSTOURETHROGRAPHY

Children

The main indication for VCU in children is *urinary tract infection*. It usually occurs in girls, and the overwhelming majority of VCUs in childhood are performed in girls under 6 years of age. *The examination is performed to determine whether vesicoureteral reflux or, more rarely, congenital anomalies of the lower urinary tract are present.* The incidence of reflux in children with urinary tract

infection is between 30% and 50%.[49–51] The VCU is usually carried out some weeks after the infection has cleared, although it may be performed during acute infection with antibiotic coverage. Formerly, it was thought that infection was the cause of reflux and that the VCU should be postponed until after the infection had subsided. However, reflux is most often a primary phenomenon caused by a congenital defect of the vesicoureteral junction.[52, 53] Since a significant number of siblings of children with marked reflux will also show reflux, consideration should be given to examining them also if adequate resources permit.[54, 55, 97, 101] Patients with reflux should be re-examined at regular intervals, perhaps every 2 years, either by VCU or a radionuclide cystogram. The latter technique is useful for follow-up evaluation, the radiation dose being much lower than in VCU.[56] The lower grades of reflux usually subside spontaneously over a period of several years.[57, 58] Patients with severe reflux should be considered for an antireflux operation.

Many authorities feel that VCU is indicated after the first occurrence of urinary tract infection in either boys or girls.[59, 60] Other indications in children include voiding difficulties such as pain on micturition, a thin stream, dribbling, frequency, and urgency. In boys, posterior urethral valves are a rare cause of dysuria, whereas bladder diverticula may result in a misleading residual urine determination, urinary stasis, and infection.

When a sonographic study of the kidneys or an excretory urogram shows abnormalities such as a dilated collecting system, an investigation by VCU often demonstrates whether obstruction or reflux is the cause of dilatation, either at the pyeloureteral or the ureterovesical junction.[61, 96] Stenosis at the pyeloureteral junction may be secondary to tortuosity and angulation of an atonic ureter due to reflux. Reflux is often found in children with ectopic kidneys,[62] and a higher rate of incidence is found in children with duplex kidneys.[63, 64] Other congenital anomalies such as meningomyeloceles,[65] sacral agenesis, and rectal anomalies are further indications for VCU.[66, 67] Among boys with hypospadias, about 15% will have vesicoureteral reflux, 30% will have meatal stenosis, and 10% will have müllerian duct remnants.[68] VCU is also recommended as a baseline study prior to lower tract surgery and for postoperative evaluation of the urethra.[69, 81]

Where bladder trauma is suspected, a cystogram is necessary. After repair of a urethral rupture, the VCU shows whether passage of contrast material through the urethra is satisfactory and whether strictures, diverticula, or false passages are present.

In cases of kidney failure in children, reflux should be excluded as a cause of the renal disease. In boys with hematuria, the VCU may on occasion demonstrate a posterior urethral valve or a polyp.

Adults

The main indications for retrograde urethrogram in males are trauma to the urethra or urethral stricture; in females, the main indication is a suspected urethral diverticulum. A cystogram is indicated in patients with significant trauma to the pelvis. In fractures of the pelvic arch, 10% to 15% are accompanied by rupture of the

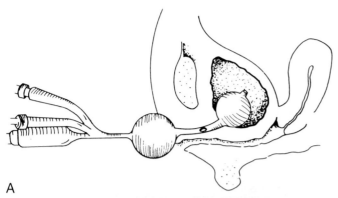

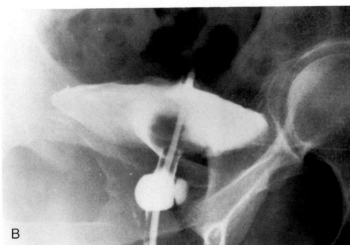

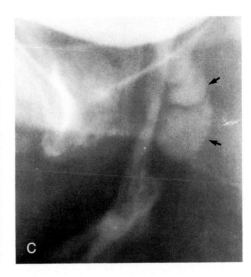

Figure 8–60. *A,* Schematic drawing of Trattner catheter. (Modified from Greenberg M et al: Female urethral diverticula: Double-balloon catheter study. AJR 136(2):259–264, © by Am Roentgen Ray Soc, 1981.) *B,* Demonstration of a urethral diverticulum with the aid of Trattner double balloon catheter. Proximal balloon occludes bladder neck; distal one occludes urethral meatus. Contrast material in urethra from opening between the two balloons demonstrates a diverticulum. *C,* VCU of the same patient also shows large urethral diverticulum *(arrows).*

bladder and/or urethra.[70] The excretory urogram may not show extravasation because of the diluted contrast material and the low pressure in the bladder. The first examination should be retrograde urethrography, which is followed by a cystogram, preferably with fluoroscopic control. The patient is usually referred from the emergency ward and may have already had a Foley catheter inserted.

A retrograde urethrogram can be performed by sliding a polyethylene feeding tube adjacent to the Foley catheter. If there is a rupture of the bladder, the VCU will usually demonstrate it, but even with this study up to 10% of bladder ruptures are missed.[71] It should be emphasized that, except in patients with trauma, retrograde urethrography is of little or no value in evaluating the posterior urethra.

Other indications for VCU in adults include urinary tract infection and signs on the urogram of reflux nephropathy of one or both kidneys. VCU is useful in the evaluation and follow-up of patients with spinal cord injury, voiding difficulties, or renal failure prior to transplant surgery. It is also valuable prior to instillation of certain irritating chemicals, such as formalin, into the bladder. Vesicoureteral reflux is uncommon in adults, but if it occurs, surgical repair to prevent repeated infections may be necessary.[98, 100] However, previous damage to the kidneys is irreversible. Male patients with voiding problems may have strictures resulting from long-forgotten childhood trauma or from instrumentation or operation.

The evaluation of the patient before renal transplant includes a VCU to demonstrate bladder capacity and the presence of vesicoureteral reflux or bladder outflow obstruction, which may have to be corrected at the time of the transplant operation.

COMPLICATIONS

If the principles of a reliable technique are scrupulously followed, the complications of cystourethrography should be few and far between. However, several complications have been reported. McAlister and coworkers listed several incidents, including two patients who died from sepsis.[72] Some of these problems resulted from faulty technique.

Infections

Bacteria may be introduced into the bladder or urethra via the catheter, and high fever can develop following cystography. Glynn and Gordon mention a 6% incidence of new or recurrent infections associated with cystography.[73]

McAlister and coworkers suggest that cystography in patients with active infections should be avoided.[72] Duckett and Bellinger claim that this practice may lead to permanent, severe bladder contractures.[105] Perhaps it is best to postpone the examination until after the infection has subsided or to perform it under antibiotic coverage. It may also be prudent to avoid performing radiographic procedures on the lower urinary tract immediately after vesicourethral instrumentation.

Trauma

Dysuria or urinary retention can result from catheterization. Using ultrasound techniques, Markle and Catena showed that the bladder mucosa can become very edematous following catheterization, sometimes even resembling a mass.[74] The procedure should be carried out by an experienced radiologist, and should not be pursued when there is difficulty introducing the catheter. A retrograde urethrogram can be performed to demonstrate the stricture; otherwise the patient can return on another day, after a urologist has inserted a catheter under suitable conditions. Gentleness is one key to a safe and satisfactory examination. Overinjection must be avoided.

Reaction to Contrast Medium

A local or systemic reaction to the contrast material may occur. The medium might have been absorbed from the bladder and from the kidneys in patients with marked vesicoureteral and intrarenal reflux (Fig. 8–61). Intravasation of contrast material flowing directly into the blood stream might also be the cause. Dermatitis may occur.[107]

Inadvertent Catheterization of the Vagina or a Ureter

Inadvertent catheterization of the vagina is possible, but it is usually harmless. Reflux into the uterus, fallopian tubes, and even peritoneal cavity has been noted without sequelae (see Fig. 8–66). The catheter can also enter a ureter with an ectopic ending (Fig. 8–62), the ureter of a double-collecting system (Fig. 8–63), or perhaps a ureter with a very dilated orifice. Dilatation of the ureter by direct filling with contrast material causes pain. This can also happen if a Foley catheter is inadvertently inserted into the ureter with inflation of the balloon. After identifying the error, the catheter should be deflated and withdrawn instantly.

Perforation of the Bladder Wall

Perforation of the bladder wall by the catheter and rupture of the bladder by overfilling have been reported.[72] During suprapubic cystography the needle may become dislodged, and the contrast material will accumulate within or around the bladder wall. The patient generally complains of severe pain, and the examination should be terminated at once.

A successful puncture of the bladder was achieved in a 45-year-old male patient in our care. However, directly after the needle was connected to an infusion set, the contrast material accumulated around the bladder (Fig. 8–64), causing severe pain to the patient and necessitating surgical intervention. Apparently, the needle had become dislodged.

Knotting of a Urethral Catheter within the Bladder

This is a possible hazard, usually when the catheter is soft and a long segment of it is introduced into the bladder.[75]

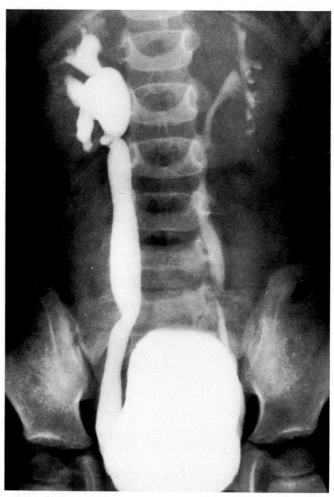

Figure 8–61. Cystogram shows that marked intrarenal reflux in the right kidney of a 5-year-old girl with urinary tract infections resulted in absorption of contrast material (and allergic reaction to it) and excretion by left kidney.

Radiation Effect

The VCU is a diagnostic procedure that inevitably exposes the gonads to some radiation. This dose should be kept to a minimum, especially in children who often undergo repeat examinations.[76] Careful attention to ensure very short screening periods, a tightly collimated x-ray beam, and the use of 70- or 105-mm photofluorography will reduce the amount of radiation to the gonads to a minimum[10, 11, 77, 82, 83] (see Table 8–1 and Chapter 3).

Autonomic Dysreflexia

In tetraplegic patients, and patients with lesions above T5, the filling of the bladder and forcible opening of the bladder neck during voiding may cause a severe reaction including severe headache, sweating, hypertension, and bradycardia. An α-adrenergic blocker prior to the VCU will prevent this complication.[79]

POTENTIAL PITFALLS AND DIFFICULTIES IN INTERPRETING RADIOLOGICAL STUDIES

When interpreting radiographic studies of the pelvis, bladder, and urethra, the external soft-tissue shadows,

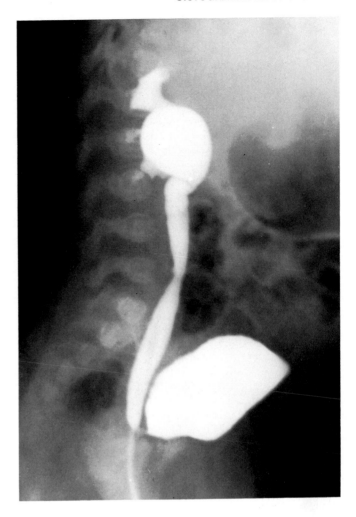

Figure 8–62. Inadvertent catheterization of ectopic ureter emptying into urethra. Catheter lies outside bladder, directly filling right collecting system.

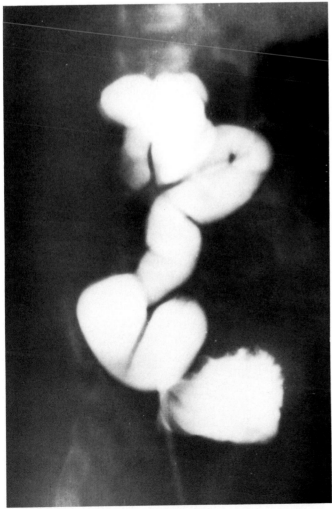

Figure 8–63. In this girl, catheter enters very dilated ureter of duplex system with ectopic ureterocele.

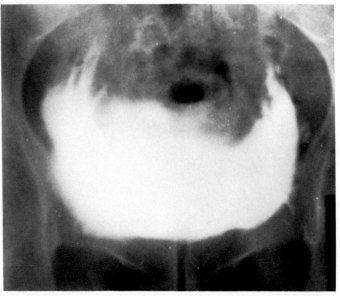

Figure 8–64. Direct percutaneous needle cystogram. Dislodgment of suprapubic needle results in accumulation of contrast material in and around bladder wall.

such as represent the penile tip (Fig. 8–65), should be easy to define.

On the urogram, the vagina may be seen to fill by retrograde backflow from the urethra. Once filled, the vagina can be distinguished from the bladder by its vertical position and small size (Fig. 8–66). Reflux from the vagina to the uterus can produce a hysterosalpingogram, and continued filling may result in opacification of the peritoneal cavity (Fig. 8–66*B*).

A Foley catheter balloon can produce a filling defect in the bladder, as shown on the urogram (Fig. 8–67). The catheter's "tail" helps to make the correct diagnosis. It may be confused with a ureterocele. An air bubble, which may have entered the bladder during instrumentation, may present the same appearance (Fig. 8–68). Air also enters the bladder during filling with contrast medium and is best visualized in the upright position. A large filling defect in the recumbent position is most often caused by a different process, such as a blood clot (Fig. 8–69) or tumor.

The appearance of a filling defect in the urethra can be the effect of an enlarged prostate compressing the posterior urethra (Fig. 8–70), of air bubbles introduced during retrograde urethrography (Fig. 8–71), or of a catheter that was not withdrawn at the start of voiding (Fig. 8–72). Spasms of the external sphincter should not

Text continued on page 294

Figure 8–65. Plain film of pelvis shows distal part of penis overlying symphysis pubis and superimposed on pelvis.

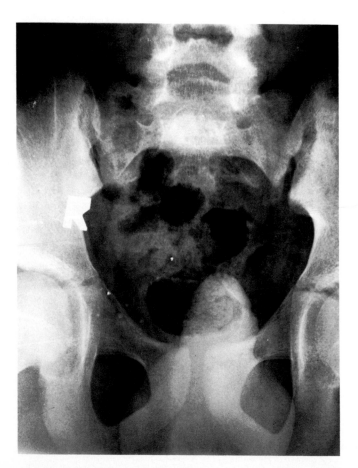

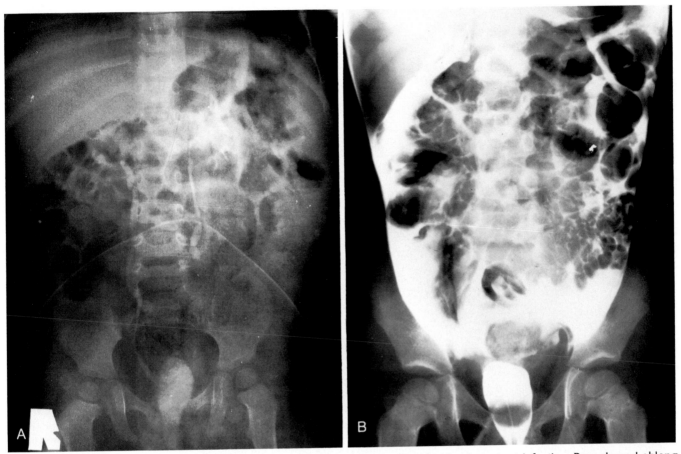

Figure 8–66. *A*, Excretory urogram showing filling of vagina in 10-month-old girl with urinary tract infection. Pear-shaped oblong cavity in lower pelvis is vagina filled retrogradely from urethra during involuntary voiding. *B*, Inadvertent catheterization of the vagina during attempted cystography in a young girl produced this striking picture of diffuse intraperitoneal extravasation of contrast material through the fallopian tubes. (From Stanfield BM, Soderdahl DW, Schamber DT: Case profile: Extravagram. Urology 7:97, 1976.)

Figure 8–67. Rounded filling defect in bladder caused by balloon from Foley catheter. Shaft of catheter is opacified and serves to differentiate balloon from other defects, such as ureteroceles.

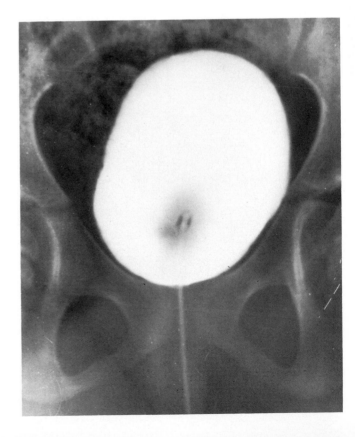

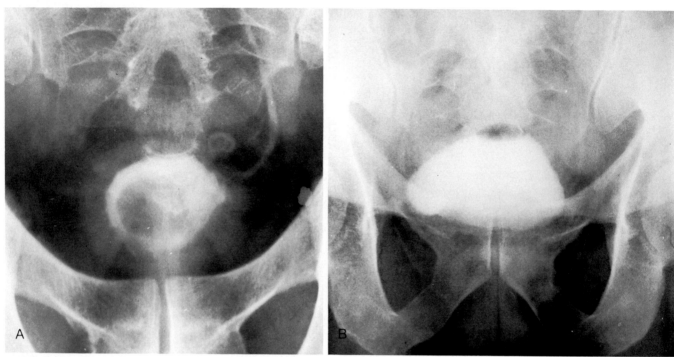

Figure 8–68. Filling defect in bladder caused by air. A 59-year-old male with hypertrophy of the prostate had undergone cystoscopy prior to urography. *A*, Air has entered bladder as demonstrated on a prone film. *B*, Erect film confirms presence of gas in the bladder. No stones or other space occupying lesions were seen by the urologist.

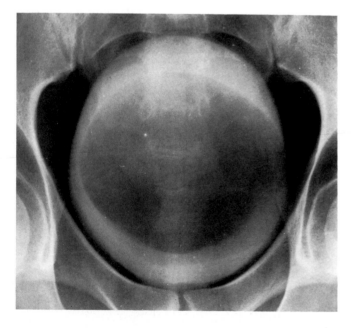

Figure 8–69. Intravesical filling defect caused by large blood clot. Urogram was taken because of macroscopic hematuria, which appeared 3 days after renal biopsy. Large blood clot within bladder was cause of filling defect encompassing almost entire bladder lumen. Repeat urogram 1 week later was normal.

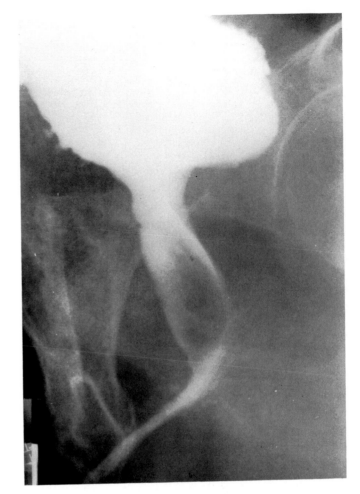

Figure 8–70. VCU. Filling defect in posterior urethra was caused by intrusion of enlarged prostate.

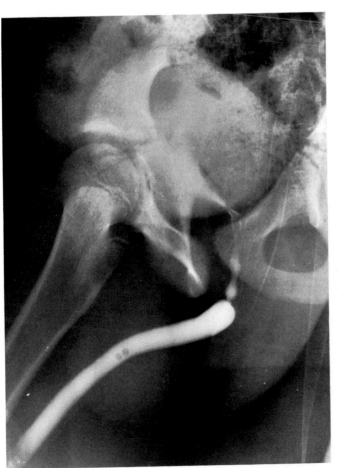

Figure 8–71. Small filling defects in the urethra caused by air bubbles introduced during retrograde injection. Defects are perfectly round and move during shifts in position, differentiating them from intrinsic lesions.

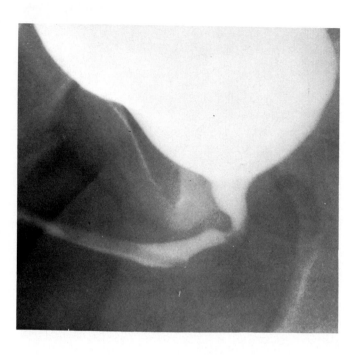

Figure 8–72. Elongated filling defect in urethra caused by incompletely withdrawn catheter.

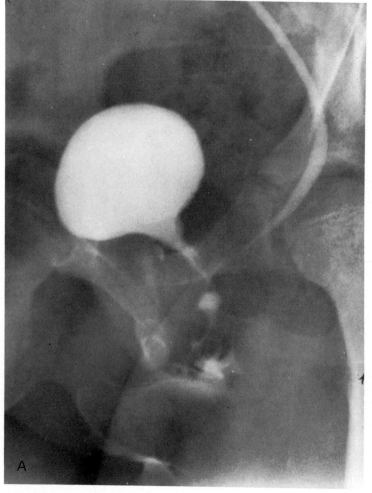

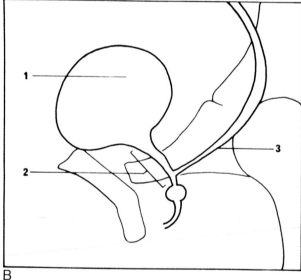

Figure 8–73. *A,* Voiding stage of VCU. Reflux is into a ureter that seems to end ectopically. However, ureter emptied orthotopically. Marked contraction of bladder base, causing descent of interureteral ridge, makes orifice appear to be ectopic. *B,* Drawing of *A* shows (1) bladder, (2) trigonal canal, and (3) ureter.

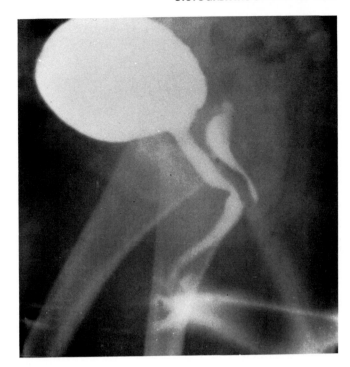

Figure 8–74. Filling of vestigial vagina in a boy. Patient has hypospadias, and urethra is therefore short.

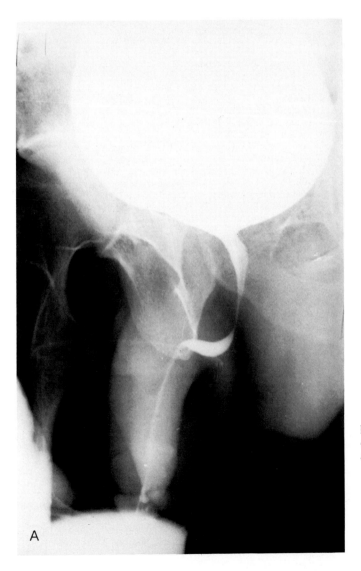

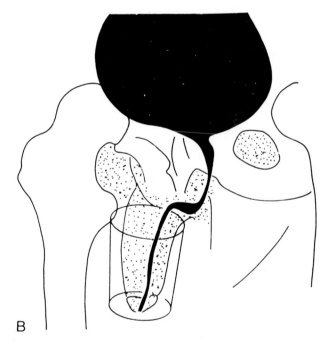

Figure 8–75. *A*, Pseudourethral stricture. Container pressing on undersurface of the penis causes narrowing of urethra and an artificial hold-up of contrast material. *B*, Diagram of *A*.

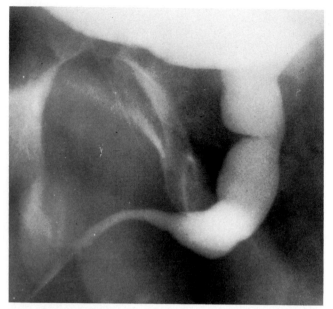

Figure 8–76. VCU reveals marked proximal dilatation and distal narrowing of urethra after operation for hypospadias. This is a bona fide lesion and not a hold-up caused by pressure from the urine receptacle.

be mistaken for a membranous urethral stricture. Marked contraction of the bladder base may cause the descent of the interureteral ridge. This phenomenon can have the appearance of the ectopic ending of a ureter in cases of reflux (Fig. 8–73).[80]

A relatively short urethra and filling of the vagina should not immediately be regarded as the normal appearance in a female child. It could, in fact, be a sign of intersex in a child with marked hypospadias (Fig. 8–74).[26, 81]

Although the distal urethra may seem somewhat narrowed during voiding (due to pressure from the urine container) (Fig. 8–75), narrowing of the anterior urethra in the absence of pressure is always pathological (Fig. 8–76). Clinically significant narrowing is almost always associated with proximal distention.

References

1. Cunningham JH: The diagnosis of stricture of the urethra by the roentgen rays. Trans Am Assoc Genitourin Surg 5:369–371, 1910.
2. Beclere H, Henry R: Quelques radiographies de retrecissements de l'uretre. J D'Urol 13:417, 1922.
3. Edling NPG: Urethrocystography in the male with special regard to micturition. Acta Radiol (Suppl)58:56–96, 1945.
4. Kjellberg SR, Ericsson NO, Rudhe U: The Lower Urinary Tract in Childhood. Chicago, Year Book Medical Publishers, 1957.
5. Burrows EH: Urethral lesions in infancy and childhood, studied by micturition cysto-urethrography. Springfield, Illinois, Charles C Thomas, 1965.
6. Shopfner CE: Roentgenological evaluation of bladder neck obstruction AJR 100:162–175, 1967.
7. Shopfner CE, Hutch JA: The normal urethrogram. Radiol Clin North Am 6:165–189, 1968.
8. Shopfner CE: Roentgenological evaluation of distal urethral obstruction. Radiology 88:222–231, 1967.
9. Shopfner CE: Cystourethrography: Methodology, normal anatomy, and pathology. J Urol 103:92–103, 1970.
10. Kaude JV, Reed JM: Gonad dose to children in voiding urethrocystography performed with 70-mm image-intensifier fluorography. Radiology 92:771–774, 1969.
11. Hertz M, Werner A: Radiation dose to the gonads during cystourethrography in adults. Isr J Med Sci 13:614–616, 1977.
12. McCallum RW, Colapinto V: Urological Radiology of the Adult Male Lower Urinary Tract. Springfield, Illinois, Charles C Thomas, 1976.
13. Davis HJ, Cian LG: Positive pressure urethrography: A new diagnostic method. J Urol 75:753–757, 1956.
14. Uray W: Die Localisation der nicht ausdehnbaren rektalen und urethralen Strikturen mit Hilfe von X Strahlen. Orvosihetil, 56, 450, 1912. Ref Urolof, Yahresbericht, 326, 1912.
15. Pfister E: Uber Rontgenbilder der mannlichen Harnrohre. Ztsch F Urol 14:281, 1920.
16. Sicard JA, Forestier J: Exploration radiographique de l'uretre au lipiodol. Bull Mem Soc Med Hop Paris 48:207, 1924.
17. Kohnstam GLS, Cave EHP: The Radiological Examination of the Male Urethra. London, Baillière, Tindall and Cox, 1925.
18. Ulm AM, Wagshul EC: Pulmonary embolization following urethrography with oily medium. N Engl J Med 263:137–139, 1960.
19. Crabtree EG: Venous invasion due to urethrogram made with lipiodol. J Urol 57:380–389, 1947.
20. Brodeur AE, Goyer RA, Melick W: A potential hazard of barium cystography. Radiology 85:1080–1084, 1965.
21. McAlister WH, Shackelford GD, Kissane J: The histologic effects of 30% Cystokon, Hypaque 25% and Renografin-30 in the bladder. Radiology 104:563–565, 1972.
22. Allen RP, Condon VR: Transitory extraperitoneal hernia of the bladder in infants (bladder ears). Radiology 77:979–983, 1961.
23. Shopfner CE, Hutch JA: The trigonal canal. Radiology 88:209–221, 1967.
24. Gray H: Anatomy of the Human Body. Goss CM(ed): Philadelphia, Lea & Febiger, 1956.
25. Kelalis PP, King LR: Clinical Pediatric Urology. Philadelphia, WB Saunders Company, 1976, p 292.
26. Shopfner CE: Radiology in pediatric gynecology. Radiol Clin North Am 5:151–167, 1967.
27. Hertz M: Cystourethrography: A Radiological Atlas. Amsterdam, Excerpta Medica, 1973.
28. Ben-Ami T, Boichis H, Hertz M: Fused labia: Clinical and radiological findings. Pediatr Radiol 7:33–35, 1978.
29. Lebowitz RL: Pseudostricture of the urethra: Urinal artifact on urethrography AJR 130:570–571, 1978.
30. Pearman RO, Muller JB: Choke voiding cystourethrography. Urology 90:481–488, 1963.
31. Nogrady MB, Dunbar JS: The value of excretory micturition cystourethrography (MCU) in the pediatric age group. Can Assoc Radiol 16:181–189, 1965.
32. Seidelman NE, Cohen WN, Bryan PJ, et al: Accuracy of CT staging of bladder neoplasms using the gas-filled method: Report of 21 patients with surgical confirmation. AJR 130:735–739, 1978.
33. Bartley D, Helander CG: Double-contrast cystography in tumors of the urinary bladder. Acta Radiol 54:161–169, 1960.
34. Bartley O, Eckerbom H: Perivesical insufflation of gas for determination of bladder wall thickness in tumors of the bladder. Acta Radiol 54:241–250, 1960.
35. Johannessen S: Pneumocystography. Dan Med Bull 12:193–196, 1965.
36. Pryles CV, Athius MD, Morse TS, Welch KJ: Comparative bacteriologic study of urine obtained from children by percutaneous suprapubic aspiration of the bladder. Pediatrics 24:983–991, 1959.
37. Omogbehin B, Willich E: Suprapubic micturition cystourethrography in infancy and childhood. Pediatr Radiol 3:20–23, 1975.
38. Thornbury JR, Wicks JD, Eckel CG: Imaging methods for evaluating the adult bladder and urethra: An overview. Semin Roentgenol 18:250–254, 1983.
39. Hu KN, Martz R, Vallandingham S: Use of the continuous flush maneuver to prevent air bubbles on the urethrogram in a male patient: Technical note. Urol Radiol 6:229, 1984.
40. Mukerjee MG, Deshon GEJr, Bruckman JA, et al: Urethrovascular reflux and its significance in urology. J Urol 112:608–609, 1974.
41. Knutsson F: On the technique of urethrography. Acta Radiol 10:437, 1929.
42. Brodny ML, Robins SA: Use of new viscous water-miscible contrast medium Rayopaque for cystourethrography. J Urol 58:182–184, 1947.
43. Henriet R: Pince "arbalete" pour urethrographie. J Urol Nephr 75:765–767, 1969.
44. Lapides J, Stone TE: Usefulness of retrograde urethrography in diagnosing strictures of the anterior urethra. J Urol 100:747–750, 1968.

45. Lucaya J: A simple technique of retrograde urethrography in male infants. Radiology 102:402, 1972.

46. Yokoyama M, Watanabe K, Iwata H, et al: Double-contrast urethrography for visualizing small lesions in distal urethra. Urology 19:440, 1982.

46a. Lang EK, Davis HJ: Positive pressure urethrography: A roentgenographic diagnostic method for urethral diverticula in the female. Radiology 72:401–405, 1959.

47. Andersen MJF: Instrument for injection urethrography in women. Acta Radiol 2:523–524, 1964.

48. Greenberg M, Stone D, Cochran ST, et al: Female urethral diverticula: double-balloon catheter study. AJR 136:259–264, 1981.

49. Kunin CM, Deutscher R, Paquin AJ: Urinary tract infection in school children: An epidemiologic, clinical and laboratory study. Medicine 43:91–130, 1964.

50. Smellie JM, Normand JCS: Urinary tract infection: Clinical aspects. In Williams DI, Johnston JH(eds): Pediatric Urology. Boston, Butterworth Scientific, 1982, pp 95–110.

51. Hertz M, Rozenman J: Cystourethrography: Technique, indications and normal findings. Appl Radiol 53:64, 1983.

52. Tanagho EA, Hutch JA: Primary reflux. J Urol 93:158–164, 1965.

53. Stephens FD, Lenaghan D: The anatomical basis and dynamics of vesicoureteral reflux. J Urol 87:669–680, 1962.

54. Lewy PR, Belman AB: Familial occurrence of non-obstructive, non-infectious vesicoureteral reflux with renal scarring. J Pediatr 86:851–856, 1975.

55. Sirota L, Hertz M, Laufer J, et al: Familial vesicoureteral reflux: A study of 16 families. Urol Radiol 8:22–24, 1986.

56. Conway JJ, Belman AB, King LR, et al: Direct and indirect radionuclide cystography. J Urol 113:689–693, 1975.

57. Edwards D, Normand JCS, Prescod NS, Smellie JM: Disappearance of vesicoureteric reflux during longterm prophylaxis of urinary tract infection in children. Br Med J 2:285–288, 1977.

58. Aladjem M, Boichis H, Hertz M, et al: The conservative management of vesicoureteric reflux: A review of 121 children. Pediatrics 65:78–80, 1980.

59. Friedland GW: Recurrent urinary tract infection in infants and children. Radiol Clin North Am 15:19–35, 1977.

60. Saxena SR, Laurence BM, Shaw DG: The justification for early radiological investigation of urinary tract infection in children. Lancet 2:403–404, 1975.

61. Willi UV, Lebowitz RL: The so-called megaureter, megacystis syndrome. AJR 133:409–416, 1979.

62. Kelalis PP, Malek RS, Segura JW: Observations on renal ectopia and fusion in children. J Urol 110:588–592, 1973.

63. Ambrose SS, Nicolson WP: Ureteral reflux in duplicated ureters. J Urol 92:439–444, 1964.

64. Caldamone AA: Duplication anomalies of the upper tract in infants and children. Urol Clin North Am 12:75–91, 1985.

65. Magnus RV: Vesicoureteral reflux in babies with myelomeningocele. J Urol 114:122–125, 1975.

66. Rickwood AM, Spitz L: Primary vesicoureteric reflux in neonates with imperforate anus. Arch Dis Child 55:149–150, 1980.

67. Parrot TS: Urologic implications of anorectal malformations. Urol Clin North Am 12:13–21, 1985.

68. Rozenman J, Hertz M, Boichis H: Radiological findings of the urinary tract in hypospadias: A report of 110 cases. Clin Radiol 30:471–476, 1979.

69. Shafir R, Hertz M, Borenstein R, Tzur H: Cystourethrography as an aid in the evaluation of hypospadias and its complications. J Plast Reconstr Surg 62:722–726, 1978.

70. Bonavita JA, Pollack HM: Trauma of the adult bladder and urethra. Semin Roentgenol 18:299–306, 1983.

71. Lieberman AH, Walden TB, Bogash M, et al: Negative cystography with bladder rupture: Presentation of two cases and review of the literature. J Urol 123:428–430, 1980.

72. McAlister WH, Cacciarelli A, Shackelford GD: Complications associated with cystography in children. Radiology 111:167–172, 1974.

73. Glynn B, Gordon IR: The risk of infection of the urinary tract as a result of micturition cystourethrography in children. Ann Radiol 13:283–287, 1970.

74. Markle BM, Catena L: Bladder pseudomass following cystography-related trauma. Radiology 159:265, 1986.

75. Gaisie G, Bender TM: Knotting of urethral catheter within bladder: An unusual complication of cystourethrography. Urol Radiol 5:271–272, 1983.

76. Fendel H: Radiation exposure due to urinary tract disease. In Kaufman HJ(ed): Progress in Pediatric Radiology, Vol 3. Chicago, Year Book Medical Publishers, 1970, pp 116–135.

77. Kaude JV, Reed JM: Voiding urethrocystography by means of 70 mm image intensifier fluorography. Radiology 92:768, 1969.

78. Hertz M, Werner A: Radiation dose to the gonads during cystourethrography. Isr J Med Sci, 13:614–616, 1977.

79. Friedland GW, Perkash J: Neuromuscular dysfunction of the bladder and urethra. Semin Roentgenol 18:255–266, 1983.

80. Lebowitz RL, Avni FE: Misleading appearances in pediatric uroradiology. Pediatr Radiol 10:15–31, 1980.

81. Hertz M, Rozenman J, Boichis H, Shafir R: Hypospadias before and after repair: A radiological evaluation. Ann Radiol (Paris) 24:147–150, 1981.

82. Aspin A: The gonadal x-ray dose to children from diagnostic radiographic technics. Radiology 85:944–951, 1965.

83. Gross KE, Sanderson SS: Cineurethrography and voiding cinecystography, with special attention to vesico-ureteral reflux. Radiology 77:573–586, 1961.

84. Wulff P: Verwendbarkeit der X Strahlen fur die diagnose der Blasendifformitaten. Fortschr Geb Rontgenstr Nuklearmed Erganzungsband 8:193, 1904–1905.

85. Coe FO, Arthur PS: A new medium for cystourethrography. AJR 56:361–365, 1964.

86. Kaufman JJ, Russell M: Cystourethrography: Clinical experience with the newer contrast media. AJR 75:884–892, 1956.

87. Richards CE: Visco-Rayopake in cystourethrography. J Urol 58:185–191, 1947.

88. Shopfner CE: Clinical evaluation of cystourethrographic media. Radiology 88:491–497, 1970.

89. Berger RM, Maizels M, Moran GC, et al: Bladder capacity (ounces) equals age (years) plus 2 predicts normal bladder capacity and aids in diagnosis of abnormal voiding patterns. J Urol 129:347–349, 1983.

90. Boltuch RL, Lalli AF: A new technique for urethrography. Radiology 115:736, 1975.

91. Elebute EA, Veiga-Peres JA: Urethrographic diagnosis of bladder neck contraction. AJR 95:442–446, 1965.

92. Hillman BJ, Silvert M, Cook G, et al: Recognition of bladder tumors by excretory urography. Radiology 138:319–323, 1981.

93. Koff SA: Estimating bladder capacity in children. Urology 21:248, 1983.

94. Steinhardt GF, Landes RR: Counteraction retrograde urethrography in women: An improved diagnostic technique. J Urol 128:936–937, 1982.

95. Wolin LH: Voiding patterns in young healthy women. J Urol 106:923–926, 1971.

96. Alton DJ: Pelviureteric obstruction in childhood. Radiol Clin North Am 15:61–70, 1977.

97. Burger RH: Familial and hereditary vesicoureteric reflux. JAMA 216:680–683, 1971.

98. Kontturi MJ, Koskela EA: Active surgical management of primary vesicoureteral reflux in adults. Scand J Urol Nephrol 11:239–244, 1977.

99. Levine JI, Crampton RS: Major abdominal injuries associated with pelvic fracture. Surg Gynecol Obstet 116:223–226, 1963.

100. Neves RJ, Torres VE, Malek RS, Svensson J: Vesicoureteral reflux in the adult. Medical versus surgical management. J Urol 132:882–885, 1984.

101. Screening for reflux (editorial). Lancet Jul 1:23–24, 1978.

102. Seidelman FE, Cohen WN, Bryan PJ: Computed tomography staging of bladder neoplasma. Radiol Clin North Am 15:419–440, 1977.

103. Brodny ML: New Instrument for Urethrography in Male. J Urol 46:350–354, 1941.

104. Williams DI, Johnston JH: Paediatric Urology, 2nd Ed. Boston, Butterworth Scientific, 1982.

105. Duckett JW, Bellinger MF: Cystographic grading of primary reflux as an indicator of treatment. In Johnston JH: Management of Vesicoureteral Reflux. Baltimore, Williams & Wilkins, 1984, p 99.

106. Saxton HM, Borzyskowski M, Munday AR, Vivian GC: Spinning-top urethra: Not a normal variant. Radiology 168:147, 1988.

107. Wood BP, Lane AT, Rabinowitz, R: Cutaneous reaction to contrast material. Radiology 169:739, 1988.

9

Radiology of Vesical and Supravesical Urinary Diversions

DAVID B. SPRING □ GEORGE E. DESHON, Jr.

Urinary diversions are surgical interventions created to redirect urine flow and to preserve renal function. Most diversions are placed to relieve urinary tract obstruction or incontinence secondary to congenital, traumatic, or neoplastic bladder dysfunctions. These diversions may be classified variously as intubated or nonintubated, percutaneously placed or surgically placed, single-staged or multistaged, and incontinent or continent. The many forms of urinary diversions reflect a diversity of patient needs, the imagination of the urological surgeon, and, ultimately, the limitations of each diversion.

The radiographic evaluation of the diverted urinary tract requires an understanding of the surgical procedure and altered function of the urinary tract. Although the excretory urogram remains the cornerstone of the evaluation of a patient, other imaging modalities may help in problem solving. A tailored study, directed to answering specific, clinically important questions, is the ideal examination. Such an examination may include plain film tomography, urography, retrograde or antegrade pyelography, sonography, radionuclide imaging, computed tomography (CT), or magnetic resonance imaging (MRI).

A classification of the sites of the diversion is provided in Table 9–1.

This classification scheme is necessarily incomplete. Urinary diversions have many major and minor variations that should be understood in order to interpret radiographs when studies are performed. Consultation between a urologist familiar with the variations used in a particular instance and the physician performing and interpreting an imaging study can help to clarify otherwise confusing findings.

RENAL DIVERSION

Nephrostomy

A large-bore drainage tube left in the renal pelvis and brought out through the renal parenchyma after open surgery can be a practical approach to an obstructed kidney. These open nephrostomies, still quickly and easily inserted after open renal surgery, are the precursors of the now common, percutaneously placed nephrostomies. Complications of nephrostomies include tube dislodgment, tube encrustation, and inconvenience to the patient of an externally draining tube.

Radiographic evaluation of a nephrostomy (the "nephrostogram") is relatively simple (Fig. 9–1). Plain films are obtained prior to examination so as not to overlook interval development of urolithiasis or other pathologic conditions. Fluoroscopy can aid in obtaining optimal radiographs and in delineating distal ureteral pathology, if present. After first withdrawing urine from the collecting system, low-pressure, passive filling of the collecting

system with the patient in the prone position is performed. This is done by instilling 15% to 30% contrast material by gravity drainage into a syringe attached to the drainage tube and held approximately 10 cm above the patient. The amount of contrast material used depends on the tube size, the degree of hydronephrosis of the pyelocalyceal system, and the length and/or continuity of the remaining ureter.

Pyelostomy

A nephrostomy is to be distinguished from a pyelostomy, in which the drainage tube exits directly from the renal pelvis to the exterior, bypassing the renal parenchyma. Pyelostomy is fraught with the danger of tube dislodgment and difficulty in changing the tube, as contrasted with nephrostomy. It is rarely performed.

URETERAL DIVERSIONS

Cutaneous Ureterostomy

End cutaneous ureterostomy is a method of urinary diversion sometimes used when an adequate length of

Table 9–1. Classification of Urinary Diversions

Renal Diversion
A. Nephrostomy
B. Pyelostomy

Ureteral Diversion
A. Directly to skin: cutaneous ureterostomy
B. To the contralateral ureter: transureteroureterostomy, with or without cutaneous ureterostomy
C. To bowel
  1. Intact anal sphincter: ureterosigmoidostomy (without or with sigmoid colostomy)
  2. To redirected bowel (with cutaneous stoma)
    a. Conduits: Ureteroileal cutaneous (ileal loop); sigmoid; other colon conduits (ileocecal, transverse colon)
    b. Continent urinary diversions (reservoirs): Kock pouch; Mainz pouch; LeBag (ileocolonic pouch); Indiana pouch
  3. To urethral sphincter through bowel segment (bladder replacement)
    a. Bladder replacement: ileocystoplasty (Camey procedure; hemi-Kock pouch; Melchior ileal pouch)
    b. Ileocecocystoplasty (modified leBag)

Bladder Diversion
A. Suprapubic cystostomy
B. Cutaneous vesicostomy
C. Continent vesicostomy
D. Abdominal neourethrostomy
E. Continent appendicovesicostomy (Mitrofanoff procedure)

Undiversions

Miscellaneous Other Diversions
A. Ureteral replacement
B. Continent perineal stoma

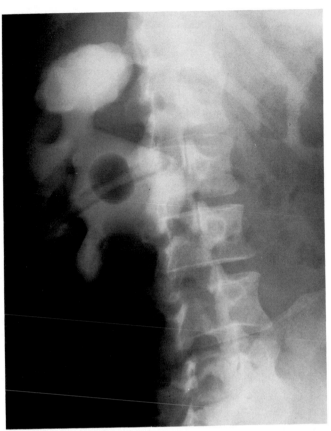

Figure 9–1. Permanent nephrostomy with indwelling Foley catheter. Hydronephrosis and ureteral injuries predated the nephrostomy by many years. Ureter is occluded and no contrast material flows beyond the renal pelvis.

dilated ureter is available to bring to the skin. Le Dentu first performed this procedure in 1899.[8] Subsequent experience has revealed that stricture formation frequently occurs in patients with preoperative irradiation, flush stomas, or a ureteral diameter of less than 8.0 mm.[18] Conversely, the rate of stricture formation has been noted to be least when a protruding nipple-like stoma was constructed and when the preoperative ureter exceeded 8.0 mm in diameter.

Loop cutaneous ureterostomy is frequently the diversion of choice when a chronically dilated and obstructed, redundant ureter is diagnosed. This type of ureterostomy allows the ureter to remain in continuity with the lower urinary tract while being brought to the skin. An advantage of this arrangement is that the upper tract can be evaluated in a retrograde manner while the lower tract is simultaneously evaluated in an antegrade fashion.

Excretory urography remains the first consideration in assessment of the urinary tract for cutaneous ureterostomies. Retrograde studies, using a 5- or 6-F whistle-tipped ureteral catheter, which usually passes readily, are easily performed when necessary. Sonography and radionuclide studies provide alternatives for assessing upper tract morphology.

Transureteroureterostomy

Transureteroureterostomy is a valuable reconstructive urological procedure that was first reported by Higgins in 1935.[16, 31] The technique is particularly suitable for anastomosis of the middle-third ureters (Fig. 9–2). Remarkable success with the procedure has been reported, with normal ureters remaining normal in most instances.[32, 74] There is reluctance, however, to perform the procedure in patients with large-field radiotherapy for bladder, bowel, or gynecological carcinomas, in patients with urolithiasis, and in patients with tuberculous infection or severe chronic pyelonephritis.[74] Transureteroureterostomy may be combined with cutaneous ureterostomy.[80] Because there is only a single stoma, long-term care is easier than in bilateral cutaneous ureterostomies.[76] The major drawback of transureteroureterostomy, of course, is that it places both ureters at risk to salvage one.

Excretory urography allows evaluation of the entire urinary tract. Oblique films may be particularly helpful because of the ureteral segment that passes anterior to the spine and great vessels. If precise visualization of any segment of the ureter (e.g., for delineation of a fistula) is required, retrograde or antegrade pyelography can provide the necessary detailed information.

Ureterosigmoidostomy

Anastomosis of the ureters to the intact sigmoid colon became the most common form of urinary drainage into bowel soon after it was first used by Simon in 1852 for a

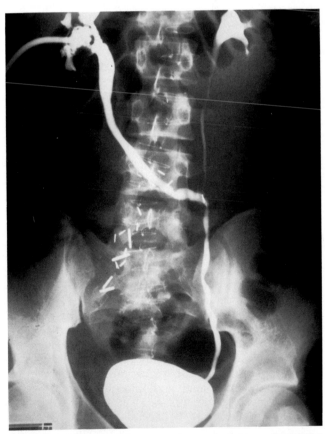

Figure 9–2. Right-to-left transureteroureterostomy (TUU). This 19-year-old male suffered a gunshot wound to the right iliac vessels. The ureter, also, was badly damaged, necessitating the right-to-left TUU. The end-to-side anastomosis lies near the lumbosacral junction and can often be seen most clearly with oblique projections.

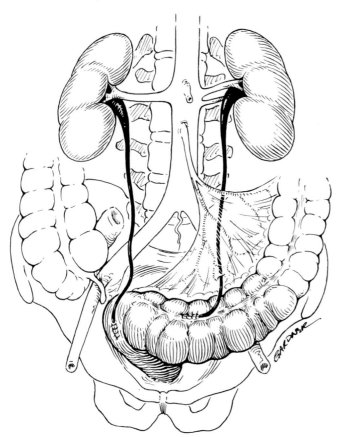

Figure 9–3. Ureterosigmoidostomy, diagram. Distal ureters enter the muscular wall of the sigmoid colon in tunnels at the taenia.

patient with bladder exstrophy.[60, 65] Ureterosigmoidostomy can be an ideal form of urinary diversion, if there is evidence of normal rectal continence, normal upper urinary tracts, and no previous history of bowel irradiation or significant bowel disease.

Free fecal reflux was possible in early ureterosigmoidostomies, but antirefluxing modifications in the ureteral anastomoses have helped to overcome this (Fig. 9–3).[24, 56] The reported incidence of pyelonephritis, formerly a common complication of ureterosigmoidostomy, has since dropped dramatically from 69.9% to 11.8%.[9, 27]

A serious long-term complication of ureterosigmoidostomy is the development of colonic carcinomas at the site of the ureterosigmoid anastomosis.[62, 70, 79] The risk of developing colonic carcinoma has been estimated at from 5% to 11% when patients are followed for 15 years or more.[70, 79] The latency period for the development of these colonic neoplasms is 15 to 25 years in patients with underlying benign disease (e.g., bladder exstrophy) and 7 to 10 years for patients with underlying malignancies.

Although excretory urography adequately evaluates the upper urinary tract, such studies rarely outline satisfactorily the ureterosigmoid anastomoses, although sporadic filling of the distal ureters may suggest the sites of the anastomoses (Fig. 9–4).

Because of the high incidence of colonic carcinomas, the colon should be carefully scrutinized for abnormal masses in any patient with a ureterosigmoidostomy present for several years (Fig. 9–5). Flexible sigmoidoscopy should be performed at regular intervals; however, barium enemas should be avoided, if at all possible, in the

presence of refluxing anastomoses. Even if the ureterosigmoidostomy is converted to a cutaneous form of diversion, colonic carcinoma may still develop at the site of the prior anastomosis.[63] Screening for benign and malignant colonic masses must continue throughout the patient's lifetime.

Ureterosigmoidostomies were once abandoned as a common form of diversion because of a high incidence of pyelonephritis and upper tract deterioration. With the introduction of antirefluxing ureterocolonic anastomoses, the incidence of pyelonephritis dropped substantially. Despite this reduction in clinical pyelonephritis, another serious long-term complication, the development of colonic carcinoma, has dampened enthusiasm for this procedure once again.

Ureteroileal Cutaneous Conduit (Cutaneous Ureteroileostomy, Ileal Conduit, Ileal Loop)

An extremely important form of permanent supravesical urinary diversion is the ureteroileal anastomosis and cutaneous ileostomy (ileal conduit, ileal loop) introduced by Bricker in 1950.[7] Its popularity stems from its acceptance by both patients and surgeons as a compromise between its success as a diversion and the inherent incon-

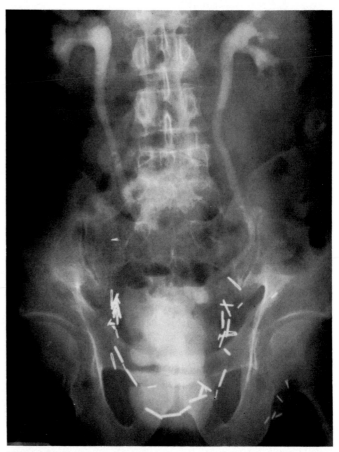

Figure 9–4. Ureterosigmoidostomy. Distal ureters at ureterosigmoid anastomoses are poorly seen in the absence of obstruction. Contrast material may occasionally be seen passing retrograde throughout much of colon. Here, only the rectosigmoid has intraluminal contrast material that is easily seen.

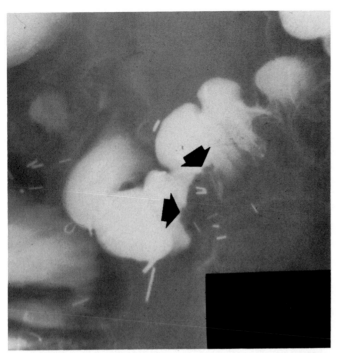

Figure 9–5. Ureterosigmoidostomy. Barium enema examination demonstrates mass *(arrows)* in wall of sigmoid colon near site of ureterosigmoid anastomosis in a patient with history of bladder carcinoma and past radical cystectomy. Biopsy and local resection confirmed a hemorrhagic benign neoplasm, rather than the more common colon carcinoma. (Courtesy R. Thoeni, M.D.)

veniences of stomas and drainage devices. Despite a significant rate of long-term complications, it remains the standard by which other forms of supravesical urinary diversions are compared.

Surgical Technique

The ileal loop is formed from a surgically isolated 15 to 25 cm segment of distal small bowel.[59] The butt, or proximal end, is closed and anchored to the sacral promontory near the aortic bifurcation (Fig. 9–6). The ileal loop passes medial to the cecum and caudad to the small bowel mesentery (Fig. 9–7). The distal end of the loop is brought to the right abdominal wall and placed at a convenient site near the lateral border of the rectus abdominus muscle.

Radiographic Evaluation[2, 34, 40, 41, 55]

Excretory urography is the standard technique used to evaluate patients with ileal loops. Routine postoperative studies should be obtained 3 months after surgery.[2] Because obstruction and other complications may be silent, limited follow-up studies should then be obtained at yearly intervals. This usually consists of excretory urography (Figs. 9–7A and 9–8A). Sonography and radionuclide studies may be substituted.[10]

When performing excretory urography in these patients, several technical aspects are important. First, gas in the upper urinary tract is often seen because of free reflux from the ileal loop.[61] Second, plain film tomography may be necessary to exclude the presence of renal calculi.

Third, oblique and prone positioning may be necessary to adequately visualize the ureters and loop.[17, 25, 69]

Should further evaluation of the loop itself be necessary, an ileostoureterogram ("ileal loopogram") should be performed (Figs. 9–7B, 9–8B, and 9–9). This procedure may be carried out with fluoroscopic monitoring, and sufficient spot films obtained in oblique projections to visualize the entire loop. A Foley catheter with a 5-ml balloon is passed retrograde through the stoma and then carefully inflated. Gentle tension on the catheter occludes the stoma. Gravity filling of the loop with 15% to 30% contrast material will identify ureteral reflux during ileal loopography. If one or both ureters fail to fill, but there has been good filling of the loop, one must explain whether the absence of reflux is due to a technically inadequate study or to pathological obstruction (Fig. 9–9). There may be delayed filling of the left ureter, owing to its course over the vessels at the sacral promontory. At the conclusion of the procedure, drainage films should be obtained to evaluate the adequacy of emptying of the kidneys and ureters, as well as the loop itself.

A loopogram is not always an innocuous procedure. Serious bacteremia or autonomic dysreflexia may occur. Since the loopogram often entails some increased pressure, Stamey recommends that it be preceded by a single IM or IV dose of an aminoglycoside.[72] Barbaric has cautioned that the loop must not be overdistended during loopography in patients with spinal cord injuries at or above T7 because of autonomic dysreflexia with resultant rapid development of severe hypertension.[3] Reported complications have included convulsions, cerebral hemorrhage, retinal hemorrhage, renal failure, and death.

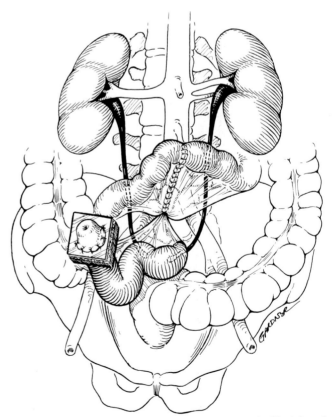

Figure 9–6. Ureteroileal cutaneous anastomosis (ileal loop), diagram. Butt end of ileal loop is anchored near aortic bifurcation. Reanastomosed ileum passes craniad to loop, which lies medial to the cecum. A nipple stoma is at the skin.

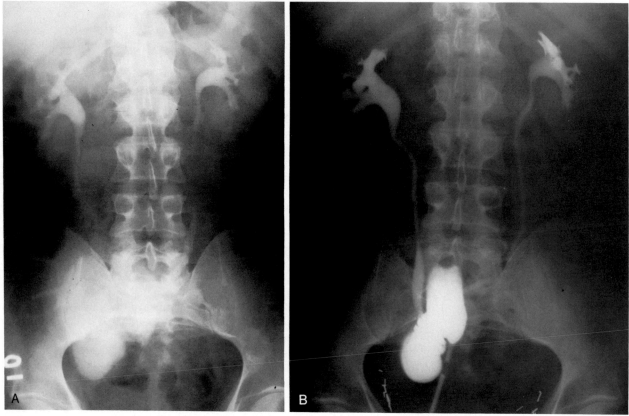

Figure 9–7. Ureteroileal cutaneous anastomosis (ileal loop). *A,* Excretory urogram shows normal upper tracts, but loop, overlying sacrum, is difficult to see clearly. Oblique films are particularly helpful. *B,* Retrograde "loopogram" shows distal ureteroileal anastomoses at their points of entry into ileal loop. One normally expects to identify bilateral reflux of contrast-laden urine in ureters and renal pelves. Note atypical near-midline location of stoma.

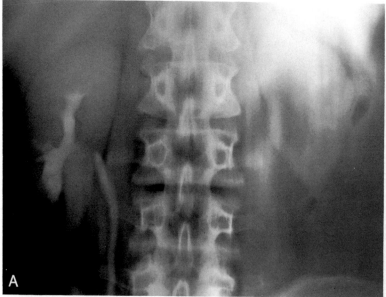

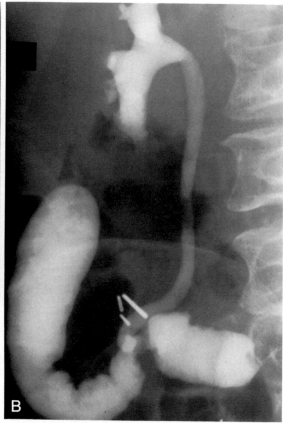

Figure 9–8. Ureteroileal cutaneous anastomosis (ileal loop). *A,* Tomogram from excretory urogram shows left hydronephrosis as a central defect with a markedly delayed nephrogram in a shrunken kidney. *B,* Loopogram demonstrates nonfilling of left ureter secondary to a benign ureteroileal anastomotic stricture. Right side is normal.

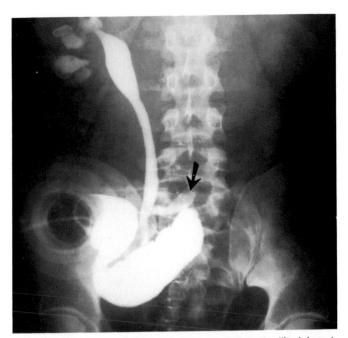

Figure 9–9. Ureteroileal cutaneous anastomosis (ileal loop). Loopogram shows filling of right ureter and renal pelvis (which contains numerous calculi obscured by contrast material). Left ureter fills only in its most distal portion, where a faint, obstructing calculus (*arrow*) overlies lower lumbar spine. (Courtesy A. J. Palubinskas, M.D.)

Kilcheski and Pollack have employed gas for loopography in patients with documented severe sensitivity to iodinated contrast.[36]

Additional imaging techniques are frequently necessary to evaluate specific aspects of renal physiology and anatomy. Radionuclide imaging of the ileal loop diversion can quantify upper tract function and provide considerable morphological detail. Radioisotope loopography has been advocated as being more physiological than iodinated radiographic contrast material instilled in the routine ileal loopogram.[77] Sonography is an excellent technique to evaluate upper tract morphology and to examine for the presence of hydronephrosis; however, it cannot satisfactorily evaluate the lower ureters, the ileal loop, or adjoining abdominal structures. Recognition of apparent hydronephrosis must be carefully correlated with other studies, inasmuch as dilatation preceding urinary diversion may persist and reflux from the ileal loop may simulate fullness of the upper tract. CT in specific circumstances may prove valuable in the assessment of ileal loop diversions. It is important to recognize the normal transaxial relationship of the loop to the sacral promontory, the aortic bifurcation, the cecum, and the anterior abdominal wall (Fig. 9–10). In rare instances, retrograde installation of 2% radiographic contrast material into the loop ("CT loopography") for better CT evaluation proves helpful.[71]

Complications

As previously noted, routine follow-up studies are usually not obtained until 3 months postoperatively in order to allow resolution of the mild ureteroileal obstruction seen during the initial postoperative period. It is, however, extremely important for the radiologist to be familiar with an array of complications in order that appropriate studies can be obtained.

Early complications of ileal loop diversions may be related to the primary surgical site (the cystectomy bed), the ureters, the ureteroileal anastomoses, or the ileal conduit itself. When infection or hemorrhage in the bladder bed is clinically suspected, CT may be particularly valuable in the identification of postoperative pelvic collections.[46] Needle aspiration and drainage with CT guidance can be therapeutic.[71]

Mild obstruction at the ureteroileal anastomoses is common in the immediate postoperative period. This may persist for up to 3 months. If there is clinical suspicion of ureteroileal obstruction, careful monitoring for progression of hydronephrosis with sonography or radionuclide studies is warranted.

Loop ischemia occasionally develops in the early or late postoperative period. This may be caused by excess tension on, or a hematoma in, the loop mesentery, by vascular injury, or by venous insufficiency.[2, 51]

Urinary leakage at the ureteroileal anastomosis is a dreaded complication with a mortality rate, in the past approaching 50%[30] (Fig. 9–11). Hensle and colleagues[30] identified two distinct groups of patients with ureteroileal anastomotic leaks: those with an early postoperative leak in the first 24 hours, and those with a second type of leak 6 to 12 days postoperatively. They noted that a persistent postoperative rise of the serum blood urea concentration without a concomitant rise in serum creatinine level is a specific indicator of urinary extravasation warranting further clinical investigation. An elevated serum ammonia without clinical hepatic failure also warrants investigation of a possible anastomotic leak. The authors noted that the second group in whom the diagnosis of a loop leak was delayed had a poorer prognosis.

Although excretory urography is usually diagnostic of a ureteroileal leak when extravasation of contrast material is noted in the area of the anastomosis, retrograde loopography helps to confirm and localize the leak. CT loopography is occasionally helpful.[71] After initial evaluation without any contrast material, dilute (1% to 2%) contrast material is used to fill the loop through a Foley catheter. Scanning is then repeated in the region of the loop.

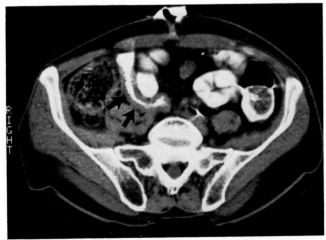

Figure 9–10. Ureteroileal cutaneous anastomosis (ileal loop). CT scan shows ileal loop (*arrows*) passing medial to cecum.

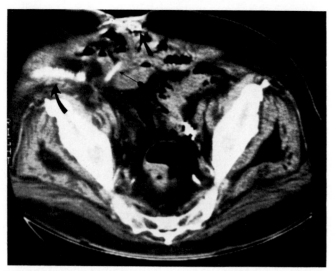

Figure 9–11. Ureteroileal cutaneous anastomosis (ileal loop). CT scan shows extravasation of radiographic contrast material (*arrow*) from loop (*curved arrow*) into abdominal incision (*large arrow*) during early postoperative period.

Percutaneous techniques have aided in pinpointing the source of ureteroileal anastomotic leaks and obstructions.[6, 19]

Late complications of ileal loop surgery include ureteroileal anastomotic strictures, urolithiasis, pyelonephritis, midloop stenosis, and stomal stenosis—all of which can result in significant renal deterioration (Fig. 9–12). Because of these complications, the incidence of which, Dunn noted,[15] increases with time, careful continued radiographic follow-up is imperative. Excretory urography is the study of choice, since renal calculi, chronic pyelonephritis (reflux nephropathy), and obstruction are all readily diagnosed by this modality.

In adults with diversions performed for pelvic malignancies, recurrent neoplastic disease often intervenes before long-term complications can develop.

Sigmoid Conduit [35, 60, 66]

Because many of the long-term complications of ileal loops are secondary to reflux, nonrefluxing colon conduits were introduced by Mogg in 1967.[53] Advantages of ureterosigmoid cutaneous diversions include ureteral tunneling in the colonic taenia, which prevents ureteral reflux, and a large stoma, which decreases the likelihood of stomal stenosis.[67]

Surgical Technique

A loop of sigmoid colon is isolated on its vascular pedicle and is brought either anteriorly or posteriorly to the descending colon (Figs. 9–13 and 9–14).

Radiographic Evaluation [78]

Preoperatively, the urinary tract should be evaluated with excretory urography or sonography, and the bowel should be studied with a barium enema or endoscopy. Diverticulosis or colonic neoplasms usually preclude the use of involved segments of bowel as conduits.

Postoperative assessment is similar to assessment of ureteroileal cutaneous diversion, with routine follow-up being delayed until 3 months to allow resolution of mild perioperative obstructive changes. Early complications, which are similar to those seen with ileal loops, are studied in a similar manner. One of the most common late complications is stenosis and obstruction at the ureterosigmoid anastomosis. This is best evaluated by excretory urography or percutaneous puncture and antegrade pyeloureterography. Retrograde studies of the loop do not aid in the diagnosis of upper tract pathology because of the absence of reflux; however, they may be useful in the evaluation of the loop itself.

Other Colon Conduits

When the sigmoid colon is not available for conduit construction, other segments of colon may be used in a similar fashion. Hradec reviewed the use of various bowel segments for bladder replacement and concluded that ileocolic or sigmoid segments were superior to small bowel segments.[33]

Beckley and colleagues described using a transverse colon loop for patients in whom pelvic irradiation complicates attempts to perform other types of diversion.[5] Preoperative and postoperative radiographic evaluation of these patients is the same as for patients with sigmoid loops.

Continent Urinary Diversions

Urinary continence is an important goal for urinary diversions since continent diversions are much more socially and psychologically agreeable to the patient than ordinary conduits.[26] Goldwasser and Lieskovsky have reviewed many of these surgical approaches.[21] Hinman has elegantly outlined the physical and physiological characteristics that are important considerations in the selection of intestinal segments for bladder substitution.[88] Each of these variations has its advantages and proponents. The importance of some of the procedures remains to be proven with long-term patient follow-up.

Kock Continent Ileal Reservoir

Kock initially developed the intra-abdominal reservoir or continent ileostomy for patients undergoing proctocolectomy for ulcerative colitis.[37, 38] Modifications have resulted in applications to the urinary tract.[21, 57, 67, 68] Initial patient acceptance appears high, although the frequency of complications may reduce the long-term acceptance of this surgical technique. Skinner and associates reported 250 patients undergoing a modified Kock continent ileal reservoir, most often for pelvic malignancy.[81] The Skinner modification of the Kock pouch utilizes Marlex mesh and staples to stabilize the intussuscepted nipple valves, which are the key to preventing reflux and insuring continence (Fig. 9–15). The resultant continent ileal reservoir is, with time, more capacious than the ileal loop and requires catheterization approximately every 4 to 8 hours.[39]

Ralls and colleagues have described well the surgical techniques and radiographic evaluation of the Kock pouch.[57] At the time of surgical formation of the Kock

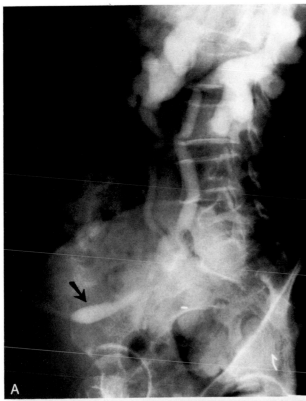

Figure 9–12. Ureteroileal cutaneous anastomosis. *A*, Right posterior oblique projection from an excretory urogram shows dilated upper tracts with a poorly distensible ileal loop (*arrow*). Loop stenosis was confirmed by loopography. *B*, CT loopogram shows position of Foley catheter (*arrow*) in ileal loop medial to ascending colon. *C*, CT section slightly more craniad shows butt end of contrast-filled ileal loop (*arrow*) and distal ureters near anastomoses. Incidentally identified parastomal hernia is present at right anterior abdominal wall.

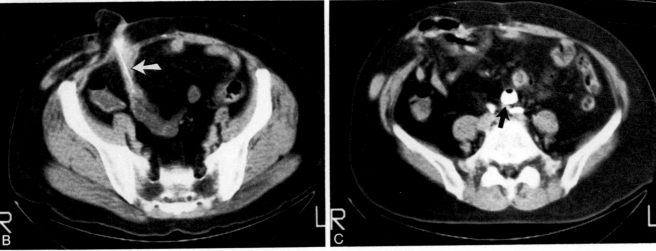

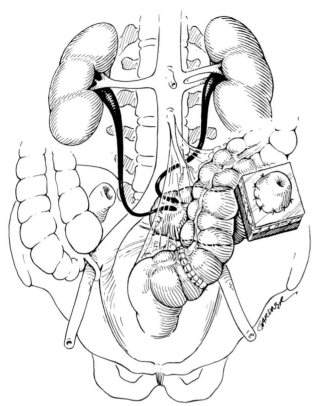

Figure 9–13. Sigmoid loop, diagram. Retrocolic placement of sigmoid loop with butt end anchored near sacral promontory and anterior end, near lateral wall of left rectus abdominus muscle.

pouch, No. 8 polyethylene feeding-tube stents are placed from the Kock reservoir through the afferent nipple valve and ureteroileal anastomoses into the renal pelves. A No. 30 Medina tube is placed through the efferent nipple into the reservoir. Kock pouch cystography is performed 3 weeks after surgery. Cystography precedes intravenous urography in order to exclude reservoir-ureteral reflux (Fig. 9–16A). Rall's technique uses gravity infusion of water-soluble contrast medium through the Medina tube from 36 inches above the patient. This is stopped when the patient experiences fullness, usually after infusion of 100 to 300 ml of contrast medium. Standard intravenous urography follows to assess the upper tracts. If no complications are identified, the Medina tube is withdrawn and afferent limb stents are removed endoscopically.

The "mature" pouch has a greater reservoir capacity (up to 1000 ml) and studies after 6 months routinely use 500 ml to distend the pouch and search for leaks or reflux (Figs. 9–16B and 9–17). Gravity filling of the pouch through a soft rubber catheter on these follow-up studies is followed by anteroposterior and oblique films with distention and then postdrainage films. The examination is tailored appropriately with additional films and fluoroscopy if suspicious findings are identified. Routine urography follows for assessment of the kidneys and ureters. Calculus formation within the pouch appears to be more frequent with this procedure than with other forms of diversion. Ralls and associates have reported that formation of calculi within the pouch has been associated with exposed staples.[57] Where staples are not used or are buried submucosally, calculus formation is much less

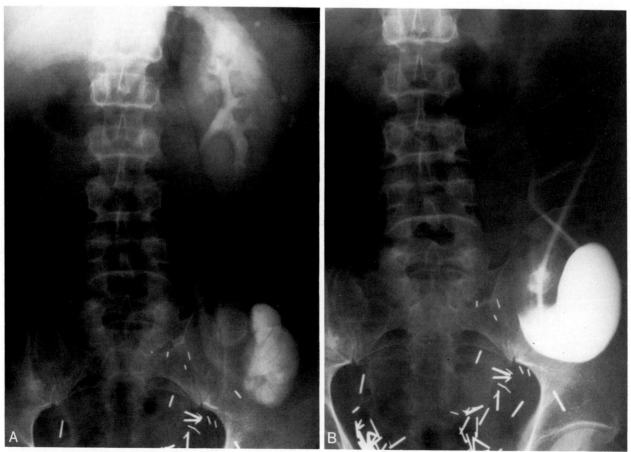

Figure 9–14. Sigmoid loop. A, Excretory urogram shows normal left upper tract. Right kidney and ureter have been removed. B, Sigmoid loopogram shows absence of reflux, but satisfactory loop detail.

likely. Evaluation of the Kock pouch by CT has been described by Mirvis and associates.[89]

Ghoneim and colleagues have reported a further modification of the Kock pouch to allow it to be anastomosed directly to the urethra ("hemi-Kock"), eliminating the need for an efferent value.[84] Similar direct anastomoses of other types of reservoirs have also been proposed.

Mainz Pouch

Thuroff and colleagues recently reviewed their experience with mixed-augmentation ileum and cecum (Mainz pouch) for continent diversion.[73] The Mainz pouch utilizes the cecum and two ileal loops (Fig. 9–18), resulting in substantial reservoir capacity. Important functional features besides the large-capacity low-pressure reservoir include antirefluxing submucosal tunneling of the ureteral segments and continence, both of which are achieved with an isoperistaltic ileoileal anastomotic segment at the skin stoma or with the intact urinary sphincter when anastomosed to the bladder remnant.

Indiana Pouch

Rowland and associates at the University of Indiana have reviewed their early experience with 29 cecal pouches, utilizing the terminal ileum as a continence mechanism.[82] The diverted ureters are tunneled posterior to the cecum in the taenia to prevent pouch-ureteral reflux. The ascending colon may be capped with a short segment of additional distal ileum (eliminating high-frequency colonic contractions); alternatively, the ascending

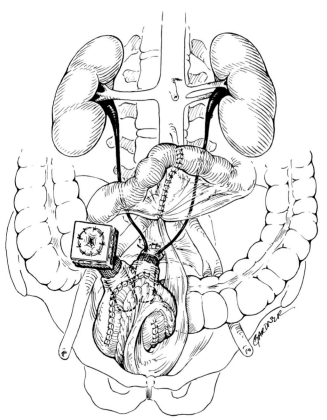

Figure 9–15. Kock pouch, diagram. Intussuscepted limbs of Kock pouch allow urine to collect without developing ureteral obstruction, reflux, or incontinence. Stoma must be catheterized every 4 to 8 hours to empty collected urine.

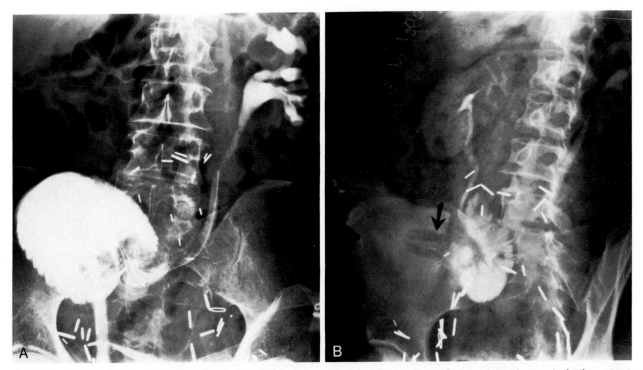

Figure 9–16. Kock pouch. *A*, Ureteral reflux from an "immature" pouch, common in early postoperative period when stents are still in place. *B*, Excretory urogram in a "mature" pouch shows kidneys and ureters entering the afferent, intussuscepted limb of the pouch (*arrow*). Stoma opens onto anterior abdominal wall near site of surgical clips (*curved arrow*). (Courtesy Phillip W. Ralls, M.D.)

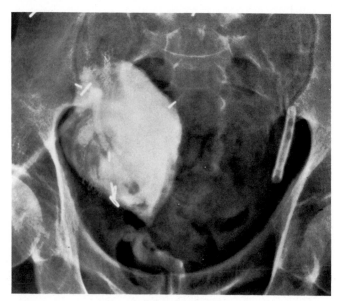

Figure 9–17. Kock pouch. Extravasation from base of pouch to vagina. Fistula formation to gastrointestinal tract or skin may also develop in any of the urinary diversions. (Courtesy Phillip W. Ralls, M.D.)

colon may be folded down upon itself (Heineke-Mikulicz reconstruction).

A pouchogram and an excretory urogram are performed 3 weeks postoperatively to evaluate for leakage, reflux, and upper tract obstruction. Follow-up studies include period pouchograms and excretory urograms.

Mean pouch capacity has been reported to be approximately 0.5 L, which is comparable to intact bladder capacities. Antegrade urography, ultrasonography, and pouch studies all provide useful morphological information about these diversions. Bladder capacity is readily assessed on a daily basis when the pouch is self-catheterized (Fig. 9–19).

LeBag (Ileocolonic Pouch)

Light and Engelmann recently reported a variation of the ileocolonic pouch, which is anastomosed to the urethral remnant to create a continent neobladder.[48] This diversion is similar to the Mainz pouch in that the ureters are implanted into sigmoid taenia in a nonrefluxing manner and the ileocolonic pouch is fashioned to create a large-capacity, highly compliant reservoir with low filling pressure. The pouch is anastomosed to the urethral remnant and relies on the membranous urethra for continence. If the continent mechanism is insufficient, an artificial sphincter can be utilized to ensure continence.

Radiographic evaluation of continent diversions differs from that of loop diversions in that retrograde studies of the pouch or neobladder are obtained at 3 weeks to ensure that adequate healing has occurred. Subsequent follow-up studies, including excretory urography and sonography are employed to evaluate the upper urinary tract. Retrograde studies of the neobladder are used to ensure the competence of the intussuscepted ileal segments in the Kock and Mainz pouches and the integrity of the ureteral anastomoses in all three diversions.

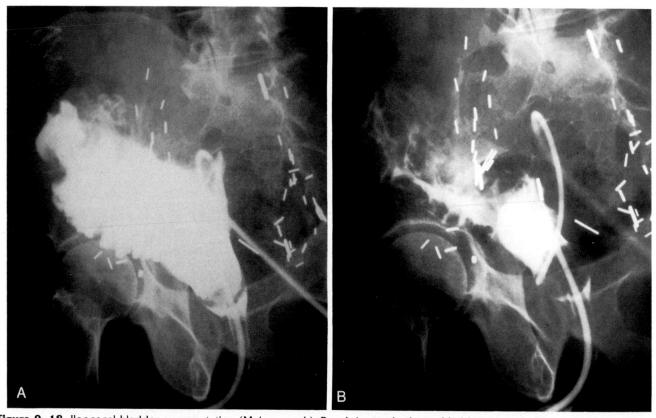

Figure 9–18. Ileocecal bladder augmentation (Mainz pouch). Pouch is attached to a bladder remnant. Alternatively, pouch may be brought to an abdominal wall stoma. *A,* Six-week pouch study through a suprapubic catheter shows adequate distention and no leakage. *B,* Post-drainage film confirms pouch is intact and functioning adequately. (Courtesy Perinchery Narayan, M.D.)

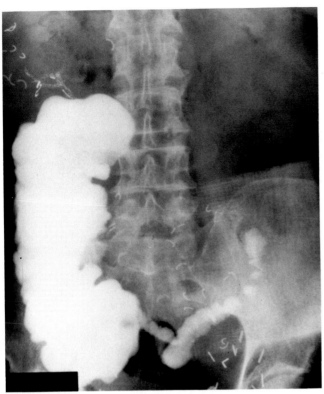

Figure 9–19. Indiana pouch. Pouch opacified through cecostomy (not shown). Note absence of ureteral reflux. (Courtesy Eli Glatstein, M.D.)

Ileocystoplasty (Camey Procedure)

Camey recently reviewed 25 years of experience with his procedure of ileocystoplasty in males who had undergone cystoprostatectomy for bladder carcinoma.[49] A diurnally continent bladder substitute is created from a 40-cm loop of distal small bowel. Antirefluxing ureteroileal anastomoses are created surgically at the lateral limbs of the loop of bowel. The midpoint of the antimesenteric border of the loop is anastomosed to the urethral stump. Incontinence, especially nocturnal incontinence, is a common problem, inasmuch as the storage of urine is dependent entirely on an intact external sphincter.

Melchior Ileal Bladder

Melchior and associates recently reported a new variation that appears to have the advantages of a Camey procedure (i.e., relative ease of construction) and the continence of more complicated pouches.[85] A 40-cm segment of ileum is partially opened along the antimesenteric border, then closed to form a larger-capacity reservoir. Both ureters are implanted into an intussuscepted end of the ileum to prevent reflux. Radiographic evaluation is similar to the Camey procedure.

BLADDER DIVERSIONS

Suprapubic Cystostomy

The surgically or percutaneously placed suprapubic tube remains one of the most common types of temporary diversion for patients who have sustained lower urinary tract trauma or undergone lower urinary tract surgery. It is less commonly used for permanent diversion, since long-term suprapubic drainage may be associated with chronic infection, stone formation, and reflux.

Radiographic evaluation of suprapubic cystostomy consists of low-pressure filling of the bladder through the cystostomy tube. The use of fluoroscopic monitoring, whenever possible, is recommended. Filling may be accomplished by gravity or careful hand injection. The sensation of bladder fullness is taken as the usual end point. Distention and drainage films are obtained, with oblique views taken during filling.

Cutaneous Vesicostomy

Cutaneous vesicostomy has been a popular form of temporary diversion, especially for selected infants and children, because it is simple, tubeless, and easily reversible.[44, 45, 54] It is not acceptable for long-term, upper tract drainage but is an excellent temporary form of diversion in newborns. The location allows drainage into a diaper and the long-term complications associated with other types of permanent drainage have not been found.[4] Urographically, the urinary bladder may be obscured by the overlying collection bag and incomplete bladder filling. Urographic evaluation of the urinary tract may thus be limited to kidneys and ureters. Renal function may best be assessed simply with serum creatinine.[75] Sonography is a simple way to assess upper tract deterioration by detecting hydronephrosis or progression of focal renal scarring. Deterioration may be an indication for higher diversion.

Continent Vesicostomy

Schneider and colleagues describe the use of a valvelike intussusception from an anterior bladder flap, which then communicates with a stoma on the anterior abdominal wall.[64] The technique requires a bladder capacity of at least 200 ml. They used this form of bladder diversion primarily in adult patients with neurogenic bladders. As with the pouch type of continent diversions, with continent vesicostomy the bladder is emptied by means of self-catheterization.

Abdominal Neourethrostomy. A variant of the continent vesicostomy is a continent bladder tube, or abdominal neourethrostomy.[42, 43] This utilizes a bladder flap and skin segment. Small bladders may be augmented with portions of the sigmoid colon. Unlike the cutaneous vesicostomy, which is designed for constant urinary drainage, the neourethrostomy with its umbilicus-like stoma requires intermittent catheterization and is well tolerated by growing children and adults.[43]

Continent Appendicovesicostomy

Another form of continent vesicostomy is the continent appendicovesicostomy. Mitrofanoff in 1980 proposed the use of the isolated appendix as a urinary conduit from the augmented bladder to the skin in children (Fig. 9–20).[14, 52] Similarly, Mitrofanoff has described using a segment of ureter as a conduit from the bladder to the skin. In both cases, children with urethral incontinence

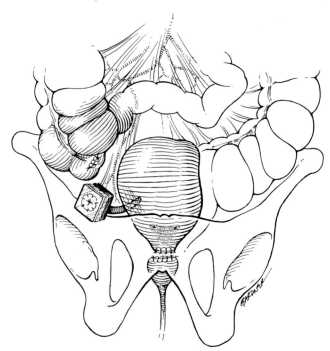

Figure 9–20. Continent appendicovesicostomy (Mitrofanoff procedure), diagram. Incontinent vesicourethral outlet has been surgically closed. Transplanted vermiform appendix acts as a continent urinary conduit.

who cannot undergo urethral reconstruction are candidates for this procedure. Early results are encouraging.

Radiographic evaluation of the appendicovesicostomy is performed with excretory urography. Because the bladder is continent, it fills and may be well seen. A retrograde examination with dilute radiographic contrast material performed through the stoma and appendiceal or ureteral conduit can be performed in the same manner as one would otherwise catheterize the urinary bladder.

UNDIVERSIONS

A urinary diversion may at a later date be surgically altered if patient condition or surgical therapies change.[29] Hendren has used the term *undiversion* to describe returning the surgically diverted urinary tract to a more normally functioning system, incorporating the urinary bladder. Gonzales and colleagues[23] recently reported excellent results with undiversion in children and young adults with neurogenic bladder dysfunction in both those with severe renal failure from such processes as posterior urethral valves, and those with normal renal function in processes such as vesicoureteral reflux. Many years of bladder disuse does not necessarily preclude a successful refunctionalization of that organ. As part of the evaluation of bladder function, cystography to evaluate for the presence of bladder diverticula, urethral valves, and reflux into ureteral stumps must be undertaken. The investigation of these undiversions, once surgically performed, must be directed to specific problems with an awareness of the altered course of the urinary tract. The radiology of urinary undiversions in children is considered more fully in Chapter 99.

MISCELLANEOUS DIVERSIONS

Ureteral Replacement[12, 13]

In the presence of irreparable damage to one or both ureters when the bladder and kidneys are otherwise normal, an isolated segment of ileum may be interposed between kidney and bladder. DeWeerd has described the use of bilateral loops of ileum attached as a roux-en-Y conduit.[12, 13]

Excretory urography, sonography, and radionuclide studies all may prove useful in following patients with ileal substitution; in general, however, the most informative study is cystography, since there is almost always free reflux to the kidney. Ileal mucus production may cause nonopaque bladder masses; bladder stone formation may result in the presence of chronic infection.

Continent Perineal Stoma

Perineal stomas utilize the intact anal sphincter, through which two separate ostia are brought in order to maintain continence and yet to separate the fecal and urinary streams. The radiologist must be aware of the specific type of surgery performed to understand the relationships among the ureters, rectal bladder, and repositioned rectum. Goldwasser and Webster[21] reviewed methods that divert the urinary stream through the anal sphincter utilizing a rectal bladder; Gersuny[20] mobilized the descending colon and brought it down between the internal and external anal sphincter, implanting it anterior to the rectum as a perineal sigmoidostomy; Heitz-Boyer and Hovelaque[28] brought the sigmoid colon behind the rectum to open within the anal sphincter; Ashken and colleagues[1] brought an ileocecal segment anterior to the rectum to utilize the anal sphincter. In all of these cases, the rectal bladder can be studied by inserting a Foley catheter through the anus and gently filling the rectal pouch with contrast material. As with most urinary diversions, the most informative results are obtained when the procedure is performed under fluoroscopic control. The upper urinary tracts can be evaluated using standard techniques.

References

1. Ashken MH: Urinary reservoirs. *In* Ashken MH (ed): Urinary Diversion. New York, Springer-Verlag, 1982, p 112.
2. Banner MP, Pollack HM, Bonavita JA, Ellis PS: The radiology of urinary diversions. RadioGraphics 4:885–913, 1984.
3. Barbaric ZL: Autonomic dysreflexia in patients with spinal cord lesions: Complication of voiding cystourethrography and ileal loopography. AJR 127:293–295, 1976.
4. Bauer SB: Editorial. Management of neurogenic bladder dysfunction in children. J Urol 132:544–545, 1984.
5. Beckley S, Wajsman Z, Pontes JE, Murphy G: Transverse colon conduit; a method of urinary diversion after pelvic irradiation. J Urol 128:464–468, 1982.
6. Bettmann MA, Murray PD, Perlmutt LM, et al: Ureteroileal anastomotic leaks: Percutaneous treatment. Radiology 148:95–100, 1983.
7. Bricker EM: Bladder substitution after pelvic evisceration. Surg Clin North Am 30:1511–1521, 1950.

8. Claman M, Shapiro AE, Orecklin JR: Cutaneous ureterostomy, the preferred diversion of the solitary functioning kidney. Br J Urol 51:352–356, 1979.

9. Clarke BG, Leadbetter WF: Ureterosigmoidostomy: Collective results in 2897 reported cases. J Urol 73:999–1008, 1955.

10. Cronan JJ, Amis ES, Scola FH, Schepps B: Renal obstruction in patients with ileal loops: US evaluation. Radiology 158:647, 1986.

11. Ehrlich RM, Skinner DG: Complications of transureteroureterostomy. J Urol 113:467–473, 1975.

12. DeWeerd JH: Urologic dilemmas resolved by the ileal conduit. JAMA 178:983–988, 1961.

13. DeWeerd JH: Urinary diversion. In Witten DM, Myers GH, Utz DC (eds): Clinical Urography, Vol 3, 4th Ed. Philadelphia, WB Saunders Company, 1977, p 2120.

14. Duckett JW, Snyder HM: Continent urinary diversion: Variations on the Mitrofanoff principle. J Urol 136:58–62, 1986.

15. Dunn M, Roberts JBM, Slade N: The longterm results of ileal conduit urinary diversion in children. Br J Urol 51:458–461, 1979.

16. Ehrlich RM, Skinner DG: Complications of transureteroureterostomy. J Urol 113:467–473, 1975.

17. Elkin M: The prone position in intravenous urography for study of the upper urinary tract. AJR 76:961–967, 1961.

18. Feminella JG Jr, Lattimer JK: A retrospective analysis of 70 cases of cutaneous ureterostomy. J Urol 106:538–540, 1974.

19. Fowler JE, Jr, Raife MJ, Sennott R: A method for placement of a ureteral stent following supravesical intestinal diversion. J Urol 124:547–549, 1980.

20. Gersuny R: Cited by Foges: Officielles protokoll der K.K. Gesellschraft der Hertze in Wein. Wein Klin Wschr 11:989, 1898.

21. Goldwasser B, Webster GD: Continent urinary diversion. J Urol 134:227–236, 1985.

22. Goldwasser B, Webster GD: Augmentation and substitution enterocystoplasty. J Urol 135:215–224, 1986.

23. Gonzalez R, Sidi AA, Zhang G: Urinary undiversion: Indications, technique and results in 50 cases. J Urol 136:13–16, 1986.

24. Goodwin WE, Harris W, Kaufman JJ, Beal JM: Open, transcolonic ureterointestinal anastomosis. A new approach. Surg Gynecol Obstetr 97:295–300, 1953.

25. Handel J, Schwartz S: Value of the prone position for filling the obstructed ureter in the presence of hydronephrosis. Radiology 71:102–103, 1958.

26. Hanley HG: The rectal bladder. Br J Urol 39:693–695, 1967.

27. Harvard RM, Thompson GJ: Congenital exstrophy of the bladder: Late results of treatment by the Coffey-Mayo method of ureterointestinal anastomosis. J Urol 66:223–234, 1951.

28. Heitz-Boyer M, Hovelaque A: Creation d'une nouvelle vessie et un nouvel uretre. J Urol Nephrol 1:237–258, 1912.

29. Hendren WH: Urinary undiversion: Refunctionalization of the previously diverted urinary tract. In Walsh PC, Gittes RF, Perlmutter AD, Stamey TA (eds): Campbell's Urology, Vol II, 5th ed. Philadelphia, WB Saunders Company, 1986, pp 2137–2158.

30. Hensle TW, Bredin HC, Dretler SP: Diagnosis and treatment of a urinary leak after ureteroileal conduit for diversion. J Urol 116:29–31, 1976.

31. Higgins CC: Transuretero-ureteral anastomosis: Report of a clinical case. J Urol 34:349–355, 1935.

32. Hodges CV, Moore RJ, Lehman TH, Benham AM: Clinical experience with transuretostomy. J Urol 90:552–562, 1963.

33. Hradec EA: Bladder substitutions and results in 114 operations. J Urol 94:406–417, 1965.

34. Jude JR, Lusted LB, Smith RR: Radiographic evaluation of the urinary tract following urinary diversion to ileal bladder. Cancer 12:1134–1141, 1959.

35. Kelalis PP: Urinary diversion in children by the sigmoid conduit: Its disadvantages and limitations. J Urol 112:666–672, 1974.

36. Kilcheski TS, Pollack HM: Gas contrast radiography of ileal conduits. Radiology 129:242, 1978.

37. Kock NG: Continent ileostomy. Prog Surg 12:180–201, 1973.

38. Kock NG: Intra-abdominal "reservoir" in patients with permanent ileostomy. Preliminary observations on a procedure resulting in fecal "continence" in five ileostomy patient. Arch Surg 99:223–231, 1969.

39. Kock NG, Nilson AE, Nilsson LO, et al: Urinary diversion via a continent ileal reservoir: Clinical results in 12 patients. J Urol 128:469–475, 1982.

40. Koehler PR, Bowles WT: Radiologic evaluation of upper urinary tract following ileal loop urinary diversion. Radiology 86:227–237, 1966.

41. Koehler PR, Bowles WT, McAlister WH: Roentgenographic evaluation of late results of ileal loop diversion in infants and children. AJR 100:177–185, 1967.

42. Koff SA: The abdominal neourethra in children: Technique and long-term results. J Urol 133:244–247, 1985.

43. Lapides J: Evacuation of bladder via abdominal urethrostomy (editl). J Urol 133:253, 1985.

44. Lapides J, Ajemian EP, Lichtwardt JR: Cutaneous vesicostomy. J Urol 84:609–614, 1960.

45. Lasakowski TZ, Scott FB: Cutaneous vesicostomy as means of urinary diversion: 3 years' experience. J Urol 94:549–555, 1965.

46. Lee JKT, McClennan BL, Stanley RJ, Levitt RG, Sagel SS: Use of CT in evaluation of postcystectomy patients. AJR 136:483–487, 1981.

47. Lieskovsky G, Skinner DG: Use of intestinal segments. In Walsh PC, Gittes RF, Perlmutter AD, Stamey TA (eds): Campbell's Urology, Vol III, 5th ed. Philadelphia, WB Saunders Company, 1986, pp 2620–2638.

48. Light JK, Engelmann UH: Le Bag: Total replacement of bladder using ileocolonic pouch. J Urol 136:27–31, 1986.

49. Lilien OM, Camey M: 25-year experience with replacement of the human bladder (Camey procedure). J Urol 132:886–891, 1984.

50. Mauclaire P: De quelques essais de chirurgie experimentale applicables au traitement de l'extrophie de la vessie et des anus contre nature complexes. Ann Malad Org Genurin 13:1080, 1895.

51. Mitchell ME, Yoder IC, Pfister RC, et al: Ileal loop stenosis: A late complication of urinary diversion. J Urol 118:957–961, 1977.

52. Mitrofanoff P: Cystostomie continente trans-appendiculaire dans le traitement des vessies neurologiques. Chir Ped 21:297, 1980.

53. Mogg RA: The treatment of urinary incontinence using the colon conduit. J Urol 97:684–692, 1967.

54. Noe HN, Jerkins GR: Cutaneous vesicostomy experience in infants and children. J Urol 134:301–303, 1985.

55. Nogrady MB, Petitclerc R, Moir JD: The roentgenologic evaluation of supravesical permanent urinary diversion in childhood (ileal and colonic conduit). J Can Assoc Radiol 122:154–157, 1969.

56. Politano VA, Leadbetter WF: An operative technique for the correction of vesicoureteral reflux. J Urol 79:932–941, 1958.

57. Ralls PW, Barakos JA, Skinner DB, et al: Radiology of the Kock continent ileal urinary reservoir. Radiology 161:477–483, 1986.

58. Retik AB, Perlmutter AD: Temporary urinary diversion in infants and young children. In Walsh PC, Gittes RF, Perlmutter AD, Stamey TA (eds): Campbell's Urology, Vol III, 5th ed. Philadelphia, WB Saunders Company, 1986, p 2117.

59. Richie JP, Skinner DG: Ureterointestinal diversion. In Walsh PC, Gittes RF, Perlmutter AD, Stamey TA (eds): Campbell's Urology, Vol III, 5th ed. Philadelphia, WB Saunders Company, 1986, pp 2601–2619.

60. Richie JP, Skinner DG: Urinary diversion: The physiological rationale for nonrefluxing colonic conduit. Br J Urol 47:269–273, 1975.

61. Rittenberg GM, Warren E: Air in the pelvicalyceal system: A normal finding in patients with ureteroileostomies. AJR 128:311–312, 1977.

62. Rivard JY, Bedard A, Dionne L: Colonic neoplasms following ureterosigmoidostomy. J Urol 113:781–786, 1975.

63. Schipper H, Decter A: Carcinoma of the colon at ureteral implant sites despite early external diversion: Pathogenetic and clinical implications. Cancer 47:2062–2065, 1986.

64. Schneider KM, Ried RE, Fruchtman B: The continent vesicostomy: Clinical experiences in the adult. J Urol 117:571–572, 1977.

65. Simon J: Ectopia vesicae (absence of the anterior walls of the bladder and pubic abdominal parietes); operation for directing the orifices of ureters into the rectum: temporary success: subsequent death: autopsy. Lancet 2:568, 1852.

66. Skinner DG, Boyd SD, Lieskovsky G: Clinical experience with the Kock continent ileal reservoir for urinary diversion. J Urol 132:1101–1107, 1984.

67. Skinner DG, Gottesman JE, Richie JP: The isolated sigmoid segment: Its value in temporary urinary diversion and reconstruction. J Urol 118:614–618, 1975.

68. Skinner DG, Lieskovsky G, Boyd SD: Technique of creation of a continent internal ileal reservoir (Kock pouch) for urinary diversion. Urol Clin North Amer 11:741–749, 1984.

69. Solovay J: Advantages of the prone position for the excretory urogram in ileal conduit urinary diversion. J Urol 111:530–533, 1974.

70. Sooriyaarachchi GS, Johnson RO, Carbone PP: Neoplasms of the

large bowel following ureterosigmoidostomy. Arch Surg 112:1174–1177, 1977.

71. Spring DB, Moss AA: Computed tomography of ileal loop urinary diversion in adults. J Comp Assist Tomogr 8:866–870, 1984.

72. Stamey T: Personal communication.

73. Thuroff JW, Alken P, Riedmiller H, et al: The Mainz pouch (mixed augmentation ileum and cecum) for bladder augmentation and continent diversion. J Urol 136:17–26, 1986.

74. Udall DH, Hodges CV, Pearse HM, Burns AB: Transureteroureterostomy: A neglected procedure. J Urol 109:817–820, 1973.

75. Warshaw BL, Hymes LC, Trulock TS, Woodward JR: Prognostic features in infants with obstructive uropathy due to posterior urethral valves. J Urol 133:240–243, 1985.

76. Weiss RM, Beland GA, Lattimer JK: Transuretero-ureterostomy and cutaneous ureterostomy as a form of urinary diversion in children. J Urol 96:155–160, 1966.

77. Woodside JR, Boorden TA, Damron JR, Kiker JD: Isotope loopography, a new test: Comparison with standard loopography and its relationship to renal function in patients with ileal conduit urinary diversion. J Urol 119:31–34, 1978.

78. Yoder IC, Pfister RC: Radiology of colon loop diversion: Anatomical and urodynamic studies of the conduit and ureters in children and adults. Radiol 127:85–92, 1978.

79. Zabbo A, Kay R: Ureterosigmoidostomy and bladder exstrophy: A long-term followup. J Urol 136:396–398, 1986.

80. Zincke H, Malek RS: Experience with cutaneous and transureteroureterostomy. J Urol 111:760–763, 1974.

81. Skinner DG, Lieskovsky G, Boyd SD: Continuing experience with the continent ileal reservoir (Kock pouch) as an alternative to cutaneous urinary diversion: An update after 250 cases. J Urol 137:1140–1145, 1987.

82. Rowland RG, Mitchell ME, Bihrle R, et al: Indiana continent urinary diversion. J Urol 137:1136–1139, 1987.

83. Kock NG, Nilson AE, Nilsson LO, et al: Urinary diversion via a continent ileal reservoir: Clinical results in 12 patients. J Urol 128:469–475, 1982.

84. Ghoneim MA, Kock NG, Lycke G, Shehab El-Din AB: An appliance-free, sphincter-controlled bladder substitute: The urethral Kock pouch. J Urol 138:1150–1154, 1987.

85. Melchior H, Spehr C, Knop-Wagemann I, et al: The continent ileal bladder for urinary tract reconstruction after cystectomy: A survey of 44 patients. J Urol 139:714–718, 1988.

86. Thuroff JW, Alken P, Riedmiller H, et al: 100 cases of Mainz pouch: Continuing experience and evolution. J Urol 140:283–288, 1988.

87. Amis ES Jr, Newhouse JH, Olsson CA: Continent urinary diversions: Review of current surgical procedures and radiologic imaging. Radiology 168:395–401, 1988.

88. Hinman F Jr: Selection of intestinal segment for bladder substitution: Physical and physiological characteristics. J Urol 139:519–523, 1988.

89. Mirvis SE, Whitley NO, Javadpour N, Young JD: Computed tomography of Kock and modified Kock continent ileal reservoir. Urology 29:361, 1987.

10 Seminal Vesiculography and Vasography

IRWIN GOLDSTEIN □ ROBERT J. KRANE □ ALAN J. GREENFIELD

Belfield in 1913 performed the first seminal vesiculogram. He surgically exposed the vas deferens in the scrotum and by injecting 5% collargol into the vas, was able to demonstrate the abdominal portion of the vas, the seminal vesicles, and the ejaculatory ducts.[1] Subsequently, large series of cases were collected, and the results published by Sargent,[2] Pereira,[3] and Vestby.[4] In 1935, Boreau published a beautifully illustrated textbook and atlas of seminal vesiculography.[5] Most of the early studies were concerned with the appearance of the seminal vesicles in chronic inflammatory disease, while a few detailed the changes found in benign prostatic hyperplasia and carcinoma of the prostate.[4, 5]

Young and Waters[6] were the first to successfully catheterize the ejaculatory ducts in a retrograde fashion, but this technique proved to be difficult and unreliable and was discarded by most who attempted it for vesiculography.

INDICATIONS

The indications for seminal vesiculography have narrowed sharply in the last decade. Carcinoma of the prostate and benign hyperplasia are much more readily and reliably imaged by CT, ultrasonography, and MRI, while the concept of seminal vesiculitis as an important clinical problem has been largely abandoned. Parenthetically, it is noted that Dunnick and colleagues have shown seminal vesiculography to be unreliable in the diagnosis of this condition, as shown by an unacceptably large number of false-negative as well as false-positive studies.[7] Operative procedures for the removal of the seminal vesicles, once popular, are now rarely performed. Currently, it is thought that many patients who once would have undergone vesiculography and removal of the seminal vesicle for various pain syndromes now fall into the category of functional disturbances that includes voiding dysfunction. Increasing knowledge of the neurophysiological and psychological aspects of voiding dysfunction has formed the basis for more physiological explanations of these clinical problems, and the few patients whose symptoms are actually attributable to bona fide infections of the seminal tract are usually treated effectively with antibiotics. As urodynamic investigations become more sophisticated, and with the development of ancillary imaging modalities, only a vanishing small number of patients remain who would benefit from seminal vesiculography.

At present, the most common indication for vasovesiculography is the evaluation of male infertility—specifically in patients suspected of having obstructive azoospermia.

DIAGNOSTIC EVALUATION

A useful algorithm for the evaluation of azoospermia begins with a follicle-stimulating hormone (FSH) level. If primary testicular failure is not proven, a testis biopsy should be performed under local anesthesia. Should normal seminiferous tubular tissue be found in the presence of azoospermia, and should the FSH level be normal, the patient is considered for vasography and seminal vesiculography. This study is usually performed in conjunction with scrotal exploration.

As indicated, vesiculography by the retrograde approach is now rarely performed. For all practical purposes, the procedure is carried out exclusively through a vasotomy. A scrotal incision is fashioned identical to that used during a routine vasectomy. Care should be taken, however, not to disturb the perivasal neurovascular structures while isolating the vas deferens. A small vasotomy is subsequently performed with the use of a No. 11 blade. A blunt-tipped 25-gauge needle is then placed through the vasotomy into the lumen of the vas. Care should be taken that it is placed directly into the lumen and not through the vasal musculature. The entire procedure should be performed very delicately so as to obviate any subsequent stricture formation of the vas deferens by either damage from the needle or extravasation of contrast medium. A simple injection of approximately 1 to 2 cc of 60% water-soluble contrast medium should be enough to perform the entire study (Fig. 10–1). It is usually not necessary to perform bilateral vasograms. If the vasogram is normal on the side ipsilateral to the testis biopsy and if contrast medium can be seen leaving the ejaculatory duct and flowing back to the urinary bladder, one has effectively ruled out the possibility of obstruction at the level of the seminal vesicle or ejaculatory duct as a cause for azoospermia. To rule out obstruction at the level of the epididymis or vasoepididymal junction, one can inject with the same needle in a distal orientation to visualize the distal vas and epididymis. At the termination of the procedure, the vasotomy generally is closed with one 7-0 suture. As mentioned before, care should be taken to avoid destroying any perivasal tissue that contains important neurovascular structures. If necessary, the vas cannulation may be performed under the operating microscope.

NORMAL ANATOMY

The normal anatomy of the male seminal tract has been nicely summarized by Banner and Hassler (Fig. 10–2).[8] The vas deferens enters the abdomen through the

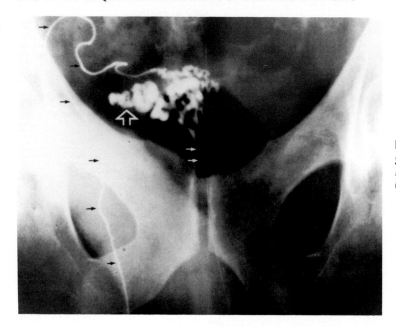

Figure 10–1. A normal vasogram and seminal vesiculogram demonstrating the vas deferens (*small black arrows*), seminal vesicle (*large arrow*), and ejaculatory duct (*small white arrows*).

Figure 10–2. Diagram of normal male seminal tract as seen by means of seminal vesiculography (AP view with slight caudal angulation). *1*, Vas deferens. *2*, Ampullary-vasal junction. *3*, Ampulla of the vas deferens. *4*, Ampullary neck. *5*, Junction of ducts of vas and seminal vesicle. *6*, Excretory duct. *7*, Seminal vesicle. *8*, Ejaculatory duct. *9*, Urinary bladder. (Courtesy Dr. Marc P. Banner.)

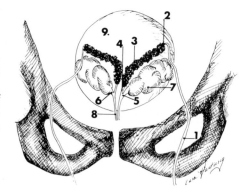

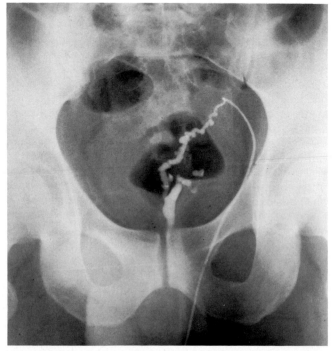

Figure 10–3. An abnormal vasogram and seminal vesiculogram performed in patient with azoospermia, demonstrating an obstructed ejaculatory duct.

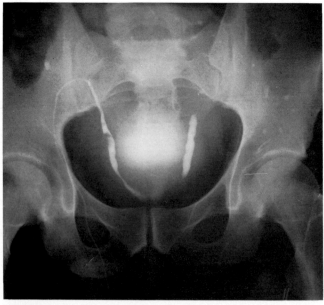

Figure 10–4. An abnormal vasogram performed in patient with azoospermia demonstrating congenital absence of the seminal vesicles.

internal inguinal ring, follows the lateral pelvic wall, and then curves downward, backward and medially. It is 30 to 40 cm in length, and its lumen, which is uniform, is approximately 1 mm in diameter. It becomes convoluted as it passes alongside the upper medial border of the seminal vesicle, where its diameter widens significantly as it forms the ampulla of the vas deferens. The seminal vesicle, which is actually a diverticulum of the vas, is variable in appearance. It is highly convoluted, roughly ovoid, and lateral to the ampulla. The vesicle narrows medially as it joins the ampulla to form the ejaculatory duct at the upper surface of the prostate gland. The thin ejaculatory duct, about 16 mm long and 1.5 mm wide, runs a straight, sometimes slightly curved course to open on either side of the verumontanum, in the region of the utricle. Normally, contrast medium leaving the ejaculatory ducts flows back into the bladder.

THE ABNORMAL VESICULOGRAM

Visualization of the specific architecture of the seminal vesicle has become less important in recent years, as noted. Changes such as tubular dilatation and tubular fusion, purportedly the hallmarks of infection, have largely lost their importance.[9] However, obstruction of the ejaculatory ducts, a relatively uncommon cause of azoospermia, can be diagnosed rather clearly by vesiculography (Fig. 10–3). In addition, rare congenital anom-alies, such as absence of the seminal vesicles and seminal vesicle cysts, can also be recognized (Fig. 10–4). Acquired vasal obstruction from infectious disease such as tuberculosis[10] can be diagnosed by vasography, although these conditions are now essentially unseen in the United States.

References

1. Witten DM, Myers GH, Utz DC (eds): Clinical Urography. 4th ed. Philadelphia, WB Saunders, 1977, p 76.
2. Sargent JC: Interpretation of seminal vesiculograms. Radiology, 12:472, 1929.
3. Pereira A: Roentgen interpretation of vesiculograms. AJR, 69:361, 1953.
4. Vestby GW: Vaso-seminal vesiculography in hypertrophy and carcinoma of the prostate with special reference to the ejaculatory ducts. Acta Radiol (Suppl):199, 1960.
5. Boreau J: Les Images des Voies Seminales. Basel, S. Karger, 1974.
6. Young HH, Waters CA: X-ray studies of the seminal vesicles and vasa deferentia after urethroscopic injection of the ejaculatory ducts with Thorium, a new diagnostic method. Bull Johns Hopkins Hosp, 31:12, 1920.
7. Dunnick NR, Ford K, Osborne D, et al: Seminal vesiculography: limited value in vesiculitis. Urology, 20:454, 1982.
8. Banner MP, and Hassler R: The normal seminal vesiculogram. Radiology, 128:339, 1978.
9. Golgi H: Clinical value of epididymovesiculography. J Urol, 78:445, 1957.
10. Mygind HB: Urogenital tuberculosis in the human male. Vesiculographic and urethrographic studies. Dan Med Bull, 7:13, 1960.

Cavernosography

DAVID R. STASKIN

Corpus cavernosography is a simple and occasionally useful technique for the direct visualization of the corpora cavernosa (Figs. 11–1 and 11–2). Cavernosography may be viewed as either *static*, when used primarily to obtain anatomical information, or *dynamic*, as when combined with pressure-flow measurements in the investigation of erectile dysfunction (Chapter 78). The instillation of contrast into the corpora cavernosa of the penis was initially reported as an access route for demonstration of the pelvic venous system.[1,2] May and Hirtl[3] and Molnar and Hajos[4] described specific abnormalities of the corpora before the initial reports of Fetter and colleagues in the English radiological literature in 1963.[5] Since that time, cavernosography has been used to visualize the anatomy of penile trauma[6-13] and penile deformity[11-18] (Peyronie's disease, corporal hypoplasia, megaphallus); it has also been used in the evaluation of erectile impotence or priapism[19-22] (postpriapism, prosthetic implant sizing, venous incompetence) and in the staging of primary and metastatic carcinoma of the penis.[23-25] The recommended technique for cavernosography is summarized in Table 11–1. The injection site should be contralateral to the side of suspected disease. The normal side-to-side intercavernosal communications assure that contrast medium injected into one corpus will opacify both sides.

PENILE TRAUMA [6-13]

Cavernosography has been reported to be useful in the assessment of acute penile trauma. Radiographic examination can be utilized to establish the integrity of the cavernosal bodies and tunica albuginea, eliminating the need for surgical exploration. In the event of corporal rupture, the specific site and extent of the injury may be identified, simplifying exploration and surgical repair (Fig. 11–3). By establishing the absence of cavernosal injury, surgical therapy may be avoided.

Injury to the penis is rare, owing to the mobility, well-guarded position, and flexibility of the organ in the flaccid state. The history of the etiology of the trauma is sometimes useful. Acute rupture of the corpora cavernosa may occur from blunt trauma to the erect penis. Trauma during sexual activity is responsible for approximately one-third of all cases. Classically, a "cracking" or "snapping" is heard, accompanied by the onset of pain. A large but often localized hematoma may form on the affected side of the penis and is associated with marked ecchymosis and deformity. Although conservative therapy has been employed, immediate repair of the fascial injury is generally recommended to relieve the symptoms, as well as

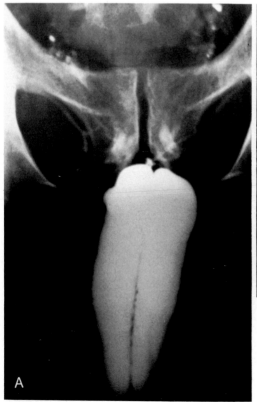

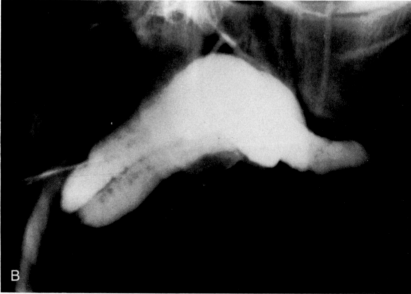

Figure 11–1. Normal static cavernosography in the flaccid state. *A*, Anteroposterior view; *B*, Oblique view. Both corpora cavernosa are fully opacified. Note the intercavernous septum and the venous filling, which is normal in the flaccid state. (From Gray R, Grosman H, St Louis EL, Leekam R: The uses of corpus cavernosography. A review. J Can Assoc Radiol 35:338–342, 1984.)

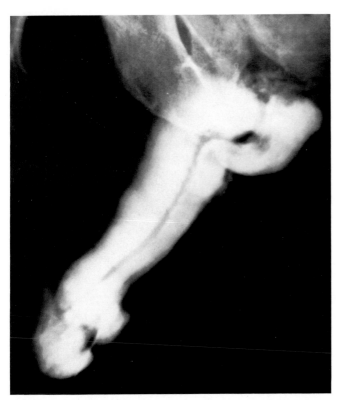

Figure 11–2. Filling of the glans and corpus spongiosum during cavernosography. Although the injection of contrast material was made into one of the corpora cavernosa, opacification of both corpora and the glans is seen. Although this occurrence is normal in the flaccid state, in the erect state it indicates an abnormal venous leak and may be a cause of impotence.

decrease the incidence, of postoperative impotence.[26–30] Blood from the urethra can be seen in up to 30% of cases. Prior retrograde urethral studies should be performed in order to avoid diagnostic problems related to retained cavernosal contrast medium.

Industrial accidents, gunshot wounds, or other causes of forcible breaking of the erect penis may be encountered. The site of formation of a urethrocavernosal or cavernosospongiosal fistula from external trauma or from the erosion of a penile implant may also be identified.

ERECTILE IMPOTENCE

The most common current use of cavernosography is for the evaluation of erectile impotence. Advances in the understanding of the pathophysiology of impotence have placed more emphasis on the recognition of abnormal corporal venous drainage during erection in a subset of patients. In conjunction with cavernosometry (intracorporal pressure monitoring), and by employing pharmacologically induced erections, dynamic-infusion cavernosometry and cavernosography (DICC) can be used to demonstrate intracorporal anatomy, filling and storage pressures, and physiologically abnormal cavernosal venous drainage (This subject is discussed in detail in Chapter 78).

Although an accurate diagnosis of corporal venous leak cannot be made without a DICC study, impotence secondary to a cavernosospongiosal venous leak, resulting from a prior shunt procedure for priapism,[31] or iatrogenic trauma (urethrotomy or sphincterotomy) may be grossly evident by simple cavernosography (Fig. 11–4).

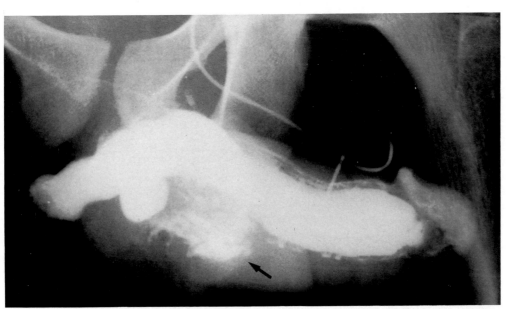

Figure 11–3. Cavernosography in rupture of the corpus cavernosum. This patient heard a loud "crack" during intercourse followed by pain and detumescence. Cavernosography demonstrates extravasation of contrast material into the penile soft tissues (*arrow*), indicating a laceration of the tunica albuginea requiring surgical repair.

Table 11–1. Technique for Cavernosography

Position	1. Patient is in supine position with legs spread.
	2. Penis is prepped and placed on mild traction.
Anesthetic	1. Lidocaine 2%, *without* epinephrine is applied at injection site.
	2. Another alternative is regional block, with 5 ml placed circumferentially at the base of the penis, superficial to the tunica albuginea.
Injection	1. Combine with prior retrograde urethrography, if urethral trauma is suspected.
	2. Injection site is *opposite* side of injury or suspected disease. Avoid urethra ventrally; avoid artery, nerve, and vein dorsally.
	3. A single 18- to 23-gauge needle is placed at dorsolateral aspect of penis, 1 cm proximal to the glans. This is sufficient to evaluate both corpora (except in epispadias). A palpable "give" is felt as the tunica albuginea is being pierced.
	4. *Dilute* contrast medium (e.g., 30% diatrizoate meglumine or iohexol) must be used *(full-strength contrast may cause priapism secondary to hyperosmolarity)*.
	5. Injection of 0.5 ml displays spongy pattern of corpus cavernosum, confirming position of needle.
	6. Injection of approximately 60 ml of diluted contrast medium over 1 minute under fluoroscopy. Frontal and 30-degree posterior oblique projections are obtained, with the penis extended over the ipsilateral thigh.
	7. Avoid extravasation of contrast medium (subcutaneous edema results and resolves in 24 hours).
	8. Injection should be terminated, if the patient experiences pain.
	9. Treatment of a prolonged erection is performed by aspiration (18-gauge butterfly needle), very thorough irrigation with heparinized (1 unit/ml) normal saline, and injection of 0.3 ml to 0.4 ml of phenylephrine (1 ml of 1% phenylephrine (10 mg) diluted to 10 ml).
	10. Plain abdominal film is taken at conclusion of study, to demonstrate urinary tract, if indicated.

Priapism may be associated with leukemia, gout, sickle cell anemia, penile malignancy, medications, inflammatory lesions, and tumors of the central, spinal, or peripheral nervous system. Cavernosal fibrosis resulting from priapism may also be visualized. In addition, *cavernosography has been implicated as a cause of priapism. These instances have generally been associated with the use of concentrated contrast media.*

CORPORAL ANATOMY[19–21]

Cavernosography may be useful in assessing the amount of cavernosal tissue remaining after traumatic loss of the penis, aiding in the decision between a lengthening procedure or phalloplasty. Congenital curvatures, corporal hypoplasia, and "megacopora" (megaphallus) following priapism can be demonstrated prior to corporoplasty (Fig. 11–5).

PEYRONIE'S DISEASE[14, 17]

The anatomical deformity associated with Peyronie's disease is also demonstrable by cavernosography (Fig. 11–6). The development of a fibrous tissue plaque in the tunica albuginea or intercavernous septum is evident on the dorsal surface of the penis. The plaque may extend laterally and may be significantly larger than the clinical examination suggests. Radiographically, the plaques appear as constricting filling defects in the contour of the corpora, along with widening of the intracorporal septum. Calcification may be evident in 20% of cases.

Demonstration of the anatomy has been proposed for use in planning corporal plications prior to the placement of a prosthetic device, the excision of the plaque with grafting, or the ligation of the associated venous drainage

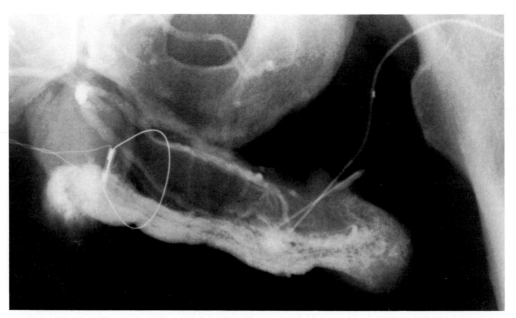

Figure 11–4. Cavernosography following cavernosospongiosal shunt. A Winter cavernosospongiosal shunt had previously been performed for intractable priapism. Injection of contrast material into the corpus cavernosum reveals immediate filling of the glans and corpus spongiosum, indicating patency of the shunt. Note early filling of the large draining veins.

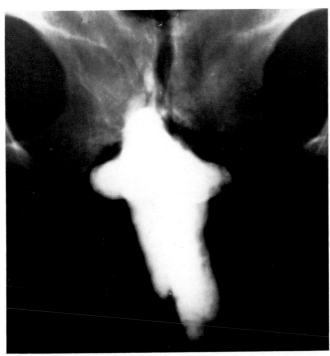

Figure 11–5. Corporal hypoplasia. Cavernosography demonstrates both corpora cavernosa to be diminutive, consistent with microphallus. Cavernosography is helpful in assessing the amount of cavernosal tissue prior to phalloplasty. (From Gray R, Grosman H, St Louis EL, Leekam R: The uses of corpus cavernosography. A review. J Can Assoc Radiol 35:338–342, 1984.)

abnormalities. Cavernosography is often replaced with photographic documentation by the patient and an intraoperative artificial erection using a saline injection and a tourniquet around the base of the penis.

CARCINOMA[23, 25]

Cavernosography may be useful in differentiating Stage-I (tumor limited to the glans penis, and/or prepuce) from Stage-II (invasion of the shaft or corpora) carcinoma of the penis.[23] Intraoperative sectioning and histopathologic examination are necessary for determining the final surgical margin during penectomy.[32] Preoperative cavernosography may elucidate the filling defect in the corporal shaft, if tumor infiltration is present, and may be useful for suggesting the extent of the proximal section of the penis during surgery.

Metastatic disease to the corpora is rare[25] (271 cases reported) and is usually a result of direct extension from the prostate and bladder (over one-half of cases) or the rectosigmoid. *Malignant priapism*, most likely secondary to venous thrombosis and neural irritation, is a common presenting symptom. Metastatic penile disease is infrequently diagnosed before the primary tumor is recognized and is usually noted 1 to 2 years after the initial diagnosis. Metastatic penile tumor indicates widespread metastases in 80% to 90% of patients, with a poor 1-year survival. Owing to the ease in palpating nodular metastases, needle biopsy or fine aspiration can usually be performed without cavernosography and fluoroscopic guidance.

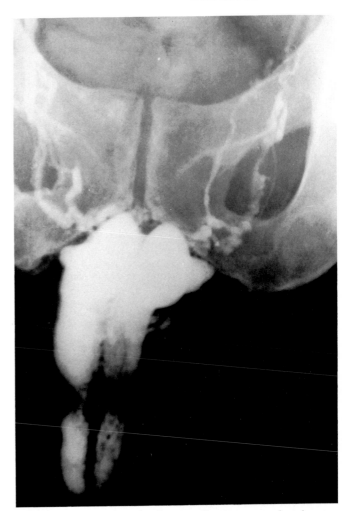

Figure 11–6. Peyronie's disease. Cavernosography demonstrates marked constriction of both corpora, secondary to fibrous plaques in the tunica albuginea and Buck's fascia. Note the widening of the intercavernosal septum. (From Gray R, Grosman H, St Louis EL, Leekam R: The uses of corpus cavernosography. A review. J Can Assoc Radiol 35:338–342, 1984.)

Cavernosography was utilized to study the periglandular venous pattern in patients with prostatic carcinoma.[24] Visualization of the periprostatic venous pattern by this method does not appear to add significant information about tumor staging, when compared with other commonly employed diagnostic modalities.

CONCLUSION

Currently, cavernosography is primarily used in combination with measurements of corporal drainage pressures in evaluating erectile dysfunction that results from physiologically abnormal venous drainage (dynamic cavernosography). Simple cavernosography is occasionally useful to evaluate and document corporal anatomy and integrity in cases of penile trauma and deformity. Its simplicity and low morbidity will continue to prompt physicians to look for new applications of the technique.

References

1. De la Pena A: Flebografia de plexos e vasos palvianos en el vivo. Revista Espanola de Cirugia, Traumatologia y Ortopedia 4:245–251, 1946.
2. Motta A de I: Urologic aspects of pelvic phelbography. J Internat Coll Surg 25:578–582, 1956.
3. May F, Hirtl H: Das Cavernogramm. Urol Intern 2:120–134, 1955.
4. Molnar J, Hajos E: Kavernosogramme. Zeit Urol 53:441, 1960.
5. Fetter TR, Yunen JR, Dodd G: Application of cavernosography in the diagnosis of lesions of the penis. AJR 90:169–175, 1963.
6. Cass AS: Immediate radiological evaluation and early surgical management of genitourinary injuries from external trauma. J Urol 122:772–774, 1979.
7. Abrahamy R, Leiter E: Post traumatic segmental corpus cavernosum fibrosis: The diagnostic value of cavernosography and the surgical correction by cavernosum-cavernosum shunt. J Urol 123:289–290, 1980.
8. Grosman H, Gray RR, St Louis EL, et al: The role of corpus cavernosography in acute fracture of the penis. Radiology 144:787–788, 1982.
9. Gross H: The role of corpus cavernosography in acute fracture of the penis. Radiology 144:787, 1982.
10. Dever DP, Saraf PG, Catanese RP, et al: Penile fractures: Operative management and cavernosography. Urology 22:394–395, 1983.
11. Gray R, Grosman H, St Louis EL, Leekam R: The uses of corpus cavernosography. A review. J Can Assoc Radiol 35:338–342, 1984.
12. Data NS: Corpus cavernosography in conditions other than Peyronie's disease. J Urol 118:588–590, 1977.
13. Ney C, Miller H, Friedenberg RM: Various applications of corpus cavernosography. Radiology 119:69–73, 1976.
14. Bystrom J, Johnsson B, Edgren J, et al: Induration penis plastica (Peyronie's Disease). Cavernosography in assessment of the disease process. Scand J Urol Nephrol 118:588–590, 1977.
15. Datta NS: Megalophallus in sickle cell disease. J Urol 117:672, 1977.
16. Datta NS: Silicone granuloma of the penis. J Urol 109:840, 1977.
17. Hamilton RW, Swann JC: Corpus cavernosography in Peyronie's Disease. Br J Urol 39:409, 1967.
18. Fitzpatrick TJ: Hemihypertrophy of the human corpus cavernosum. J Urol 115:560, 1976.
19. Goldstein I, Krane RJ, Greenfield AJ: Vascular diseases of the penis: Impotence and priapism. In Pollack HM (ed): Clinical Urography. Philadelphia, WB Saunders, 1990.
20. Datta NS: Corpus cavernosography prior to insertion of penile prosthesis. Urology 10:142, 1977.
21. Dimorpoulos C: Priapism: Successful treatment and post-operative cavernosogram. Br J Radiol 52:75, 1979.
22. Fitzpatrick TJ: Spongiosograms and cavernosograms: A study of their value in priapism. J Urol 109:843, 1973.
23. Raghavaiah NV: Corpus cavernosogram in the evaluation of carcinoma of the penis. J Urol 120:423, 1978.
24. Proca E, Lucan M: Cavernosography in the management of prostatic cancer. Br J Urol 51:397, 1979.
25. Escribiano A, Allona A, Bursos FJ, et al: Cavernosography in diagnosis of metastatic tumors of the penis: 5 new cases and a review of the literature. J Urol 138:1174–1177, 1987.
26. Gross M, Arnold TL, Waterhouse K: Fracture of the penis. Rationale of surgical management. J Urol 126:708–710, 1971.
27. Nicolaisen GS, Melamud A, Williams RD, et al: Rupture of the corpus cavernosum: Surgical management. J Urol 130:917–919, 1983.
28. Palomar JM, Halikiopoulas H, Palanco E: Primary surgical repair of the fractured penis. Ann Emerg Med 9:260–261, 1980.
29. Pryor JP, Hill JT, Packham DA, Yates-Bell AJ: Penile injuries with particular reference to injury to the erectile tissue. Br J Urol 53:42, 1981.
30. Zenteno S: Fracture of the penis; plastic and reconstruction surgery. Surgery 52:559, 1973.
31. Cosgrove MD, LaRocque MA: Shunt surgery for priapism. Review of results. Urology 4:1, 1974.
32. deKernion JB, Tynbers P, Persky L, Fegen JP: Carcinoma of the penis. Cancer 32:1256, 1973.

12 Ultrasonography of the Urinary Tract

ARTHUR T. ROSENFIELD □ CHRISTOPHER M. RIGSBY □ PETER N. BURNS □ ROBERTO ROMERO

In most institutions, ultrasonography has become the most commonly performed examination for evaluating the urinary tract. This is because of its speed and safety, relatively low cost, widespread availability, noninvasiveness and lack of ionizing radiation, and high accuracy in identifying anatomical abnormalities. For patients undergoing renal failure, hydronephrosis can be identified or excluded, and medical renal disease can be defined. Clots can be identified in the inferior vena cava or renal veins. In many of these patients, Doppler ultrasonographic studies can also aid in looking at renal blood flow. The renal cystic diseases can be readily identified by ultrasound techniques. Furthermore, in children with vesicoureteral reflux, ultrasonography is an ideal way to assess the size of the renal collecting system without using contrast medium. Renal transplants can be evaluated as to size, presence or absence of hydronephrosis, textural analysis, and blood flow. Ultrasonography can be used to guide the puncture of hydronephrotic collections in order to diagnose pyonephrosis and perform antegrade pyelography or percutaneous nephrostomy.

Ultrasonography can be used to identify masses and is the technique of choice for discriminating between cysts and tumors. In the renal sinus, ultrasonography can help to distinguish among the various causes of filling defects in the renal pelvis, although computed tomography (CT), as well, has recently assumed a major role in this endeavor.

Ultrasonography has come to play a primary role in the evaluation of abdominal, particularly renal, infection. The safety of the study has permitted it to be used in all patients, including those in renal failure. Scans can be performed at the bedside or in the laboratory. Ultrasonography can identify acute focal bacterial nephritis (lobar nephronia), diffuse pyelonephritis, abscesses and changes related to chronic renal infection such as xanthogranulomatous pyelonephritis or tuberculosis. Serial scans can be readily performed to follow lesions. Abscesses and infected cysts can be punctured using sonographic guidance.

The lower urinary tract and genital systems are also readily accessible to sonographic imaging using a variety of instrumentation.

Renal ultrasonography utilizes imaging properties totally different from those of radiography. In fact, it is the only technique in which artifacts are carefully searched for and routinely used in formulating a diagnosis. In addition, the changes in parenchymal acoustic properties, and therefore in echogenicity, that accompany disease are unique to ultrasound imaging and provide a different way of recognizing pathological conditions. This chapter stresses (1) the role of ultrasonography in solving various clinical problems, (2) the diagnostic criteria that are utilized for each of these problems, (3) the difference between ultrasonography and other imaging techniques in evaluating these problems, (4) the coordinated approach, using multiple techniques to make diagnoses, and (5) the pitfalls that are encountered in ultrasonography. It is worthwhile for clinicians and imagers to remember these pitfalls so that the limits of ultrasonography can be appreciated and the results of the study are not applied inappropriately.

HISTORY

Clinical ultrasound imaging has its origin in the wake of the Titanic disaster of 1912, when efforts began to develop a method of detecting undersea obstacles. The idea of transmitting a "beam" of sound under water and listening for echoes from distant objects was pursued with vigor during World War I, and in 1917, Paul Langevin in England developed a method of detecting submerged submarines. His work laid the foundation for sonar (sound navigation and ranging) and later for ultrasonic imaging.

Although the theory of the propagation of high-frequency sound in liquids and solid materials had been well understood since Lord Rayleigh's comprehensive mathematical treatise on sound was published in 1877, it was not until 1946 that the first ultrasonic pulse-echo systems were developed. Although these were designed for the nondestructive testing of industrial materials, it was not long before the method was applied to living tissue. The first A-scan signals from human subjects were reported in 1950 by Reid and Wild, among others. The one-dimensional display that they employed was borrowed from the more highly evolved radar technology and was quickly supplemented by two-dimensional brightness-modulated displays, forming a somewhat crude cross-sectional image of tissue boundaries. The works of pioneers such as Howry, Kossoff, Donald, and White demonstrated the potential of the technique for imaging the brain, the fetus, and the abdominal structures. In 1957, Satomura in Japan added the ultrasonic Doppler technique as a sensitive method for detecting moving structures, including blood. By 1969, instruments combining the Doppler and pulse-echo methods had been developed, making available to clinical investigators, for the first time, the noninvasive interrogation of small selected volumes of soft tissue (such as in the heart) for the detection of movement and in some cases the measurement of blood flow velocity.

During the 1960s and early 1970s, strides were made in the design and manufacture of transducers using synthetic materials and in storage techniques for the display of images. These advances culminated in 1972 with the first gray-scale images, in which a wide range of echo intensities, from those of the weakest scatterers to the strongest reflectors, could be seen on the same image. This innovation consolidated the developing role of ultrasound in imaging organs of the upper abdomen, pelvis, and retroperitoneum.

More recently, real-time scanning, introduced in the

middle 1970s and using both mechanically swept transducers and electronically controlled transducer arrays, has largely supplanted the earlier "static" B-scan techniques. The compromises in image quality apparent in the earlier real-time instruments are offset by more advanced techniques in beam-forming, using arrays of transducers. These techniques have also relied on the parallel development of high-speed digital computing technology, which is now the basis of commercially produced ultrasonographic instruments. The versatility of such technology is apparent in the most recent development in ultrasound, in which color-coded Doppler information is superimposed on the cross-sectional images, showing blood flow and soft-tissue forms together in real time.

Improvements in the technical performance of ultrasound instruments are likely to be incremental compared with the dramatic advances made in the early part of the 35-year history of clinical ultrasound, but the steady innovation of clinical applications for its techniques will certainly assure its continued, ample use by diagnosticians.

PHYSICAL PRINCIPLES

Ultrasound imaging is based on the pulse-echo principle, in which a short burst of ultrasound is emitted from a transducer and directed into tissue. Echoes are produced as a result of the interaction of sound with tissue, and some of these travel back to the transducer. By timing the elapsed period between the emission of the pulse and the reception of the echo, the distance between the transducer and the echo-producing structure can be calculated (Fig. 12–1), and an image formed (Fig. 12–2). In diagnostic imaging of the genitourinary system, frequencies of 1 to 5 MHz (megahertz) are used, except for superficial structures such as the scrotum and penis. At these frequencies, ultrasound has a wavelength of between 1.5 and 0.3 mm, a dimension that sets a fundamental limit on the potential spatial resolution of the resulting image. Better resolution is associated with a higher ultrasound frequency, but attenuation of ultrasound in tissue also increases with frequency. Optimum imaging is obtained by choosing the highest frequency transducer that permits acoustic penetration adequate to identify the region of interest.

Echoes arise when a burst of ultrasound (which travels through tissue at about 2000 mph) encounters an interface between structures of differing acoustic impedance. Acoustic impedance reflects mechanical properties of tissues such as density and stiffness. If the difference in impedance is small (as it is in soft-tissue interfaces), only a tiny proportion of the ultrasound pulse is reflected back toward the transducer; most of it is transmitted and continues on to the next interface. Echoes arrive back at the transducer, separated by a time period proportional to the distance between interfaces. These are displayed in a one-dimensional trace, with echo amplitude on the vertical axis and depth on the horizontal axis: this is known as the *A scan* (Fig. 12–1).

The echoes can also be displayed as dots in a straight line, with brightness proportional to echo amplitude (Fig. 12–2A). The transducer can then be mounted on a position sensing arm so that the line of view of the acoustic beam corresponds to the orientation of the brightness-modulated A-scan line on the display screen.

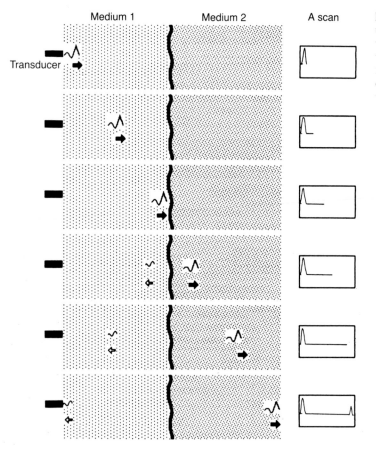

Figure 12–1. The pulse-echo principle is used to produce an ultrasound A scan. A pulse is emitted from the transducer at the same time that a dot is set in motion from left to right on the A-scan screen. When an echo reaches the transducer, the received signal causes a vertical deflection of the trace. The distance between deflections on the A scan corresponds to the depth of the interface from the transducer.

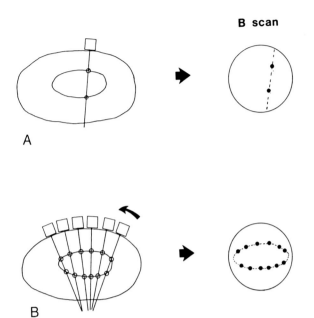

B scan

Figure 12–2. B scanner. *A,* Echoes displayed by an A-scan line are encoded as brightness-modulated dots. The line is then displayed with the same orientation on the screen as the beam scans the patient. *B,* Transducer is moved across the patient, resulting in a series of echoes being written on the screen, thus forming a gray-scale image of the interface.

Moving the arm across the skin surface will then produce a series of dots corresponding to the cross section of the interface within tissue (Fig. 12–2B).[1] Thus, an image of this interface is formed, known as a *B scan*.

Variations in acoustic impedance may take the form of a smooth surface (such as the bladder wall), in which case the reflection of ultrasound is *specular* (Fig. 12–3A), an effect that is analogous to light striking a glass interface. Echoes are seen only if the beam is almost perpendicular to the surface (Fig. 12–3B). Older "bistable" ultrasound equipment was able to demonstrate only these strong, specular echoes. They are seen at interfaces of organs as well as at brightly reflecting smooth areas such as the walls of major vessels. Other interfaces may be irregular, in which case specular reflection takes place over many angles within the ultrasound beam (which is some millimeters in width), and echoes are produced in many directions. Such *scattering* gives rise to an echo that travels back to the transducer over a range of angles of incidence (Fig. 12–4A). The diaphragm is an example of such a structure in the body. Finally, small variations in acoustic impedance are in the tissue parenchyma itself, and these give rise to low-level, isotropic scattering (Fig. 12–4B). The small proportion of this *backscattered* echo is received by the transducer. If these weak echoes are displayed by the gray scale of the ultrasound imaging system, the parenchyma of an organ is characterized by a distinct shade of gray. The structure and intensity of backscattered parenchymal echoes form the basis of gray-scale ultrasonography. In fact, such backscattered echoes are coherent in phase and interfere with each other just as ripples on water caused by many small disturbances combine to form a pattern of crests and troughs. In ultrasound this stationary interference pattern corresponds to the *speckle* of a gray-scale image, a factor that determines the apparent texture of an organ seen sonographically. Different organs have characteristic textures. Although the absolute intensity (or *echogenicity*) and

(A) Reflection

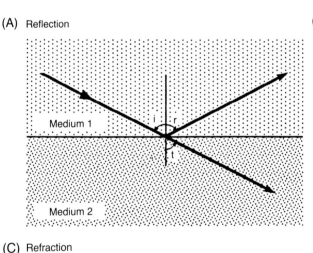

(B) Reflection: orthogonal beam

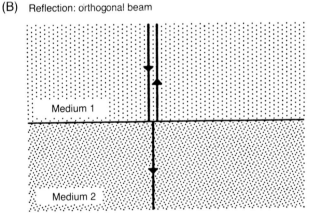

(C) Refraction

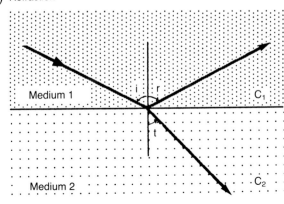

Figure 12–3. Ultrasound pulse encounters an interface between soft tissues of differing acoustic impedance. *A,* Specular reflection. A small portion of the ultrasound beam is reflected, but most passes across the interface undeviated. Angle of incidence (i), angle of reflection (r), and angle of transmission (t) are all equal. *B,* Normal incidence. In this special case of specular reflection, the angle of incidence is zero and the echo is received by the transmitting transducer. *C,* Refraction. If the velocity of sound is different in the two media, the angle of transmission will differ from the angle of incidence.

(A) Irregular interface

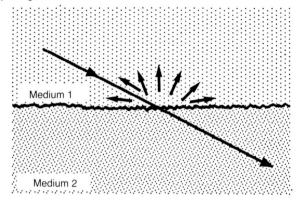

(B) Inhomogeneous medium

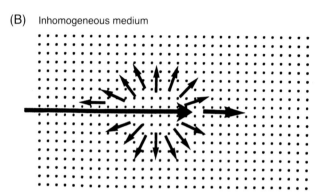

Figure 12–4. Scattering of ultrasound. *A,* Specular reflections from a multiplicity of irregularly oriented interfaces cause echoes that represent a range of angles. *B,* As sound propagates through the parenchyma of an organ that contains microscopic fluctuations in acoustic impedance, small quantities of ultrasound are scattered in all directions, including back toward the transducer. This scattering is responsible for the gray-scale appearance of the organ.

texture cannot be used to obtain tissue-characterizing information, since texture is determined primarily by a combination of the acoustic characteristics of the ultrasound beam and the mechanical structure of tissue, the relative appearance of different organs is constant, thus allowing the diagnosis of abnormality. The normal cortex of the kidney, for example, is characterized by parenchymal echoes less intense than those of the contiguous liver, spleen, and pancreas (Fig. 12–5). The parenchymal texture of these organs is also different (Fig. 12–5). In addition, specular echoes from the renal sinus in the adult are more intense than those from within the cortex.

One source of artifact in ultrasound imaging is the phenomenon of *refraction*. Among the factors that influence the acoustic impedance of a tissue is the velocity at which sound travels in it. Thus, an interface between two tissues of differing velocity gives rise to an echo by reflection. However, as the transmitted portion of the pulse continues into the deeper tissue, its path is deviated at the interface (Fig. 12–3C). The degree of deviation from a straight line depends on the difference in velocities across the interface: this may be negligible between renal cortex and sinus, for example, but can be significant between fat and collagen. Because, according to the pulse-echo principle, sound propagates in a straight line, refracting interfaces will degrade or distort an ultrasound image.

Attenuation of the ultrasound beam in normal tissue is primarily a result of the absorption of the acoustic wave motion producing an immeasurably small quantity of heat. Scattering is thought to contribute a negligible amount of attenuation. Attenuation is strongly dependent on frequency and reduces the intensity of the beam exponentially as it travels through tissue. For example, the intensity of a 5 MHz beam is reduced by half in 6 mm of liver, 2 mm of muscle, or 0.3 mm of bone. Gas and bone attenuate ultrasound rapidly: in addition, their acoustic impedance results in almost total reflection from interfaces with soft tissue. The effect of attenuation on returning echoes is seen as a dramatic reduction in the intensity of echoes from deeper structures. To compensate for this effect, the gain of the receiver is increased logarithmically as echoes arrive from progressively deeper structures. When the last echo arrives, the next pulse of ultrasound is emitted from the transducer and the gain is reset to its lowest level for reception of the first echo. The gain is automatically increased throughout the subsequent period in which echoes from deeper structures arrive. In this way, equal-strength echoes from different depths are displayed with the same intensity on the screen. The control of this time gain compensation (TGC) is at the operator's disposal and must be set properly in order to assess the relative echogenicity of organs at various depths. Inappropriate setting of the TGC curves can cause the appearance of artifactual lesions; conversely, incorrect settings may obscure real lesions.

Because the difference in echo intensity between the bright specular reflector and the weakest parenchymal

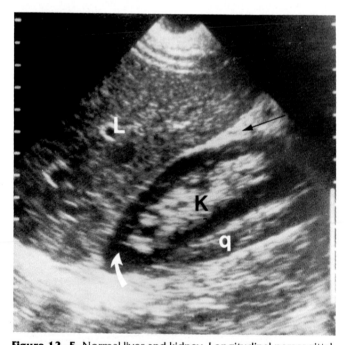

Figure 12–5. Normal liver and kidney. Longitudinal parasagittal section through the right upper quadrant demonstrates the liver (L) with homogeneous low-level backscattered echoes. Posterior to the liver is the right kidney (K). Cortex of the right kidney (*curved arrow*) produces less intense backscattered echoes than does the liver. Renal sinus is seen as an ovoid echogenic structure in the central portion of the kidney on this section. Straight arrow indicates fat in the retroperitoneum between liver and kidney. In this patient, the fat is highly reflective, although it can be of variable echogenicity. (q = quadratus lumborum muscle.)

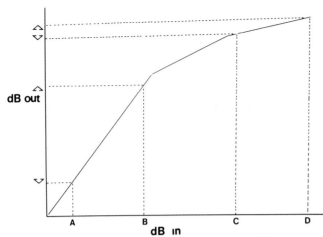

Figure 12–6. Compression amplification curve demonstrates the relationship between the echo amplitude returning to the transducer (dB in) and the echo amplitude that is displayed (dB out). Note that the echo data show a constant difference between A and B and between C and D. This difference is preserved for low-level echoes, but it is decreased for large ones. (From Taylor KJW, Jacobsen P, Jaffe CC: Lack of acoustic shadow on scans of gallstones: A possible artifact. Radiology 131:463–464, 1979.)

scatter may be as much as 60 dB, and since a television screen may be capable of displaying no more than 30 dB, some compression of the range of echo amplitudes is necessary. This is achieved by amplifying the low-level echoes linearly and the high-level echoes in a manner that compresses them into a narrow dynamic range (Fig. 12–6).[2, 3] This characteristic (known as the display compression or postprocessing curve) may be adjusted to enhance the contrast between a lesion and surrounding tissue of almost similar echo intensity. Thus, in Figure 12–6, the intensity between echoes A and B, and between echoes C and D are similar, but the display contrast between A and B is greater than that between C and D.[3] Additional enhancement of edges may be provided by electronic differentiation of the demodulated signal, a processing facility built into many modern abdominal scanners. In selecting postprocessing characteristics, one should attempt to optimize the contrast between structures of interest without sacrificing the dynamic range (i.e., the range of gray shades) in the display.

The process of moving a transducer attached to an arm has been largely replaced in modern *real-time* scanners by the movement of a transducer using a mechanical rotator or translator, driven under servo control, such that the display of a scan line is moved in exact correspondence with the position of the beam (Fig. 12–7). The beam is swept with speed sufficient to produce an entire image in a fraction of a second, so that independent images may be acquired at a rapid rate. The display of these images in quick succession and the elimination of flicker by alternating between image memories create a device capable of visualizing structures that are moving in real time. The assessment of the movement of tissue in the abdomen yields additional diagnostic information unique to ultrasound imaging. Movement of a lesion during respiration can identify it as arising from the peritoneal or retroperitoneal space. For example, fluid-filled structures that pulsate may be identified as arteries and ureteric jets may be visualized directly with real-time

ultrasound as they empty into the bladder (see Fig. 12–69B). Dynamic information may be recorded on videotape or "frozen" by an operator control and stored in an image memory. Review of a real-time ultrasound examination of the abdomen can, however, be a problem, as the hand-eye coordination of the scanning process is impossible to record and because it is often difficult to appreciate in retrospect the precise plane of visualization. Multiple views in standard planes, however, although lending predictability to the images produced, result in the sacrifice of many of the qualities unique to real-time ultrasound imaging.

A variety of techniques may be used to steer the ultrasound beam in a real-time scanner. In the *mechanical-sector* scanner (Fig. 12–7A), the beam from a single transducer is moved by the rotation of the ceramic element itself, or of acoustic mirrors within the beam. In the *linear array* a large number of small, discrete transducer elements are arranged in a line (Fig. 12–7B), and a small number are excited together to form a beam. When all the echoes have been received along the resulting line of sight, the next pulse is issued from the adjacent series of elements, and so on. The beam is swept rapidly from one end of the transducer array to the other, thereby forming an image. The frame rate of such an image is determined by a combination of the number of lines within the field of view (this is related to the image resolution) and the time taken for the last echo to return to the transducer, once the pulse has been transmitted

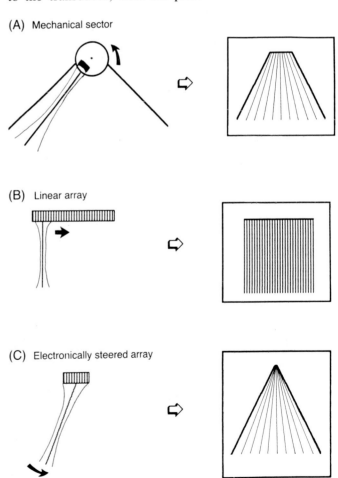

(A) Mechanical sector

(B) Linear array

(C) Electronically steered array

Figure 12–7. A–C, Three configurations of an ultrasound scanner that permit echoes to be obtained at sufficient speed to produce real-time images.

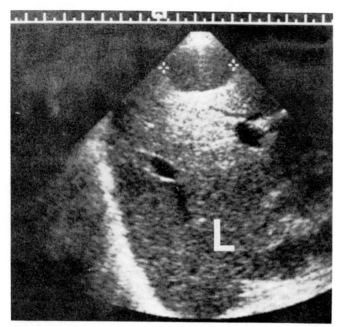

Figure 12–8. A superficial lesion (between the cursors), normally hidden by near-field artifact when a fixed focus transducer is used, is clearly defined when a swept-focus electronically steered array is used. Note that there is no sacrifice of the middle-field and far-field focus (L = liver). (From Maslak SH: Computed sonography. *In* Sanders RC, Hill MC (eds): Ultrasound Annual, 1985. New York, Raven Press, 1985.)

(this is related to the maximum depth of the field of view). Thus, the size of the field of view, the frame rate, and the resolution of the image are all related in a real-time scanner. The optimum choice of those parameters is inevitably a matter of compromise. Electronic switching precludes the need for moving parts in the linear-array scanner. One of the limitations of this configuration is that it requires a relatively large transducer and therefore cannot be applied to intercostal scanning or scanning through other small acoustic windows (a *window* refers to a superficial area through which deeper structures can be visualized and that is not composed of structures such as gas or bone that attenuate the ultrasound beam). On the other hand, the linear array has proved ideal for scanning areas with large windows and a smooth abdominal surface such as the pregnant uterus. Linear-array transducers are also relatively inexpensive.

Finally, in the electronically steered or *phased-array* scanner (Fig. 12–7C) the sector format is produced by precise control of the instant at which each element in a small rectangular array of transducers is excited. Here all the elements (there may be 64 or 128) are excited together, but with a small, progressive phase difference from one side to the other. The size and direction of this difference determines the direction in which the main lobe of the ultrasound beam emerges. By controlling this phase between successive bursts, the beam may be "steered" electronically. Applying delays to the signal received by each element in the array enables the beam to also be manipulated to receive and transmit in the same direction. The advantages of the electronically steered arrays are their lack of moving parts, the relatively small size of the transducer footprint (perhaps 2 cm²), and their ability to produce beams for which focus may be controlled electronically. Electronically focused beams

improve the uniformity of image quality at different depths, especially enhancing visualization of structures near the transducer face (Fig. 12–8). Receiving with a larger number of elements, in either a linear or phased array, allows the electronic focus to sweep downward as echoes arrive from progressively deeper structures. Figure 12–8 illustrates the ability of such a scanner to produce a clear image of a superficial lesion, while still maintaining resolution of more distal structures. Figure 12–9 shows the performance of the scanner using a standard ultrasound tissue phantom. The dots correspond to nylon wire target elements. Note the uniformity of their size over the field of view.

A hybrid of the mechanical-sector scanner and the phased array, the *annular-array* system, allows the electronic focusing of mechanically manipulated transducer elements. These are particularly useful at higher ultrasound frequencies, where the electronic beam-steering technology performs less well. High frequencies may be used where high-resolution imaging of superficial structures is necessary, such as in the testes, and here the

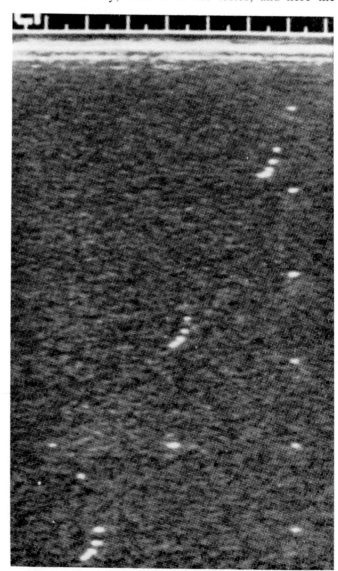

Figure 12–9. Nylon wires in a tissue-mimicking phantom are imaged, using a swept-focus array. Note the uniformity of resolution throughout the field of view. (From Maslak SH: Computed sonography. *In* Sanders RC, Hill MC (eds): Ultrasound Annual, 1985. New York, Raven Press, 1985.)

annular-array mechanical-sector scanner may be particularly advantageous.

Ultrasound transducers have been produced in a wide variety of sizes and shapes. Transducers designed for transrectal scanning have been built using linear-array or rotating mechanical-sector designs. These are used routinely for prostate and bladder imaging. Transurethral transducers are also used in some institutions to examine the walls of the bladder in order to stage bladder carcinoma; small electronically steered sectors or high-frequency linear-array systems have been designed for intraoperative use. Transducers of all types are also available with attachments to guide a biopsy needle under ultrasound imaging control.

Developments in current technology also permit the combination of real-time, electronically steered ultrasound images with simultaneous Doppler blood flow information. Here, the Doppler flow information is color coded on the image, providing a real-time map of venous and arterial flow elements and their location within the imaging plane. These so-called *color Doppler* imaging systems are currently under intensive development and are undergoing evaluation in cardiac and peripheral vascular imaging, and they are likely additions to the ultrasound armamentarium of the future.

NORMAL ANATOMY AND VARIANTS

The renal sinus represents the portion of the kidney that contains the calyces and infundibula, as well as arteries, veins, and lymphatics, and part of the renal pelvis. It consists primarily of fibrous tissue and fat. The renal parenchyma is the portion of the kidney peripheral to the renal sinus; a membrane defines the junction between renal parenchyma and sinus. Connecting the papillary tips on an excretory urogram provides a general indicator of this line of demarcation.[4] Two major zones are seen in the renal parenchyma: the glomerular-bearing cortex is at the periphery; the medulla or pyramids are more central and are contiguous with the calyces. The pyramids are defined medially by the renal sinus and laterally by the cortex, and are separated from each other by protrusions of the renal cortex (the septa of Bertin). At the corticomedullary junction, the arcuate vessels (artery and vein) can be identified. In most kidneys, some pyramids are fused. At these points of fusion, larger vessels, called the subsidiary interlobar arteries and veins, are identified at the junction between cortex and medulla.[4] On sonographic examination, the cortex of the kidney produces low-level, backscattered echoes and the medullary region is echo poor or echo free (Fig. 12–10).[5] The septa of Bertin have a consistency similar to that of the peripheral renal cortex. On cadaver specimens examined sonographically, the arcuate vessels can be seen.[5] They are identified as intense, specular echoes (Fig. 12–11A). These vessels are generally imaged in cross section, as can be seen from the corresponding cadaver slice (Fig. 12–11B), and they appear as echogenic punctate regions, although longer portions are occasionally seen. The arcuate vessels are similarly identified during routine patient scanning (Fig. 12–10).

Changing the transducer frequency changes the appearance of the cortex as well as the depth of penetration

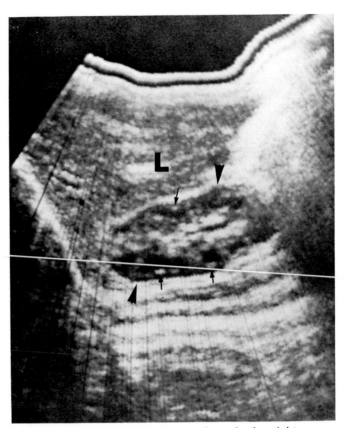

Figure 12–10. Longitudinal scan through the right upper quadrant of a 6-year-old child demonstrates the liver (L) and right kidney (*arrowheads*). The renal sinus is seen as an echogenic central zone, with fluid in the renal sinus being echo free. The cortex is hypoechoic and the pyramids are echo free. At the corticomedullary junction, punctate echoes corresponding to the arcuate artery and vein in cross section are seen (*arrows*). (From Rosenfield AT, Richman T: The Urinary Tract. *In* Taylor KJW (ed): Atlas of Ultrasonography, 2nd Ed. New York, Churchill-Livingstone, 1984. By permission.)

(Fig. 12–12). The higher the frequency of the transducer, the better the resolution, but the less the penetration. The kidney can be visualized in vivo on standard scans in any projection including longitudinal, transverse, and oblique sections. The patient can be scanned in the supine, prone, or decubitus position. Cortex, medulla, and arcuate vessels are routinely identified in all but the largest patients,[6] in whom the resolution is limited, since lower frequency transducers must be used. Fat refracts the ultrasound beam and may degrade image quality in obese subjects. Anatomical detail of the right kidney is seen optimally when the patient is supine and the liver is used as a window (Fig. 12–10). The anatomy of the left kidney is best seen with the patient in the right-side-down decubitus position (Fig. 12–13). Using this technique, the scanning must often be performed through intercostal spaces. Thus, multiple scans may be required to demonstrate the entire kidney in the longitudinal plane. The kidneys can be well visualized at any age and, in fact, are easiest to see in infants and children, who are smaller and have the least body fat, permitting the use of high ultrasound frequencies. They are well seen in the fetus in utero. The renal cortex in the adult is generally less bright than the renal sinus or contiguous liver (Fig. 12–10).[6] In the neonate, the renal cortex may be relatively brighter

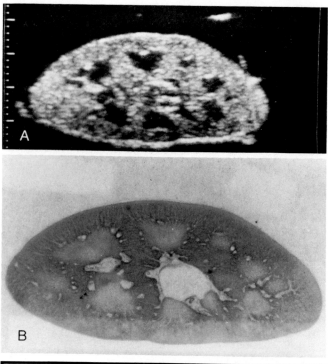

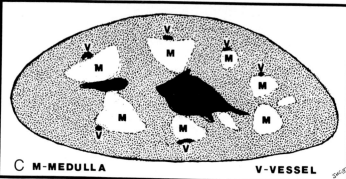

Figure 12–11. Sonogram of the normal cadaver kidney from a 9-year-old boy who died in an automobile accident. *A,* Longitudinal scan through the cadaver kidney demonstrates that the cortex contains homogeneous backscattered echoes and that the pyramids are echo free. At the corticomedullary junction, punctate echoes correspond to the arcuate artery and vein in cross section. *B,* Thin section through the cadaver kidney at the same level demonstrates this anatomy. *C,* Schematic drawing of *A* and *B*. (From Cook JH III, Rosenfield AT, Taylor KJW: Ultrasonic demonstration of intrarenal anatomy. AJR 129(5):831–835, 1977, © Am Roentgen Ray Soc, 1977.)

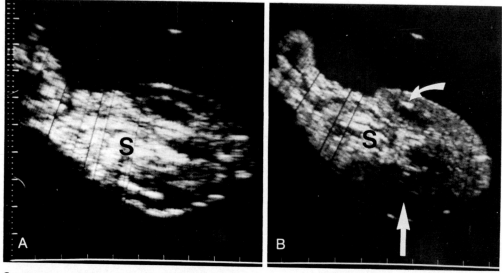

Figure 12–12. Sonograms of the normal adult cadaver kidney. *A,* Transverse section through an adult cadaver kidney demonstrating the entire kidney, including cortex and medulla. The scan was performed at 2.25 MHz. *B,* Scan of the same kidney using a higher frequency transducer at 5 MHz demonstrates better-defined echoes within the cortex. Arcuate vessels in the anterior portion of the kidney (*curved arrow*) are also better demonstrated. Note, however, the loss of echoes in the posterior portion of the kidney (*straight arrow*). Thus, the 5-MHz transducer is not adequate to insonify the entire kidney, although it would be optimal for lesions in the anterior portion. Note that in both sections the renal sinus (S) of the adult contains more intense echoes than that of the child (compare with Figure 12–11).

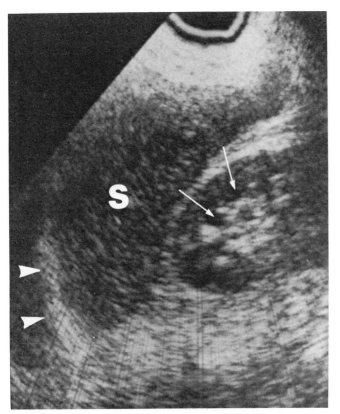

Figure 12–13. Sonogram of the normal left upper quadrant. Coronal scan through the left upper quadrant demonstrates the diaphragm (*arrowheads*), spleen (S) and left kidney. The pyramids of the left kidney are well identified (*arrows*), although the entire left kidney is not insonified, and other scans were required to demonstrate the lower portion of the kidney.

measured on a radiograph. In one series, the mean right sonographic length was 10.74 (± 1.35 SD) and that of the left 11.10 (± 1.15 SD).[16] Nomograms for renal length in the child have been determined.[12–14] Since the major role of ultrasound has been to evaluate renal growth in serial studies, the most important technical factor is to obtain the maximum length of the kidney.

Renal Sinus

Sonographically, the appearances of the renal sinus vary.[17, 18] In most individuals, the renal sinus is an ovoid single echogenic structure (Figs. 12–10, 12–13), although in some two echogenic structures may be identified (see Figs. 12–50, 12–51 and related discussion). Figure 12–16 is a coronal scan through the left upper quadrant showing normal calyces within the renal sinus of the upper portion of the right kidney. The echogenic urothelium of these calyces and infundibula merge with the echogenic fat and fibrous tissue of the renal sinus. In individuals who are well hydrated, the collecting system may be seen to be slightly distended by echo-free urine. The echogenic urothelium defines this slightly distended collecting system.

On transverse images, the anatomical relationship between the renal sinus and the renal parenchyma varies with the level that is being scanned. On scans through the upper and lower portions of the kidney, the renal sinus is central. However, on scans through the middle portion of the kidney, the renal sinus exits medially.

The normal ureter is generally not identifiable, but mild ureterectasis is readily appreciated. On coronal scans, a dilated ureter can frequently be traced down into the true pelvis to the bladder. However, overlying structures frequently prevent optimal delineation of the entire ureter.

than the liver (Fig. 12–14).[7–9] In addition, the neonate renal sinus is less echogenic than that of the adult, since it contains less fibrous tissue and fat. Thus, the brightness of the cortex may appear similar to that of the renal sinus at this age. The intensity of echoes in the renal cortex is related to maturity, being greatest in premature infants and decreasing as the child grows older. Hricak has speculated that the brightness of the cortex in infants results from the full complement of glomeruli, which are most responsible for renal echogenicity, being present at birth when there is less interstitium between them.[9] The progressive decrease in cortical echogenicity may result from the less echogenic interstitium occupying a relatively greater region.

It should be noted that ultrasound scans of the abdomen are displayed with a uniform format from institution to institution. On longitudinal scans, cranial is to the left and caudad is to the right. On transverse scans, one views the patient as if looking up from below, in a manner similar to viewing CT scans. The scans can be written as either black dots on a white background or white dots on a black background (Fig. 12–15). Both approaches have proved acceptable, although it is difficult for an interpreter to change from one to the other. Sonography has been used to determine renal size using either renal length or estimated renal volume.[10–16] Although a variety of disparate numbers for normal renal length are presented in the literature, a reasonably accurate estimation of renal size in the adult is approximately 15% less than that

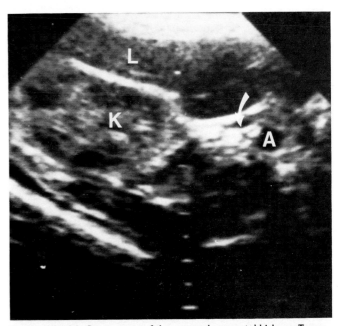

Figure 12–14. Sonogram of the normal neonatal kidney. Transverse scan through the right upper quadrant shows the liver (L) and the right kidney (K). The echogenicity of the cortex of the kidney is slightly greater than that of the liver, and the pyramids are well seen. More intense echoes are seen within the renal cortex in the neonatal and infant kidney than are seen later in life. (A = aorta. Curved arrow = inferior vena cava.)

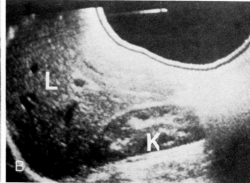

Figure 12–15. Longitudinal sonographic scans through the right upper quadrant, with the patient supine, demonstrating liver (L) and right kidney (K) in a normal patient. *A,* Scan is done with black dots on a white background. *B,* Scan is a reversal of the same picture, showing white dots on a black background. Information obtained by these approaches is identical.

Perinephric Space

The normal perinephric space is typically composed of echogenic fat (Fig. 12–5), although in some individuals it can be extremely hypoechoic. Gerota's fascia may be appreciated in this latter situation as an echogenic line separating the perinephric from paranephric fat (Fig. 12–17).[19] Perinephric fluid can be recognized as an echo-free or echo-poor collection about the kidney (Fig. 12–18).[20]

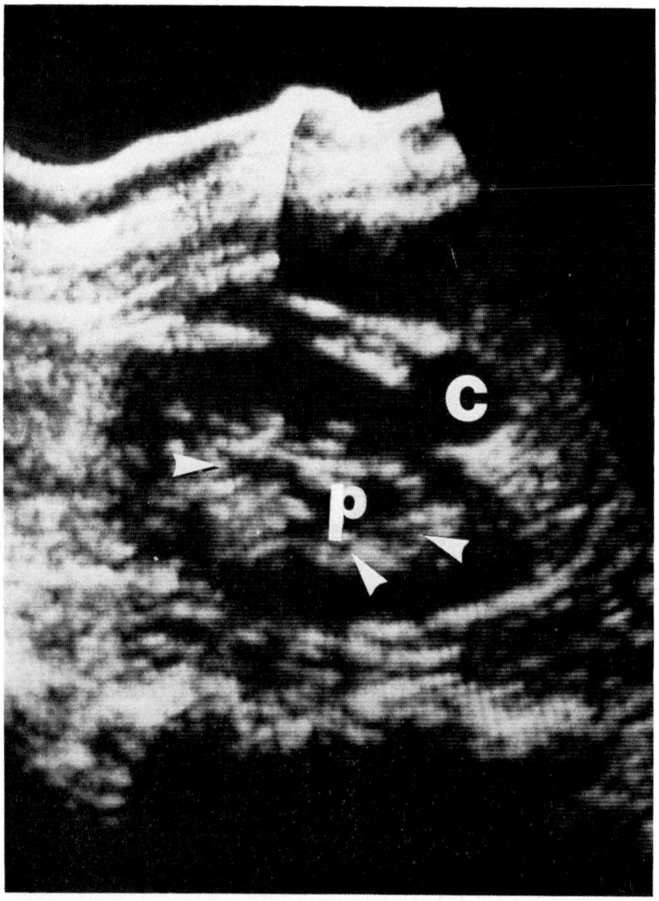

The renal vessels can be routinely identified and information about them can be obtained. The normal renal vessels can be well seen in the transverse scan (Fig. 12–19), as well as in cross section on longitudinal projection. On the transverse scan, the inferior vena cava at the level of the kidneys is anterior to the renal artery (Fig. 12–19). The left renal vein can be seen exiting the left kidney and extending between the superior mesenteric artery and aorta, subsequently coursing into the inferior vena cava. It may be narrowed between the aorta and superior mesenteric arteries with distention of its proximal portion (the "nutcracker" phenomenon).[21] The left renal artery extends from the aorta to the left kidney behind the level of the left renal vein. The right renal artery extends behind the inferior vena cava into the right kidney. Doppler ultrasound may be used to make a positive identification of blood flow in a vessel. A potential pitfall

Figure 12–16. Coronal sonographic scan through the left upper quadrant, performed with a low gain, demonstrates the normal calyceal cups (*arrowheads*) and the renal pelvis (p). An incidental renal cyst (C) is noted. (From Rosenfield AT, Taylor KJW: Grey-scale ultrasound in the imaging of urinary tract disease. Yale J Biol Med 50:335–353, 1977.)

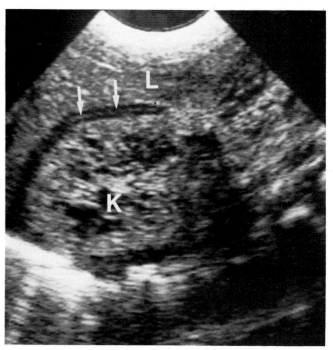

Figure 12–17. Longitudinal sonogram of the right upper quadrant in a child with autosomal dominant polycystic kidney disease. The abnormal kidney (K) has ill-defined internal cysts and the liver (L) is normal. Note Gerota's fascia (*arrows*) dividing perinephric and anterior paranephric spaces.

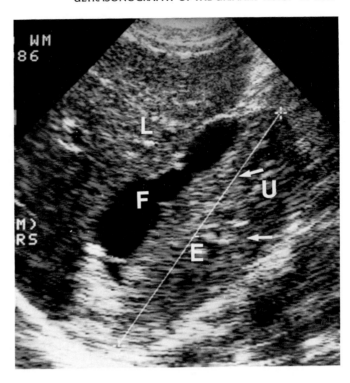

Figure 12–18. Perinephric fluid. A longitudinal sonographic scan through the right upper quadrant in a patient with perinephric fluid verified by computed tomography demonstrates the fluid (F) anterior to the right kidney. Note that the portion of the kidney behind the fluid (E) is significantly brighter than the remainder of the kidney (U). A straight line (*arrows*) separates these two regions. Area E is enhanced by good transmission of the sound beam, while the remainder of the kidney remains unenhanced. Thus, renal echogenicity is dependent, to a great degree, on the structures traversed by the ultrasound beam before it reaches the kidney. (L = liver. The cursors are connected by a straight line to designate the uppermost and lowermost limits of the right kidney on this section.)

in retroperitoneal imaging is to mistake the right crus of the diaphragm (Fig. 12–19) for one of the vessels. The crura are hypoechoic[22] but, unlike the vessels, extend behind the cava and in front of the aorta. Not only can they mimic vessels but, when large, can mimic adenopathy on either ultrasonography or CT. Retroperitoneal anatomy can be identified in different planes; of particular interest is the use of the coronal scan (Fig. 12–20) to identify the great vessels and associated structures, such as the crura, and to identify adenopathy and vascular aneurysms.

Besides the pitfall of hypoechoic perinephric fat mimicking a fluid collection or other abnormality, the quadratus lumborum muscle behind the kidney may similarly be hypoechoic (Fig. 12–19).[23] The characteristic appear-

ance of this muscle on the longitudinal scan as well as a typical position on both transverse and longitudinal scans should permit recognition of this abnormality. Occasionally, the psoas muscle may be large and hypoechoic. Again, this should not be confused with an abnormality. Venous anomaly, such as circumaortic or retroaortic left renal vein (Fig. 12–21) can be identified at sonography and should not be mistaken for a mass.

Malrotation of the kidney can be appreciated, because in that case the renal sinus exits from an abnormal location (Fig. 12–22). Ultrasonography is also routinely used to identify the presence or absence of a kidney, as well as to identify an ectopic kidney (Fig. 12–23). Pitfalls abound in attempting to use ultrasonography for the former purpose. This is because ultrasonography does

Figure 12–19. Normal sonographic anatomy. Transverse scan through the upper abdomen at the level of the pancreas demonstrates the liver (L) and pancreas (*arrowheads*). Both kidneys are seen (K), as well as the spine (S), inferior vena cava (c), and aorta (a). The quadratus lumborum muscles are noted behind the kidney (1). These can be hypoechoic and can mimic posterior paranephric collections. Among the vessels that can be seen are the portal vein (2), as it is formed from the superior mesenteric and splenic veins; the splenic vein (4); the superior mesenteric artery (3); the left renal vein (8); the right renal artery (6); and the left renal artery (5). Note that the more proximal left renal vein is distended by the nutcracker effect between the aorta (a) and superior mesenteric artery. Note also the right crus of the diaphragm (7), which is hypoechoic and could be mistaken for a renal vessel. Its position behind the cava and medial to the right kidney (rather than into the hilum of the kidney) distinguishes it from a renal vessel.

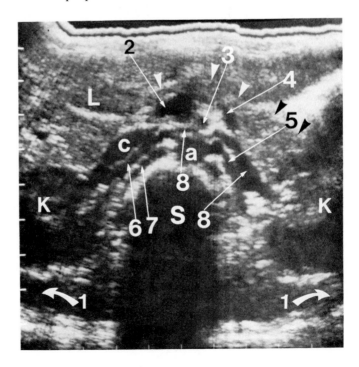

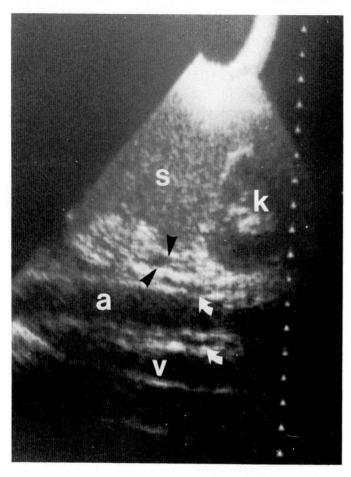

Figure 12–20. Coronal sonographic scan through the left upper quadrant demonstrates spleen (s), kidney (k), aorta (a), and vena cava (v). The left adrenal (*arrowheads*) can be seen between the spleen and left crus (upper curved arrow indicates the left crus). In the left adrenal, note the echogenic linear central zone, representing the medulla, and the more hypoechoic peripheral region, representing the cortex. The lower curved arrow demonstrates the right crus between the aorta and vena cava.

not take advantage of the way in which renal parenchyma functions (it is the only technique used routinely for renal imaging that does not). For this reason, contrast agents are being developed for ultrasonography, using a new generation of stable small particles capable of passing through the capillary circulation. In adults, the greatest pitfall is identifying the anatomical splenic flexure as the

left kidney or the anatomical hepatic flexure as the right kidney. In infants, the normally large neonatal adrenal gland may be mistaken for a kidney. In cases of renal agenesis or ectopia, the anatomical splenic flexure occupies the left renal fossa,[24, 25] and the anatomical hepatic flexure occupies the right renal fossa.[26] When folded upon itself or if fluid-filled with feces in the center, this structure

Figure 12–21. Retroaortic left renal vein. The left renal vein (*straight arrows*) can be seen behind the aorta (A). (V = vena cava. Curved arrow indicates superior mesenteric artery.)

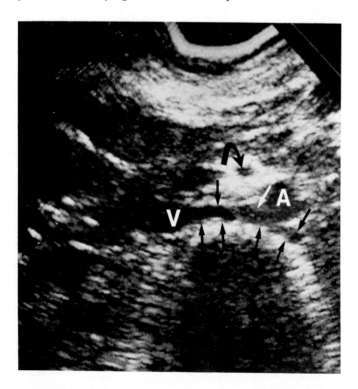

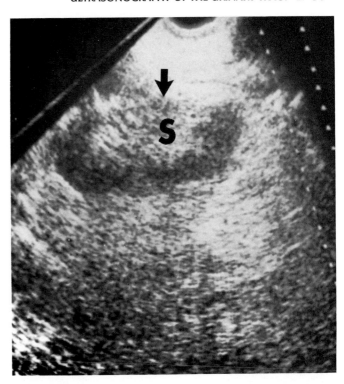

Figure 12–22. Malrotation of the kidney. Coronal sonographic scan through the left upper quadrant shows the renal sinus (S) of the left kidney exiting laterally (*arrow*).

may mimic exactly the appearances of a left kidney (Fig. 12–24).[27] A similar phenomenon may occur on the right.[28] In other circumstances, a cystic or solid structure in the renal fossa may be mimicked. The identification of the position of the anatomical splenic flexure medially rather than under the spleen on barium studies or standard radiographs, particularly when taken with the patient prone, can permit the correct diagnosis.[27] In this regard, it should be noted that the anatomical splenic flexure does not change in position when a standard flank nephrectomy is performed. However, following an abdominal nephrectomy it may be positioned medially.[25] Thus, obtaining the correct clinical history is important in the

application of this sign. In general, the optimal information about the presence or absence of a kidney is obtained by CT.

Adrenal Gland

The normal adrenal gland can be identified ultrasonographically, although it is visualized more easily on CT. The standard technique to identify the adrenal glands as described by Sample[29, 30] is to image them in the decubitus position using the liver and spleen as windows (see Fig. 12–20). The right adrenal is also well seen using transverse

Figure 12–23. Pelvic kidney. A longitudinal sonographic scan through the right side of the true pelvis demonstrates a pelvic kidney (K). (B = bladder. Arrows indicate the right ovary.)

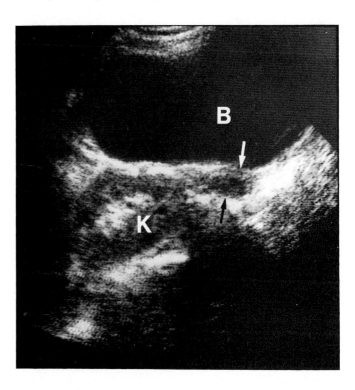

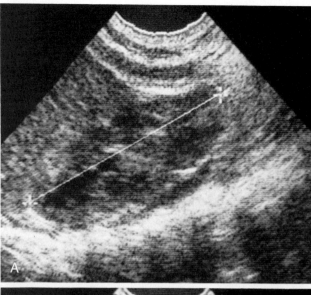

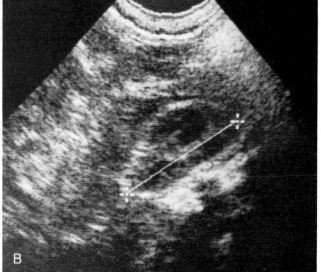

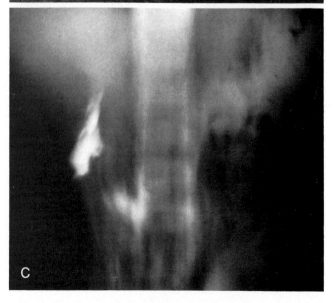

Figure 12–24. Anatomical splenic flexure as a renal impostor. *A*, Longitudinal sonographic scan through the right upper quadrant in a supine patient demonstrates the right kidney, the length of which is shown by the superimposed line. *B*, Coronal scan through the left upper quadrant portrays an apparent kidney that is smaller than the one on the right. The superimposed line shows the length of this structure. *C*, Representative tomogram from an excretory urogram demonstrates crossed-unfused renal ectopia. No kidney is present in the left renal fossa. The anatomical splenic flexure created the apparent pseudokidney.

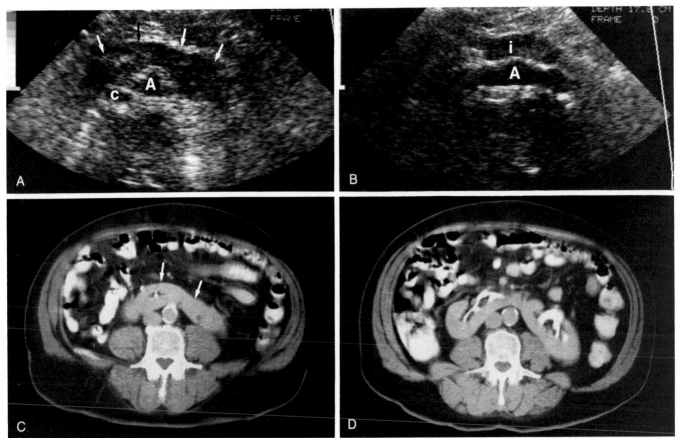

Figure 12–25. Horseshoe kidney mimicking adenopathy. *A,* Transverse ultrasonic scan through the retroperitoneum demonstrates an apparent mass of lymph nodes (*arrows*) anterior to the cava (c) and aorta (A). *B,* Longitudinal scan through the aorta (A) once again demonstrates an abnormality anterior to it, which represents the isthmus (i) of the horseshoe kidney but mimics nodes or other masses. *C,* Transverse CT scan at the same level as *A* demonstrates the isthmus of a horseshoe kidney (*arrows*) in front of the aorta and cava. *D,* CT scan at a higher level than *C* demonstrates the pelves exiting from the horseshoe kidney. Note that the bowel anterior to the pelves and the spine posterior to them preclude visualization of this region sonographically.

scans with the individual lying supine. The adrenal is relatively large compared with the kidney in the fetus[31] and neonate[32] and is particularly well visualized in these age groups. The medullary region produces more intense echoes than does the adrenal cortex.

Retroperitoneum

The retroperitoneum is easier to scan using CT and magnetic resonance imaging (MRI) because bowel gas anteriorly and the spine posteriorly limit the field of view on ultrasonography. However, ultrasonography is routinely used to evaluate the aorta for abdominal aortic aneurysm, and the other techniques are generally reserved for cases in which an optimal study cannot be obtained. Similarly, ultrasound can identify retroperitoneal adenopathy or retroperitoneal fibrosis.[33] A major pitfall in examining this region is to mistake the isthmus of a horseshoe kidney for adenopathy (Fig. 12–25).[34] The abnormal axis of the kidney in this situation should alert one to the correct diagnosis.

APPLICATIONS OF ULTRASONOGRAPHY

Ultrasonography has many advantages over competitive techniques. It is extremely safe and does not use

ionizing radiation, as do standard radiography and CT. In addition, no contrast media are needed so that the risk of contrast reactions is eliminated. The high-frequency sound waves used in imaging do not travel through the air far enough to affect the sonographer at all. As for the patient, many in vitro animal and clinical studies have been performed in an attempt to identify any adverse bioeffects. The general conclusion of all of these studies is that high-frequency sound waves utilized in short pulses are not carcinogenic or teratogenic, nor do they cause major abnormalities in tissues at diagnostic intensities.[35] This is related, to a great extent, to the short pulse of ultrasound used. For most of the scanning time the transducer is receiving the returning ultrasound beam. While one should never scan the fetus unnecessarily, ultrasound is considered safe in pregnancy and is routinely used for the evaluation of the fetus and surrounding structures.

The rapidity of ultrasound is a major advantage as compared with a conventional excretory urogram or with CT. Images are obtained instantaneously and on real-time equipment dynamically as well. Needle aspiration procedures are much more rapidly performed than with CT. Organ motion is instantaneously appreciated, and the relationship of one structure to another can be determined in any plane in seconds. In addition to the ability to scan rapidly, the equipment is portable. Scans can be performed at the bedside, and patients who are extremely ill need not be moved. In fact, procedures such as needle aspiration can be guided by portable ultrasound as easily as in the ultrasound suite.

Ultrasonography is relatively inexpensive. Although the price of different types of equipment is extremely variable, ultrasound scanners cost one-tenth to one-thirtieth the price of CT or MRI equipment. In a cost-conscious era, this factor cannot be overlooked. It is far less expensive to screen with ultrasonography than with CT or MRI.

A major distinction between ultrasonography and x-ray techniques, including CT, is that the performance of the ultrasound study is not affected by renal function. Contrast media are not required to identify urinary tract dilatation. Ultrasonography, therefore, is routinely used to evaluate patients in renal failure and excellent scans are generally obtained in this situation, unless the kidney is so small and fibrotic that clear delineation is impossible. For most ultrasonographic examinations of the urinary tract, no preparation is necessary. Hydration is, however, routinely required to examine the bladder and adjacent pelvic organs and may be needed to identify partial obstruction.

These advantages of ultrasound account for its popularity. However, its disadvantages must be borne in mind. First, the ultrasound beam does not adequately penetrate gas or bone, which leads to a number of problems. Structures such as ribs or gallstones may obscure part of the kidney (Fig. 12–26). As noted above, the normal nondistended ureter is not seen. The small field of view created by scanning in a narrow window defined by areas of gas and bone can lead to major diagnostic errors (see Fig. 12–25).

Equally important, ultrasound is operator dependent. Innumerable pitfalls exist, even for the experienced sonologist, and these are magnified when an inexperienced person is performing the study. Many of these are detailed in this chapter. In contrast, techniques such as CT are generally operator independent. In addition, the real-time ultrasound examination is difficult to review in retrospect. Since the images demonstrate a narrow field of view, one must trust that the person who performed the study correctly placed the transducer to create the image. With techniques such as CT and MRI, orienting landmarks are present, and the field of view is wide. In addition, when these scans are repeated with identical technique, similar pictures are produced. However, if different technicians perform sequential ultrasonographic studies, different images may be obtained for identical pathologic conditions.

These factors clearly define the role of ultrasonography in evaluating the urinary tract and the adjacent structures. As a screening technique for patients suspected of a particular disease, ultrasonography has taken on the major imaging role. It is inexpensive, provides excellent anatomical information, and, when a good study is obtained, generally identifies or excludes the abnormality. If an abnormality is identified, or if an optimal study cannot be obtained, other imaging techniques, particularly CT, can be of great value. Ultrasonography also is useful in guiding needle and catheter placement in the upper and lower urinary tract. It is of less value in the retroperitoneum and in applications that take advantage of renal function, such as discriminating between pseudotumor and true lesions. Although the ultrasonographic texture of a pseudotumor such as a septum of Bertin is similar to the normal parenchyma, contrast-enhanced CT is more definitive, because pseudotumors are seen as functioning and true lesions are not.[35a]

RENAL ULTRASONOGRAPHY: INDICATIONS AND PITFALLS

The indications and pitfalls related to renal ultrasonography are defined in Table 12–1 and are discussed in detail below. Because this book is organized by clinical problems and diseases, this section emphasizes diagnostic features unique to ultrasonography.

Lesions of the Renal Sinus

On ultrasound study, the renal sinus is typically seen as a zone of specular echoes that is oval on longitudinal sections and round on transverse scans. As noted below, because of the formation of the kidney from two renunculi, anterosuperior and posteroinferior extensions of the renal sinus may be identified. In addition, the echogenicity of the renal sinus is variable, being much less prominent in infants and young children who have much less fat and fibrous tissue in that area than adults. The urothelium of the renal sinus is highly reflective.[36] With severe submucosal edema, such as in transplant rejection, thickening associated with a hypoechoic zone beyond the echogenic rim may be identified.[37]

Ultrasound is routinely used to identify and exclude hydronephrosis. Hydronephrosis is identified as a separation of the walls of the collecting system by fluid-filled urine.[38] The dilated pelvis may predominate as a central fluid-filled structure, or the dilated calyces may be seen

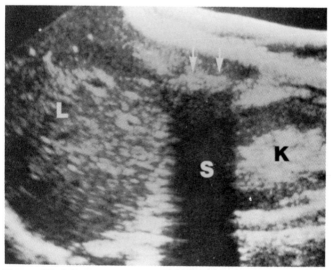

Figure 12–26. Acoustic shadowing, obscuring the upper pole of the right kidney. Longitudinal scan through the right upper quadrant demonstrates the liver (L) and right kidney (K). The gallbladder is contracted and within it are zones of intense echoes, attributable to gallstones (*arrows*), with associated acoustic shadowing (S) behind them. The upper pole of the right kidney is not seen on this scan because of the acoustic shadow. (From Rosenfield AT, Hobbins JC, Taylor KJW, Cook JH III: Renal ultrasound. *In* Rosenfield AT, Glickman MG, Hodson J (eds): Diagnostic Imaging in Renal Disease. New York, Appleton-Century-Crofts, 1979.)

Table 12–1. Renal Ultrasonography: Indications and Pitfalls

Clinical Problem	Diagnosis by Ultrasonography	Findings	Pitfalls
Renal failure	Obstructive uropathy	Dilated collecting system	Lesions mimicking obstructive uropathy
	Medical/renal disease	High-level cortical echoes (bilateral)	Acoustic enhancement of normal cortex when scanning through fluid-filled structure
	Transplant rejection	Pulsatile arterial flow in all vessels (Doppler) = vascular rejection	Normal Doppler study in nonvascular rejection
		Nephromegaly	
		Increased cortical echoes with prominent pyramids	
		Loss of corticomedullary definition	
		Focal decrease in cortical echoes (focal infarct)	
		Decreased echogenicity in renal sinus	
	Congenital renal cystic disease	See Chapter 109	
	Acute tubular necrosis	1. "Ischemic"—normal sonogram 2. Drug-induced or secondary to myoglobinuria high-level cortical echoes 3. Secondary to intratubular block from precipitation of Tamm-Horsfall protein—echogenic pyramids	
Renal mass or infection	Dystrophic calcification or nephrolithiasis	Echogenic focus with "clean" shadow	No shadow with small stone outside focal zone of transducer
	Cyst	1. Echo-free 2. Posterior acoustic enhancement 3. Refraction artifact 4. Smooth wall	Artifactural internal echoes due to 1. Reverberation artifact 2. Positioning small cyst outside of focal zone 3. Too high a gain 4. Ca^{++} renal cysts attenuate the beam
	Solid mass	1. Mass with variable echogenicity 2. No artifacts associated with cysts	Cannot distinguish benign from malignant lesions (except angiomyolipoma)
	Angiomyolipoma	1. Echogenic mass 2. Speed-propagation artifact	Some do not have enough fat to be echogenic or demonstrate speed propagation artifact
	Acute focal pyelonephritis (lobar nephronia)	Echo-poor mass	1. May be mistaken for tumor or abscess 2. Hemorrhagic pyelonephritis is echogenic
	Acute pyelonephritis	Diffuse decrease in cortical echogenicity	Acute renal vein thrombosis can give identical findings
	Intrarenal abscess	1. Mass with variable echogenicity 2. Artifacts associated with cystic lesions 3. Gas—echogenic focus with dirty shadow	May be confused with acute focal bacterial nephritis or tumor
	Perinephric abscess	Perinephric collection with variable echogenicity	1. Echo-poor perinephric or paranephric fat may mimic fluid (verify presence of collection with CT) 2. Quadratus lumborum muscle may be mistaken for collection
	Pyonephrosis	Debris in a dilated collecting system	Blood in collecting system can cause identical appearances

Table continued on following page

Table 12–1. Renal Ultrasonography: Indications and Pitfalls *Continued*

Clinical Problem	Diagnosis by Ultrasonography	Findings	Pitfalls
Unilateral nonfunctioning kidney	Unilateral renal vein thrombosis	1. Clot in renal vein 2. Loss of transmitted pulsations in renal vein 3. Abnormal flow (Doppler) 4. Textural change, unilateral decrease in cortical echoes (early) 5. Unilateral increase in cortical echoes (subacute and chronic)	Too high a gain leading to artifactual echoes in renal vein Flow in renal vein difficult to evaluate by Doppler
	Obstructive uropathy	(See above)	
	Acute renal infarction	Variable findings—globally echo-poor or echogenic kidneys may be seen	Sonogram may be normal when CT or angiography is abnormal
	Renal agenesis	No kidney in renal fossa	Anatomic splenic or hepatic flexure can mimic kidney or mass
	Renal infection or mass	(See above)	
Guide cyst puncture, biopsy, antegrade pyelography			Parapelvic cyst or calyceal diverticulum may be mistaken for collecting system

as rounded intercommunicating fluid-filled structures (Fig. 12–27). It is important to realize that echo-free urine within the collecting system is frequently not identified to a significant extent in the fluid-restricted patient, whereas the collecting system can be quite capacious, even in normal patients who are well hydrated. Also, in infants and children, the collecting system may distend significantly when the bladder is full and a repeat study with an empty bladder must be done to determine whether the phenomenon is physiological.

When partial obstruction to either the entire collecting system or a portion of it is suspected, scans must be obtained both before and after fluid challenge.[19, 39] The challenge can be done by having the patient drink at least a pint of water or by utilizing a diuretic such as furosemide. Following the fluid load, dilatation of the collecting system not previously apparent may be seen (Fig. 12–28).

A number of potential pitfalls exist in evaluating the collecting system for hydronephrosis. The normal echo-free pyramids may be confused with dilated calyces by the inexperienced ultrasonologist. The characteristic location of the pyramids defined by cortex on three sides and the renal sinus centrally, as well as the presence of the punctate echoes of the arcuate vessels of the cortico-medullary junction, should prevent this error. It may also be difficult at times to discriminate between renal parenchymal cysts and urinary tract dilatation. The most important sign that one is observing parenchymal cysts is the inability to connect the cystic structures[40] as well as the general presence of a small but defined reflective sinus in the center of the kidney. Parapelvic cysts may completely mimic hydronephrosis on ultrasonography (as well as on other studies such as non–contrast-enhanced CT) (Fig. 12–29),[41] while normal papillae can simulate pathological filling defects in dilated calyces.[41a] Radiographic studies such as excretory urography or contrast-

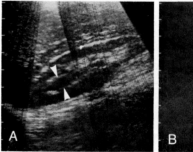
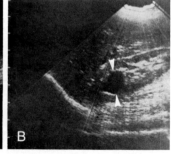

Figure 12–27. Obstructive uropathy. Coronal sonographic scan through the left upper quadrant shows a dilated pelvis (p) and blunted calyces (*arrows*). (From Rosenfield AT, Taylor KJW, Crade M, DeGraaf CS: Anatomy and pathology of the kidney by gray scale ultrasound. Radiology 128:737–744, 1978.)

Figure 12–28. Sonograms of partial obstruction demonstrated by a fluid challenge. The 24-year-old woman had a history of intermittent right flank pain that began in childhood, occurring whenever she drank large amounts of fluid. *A,* Longitudinal scan of the right upper quadrant during fluid restriction. Slight separation of the walls of the upper-pole calyx (*arrowheads*) of the right kidney is seen. *B,* Similar scan after fluid challenge. The patient was asked to drink enough water to reproduce her right flank pain. Significant hydronephrosis to the upper-pole collecting system (*arrowheads*) is seen. At surgery, obstruction of the calyx due to a crossing vessel was found. (From Rosenfield AT, Taylor KJW, Dembner AG, Jacobsen P: Ultrasound of the renal sinus: New observations. AJR 133(3):441–448, 1979, © Am Roentgen Ray Soc, 1979.)

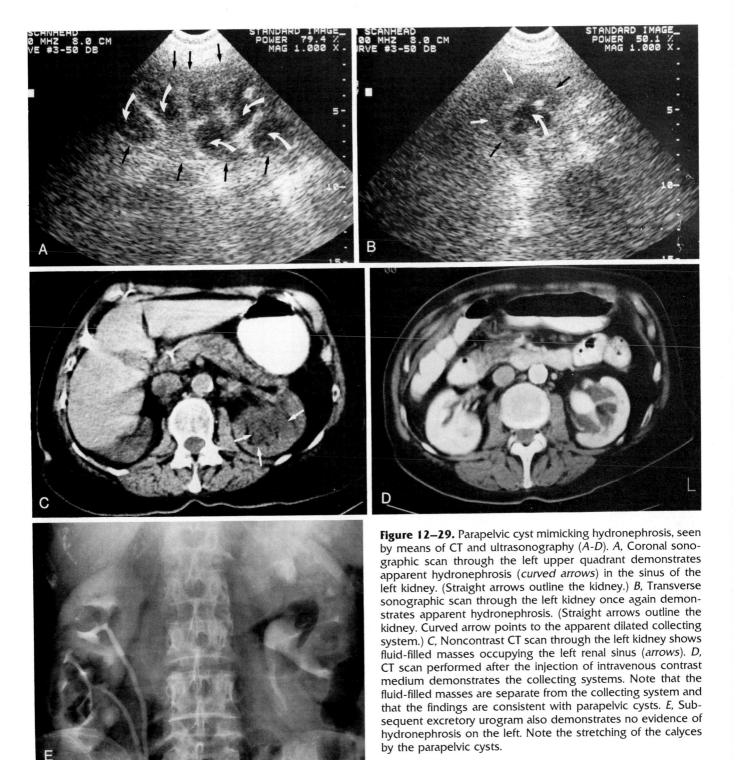

Figure 12–29. Parapelvic cyst mimicking hydronephrosis, seen by means of CT and ultrasonography (*A-D*). *A*, Coronal sonographic scan through the left upper quadrant demonstrates apparent hydronephrosis (*curved arrows*) in the sinus of the left kidney. (Straight arrows outline the kidney.) *B*, Transverse sonographic scan through the left kidney once again demonstrates apparent hydronephrosis. (Straight arrows outline the kidney. Curved arrow points to the apparent dilated collecting system.) *C*, Noncontrast CT scan through the left kidney shows fluid-filled masses occupying the left renal sinus (*arrows*). *D*, CT scan performed after the injection of intravenous contrast medium demonstrates the collecting systems. Note that the fluid-filled masses are separate from the collecting system and that the findings are consistent with parapelvic cysts. *E*, Subsequent excretory urogram also demonstrates no evidence of hydronephrosis on the left. Note the stretching of the calyces by the parapelvic cysts.

enhanced CT may be required to make this determination.

Ureteral compression can be used to distend the collecting system, but it is indicated only in selected situations, such as to distend the collecting system when looking for transitional cell carcinoma (in a patient sensitive to intravenous contrast medium) or in order to discriminate between a distended collecting system and adjacent cystic structures. Although the normal ureter is not generally identified sonographically, a dilated ureter may be appreciated when obstruction is present at a level below the ureteropelvic junction.[42] The identification of a dilated ureter is of value in determining the level of obstruction. Coronal scans in the decubitus position may be necessary to trace the course of the dilated fluid-filled ureter. The area behind the fluid-filled bladder should also be searched for ureteral dilatation as well as for the cause of this dilatation, such as ureterocele, stone, or tumor.

In general, only a limited amount of information about the hydronephrotic system can be obtained sonographically. Because motion of fluid is so slow within a dilated collecting system, Doppler ultrasonography has not been successfully used to discriminate between obstructive and nonobstructive dilatation (although ultrasonography can be used to guide needle puncture for antegrade pyelography and pressure studies as well as for percutaneous nephrostomy).[43, 44] However, debris appearing as widespread echogenicity within the fluid or as a debris-fluid level may be seen within a dilated collecting system when pyonephrosis (infection of the dilated collecting system) is present.[45–47] In a patient with fever, a debris-fluid level is characteristic of pyonephrosis; if focal pyonephrosis is present, a focal debris-fluid level can be seen, such as in tuberculosis (Fig. 12–30).[18] Echogenic fluid was found in

most cases of pyonephrosis in one series,[45] but in less than half of the patients in another.[46] Needle aspiration of the fluid may be necessary for diagnosis. It can also provide a means of percutaneous drainage if pus is obtained. Debris within a dilated collecting system may also be due to blood, as may a debris-fluid level (Fig. 12–31).[18] In a patient with hematuria, if debris within the collecting system is identified ultrasonographically, serial sonograms should be obtained. Urography, which is generally indicated, should be delayed until the debris is cleared; otherwise, the study may have to be repeated unnecessarily.

Transitional cell carcinoma in the collecting system generally has low-level echoes (Fig. 12–32)[48] and rarely calcifies. A fungus ball may also appear as an echogenic mass within the collecting system[49] or may lead to echogenic fluid.

Stones within the collecting system lead to echogenic foci with acoustic shadowing (Fig. 12–33).[50, 51] If hydronephrosis is not present, the echogenic focus may be obscured by the echogenic renal fat. Thus, proper technique is crucial to identifying the artifact, represented by the acoustic shadow. Using standard transducers, the ultrasound beam is focused (Fig. 12–34) so that it is narrow in the focal zone and wider in the near and far fields. Since the acoustic shadow depends on the stone occluding the beam, it may not be seen when a stone is in the near field or far field (Fig. 12–35).[3, 18] With the stone in the focal zone, the shadow will appear. Thus, in order to avoid missing small stones, the renal sinus must be within the focal zone of the transducer. In addition, the proper gain must be used, since a high far gain may obscure the acoustic shadow.[3] Approaching the stone from many angles also aids in finding the acoustic shadow. It is not uncommon for small changes in scanning tech-

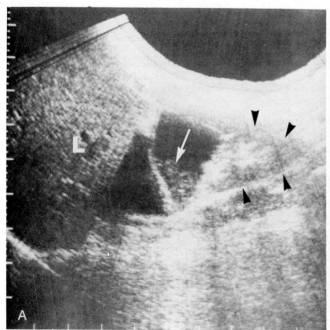

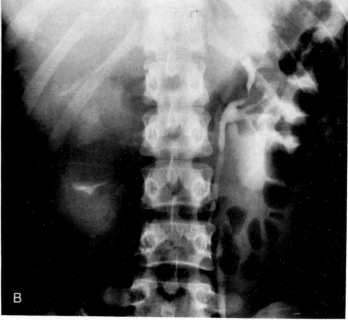

Figure 12–30. Focal pyonephrosis, secondary to tuberculosis. *A*, Longitudinal sonographic scan through the right upper quadrant shows the liver (L) cranial to the right kidney. The lower pole of the right kidney is unremarkable (*arrowheads*). The upper pole of the right kidney is a partially septated fluid-filled zone that is consistent with focal hydronephrosis. The arrow indicates debris layering out, also consistent with focal pyonephrosis. This condition, especially in the presence of calcification, is typical of tuberculosis. *B*, Excretory urogram in the same patient shows focal hydronephrosis in the upper pole of the right kidney, with excretion into the dilated collecting system. The left kidney is unremarkable. (From Rosenfield AT, Hodson CJ, Glickman M: *Diagnostic Imaging in Renal Disease.* New York, Appleton-Century-Crofts, 1979.)

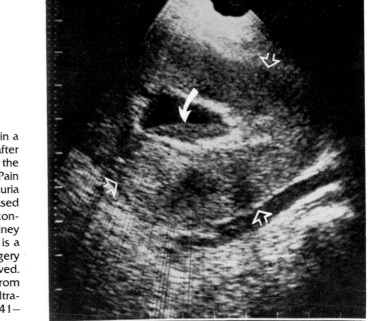

Figure 12–31. Urinary tract obstruction due to blood clot in a patient experiencing renal transplant rejection. Two years after renal transplant, this 19-year-old man developed pain in the region of the allograft on the evening before admission. Pain was followed by marked gross hematuria and complete anuria by the time of the admission. Cortical echogenicity is increased with preservation of corticomedullary definition, findings consistent with renal transplant rejection. (The transplanted kidney is outlined with open arrows.) The renal sinus abnormality is a debris-fluid level (*curved arrow*) in a dilated pelvis. At surgery 3 days later, a kidney undergoing acute rejection was removed. Old blood was found within the collecting system. (From Rosenfield AT, Taylor KJW, Dembner AG, Jacobsen P: Ultrasound of the renal sinus: New observations. AJR 133(3):441–448, 1979, © Am Roentgen Ray Soc.)

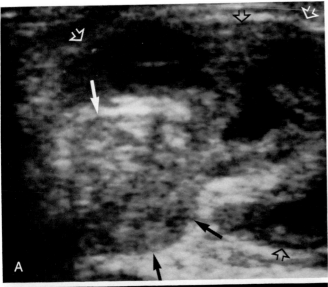

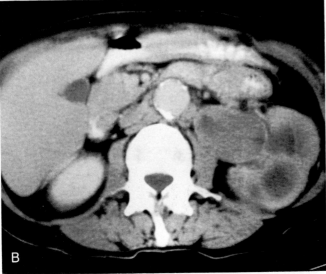

Figure 12–32. Transitional cell carcinoma of the renal pelvis. *A,* Coronal sonographic scan through the left upper quadrant shows a solid mass (*solid arrows*) filling the renal pelvis and separating its walls (open arrows indicate the left kidney). Note preservation of corticomedullary definition, indicating that this portion of the visualized parenchyma is uninvolved. *B,* CT scan of the same patient demonstrates a solid mass within the left renal pelvis. Note the less intense nephrogram on the left, as compared with the right, due to functional impairment secondary to obstruction by the tumor.

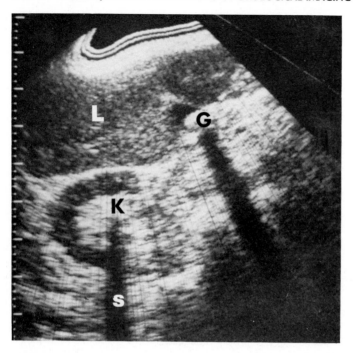

niques to make inapparent shadows visible (Fig. 12–36). This point is important because ultrasonography can potentially discriminate between a transitional cell tumor of the renal pelvis and a stone by the presence of an acoustic shadow in the latter but not the former. The study is limited in this regard by technical variables.

It should also be appreciated that acoustic shadowing is not specific for or diagnostic of nephrolithiasis. Acoustic shadowing may be seen in a number of situations related to lesions of both the renal sinus and the renal parenchyma, including nephrolithiasis, nephrocalcinosis, and dystrophic calcification. All of these shadows are typically "clean shadows" without significant internal echoes.[52] Shadowing can also be seen from gas in the renal sinus. Gas typically produces a "dirty shadow,"[52] which is a shadow containing low-level internal echoes (see Fig. 12–58). This is probably due to reverberation between the transducer and skin. Significant shadowing may be seen with refraction or scattering caused by fat (as is seen behind the ligamentum teres of the liver) or with certain

Figure 12–33. Nephrolithiasis and cholelithiasis. Transverse sonographic scan through the right upper quadrant, demonstrating the liver (L), gallbladder (G), and kidney (K). In the kidney, there is an intense zone of echogenicity and an acoustic shadow (s) behind the renal sinus. Similarly, a zone of intense echoes is seen within the gallbladder and an acoustic shadow is distal to it. Note that the shadows have very few internal echoes ("clean shadows"), a phenomenon typical of stones (with or without calcification) and other similar structures.

tumors that have a high attenuation coefficient and hence absorb the ultrasound beam (Fig. 12–37). Refraction of the ultrasound beam at the edge of a cyst may also lead to an acoustic shadow (see below).[53] Thus, an acoustic shadow is a nonspecific sign and should not be taken as diagnostic of a specific entity. Figure 12–38 is a diagrammatic representation of the different causes of acoustic shadowing at ultrasonography.

Ultrasound is appropriately used in patients with chronic renal failure to exclude obstructive uropathy as the cause.[54, 55] In general, only retroperitoneal fibrosis leads to chronic renal failure due to obstruction, without urinary tract dilatation (Fig. 12–39) or some other sonographic abnormality.[18, 56] Occasionally with staghorn calculi, significant hydronephrosis may be absent behind the stone when it is responsible for renal failure without associated dilatation.[55] Identification of the characteristic acoustic shadow from the large stone should lead to the correct diagnosis.

Ultrasound may be over-utilized in patients with acute

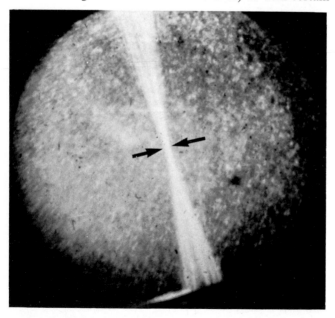

Figure 12–34. Schleiren photograph demonstrating the beam of a focused transducer. The focal zone (*arrows*) is clearly demarcated. (From Rosenfield AT, Taylor KJW, Jaffe CC: Clinical applications of ultrasound tissue characterization. *In* James AE: Advances in Ultrasonography. Radiol Clin North Am 13:31–58, 1980.)

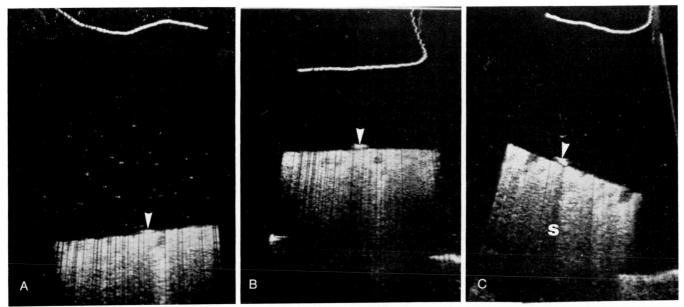

Figure 12–35. Beam focusing and shadowing. A gallstone was placed on a surgical sponge and examined within a water bath in vitro. *A,* The gallstone (*arrowhead*) is in the far field of the transducer. No acoustic shadow is seen. *B,* When the gallstone (*arrowhead*) is in the near field of the transducer, no acoustic shadow is delineated. *C,* With the gallstone (*arrowhead*) in the focal zone of the transducer, a definite acoustic shadow (s) is demonstrated. (From Rosenfield AT, Taylor KJW, Dembner AG, Jacobsen P: Ultrasound of the renal sinus: New observations. AJR 133(3):441–448, 1979, © Am Roentgen Ray Soc.)

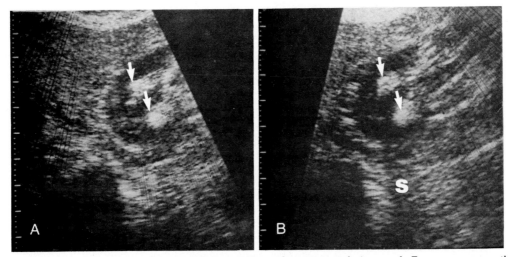

Figure 12–36. Sonographic recognition of nephrolithiasis. Effect of varying techniques. *A,* Transverse scan through the right upper quadrant demonstrating the liver and the right kidney in a patient known to have right nephrolithiasis. Intense echoes from the stone (*arrows*) are similar to those in the renal sinus, given the technical factors being used. The stones are not in the focal zone of the transducer. *B,* The stones (*arrows*) are in the focal zone of the transducer, and a lower far gain is used; an acoustic shadow (s) is identified. Technical factors are crucial in the identification of the acoustic shadow when it is associated with nephrolithiasis. (From Rosenfield AT, Taylor KJW, Dembner AG, Jacobsen P: Ultrasound of the renal sinus: New observations. AJR 133(3):441–448, 1979, © Am Roentgen Ray Soc.)

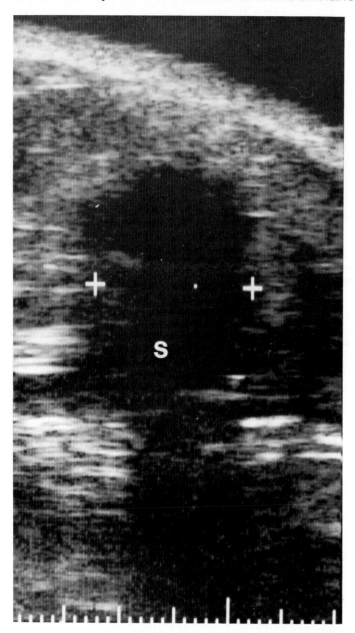

Figure 12–37. An ultrasound examination of a breast tumor (between the two cursors) demonstrates a relatively echo-free tumor. An acoustic shadow (s) is seen because of the high absorption of the ultrasound beam by the tumor. (From Rosenfield AT, Taylor KJW, Jaffe CC: Clinical applications of ultrasound tissue characterization. Radiol Clin North Am 18:31–58, 1980.)

Figure 12–38. Diagram of potential causes of acoustic shadowing.

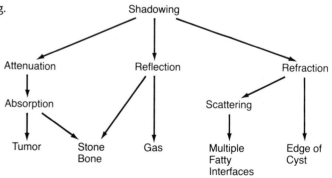

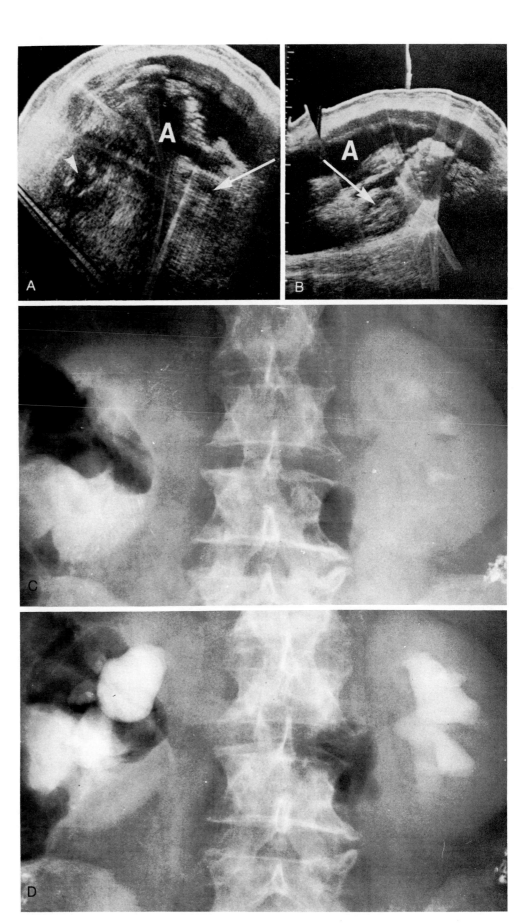

Figure 12–39. Retroperitoneal fibrosis secondary to metastatic breast carcinoma. *A,* Transverse sonographic scan through the abdomen at the level of the kidneys with the patient supine demonstrates significant ascites (A). There is dilatation of the right collecting system (*arrowhead*) but the left renal sinus (*arrow*) is a dense zone of echoes without evidence of hydronephrotic change. *B,* Longitudinal scan through the left hemiabdomen demonstrates ascites (A) and the renal sinus of the left kidney without dilatation (*arrow*). *C,* Three-minute film from an excretory urogram demonstrates right hydronephrosis without significant fullness to the opacified portion of the left collecting system. *D,* At 10 minutes, which is the height of the osmotic diuresis, there is marked right hydronephrosis and now significant left hydronephrosis can be seen. Note the change in calyceal size from the earlier 3-minute film. Since sonography was performed without applying fluid stress, no dilatation of the left collecting system was present. (From Rosenfield AT, Taylor KJW, Dembner AG, Jacobsen P: Ultrasound of the renal sinus: New observations. AJR 133(3): 441–448, 1979, © Am Roentgen Ray Soc.)

obstruction.[56a] Falsely normal studies occur if patients are scanned before significant dilatation of the urinary tract, in instances of renal colic or in other situations such as rupture of a fornix that decompresses the system.[57] Although the approach to acute renal failure is controversial, we believe that urography is the best technique to exclude acute urinary tract obstruction if renal function is adequate.

The presence of a dilated urinary tract is not indicative of obstructive uropathy and can be seen in a number of situations including high flow (e.g., diabetes insipidus), vesicoureteral reflux, papillary necrosis, and postobstructive atrophy.[57]

Disproportionate ureterectasis, as compared with pyelectasis, is typically seen with decreased ureteral motility (such as in prune belly syndrome),[58] with vesicoureteral reflux, and in most cases of primary megaureter.

Medical Renal Disease and Other Global Parenchymal Abnormalities

Ultrasound produces information different from that which is available by CT or urography. In particular, the acoustic properties of the tissues being interrogated are identified. The apparent echogenicity of the structure being examined is dependent on the frequency and shape of the beam as well as on the tissues through which it must travel before reaching the structure and is not an absolute number (see Fig. 12–18). Since all texture is relative on standard B scans, contiguous areas are generally compared. Because after the neonatal period the echogenicity of the renal cortex is less than that of the adjacent liver, it has become a standard place to evaluate echogenicity.[5, 6, 59–61]

Renal ultrasound patterns can be divided into two groups: (1) those that lead to an increase in cortical echogenicity with preservation of corticomedullary definition, and (2) those that distort corticomedullary definition in a diffuse, focal, or multifocal pattern.[6] The first type (Type I) is a relatively distinct pattern that can be identified only by ultrasonography and can be of aid in differential diagnosis.[59–68] In medical renal diseases, both acute and chronic, such as acute or chronic glomerulonephritis, the echo intensity of the cortex increases with preservation of corticomedullary definition (Fig. 12–40).[59–64] This pattern is nonspecific and can be seen in any medical renal disease. In one series, the most intense echogenicity was seen with active cellular infiltration, whereas less intense echoes were seen with interstitial scarring.[60] However, one cannot predict the underlying disease being studied.[59] For example, glomerulonephritis and leukemia can produce identical pictures.

Nonetheless, this is a readily recognizable pattern, which when bilateral leads to a specific differential diagnosis of three groups of diseases: (1) the medical renal diseases,[59–61] (2) infiltrative diseases—amyloidosis[62] and leukemic infiltration,[63, 64] and (3) diseases that cause cortical nephrocalcinosis (Fig. 12–41)[61, 65–67] even before calcification is identifiable on the radiograph (these diseases include Alport's disease,[61] chronic glomerulonephritis, oxalosis,[65–67] and renal cortical necrosis). Oxalosis may alternatively lead to increased echoes in both cortex and medulla.[67] A unilateral increase in cortical echogenicity

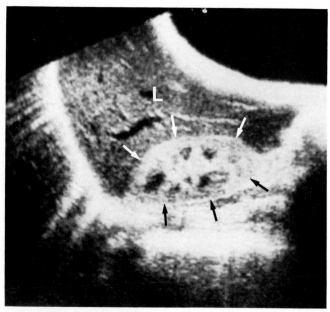

Figure 12–40. Medical renal disease (diabetic glomerulosclerosis). Longitudinal sonographic scan through the right upper quadrant shows the liver (L) and right kidney (*arrows*). Note that there is a reversal of the normal ratio of echogenicity, with the kidney being much more echogenic than the liver and the echoes in the cortex being equal to those in the renal sinus. High-level echoes in the kidney with preservation of corticomedullary definition is typical of medical renal disease. The left kidney was of similar appearance.

with preservation of corticomedullary definition is generally limited to subacute renal vein thrombosis (a stage reached after approximately 10 days and lasting from months to years),[68] but occasionally it is seen in acute pyelonephritis. Ultrasonography can be used to follow patients with medical renal disease when they are undergoing therapy to see whether improvement occurs. Cortical echogenicity will decrease with such improvement.[60] At times, a specific diagnosis can be suggested. For example, in a patient with hemoptysis and pulmonary infiltrates, this Type-I ultrasound pattern is typical of Goodpasture's syndrome.

An entirely different pattern of density is that of intense echoes within the pyramids (Type II). This is the reverse pattern of medical renal disease in which intense echoes occur within the cortex. The pyramids will be visualized as rounded or triangular echogenic structures (Fig. 12–42). This pattern is typically seen in conditions that produce medullary nephrocalcinosis,[69–71] a group that is composed primarily of diseases that cause hypercalcemia and/or hypercalciuria. Early medullary nephrocalcinosis can be seen as echogenic pyramids before the identification of calcium on standard radiographs.[71] Later, the pyramids become highly reflective and may have associated acoustic shadowing. Another cause of echogenic pyramids is dehydration in infancy with subsequent precipitation of Tamm-Horsfall protein in the tubules.[72] In addition, autosomal-recessive (infantile) polycystic kidney disease, which typically causes marked increase in central echoes with a thin hypoechoic rim,[73] can in a minority of cases lead to echogenic pyramids (Fig. 12–43).[74]

The ability to define global renal diseases by their sonographic pattern is important, because it is unique information. Besides the Type-I pattern and increased

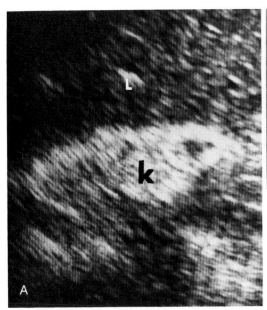
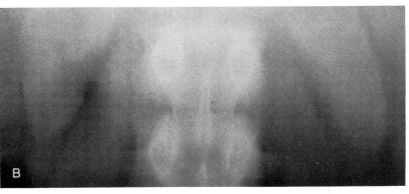

Figure 12–41. Cortical nephrocalcinosis secondary to chronic glomerulonephritis. *A,* Longitudinal scan through the right upper quadrant shows the kidney (k) and liver (L). Note the intense echoes in the cortex of the kidney, as compared with those in the liver. *B,* Linear tomography without intravenous contrast medium demonstrates the kidneys to be small and very dense (with the periphery most dense of all), consistent with cortical nephrocalcinosis.

medullary echoes, other patterns can also lead to a limited differential diagnosis. For example, a unilateral global decrease in cortical echogenicity with loss of cortico-medullary definition when identified in a patient with acute symptoms should lead to a differential diagnosis of only two entities: acute renal vein thrombosis[68] and acute pyelonephritis.[75] Occasionally, this pattern may also be seen with renal infarction in the acute to subacute phase, although infarction may also produce an echogenic focus within the parenchyma.[76] When a global decrease in cortical echogenicity with loss of corticomedullary definition is seen in a patient without acute symptoms, infiltrative tumors such as lymphoma as well as diffuse chronic inflammatory diseases such as xanthogranuloma-tous pyelonephritis[77] and malacoplakia[78] all should be considered in the differential diagnosis. Nonetheless, a relatively limited number of diseases produce this pattern. In approaching the renal sonogram, it is therefore nec-

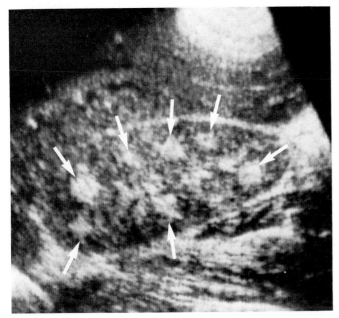

Figure 12–42. Medullary nephrocalcinosis. Longitudinal so-nographic scan through the right kidney of a patient with hypercalcemia demonstrates echogenic foci (*arrows*) within the pyramids. The other kidney was similar in appearance. In medullary nephrocalcinosis, echogenic pyramids can be seen earlier than calcium can be visualized with standard radiography. When the calcification is more pronounced, there may be associated acoustic shadowing from the pyramid.

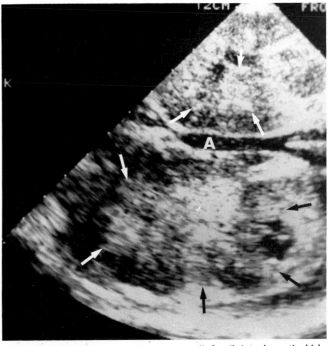

Figure 12–43. Autosomal-recessive (infantile) polycystic kid-ney disease (APKD) with dense pyramids. Coronal scan through the abdomen of a child with APKD demonstrates nephrome-galy. The kidneys are seen on both sides of the aorta (A). The pyramids contiguous with the renal sinus are echogenic (*ar-rows*), while the peripheral cortex is hypoechoic.

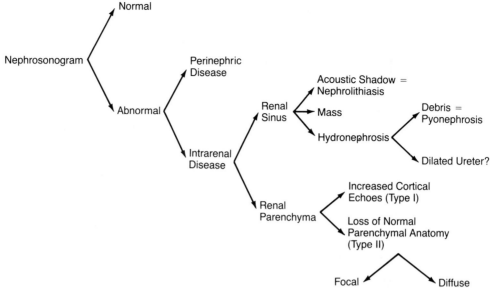

Figure 12–44. Logical approach to the renal sonogram. An approach to renal ultrasonography requires one to determine whether an abnormality is present in the perinephric tissues or in the kidney itself. Lesions of the kidney can be divided into those that are in the renal sinus and those that are in the renal parenchyma. All renal parenchymal diseases can be further divided into two groups: those that produce increased cortical echoes with preservation of cortical medullary definition (Type I) and those that cause a loss of normal parenchymal anatomy in a focal or diffuse manner (Type II). (From Rosenfield AT, Taylor KJW, Crade M, DeGraaf CS: Anatomy and pathology of the kidney by gray scale ultrasonography. Radiology 128:737–744, 1978.)

essary to define whether one is dealing with disease of the renal sinus or of the renal parenchyma. If hydronephrosis is present, one must try to identify whether the ureter is dilated or whether internal echoes or masses are within the hydronephrotic system. If renal parenchymal disease is present, one must determine whether it is global or focal, whether corticomedullary definition is preserved or lost, and whether there is an increase or decrease in echogenicity as compared with normal renal parenchyma in the area of abnormality. By so doing, a relatively narrow differential diagnosis is frequently possible. When the sonogram is combined with other imaging studies and the clinical history, a specific diagnosis can usually be made. Our approach to the renal sonogram is defined in Fig. 12–44.

Cysts and Echo-Poor Masses

The typical cyst is recognized sonographically by its intrinsic properties and by the artifacts associated with it. As noted in experimental and clinical work, a cyst is generally echo free and has a smooth back wall (Figs. 12–45 to 12–48).[81, 82] The absence of echoes within the cyst is due to the lack of interfaces to reflect the ultrasound beam. However, echoes may be seen in the anterior portion of the cyst due to the *reverberation artifact*.[83] This artifact should not be confused with internal echoes. It is due to the delayed return of echoes that have been reflected back and forth within a structure being interpreted by the scanner as originating from a deeper structure. The echo is thus depicted in the wrong location. Multiple reverberations cause multiple, entirely separate echoes. This artifact exactly recapitulates the soft tissues anterior to the cyst, but with lower intensity (Fig. 12–48). In addition, imaging from a different direction fails to reproduce these echoes in a similar location. Two artifacts are crucial in the identification of cysts, particu-

larly when the cystic structure is complicated and has internal echoes. The first artifact is enhancement posterior to the cyst (good through transmission) (Figs. 12–45, 12–46).[84] The ultrasound scanner is manually adjusted by the

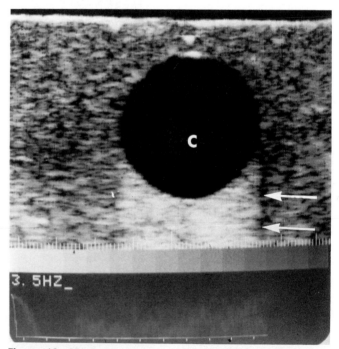

Figure 12–45. Cystic mass and tissue-equivalent phantom. A cystic mass (C) is seen within a tissue-equivalent phantom. The mass is echo free, a finding typical of a cyst. The brightness of the echoes behind the cyst is greater than that behind the adjacent tissue, increased through transmission because there is less attenuation of the beam by the cystic mass. Emanating from the junction of the cystic mass and solid tissue is an acoustic shadow (*arrows*). This shadow (the "refractive artifact") is due to refraction caused by the difference between the speed of sound in the fluid and that in the adjacent soft tissue.

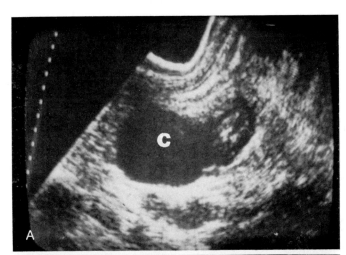

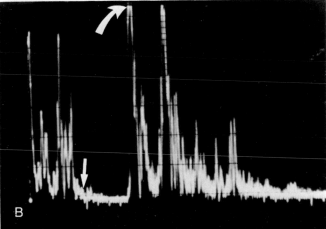

Figure 12—46. Left renal cyst. *A,* Coronal sonographic scan through the left upper quadrant shows a cyst (c) extending from the top of the left kidney. Note that the echoes behind the cyst are more intense than the echoes behind adjacent solid tissue at a comparable distance from the transducer. *B,* A-mode tracing through the renal cyst. Note that there are more intense echoes from the back wall of the renal cyst (*curved arrow*) than from the front wall. Note also the low-level internal echoes in the anterior portion of the cyst (*straight arrow*) representing a reverberation artifact.

TGC curve to increase the intensity of distal echoes as compared with proximal ones in order to offset the attenuation of the ultrasound beam in tissue; consequently, the lack of attenuation through the cyst leads to artifactual enhancement of the echoes behind it. The second major artifact is the *refraction* artifact discussed earlier in this chapter.[55] An acoustic shadow can frequently be seen at the junction of cystic and solid structures (Figs. 12–45, 12–47). This artifact is thought to be due to the differing speeds of sound in fluid and soft tissues and must be searched for with meticulous scanning techniques.

Although ultrasonography is the most accurate technique for discriminating between cystic and noncystic structures, a number of pitfalls exist. The accuracy of ultrasonography in identifying cysts is directly related to the experience of the person performing the examination. The following problems can arise:[85]

1. Reverberation can occur from the skin transducer interface and also from specular reflectors anterior to the cyst as described above. These lines can be verified to be artifacts by having the beam strike the reflector at a

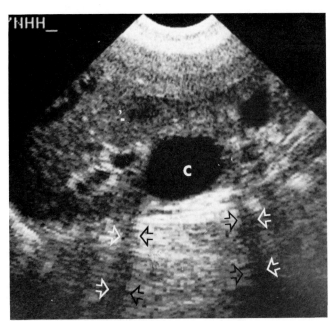

Figure 12—47. Refractive artifact. A cystic mass (c) is seen on the longitudinal scan through the right upper quadrant. This cyst demonstrates excellent through transmission with intense echoes behind it. Also, note the refractive shadow from the edges of the cyst (*open arrows*).

different angle or by scanning the cyst from a different approach.

2. Artifactual echoes in small cysts occur if they are not in the focal zone of the transducer. The ultrasound beam is typically focused by the transducer leading to the narrowest width of the beam in the focal zone (Fig. 12–34), whereas the beam is wider in the near and far fields.

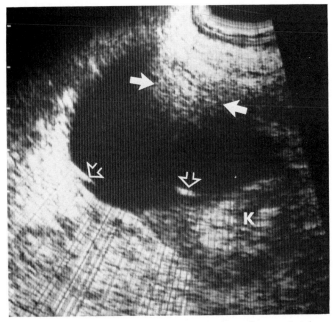

Figure 12—48. Simple, partially septated renal cyst. A transverse sonographic scan through the left kidney (K) demonstrates a cyst protruding lateral to the kidney. Note the partial septation (*open arrows*) within the cyst. Note also the reverberation artifact in the anterior portion of the cyst (*solid arrows*). Scanning from other projections demonstrated that the reverberation artifact was not a constant finding. The cyst is otherwise echo free. It has a smooth back wall and demonstrates good through transmission.

The beam at its origin is no narrower than the diameter of the transducer face, although it may narrow considerably at the focal point. Beyond the focal point, there is divergence of the beam width in the far field. Thus, off-axis reflectors can be projected as being within the beam, if the observed lesion is not in the focal zone of the transducer (12–49A,B). For a 1-cm cyst being interrogated by a medium internally focused transducer of 19 mm in diameter, only the portion of the beam 3 to 12 cm from the transducer will be equal to or smaller than the cyst; in other regions, even low-level reflectors adjacent to the cyst will contribute artifactual echoes that seem to

be within the cyst. In addition, the reflective characteristics of the adjacent tissue determine the extent to which this beam width artifact plays a role. A small cyst within the normally hypoechoic renal cortex is more resistant to off-axis reflectors than cysts in the substance of the liver that are surrounded by tissue of higher echogenicity. One solution to this problem is to employ swept-focus electronic arrays, such as the linear or phased arrays, and to avoid the use of a fixed-focus transducer in this application. Figure 12–8 shows an example of a cyst that is close to the transducer face but is shown clearly because this electronically steered array employs swept focusing. This

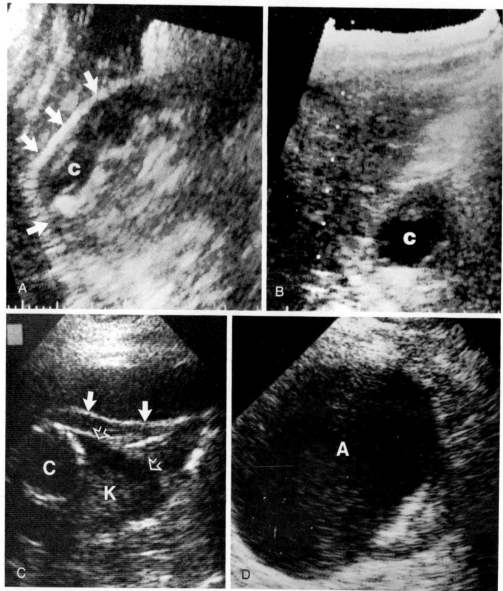

Figure 12–49. Problems in accurately identifying renal lesions. *A,* Renal cyst. With the cyst (C) in the near field of the transducer, artifactual internal echoes prevent characterization of the lesion. (Arrows indicate fat between the liver and right kidney.) *B,* When the patient is repositioned so that the renal cyst is within the focal zone of the transducer, the lesion is seen to be echo free. (*A, B,* from Rosenfield AT, Taylor KJW, Jaffe CC: Clinical applications of ultrasound tissue characterization. *In* James AE (ed): Advances in Ultrasonography. Radiol Clin North Am 18:34–58, 1980.) *C,* Calcified renal cyst. Coronal scan through the left kidney (K) shows the calcified cyst (C). Note that the walls of the cyst are highly reflective. Attenuation of the ultrasound beam by calcium in the walls leads in this case to some degree of acoustic shadowing distal to the cyst. (Open arrows define the lateral border of the kidney. Solid arrows define Gerota's fascia.) *D,* Renal abscess. A transverse scan through the kidney of a patient with fever demonstrates a mass (A) containing low-level echoes. There is good transmission through the mass. Complex cystic masses with internal echoes can be caused by a number of disorders, including abscess, hemorrhagic cyst, infected cyst, and necrotic tumor.

technique enables visualization of the lesion without sacrificing detail of the more distant structures. Such a structure may be lost in the near-field artifacts of a fixed focus abdominal scanner.

3. Conversely, an absence of echoes may be seen in a number of situations in which the lesion is not cystic. This is true because some solid masses may appear hypoechoic or even anechoic if they produce substantial acoustic absorption. This will be recognized on the ultrasound scan by an absence of acoustic enhancement distal to the lesion or, at times, some degree of acoustic shadowing (see Fig. 12–37).

4. Acoustic enhancement behind a cyst is a major finding indicating a fluid-filled lesion. This is true even in the presence of internal echoes, which are seen with some complex fluid collections. However, acoustic enhancement is an artifact resulting from the manual setting of the conventional TGC curves for the expected attenuation of solid tissues. Since tissue attenuation increases with acoustic frequency, one must increase the slope of the TGC curve when the frequency is increased, in order to penetrate adequately through tissue. Consequently, for a small cyst the distal sonic enhancement is most visible at higher frequencies.[85] In addition, in the focal zone, the beam intensity is concentrated over smaller areas and is greater. When the cyst is in the focal zone, the tissues distal to it demonstrate greater sonic enhancement in addition to the effect of the TGC slope. If a cyst is calcified, the attenuation of the beam by the calcium eliminates the expected enhancement behind the cyst (and may even produce acoustic shadowing behind the cyst (Fig. 12–49C). CT is required to evaluate calcified cysts.

Therefore, small cysts can be misinterpreted as solid masses without meticulous attention to technique. Ideally, the mass should be within the focal zone of the transducer, since this is the region in which the cyst will be most resistant to artifactual off-axis signals. The clinician and imager should be aware that *the larger the mass, the greater the likelihood that the ultrasound characterization will be accurate.*

When a mass containing low-level echoes is identified in the kidney, the initial determination must be made of whether it is a cyst or a solid structure (Fig. 12–49D). For this reason, one must carefully search for the artifacts described above. If the lesion is solid, a number of causes are possible, including tumor and focal infection. A CT scan can aid in discriminating among these possibilities.[86] A tumor will typically be a focal solid mass (see Figs. 12–54, 12–55). Acute focal bacterial nephritis (lobar nephronia), which is usually an echo-poor mass[87, 88] (see Fig. 12–59), will present as a wedge-shaped or inhomogeneous mass leading to a defect in the nephrogram. Frequently associated wedge-shaped lucencies appear in other parts of the kidneys.[89] In addition, a delayed CT scan may show contrast medium within the mass at a time when the nephrogram is clearing in the rest of the kidney.[90] Slow flow to the affected portion of the kidney, which nonetheless consists of functioning renal parenchyma, accounts for this pattern. Gallium scanning, in our experience, typically shows intense activity within the mass and also frequently shows activity within the remainder of the affected kidney and/or within a contralateral kidney.[87] However, one should be aware that renal cell carcinoma can occasionally be, and that lymphoma typically is, gallium avid. Sequential ultrasound scans showing disappearance of the mass following therapy is required for a firm diagnosis. Thus, coordinated imaging plays an important role in defining the echo-poor mass. In difficult diagnostic cases, needle aspiration under sonographic or CT guidance can be performed for a firm diagnosis.

The Echogenic Focus

The evaluation of an echogenic mass by means of ultrasonography differs markedly from that using other techniques and serves as an excellent example of the sonographic approach. When examining a mass sonographically, careful dynamic scanning to trace the exact location of the mass is needed. In addition, artifacts are important to the process of characterizing the mass and in deciding on the next diagnostic study.

As noted above, the *renal sinus* is typically an ovoid echogenic central structure. Several variants of the sinus occur and must be appreciated. In some patients, two separate renal sinuses can be seen (Fig. 12–50). Although it has been suggested in the literature that patients with a nonobstructed duplicated collecting system will have two separate renal sinuses,[91] in a review of material in our institution, we found that most kidneys with a nonobstructed duplicated collecting system had a single renal sinus, whereas most patients with two separate echogenic foci representing the renal sinus had a single bifid col-

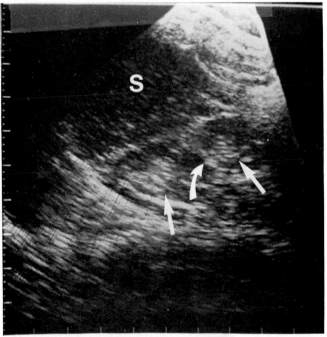

Figure 12–50. Longitudinal sonographic section through the left kidney demonstrates the renal sinus to consist of two echogenic foci (*straight arrows*). By means of urography, a single bifid collecting system was seen in this kidney. In our experience, most of these kidneys have a bifid collecting system, rather than a completely duplicated system. Although some patients with a duplicated collecting system have two separate renal sinuses, most have a single renal sinus. Note the oblique line between the two portions of the kidney, representing an edge of the junctional parenchymal defect (*curved arrow*) (see Fig. 12–51). (S = spleen.)

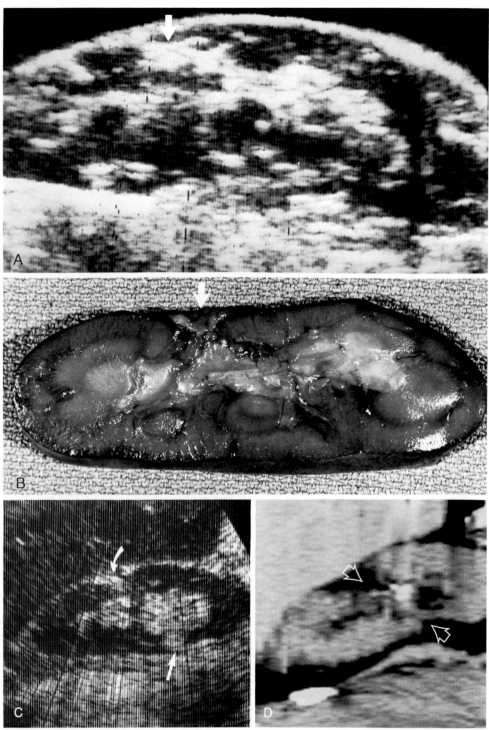

Figure 12–51. Junctional parenchymal defect. *A,* Sagittal sonogram of a cadaver kidney in a water bath demonstrates the anterior echogenic defect (*arrow*) in the parenchyma. *B,* Sagittal section of the same cadaver kidney demonstrated in *A* shows a triangle of fat (*arrow*) extending to the renal sinus and corresponding to the echogenic focus shown in *A. C,* Sagittal sonogram of a normal right kidney possessing both the anterior (*curved arrow*) and posterior (*straight arrow*) junctional parenchymal defects. The anterior junctional parenchymal defect in this case may mimic a scar, whereas the posterior junctional parenchymal defect may mimic an echogenic mass such as angiomyolipoma. *D,* Sagittal reformation of a CT scan performed on the same patient demonstrated in *C.* Fat (*open arrows*) contiguous with the sinus and perinephric fat accounts for the echogenic nature of the junctional parenchymal defect. (From Carter AR, Horgan JG, Jennings TA, Rosenfield AT: The junctional parenchymal defect: A sonographic variant of renal anatomy. Radiology 154:499–502, 1985.)

lecting system.[92] Thus, ultrasonography cannot be used prior to gastrointestinal or gynecological surgery to determine whether the collecting system is single or duplicated. Urography is required for this purpose.

Another major normal variant of renal anatomy is the *junctional parenchymal defect*.[93, 94] In many patients, sagittal scans of the right kidney demonstrate a triangular echogenic mass located in the anterior aspect of the upper-pole parenchyma (Fig. 12–51), and in some patients, a similar structure can be identified in the posterior aspect of the lower-pole parenchyma.[93] Although these echogenic foci are typically triangular, simulating cortical scars, round foci can mimic a small angiomyolipoma (Fig. 12–51). We believe that this normal variant of renal anatomy is related to the formation of the kidney in utero by fusion of upper- and lower-pole parenchymal masses.[95] These two masses or renunculi typically fuse so that the renal sinus is facing in the same direction. However, in some patients, as noted on routine CT, the upper-pole renal mass has the sinus facing medially or posteromedially. The renal vein typically enters the upper-pole sinus, and the renal pelvis exits the lower-pole sinus. As one traces the renal sinus on transverse sections from upper to lower pole, the sinus in these patients turns in a corkscrew fashion from an oblique anteroposterior axis to a transverse axis. A spectrum of fusion of the renal parenchyma is seen in the adult kidney. Just as fetal lobations are variably encountered, distinct renunculi with an associated junctional parenchymal defect are not constant findings. The diagnosis of this normal variant is made by careful scanning so that one can note the characteristic location and trace it into the renal sinus.

A *renal cortical scar* produces a loss of parenchyma with associated echogenicity within the affected parenchyma beneath the scar. This occurs typically after renal infarction or chronic atrophic pyelonephritis (Fig. 12–52).[95] In these situations, the echogenicity within the parenchyma is presumably due to the collagen deposit within the associated scar.

Crossed renal ectopia represents an uncommon congenital abnormality, in which both kidneys are situated on the same side of the abdomen; however, one of the two ureters crosses the midline to the vesicle orifice on the contralateral side. The kidneys may be nonfused or fused. This lesion can produce several abnormalities regarding echogenic foci in the kidney.[96] First, two separate collecting systems may be seen, and thus a duplicated collecting system may be mimicked (Fig. 12–53A). Second, with either a crossed fused renal ectopia or a crossed nonfused renal ectopia, a major problem relates to the empty renal fossa. As noted above, in cases of renal agenesis or ectopia, the anatomical splenic flexure occupies the left renal fossa, and the hepatic flexure occupies the right renal fossa. Bowel in the renal fossa may simulate a mass replacing the kidney. In some such cases, a kidney may be mistakenly identified as normal (the echogenic feces may mimic a normal renal sinus with the less echogenic fluid around it mimicking renal parenchyma), or fat between the loops of colon may mimic the renal sinus (Fig. 12–53B). Recognition of the crossed kidney is necessary to make the correct diagnosis. In most cases of crossed fused renal ectopia, the kidney is larger than normal. In addition, there is a characteristic echogenic notch anteriorly and/or posteriorly, where the two fused kidneys join (Fig. 12–53A). The notch, which is a significant clue to crossed fused renal ectopia, will not be contiguous with the renal sinus as is the junctional parenchymal defect.

Renal cell carcinoma may produce either a mass that is echo poor or one that is echogenic (Fig. 12–54).[97, 98] The typical findings of a solid mass will be seen with none of the artifacts noted below that are associated with fluid. Although attempts have been made to determine the nature of the solid mass based on its echogenicity, no definitive tissue characterization can currently be performed using ultrasonography. *Wilms's tumor* usually produces a homogeneously echogenic mass (Fig. 12–55).[99] There may be necrosis within it.

The *angiomyolipoma* is a mass that typically is very bright.[101, 102] The high reflectivity of this lesion is a strong clue to the presence of fat and should lead one to obtain a CT scan to confirm the lesion. Small angiomyolipomas

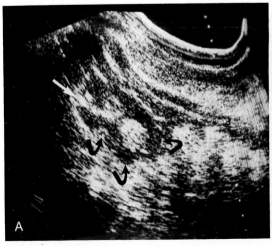
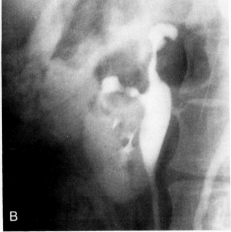

Figure 12–52. Chronic atrophic pyelonephritis (reflux nephropathy). *A,* Longitudinal sonographic scan through the kidney demonstrates loss of parenchyma in the upper pole with extension of the calyx and renal sinus to the edge of the kidney (*straight arrow*). The parenchyma about the calyx is echogenic. Curved arrows outline the unscarred lower pole. The finding of an echogenic focus associated with loss of parenchyma and continuity of the renal sinus is typical of scarring. *B,* Corresponding excretory urogram. (From Kay CJ, Rosenfield AT, Taylor KJW, Rosenberg MA: Ultrasound grey-scale characteristics of chronic atrophic pyelonephritis. AJR 132(1):47–49, 1979, © Am Roentgen Ray Soc.)

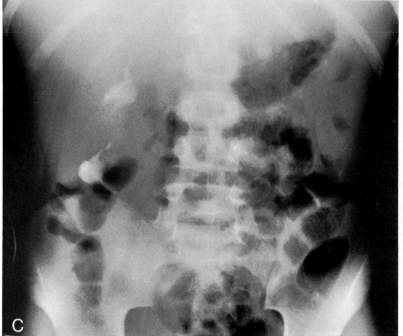

Figure 12–53. Crossed fused renal ectopia. *A,* Longitudinal scan through the right renal fossa demonstrates a reniform structure with an echogenic notch *(curved arrow)* (L = liver). *B,* Coronal scan through the left renal fossa demonstrates the spleen (S). The reniform-like structure *(curved arrows)* with a central echogenic zone is the anatomical splenic flexure. This could be mistaken for an abnormal kidney. Note also the acoustic shadowing distal to the central echogenic zone and the echogenic notch *(open arrow). C,* Corresponding film from an excretory urogram demonstrates crossed fused renal ectopia. The anatomical splenic flexure is medial in position. (From McCarthy SM, Rosenfield AT: Ultrasonography in crossed renal ectopia. J Ultrasound Med 3:107–112, 1984, by the American Institute of Ultrasound in Medicine.)

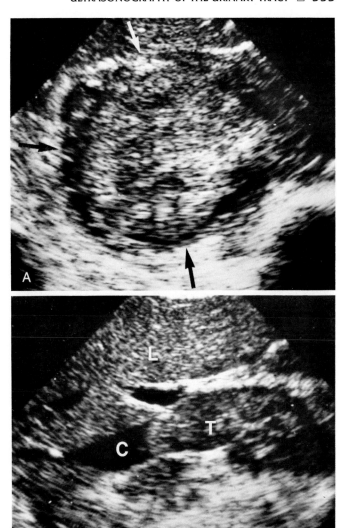

Figure 12–54. Renal cell carcinoma with tumor within the inferior vena cava. *A,* Longitudinal sonographic scan through the upper pole of the right kidney demonstrates a large solid echogenic mass (*arrows*). This represents an example of an echogenic mass in the kidney from renal cell carcinoma. Renal cell carcinoma may also be hypoechoic. *B,* Longitudinal scan through the inferior vena cava demonstrates an echogenic mass within the cava which represented tumor (T). (C = inferior cava above the tumor. L = liver.)

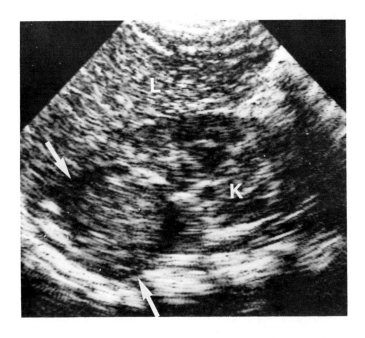

Figure 12–55. Wilms' tumor. An echogenic mass (*arrows*) is seen in the posteroinferior aspect of the right kidney representing Wilms' tumor. Note the hypoechoic rim about the mass, most likely representing a capsule or pseudocapsule. (K = remainder of the right kidney. L = liver.)

are not uncommon incidental findings. In some large angiomyolipomas, a characteristic artifact, the *speed propagation artifact*, may be present. Since the speed of sound in fat is significantly slower than that in soft tissue, specular reflectors posterior to the angiomyolipoma will be written more distally than expected, as compared with structures posterior to soft tissue. This is because it takes longer for the sound beam to traverse the fatty mass, both going and returning. Since the time it takes for the echo to return to the transducer determines its position in the picture, this artifact results.[101] Figure 12–56 demonstrates a myelolipoma of the adrenal with a speed propagation artifact.

Renal abscesses may be echo free, may contain low-level echoes (Fig. 12–49), or may be highly reflective. When echo free, they are readily recognized as cystic structures. When they contain an echogenic material, particularly when they are highly reflective, sonographic artifacts are used to determine their cystic nature. The two major artifacts are good through transmission and a refractive shadow. The identification of enhanced transmission behind the mass and/or a refractive shadow is strong evidence that one is dealing with a fluid-containing mass and not solid tissue (Fig. 12–57). In the proper clinical setting, this finding should lead to puncture both for diagnosis and for therapy. Gas may be present within the abscess. As noted previously, gas produces a "dirty" acoustic shadow due to reverberation between the transducer and skin (Fig. 12–58).[55] At times a solid streak or series of parallel bands radiating away from gas may be seen ("ring-down" artifact). The ring-down artifact has been postulated to be secondary to resonance traveling back to the transducer from a horn-shaped fluid collection trapped by the air bubbles.[103]

Blood within the renal parenchyma is of variable echogenicity, but at some stage it is highly reflective. An acute *renal infarct* can produce a highly reflective mass[78] as can *hemorrhagic pyelonephritis* (Fig. 12–59).[104] Correlation with CT is extremely useful because blood at this stage is frequently of higher attenuation on a noncontrast scan than is normal renal parenchyma. Thus, hemorrhagic focal pyelonephritis, as well as acute renal hemorrhagic infarction, can cause echogenic masses seen with ultrasonography.

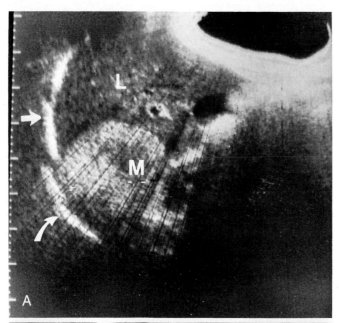

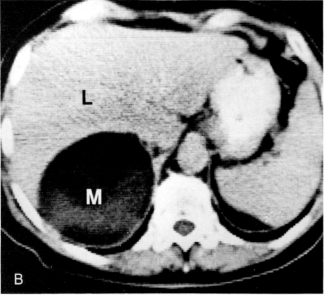

Figure 12–56. Adrenal myelolipoma demonstrating *speed propagation artifact. A,* Longitudinal scan through the right upper quadrant demonstrates an echogenic mass (M) behind the liver (L). The mass is highly reflective, consistent with it being of fatty density. Note that the portion of the diaphragm behind the liver (*straight arrow*) is closer to the transducer face than the portion of the diaphragm behind the mass (*curved arrow*). This artifact is due to the slower speed of sound in the fatty mass than in the liver. *B,* CT scan verifies the fatty adrenal masses (M). (L = liver). These findings are typical of a myelolipoma when seen in the adrenal. Similar findings in the kidney occur with angiomyelolipomas. (From Richman TS, Taylor KJW, Kremkau FW: Propagation speed artifact in a fatty tumor (myelolipoma): Significance for tissue differential diagnosis. J Ultrasound Med 2:45–47, 1983, by the American Institute of Ultrasound in Medicine.)

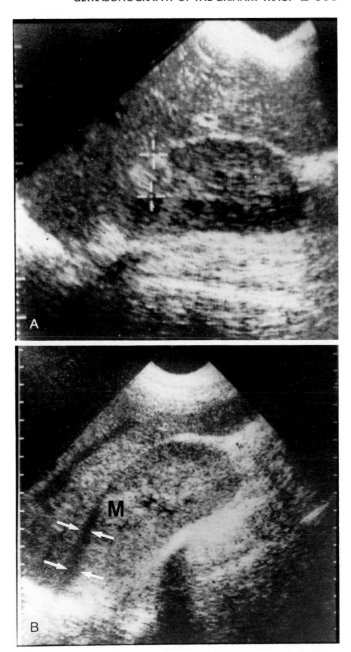

Figure 12–57. Refractive artifact. An abscess containing echogenic fluid. *A,* Longitudinal sonographic scan through the right kidney demonstrates a small echogenic focus in a patient with fever. Cursors identify the echogenic focus. *B,* Real-time sonographic scan demonstrates a refractive shadow (*arrows*) at the junction of the echogenic mass and solid tissue that is most consistent with a mass that contains echogenic fluid. At surgery, a small renal abscess was identified in this location. (M = renal mass.)

Calcium within the parenchyma, either dystrophic or as part of nephrocalcinosis, produces intense echoes and may be associated with acoustic shadowing.

The sonographic findings in echogenic masses are summarized in Table 12–2.

LOWER URINARY TRACT ULTRASONOGRAPHY

The Bladder

The bladder conforms to a great extent to surrounding tissues. On transverse scans, the male bladder is seen as a fluid-filled structure superior and anterior to the prostate and extending superior to the seminal vesicles as well (Fig. 12–60). The iliopsoas muscles can be seen lateral to the bladder. In the female, the uterus and the adnexal regions are well seen posterior to the bladder (Fig. 12–61). During the typical ultrasound examination, the blad-

der is used as a sonographic window to examine the genital tract and the pelvis for masses. However, lesions of the bladder itself can be identified and to some extent staged. Of equal importance, the bladder can create major pitfalls during the ultrasonic study. This is primarily because contrast medium, ascites, fluid in the bladder, blood, and cystic masses may all have a similar location and appearance.[104a] The bladder can be scanned through the anterior abdominal wall (Fig. 12–61), per rectum or per urethra using an intracavitary probe (Fig. 12–62) in the bladder.

Indications. The urinary bladder is easily identified when fluid filled. Therefore, ultrasonically guided suprapubic urinary bladder aspiration is a rapid and simple technique to obtain urine for bacteriologic examination.[105] The distance from the skin, as well as the angle of the needle can readily be determined sonographically.

Ultrasonography also permits an estimation of bladder volume. A recommended approach to the volume is to use the formula (0.625 ht $\times$ w $\times$ d).[106] This has been

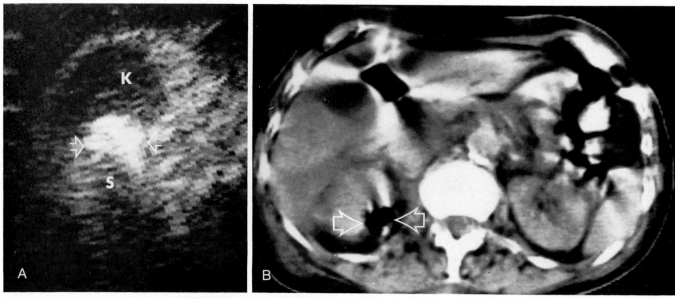

Figure 12–58. Gas-containing renal infection in a diabetic. *A,* Transverse sonographic scan through the right kidney (k) with the patient prone. An area of intense echoes (*open arrows*) is seen in the posterior portion of the right kidney. Note the acoustic shadow (s) distal to this focus. There are internal echoes within the acoustic shadow (a "dirty shadow"), a phenomenon commonly seen when gas is the cause of this artifact. *B,* CT scan of the same patient verifies the gas (*open arrows*).

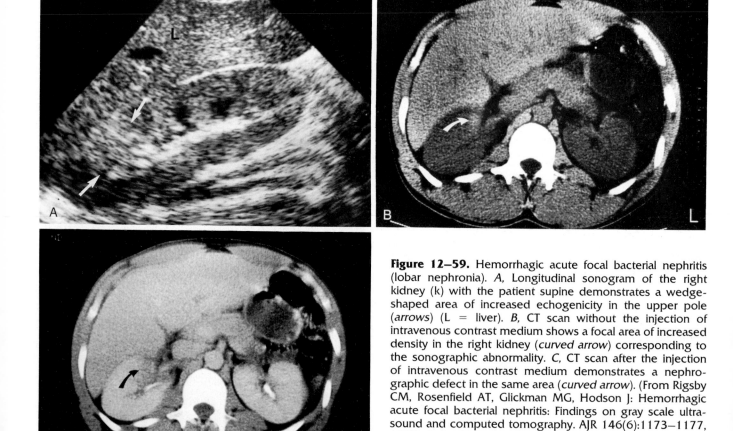

Figure 12–59. Hemorrhagic acute focal bacterial nephritis (lobar nephronia). *A,* Longitudinal sonogram of the right kidney (k) with the patient supine demonstrates a wedge-shaped area of increased echogenicity in the upper pole (*arrows*) (L = liver). *B,* CT scan without the injection of intravenous contrast medium shows a focal area of increased density in the right kidney (*curved arrow*) corresponding to the sonographic abnormality. *C,* CT scan after the injection of intravenous contrast medium demonstrates a nephrographic defect in the same area (*curved arrow*). (From Rigsby CM, Rosenfield AT, Glickman MG, Hodson J: Hemorrhagic acute focal bacterial nephritis: Findings on gray scale ultrasound and computed tomography. AJR 146(6):1173–1177, 1986, © Am Roentgen Ray Soc.)

Table 12–2. Sonography of the Echogenic Focus

Etiology	Cause of Echogenicity	Findings
Renal cell carcinoma	Solid tissue (collagen)	Attenuation similar to contiguous solid tissue
Angiomyolipoma	Fat	Speed propagation artifact
Echogenic abscess	Debris	Refraction artifact enhancement posterior to lesion
Echogenic abscess	Gas	"Dirty shadow" "Ring-down" artifact
Calcified mass or stone	Calcium	"Clean shadow"
Junctional parenchymal defect	Normal anatomical variant (fat)	Anterosuperior or defect posteroinferior focus contiguous with renal sinus
Crossed fused renal ectopia	Indentation at junction of kidneys (fat and fibrous tissue)	Anterior or posterior indentation not contiguous with renal sinus
Scar (secondary to infarction or infection)	Collagen	Loss of parenchyma and increased echogenicity of contiguous renal parenchyma
		Calyceal blunting if etiology is reflux nephropathy
Hemorrhage (infarct, trauma, or hemorrhagic lobar nephronia)	Blood	Increased echogenicity, without posterior enhancement or refraction
Hemorrhagic cyst	Blood or high protein	Increased echogenicity, posterior enhancement refraction

found to be reasonably accurate in an estimate of residual volume. Other methods have also been advocated.[107]

Ultrasonography can be used as a screening test for bladder carcinoma.[108, 109] Information similar to that obtained on urography is obtained sonographically.[108] A number of lesions including blood clot (Fig. 12–63A), benign prostatic hypertrophy, focal cystitis, and bladder diverticula can mimic bladder tumors.[108, 110]

Other lesions of the bladder can also be identified. Stones will appear as echogenic foci that shift in position and demonstrate acoustic shadowing (Fig. 12–63B).[111] A ureterocele can be seen as a fluid-filled structure contiguous with the ureter (Fig. 12–64). The dilated ureter leading to the ureterocele (Fig. 12–64) may also be identified. Diffuse cystitis will appear as a thickening of the bladder wall (Fig. 12–65). A similar thickening can be seen with other entities such as obstruction to bladder outflow with secondary hypertrophy and spastic neurogenic bladder. Extrinsic masses such as lymph nodes (Fig. 12–66), aneurysms, or pelvic lipomatosis (Fig. 12–67) can also be identified. Lymph nodes are solid but hypoechoic, aneurysms may pulsate and/or demonstrate flow on Doppler ultrasonography, and pelvic lipomatosis is identical in texture to normal fat around the bladder.

Pitfalls Relating to the Urinary Bladder During Pelvic Ultrasonography. Vick and associates have described a number of pitfalls related to the urinary bladder that may be encountered during the study of the pelvis.[104a] Fluid-filled masses can mimic the bladder when they are large enough to obscure visualization of the bladder. If two fluid-filled masses are seen within the pelvis, such as a lymphocele and bladder, it is necessary to pass a catheter or to have the patient void in order to determine which lesion is lymphocele and which lesion is bladder (Fig. 12–68). A rectus sheath hematoma is another example of a fluid-filled mass that may mimic the bladder (Fig. 12–69A).

A classic pitfall is the diagnosis of an enlarged bladder as a pelvic mass. This occurs generally when the patient is unable to void a significant amount of urine.[104a] Catheterization of the bladder may be necessary to verify that the lesion is bladder and not a pelvic mass. A major limitation of ultrasonography is the general lack of specific signs that discriminate among fluid-filled masses, such as a lymphocele, urinoma, or hematoma. As noted above, it is also crucial to identify the mass and the bladder. Another potential pitfall relates to the normal ureteral jet effect. Care must be taken not to misinterpret the echogenic jet of urine for the outlines of an intravesical mass (Fig. 12–69B).[111a]

The most significant artifact related to the bladder during pelvic ultrasonography is the reverberation artifact. The concept of reverberation is described on page 346. The anterior portion of the bladder may be filled with echoes due to reverberation between the bladder wall and overlying tissue layers. As shown in Figure 12–70, a bladder duplication artifact can be created behind the bladder by reverberation. This is produced by the total reflection of sound at the interface between the posterior bladder and the gas in the adjacent rectosigmoid colon.[112, 113] Reverberated echoes, which are detected later than the initially returning echoes, are interpreted by the instrument as having arisen from deeper within the body. This may lead to a mass that either seems cystic or contains echoes. Multiple masses may be seen as the process is repeated. Emptying some fluid from the bladder can eliminate this artifact.

The Prostate and Seminal Vesicles

The region of the prostate and seminal vesicles is well insonated transabdominally but is seen to even better advantage transrectally.[114–116] Transabdominally, the pros-

Text continued on page 363

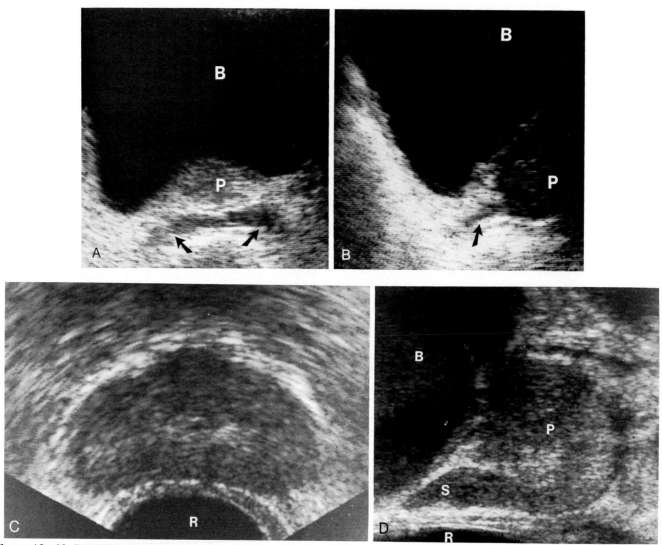

Figure 12–60. Prostate and seminal vesicles. *A,* Transverse abdominal sonogram through the true pelvis shows a slightly enlarged prostate gland (P). Note the seminal vesicles (*arrows*) behind the prostate. (B = bladder.) *B,* Longitudinal scan through the right pelvis in the same patient demonstrates the bladder (B) and hypertrophy of the prostate (P). Note the right seminal vesicle extending cranially (*straight arrow*). In both *A* and *B* the seminal vesicle angles are well seen and they contain echogenic fat. *C,* Axial endorectal sonogram of the prostate demonstrates the size and consistency of the prostate nicely. (R = rectum.) *D,* Longitudinal, endorectal sonogram of the prostate (P) demonstrates its relationship to the rectum (R) and seminal vesicle (S). (B = bladder.) (*C, D,* courtesy Matthew D. Rifkin, M.D., Philadelphia.)

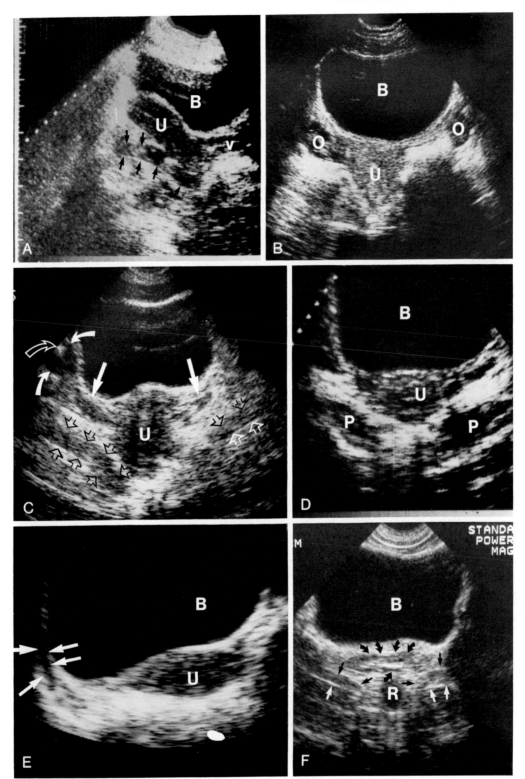

Figure 12–61. Normal female pelvis. Multiple sonograms of various female patients, demonstrating normal pelvic anatomy. The structures labeled on these scans can generally be identified, which can be useful in staging bladder and gynecological tumors. *A*, Longitudinal scan through the true pelvis of a normal patient demonstrates the bladder (B) with the uterus (U) behind it. The longitudinal bright line in the center of the uterus represents mucus within the endometrial cavity. The vagina (v) is identified in the caudad portion of the scan with a central linear echogenic line, also typical of mucus. The arrows outline bowel behind the uterus. *B*, Transverse scan through the normal female pelvis demonstrates the bladder (B) with the uterus (U) posterior to it. The ovaries (O) are well seen. Note the multiple ovarian cysts in the right ovary. *C*, Transverse scan through the pelvis demonstrates the uterus (U) behind the fluid-filled bladder. Solid straight arrows denote the ovaries. Open straight arrows outline the piriformis muscles. Solid curved arrows demonstrate the right iliopsoas muscle. Open curved arrow demonstrates the echogenic fat about the femoral nerve sheath. *D*, Transverse scan through the true pelvis demonstrates the bladder (B) with the uterus (U) behind it. Note the piriformis muscles (P), well seen behind the uterus. *E*, Oblique transverse scan through the true pelvis demonstrates the bladder (B) and uterus (U). Note the right internal obturator muscle (*arrows*). *F*, Transverse scan at the level of the vagina (*curved arrows*). Note the linear echogenic line in the center of the vagina, representing mucus. The levator ani muscles are well seen (*straight arrows*). (B = bladder. R = rectum.) (*A–F*, courtesy Linda Batista R.T., R.D.M.S., and Sheri Wood, R.T., R.D.M.S.)

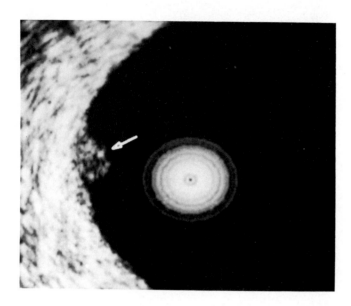

Figure 12–62. Transurethral intravesical sonogram demonstrating a noninvasive low-grade transitional cell carcinoma. A transurethral intravesical sonogram of the fluid-filled urinary bladder demonstrates a lesion (*arrows*) protruding from the wall of the bladder. The wall itself is intact with no evidence of invasion. (The central circular density within the bladder is the probe.) (From Rifkin M: Diagnostic Imaging of the Lower Genitourinary Tract. Raven Press, 1985.)

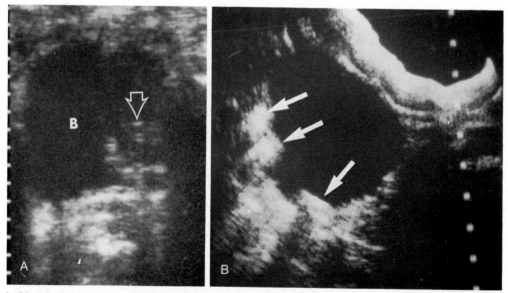

Figure 12–63. *A,* Blood clot within the bladder shown in stop frame from real-time linear-array scans, transverse image. An echogenic mass (*open arrow*) rests against the posterior bladder wall (B = bladder) without acoustic shadowing. When the patient changes position the mass may shift, suggesting the presence of blood clot. (From Zeman RK, Taylor KJW, Rosenfield AT: Sonographic features of kidney, adrenal, and bladder tumors. *In* Kossoff G, Fukuda M: Ultrasonic Differential Diagnosis of Tumors. New York, Igaku-Shoin, 1984. *B,* Bladder calculi. Longitudinal sonographic section through the bladder demonstrates echogenic foci with distal acoustic shadowing (*arrows*). When the patient changed position, these echogenic foci shifted, a finding typical of bladder calculi. (From Rosenfield AT, Taylor KJW, Weiss RM: Ultrasound evaluation of bladder calculi. J Urol 121:955–960, 1979.)

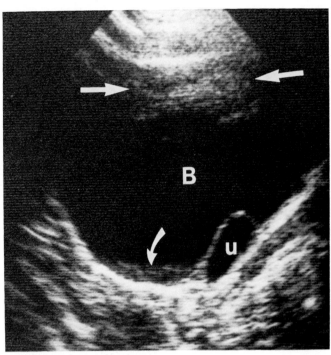

Figure 12–64. Ureterocele. Transverse sonographic section through the bladder of a woman subsequently shown to have an ectopic ureterocele from a nonfunctioning upper pole demonstrates the left-sided ureterocele (u). A reverberation artifact is seen in the anterior portion of the bladder (*straight arrows*). Note also debris layering in the dependent portion of the bladder (*curved arrows*), a common and generally not significant finding.

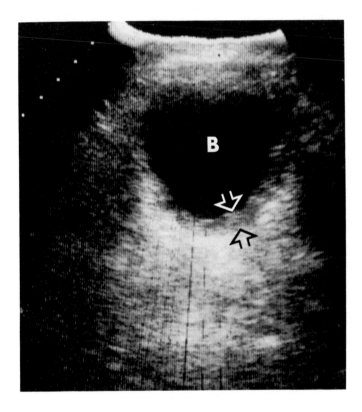

Figure 12–65. Cyclophosphamide (Cytoxan) cystitis. Transverse sonographic scan through the bladder (B) in a patient being treated with cyclophosphamide and other drugs for lymphoma. Note the bladder wall thickening (*open arrows*) secondary to the cystitis.

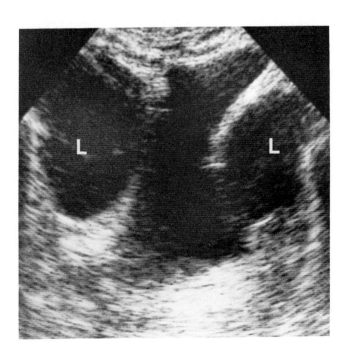

Figure 12–66. Enlarged pelvic lymph nodes. Transverse scan through the true pelvis in a patient with lymphoma demonstrates large lymph nodes (L) compressing the bladder from the two sides. Lymph nodes are typically hypoechoic, as in this case.

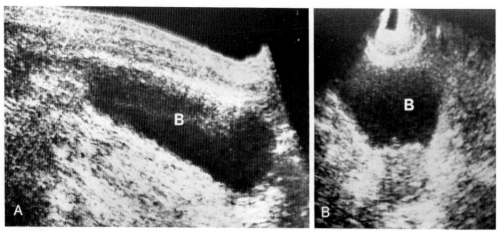

Figure 12–67. Pelvic lipomatosis. *A,* Longitudinal sonographic scan through the bladder of a patient whose bladder was indented and elongated on excretory urography demonstrates the elongated bladder (B). *B,* Transverse scan through the bladder demonstrates the relatively narrowed waist of the bladder. Note that only pelvic fat is seen about the bladder, without evidence of mass. CT confirmed the presence of fat without an external mass. (From Rosenfield AT, Richman T: The urinary tract. *In* Taylor KJW (ed): Atlas of Ultrasonography, 2nd Ed. New York, Churchill Livingstone, 1985, pp. 733–838, by permission.)

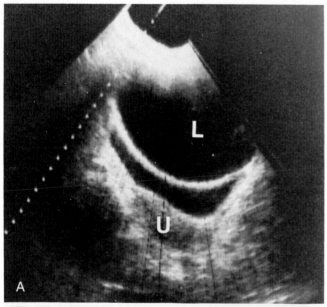

Figure 12–68. Lymphocele simulating the bladder. *A,* Longitudinal sonographic scan through the pelvis demonstrates two fluid-containing structures, the largest of which (L) simulates the bladder (U = uterus). *B,* A post-void study definitively identifies the smaller collection as the bladder. The larger collection (L) proved to be a lymphocele. (From Vick CW, Viscomi GN, Mannes E, Taylor KJW: Pitfalls related to the urinary bladder and pelvic sonography: A review. Urol Radiol 5:253–259, 1983.

whereas prostatic carcinoma appears as a mass of variable echogenicity (Fig. 12–71).[114–116]

Transrectal Prostate Ultrasonography. Transrectal ultrasonography has been shown to be a useful modality for detecting small lesions and textural changes of the prostate produced by benign and malignant disease.[114–116a] It can also provide accurate guidance for percutaneous transperineal biopsy of suspicious prostatic lesions.[115, 116b,c]

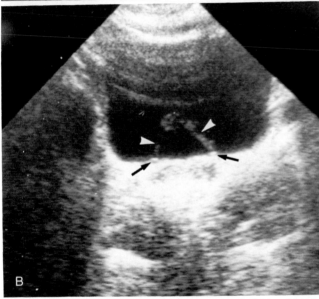

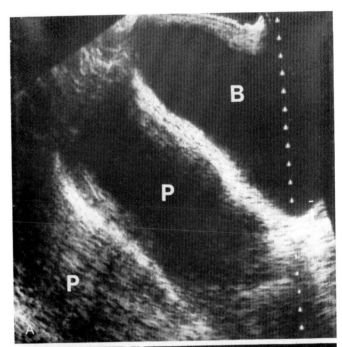

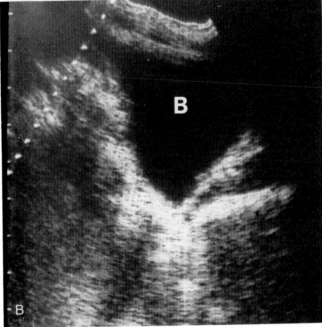

Figure 12–69. *A,* Rectus sheath hematoma mimicking bladder in 65-year-old man with pelvic mass 5 days after institution of intravenous heparin therapy. Transverse sonographic scans through the pelvis show two fluid-filled structures, the more anterior one of which (H) proved to be a rectus sheath hematoma. (b = bladder.) (From Vick CW, Viscomi GN, Mannes E, Taylor KJW: Pitfalls related to the urinary bladder and pelvic sonography: A review. Urol Radiol 5:253–259, 1983.) *B,* Ureteral jet creating a pseudobladder lesion. The ureteral jets are seen as echogenic lines (*arrowheads*) beginning at the mucosal elevations (*arrows*) that represent the ureteral orifices. These lines create an apparent bladder lesion. Rescanning a few moments later will demonstrate that these findings are not constant. (Courtesy Pinchus Lebenshardt, M.D., Hadassah Hospital, Jerusalem, Israel.)

tate is seen as a rounded structure with homogeneous echoes inferior to and posterior to the bladder (Fig. 12–60*A*,*B*). On longitudinal studies, a line may be seen within the prostate, representing the urethra. On transverse scans, this appears as an echogenic focus within the prostate.[215] The seminal vesicles can be readily identified on both transverse and longitudinal scans behind and extending cranial to the prostate. Benign prostatic hypertrophy leads to symmetrical enlargement of the gland,

Figure 12–70. Reverberation artifact creating pseudomass behind the bladder. *A,* Longitudinal sonographic scan through the true pelvis shows the bladder (B) with an apparent mass (pseudomass) (P) behind it. Note a similar mass behind the pseudomass. *B,* With the bladder (B) less full, the pseudomass is not identified. The pseudomass was created by the reverberation artifact from the highly echogenic gas behind the back wall of the bladder. (From Vick CW, Viscomi GN, Mannes E, Taylor KJW: Pitfalls related to the urinary bladder and pelvic sonography: A review. Urol Radiol 5:253–259, 1983.)

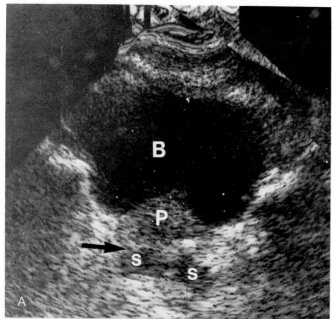

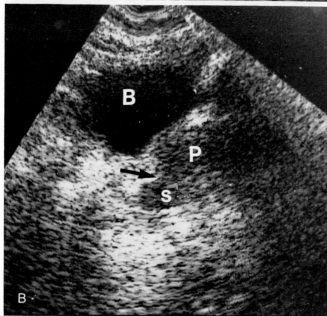

Figure 12–71. Adenocarcinoma of the prostate involving the right seminal vesicle. *A,* Transverse sonographic scan through the true pelvis demonstrates an enlarged irregular prostate (P) impinging on the bladder (B). The seminal vesicles are clearly identified (S). Note that the seminal vesicle angle on the left is well preserved, while the seminal vesicle angle on the right (*arrow*) is effaced. *B,* Longitudinal scan through the right true pelvis once again demonstrates the bladder (B) and prostate (P), as well as the right seminal vesicle (s). Note the irregular loss of angle between the prostate and seminal vesicle (*straight arrow*). (Courtesy Lincoln Russin, M.D., Westfield, Massachusetts.)

Anatomically, the prostate is divided into two regions, surrounded by a thin, fibrous capsule. The peripheral zone occupies the posterior, lateral, and apical portions of the gland and consists of glandular tissue. The central zone represents the central gland, extending from the bladder neck to the area of the verumontanum. It, too, is glandular, but the glands differ structurally and biochemically from those of the peripheral zone. Surround-

ing the urethra is a transition zone that consists of periurethral mucosal and submucosal glands.

An exam is performed with a transrectal ultrasound probe equipped with either an axial (Fig. 12–60C) or a longitudinal oriented (Fig. 12–60D) linear-array scanner producing images in a transverse or longitudinal plane, respectively. Biplanar probes are also available. High-frequency (5 to 10 MHz) transducers are required to produce high-resolution images.

Prostate cancer typically develops in the peripheral glandular tissue. The sonographic appearance of malignant lesions varies among reports.[114–116a] In one study, all cancerous lesions were hypoechoic.[115] In another study, 76% of such lesions were echopenic or hypoechoic, with the remainder of malignant lesions being isoechoic.[116] In contrast to these results, another study reported a majority of malignant lesions (69%) to be hyperechoic with only 3% being hypoechoic.[114] A similar discrepancy in the reported appearances of benign lesions also exists. Furthermore, there is considerable overlap in the sonographic appearances of benign and malignant lesions.[114, 116a] Therefore, biopsy of all suspicious lesions should be performed.[114, 116, 218] Transrectal ultrasonography can help to determine which areas should be biopsied as well as to guide accurate biopsy needle placement (see Fig. 12–92),[115, 116b,c, 219] but its diagnostic usefulness in the detection of prostatic carcinoma is hampered by a relatively high number of false-negative and false-positive studies.[116d,e] The subject is covered fully in Chapter 47.

The Scrotum

High-resolution, high-frequency ultrasound images of the scrotum have assumed a significant role in the evaluation of both acute and chronic scrotal lesions. This safe and rapid technique produces information that is complementary to the clinical history and examination and to physiological studies such as radioisotope scanning or Doppler ultrasonography. Successful images can be obtained with dynamic or static scanning and can be performed using either contact scanning of the scrotum or a water bath to permit the transducer to stand off from the scrotum. Frequencies between 7.5 and 20 MHz are generally employed.

Normal Anatomy

The testis is identified as a homogeneously echogenic structure (Fig. 12–72). The lobes of the testis cannot be defined sonographically. The fibrous tunica albuginea encompasses the testis and is not identified as a separate structure, except where it enters the testis itself as the mediastinum testis.[117] The mediastinum is seen as a bright line when imaged in a longitudinal section (Fig. 12–73), but portions may be imaged in other planes, creating bright foci. The head, body, and tail of the epididymis can be identified as contiguous with the testis. This structure is at least as brightly reflective as the testis. The multiple individual layers of scrotal skin are generally seen as a single echogenic band; differences in skin thickness between the two sides are an important sonographic finding. Among the small structures that are frequently seen are the normal veins of the pampiniform

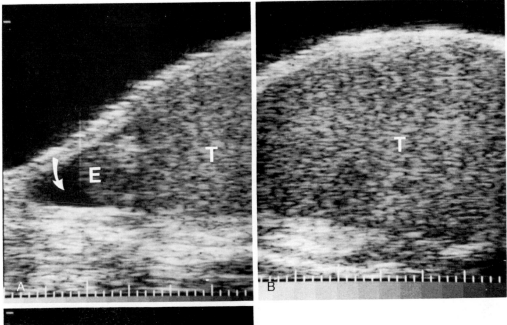

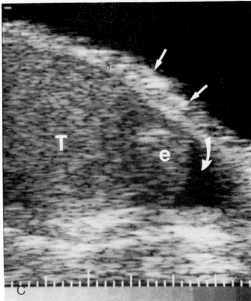

Figure 12–72. Normal scrotum as seen on a high-resolution ultrasound scanner. *A,* Scan through the upper portion of the right hemi-scrotum demonstrates the head of the epididymis (E) and testis (T). Note that the testis has homogeneous echoes and the individual lobes of the testis are not able to be differentiated. A small amount of fluid (*curved arrow*) is seen above the epididymis. This amount of fluid is within normal limits. *B,* Scan through the mid portion of the testis (T) shows the testis as a homogeneously echogenic structure. *C,* Scan through the inferior portion of the scrotum demonstrates the testis (T) and tail of the epididymis (e). A small amount of fluid is noted inferior to the tail of the epididymis (*curved arrow*). Note also the hair seen extending from the skin (*straight arrows*).

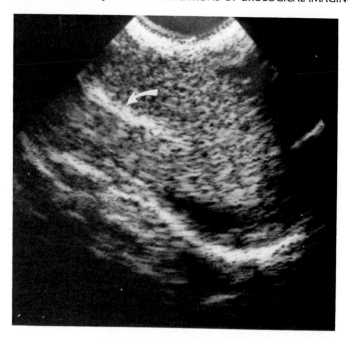

Figure 12–73. Mediastinum testis. Sonographic scan through a normal testis demonstrates a mediastinum testis as a linear echogenic line (*curved arrow*). At times, portions of the mediastinum may be seen on transverse scans, mimicking an echogenic focus.

plexus as well as the appendix of the testis or epididymis, which may be identified as a punctate echogenic focus.

Scrotal Masses

Extratesticular Masses. In patients who present with swelling of the scrotum, ultrasonography is an excellent initial step to define whether the lesion is extratesticular or intratesticular and to characterize the lesion.[118-120] A hydrocele is a collection of fluid within the layers of the tunica vaginalis, which encompasses the anterior portion of the testis (Fig. 12–74). A small amount of fluid is normal. Larger amounts of fluid are seen as echo free or occasionally as echogenic enlargement of the region of

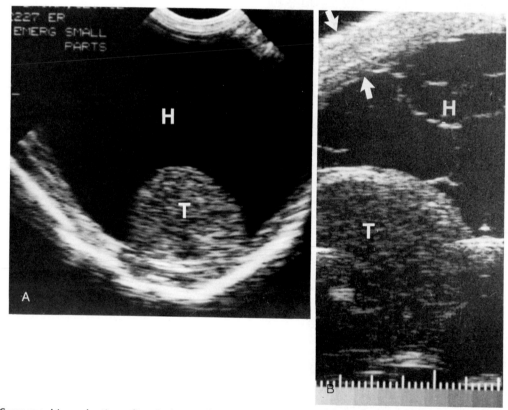

Figure 12–74. Sonographic evaluation of testicular swelling secondary to a hydrocele. *A*, Hydrocele with no underlying pathology. Transverse scan through the scrotum in a patient with a large hydrocele (H). Note that the testis (T) is surrounded on three sides by the hydrocele but is fixed to surrounding tissues posterolaterally. The hydrocele represents fluid within the layers of the tunica vaginalis. Sonography can be of value to exclude underlying testicular pathology. *B*, Hydrocele associated with testicular torsion. Transverse scan through the right hemiscrotum in a patient with acute right scrotal swelling and pain. The testis (T) is hypoechoic. Note the hydrocele (H) with multiple septa. Note also the skin thickening (*arrows*). Skin thickening is more commonly seen with benign than with malignant processes.

the tunica. Ultrasonography can be a valuable aid in distinguishing between an idiopathic hydrocele, which will have no associated findings, and one associated with underlying disease (symptomatic hydrocele).

A varicocele can be identified as a collection of distended veins (Fig. 12–75). The varicocele is most distended and best seen with the patient erect. Cysts and spermatoceles of the epididymis are readily identified as cystic structures in the epididymis. Spermatoceles may have a central echogenic focus, thought to be related to clumped sperm, that moves with a shift in patient position.

Scrotal hernias may be identified as masses that typically have highly reflective regions due to the echogenic fat in the bowel wall or to intraluminal gas.[121] On dynamic scanning, the observation of peristalsis within the mass is confirmatory.

Fibrous plaques related to the tunica albuginea as well as areas of scarring and fibrosis can be identified as focal echogenic lesions. Occasional rare tumors, such as the adenomatoid tumor of the epididymis, can be seen as masses that may be either echogenic or echo poor; other uncommon lesions can arise from any extratesticular tissues.

Intratesticular Masses. Germ-cell tumors are solid neoplasms in young adult men. Seminomas tend to be hypoechoic, whereas nonseminomatous tumors tend to be of mixed echogenicity.[122] Ultrasonography can be used to identify a tumor within a testis, particularly in the situation where a hydrocele is present and the testis itself cannot readily be palpated. Hypoechoic testicular masses in older men are most likely to be lymphoma. Ultrasonography has also been a useful technique to identify nonpalpable testicular tumors when metastatic disease of a cell type consistent with a testicular primary is identified.[123, 124]

Masses that do not represent malignancies may be identified sonographically in the testis. Simple testicular cysts can occur and have the characteristic signs of a cystic lesion.[125] Unlike neoplastic cystic lesions, such as teratoma, these simple cysts should not have any associated solid tissue. Epidermoid cysts, which are a separate entity with malignant potential, also occur; they have been described as cystic but with central echo-producing regions.[126] Following torsion of the testicle[127] or infarction from other causes,[128] hypoechoic masses may be identified within the testis. In our experience, these have been indistinguishable from neoplastic lesions.[128] Hypoechoic masses may occur in the testicle during or following orchitis. These masses may take months to resolve and, once again, are indistinguishable from tumor.

The Acute Scrotum

In patients with acute scrotal pain, the major differential diagnosis is between testicular torsion and inflammatory disease such as epididymitis or epididymo-orchitis. A physiological study is generally the first one that should be performed. Both radioisotope flow studies and Doppler ultrasonography (see later discussion) have been used for this purpose. Inflammatory disease shows normal to increased flow, whereas torsion of the testis leads to an absence of flow within the testis. B-scan ultrasonography is a valuable complement to the radioisotope scan for defining the anatomy in order to determine whether an area that has no flow is the testicle itself or is an abnormal structure such as a hydrocele.

Although B-scan ultrasonography is a secondary test performed to exclude torsion and to distinguish between testicular torsion and epididymitis, the findings seen with testicular torsion and epididymitis have been defined, and one should be aware of them.[127, 129] The sequence of events in testicular torsion is characterized by enlargement of the testis with decreased echogenicity after a few hours of symptoms. The epididymis also enlarges and contains a mixture of high- and low-level echoes. The testis remains enlarged for approximately 10 days, while the epididymis becomes homogeneously echogenic. After 10 days to 2 weeks, the affected testis becomes smaller than the unaffected side, and the epididymis tends to remain homogeneously echogenic. We have found that after 6 hours of symptoms a normal sonogram can reliably exclude torsion.[127] Experimental work supports this con-

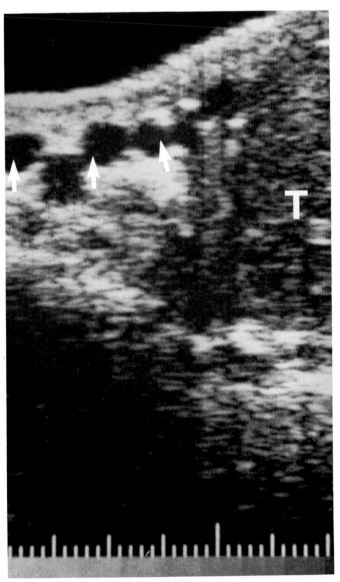

Figure 12–75. Varicocele. Longitudinal sonographic scan through the superior aspect of the scrotum, using a high-resolution scanner, demonstrates a dilated tortuous vein in the pampiniform plexus (*straight arrows*), which is part of a varicocele. (T = testis).

cept.[129] In addition, we believe that ultrasonography is extremely valuable for identifying missed torsion when the initial insult was remote in time, since collateral vessels may cause falsely normal radioisotope flow studies. It is important to identify missed torsion since a bilateral, congenital "bell-clapper" deformity is generally present in this entity, and contralateral orchiopexy is usually indicated to prevent contralateral torsion.

Sonographically, the epididymis is typically enlarged and hypoechoic in pure epididymitis. The testis is normal in appearance. If orchitis is also present, a completely hypoechoic testis may be seen or focal hypoechoic masses may be identified within the testis. These abnormalities within the testis may persist for months after the symptoms have resolved, which results in a major pitfall of scrotal imaging.[130] In addition, because the blood supply to the testis travels in close proximity to the head of the epididymis, epididymitis, through compression of the spermatic vessels, can lead to focal or diffuse infarction of the testis with associated global or focal hypoechoic textural abnormality.[128] Ultrasound is valuable to define the anatomy in this situation to determine whether the echo-poor area represents the testis itself or some other abnormality, such as focal hydrocele.

Ultrasonography is also useful in regard to the traumatized testis. The main question in evaluating the patient with scrotal trauma is whether the testis is intact, because if not, surgery is required. Ultrasonography can be used to demonstrate testicular rupture or to exclude it.[131]

Undescended Testes

Results of experiences using ultrasonography to detect undescended testes have been mixed.[132-134] Wolverson and coworkers have found ultrasound to be extremely reliable for this purpose,[133] but our results have been less salutary.[132] Although most inguinal testes can be reliably identified by ultrasonography, they can also be detected clinically, perhaps with even greater accuracy. Abdominal testes, however, are generally not detectable by ultrasound. In our experience, false-positive studies are generally attributable to mistaking the distal bulbous portion of the gubernaculum testis (the pars infravaginalis gubernaculi) for the testis proper. Perhaps the major role of ultrasonography in cryptorchism lies in its ability to confirm the existence of a suspected inguinal testicle. If the mediastinum testis is identifiable by its characteristic bright echoes, there is little doubt of the diagnosis. If it is not detected, it cannot be inferred that the structure is not testis, however, since the mediastinum is not always identified in atrophic testes. CT supplemented by testicular phlebography continues to produce the most reliable studies in the search for a nonpalpable testis. MRI has the potential to replace CT as the technique of choice.[134a]

Approach to Scrotal Ultrasonography

The role of ultrasound in scrotal imaging as defined in this chapter is noted in Table 12–3. It is important to recognize the nonspecificity of most B-scan ultrasound findings. Solid masses in the testis can be neoplasms (and in fact are generally germ-cell tumors in the young adult and lymphoma in the older adult) but may also be related to infarction or to inflammatory disease. Although skin

Table 12–3. Role of Ultrasound in Scrotal Imaging

Evaluation of scrotal masses
    Testicular versus extratesticular
    Cystic versus solid

Evaluation of patients with hydrocele for underlying lesion

Identification of occult primary tumors in patients with metastatic disease

Evaluation of the acute scrotum
    Radioisotope flow study or Doppler ultrasound for physiology
    B-scan ultrasonography for anatomy

Evaluation of the traumatized scrotum for testicular integrity

To identify varicoceles in infertility work-up

To complement computed tomography in the evaluation of the undescended testis

Modified from Bird K, Rosenfield AT: Testicular imaging. *In* Putman C, Ravin C (eds): Textbook of Diagnostic Imaging. Philadelphia, WB Saunders Company, 1988, p 1369.

thickening and an abnormal epididymis were once thought to be typical of benign disease, it is now thought that these findings cannot be used alone as a criterion to differentiate malignant from nonmalignant states.[135] Extratesticular masses are generally benign, but any of the elements of the scrotum can produce a corresponding extratesticular malignant tumor. Pure extratesticular cysts are invariably benign, but concern still exists about ignoring intratesticular cysts.[136] Similarly, in the acute scrotum some B-scan findings for epididymo-orchitis overlap with those for torsion so that a physiological study is crucial for initial evaluation.[137] Thus, B-scan ultrasonography of the scrotum is, for the most part, an extremely rapid, relatively inexpensive imaging technique that presents excellent definition of anatomy. It is highly sensitive for disease, and a normal sonographic study is a reasonable indication that major scrotal abnormality is not present (with the exception of a sonogram performed in the first few hours of testicular torsion). A positive sonogram must be evaluated in conjunction with the other imaging studies, the clinical history, and the physical examination. Although in most situations this coordinated approach to diagnosis leads to the probable cause of the findings and/or symptoms, in some cases of acute disease and of scrotal masses exploratory surgery is required for diagnosis.

The Penis

High-resolution ultrasonography is ideally suited to image the penis. The corpus cavernosum and spongiosum, as well as the urethra, are readily identified (Fig. 12–76). While the patient is voiding, the echogenic urethra is separated by the urine (Fig. 12–73). Strictures can be demonstrated.[220] Ultrasonography has been used to identify Peyronie's plaques, which are deposits of fibrous tissue in the penis leading to deviation during erection.[138] The plaques can be followed during therapy to determine to what degree they are changing. An important potential role for ultrasonography is in the evaluation of penile trauma.[139] The integrity of the corpora of the penis can

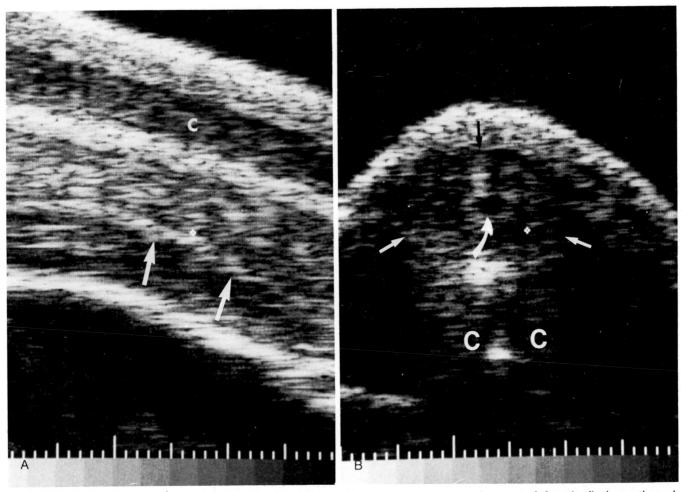

Figure 12–76. Sonographic scans of the normal penis, utilizing a high-resolution ultrasound scanner. *A,* Longitudinal scan through a portion of the penis. The urethra is seen as a linear echogenic line (*arrows*) within the corpus spongiosum. Dorsal to the corpus spongiosum, one of the corpora cavernosa is seen (c). Note the echogenic tissue between the two corpora (tunica albuginea). *B,* Transverse scan of the penis in the same patient during voiding. This study was performed with the transducer on the urethral side of the penis. Note the urine-filled urethra (*curved arrow*) in the center of the corpus spongiosum (*straight arrows*). The corpora cavernosa (C) are not optimally visualized with this high frequency.

be determined, and ultrasonography can therefore be used to replace more invasive techniques.

DOPPLER ULTRASONOGRAPHY

Doppler ultrasonography is a noninvasive technique that permits evaluation of arterial and venous blood flow. The ability to observe and measure the difference in frequency (frequency shift) between a transmitted ultrasound signal and that reflected from moving blood particles allows detection and characterization of blood flow in intact vessels. Since the first medical application of Doppler ultrasound in 1959,[140] improved technology and signal display have produced an increase in the number of areas in which this technique is clinically useful, including the genitourinary system.

Principles

In 1842 Johann Christian Doppler first described the effect that bears his name. He showed mathematically that the frequency of a traveling wave appears to increase to an observer who is moving toward its source and to decrease to an observer who is moving away from the source. The Doppler effect was confirmed in a rather picturesque experiment of 1845 in which the Dutch government was persuaded to lend a steam locomotive. A trumpeter standing on its footplate played a steady note while the train approached a station platform on which a second trumpeter stood playing the same note. The pitch of the moving trumpeter's note was heard to be higher as the locomotive approached the station, and lower as it passed. In our own time, the sound of the changing pitch of a passing ambulance siren is a more familiar experience.

In medical ultrasound, a ceramic transducer element produces a beam of sound at a frequency of between 2 and 15 MHz, depending on the penetration required. The same echoes as those responsible for a B-scan image, arising from discontinuities in acoustic impedance, are reflected or scattered back to the transducer. In continuous wave (CW) Doppler instruments, a second element is used as a receiver. The two beams overlap to form a sensitive volume, which is defined by their spatial product. If a moving target lies within this region, the frequency of received sound will differ from that of the transmitted sound by an amount determined by the Doppler equation:

$$f_D = \frac{2\ fv\cos\theta}{c}$$

The change in the ultrasonic frequency is f_D, known as the Doppler shift frequency; f is the frequency of the incident ultrasound; v is the relative velocity between the transducer and the target; θ is the angle between the beam and the direction of movement of the target and c is the velocity of sound in the medium. Velocities are measured in meters per second and frequency in hertz (cycles per second).

It happens that for the range of ultrasonic frequencies used and the range of tissue velocities encountered in the human body, the frequency f_D lies within the audible range. It is convenient, then, for a Doppler flow meter to convert this shift frequency into an audible signal that can be monitored by the operator through a loudspeaker. Although, as we will see, modern techniques require electronic analysis of this Doppler signal, experienced operators are capable of subtle discrimination of the sound by using their ears alone.

Pulsed Doppler combines the velocity detection of the continuous-wave Doppler device with the range discrimination of a pulse-echo system. Short bursts of ultrasound are transmitted at regular intervals, and the echoes are examined for Doppler frequency shifts. The range of the target can be determined from the elapsed time between the transmission of the pulse and the reception of its echoes. By adjusting an electronic gate, only echoes originating from a certain time interval (corresponding to a certain range of depths) are sampled. The axial dimension of this "sample volume" is governed by the length of the gate and may vary between 1 and 15 mm; often this is controlled by the operator. The lateral dimensions depend on the beam width and are therefore a consequence of transducer frequency and design, as well as distance from the transducer face. Unlike the CW Doppler, a pulsed Doppler never transmits and receives at the same time, so that only one element is necessary.

In a duplex system, the pulsed Doppler is interfaced with a real-time ultrasonic imaging system that allows the source of the vascular signal to be visualized. The direction of the interrogating Doppler beam is displayed on the real-time image and can be adjusted by the operator. The gate length and the depth of interest are also selected under ultrasonic guidance. Duplex scanners based on mechanical sector scanners, electronically steered sector scanners, and linear arrays are now available. Other Doppler instruments include the pulsed or CW flow imaging systems that can be used to map the spatial location of Doppler signals; multigate or "infinite-gate" systems, which are capable of interrogation of more than one site simultaneously, without loss of spatial resolution; and combined-flow imaging and duplex scanners, which can map the location and direction of flow on a B-mode image, sometimes in real time.[141]

Although the movement of the single target gives rise to a Doppler signal of one frequency with a pitch proportional to the target velocity, the sample volume of a pulsed Doppler (or the beam of a CW Doppler) usually insonates blood cells moving at a large number of differing velocities, sometimes even in opposite directions within the same vessel. The Doppler signal is therefore perceived by the operator as a complex and changing set of sounds. The successful application of the technique in a clinical situation relies to a great extent on the appropriate choice of subsequent processing and measurement made on this signal. To this end, a variety of signal processing tech-niques are available, some of which are now incorporated routinely into commercial instruments.

The combination of different Doppler shift frequencies within the signal provide information; therefore, it is natural that the fundamental tool for processing Doppler signals is the frequency (or spectrum) analyzer. This instrument provides a display of the frequency components in the signal at a given time. Dedicated arithmetic processors can perform the necessary calculations fast enough to accept the next period to be analyzed as it arrives, thereby producing a series of spectra in real time. These spectra are in fact graphs showing the relative power of each of the frequency components constituting the Doppler signal. If the target is blood flowing in a vessel, the power at a given frequency relates to the quantity of blood flowing at the corresponding velocity. The spectra are usually displayed as a *sonogram*, in which a single spectrum is depicted as a vertical line on whose axis lies frequency, brightness-modulated to represent power. Subsequent spectra are displayed as vertical lines a fixed distance apart, creating an image that scrolls from left to right with time. The three variables—time, frequency and power—are thus shown in real time as the signal is heard. Information can be gleaned from inspection of this spectral display alone. Thus, if the sample volume is situated in an artery in which all the cells are moving at the same velocity, the spectrum will show a concentration of power at one Doppler shift frequency that varies over the cardiac cycle. An example is the plug flow of the normal main renal artery (Fig. 12–77). The "window" seen in the display within the systolic portion of the cycle is typical of such flow in a large vessel. Turbulence downstream to a stenosis will cause a range of velocities to be present across the vessel lumen, thereby broadening the display in a vertical direction. When the stenosis is severe, there is also an increase in peak systolic velocity as the blood flows through the narrowed lumen; the Doppler technique is particularly sensitive to this phenomenon.

The outline of the Doppler waveform represents the variation of the maximum Doppler shift frequency (corresponding to the center stream velocity) with time. As long as the conditions in the proximal circulation remain constant,[140] the shape of this maximum-frequency envelope has been shown to depend on the impedance of the distal vascular bed supplied by the artery, varying with the presence of occlusive lesions in the distal circulation. Simple indices of pulsatility have been defined, and this form of assessment enables the Doppler technique to be used to differentiate the low-resistance from the high-resistance renal vascular bed.

Clinical Applications of Doppler Ultrasonography in the Genitourinary System

Native Kidneys

Doppler interrogation of the renal arterial and venous systems can be performed, although evaluation of the main renal artery and vein may often be limited by the presence of bowel gas, particularly on the left. Doppler signals can be obtained from the main renal artery as well as the intrarenal arterial system, including segmental, interlobar, and arcuate arteries[142] (Fig. 12–77). With the

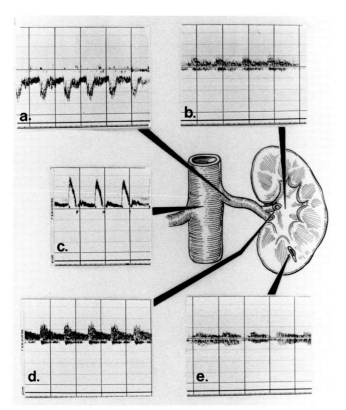

Figure 12–77. Doppler signals from a normal kidney obtained from *A*, main renal artery, *B*, midzone of kidney, *C*, abdominal aorta, *D*, segmental artery, and *E*, arcuate artery. Time is recorded on the x-axis and Doppler shift frequency, which is proportional to blood flow velocity, on the y-axis. (From Taylor KJW, Burns PN, Woodcock JP, Wells PNT: Blood flow in deep abdominal pelvic vessels: Ultrasonic pulsed Doppler analysis. Radiology 154:587, 1985.)

exception of the main renal artery, these vessels are usually too small to be identified on the real-time B-scan image. However, the gated cursor can be positioned in the corresponding anatomical location until spectra from the appropriate vessel are obtained.

Normal renal arterial Doppler signals have a rapid-forward phase in systole followed by persistent antegrade flow throughout diastole (Fig. 12–77),[142] which reflects a low peripheral impedance. At the level of the main renal artery, a spectral "window" is present in systole resulting from near-uniform blood flow velocity[143] with a blunted parabolic profile.[142] Doppler signals from the renal veins show flow in a direction opposite to that of arterial flow. Venous flow is continuous in the small vessels, and mild respiratory and cardiac variation may be seen in the main renal vein. Pulsed Doppler may be useful in differentiating hypervascular renal carcinomas from other tumors.[221]

Doppler Measurement of Renal Artery Blood Flow

Two groups of investigators have studied the application of Doppler ultrasonography in measuring renal artery blood flow.[144, 145] However, the difficulty in obtaining accurate arterial lumen diameter and in determining probe-vessel angle, as well as the inability to consistently visualize the renal arteries, appears to limit the clinical use of this modality.

Vascular Occlusion

The absence of arterial or venous Doppler signals throughout a kidney suggests the diagnosis of renal artery or venous occlusion, respectively.[142] The identification of such signals does not necessarily exclude thrombosis but virtually excludes total vascular occlusion. One report, however, had two false-negative results for renal artery occlusion in a group of three patients with this complication, which was confirmed by angiography.[143] These investigators limited their Doppler examination to the main renal artery without attempting to identify intrarenal arterial flow.

Renal Artery Stenosis

Nichols and coworkers reported success using pulsed Doppler for evaluation of renal artery stenosis.[143] In their series, 90% of 84 arteries examined by arteriography had technically adequate studies by Doppler interrogation. The reported sensitivity for stenosis was 83%, with 97% specificity and 92% overall accuracy. Criteria for stenosis included irregularity of the waveform, with a rounded or nondistinct peak, and absence of a window in systole indicating disruption of laminar flow. A sharp rise in peak frequency coupled with a frequency drop distal to the stenosis was seen in cases of severe stenosis. Our own experience of evaluating patients for renal artery stenosis has been somewhat less favorable, in part because of the propensity of bowel gas to obscure portions of the retroperitoneum, precluding a complete evaluation of the renal arteries, particularly on the left.

Renal Allografts

There are multiple causes of post-transplant renal failure, which include acute and chronic rejection, acute tubular necrosis (ATN), obstruction of the collecting system, vascular occlusion, renal artery stenosis, infection, and cyclosporin toxicity.

Duplex ultrasonography is a useful modality in the work-up of allograft dysfunction. It is easily performed because of the superficial location of the transplanted kidney and the absence of interposed loops of bowel between the organ and overlying skin. Furthermore, a Duplex study can be performed portably, at the patient's bedside. The utility of B scanning for morphological evaluation of renal allografts is well established (see Table 12–1; see also Chapter 108).[146–155] Doppler ultrasonography can detect vascular changes that often occur in acute rejection[156–160] and evaluate the renal arterial and venous system to exclude vascular occlusion[157, 158, 161] and stenosis.[142, 162, 163]

Normally, signals can be obtained with pulsed Doppler from the main anastomosed renal artery as well as the intrarenal arterial system, including segmental, interlobar, and arcuate vessels (Fig. 12–78).[142, 160] The normal arterial signal has a rapid rise in frequency shift during systole followed by a gradual fall in diastole, reflecting persistent antegrade flow in a low-impedance microcirculation (Fig. 12–79).[142, 156–158, 160, 162] Time-velocity spectra of the intrarenal arteries resemble those obtained from normal native kidneys. However, signals from the allograft main renal artery differ slightly. The difference in

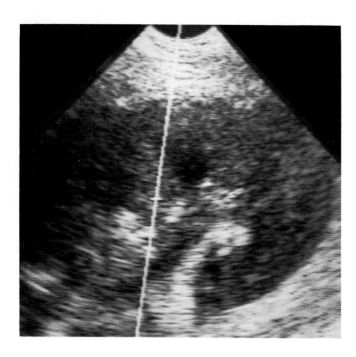

Figure 12–78. Frozen real-time image of a renal allograft. The gated cursor (*small white bar*) was positioned in a column of Bertin, where Doppler signals from an interlobar artery were obtained in a renal transplant.

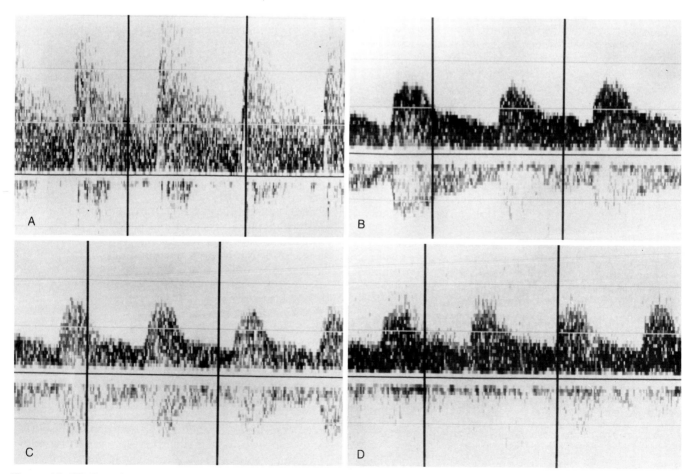

Figure 12–79. Doppler signals obtained in a normal renal allograft from *A*, main renal artery; *B*, segmental artery; *C*, interlobar artery; *D*, Arcuate artery. A peak blood flow velocity in systole is followed by persistent flow throughout diastole in all vessels.

the source of arterial input for a native and transplanted kidney constitutes one theoretical cause for this disparity. Arterial input is from the abdominal aorta in the former and from the anastomosed iliac artery in the latter. Additionally, the presence of mild turbulence in the Doppler signal obtained at the anastomosis of the allograft main renal artery can often be identified. Doppler signals from the renal veins show flow in a direction opposite to that of arterial flow. Venous flow is continuous in the small vessels, and mild respiratory variation may be seen in the main renal vein.

Acute Renal Allograft Rejection

Renal transplant arterial flow was first studied by Sampson using a Doppler flow meter.[164] He demonstrated a reduction in blood flow velocity to the allograft in episodes of rejection, expressed by a decrease in the ratio of peak renal-artery to femoral-artery frequency shift. An increase in this ratio was observed when patients responded to antirejection therapy. The study was limited, however, primarily by the inability to maintain a constant angle between the transducer and vessel for all recordings. In a second study, Sampson and associates employed a device that maintained a constant probe-vessel angle and showed good correlation between transplant renal artery blood-flow measurements determined by indwelling electromagnetic and external Doppler flow meters in canine allografts.[165] However, regulation of a constant probe-vessel angle is not possible for clinical use.

Subsequent investigation concentrated on analysis of the Doppler waveform, examining the relative change of diastolic to peak systolic frequency shift. This method offers the advantage of being unaffected by a relatively wide variation in the probe-vessel angle. In episodes of acute rejection, there is a relative decrease in diastolic to peak systolic frequency shift, reflecting decreased diastolic blood flow velocity (Fig. 12–80).[142, 157, 158, 160] In episodes of severe rejection, diastolic flow is obliterated (Fig. 12–81) or reversed. These changes result from increased vascular impedance in the allograft microcirculation.[142, 157–160] This increased peripheral resistance is believed to result from an endovasculitis with endothelial cell swelling and proliferation seen in episodes of acute vascular rejection.[160] In interstitial rejection there are no intrinsic arterial or arteriolar changes. The elevated microvascular impedance in these patients may result from external

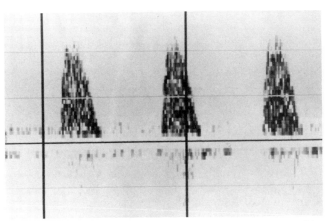

Figure 12–81. Doppler signal in severe acute rejection. Diastolic flow is obliterated.

factors such as interstitial edema[157, 159] or vasomotor constriction.[157] Improved diastolic flow can be identified in patients who respond to antirejection therapy.[157, 160]

In a prospective study, Rigsby and associates qualitatively analyzed 69 Doppler waveforms in 24 renal transplant patients.[160] The sensitivity of the Doppler technique for detection of all forms of acute rejection was 60%, and for acute rejection with a vascular component it was 82%. Specificity was 95% and 96% respectively. Acute rejection was diagnosed in three patients less than 48 hours following transplantation. This is important in that poor graft function in the immediate post-transplantation period is typically believed to result from ATN.

Preliminary results concerning Doppler differentiation of acute rejection from other causes of transplant dysfunction are inconclusive. Rigsby and coworkers reported normal Doppler waveforms in one patient with ATN and two patients with hydronephrosis. However, Berland and associates observed abnormal, pulsatile signals in some patients with ATN, whereas others had normal signals.[158]

At the present time, Doppler evaluation of renal transplants has a relatively poor sensitivity for detection of acute rejection. Sensitivity, however, is good when vascular rejection is present. Vascular rejection correlates with a poorer prognosis and often is treated more aggressively. The specificity of the Doppler technique is excellent, and the abnormal signals may permit prompt antirejection therapy without biopsy. Early Doppler changes indicating acute rejection can also be identified and allow early treatment for improved graft survival. Furthermore, normalization of Doppler signals after documented rejection correlates with successful response to therapy.

Vascular Occlusion

Vascular occlusion following renal transplantation represents a major complication requiring surgical intervention. Graft viability at the time of detection is infrequent, and allograft nephrectomy is usually indicated.

A diagnosis of arterial occlusion is made when one is unable to obtain Doppler signals from the main renal or intrarenal arteries.[157, 158, 161] In our experience, arterial thrombosis usually results from severe acute rejection but may also occur at the site of a technically difficult surgical anastomosis.

In the presence of renal vein occlusion or significant stenosis, Wood and Nasmyth reported increased pulsatil-

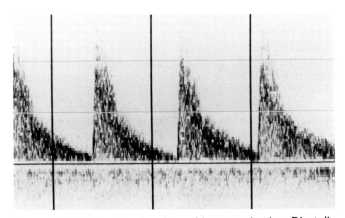

Figure 12–80. Doppler signal in mild acute rejection. Diastolic blood flow velocity is reduced.

ity of the Doppler arterial waveform from intraoperative studies in canine autografts.[163] An increased pulsatility index (PI) correlated with experimentally produced venous outflow obstruction of greater than 88% of original venous diameter. Clinically, this complication may result from kinking of the venous anastomosis or as a secondary event subsequent to thrombosis of the anastomosed iliac artery.

Transplant Renal Artery Stenosis

Transplant renal artery stenosis occurs in 1.6% to 16% of allograft recipients.[166] This complication represents one cause of post-transplant hypertension and should be suspected when elevated blood pressure is seen in association with a decline in graft function. The presence of a bruit over the transplant renal artery is a suggestive but inconsistent finding. Doppler interrogation of the main renal artery in one study demonstrated increased peak frequency at the site of stenosis with spectral broadening, disorganization of flow, and distal decreased peak frequency.[162] In that series of seven patients, Doppler analysis provided five true positive diagnoses of stenosis and two true negatives. Another report described the combination of high-velocity blood flow and distal turbulence as characteristic Doppler features of stenosis (Fig. 12–82).[142] It should be noted, however, that the relationship between the Doppler spectrum and the presence of flow disturbance or turbulence in the renal artery is complicated by a number of methodological factors. The Doppler diagnosis of renal artery stenosis is less well defined than, for example, carotid artery stenosis. Attempts must be made to examine the entire length of the main renal artery in that these abnormal flow patterns may exist in only a short segment of the vessel. Additionally, flow disturbance does not alone indicate stenosis and may exist normally to a mild degree at the site of anastomosis. Comparison with a baseline study is useful in the interpretation of such a finding. A decrease in PI has been reported to correlate with the presence of stenoses greater than 78% of arterial diameter in intraoperative canine studies.[163]

Doppler evaluation of transplant renal arteries should be performed as a screening for stenosis in patients in whom the diagnosis is suspected. It is noninvasive and avoids the risk of contrast toxicity.

Spermatic Cord—Acute Torsion (see Chapter 73)

Acute torsion of the spermatic cord represents a surgical emergency. Patients typically experience acute onset of unilateral scrotal pain followed by swelling, inflammation, and tenderness of the corresponding testis. However, the clinical presentation may often be unclear, and exclusion of other causes of acute scrotal pain, such as epididymitis or torsion of the appendix testis, may be difficult. Doppler ultrasonography offers an alternative modality to scintigraphy to evaluate blood flow to the testis.

Continuous-wave (CW) Doppler evaluation of the testis in episodes of acute scrotal pain has been reported.[167–174] Determination of the absence or presence of testicular blood flow has been used to distinguish torsion from other causes of this acute presentation. Early reports using this

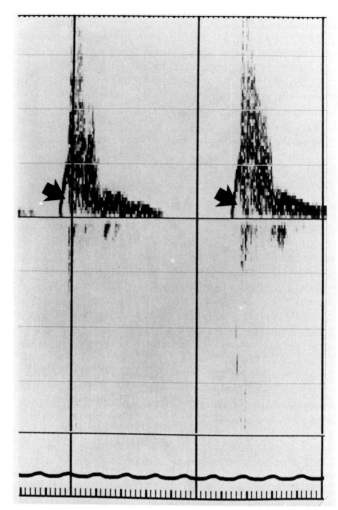

Figure 12–82. Example of a spectral display of turbulent flow distal to a renal artery stenosis. Plug flow is seen in early systole as a "window" (*arrows*) below the time velocity spectrum. As the velocity increases, turbulence suddenly appears as a broad spectrum, with an irregular spectral outline and simultaneous forward and reverse flow. Note that laminar flow is re-established in diastole.

modality were encouraging and demonstrated good correlation with surgical findings.[167–170] Absent or significantly diminished Doppler signals were observed over the testis in episodes of torsion. Normal or intensified signals were noted following spontaneous or surgical detorsion. In patients with epididymitis or torsion of the appendix testis, Doppler signals were normal or increased, compared with the contralateral testis. Subsequently, however, occasional false-negative results of the CW Doppler technique were reported, with normal or increased arterial signals registered over testes with surgically documented torsion.[171–173] The adjacent hyperemia surrounding the testis was believed to be responsible for mimicking testicular flow in many of these patients. In the immediate post-torsion period, arterial pulsations may persist despite venous stasis, and this too may cause a false-negative Doppler study. Additionally, increased scrotal wall blood flow can be misinterpreted as testicular flow. Manual compression of the spermatic cord in the inguinal canal, however, should obliterate testicular signals while scrotal flow persists, thus avoiding this potential pitfall.[167] Rodriguez and colleagues employed this compression test in evaluating 47 patients with an acute scrotum.[174] Persistence of signals following compression in 19% of the patients constituted an indeterminate study. Doppler findings correlated with 62% of patients with torsion and 85% of those without torsion. Overall accuracy was 79%. Radionuclide scintigraphy correlated 100% with surgical findings in the 20 patients of the group studied by means of this modality.

In conclusion, CW Doppler evaluation of the testis in patients with acute scrotal pain appears limited. Identification of arterial signals over the involved testis cannot reliably exclude torsion of the spermatic cord. However, no false-positive results have yet been reported. Absent or significantly decreased signals over the testis would appear to indicate torsion.

Duplex ultrasonography using pulsed Doppler theoretically offers much promise in the work-up of the acute scrotum. Precise location of the Doppler cursor and control of sample volume size would avoid the pitfalls of obtaining signals from the peritesticular tissue, scrotal wall, or spermatic cord proximal to the site of torsion. Hricak and associates reported the absence of Doppler signals using a duplex system in four dogs with surgically created torsion.[129] Color Doppler may also prove valuable.[222]

Varicocele and Internal Spermatic Vein Reflux

A varicocele consists of dilated veins in the pampiniform plexus and occurs almost exclusively on the left side. This is believed to result from reflux in the internal spermatic vein secondary to incompetent valves and is the most common surgically correctable cause of subfertility in men.[175]

Greenberg and coworkers were the first investigators to use Doppler in evaluating patients with known or suspected varicocele.[176] A directional CW Doppler device detected Valsalva-induced regurgitant blood flow over the testicular hilus in all patients with a clinically palpable varicocele. In patients with clinically suspected but nonpalpable varicoceles, Doppler identified regurgitant flow in patients with oligospermia. This suggested that Doppler might be able to identify subclinical varicoceles. Perrin and associates subsequently reported similar results.[177] Venous reflux was demonstrated by Doppler in all patients with known varicocele, and in most patients when it was suspected but not palpable. However, Hirsh and associates reported Valsalva-induced reflux on the left in 83% and on the right in 59% of 118 patients without clinical evidence of varicocele, with no significant difference in incidence between fertile and infertile subjects.[178] Therefore, the significance of Valsalva-induced reflux detected by Doppler, and its association with male infertility, remains unclear in patients without palpable varicocele. In patients with clinical varicocele, the degree or pattern of venous reflux did correlate with varicocele size and the diameter of the internal spermatic vein but showed no relationship with sperm count or state of spermatogenesis on testicular biopsy.

Arteriogenic Impotence

Penile arterial insufficiency is a potentially correctable cause of impotence. The Doppler technique has been applied for assessment of this problem to assist in the work-up and evaluation of the impotent patient.[179–186]

Early work using a Doppler flow meter compared Doppler signals obtained from the dorsal and deep penile arteries with those obtained from a radial artery, which served as a control.[179] Using a scored grading system, a difference between potent and impotent subjects was observed, although the difference was narrow. Velcek and colleagues evaluated Doppler waveforms, calculating an average penile artery acceleration relative to the radial artery acceleration, expressed as the penile flow index.[180] A high penile flow index correlated with pelvic arterial disease demonstrated by arteriography, and erectile failure. Jevtich qualitatively evaluated penile arterial Doppler signals and noted evidence of obstructive blood flow in the penis in 44% of 93 impotent men.[181] An accuracy rate of 95% was reported in patients who had correlative penile angiography results. Other investigators have utilized a Doppler velocimeter and pneumatic cuff to measure penile systolic pressure, which was compared with brachial systolic pressure.[182–185] Abelson reported a penile-brachial systolic gradient (PBSG) of less than 30 mmHg in potent patients.[182] Engel and colleagues reported a ratio of penile systolic pressure to brachial systolic pressure (penile brachial index; PBI) being at least 0.833 in potent males with a significant difference (p < 0.05) in mean indices between potent and impotent subjects.[183] In a study by Kempczinski, a PBSG less than 40 mmHg or a PBI greater than 0.75 with a fair to good penile volume waveform suggested adequate penile blood flow and a nonvascular cause of impotence when such results were observed in patients with erectile dysfunction.[184] A PBSG greater than 60 mmHg or a PBI less than 0.6 was consistent with arteriogenic impotence but was nonspecific in view of the considerable overlap of results in elderly potent and impotent patients. Lane and associates correlated PBSG and PBI in potent and impotent males and reported 10 cases of false-positive Doppler results, when compared with photoplethysmography, resulting from difficulty in insonating the penile arteries.[185]

Recently, Lue and associates reported their experience using duplex ultrasonography with pulsed Doppler in evaluating normal subjects and impotent patients.[186] In the erectile state, induced by intracavernosal injection of papaverine in the impotent males, an interval increase in the diameter of the deep arteries was observed, when compared with vessel size in the flaccid state. Little or no change was detected in patients with poor tumescence. Calculation of blood flow was attempted, but variations in penile size prevented determination of a normal range in this small population.

ULTRASONOGRAPHY OF THE FETAL URINARY TRACT

Normal Anatomy of the Fetal Urinary Tract

It is thought that the first nephrons begin to function at about the eleventh week of gestation.[187] The kidneys are usually visualized sonographically after the fifteenth week. In early pregnancy, the kidneys appear as hypoechogenic oval structures in the posterior midabdomen. As the kidney matures, the pyelocalyceal system becomes apparent as an echo-poor structure (Fig. 12–83). The capsule becomes more clearly visible, and the distinction between the pyramids and the cortex becomes apparent.

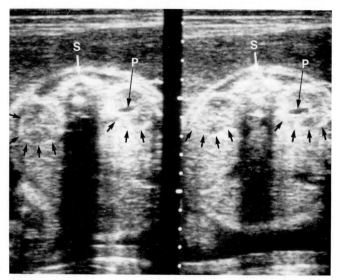

Figure 12–83. Cross section of the normal fetal abdomen in the third trimester. The kidneys appear as hypoechogenic structures (*black arrows*) on both sides of the spine (S). Renal pelvis is clearly visible in one kidney (P).

With high-resolution equipment, the arcuate arteries can be identified quite readily.[188–191] The renal length is measured from the upper pole to the lower pole of the kidney in a longitudinal section of the fetus in a scan that is parallel to the long axis of the aorta. The thickness, width, and perimeter of the kidney are values for kidney biometry and are displayed in Table 12–4. Caliper positioning can be challenging because of the low contrast between the renal parenchyma and the surrounding tissues. Respiratory movements, when present, are extremely helpful in defining the cleavage plane between the kidney and the adrenal glands, spleen, liver, and bowel. The ratio of the kidney perimeter to the abdominal perimeter can be utilized to detect fetal nephromegaly.[190] This ratio is constant throughout gestation; thus, it is more convenient to remember the range of this ratio than to refer constantly to a table for kidney biometry.

The kidney-to-abdominal perimeter ratio is computed as follows:

$$\text{Ratio} = \frac{\text{Kidney width } + \text{ Kidney thickness}}{\text{Anterior abdominal diameter } + \text{ Transverse abdominal diameter}}$$

The ratio is constant and is equal to 23% ± 5% for the 5th and 95th percentiles; the normal range is, therefore, between 18% and 28%.

The normal fetal bladder can be visualized as early as the thirteenth week of gestation. Changes in the size of this organ are generally apparent during the course of a sonographic examination, because the fetus empties his or her bladder every 30 to 45 minutes. A technique for the calculation of fetal bladder volume has been proposed by Campbell and others.[192] They obtained three bladder diameters and utilized the formula:

Bladder volume =

$$\frac{4}{3} \times \pi \times \text{Diameter } \frac{a}{2} \times \text{Diameter } \frac{b}{2} \times \text{Diameter } \frac{c}{2}$$

Diameter a is obtained from the bladder fundus to the bladder neck, diameter b is the maximum transverse diameter and diameter c is the maximum anteroposterior diameter. Hourly urinary output was calculated by doing serial examinations at 15- to 30-minute intervals. The

Table 12–4. Values for Fetal Kidney Biometry*

Age	Kidney Thickness			Kidney Width			Kidney Length			Kidney Volume		
	5th	50th	95th	5th	50th	95th	5th	50th	95th	5th	50th	95th
16	2	6	10	6	10	13	7	13	18	—	0.4	2.6
17	3	7	11	6	10	14	10	15	20	—	0.6	2.8
18	4	8	12	6	10	14	12	17	22	—	0.7	2.9
19	5	9	13	7	10	14	14	19	24	—	0.9	3.1
20	6	10	13	7	11	15	15	21	26	—	1.1	3.3
21	6	10	14	8	12	15	17	22	28	—	1.4	3.6
22	7	11	15	8	12	16	19	24	29	—	1.7	3.9
23	8	12	16	9	13	17	21	26	31	—	2.1	4.3
24	9	13	17	10	14	18	22	28	33	0.3	2.5	4.7
25	10	14	18	11	15	19	24	29	34	0.8	3.0	5.2
26	11	15	19	12	16	19	25	31	36	1.3	3.5	5.7
27	11	15	19	12	16	20	27	32	37	1.9	4.1	6.3
28	12	16	20	13	17	21	28	33	38	2.5	4.7	6.9
29	13	17	21	14	18	22	29	35	40	3.2	5.4	7.6
30	14	18	22	15	19	23	31	36	41	3.9	6.1	8.3
31	14	18	22	16	20	24	32	37	42	4.6	6.8	9.0
32	15	19	23	17	20	24	33	38	43	5.4	7.5	9.7
33	16	20	23	17	21	25	34	39	44	6.1	8.3	10.5
34	16	20	24	18	22	26	35	40	45	6.8	9.0	11.2
35	17	21	25	18	22	26	35	41	46	7.4	9.6	11.8
36	17	21	25	19	23	27	36	41	47	8.1	10.2	12.4
37	18	22	26	19	23	27	37	42	47	8.6	10.8	13.0
38	18	22	26	19	23	27	37	43	48	9.0	11.2	13.4
39	19	23	27	19	23	27	38	43	48	9.4	11.6	13.8
40	19	23	27	19	23	27	38	44	49	9.6	11.8	14.0
	mm	mm	mm	mm	mm	mm	mm	mm	mm	cm³	cm³	cm³

*Values are given as percentiles.

urinary output increased with progressive gestational age from a mean of 12.2 ml/hour at 32 weeks to 28 ml/hour at 40 weeks. The bladder walls are normally thin, but in the presence of obstruction, they may undergo hypertrophy.

Diagnosis of Congenital Anomalies[192a]

Ultrasound has been used in the prenatal diagnosis of congenital anomalies of the urinary tract including renal agenesis, infantile polycystic kidney disease, adult polycystic kidney disease, multicystic kidney disease, obstructive uropathy and renal tumors.

The pathogenesis of the different anomalies of the kidneys is poorly understood. It is thought that if the insult occurs within 5 weeks of conception, failure of communication between the ureteral bud and mesonephric blastema results in renal agenesis. Disturbances occurring immediately after union of these two structures would result in dysplastic cystic kidneys. If the insult takes place after most of the structural development of the kidney has occurred, then a milder form of cystic kidney disease (Potter syndrome Type IV) or hydronephrosis will ensue.[187]

Bilateral Renal Agenesis

Bilateral renal agenesis (BRA) occurs in between 0.1 and 0.3 per 1,000 births and is a uniformly fatal disorder. BRA can be an isolated finding or, less commonly, it can be part of a syndrome. Syndromic BRA can present in conjunction with chromosomal disorders, mendelian disorders, or other congenital syndromes inherited without a mendelian pattern. BRA can also occur sporadically and in association with teratogens (i.e., diabetes mellitus). Nonsyndromic BRA can be inherited with autosomal recessive, X-linked recessive, and multifactorial patterns.[193]

BRA is associated with other anomalies in what has been termed the Potter sequence, Potter syndrome, or oligohydramnios sequence. They include pulmonary hypoplasia, typical facies (low-set ears, redundant skin, prominent fold arising at inner canthus of each eye, parrot-beak nose and receding chin), and aberrant hand and foot positioning. Severe oligohydramnios is thought to be responsible for this phenotype.

Prenatal diagnosis of BRA has been reported several times in the literature.[194, 195] Criteria for a positive diagnosis include absence of a fetal bladder, bilateral absence of the kidneys, and oligohydramnios. Failure to visualize a fetal bladder in a patient with severe oligohydramnios should raise the suspicion for the diagnosis. On occasion, demonstration of the fetal bladder may be hampered by breech presentation or when the fetal spine is up. Although a conclusive diagnosis of BRA should be reached by demonstrating absence of renal shadows, this may be extremely difficult in practice (Fig. 12–84). Indeed fetal adrenal glands have been confused with kidneys, as the normal adrenal and the kidney of the second trimester fetus are of comparable size (Fig. 12–85). The differential diagnosis is based on the visualization of a well-defined renal capsule and renal pelvis. In some cases, it is impos-

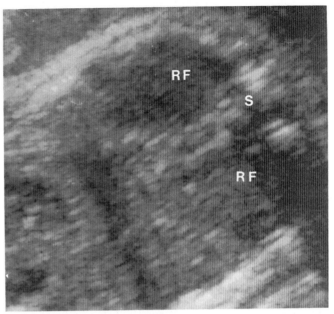

Figure 12–84. Transverse sonogram of the fetal abdomen in a case of bilateral renal agenesis. The renal fossae (RF) are empty. Oligohydramnios hampers a clear visualization of fetal structures. (S = spine.)

sible to differentiate between kidneys and adrenals. A method that can be utilized to improve visualization of the renal fossae is the instillation of warm saline (37°C) into the amniotic cavity.

A second technique used in the prenatal assessment of renal function is the furosemide test. An intravenous dose of 20 to 60 mg of furosemide is given to the mother and filling of the fetal bladder is monitored during the next 2 hours. A distended bladder would obviously indicate the presence of functioning kidneys. Despite the logical basis for this test, several authors have reported the failure of

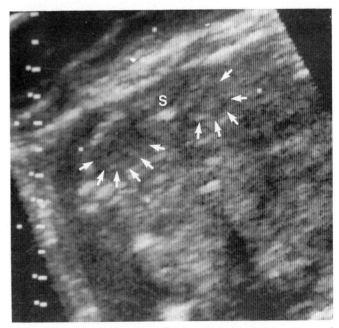

Figure 12–85. In this case of bilateral renal agenesis, the renal fossae are occupied by the adrenal glands (*white arrows*). Differentiation between these organs and the kidney is difficult and in some cases impossible. (S = spine.)

the furosemide test to reliably distinguish BRA from other causes of intrauterine renal failure.[195–199] Indeed, a case has been reported in which an infant with severe oligohydramnios that failed to respond to furosemide was found after delivery to have renal failure requiring peritoneal dialysis.[199]

The differential diagnosis should include the other renal malformations that can give rise to oligohydramnios and nonvisualization of the bladder (polycystic kidneys, multicystic kidneys, fibrous renal dysplasia, obstructive uropathy).

An accurate diagnosis of BRA does not seem possible with ultrasound at this time in all cases. It is extremely difficult to establish the differential diagnosis between BRA and a functional cause of in utero renal failure.

Infantile Polycystic Kidney Disease

Infantile polycystic kidney disease (IPKD) is bilateral and exhibits symmetrical enlargement of the kidneys with polycystic involvement. It is inherited with an autosomal recessive pattern, and its incidence is 1 in 55,000 infants. The disease has been classified into four groups, according to the patient's age at the time of clinical presentation: perinatal, neonatal, infantile, and juvenile (see Chapter 37, Autosomal Recessive Polycystic Disease). Sonographic criteria for the diagnosis include bilaterally enlarged hyperechoic kidneys, oligohydramnios, and an absent fetal bladder (Fig. 12–86). As IPKD presents with

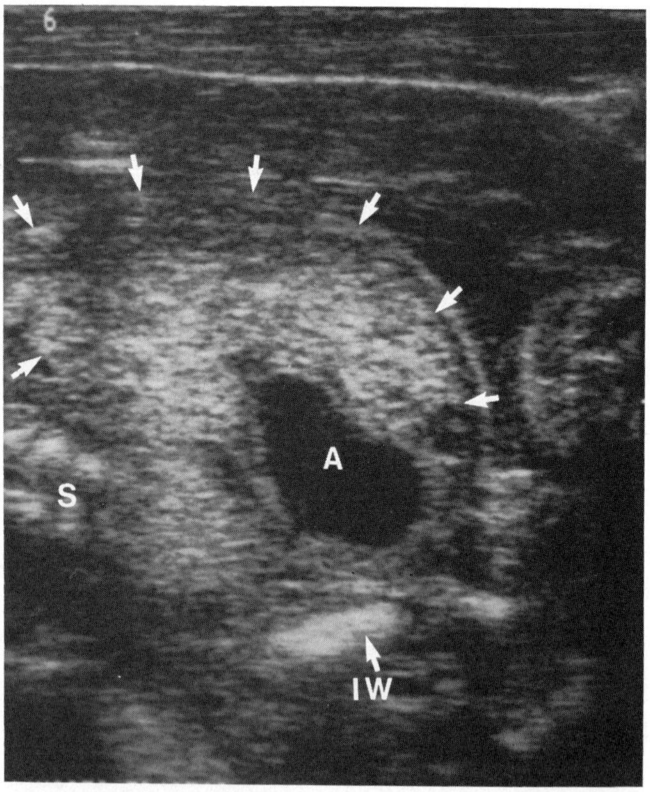

Figure 12–86. Longitudinal sonogram of the abdomen in a third-trimester fetus with infantile autosomal recessive polycystic kidney disease. The huge, highly echogenic left kidney is visible (*arrows*) in this section. The fluid-filled structure visible in the lower abdomen is not the bladder, but a collection of ascitic fluid (A). (IW = iliac wings. S = spine.)

a broad spectrum of renal compromise, the in utero diagnosis may be limited to the severe forms in which the signs can often be identified prior to the twenty-fourth week of gestation. In some cases, diagnosis may be possible until the third trimester or not at all.[200, 201]

Adult Polycystic Kidney Disease

Adult polycystic kidney disease (APKD) is an autosomal dominant disease characterized by replacement of renal parenchyma with multiple cysts of variable size due to dilatation of collecting tubules and other tubular segments of the nephrons. There are seven documented cases of prenatal diagnosis of this condition at the time of this writing.[214] The sonographic appearance has been described as enlarged kidneys with increased parenchymal echogenicity or multiple cysts.[214] The amount of amniotic fluid has been reported to be normal in the two cases reported on to date. In no instance has the disease been diagnosed before 24 weeks of gestation. In two cases in which serial examinations were performed, the dimensions and appearance of the kidneys were normal in the midtrimester, and abnormalities were first detected at 30 and 36 weeks. In the other two cases, diagnosis was made at 32 and 33 weeks of gestation. In some cases the gross lesions may be more prominent in one kidney. APKD in the fetus should be suspected when cystic enlarged kidneys are detected in the presence of a normal amount of amniotic fluid.[202, 203]

Multicystic Kidney Disease

Multicystic kidney disease (MKD) is a congenital renal disorder characterized by cystic lesions that correspond primarily to dilated collecting tubules. MKD is generally a sporadic condition. Familial occurrence is rare. MKD can be bilateral, unilateral, or limited to a localized portion of a kidney.

Multicystic kidneys have a typical appearance on ultrasound, and their antenatal diagnosis has been reported on numerous occasions for both the unilateral and the bilateral forms. Ultrasound criteria for the diagnosis of bilateral multicystic kidneys include cystic kidneys, failure to visualize a fetal bladder, and oligohydramnios. The renal cysts are multiple, peripheral, round, and of variable size (Fig. 12–87). In most instances, the kidneys will be enlarged (Type IIA), but in some cases, they will be small and hyperechoic (Fig. 12–88). The enlarged kidneys may fill a significant portion of the abdomen and may have a lobulated shape or "cluster of grapes" appearance. The differential diagnosis includes infantile polycystic kidney (IPK) and ureteropelvic junction (UPJ) obstruction. UPJ obstruction is suggested by visible renal parenchyma, cystic lesions that are nonspherical in shape and radiating from the kidney to the pelvis, a dilated ureter or a single large cyst (multicystic kidney can present as a single cyst as well), and visualization of cysts that communicate with the renal pelvis.[195, 204]

In unilateral MKD, the only signs of the disease are renal in origin. The bladder and contralateral kidney may be completely normal. This disorder is diagnosed only when attention is paid to the size and morphology of kidneys in routine scans.[204]

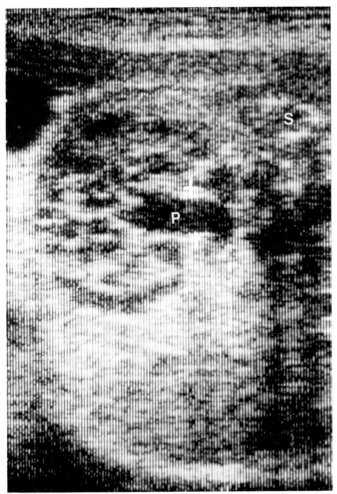

Figure 12–87. Transverse sonogram of a third-trimester fetal kidney with multicystic kidney disease. The kidney is enlarged and filled with multiple cysts of various dimensions ("cluster of grapes" image). (P = renal pelvis. S = spine.)

Obstructive Uropathy

The two major types of obstructive uropathies in the fetus include UPJ obstruction and posterior urethral valves.

The diagnosis of UPJ obstruction depends on the demonstration of a dilated renal pelvis (Fig. 12–89).[205] The two problems with the diagnosis of UPJ obstruction are (1) the criteria employed to classify a renal pelvis as dilated and (2) the natural history of the disease in utero.

At this time there is no available nomogram of renal pelvis size and gestational age. Two criteria of renal pelvis measurements have been proposed: (1) Anteroposterior diameter—renal pelves of less than 5 mm are normal, whereas those between 5 and 10 mm are normal in most instances but may require follow-up. In a recent study of eight fetuses with a 10-mm renal pelvic diameter, seven had an anatomical abnormality at postnatal examination to account for the dilatation.[205a] (2) Ratio between the maximum transverse pelvic diameter and the renal diameter at the same level—ratios above 50% would suggest hydronephrosis. However, diagnostic indices with this criterion are not available.

Several cases have been reported in which a diagnosis of hydronephrosis, either unilateral or bilateral, was ini-

tially made in utero, but follow-up scans in utero and postnatally failed to confirm the finding. Interpreting these reports of transitory hydronephrosis is difficult, because authors have not described the dimensions of the renal pelvis. However, such evidence suggests that serial ultrasound scans are needed to predict trends in amniotic fluid volume and in hydronephrosis severity. Allen and associates were unable to increase the diameter of the fetal renal pelvis by maternal hydration.[205b]

Most UPJ obstructions are unilateral, and the amount of amniotic fluid as well as bladder dynamics should be normal. In cases of unilateral UPJ obstructions, the presence of severe oligohydramnios should raise the suspicion of contralateral renal agenesis or dysplasia. In patients with bilateral dilatation of the renal pelvis, the amount of amniotic fluid can provide information about the severity of the obstruction. If the amount of fluid is normal and/or the bladder is visible, the obstruction is either of recent onset or of an intermittent nature. A normal-to-increased amount of amniotic fluid may coexist with bilaterally poor renal function in patients with associated anomalies that lead to polyhydramnios, such as diaphragmatic hernia, congestive heart failure, or gastrointestinal atresia.

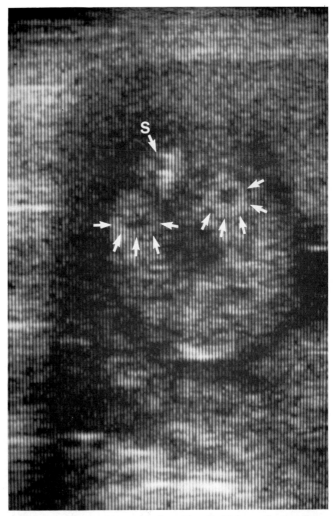

Figure 12–88. In this case of multicystic kidney disease Type IIB, the dysgenetic kidneys (*arrows*) appear as small, hyperechoic areas on both sides of the spine (S).

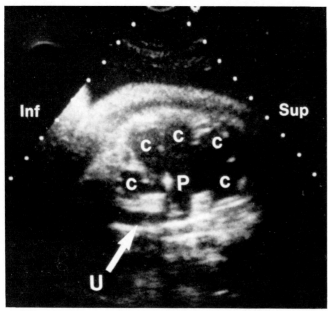

Figure 12–89. Longitudinal sonogram of the kidney in a case of ureterovesical junction obstruction. The sonographic image of the dilated pelvis (P) and calyces (c) resembles that of UPJ (ureteropelvic junction) obstruction. However, the ureter can be clearly visualized (U), allowing the differential diagnosis to be made. (Inf = inferior. Sup = superior.)

Posterior Ureteral Valves

Posterior ureteral valves (PUV) consist of obstruction caused by a membrane-like structure in the posterior urethra. The disorder is usually sporadic. However, some familial cases have been reported in the literature in twins and in siblings. Visualization of the urethral valves with ultrasound is not possible because of their small size. A diagnosis of PUV should be suspected in the presence of sonographic signs of lower urinary tract obstruction (dilated bladder, hydroureter, and hydronephrosis) in a male

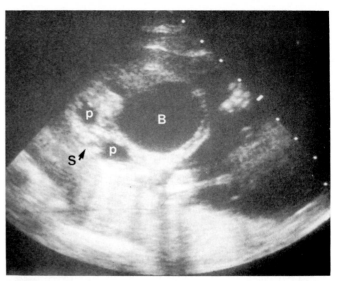

Figure 12–90. Typical sonographic appearance of posterior urethral valves. Dilated bladder (B) and renal pelves (p) are visible in this transverse scan. (S = spine.)

infant (Fig. 12–90).[205] In severe cases, it is possible to demonstrate the dilated posterior urethra proximal to the valves. Sex determination is important, as PUV does not occur in female infants. Causes of lower urinary tract obstruction in females may include agenesis of the urethra and variants of the caudal regression syndrome.

Another sign of PUV occurs when the bladder is distended, and its wall may be hypertrophic (Fig. 12–91). In severe cases, the entrance of the ureters into the bladder wall can be observed. Vesical rupture leads to ascites and decreases bladder size. The ureters are characteristically dilated and tortuous. The degree of dilation of the renal pelvis is in the absence of marked distention of the renal pelvis. This can be explained by one of the following reasons: (1) renal dysplasia has decreased urinary production, (2) rupture at the level of

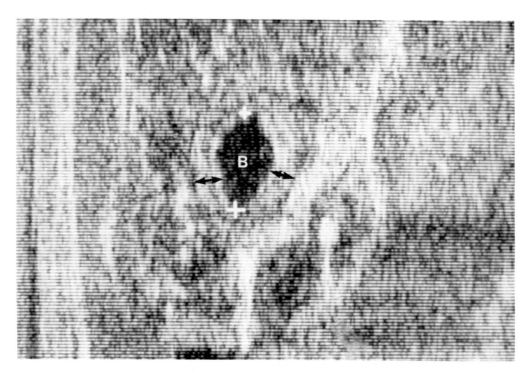

Figure 12–91. Coronal sonogram of fetal abdomen in a long-standing lower urinary tract obstruction. Even if the oligohydramnios hampers a clear visualization of the fetal structures, the thickened bladder wall (*black arrows*) can be seen. (B = bladder.)

Table 12-5. Diagnostic Indices of Sonographic Criteria for the In Utero Identification of Renal Dysplasia in Obstructive Uropathy

	Sensitivity	Specificity	PPV	NPV
Renal cysts	44%	100%	100%	44%
Hyperechogenic renal parenchyma	73%	80%	89%	57%
Hydronephrosis	41%	73%	78%	35%

PPV = Positive predictive value
NPV = Negative predictive value

the bladder or extravasation at any other point along the urinary tract has resulted in decompression of the renal pelvis, (3) there is pyeloureteral atresia.

The most important consideration in regard to the kidney involves the prenatal detection of renal dysplasia.[206] Renal dysplasia can occur with both small and enlarged kidneys. The most important sonographic signs of renal dysplasia are multiple cysts and hyperechogenicity of the renal parenchyma. Table 12-5 displays the diagnostic indices of renal dysplasia. The renal cysts are difficult to detect with ultrasound, but their identification is 100% specific for dysplastic kidneys. Renal echogenicity is more sensitive but is also less specific, with a 20% false-positive rate. Hydronephrosis is the weakest of the renal signs in the prediction of renal dysplasia.

Oligohydramnios is not an invariable finding and is related to the severity and the duration of the obstruction. Severe oligohydramnios is considered a poor prognostic sign; conversely, a normal amount of amniotic fluid is a good prognostic sign.

The differential diagnosis includes other obstructive uropathies such as UPJ or UVJ obstruction, primary megaureter, and massive vesicoureteral reflux. In both UPJ and UVJ obstructions, the bladder should not be dilated. The differential diagnosis between posterior urethral valves and other causes of low urinary tract obstruction, such as absence of the urethra or detrusor hypertrophy, may not be possible in all cases.

A critical aspect of the evaluation of the fetus with obstructive uropathy is the assessment of renal reserve.[207] Infants with bilateral dysplastic kidneys have a uniformly poor prognosis. Although sonographic detection of cortical cystic changes has excellent specificity in the prenatal diagnosis of renal dysplasia, its sensitivity is relatively poor. Therefore, infants whose kidneys appear normal on ultrasound can be born with nonfunctioning kidneys. Management decisions such as pregnancy termination and in utero surgery rely on the assessment of renal reserve. For example, a diagnosis of renal dysfunction, even in the absence of sonographic findings, would render prenatal surgery useless.[207a] This has been accomplished with the use of several parameters outlined in Table 12-6.

Table 12-6. Prognostic Signs in Congenital Renal Disease in the Fetus

Poor Prognostic Signs	Good Prognostic Signs
1. Severe oligohydramnios	1. Normal amniotic fluid
2. Cystic kidneys	2. Normal kidneys
3. Na > 100 mEq/ml	3. Na < 100 mEq/ml
4. Cl > 90 mEq/ml	4. Cl < 90 mEq/ml
5. Osmolarity > 210 mosm	5. Osmolarity < 210 mosm
6. Urinary output of < 2 ml/hr	6. Urinary output > 2 ml/hr*

*Urinary output was measured by exteriorizing the fetal bladder with an indwelling catheter for several hours.

Table 12-7. Interventional Procedures in the Genitourinary Tract Aided by Ultrasound

Procedure	Indication
1. Renal cyst puncture	Evaluate atypical cyst to exclude malignancy
2. Renal mass biopsy	Determine if renal mass is a second primary or metastatic lesion in a patient with known extrarenal malignancy
	Document malignancy if such a diagnosis renders lesion inoperable
3. Renal biopsy	Provide etiology of renal insufficiency
4. Renal abscess aspiration and drainage	Document abscess and establish percutaneous drainage for therapy
5. Perinephric fluid aspiration and drainage	Distinguish abscess from hematoma or other fluid collection and provide drainage if infected
6. Antegrade pyelography	Use as an alternative to retrograde pyelography
7. Percutaneous nephrostomy	Management of obstructive uropathy and pyonephrosis
8. Adrenal mass biopsy	Evaluate for malignancy if mass is large or suspicious on initial presentation or demonstrates an increase in size on follow-up examination
9. Prostate biopsy	Evaluate a suspicious area or mass for malignancy
10. Bladder aspiration or cystostomy	Use to obtain urine specimens for microbiology or to place cystostomy tube

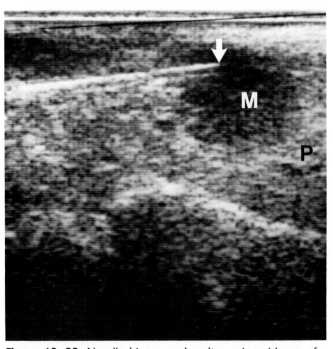

Figure 12-92. Needle biopsy under ultrasonic guidance of a prostatic mass (M), endorectal sagittal sonogram. The needle tip (*arrow*) is seen to be within the mass, which has an abnormally low echogenicity compared with the texture of the remainder of the prostate gland (P). The needle aspiration yielded cytological findings positive for malignancy.

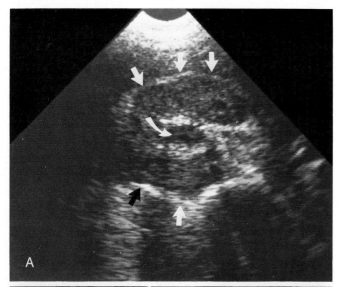

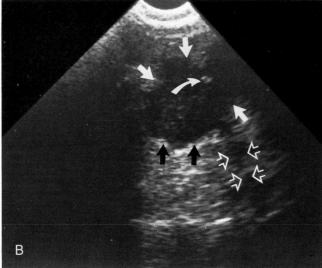

Figure 12–93. Drainage of perinephric abscess under sonographic guidance. *A,* Transverse scan through the right kidney (*arrows*) in a patient with fever demonstrates mild dilatation of the collecting system with internal echoes within it (*curved arrow*). The finding of debris within a dilated system is typical of pyonephrosis. *B,* Transverse scan through a perinephric abscess on the same patient as in *A.* (Solid arrows indicate the abscess.) A drainage catheter has been placed under sonographic guidance. Note that both walls of the catheter (*curved arrow*) can be seen in this axial image. Note also the acoustic shadow (*open arrows*) distal to the catheter. The patient also had a percutaneous nephrostomy under sonographic guidance to treat the underlying pyonephrosis.

INTRAOPERATIVE ULTRASONOGRAPHY

Intraoperative applications of ultrasound have been reported using B-scan and Doppler techniques.

Intraoperative B scanning has been used for calculus and tumor localization.[208–210a] Using a high-frequency transducer (7.5 to 10 MHz), calculi as small as 2 mm to 3 mm can be identified. Precise localization of stones permits relatively small nephrotomy incisions, reduced search time, and tissue manipulation. Ultrasonography can identify retained fragments after removal of staghorn calculi, and it offers the advantage of visualizing stones

that are nonopaque on radiographs. Gilbert and coworkers have used intraoperative sonography successfully to locate renal cell carcinomas, which were deep within the kidney and could not be seen or felt.[210a]

Intraoperative Doppler ultrasonography has been used to identify anatrophic planes in the kidney for nephrotomy to remove large or dendritic calculi.[211] This reduces blood loss and operative time. The Doppler technique can localize intrarenal arteriovenous fistulas prior to excision, document blood flow before wound closure following procedures with prolonged ischemia, and determine parenchymal viability in patients with segmental obstruction.[212] The technique can also prove useful in localizing the main renal artery and vein when the anatomy of the renal hilum or pedicle is obscured by inflammation, previous surgery, or tumor invasion.[212]

INTERVENTIONAL ULTRASONOGRAPHY

Multiple interventional procedures of the genitourinary tract can be performed percutaneously, using high-resolution real-time ultrasound guidance. Table 12–7 lists many of these procedures and their indications. A more thorough discussion can be found in the review by Coleman and Pollack.[213]

The needle position can be ascertained following puncture to verify its location in the lesion (Figs. 12–92 and 12–93).

References

1. Taylor KJW, Hill CR: Scanning techniques in grey-scale ultrasonography. Br J Radiol 48:918, 1975.
2. Kossoff G: Display techniques in ultrasound pulse echo investigations: A review. J Clin Ultrasound 2:61, 1974.
3. Taylor KJW, Jacobson P, Jaffe CC: Lack of acoustic shadow on scans of gallstones: A possible artifact. Radiology 131:463, 1979.
4. Hodson CJ: The renal parenchyma and its blood supply. Curr Probl Diagn Radiol 7:3, 1978.
5. Cook JH III, Rosenfield AT, Taylor KJW: Ultrasonic demonstration of intrarenal anatomy. AJR 129:831, 1977.
6. Rosenfield AT, Taylor KJW, Crade M, et al: Anatomy and pathology of the kidney by grey-scale ultrasound. Radiology 128:737, 1978.
7. Haller JO, Berdon WE, Friedman AP: Increased renal cortical echogenicity—a normal finding in neonates and infants. Radiology 142:173, 1982.
8. Scheible W, Leopold GR: High-resolution real-time ultrasonography of neonatal kidneys. J Ultrasound Med 1:133, 1982.
9. Hricak H, Slovis TL, Callen CW: Neonatal kidneys: Sonographic anatomic correlation. Radiology 147:699, 1983.
10. Jones TB, Riddick LR, Harpen MD, et al: Ultrasonographic determination of renal mass and renal volume. J Ultrasound Med 2:151, 1983.
11. Rasmussen SN, Haase L, Kjeldsen H, Hancke S: Determination of renal volume by ultrasound scanning. J Clin Ultrasound 6:160, 1978.
12. Moskowitz PS, Carroll BA, McCoy JM: Ultrasonic volumetry in children. Radiology 134:61, 1980.
13. Rosenbaum DM, Korngold E, Teele RL: Sonographic assessment of renal length in normal children. AJR 142:467, 1984.
14. Haugstvedt S, Lundberg J: Kidney size in normal children measured by sonography. Scand J Urol Nephrol 14:251, 1980.
15. Rasmussen SN, Haase L, Kjeldsen H, Hancke S: Determination of renal volume by ultrasound scanning. J Clin Ultrasound 6:160, 1978.
16. Brandt D, Neiman HL, Dragowski MJ, et al: Ultrasound assessment of normal renal dimensions. J Ultrasound Med 1:49, 1982.
17. Sanders RC, Conrad MR: The ultrasonic characteristics of the renal pelvocalyceal echo complex. J Clin Ultrasound 5:373, 1977.

18. Rosenfield AT, Taylor KJW, Dembner AG, et al: Ultrasound of renal sinus: New observations. AJR 133:441, 1979.
19. Weill FS, Perriguey G, Rohmer P: Sonographic study of the juxtarenal retroperitoneal components. J Ultrasound Med 1:307, 1982.
20. Conrad MR, Freedman M, Weiner C, et al: Sonography of the Page kidney. J Urol 116:293, 1976.
21. Buschi AJ, Harrison RB, Brenbridge ANAG, et al: Distended left renal vein: CT/sonographic normal variant. AJR 135:339, 1980.
22. Callen PW, Filly RA, Sarti DA, Sample F: Ultrasonography of the diaphragmatic crura. Radiology 130:721, 1979.
23. Callen PW, Filly RA, Marks WM: The quadratus lumborum muscle: A possible source of confusion in sonographic evaluation of the retroperitoneum. J Clin Ultrasound 7:349, 1979.
24. Meyers MA, Whalen JP, Evans JA, et al: Malposition and displacement of the bowel in renal agenesis and ectopia: New observations. AJR 117:323, 1973.
25. Moscatello V, Lebowitz RL: Malposition of the colon in left renal agenesis and ectopia. Radiology 120:371, 1976.
26. Curtis JA, Sudhu V, Steiner RM: Malposition of the colon in right renal agenesis, ectopia, and anterior nephrectomy. AJR 129:845, 1977.
27. Teele RL, Rosenfield AT, Freeman GS: The anatomic splenic flexure: An ultrasonic renal imposter. AJR 128:115, 1977.
28. Rosenfield AT, Berg GR, Taylor KJW: Anuria and palpable left upper quadrant mass in a four-year-old. In Rosenfield AT (ed): Genitourinary Ultrasonography. Clinics in Diagnostic Ultrasound, Vol 2. New York, Churchill Livingstone, 1970.
29. Sample WF: A new technique for the evaluation of the adrenal gland with gray scale ultrasonography. Radiology 124:463, 1977.
30. Sample WF: Adrenal ultrasonography. Radiology 127:462, 1977.
31. Rosenberg ER, Bowie JD, Andreotti R, Fields SI: Sonographic evaluation of fetal adrenal glands. AJR 139:1145, 1982.
32. Oppenheimer DA, Carroll BA, Yousem S: Sonography of the normal neonatal adrenal gland. Radiology 146:157, 1983.
33. Sanders RC, Duffy T, McLoughlin MG, et al: Sonography in the diagnosis of retroperitoneal fibrosis. J Urol 118:944, 1977.
34. Mendelson DS, Mitty HA, Janus C, Cohen BA: Horseshoe kidney mimicking adenopathy. Urol Radiol 5:121–122, 1983.
35. Nyborg WL, Ziskin MC (eds): Biological effects of ultrasound. Clinics in Diagnostic Ultrasound, Vol 16. New York, Churchill Livingstone, 1985.
35a. Simpson EL, Mintz MC, Pollack HM, et al: Computed tomography in the diagnosis of renal pseudotumors. Comput Tomogr 10:341, 1986.
36. Cook JH, Lytton B: Intra-operative localization of renal calculi during nephrolithotomy by ultrasound scanning. J Urol 117:543–546, 1977.
37. Birnholz JC, Merkel FK: Submucosal edema of the collecting system: new ultrasonic sign of severe, acute renal allograft rejection: Clinical note. Radiology 154:190, 1985.
38. Sanders RC, Bearman S: B-scan ultrasound in the diagnosis of hydronephrosis. Radiology 108:375, 1973.
39. Haasch E: Changes in renal pelvic size in children after fluid intake demonstrated by ultrasound. Ultrasound Med Biol 2:287, 1977.
40. Sanders RC, Hartman DS: The sonographic distinction between neonatal multicystic kidney and hydronephrosis. Radiology 151:621, 1984.
41. Cronan JJ, Amis ES Jr, Yoder IC, et al: Peripelvic cysts: An imposter of sonographic hydronephrosis. J Ultrasound Med 1:229–236, 1982.
41a. Dillard JP, Talner LB, Pinckney L: Normal renal papillae simulating calyceal filling defects on sonography. AJR 148:895, 1987.
42. Chopra A, Teele RL: Hydronephrosis: Narrowing the differential diagnosis with ultrasound. J Clin Ultrasound 8:473, 1980.
43. Zegel HG, Pollack HM, Banner MP, et al: Percutaneous nephrostomy: Comparison of sonographic and fluoroscopic guidance. AJR 137:925, 1981.
44. Holm HH, Pederson JF, Kristensen JK, et al: Ultrasonically guided percutaneous puncture. Radiol Clin North Am 13:493, 1975.
45. Subramanyam BR, Raghavendra BN, Bosniak MA, et al: Sonography of pyonephrosis: A prospective study. AJR 140:991, 1983.
46. Yoder IC, Pfister RC, Lindfors KK, et al: Pyonephrosis: Imaging and intervention. AJR 141:735, 1983.
47. Coleman BG, Arger PH, Mulhern CB, et al: Pyonephrosis: Sonography in the diagnosis and management. AJR 137:939, 1981.
48. Arger PH, Mulhern CB, Pollack HM, et al: Ultrasonic assessment of renal transitional cell carcinoma: Preliminary report. AJR 132:407, 1979.
49. Stuck KJ, Silver TM, Jaffe MH, et al: Sonographic demonstration of renal fungus balls. Radiology 142:473, 1981.
50. Edell S, Zegel H: Ultrasonic evaluation of renal calculi. AJR 130:261, 1978.
51. Pollack HM, Arger PH, Goldberg BB, et al: Ultrasonic detection of nonopaque renal calculi. Radiology 127:235, 1978.
52. Sommer FG, Taylor KJW: Differentiation of acoustic shadowing due to calculi and gas collections. Radiology 135:399–403, 1980.
53. Sommer FG, Filly RA, Minton MJ: Acoustic shadowing due to refractive and reflective effects. AJR 132:973, 1979.
54. Ellenbogen PH, Scheible WF, Talner LB, et al: Sensitivity of gray scale ultrasound in detecting urinary tract obstruction. AJR 130:731, 1978.
55. Talner LB, Scheible WF, Ellenbogen PH, et al: Ultrasound diagnosis of hydronephrosis in azotemic patients. Urol Radiol 3:1, 1981.
56. Lalli AF: Retroperitoneal fibrosis and inapparent obstructive uropathy. Radiology 122:339, 1977.
56a. Laing FC, Jeffrey RB Jr, Wing VW: Sonography versus excretory urography in evaluating acute flank pain. Radiology 154:613, 1985.
57. Amis ES, Cronan JJ, Pfister RC, et al: Ultrasonic inaccuracies in diagnosis of renal obstruction. Urology 19:101, 1982.
58. Garris J, Kangarloo H, Sarti D, et al: The ultrasound spectrum of prune belly syndrome. J Clin Ultrasound 8:117, 1980.
59. Hricak H, Cruz C, Romanski R, et al: Renal parenchymal disease: Sonographic-histologic correlation. Radiology 144:141, 1982.
60. Rosenfield ATR, Siegel N: Renal parenchymal disease: Histologic-sonographic correlation. AJR 137:793, 1981.
61. LeQuesne GW: Assessment of glomerulonephritis in children by ultrasound. In White D, Lyons EA (eds): Ultrasound in Medicine, Vol 4. New York, Plenum Press, 1978.
62. Sanders RC: Examination of kidneys not seen at excretion urography. In Resnick MI, Sanders RC (eds): Ultrasound in Urology. Baltimore, Williams & Wilkins, 1979.
63. Goh TS, LeQuesne GW, Wong KY: Severe infiltration of the kidneys with ultrasound abnormalities in acute lymphoblastic leukemia. Am J Dis Child 132:1204, 1978.
64. Finberg AJ, Hillman B, Smith EH: Ultrasound in the evaluation of the non-functioning kidney. In Rosenfield AT (ed): Genitourinary ultrasonography. Clinics in Diagnostic Ultrasound 2. New York, Churchill-Livingstone, 1979, p 105.
65. Wilson DA, Wenzel JE, Altshuler GP: Ultrasound demonstration of diffuse cortical nephrocalcinosis in a case of primary hyperoxaluria. AJR 132:659, 1979.
66. Rosenfield AT: Ultrasonic diagnosis of primary hyperoxaluria in infancy (letter). Radiology 148:578, 1983.
67. Brennan JW, Diwan RV, Makker SP, et al: Ultrasonic diagnosis of primary hyperoxaluria of infancy. Radiology 145:147, 1982.
68. Rosenfield AT, Zeman RK, Cronan JJ, Taylor KJW: Ultrasound in experimental and clinical renal vein thrombosis. Radiology 137:735, 1980.
69. Foley CL, Luisiri A, Graviss ER, et al: Nephrocalcinosis: Sonographic detection in Cushing's syndrome. AJR 139:610, 1982.
70. Patriquin H, O'Regan S: Medullary sponge kidney in childhood. AJR 145:315, 1985.
71. Glazer GM, Callen PW, Filly RA: Medullary nephrocalcinosis: Sonographic evaluation. AJR 138:55, 1982.
72. Avni EF, Spehl-Robbereet D, Gomes H, et al: Transient acute tubular disease in the newborn: Characteristic ultrasound pattern. Ann Radiol 26:175, 1983.
73. Hayden CK, Swischuk LE, Smith TH, Armstrong EA: Renal cystic disease in childhood. RadioGraphics 6:97–116, 1986.
74. Wernicke K, Heckemann R, Bachmann H: Sonography of infantile polycystic kidney disease. Urol Radiol 7:138, 1985.
75. Edell SL, Bonquita JA: The sonographic appearance of acute pyelonephritis. Radiology 132:683–685, 1979.
76. Erwin BC, Carroll BA, Walter JF, Sommer FG: Renal infarction appearing as an echogenic mass. AJR 138:759, 1982.
77. Hartman DS, Davis CJ Jr, Goldman SM, et al: Xanthogranulomatous pyelonephritis: Sonographic–pathologic correlation of 16 cases. J Ultrasound Med 3:481, 1984.
78. Pamilo M, Kulatunga A, Martikainen J: Renal parenchymal malakoplakia: A report of two cases. The radiologic and ultrasound images. Radiology 155:272, 1985.
79. Leopold GR, Talner LB, Asher WM, et al: Renal ultrasonography:

An updated approach to the diagnosis of the renal cyst. Radiology 109:671, 1973.

80. Green WM, King DL, Casarella WJ: A reappraisal of sonolucent renal masses. Radiology 121:163, 1976.

81. Bree RL, Silver TM: Differential diagnosis of hypoechoic and anechoic masses with gray scale sonography: New observations. J Clin Ultrasound 7:249–254, 1979.

82. Conrad MR, Sanders RC, James AE: The sonolucent "light bulb" sign of fluid collections. J Clin Ultrasound 4:409–419, 1976.

83. Wells PNT: Biomedical Ultrasonics. New York, Academic Press, 1977.

84. Birnholz JC: Sonic differentiation of cysts and homogeneous solid masses. Radiology 108:699–702, 1973.

85. Jaffe CC, Rosenfield AT, Sommer G, et al: Technical factors influencing the imaging of small anechoic cysts by B-scan ultrasound. Radiology 135:429, 1980.

86. Zeman RK, Cronan JJ, Viscomi GN, et al: Coordinated imaging in the detection and characterization of renal masses. CRC Crit Rev Diagn Imag 15:273–318, 1981.

87. Rosenfield AT, Glickman MC, Taylor KJW, et al: Acute focal bacterial nephritis (acute lobar nephronia). Radiology 132:552, 1961.

88. Lee JKL, McClellan BL, Melson GL, et al: Acute focal bacterial nephritis: Emphasis on gray scale sonography and computed tomography. AJR 135:87, 1980.

89. Rauschkolb EW, Sandler CM, Patel S, et al: Computed tomography of renal inflammatory disease. J Comput Assist Tomogr 6:502, 1982.

90. Ishikawa I, Saito Y, Onouchi Z, et al: Delayed contrast enhancement in acute focal bacterial nephritis: CT features. J Comput Assist Tomogr 9:894, 1985.

91. Schaffer RM, Shih YH, Becker JA: Sonographic identification of collecting system duplications. J Clin Ultrasound 11:309, 1983.

92. Horgan JG, Rosenfield NS, Weiss RM, Rosenfield AT: Is renal ultrasound a reliable indicator of a nonobstructed duplication anomaly? Ped Radiol 14:388, 1984.

93. Carter AR, Horgan JG, Jennings TA, Rosenfield AT: The junctional parenchymal defect: A normal sonographic variant of renal anatomy. Radiology 154:499, 1985.

94. Hoffer FA, Hanabergh AM, Teele RL: Interrenicular junction: A mimic of renal scarring on normal pediatric sonograms. AJR 145:1075, 1985.

95. Kay CJ, Rosenfield AT, Taylor KJW, et al: Ultrasound gray-scale characteristics of chronic atrophic pyelonephritis. AJR 132:683, 1979.

96. McCarthy S, Rosenfield AT: Crossed fused renal ectopia. J Ultrasound Med 3:107, 1984.

97. Coleman BG, Arger PH, Mulhern CB, Jr, et al: Gray-scale sonographic spectrum of hypernephromas. Radiology 137:757, 1980.

98. Maklad NF, Chuang VP, Doust BD, et al: Ultrasonic characterization of solid renal lesions: Echographic angiographic and pathologic correlation. Radiology 123:733, 1977.

99. Hartman DS, Sanders RC: Wilms' tumor versus neuroblastoma: Usefulness of ultrasound in differentiation. J Ultrasound Med 1:117, 1982.

100. Richman TS, Taylor KJW, Kremkau FW: Propagation speed artifact in a fatty tumor (myelolipoma): Significance for tissue differential diagnosis. J Ultrasound Med 2:45, 1983.

101. Hartman DS, Goldman SM, Friedman AC, et al: Angiomyolipoma: Ultrasonic-pathologic correlation. Radiology 139:451–458, 1981.

102. Lee TG, Henderson SC, Freency PC, et al: Ultrasound findings of renal angiomyolipoma. J Clin Ultrasound 6:150–155, 1977.

103. Avruch L, Cooperberg PL: The ring-down artifact. J Ultrasound Med 4:21, 1985.

104. Rigsby C, Rosenfield AT, Glickman M, Hodson CJ: Acute hemorrhagic focal bacterial nephritis. Findings on gray scale sonography and CT. AJR 146:1173–1177, 1986.

104a. Vick CW, Viscomi GN, Mannes E, Taylor KJW: Pitfalls related to the urinary bladder in pelvic sonography: A review. Urol Radiol 5:253, 1983.

105. Goldberg BB, Meyer H: Ultrasonically guided suprapubic urinary bladder aspiration. Pediatrics 51:70, 1973.

106. Hakenberg OW, Ryall RL, Langlois SL, Marshall VR: The estimation of bladder volume by sonocystography. J Urol 130:249, 1983.

107. Allen HA III, Walsh JW, Brewer WH, et al: Sonography of emphysematous pyelonephritis. J Ultrasound Med 3:533, 1984.

108. Abu-Yousef M, Narayana AS, Franken EA, et al: Urinary bladder tumors studied by cystosonography. Radiology 153:223, 1984.

109. Cronan JJ, Simeone JF, Pfister RC, et al: Cystosonography in the detection of bladder tumors: A prospective and retrospective study. J Ultrasound Med 1:237, 1981.

110. Rifkin M, Kurtz AB, Pasto ME, et al: Unusual presentations of cystitis. J Ultrasound Med 1:25, 1983.

111. Rosenfield AT, Taylor KJW, Weiss RM: Ultrasound evaluation of bladder calculi. J Urol 121:119, 1979.

111a. Dubbins PA, Kurtz AB, Darby J, Goldberg B: Ureteric jet effect: The echographic appearance of urine entering the bladder. Radiology 140:513–515, 1981.

112. Taylor KJW, Jacobson P, Talmont CA, Winters R: Artifacts and Pitfalls. In Manual of Ultrasonography. New York, Churchill Livingstone, 1980, pp 35–37.

113. Sarti DA, Sample WF (eds): Diagnostic Ultrasound Text & Cases. Boston, GK Hall & Co, 1980.

114. Rifkin MD, Friedland GW, Shortliffe L: Prostatic evaluation by transrectal endosonography: Detection of carcinoma. Radiology 158:85, 1986.

115. Lee F, Gray JM, McLeary RD, et al: Prostatic evaluation by transrectal sonography: Criteria for diagnosis of early carcinoma. Radiology 158:91, 1986.

116. Dahnert WG, Hamper UM, Eggleston JC, et al: Prostatic evaluation by transrectal sonography with histopathologic correlation: The echopenic appearance of early carcinoma. Radiology 258:97, 1986.

116a. Burks DD, Drolshagen LF, Fleischer AC, et al: Transrectal sonography of benign and malignant prostatic lesions. AJR 146:1187, 1986.

116b. Rifkin MD, Kurtz AB, Goldberg BB: Sonographically guided transperineal prostatic biopsy: Preliminary experience with a longitudinal linear-array transducer. AJR 140:745, 1983.

116c. Rifkin MD, Kurtz AB, Goldberg BB: Prostate biopsy utilizing transrectal ultrasound guidance: Diagnosis of nonpalpable cancers. J Ultrasound Med 2:165, 1983.

116d. Sanders RC, Hamper UM, Dahnert WF: Update on prostatic ultrasound. Urol Radiol 9:110, 1987.

116e. Rifkin MD: Endorectal sonography of the prostate: Clinical implications. AJR 148:1137, 1987.

117. Rifkin MD, Fory PM, Goldberg BB: Scrotal ultrasound: Acoustic characteristics of the normal testis and epididymis defined with high resolution superficial scanners. Med Ultrasound 8:91, 1984.

118. Sample WF, Gottesman JE, Skinner DG, et al: Gray scale ultrasound of the scrotum. Radiology 127:225, 1978.

119. Willscher MK, Conway JF, Daly KJ, et al: Scrotal ultrasonography. J Urol 130:931, 1983.

120. Arger PH, Mulhern CB, Coleman BG, et al: Prospective analysis of the value of scrotal ultrasound. Radiology 141:763, 1981.

121. Subramanyam BR, Balthazar EJ, Raghavendra BN, et al: Sonographic diagnosis of scrotal hernia. AJR 139:535, 1982.

122. Nachtsheim DA, Scheible WF, Gosink B: Ultrasonography of testis tumors. J Urol 129:978, 1983.

123. Glazer HS, Lee JKT, Melson GL, McClennan BL: Sonographic detection of occult testicular neoplasms. AJR 138:673, 1982.

124. Stoll S, Goldfinger M, Rothberg R, et al: Incidental detection of impalpable testicular neoplasm by sonography. AJR 146:349, 1986.

125. Rifkin MD, Jacobs JA: Simple testicular cyst diagnosed preoperatively by ultrasound. J Urol 129:982, 1983.

126. Caravelli JF, Peters BE: Sonography of bilateral testicular epidermoid cysts. J Ultrasound Med 3:273, 1984.

127. Bird K, Rosenfield AT, Taylor KJW: Ultrasonography in testicular torsion. Radiology 147:527, 1983.

128. Bird K, Rosenfield AT: Testicular infarction secondary to acute inflammatory disease: Demonstration by B-scan ultrasound. Radiology 152:785, 1984.

129. Hricak H, Lue T, Filly RA, et al: Experimental study of the sonographic diagnosis of testicular torsion. J Ultrasound Med 2:349, 1983.

130. Bird K, Rosenfield AT: B-scan ultrasonography of acute focal orchitis and its sequelae (abstr). AJR 142:239, 1984.

131. Lupetin AR, King W III, Rich PJ, et al: The traumatized scrotum: Ultrasound evaluation. Radiology 148:203, 1983.

132. Weiss RM, Carter AR, Rosenfield AT: High-resolution real-time ultrasonography in the localization of the undescended testis. J Urol 135:936, 1986.

133. Wolverson MK, Houttvin E, Heiberg E, et al: Comparison of computed tomography with high-resolution real-time ultrasound

in the localization of the impalpable undescended testis. Radiology 146:133, 1983.

134. Madrazo BL, Klugo R, Parks JA, et al: Ultrasonographic demonstration of undescended testes. Radiology 133:181, 1979.

134a. Seidenwurm D, Mathers RL, Lo RK, et al: Testes and scrotum. MR Imaging at 1.5 T. Radiology 164:393, 1987.

135. Worthy L, Miller EI, Chinn DH: Evaluation of extratesticular findings in scrotal neoplasms. J Ultrasound Med 5:261, 1986.

136. Rifkin MD, Jacobs JA: Simple testicular cyst diagnosed preoperatively by ultrasound. J Urol 129:982–983, 1983.

137. Subramanyam BR, Horii SC, Hilton S: Diffuse testicular disease: Sonographic features and significance. AJR 145:1221, 1985.

138. Gelbard M, Sarti D, Kaufman JJ: Ultrasound imaging of Peyronie's plaques. J Urol 125:44, 1981.

139. Dierks PR, Hawkins H: Sonography and penile trauma. J Ultrasound Med 2:417, 1983.

140. Satomura S: Study of flow patterns in peripheral arteries by ultrasonics. J Acoust Sci Jpn 15:151, 1959.

141. Burns PN, Jaffe CC: Quantitative flow measurements with Doppler ultrasound: Techniques, accuracy, and limitations. Radiol Clin North Am 23:641–657, 1985.

142. Taylor KJW, Burns PN: Duplex Doppler scanning in the pelvis and abdomen. Ultrasound Med Biol 11:643, 1985.

143. Nichols BT, Rittgers SE, Norris CS, Barnes RW: Noninvasive detection of renal artery stenosis. Bruit 8:26, 1984.

144. Reid MH, MacKay RS, Lantz BMT: Noninvasive blood flow measurements by Doppler ultrasound with applications to renal artery flow determination. Invest Radiol 15:323, 1980.

145. Greene ER, Venters MD, Avasthi PS, Conn RL, Jahnke RW: Noninvasive characterization of renal artery blood flow. Kidney Int 20:523, 1981.

146. Babcock DS, Slovis TL, Han BK, et al: Renal transplants in children: Long-term follow-up using sonography. Radiology 156:165–167, 1985.

147. Bartrum RJ, Smith EH, D'Orsi CJ, et al: Evaluation of renal transplants with ultrasound. Radiology 118:405–410, 1976.

148. Birnholz JC, Merkel FK: Submucosal edema of the collecting system: A new ultrasonic sign of severe, acute renal allograft rejection. Radiology 154:190, 1985.

149. Fleischer AC, James AE Jr, MacDonnell RC Jr, et al: Sonography of renal transplant patients. CRC Crit Rev Diagn Imaging 18:197–242, 1982.

150. Frick MP, Feinberg SB, Silbey R, Idstrom ME: Ultrasound in acute renal transplant rejection. Radiology 138:657, 1981.

151. Hillman BJ, Birnholz JC, Busch GJ: Correlation of echographic and histologic findings in suspected renal allograft rejection. Radiology 132:673–676, 1979.

152. Hricak H, Toledo-Pereyra LH, Eyler WR, et al: The role of ultrasound in the diagnosis of kidney allograft rejection. Radiology 132:667–672, 1979.

153. Hricak H, Cruz C, Eyler WR, et al: Acute post-transplantation renal failure: Differential diagnosis by ultrasound. Radiology 139:441–449, 1981.

154. Maklad NF, Wright CH, Rosenthal SJ: Gray scale ultrasonic appearances of renal transplant rejection. Radiology 131:711–717, 1979.

155. Slovis TL, Babcock DS, Hricak H, et al: Renal transplant rejection: Sonographic evaluation in children. Radiology 153:659–665, 1984.

156. Arima M, Ishibashi M, Usami M, et al: Analysis of the arterial blood flow patterns of normal and allografted kidneys by the directional ultrasonic Doppler technique. J Urol 122:587, 1979.

157. Arima M, Takahara S, Ihara H, et al: Predictability of renal allograft prognosis during rejection crisis by ultrasonic Doppler flow technique. Urology 19:389, 1982.

158. Berland LL, Lawson TL, Adams MB, et al: Evaluation of renal transplants with pulsed Doppler duplex sonography. J Ultrasound Med 1:215, 1982.

159. Norris CS, Barnes RW: Renal artery flow velocity analysis: A sensitive measure of experimental and clinical renovascular resistance. J Surg Res 36:230, 1984.

160. Rigsby CM, Taylor KJW, Weltin G, et al: Renal allografts in acute rejection: Evaluation using duplex sonography. Radiology 158:375, 1986.

161. Marchioro TL, Strandness DE Jr, Krugmire RB Jr: The ultrasonic velocity detector for determining vascular patency in renal homografts. Transplantation 8:296, 1969.

162. Reinitz ER, Goldman MH, Sais J, et al: Evaluation of transplant renal artery blood flow by Doppler sound-spectrum analysis. Arch Surg 118:415, 1983.

163. Wood RFM, Nasmyth DG: Doppler ultrasound in the diagnosis of vascular occlusion in renal transplantation. Transplantation 33:547, 1982.

164. Sampson D: Ultrasonic method for detecting rejection of human renal allotransplants. Lancet 2:976, 1969.

165. Sampson D, Abramczyk J, Murphy GP: Ultrasonic measurement of blood flow changes in renal allografts. J Surg Res 12:388, 1972.

166. Raine AEG, Ledingham JGG: Cardiovascular complications after renal transplantation. In Morris PJ: Kidney Transplantation—Principles and Practice, 2nd Ed. London, Grune & Stratton, 1984.

167. Pedersen JF, Holm HH, Hald T: Torsion of the testis diagnosed by ultrasound. J Urol 113:66, 1975.

168. Levy BJ: The diagnosis of torsion of the testicle using the Doppler ultrasonic stethoscope. J Urol 113:63, 1975.

169. Thompson IM, Latourette H, Chadwick S, et al: Diagnosis of testicular torsion using Doppler ultrasonic flowmeter. Urology 6:706, 1975.

170. Perri AJ, Slachta GA, Feldman AE, et al: The Doppler stethoscope and the diagnosis of the acute scrotum. J Urol 116:598, 1976.

171. Perri AJ, Morales JO, Feldman AE, et al: Necrotic testicle with increased blood flow on Doppler ultrasonic examination. Urology 8:265, 1976.

172. Nasrallah PF, Manzone D, King LR: Falsely negative Doppler examinations in testicular torsion. J Urol 118:194, 1977.

173. Brereton RJ: Limitations of the Doppler flow meter in the diagnosis of the "acute scrotum" in boys. Br J Urol 53:380, 1981.

174. Rodriguez DD, Rodriguez WC, Rivera JJ, et al: Doppler ultrasound versus testicular scanning in the evaluation of the acute scrotum. J Urol 125:343, 1981.

175. Zorgniotti AW: Testis temperature, infertility, and the varicocele paradox. Urology 16:7–10, 1980.

176. Greenberg SH, Lipshultz LI, Morganroth J, et al: The use of the Doppler stethoscope in the evaluation of varicoceles. J Urol 117:296, 1977.

177. Perrin P, Rollet J, Durand L: The Doppler stethoscope in the diagnosis of subclinical varicocele. Br J Urol 52:390, 1980.

178. Hirsh AV, Cameron KM, Tyler JP, et al: The Doppler assessment of varicoceles and internal spermatic vein reflux in infertile men. Br J Urol 52:50, 1980.

179. Malvar T, Baron T, Clark SS: Assessment of potency with the Doppler flowmeter. Urology 2:396, 1973.

180. Velcek D, Sniderman KW, Vaughan ED, et al: Penile flow index utilizing a Doppler pulse wave analysis to identify penile vascular insufficiency. J Urol 123:669, 1980.

181. Jevtich MJ: Importance of penile arterial pulse sound examination in impotence. J Urol 124:820, 1980.

182. Abelson D: Diagnostic value of the penile pulse and blood pressure: A Doppler study of impotence in diabetics. J Urol 113:636, 1975.

183. Engel G, Burnham SJ, Carter MF: Penile blood pressure in the evaluation of erectile impotence. Fertil Steril 30:687, 1978.

184. Kempczinski RF: Role of the vascular diagnostic laboratory in the evaluation of male impotence. Am J Surg 138:278, 1979.

185. Lane RJ, Appleberg M, Williams W: A comparison of two techniques for the detection of the vasculogenic component of impotence. Surg Gynecol Obstet 155:230, 1982.

186. Lue TF, Hricak H, Marich KW, et al: Vasculogenic impotence evaluated by high resolution ultrasonography and pulsed Doppler spectrum analysis. Radiology 155:777, 1985.

187. Potter EL: Normal and Abnormal Development of the Kidney. Chicago, Year Book Medical Publishers, 1972, pp 3–79.

188. Bertagnoli L, Lalatta F, Gallicchio R, et al: Quantitative characterization of the growth of the fetal kidney. J Clin Ultrasound 11:349, 1983.

189. Jeanty P, Dramaix-Wilmet M, Elkhazen N, et al: Measurement of fetal kidney growth on ultrasound. Radiology 144:159, 1982.

190. Grannum P, Bracken M, Silverman R, et al: Assessment of fetal kidney size in normal gestation by comparison of ratio of kidney circumference to abdominal circumference. Am J Obstet Gynecol 136:249, 1980.

191. Mahony BS, Filly RA: The genitourinary system in utero. Clin Diagn Ultrasound 18:1, 1986.

192. Wladimiroff JW, Campbell S: Fetal urine production rates in normal and complicated pregnancies. Lancet 1:151, 1974.

192a. Rouse GA, Kaminsky CK, Saaty HP, et al: Current concepts in sonographic diagnosis of fetal renal disease. RadioGraphics 8:119, 1988.

193. Romero R, Pilu G, Jeanty P, et al: Prenatal Diagnosis of Congenital Anomalies (in press). New York, Appleton-Century-Crofts.

194. Dubbins PA, Kurtz AB, Wapner RJ, et al: Renal agenesis: Spectrum of in utero findings. J Clin Ultrasound 9:189, 1981.

195. Romero R, Cullen M, Grannum P, et al: Antenatal diagnosis of renal anomalies with ultrasound. III. Bilateral renal agenesis. Am J Obstet Gynecol 151:38, 1985.

196. Goldenberg RL, Davis RD, Brumfield CG: Transient fetal anuria of unknown etiology: A case report. Am J Obstet Gynecol 149:87, 1984.

197. Harman CR: Maternal furosemide may not provoke urine production in the compromised fetus. Am J Obstet Gynecol 150:322, 1984.

198. Chamberlain PF, Cumming M, Torchia MG, et al: Ovine fetal urine production following maternal intravenous furosemide administration. Am J Obstet Gynecol 151:815, 1985.

199. Rosenberg ER, Bowie JD: Failure of furosemide to induce diuresis in a growth-retarded fetus. AJR 142:485, 1984.

200. Romero R, Cullen M, Jeanty P, et al: Prenatal diagnosis of renal anomalies with ultrasound. II. Infantile polycystic kidney disease. Am J Obstet Gynecol 150:259, 1984.

201. Simpson JL, Sabbagha RE, Elias S, et al: Failure to detect polycystic kidneys in utero by second trimester ultrasonography. Hum Genet 60:295, 1982.

202. Main D, Mennuti MT, Cornfeld D, et al: Prenatal diagnosis of adult polycystic kidney disease. Lancet II:337, 1983.

203. Zerres K, Volpel MC, Weib H: Cystic kidneys. Genetics, pathologic anatomy, clinical picture, and prenatal diagnosis. Hum Genet 68:204, 1984.

204. D'Alton M, Romero R, Grannum P, et al: Antenatal diagnosis of renal anaomlies with ultrasound. IV. Bilateral multicystic kidney disease. Am J Obstet Gynecol 154:532, 1986.

205. Hobbins JC, Romero R, Grannum P, et al: Antenatal diagnosis of renal anomalies with ultrasound. I. Obstructive uropathy. Am J Obstet Gynecol 148:868–877, 1984.

205a. Grignon A, Filion R, Filiatrault D, et al: Urinary tract dilatation in utero: Classification and clinical application. Radiology 160:645, 1986.

205b. Allen KS, Arger PH, Menutti M, et al: Effects of maternal hydration on fetal renal pyelectasis. Radiology 163:807, 1987.

206. Mahony BS, Filly RA, Callen PW, et al: Sonographic evaluation of fetal renal dysplasia. Radiology 152:143, 1984.

207. Glick PL, Harrison MR, Golbus MS, et al: Management of the fetus with congenital hydronephrosis. II. Prognostic criteria and selection for treatment. J Pediatr Surg 20:376, 1985.

207a. Cohen HL, Haller JO: Diagnostic sonography of the fetal genitourinary tract. Urol Radiol 9:88, 1987.

208. Cook JH III, Lytton B: Intraoperative localization of renal calculi during nephrolithotomy by ultrasound scanning. J Urol 117:543, 1977.

209. Sigel B, Coelho JCU, Sharifi R, et al: Ultrasonic scanning during operation for renal calculi. J Urol 127:421, 1982.

210. Lytton B: Intraoperative ultrasound for nephrolithotomy. J Urol 130:213, 1983.

210a. Gilbert BR, Russo P, Zirinsky K, et al: Intraoperative sonography: Applications in renal cell carcinoma. J Urol 139:582, 1988.

211. Bryniak SR, Chesley AE: The use of the Doppler stethoscope in anatrophic nephrotomy. J Urol 126:295, 1981.

212. Boyce WH: Ultrasonic velocimetry in resection of renal arteriovenous fistulas and other intrarenal surgical procedures. J Urol 125:610, 1981.

213. Coleman BG, Pollack HM: Interventional Genitourinary Sonography. In van Sonnenberg (ed): Interventional Ultrasound. New York, Churchill-Livingstone, 1987.

214. Pretorius DH, Lee ME, Manco-Johnson ML, et al: Diagnosis of autosomal dominant polycystic kidney disease in utero and in the young infant. J Ultrasound Med 6:249, 1987.

215. Hardt NS, Kaude JV, Li KC, et al: Sonography of the prostate: In vitro correlation of sonographic and anatomic findings in normal glands. AJR 151:955, 1988.

216. Littrup PJ, Lee F, Borlaza GS, et al: Percutaneous ablation of canine prostate using transrectal ultrasound guidance. Absolute ethanol and Nd:YAG laser. Invest Radiol 23:734, 1988.

217. Rifkin MD: Endorectal prostate ultrasonography. A definitive technique? Invest Radiol 23:740, 1988.

218. Rifkin MD, Choi H: Endorectal prostate ultrasound: Implications of the small peripheral hypoechoic lesions in endorectal ultrasound of the prostate. Radiology 106:619, 1988.

219. Torp-Pedersen S, Lee F, Littrup PJ, et al: Transrectal biopsy of the prostate guided with transrectal US: Longitudinal and multiplanar scanning. Radiology 170:23, 1989.

220. Gluck CD, Bundy AL, Fine C, et al: Sonographic urethrogram: Comparison to roentgenographic techniques in 22 patients. J Urol 140:1404, 1988.

221. Kuijpers D, Jaspers R: Renal masses: Differential diagnosis with pulsed Doppler US. Radiology 170:59, 1989.

222. Middleton WD, Thorne DA, Melson GL: Color Doppler ultrasound of the normal testis. AJR 152:293, 1989.

13

Computed Tomography of the Urinary Tract

LEON LOVE □ ROBERT J. CHURCHILL □ ELIAS KAZAM
YONG HO AUH □ WILLIAM A. RUBENSTEIN
JOHN A. MARKISZ □ KENNETH ZIRINSKY

COMPUTED TOMOGRAPHY OF THE UPPER URINARY TRACT

LEON LOVE □ ROBERT J. CHURCHILL

GENERAL PRINCIPLES

The role of computed tomography (CT) of the upper urinary tract is firmly established. Magnetic resonance imaging (MRI) does not yet substantially compete with CT of the body. In the future, however, the roles of MRI and CT may change, if technological advances improve MRI and if its cost decreases.

CT depicts the anatomy of the upper urinary tract and surrounding structures in unsurpassed detail. The use of intravenous contrast material in conjunction with dynamic scanning demonstrates vascular anatomy and lesion vascularity well enough that formal angiography is now unnecessary for diagnosing most surgical lesions of the kidney. The indications and applications of CT in the lower urinary tract are covered in detail elsewhere in this book.

History

The development of the first CT scanner by Sir Godfrey N. Hounsfield, a research scientist at EMI Limited in England, is one of the great advances in the field of radiology.[1] Through the years, the pioneering work of others in several disciplines, such as Radon, Oldendorf, Cormack, and Kuhl established the theoretical and practical groundwork that made it possible for Hounsfield to design and build a CT scanner.[2-4] This accomplishment was duly recognized when the Nobel Prize in Medicine was awarded to both Hounsfield and Cormack in 1980.

The first scanner was a dedicated head scanner manufactured by EMI. The first units in the United States were installed in 1973. Although manufacturers initially underestimated the impact that CT would have on the field of medicine, the industry soon began developing CT scanners capable of examining the whole body.

The first clinical body scanner was developed at Georgetown University in 1974 and was called the Automatic Computerized Transverse Axial (ACTA) scanner.[5] The scan time per slice was 5 minutes. Rapid technological improvements ensued, so that by the fall of 1975, CT scanners with scan times of 18 seconds per slice were on the market.[6-8]

Subsequent developments occurred more slowly. Nevertheless, commercially available scanners now customarily operate at speeds of 2 seconds/slice, and in some cases even more rapidly. This has largely eliminated motion artifacts, including those due to intestinal peristalsis, and has made it possible to scan patients of all ages regardless of clinical conditions.

The new scanning devices, unfortunately, were assigned generation numbers as they appeared on the market. This implied that those with higher generation numbers were significantly improved over scanners with lower generation numbers. Although this was true in some cases, it was not uniformly true. The "debuts" of the third- and fourth-generation scanners were within months of each other. Clearly, the fourth-generation scanners did not represent a logical progression in technology, compared with the third-generation scanners. Had the times of their appearances on the market been reversed, they would have simply exchanged generation numbers. Both designs are touted as theoretically superior by their various manufacturers, but no clear-cut differences in the images are apparent. The fact is that third-generation scanners virtually dominate the marketplace today. That fact might be interpreted to mean that third-generation scanners are superior to fourth-generation scanners.

The first CT scanner, manufactured by EMI, was dedicated to imaging the brain. The design geometry of the device was translate/rotate. The patient's head from the forehead up was enclosed in a rubber bag, which was filled with water. A fixed anode, air-cooled x-ray tube was positioned above the patient's head within the gantry of the scanner, and a pair of sodium iodide detectors were placed opposite the x-ray tube. A third reference detector intercepted a portion of the x-ray beam before it entered the patient. The pencil-like x-ray beam and two detectors produced two 13-mm thick tomographic slices simultaneously for each linear translate motion. The x-ray tube and detectors linearly traversed the gantry opening in tandem (translate motion). When the tube and detectors reached the opposite side, they rotated in tandem 1 degree and traversed in the opposite direction (Fig. 13–1). This translate/rotate motion took place 180 times (180 degrees) for each tomographic slice. Each detector made 160 measurements of transmitted radiation for each translation motion. Since the scanner repeated this motion 180 times, there were 28,800 linear attenua-

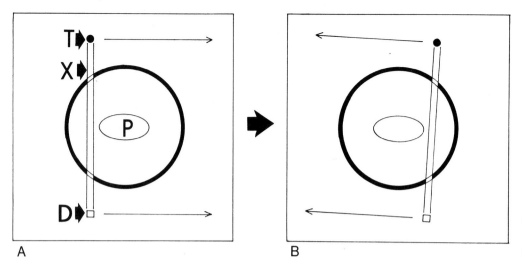

Figure 13–1. First-generation translate/rotate CT scanner. *A,* X-ray tube (T) and detector (D) translate with a linear motion across the patient (P) in the direction of the arrows. The intensity of the thin x-ray beam (X) is measured 160 times by the detector during one linear translate motion. *B,* The x-ray tube and detector rotate 1 degree, following a translate motion, and translate back in the opposite direction. There are 180 translate/rotate motions per tomographic slice.

tion coefficient measurements per tomographic slice. Attenuation is the reduction in intensity of the beam of x-rays as they pass through matter. The linear attenuation coefficient is a quantitative measurement of the amount of x-ray removed (attenuated) per centimeter of absorbing material.[2] The scan time per slice was approximately 5 minutes. By comparison, some present scanners make 1,436,640 measurements per slice during a 2-second scan. As mentioned previously, the first whole-body scanners copied this geometry and also shared the long scan time. Scanning of the torso was unacceptable at these protracted times. A variation of this geometry resulted in the second-generation scanner.

Several companies adopted second-generation geometry, which also had a translate/rotate design. This scanner used a fan-shaped x-ray beam and multiple detectors. The goal was to complete one tomographic slice during the time one breath can be held during suspended respiration. This would eliminate respiratory motion artifact. One manufacturer used a 10-degree fan width beam and 30 sodium iodide detectors (Fig. 13–2). Instead of 1-degree rotations, this scanner made 10-degree rotations, for a total of 180 degrees. The scan time for each slice took 18 seconds.[1–3, 9] The number of detectors and degrees in each rotation varied from one manufacturer to another. The fastest tomographic slice using this geometry was 10

seconds. Although 18-second scanning was fast, most radiologists using this equipment found it necessary to employ glucagon to eliminate peristaltic motion artifacts.

The next scanning geometry to be clinically introduced was the rotate/rotate design, or so-called third generation. This type of scanner uses an anode x-ray tube that is either fixed or rotating, depending on the manufacturer. Some x-ray tubes are pulsed, whereas others are on continuously. The x-ray beam has a wide-angle fan beam that encompasses the entire width of the patient. The width of the beam can be calibrated from 15 to 1.5 mm, depending on the manufacturer. The detectors are in a linear or slightly curved array on the opposite side of the gantry opening. These detectors are closely packed and their numbers vary among manufacturers, ranging from 300 to over 700. Usually, these detectors are either pressurized xenon gas ionization chambers or some variety of solid-state crystal. Both the x-ray tube and detector array rotate around the patient in tandem (Fig. 13–3). A full 360-degree rotation scan takes 2 seconds (shorter partial scans can also be obtained). Longer scans can be used to obtain more data, if desired. This detector configuration reduces the effect of scattered radiation and image noise. Low-contrast detectability is therefore superior to fourth-generation geometry. Circular or ring artifacts can occur if the detectors are not properly

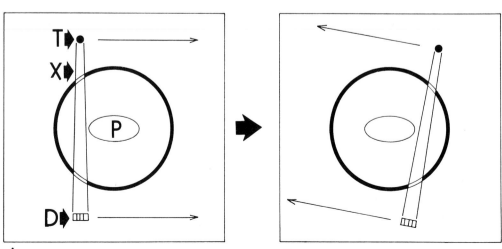

Figure 13–2. Second-generation translate/rotate CT scanner. *A,* X-ray tube (T) and detectors (D) translate linearly across the patient (P). *B,* Following the translate motion, the tube and detectors rotate 10 degrees in tandem and translate back across the patient in the opposite direction. The x-ray beam is fan shaped, and there are multiple detectors. (X = x-ray fan beam.)

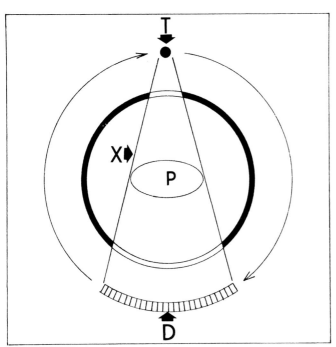

Figure 13–3. Third-generation rotate/rotate CT scanner. The x-ray tube (T) and detector array (D) rotate 360 degrees in tandem around the patient (P) during each tomographic slice. (X = x-ray fan beam.)

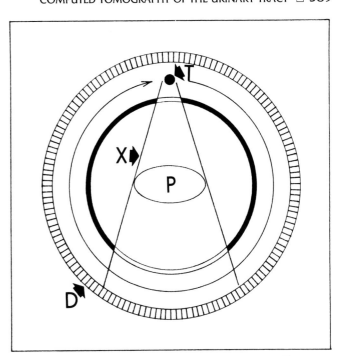

Figure 13–4. Fourth-generation rotate CT scanner. The x-ray tube (T) rotates 360 degrees around the patient (P) for each tomographic slice. The detectors (D) are mounted in a fixed ring, in the same plane as the x-ray tube, within the gantry. (X = x-ray fan beam.)

calibrated and balanced.[1–3, 9] This was an occasional problem with early scanners, but is virtually nonexistent today.

The next scanner geometry to appear was the rotating x-ray tube, fixed-detector array. This has been referred to as the fourth-generation CT scanner. The detectors are permanently mounted on a ring inside the gantry, and they completely surround the patient. The x-ray tube rotates 360 degrees around the individual on the patient side of the detector ring (Fig. 13–4). The detectors are usually some variety of scintillation crystal, such as bismuth germanate or cesium iodide. The number of detectors varies between 600 to over 2000, depending on the manufacturer. The greater the number of detectors, the more costly is the system. Dose efficiency is also a problem if the detectors are not closely spaced. The detectors are typically collimated with wide apertures so that radiation is detected over a wide angle. This can result in a scanner with high spatial resolution. The wide detector aperture also results in increased detection of scattered radiation, which decreases low-contrast detectability due to the added noise.[1–3, 9]

The problem of obtaining both high spatial resolution and efficient x-ray detection can be difficult to solve in stationary detector designs. Adding more detectors is expensive, because of the cost of both the detectors and the computer hardware needed to handle the increased amount of collected data. This can be overcome by making the detector ring smaller. The x-ray tube is mounted outside the detector ring in this design. The near detectors wobble out of the way of the x-ray beam as it rotates 360 degrees around the patient (Fig. 13–5). The motion of the ring has been described as nutating.[3] This geometry has been called fifth generation, and the first such device was the EMI 7070.

A radical departure from conventional CT design is the Imatron C-100 cine CT scanner. This scanner utilizes a

gun that fires an electron beam that is focused and deflected onto tungsten target rings by electromagnets. X-rays are generated from the tungsten target rings and collimated into a fan beam, which passes through the patient and falls on a curved stationary array of crystal detectors with photodiodes and preamplifiers. The unique

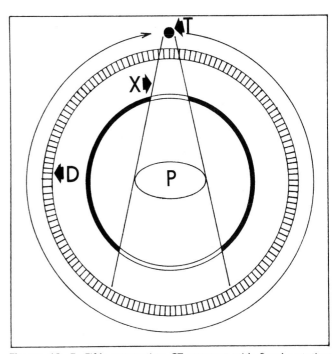

Figure 13–5. Fifth-generation CT scanner with fixed nutating detector ring. The x-ray tube (T) is mounted outside the fixed detector ring (D). The x-ray tube rotates 360 degrees around the patient (P) for each tomographic slice. The detectors adjacent to the x-ray tube nutate (wobble) out of the plane of the x-ray beam (X) as the tube rotates around the patient.

advantage of this design is its temporal resolution, because this device has scan times of 50 and 100 msec. This system eliminates artifacts due to motion and metallic objects. The scanner has both cine and flow modes of operation.[3] Measurements of renal flow,[9a] myocardial perfusion, heart wall motion, and cardiac output are a few of the applications possible, according to the manufacturer's literature. At the present time, the image quality is inferior to that obtained with conventional scanners, except when motion and metallic artifacts are a problem.

Basics

The linear attenuation coefficient measurement results from interrelated reactions that take place between x-rays and matter as the x-ray beam passes through tissue. Attenuation is affected by the energy of the x-ray beam as well as the atomic number (Z), density, and electrons per gram of the absorbing material. X-rays are attenuated by three types of interactions: coherent scattering, Compton scattering, and the photoelectric effect. Compton scattering and the photoelectric effect are the most significant interactions. However, the photoelectric effect results in greater attenuation than Compton scattering. The percentages of each of these two reactions are variable and are affected by the atomic number and number of electrons per cubic centimeter (product of the density and electrons per gram of the absorber).[2] Very simply stated, therefore, CT compares the specific gravity of tissues.

CT reconstructs a two-dimensional image of the internal anatomy of an object through the use of a complex mathematical formula (algorithm) that uses measurements of linear attenuation coefficients collected from multiple projections around the periphery of a thin tomographic slice.[1-3, 9] Most manufacturers use some form of filtered back projection or Fourier algorithm for image reconstruction.

The reconstructed image is displayed on a matrix. The matrix sizes of most contemporary scanners are 256^2, 320^2, and 512^2 pixels. Each picture element (pixel) in the two-dimensional display matrix represents the mean value of the attenuation coefficient in a volume of tissue, since the x-ray beam has a finite width. This volume element is called a voxel. The numerical values of the pixels are converted to a gray scale to produce an image. The relative linear attenuation coefficient for each pixel is normalized to the arbitrary reference materials of water and air and is transformed to a standard relative unit called a CT number (Hounsfield unit [H]). This relative density scale of numbers assigns a value of 0 to water, -1000 to air and $+1000$ to 2000 to dense bone (petrous bone). The density of a structure, as it is represented in shades of gray, is proportional to the amount of x-ray attenuation. Highly attenuating materials such as bone and contrast material have high densities, represented by lighter shades of gray, and have high CT numbers. Less attenuating materials such as bile and fat have low densities, represented by darker shades of gray, and have low or negative CT numbers. The visual representation of the attenuation characteristics of material is not textural information. Unlike ultrasound, CT data do not

impart cystic or solid characteristics to a structure. It is possible to infer such characteristics from CT data by assessing the shape, location, and density before and after contrast enhancement.

The displayed image can be manipulated to vary the number of shades of gray displayed (window width) and the number at which the window setting is centered (window level). Combinations of these settings can visually enhance the small differences in contrast between two adjacent tissues (narrow window) or can improve visualization of dense bone detail (wide window).[1-3, 9] CT is much more sensitive to small differences in contrast density than is conventional radiographic film technique. X-ray film cannot demonstrate density differences of less than 10% in contiguous structures; however, CT can demonstrate density differences of 1% or less.[2] A mass within the liver cannot be seen on a plain film of the abdomen, but it is easily seen with CT if its density varies by 1% or more from that of the liver. A mass that attenuates x-rays more than does normal liver looks lighter and is called hyperdense (with respect to liver). A mass that attenuates less than liver is termed hypodense. One that attenuates to the same degree as liver is called isodense and is imperceptible without the use of contrast media. The terms hyperdense, hypodense, and isodense are qualitative and used in relation to a particular structure. A hyperdense lesion in the kidney, for example, may be isodense with respect to the liver (Table 13–1).

The factors affecting image quality are complex and are influenced by the combined performance of the components of a CT scanner. Such factors include scan time, spatial resolution, low-contrast resolution, and artifacts.[10, 11] Spatial resolution is the ability to visualize small objects of high contrast. Related to this is the ability to differentiate between objects that are close together. Spatial resolution is affected by size of the display matrix (reconstructed pixel size), slice thickness, type of reconstruction algorithm kernel, focal spot size, size of detector aperture, and the amount of data sampling. CT manufacturers provide a variety of reconstruction kernels (also called filter functions), which modify the frequency of the measured projection data in specific ways to vary the amount of resolution and noise. These are selected by the operator to enhance specific types of information in the images. Examples of such information are bone detail, edge enhancement, and soft-tissue detail. Low-contrast

Table 13–1. CT Attenuation Values of Tissues in the Abdomen (Non–Contrast Enhanced)

Tissue	Range of CT Numbers (in Hounsfield units): scanner variations
Gas	−1000
Fat	−90 to −120
Fluid (e.g., urine, bile, simple cyst)	−5 to 15
Muscle	35 to 55
Kidney	20 to 45
Spleen	30 to 70
Liver	40 to 75
Bone	150 to 2000
Urinary calculi	75 to 400
Metal	over 2000
Oral contrast	200 to 300
IV contrast (vascular)	100 to 300
IV contrast (renal pelvis)	300 to 650

resolution is defined as the smallest object size visible at a contrast level of a given percentage. This is usually a 1% difference. Factors affecting low-contrast detectability are photon flux reaching the detector, system noise, efficiency of photon utilization, reconstruction algorithm, and matrix size. Low-contrast resolution is strongly dependent on dose.[10, 11] Low-contrast detectability can also be improved by altering subject enhancement through the use of intravenous contrast.

The radiation doses for CT scanners vary from one device to another. A wide range of possible exposures within a certain scanner may be selected by the operator of a CT scanner. Usually, three kVp settings are possible, and a wide range of mA settings is available. Scan times can also be varied. A change in any of these parameters changes the dose to the patient. The combinations of scan parameters should be tailored to the patient's size, area of the body scanned, and the expected diagnostic information. A typical surface dose for an abdominal scan is between 2 and 3 rad per slice.

Density measurements obtained with CT have been used in an attempt to make more specific diagnoses. Unfortunately, the CT numbers, or Hounsfield units, have not been shown to be extremely reliable or accurate[12] and cannot be extrapolated from one machine to another. A solution to the problem of making CT more quantitative is dual-energy scanning. The attenuation of a material is due primarily to a combination of Compton scatter and photoelectric absorption.[12, 13] By scanning an object at different x-ray energies one can, for example, determine the concentration of calcium in a lung nodule.[13] Two different techniques have been used experimentally: the postreconstruction technique and the prereconstruction method.[14] The ability to extract energy-dependent information from CT scanning will greatly expand its clinical usefulness.

Both CT and ultrasonography may be used to evaluate similar problems of the upper urinary tract. The technology of ultrasound has also improved in the last 10 years. The decision about which modality to use in evaluating the upper urinary tract should not simply be dictated by a flow chart but should be determined by a physician skilled in the urological applications of both techniques. A decision as to which examination is the first choice is based on the clinical history, patient anatomy, location of a suspected lesion, size of a lesion, possible involvement of surrounding anatomy, level of patient cooperation, and other factors. The radiology department of each institution decides how best to use each modality, based on the type and availability of equipment and the expertise of the physicians involved. It is not unusual to find different approaches to the same diagnostic problem, from one institution to another. Nor is it unusual to perform both an ultrasound examination and a CT study on the same patient for either complementary information or confirmation of an indeterminate finding.

TECHNIQUES

Positioning

Patients are supine for a routine scan of the kidneys. Patients are occasionally examined in other positions for comfort, interventional procedures, and radiotherapy planning.

Scout Film

A scout film is taken for localization of the kidneys. It is useful to have either a KUB or film from an excretory urogram on hand in case the renal outlines are not seen on the scout film. The positions of the kidneys in that instance can be related to vertebral body levels.

Scan Parameters

We use 120 kVp for routine scans. The mA is chosen according to patient size. We use a scan time of 2 seconds unless a greater mA value is needed for unusually large patients, in which case a 3-second scan is used. Some radiologists routinely use 3-second scans on a large body field of view (FOV) to obtain more views. The difference in scan speed for renal CT is usually not critical. We select a display FOV that shows the entire patient. A particular area can always be retrospectively studied as long as the scan (raw) data are available. Although a 512 × 512 matrix offers the maximum image quality and resolution, a 320 × 320 matrix that is autoenlarged is perfectly acceptable in virtually all instances. These images also occupy less room on the storage disc, and a greater number can be stored on magnetic tape. Once the data are acquired, they can be projected as coronal or sagittal views (reformatted images). Reformatted images are of limited usefulness in the urinary tract. Occasionally, the distinction between a suprarenal mass and an upper-pole renal mass can be more easily seen on a sagittal or coronal reformatted image.

Slice Width and Spacing

Renal scans are initially performed using contiguous, 1-cm-thick slices. Thinner slices (5 mm) are utilized to avoid partial volume averaging when trying to obtain a more accurate density reading of a small lesion or any time greater spatial resolution is necessary. Thin slices are also used to examine infants and children.

Oral Contrast Media

Oral contrast media are used routinely by most radiologists when examining the kidneys, particularly when renal cancer is suspected. Gastrointestinal tract opacification avoids the possibility of mistaking nonopacified loops of bowel for enlarged retroperitoneal and mesenteric lymph nodes or for other pathological masses. Two types of contrast material result in good gastrointestinal tract opacification. Historically, water-soluble iodinated contrast material (e.g., diatrizoate [Gastrografin]) was used. Although it is still utilized, many have abandoned it for the newer barium preparations made especially for CT. Commercial preparations of water-soluble contrast media are very concentrated and must be diluted. The optimal percentage of dilution may vary from one brand to another. Ten milliliters of contrast medium mixed with 400 cc of water, and some artificial flavoring added to improve palatability, has worked well. Some believe that the water-soluble agents increase both peristalsis and the likelihood of peristaltic motion artifacts. Hypersensitivity to iodinated contrast media is a valid reason to use a barium preparation, since a small amount of the water-soluble contrast is absorbed across intact bowel mucosa.[16, 17] An amount large enough to produce a urogram can be absorbed in patients with ulcerated bowel mucosa. We administer the same total volume, regardless of whether we are using dilute water-soluble contrast material or barium. The patient drinks 400 cc, waits 25 minutes, and drinks a second 400 cc immediately before the scan.

Intravenous Contrast Media

There is some controversy in the literature regarding the need to obtain a preliminary set of nonenhanced scans. Some believe that only an enhanced set of scans is necessary in evaluating a renal mass. Engelstad and associates examined 152 renal masses in this fashion, correctly diagnosing all of them.[15] They believe that nonenhanced scans are only needed in the search for calcifications, hemorrhage, and extravasation. Our belief is that most renal CT scans should be performed both before and after contrast enhancement for the following reasons: (1) Nonenhanced scans are necessary to look for parenchymal calcifications or calculi in the collecting system, because contrast in the kidney obscures them. (2) It is theoretically possible for a hematoma, depending on its age, to be isodense with either enhanced or nonenhanced renal parenchyma. Both nonenhanced and enhanced scans should be performed in order not to miss an intrarenal, subcapsular, or perinephric hematoma. (3) It is also useful to have a nonenhanced set of scans, in addition to the postcontrast scans, when evaluating a solid renal mass. Some solid renal tumors may be homogeneous and have CT numbers at the upper range, or "near water density," or slightly above. These masses may closely resemble a renal cyst on the contrast-enhanced scans. It can be very helpful to see how the density of such a mass compares with nonenhanced renal parenchyma and to measure its CT numbers on the nonenhanced scan. (4) One of the criteria used to distinguish a cyst from a solid mass is that a cyst has no significant (<10 H) change in CT numbers following administration of contrast medium. It is impossible to do this unless there is a nonenhanced set of scans for comparison. Although a postcontrast density reading near that of water usually (but not always) signifies a renal cyst, precontrast scans achieve their greatest usefulness in the cases of high-density or hemorrhagic cysts, which can easily be mistaken for neoplasms if a precontrast scan is not available to show that the lesion has not enhanced. (5) The nonenhanced scans are also used to localize a mass or other abnormality for a dynamic scan series, following a bolus injection.

There are two widely used methods of intravenous contrast administration: bolus injection and rapid drip infusion. The latter method is modified by some to run faster than gravity allows by injecting 50 to 75 cc of air into the bottle of contrast material. (Care must be taken, of course, to insure that no air gets into the intravenous line.) The purpose of a faster drip is to achieve a high intravascular concentration. Power injectors for CT scanners are also available. They offer the advantage of a constant rate of infusion. The injection rate can also be varied so that both bolus and rapid-infusion techniques can be duplicated.

Dynamic (rapid-sequence) scans following a bolus injection are particularly useful for evaluating a homogeneous low-density mass. As mentioned above, such a lesion may occasionally resemble a cyst or a complicated cyst. The "angiographic" pattern of brief enhancement that can be seen following a bolus injection can be extremely helpful in determining the solid nature of the mass. Vascular structures such as the renal vein and inferior vena cava (IVC) can be evaluated for a filling defect using this technique. A contrast medium containing 280 to 300 mg iodine/ml is usually used. The total amount for a renal CT scan normally does not exceed 100 to 150 cc. Some radiologists prefer 250 to 300 cc of a 30% material for a rapid-drip infusion. The dose is adjusted according to the package insert for children.

Scan Protocol

Nonenhanced scans are taken with contiguous, 1-cm-thick slices. Each slice is taken during suspended respiration. Scans can be taken at either the end of inspiration or end of expiration. Many think that the latter provides a more consistent lung volume from scan to scan. Contiguous 5-mm scans are used in children.

One of two conditions exists after scanning the kidneys to rule out a mass: a mass is seen, or the examination appears normal. When the scan is performed to rule out a mass, contrast medium must be injected even though a mass is not seen on the nonenhanced scans, because a small isodense intrarenal mass may be present. Bolus or rapid infusion, or a combination of both, may be used in this situation. A combination of both can be used in the following manner: A 50-cc bolus of contrast medium is injected, and a set of single-level dynamic scans are taken at the level where the kidney appears abnormal on the excretory urogram. Additional contrast material is then administered, and conventional scans through both kidneys are obtained.

We prefer the bolus method of contrast injection when a renal mass is identified. Properly performed, the renal mass, renal vein, and IVC at the level of the renal vein are all usually clearly visualized. The locations of the nonenhanced slices on which these structures are seen are noted. A 19-gauge butterfly needle or angiocath is inserted into a vein. Afterward, a prebolus localizing slice is once again taken at the table position on which the mass was seen. This slice is reconstructed and viewed to make sure the mass is in the scan plane. Fifty milliliters of contrast are injected by hand or machine. After a 12- to 15-second pause the patient is asked to suspend respiration, and five single-level dynamic scans are taken during a single breath holding. These are reviewed. If satisfactory, the sequence is repeated at the level of the renal vein, if it was not included on the first set of scans. It is important to rescan all of both kidneys following the bolus injection in order not to miss an intrarenal mass in the opposite kidney. Additional contrast material is not usually given if the total amount injected was at least 100 cc.

An alternate method used by some is a rapid-drip infusion of 100 to 150 cc of 60% contrast material or 250 to 300 cc of 30% material. It is important to obtain an adequate loading dose prior to the initiation of scanning. Dynamic scanning with preset incremental table movement can be used to scan through the kidneys. A 6- to 10-second interscan delay allows the patient to breathe between scans. The drip must be rapid enough to achieve intense opacification of the IVC.

Single-level dynamic scans clearly demonstrate the sequential enhancement of the cortex, medulla, and collecting system of the kidney (see Figs. 13–27 and 13–28). The times of peak enhancement of these structures have been established in a canine model and in humans.[16–19] The peak CT densities of these structures have also been studied using a variety of water-soluble contrast agents. Although the intensity of cortical enhancement does not change, the peak values of medulla and urine differ among the various contrast agents.[16–18]

The relationship between the time-intensity curves of the cortex and medulla have been studied with dynamic CT scanning.[19] The point in time at which the CT density curves of the cortex and medulla cross is the corticomedullary junction time.[19] This time either is prolonged or does not occur (curves do not cross) in various conditions affecting renal function.[20, 21] Some investigators have used this technique to study renal transplant rejection, whereas others have used it to predict impending diuresis in patients with acute renal failure.[20, 21] Investigators have employed dynamic renal scanning using cine CT to measure renal blood flow with a high degree of accuracy.

Aspiration and Biopsy

Biopsy, aspiration, and drainage techniques in the kidney are frequently carried out with ultrasonography because it is cheaper, faster, and generally more readily available on short notice than is CT. Most masses, cysts, and collections are readily demonstrated with ultrasonography. CT is used when the anatomy and the approach are better demonstrated with this modality. Examples of abnormalities that require intervention are abscesses in and around the kidney, hydronephrosis, pyonephrosis, complicated cysts, and masses. Although most masses are considered to be primary renal tumors in the proper clinical setting, some patients have more than one type

of malignancy. Management among these patients may differ greatly depending on the histology of the renal mass (Fig. 13–6).

CT becomes more practical as a guide for these procedures if the scan time and reconstruction times are fast. Many scanners have the option of a lower resolution scan that has a fast reconstruction time. The quality of such a scan is almost always good enough to check needle placement. The smallest needle that will obtain diagnostic tissue is used. Vascularity is first assessed with a single-level dynamic bolus scan series. All aspiration biopsy and core biopsies are performed with a cytopathologist in attendance. The procedure is terminated when a diagnosis is made. A skinny needle aspiration biopsy is performed first if the lesion is hypervascular. Core biopsies are usually obtained with needles in the 18- to 21-gauge range.

COMPUTED TOMOGRAPHY OF THE RETROPERITONEUM

On a cross-section view, the retroperitoneum is C shaped with its convexity projecting anteriorly to the axial midline. It occupies the posterior third of the abdomen and extends from the diaphragm to the pelvic brim. The anatomical features (Fig. 13–7) of the retroperitoneum are determined, for the most part, by the fixed anterior renal fascia (ARF) and posterior renal fascia (PRF) (Gerota's and Zuckerkandl's, respectively).[24–27] On axial CT sections (Fig. 13–8), these fascial layers can easily be seen extending from the upper third of the kidneys to below the lower poles of the kidneys. On direct and reformatted coronal and sagittal sections (Fig. 13–9), the fat planes and fasciae above the level of the upper third of the kidney may be demonstrated occasionally, particularly in obese patients, when faster scanning times and smaller pixel sizes are used.

NORMAL CT ANATOMY

Around the end of the nineteenth century, anatomists dissected and described the fasciae around the kid-

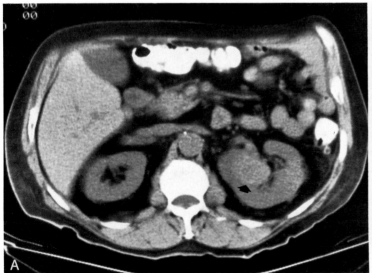
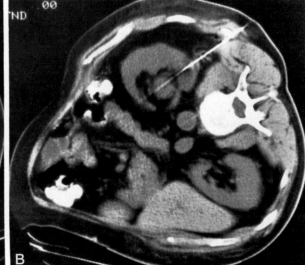

Figure 13–6. *A,* Hyperdense parapelvic mass in the left kidney (*arrow*). *B,* Patient in right lateral decubitus position. Core biopsy, obtained with an 18-gauge needle, disclosed renal cell carcinoma.

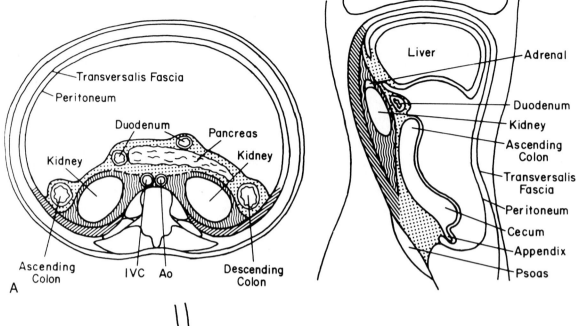

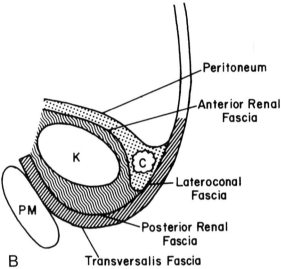

Figure 13–7. *A,* Retroperitoneal spaces. Transverse and right parasagittal sections: anterior paranephric space (*dots*), perinephric space (*wavy lines*) and posterior paranephric space (*straight lines*). *B,* Retroperitoneal fascia. Fascia forming the three compartments of the retroperitoneal space: anterior paranephric space (*dots*), perinephric space (*wavy lines*), and posterior paranephric space (*straight lines*). K = kidney. C = descending colon. PM = psoas muscle. (Modified from Meyers MA: Dynamic Radiology of the Abdomen: Normal and Pathologic Anatomy. Heidelberg, Springer-Verlag, 1982.)

ney.[28, 29] Congdon and Edson[24] added information by tracing the renal fascial planes on anatomical cross sections.

Interest in their work stimulated Mitchell[26, 30, 31] to inject these spaces in cadavers. In the 1970s Meyers and co-workers and Whalen and associates[32, 33] correlated this material and presented the information so that radiologists could approach retroperitoneal disease in a logical fashion. With the advent of high-resolution CT, radiologists were able to appreciate these fasciae as distinct anatomical structures and to expand on the anatomical, clinical and radiological data.[34–36]

Descriptions of the fascial planes vary. Descriptions by the anatomists,[24] who limited their study to dissection of the fasciae and extraperitoneal spaces, were different from those of investigators[26, 27] who injected contrast medium and then studied the extent of the fasciae and extraperitoneal spaces by radiography and cross-sectional imaging. The descriptions of the latter group are closer to the clinical material as observed on CT in patients with well-defined retroperitoneal fluid collections.

Feldberg[36] and Parienty and associates[37] independently studied 100 normal patients with axial CT to determine the extent of visualization of fasciae in subjects without renal or paranephric pathology. Their results were similar. Feldberg[36] reported that at least one CT slice demonstrated normal ARF and PRF on both sides in 56% of patients. CT failed to show any of the four fascial leaves in 11% of patients. In 10% of patients, the right ARF was the only leaf that could not be seen; in 2%, the left ARF could not be seen. Normal fascia should be about 1 to 2 mm thick.

Anterior Paranephric Space (APS)

This space lies between the posterior parietal peritoneum anteriorly and the ARF posteriorly (Figs. 13–7 and 13–8). It contains the pancreas (except for the tail, which is intraperitoneal) and the retroperitoneal portions of the alimentary tract (the descending duodenum and the ascending and descending colon).[27] The APS contains very little fat and, as a result, is difficult to evaluate by conventional radiography.[27, 32, 34] CT can demonstrate the peritoneum as a distinct structure. At the level of the pancreas, there is a potential communication across the midline. However, at the level of the renal hilus, there is apparent fusion of the ARF to connective tissue surround-

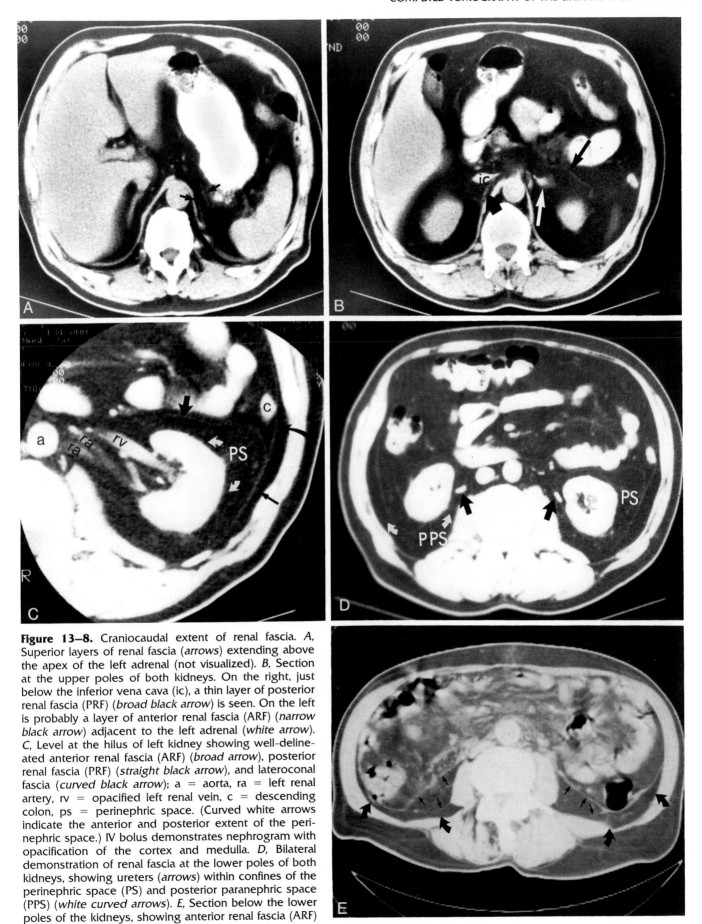

Figure 13–8. Craniocaudal extent of renal fascia. *A,* Superior layers of renal fascia (*arrows*) extending above the apex of the left adrenal (not visualized). *B,* Section at the upper poles of both kidneys. On the right, just below the inferior vena cava (ic), a thin layer of posterior renal fascia (PRF) (*broad black arrow*) is seen. On the left is probably a layer of anterior renal fascia (ARF) (*narrow black arrow*) adjacent to the left adrenal (*white arrow*). *C,* Level at the hilus of left kidney showing well-delineated anterior renal fascia (ARF) (*broad arrow*), posterior renal fascia (PRF) (*straight black arrow*), and lateroconal fascia (*curved black arrow*); a = aorta, ra = left renal artery, rv = opacified left renal vein, c = descending colon, ps = perinephric space. (Curved white arrows indicate the anterior and posterior extent of the perinephric space.) IV bolus demonstrates nephrogram with opacification of the cortex and medulla. *D,* Bilateral demonstration of renal fascia at the lower poles of both kidneys, showing ureters (*arrows*) within confines of the perinephric space (PS) and posterior paranephric space (PPS) (*white curved arrows*). *E,* Section below the lower poles of the kidneys, showing anterior renal fascia (ARF) (*upward arrows*), posterior renal fascia (PRF) (*downward arrows*) uniting at the lateroconal fascia, and posterior paranephric fat and (PPS) (*curved arrows*).

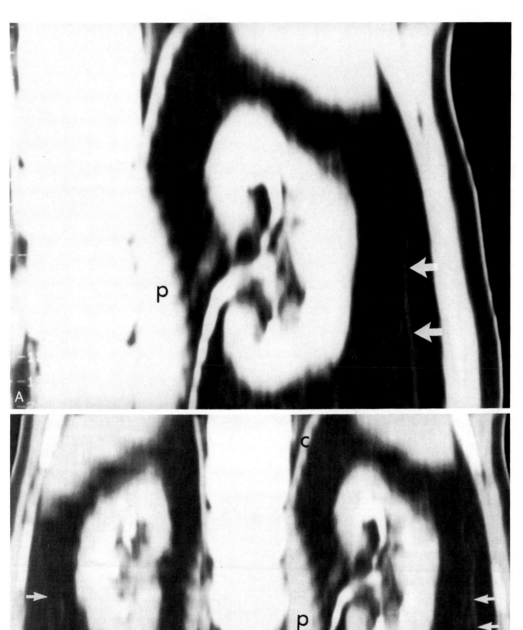

Figure 13–9. *A,* Reformatted coronal section through the hilus of the left kidney, demonstrating lateroconal fascia (*white arrows*). Proximal ureter is lateral to the psoas (P). *B,* Reformatted bilateral coronal section, showing lateroconal fascia (*white arrows*), psoas (p) extending upward toward the left diaphragmatic crus (C). Note position of the proximal left ureter lying lateral to the psoas muscle.

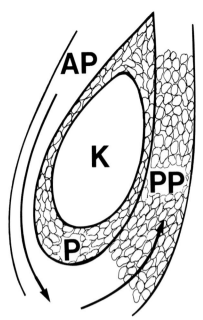

Figure 13–10. Diagram showing potential communication of the anterior paranephric space (AP) to posterior paranephric space (PP) below the cone of the renal fascia and the perinephric space (P). Kidney (K). (Modified from Meyers MA: *Dynamic Radiology of the Abdomen: Normal and Pathologic Anatomy.* Heidelberg, Springer-Verlag, 1982.)

ing the great vessels. The APS is limited on its lateral aspect by the attachment of the posterior parietal peritoneum to the lateroconal fascia (LCF). The APS extends medially and the properitoneal fat line is lateral to it in position. On the right, the ARF is posterior to the ascending colon, and the APS extends from the posterior-superior aspect of the bare area of the liver to the iliac

fossa. On the left, the ARF is posterior to the descending colon, and the APS extends cephalad toward the diaphragm. Just below the iliac crest, around the inferior margin of the cone of renal fascia, the APS is in potential communication with the posterior paranephric space (PPS) (Fig. 13–10). Communication also occurs at this level when the LCF disappears as a distinct boundary. Meyers[27] has demonstrated that in cadavers the contrast-filled APS assumes a characteristic vertical orientation, overlapping the psoas margin medially without obliterating the flank stripe, and demonstrating its lateral border to be fairly well defined by its attachment to the LCF. On CT, the fluid-filled APS shows many variations, particularly in its cranial and caudal extent. These variations may be dependent on the amount of fluid present and by impedance by contained anatomical structures of the APS. An example of a fluid collection in the APS is shown (Fig. 13–11).

Perinephric Space (PS)

The perinephric space is bounded anteriorly by the ARF and posteriorly by the PRF (Figs. 13–7 and 13–8). The PS contains the kidney, adrenal gland, proximal ureter, and renal vessels.[27] There is a variable amount of fat, most prominent posteriorly and inferiorly. Inferiorly, the layers of fascia fuse with the iliac fascia. Medially, the fascial layers blend with the periureteral connective tissue.

The anterior and posterior renal fasciae are limited medially by the connective tissue around the great vessels; therefore, collections in this space tend to remain unilateral. The PS extends over the apex of the adrenal gland on both sides. Cephalad on the right, the PS is bounded

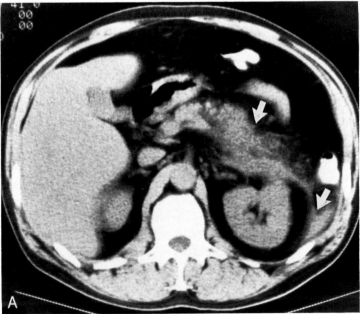

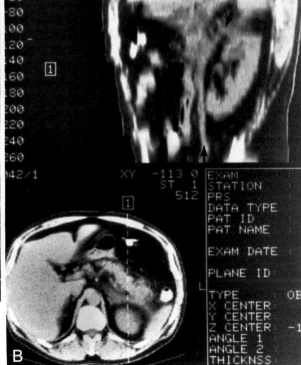

Figure 13–11. Anterior paranephric fluid collection from pancreatitis. *A*, Edematous pancreas with fluid collection extending lateral to the lateroconal fascia on the left side of the anterior paranephric space (*white arrows*). *B*, Sagittal reformat shows anterior paranephric collection (*black arrows*) extending vertically beyond the cone of renal fascia. Note that the perinephric fat, kidneys, and psoas are intact.

laterally by the posterior right lobe of the liver and medially by the right diaphragmatic crus. Cephalad on the left, the PS is bounded laterally by the medial surface of the spleen and by the left diaphragmatic crus on its medial aspect.[27] At this level, perinephric and posterior paranephric fat can rarely be differentiated.[38, 39] Perinephric gas usually will remain below the diaphragm.[27]

Mitchell[26] in 1950 injected the PS of 64 cadavers with barium and concluded the following:

1. The renal fascia is formed by a splitting of the retroperitoneal tissues to form a loose common investment for the kidney and suprarenal gland. With few exceptions, no complete septum is found between the two organs.

2. The anterior and posterior layers of renal fascia are fused superiorly and laterally. Contrary to the common view, they are also united medially and inferiorly.

3. The fusion of layers is firm above the suprarenal gland, but weak beneath the kidney. The weakest spot, through which perinephric injections or effusions escape most easily, is in the vicinity of the ureter.

4. Medially, the two layers blend with the mass of connective tissue surrounding the great vessels, in the root of the mesentery, and behind the pancreas and duodenum. Laterally, they fuse together directly.

5. The two perinephric spaces are in neither actual nor potential communication. The mass of connective tissue located in the upper part of the mesenteric root (around the vessels, behind the pancreas and duodenum in front of the vertebral column) presents an efficient barrier.

6. Fluids escaping from the PS spread downward in the retroperitoneal tissue and may invade the pelvis, but until the pressure is raised by the injection of considerable amounts of fluid, the spread is strictly unilateral.[40]

7. Extension to the opposite side occurs most often in the lumbosacral region and is infrequent above the level of the renal hilus.

8. When rupture of the PS occurs in the hilar region, the anterior layer of fascia and the attached peritoneum usually give way, permitting invasion of the peritoneal cavity.

An example of a fluid collection in the PS is shown (Fig. 13–12). Although Mitchell's conclusions are still held to be generally valid, it has more recently been shown experimentally and by CT scanning that small amounts of spread from one PS to the other may occur.

Raptopoulos and coworkers[41] have shown that, in 74 of 100 cases, the lateral junction (LCF) of the retroperitoneal fasciae tends to shift from an anterior to a posterior location as it progresses caudally. No attempt at statistical analysis of the junction of the ARF and PRF could be made above the renal hilus because of differences in shape of the lower pole of the liver and spleen. In most cases, the angle between the LCF and ARF was acute. The authors' explanation[41] for retrorenal extension of pancreatic fluid is postulated based on the presence of two layers of posterior renal fascia, rather than one. The most anterior of these two layers is continuous with the ARF, whereas the posterior layer is thought to be continuous with the LCF. In pancreatitis they assume that proteolytic enzymes permit the APS to communicate with the potential space formed by the expansion of the two layers of posterior renal fascia. Other explanations of retrorenal extension of fluid are:

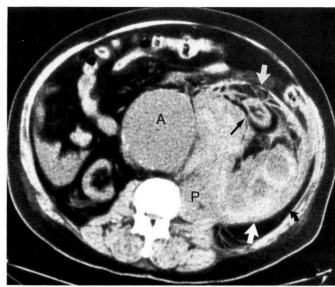

Figure 13–12. Perinephric fluid collection from ruptured abdominal aorta. Large, high-density collection of blood confined within the perinephric space (*white arrows*), arises from ruptured abdominal aortic aneurysm (A). Small left kidney (*black arrow*) markedly displaced anteriorly by the fluid collection. The left psoas (P) has lost its fat interface as a result of the hemorrhage. Posterior paranephric space (*curved arrow*) is intact.

1. Fluid confined to the PPS (Figs. 13–13 and 13–14).

2. Extension of the APS behind the kidney due to a posterior location, or absence of, the LCF (Figs. 13–15 to 13–17).

3. Extension of the peritoneal cavity retrorenally, which occasionally occurs in ascites (Figs. 13–18 to 13–21).

4. Tracking of fluid confined to the posterior dependent portion of the PS (Fig. 13–22).

Several authors have called attention to a retrorenal colon.[42–44] Hopper and associates found the frequency to

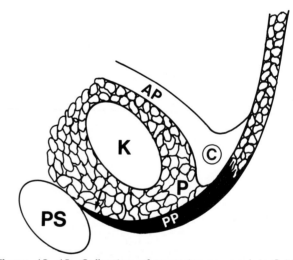

Figure 13–13. Collection of posterior paranephric fluid (PP) extending up anteriorly into the properitoneal fat. Anterior paranephric space (AP), kidney (K), descending colon (C), and perinephric space (P) are shown. Note attachment of the posterior renal fascia (*arrow*) to psoas (PS). (From Love L, Demos TC, Posniak H: CT of retroperitoneal fluid collections. AJR 145(1):87–91, 1985, © by Am Roentgen Ray Soc.)

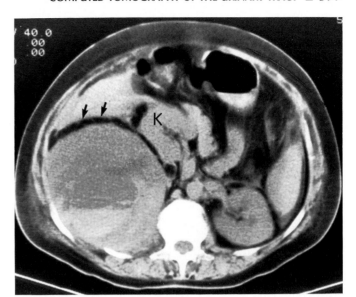

Figure 13–14. Posterior paranephric hematoma. Posterior paranephric hematoma obliterates the properitoneal fat and displaces the perinephric fat *(arrows)* and the right kidney, which is displaced anteriorly and medially (K). Note the fluid level in the posterior paranephric hematoma.

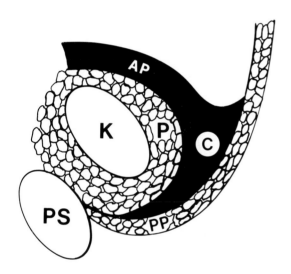

Figure 13–15. Anterior paranephric space (AP) extending behind the kidney (K) and perinephric space (P), probably the result of absence or posterior location of the lateral conal fascia. Psoas (PS), posterior paranephric space (PP), descending colon (C) are shown. (From Love L, Demos TC, Posniak H: CT of retroperitoneal fluid collections. AJR 145(1):87–91, 1985, © by Am Roentgen Ray Soc.)

Figure 13–16. Descending colon in a retrorenal position behind the left kidney. An attempt at percutaneous nephrostomy without prior knowledge of this anatomic configuration could have important implications. (From Love L, Demos TC, Posniak H: CT of retroperitoneal fluid collections. AJR 145(1):87–91, 1985, © by Am Roentgen Ray Soc.)

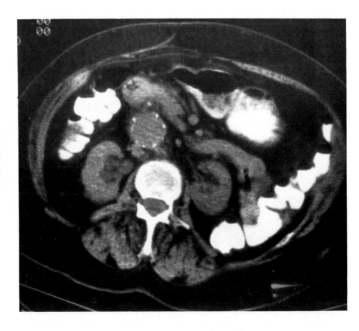

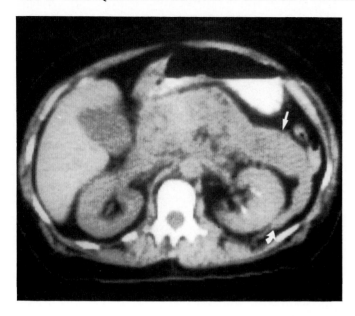

Figure 13–17. Diffuse pancreatitis involving the anterior para-nephric space *(arrow)* and extending retrorenally *(curved arrow)* is probably the result of low insertion of the lateroconal fascia (LCF) or absence of the LCF. (From Love L, Demos TC, Posniak H: CT of retroperitoneal fluid collections. AJR 145(1):87–91, 1985, © by Am Roentgen Ray Soc.)

Figure 13–18. Retrorenal extension of the peritoneal cavity in ascites. Anterior paranephric space (AP), perinephric space (P), posterior paranephric space (PP), psoas (PS), descending colon (C), and kidney (K) are shown. (From Love L, Demos TC, Posniak H: CT of retroperitoneal fluid collections. AJR 145(1):87–91, 1985, © by Am Roentgen Ray Soc.)

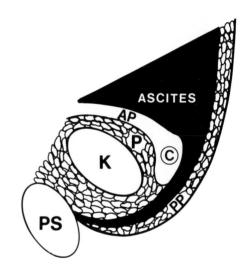

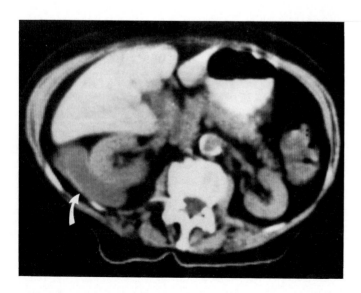

Figure 13–19. Retrorenal position of small-bowel loop. Loop of nonopacified small bowel *(curved arrow)* is behind the middle portion of the right kidney. Peritoneal extension of small bowel is shown. (From Love L, Demos TC, Posniak H: CT of retroperitoneal fluid collections. AJR 145(1):87–91, 1985, © by Am Roentgen Ray Soc.)

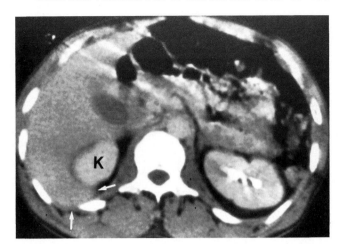

Figure 13–20. Retrorenal position of the liver. Posterior segment of the right lobe of the liver *(arrows)* in a retrorenal position. K = kidney. The liver is an intraperitoneal organ. (From Love L, Demos TC, Posniak H: CT of retroperitoneal fluid collections. AJR 145(1):87–91, 1985, © by Am Roentgen Ray Soc.)

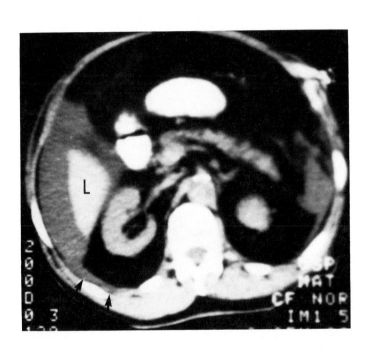

Figure 13–21. Retrorenal ascites. Liver (L) is displaced medially by ascites. Note the retrorenal extension *(arrows)* of ascites.

Figure 13–22. Tracking of fluid behind the kidney within the confines of the posterior portion of the perinephric space (P) and anterior to the posterior paranephric space (PP). Paranephric space (AP), psoas (PS), kidney (K), descending colon (C) are shown. (From Love L, Demos TC, Posniak H: CT of retroperitoneal fluid collections. AJR 145(1):87–91, 1985, © by Am Roentgen Ray Soc.)

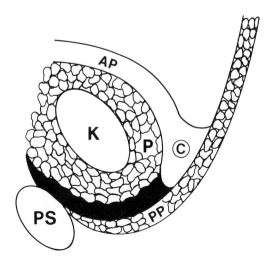

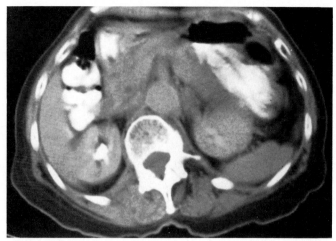

Figure 13–23. Retrorenal extension of spleen. The spleen extends posterior to the upper third of the left kidney. This relationship is not rare, even in patients with normal-sized spleens.

be 1.9% in the supine position and 4.7% in the prone position.[55] This may have practical applications when percutaneous renal surgery is contemplated. Hadar and Natan[42] pointed out that abundant perinephric fat is much more common in men than in women and that a lack of abundant perinephric adipose tissue is a major factor in permitting the colon to lie lateral to, or even to fall behind, the kidney.[42] Interventional radiologists should also be aware of the sometimes retrorenal position of the spleen (Fig. 13–23), small bowel (Fig. 13–19) and liver (Fig. 13–20).

A recent publication[45] presents a new concept of bridging septa within the PS (Fig. 13–24). Some of these septa arise from the renal capsule and extend to the perinephric fascia; other septa are attached only to the renal capsule and lie parallel to the renal surface; a third group of septa connect the anterior and posterior layers of renal fascia. McClennan and coworkers[46] believe that the consistency of these fixed groups must be considered questionable, pending further anatomical correlation. They observed a positive correlation between the amount of fat present and the presence of bridging septa. From time to time, challenges have been mounted to the classical theories of retroperitoneal anatomy,[56] but, in the main, these have been attributable to developmental variants.[57]

Posterior Paranephric Space (PPS)

This dorsal compartment lies between the PRF and the transversalis fascia (see Figs. 13–7 and 13–8D,E). It contains no organs. Fat may be seen extending anterolaterally as the flank stripe (properitoneal fat line) and continuing in an irregular fashion across the midline of the anterior abdomen.[27, 44] Superiorly, the PPS extends bilaterally to the crural surface of the diaphragm and can communicate with the mediastinum. On the right, its lateral superior border is formed by the bare area of the liver, and medially it is bounded by the right diaphragmatic crus. On the left, its lateral superior border is the medial border of the spleen, and its medial border is the left crus.[27, 38, 39] Collections within the PPS should obliterate the posterior paranephric and properitoneal fat planes (Fig. 13–14). Collections may extend into the mediastinum. In our clinical material involving fluid in the PS, the collections are similar in their configuration to those obtained by injecting fluid in cadavers. Fluid collections in clinical cases involving the APS and PPS tend not to conform with the contrast-filled spaces observed in injected postmortem studies.

Hepatic and Splenic Angles

The hepatic angle (Fig. 13–25) is an acute angle that is formed by the intersection of the border between the posterior aspect of the liver and the retroperitoneal fat and the border between the lateral edge of the liver and

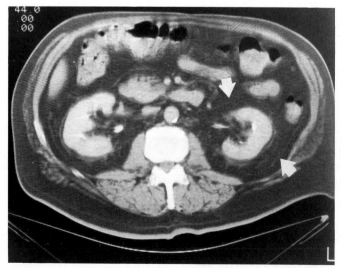

Figure 13–24. Renal fascia easily identified (arrows). Multiple strands within the perinephric space represent bridging septae.

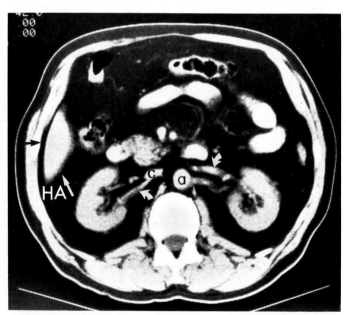

Figure 13–25. Tip of liver outlined laterally by the properitoneal fat of the posterior paranephric space (PPS) (black arrow). Medial side of hepatic angle (white arrow). Both partially opacified renal veins (curved arrows) entering into inferior vena cava (c). Aorta (a) is shown.

the properitoneal fat line. The splenic angle (see Fig. 13–26A) is formed by the intersection of the border between the posterior aspect of the spleen abutting against the retroperitoneal fat and the lateral line formed by properitoneal fat. The splenic angle is therefore dependent on the contour of the posterior inferior splenic margin. Fluid collections in the peritoneal cavity, the APS, and the PS will all cause loss of the oblique portion of these angles; however, only collections in the posterior paranephric space (PPS) extending into the flank stripe will cause loss of the vertical portion of the angles. As both the liver and spleen are capable of medial displacement from the

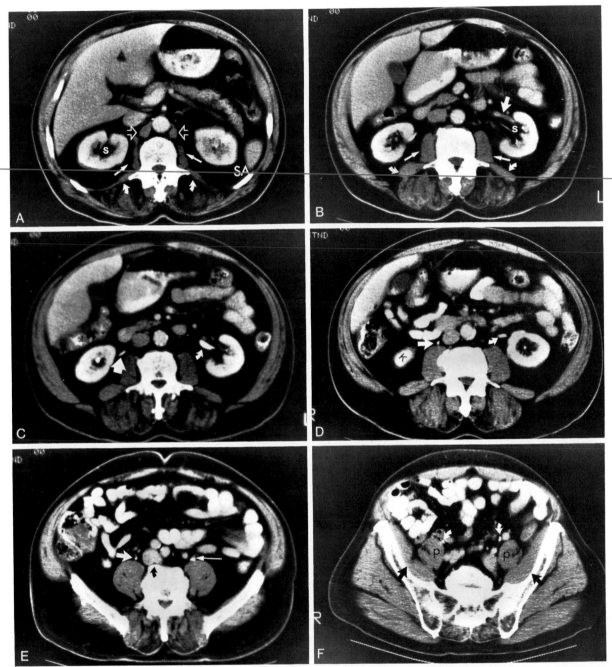

Figure 13–26. CT scans showing anatomical relationships of psoas. *A, L2 level:* inferior portion of right and left crus of diaphragm *(open arrows)* and upper fibers of the psoas *(straight white arrows)*. Quadratus lumborum *(curved arrows)*, splenic angle (SA), renal sinus (s) are indicated. *B,* Psoas, vertical portion *(straight arrows),* and quadratus lumborum *(curved arrow)*. Incidentally, nephrogram demonstrates opacification of the cortex and the medulla of both kidneys. The renal pelves are nonopacified. Left renal vein *(broad white arrow)* is indicated. *C,* Proximal right ureter *(broad arrow)* and left renal pelvis *(curved arrow)*. *D, L3 level:* lower pole right kidney (k) and middle third right ureter anterior to the psoas *(straight arrow)*. Proximal third of left ureter *(curved arrow)* is indicated. At this level the psoas muscles start to round out and are clearly separated from the quadratus lumborum by intervening fat. *E, L5 level:* distal right ureter *(broad arrow)* lateral to iliac veins *(curved arrow)*. Distal left ureter is anterior and closely associated with the left psoas *(thin arrow)*. The maximum psoas bulk occurs at the L4–L5 level. *F, S1 level:* Iliacus muscle in the iliac fossa *(straight black arrows)*. Both distal ureters lie medial to the anterior portion of the psoas *(curved arrows)*. The psoas (p) is in a more anterior location at this level.

properitoneal fat line, particularly in ascites (Fig. 13–21), the terms hepatic and splenic angles are convenient but anatomically difficult to justify.[35]

The Psoas Muscles[47]

The psoas major, minor, and iliacus are a bilateral group of muscles that arise in the abdomen and iliac regions and course downward and laterally to insert on the lesser trochanter of the femur. Distally, the muscle forms a conjoined tendon with the iliacus and courses under the inguinal ligament. The conjoined tendon lies anterior to the hip joint.[49]

Fasciae

The fascia overlying the psoas muscle is attached to the sides of the lumbar vertebrae and the upper sacrum.[49] The fascia envelops the psoas muscle and blends laterally with the anterior layer of the quadratus lumborum fascia above the iliac crest. Below the iliac crest, the psoas fascia blends with the fascia covering the iliacus muscle. At its upper end, the fascia thickens into the medial arcuate ligament, which attaches medially to the side of the body of L2 and laterally to the transverse process of L1. This medial arcuate ligament gives rise to the posteromedial muscular fibers of the diaphragm. The entry of the psoas into the posterior mediastinum is referred to as "the open end of the psoas sheath."

Anatomical Relationships

The upper psoas lies in the posterior mediastinum. Posteriorly and medially, the psoas is adjacent to the quadratus lumborum (Fig. 13–26); inferiorly, it is adjacent to the lumbar spine. Anteriorly and laterally, the psoas is related to the pancreas and the right kidney and the renal vessels, and ureters on the right side. It lies behind the ileum and inferior vena cava and on the left behind the colon.

CT Anatomy (Fig. 13–26)

The anterolateral aspects of the psoas are well delineated on CT, particularly in the presence of abundant retroperitoneal fat. Serial sections extending caudally reveal the following characteristics: From its narrow portion at the cephalad end of L1 the psoas broadens out until it reaches its maximum bulk at the level of L4 to L5. From there it tapers again until it becomes tendinous and fuses with the iliacus tendon to insert on the lesser trochanter of the femur.

Meyers[27] believes that the upper half of the psoas is usually visible because of its proximity to the fat in the PS, while the lower half is demonstrated because of its proximity to the posterior paranephric fat. The lower half of the psoas is contiguous with the abundant posterior paranephric fat and is therefore more likely to be obliterated by collections in this compartment.[27] However, this strict demarcation of the psoas has not always been confirmed by our case material.[29, 34] The posterior renal fascia may attach to the lateral border of the psoas or to the quadratus lumborum.[50] If its attachment is to the psoas, it is easy to see how pathological processes may originate in the psoas and involve the posterior paranephric and perinephric spaces and, conversely, how the psoas may become involved by remote inflammatory processes traversing fascial planes, such as ruptured diverticulitis.[35]

CT of the Kidneys

In all but the leanest patients, there is enough perinephric fat to provide adequate cross-sectional visualization of the kidneys. The CT densities of the renal cortex and renal medulla are similar, however (30 to 35 H), so that the two zones cannot ordinarily be discriminated without contrast enhancement. In fact, in many cases they cannot be differentiated after contrast enhancement, if imaging is not carried out systematically and precisely (Fig. 13–27). Corticomedullary demarcation is best obtained with a bolus injection and dynamic imaging (Fig. 13–28). Peak cortical opacification occurs normally at about 45 seconds and decreases rapidly thereafter, as contrast material accumulates in the tubules. This leads to an increasing density in the renal medulla, the values for cortex and medulla approximating each other normally at about 50 to 60 seconds after injection.

At the level of the renal hilum, the normal kidney averages 5 to 6 cm in transverse diameter, 4 cm anteroposteriorly, and 10 to 12 cm in length. The overall CT density of the renal sinus (Fig. 13–26A, B) may be affected by fat, urine in the collecting system, and blood in the

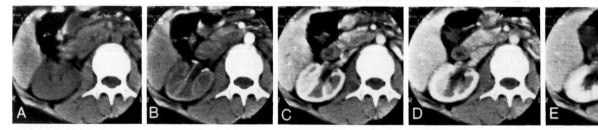

Figure 13–27. Bolus injection demonstrating corticomedullary demarcation. Following 30 cc IV of Hypaque 60 with a 10-second delay in initial scan and a 6-second interscan time between each scan, these results were obtained: A, Preliminary scan at the level of the right renal hilus. B, Scan demonstrating the right renal artery and renal cortex to be opacified by contrast medium. The medulla is not as yet opacified. The aorta has reached its peak opacification at this time. C, Scan showing increasing contrast within the cortex with beginning opacification in the medullary portion of the kidney. D, Scan showing decreased aortic density. The cortex still shows better opacification than the medulla. E, The cortex and medulla have reached equilibrium at roughly 1 minute.

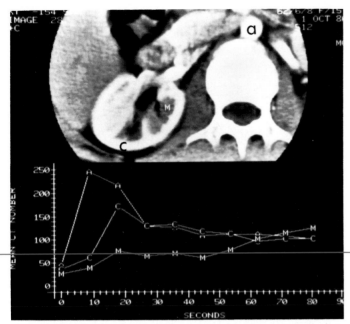

Figure 13–28. Time-density curve following bolus injection of contrast. Graph was obtained with time and level of CT numbers as designated. The crossing point of the cortex and medulla is roughly 60 seconds. a = aorta. c = cortex. m = medulla.

renal arteries and veins, as well as by calcific plaques in the renal arteries. Contrast material may be necessary to delineate the structures within the renal sinus separating renal cysts and carcinomas from vascular and other normal structures. Calyces, infundibula, renal pelves, and ureters can be visualized on nonenhanced CT images, but they are better demonstrated on scans obtained after injection of contrast media (Fig. 13–27).

On cross section, the kidney presents an almost infinite variety of appearances. Although with experience one soon learns to differentiate these normal variations from pathological lesions of somewhat similar configuration, cases occur in which even seasoned observers have difficulty separating the two. The CT appearances of these pseudotumors have been reviewed by Simpson and coworkers[53] and others.[54] Simpson and coworkers point out that if a suspected renal mass has the same base attenuation value as normal renal parenchyma and, following bolus intravenous injection of contrast material, demonstrates the same time-density changes exhibited by normal kidney tissue, the area in question represents a pseudotumor. They caution, however, that timing of the images is crucial. Whereas isoenhancement immediately after bolus injection might be seen with a vascular neoplasm as well as with normal tissue, continual enhancement over a period of several minutes—especially during the period of tubular reabsorption—can be a property of only normal renal parenchyma.

Vigneri and colleagues have made use of the normal renovertebral relationships in planning radiation treatment fields. They noted that 33% of 200 kidneys they examined by CT revealed evidence of some anterior extension beyond the anterior margin of the vertebral body and that 73% extended in some part medial to the transverse process. They emphasized the importance of these variations when laying out lateral and anteroposterior upper abdominal treatment portals.[48]

CT of the Renal Vessels[49]

Single arteries on the right and left occur in about 70% to 80% of people.[49] Renal arteries are two large trunks that branch at nearly right angles from the sides of the aorta immediately below the superior mesenteric artery. The right renal artery is longer because of the left-sided aortic position. The right artery passes posterior to the IVC, the right renal vein, the head of the pancreas and the descending part of the duodenum. The left artery is a little higher. It lies posterior to the left renal vein, the pancreatic body, and the splenic vein, and it may be crossed anteriorly by the inferior mesenteric vein (Fig. 13–8C).

The renal veins are anterior to the renal arteries and open into the IVC at almost right angles (Figs. 13–8C and 13–25). The left vein joins the IVC at a higher level than the right and is about three times longer than the right. The left vein crosses behind the splenic vein and the body of the pancreas. Near its termination it passes in front of the aorta just below the superior mesenteric artery. The left testicular or ovarian vein enters from below. The right renal vein is posterior to the descending part of the duodenum. In 2% to 4% of patients, there is either a double left renal vein (with one branch passing behind and one passing in front of the aorta) or a single retroaortic branch. In persistence of a left inferior vena cava, the left renal vein crosses to the right at the renal hilus and connects to the suprarenal portion of the right-sided inferior vena cava.[49]

CT of the Ureter

The ureter is directly continuous superiorly with the funnel-shaped renal pelvis (see Figs. 13–9A and 13–26). It turns downward in front of the psoas major, passes into the pelvic cavity, and opens into the base of the urinary bladder. It enters the lesser pelvis by crossing anteriorly to either the end of the common iliac vessel or the beginning of the external iliac vessels.[49]

On the right, the ureter is usually overlapped by the descending duodenum; in its descent it is lateral to the IVC. On the left it descends parallel to the abdominal aorta. Both ureters lie beneath the anterior renal fascia.[36]

CT of Normal Adrenals

A complete anatomical description of the adrenal glands, including their CT appearance, is to be found in the section on the adrenal gland (Chapter 83).

References

1. Hounsfield GN: Computerized transverse axial scanning (tomography). Part I: Description of the system. B J Radiol 46:1016, 1973.
2. Curry TS III, Dowdey JE, Murry RC: Christensen's Introduction to the Physics of Diagnostic Radiology, 3rd Ed. Philadelphia, Lea & Febiger, 1984.
3. Boyd DP, Parker DL: Basic principles of computed tomography. In Moss AA, Gamsu G, Genant HK: Computed Tomography of the Body. Philadelphia, WB Saunders Company, 1983.
4. Hattery RR, Williamson B Jr, Hartman GW: Computed tomography of the genitourinary tract and retroperitoneum. In Witten DM,

Myers H, Utz DC: Emmett's Clinical Urology, 4th Ed. Philadelphia, WB Saunders Company, 1977.

5. Schellinger D, DiChiro G, Axelbaum SP, et al: Early clinical experience with the ACTA scanner. Radiology 114:257, 1975.

6. Alfidi RJ, Haaga J, Meaney TF, et al: Computed tomography of the thorax and abdomen: A preliminary report. Radiology 117:257, 1975.

7. Sheedy PF II, Stephens DH, Hattery RR, Muhm JR, Hartman GW: Computed tomography of the body: Initial clinical trial with the EMI prototype. AJR 127:23, 1976.

8. Stanley RJ, Sagel SS, Levitt RG: Computed tomography of the body: Early trends in application and accuracy of the method. AJR 127:53, 1976.

9. Miraldi F: Imaging principles in computed tomography. In Haaga JR, Alfidi RJ (eds): Computed Tomography of the Whole Body. St. Louis, CV Mosby Co, 1983.

9a. Jaschke WR, Gould RG, Cogan MG, et al: Cine-CT measurement of cortical renal blood flow. J Comput Assist Tomogr 11:779, 1987.

10. General Electric Company. Medical Systems Operations: CT 9800 Evaluation Criteria. Milwaukee, 1983.

11. Hounsfield GN: Picture quality of computed tomography. AJR 127:3, 1976.

12. Cann CE: Quantitative computed tomography. In Moss AA, Gamsu G, Genant HK: Computed Tomography of the Body. Philadelphia, WB Saunders Company, 1983.

13. Cann CE, Gamsu G, Birnberg FA, Webb WR: Quantification of calcium in solitary pulmonary nodules using single and dual energy CT. Radiology 145:493, 1982.

14. Marshall WH Jr, Alvarez RE, Macouski A: Initial results with prereconstruction dual-energy computed tomography (PREDECT). Radiology 140:421, 1981.

15. Engelstad BL, McLennan BL, Levitt RG, et al: The role of pre-contrast images in computed tomography of the kidney. Radiology 136:153, 1980.

16. Poole CA, Rowe MI: Clinical evidence of intestinal absorption of Gastrografin. Radiology 118:151, 1976.

17. Eisenberg RL, Hedgecock MW, Shanser JD, et al: Iodine absorption from the gastrointestinal tract during Hypaque-enema examination. Radiology 133:597, 1979.

18. Brennan RE, Curtis JA, Pollack HM, Weinberg I: Sequential changes in the CT number of the normal canine kidney following intravenous contrast administration. I: The renal cortex. Invest Radiol 14:141, 1979.

19. Brennan RE, Curtis JA, Pollack HM, Weinberg I: Sequential changes in the CT number of the normal canine kidney following intravenous contrast administration. II: The renal medulla. Invest Radiol 14:239, 1979.

20. Brennan RE, Rapoport S, Weinberg I, et al: CT determined canine kidney and urine iodine concentrations following intravenous administration of sodium diatrizoate, metrizamide, iopamidol, and sodium ioxaglate. Invest Radiol 17:95, 1982.

21. Ishikawa I, Onouchi Z, Saito Y, et al: Renal cortex visualization and analysis of dynamic CT curves of the kidney. J Comput Assist Tomogr 5:695, 1981.

22. Fuld IL, Matalon TA, Vogelzang RL, et al: Dynamic CT in the evaluation of physiologic status of renal transplants. AJR 142:1157, 1984.

23. Ishikawa I, Masuzaki S, Saito T, et al: Dynamic computed tomography in acute renal failure: Analysis of time-density curve. J Comput Assist Tomogr 9:1097, 1985.

24. Congdon ED, Edson JN: The cone of renal fascia in the adult white male. Anat Rec 80:289–313, 1941.

25. Tobin CE: The renal fascia and its relationship to the transversalis fascia. Anat Rec 89:295–311, 1944.

26. Mitchell GAG: The renal fascia. Br J Surg 147:257–266, 1950.

27. Meyers MA: Dynamic Radiology of the Abdomen: Normal and Pathologic Anatomy. Heidelberg, Springer-Verlag, 1982.

28. Gerota D: Beitrage zur Kenntnis des Befestigungsapparates der Niere. Archives fur Anatomie und Entwicklungsgeschichte. Anatomische Abteilung, pp 265–285, 1895.

29. Zuckerkandl E: Ueber den Fixationsapparat der Nieren. Beitrage zur Anatomie des menschlichen Korpers. Gratz 1882.

30. Mitchell GAG: The spread of acute intraperitoneal effusions. Br J Surg 28:291–313, 1940.

31. Mitchell GAG: The spread of retroperitoneal effusions arising in the renal regions. Br Med J 2:1134–1136, 1939.

32. Meyers MA, Whalen JP, Peelle K, et al: Radiologic features of extraperitoneal effusions: An anatomic approach. Radiology 104:249–257, 1972.

33. Whalen JP, Berne AS, Reimenschneider PA: The extraperitoneal perivisceral fat pad. Radiology 92:466–481, 1969.

34. Love L, Meyers MA, Churchill RJ, et al: Computed tomography of the extraperitoneal spaces. AJR 136:781, 1981.

35. Love L, Demos T: Computed tomography of the retroperitoneal spaces. In Siegelmann SS (ed): Contemporary Issues in Computed Tomography, Vol 3: CT of the Kidneys and Adrenals. London, Churchill Livingstone, 1984, pp 1–29.

36. Feldberg MAM: Computed Tomography of the Retroperitoneum. Boston, Martinus Nijhoff, 1983.

37. Parienty RA, Pradel J, Picard JD, et al: Visibility and thickening of the renal fascia on computed tomograms. Radiology 139:119–124, 1981.

38. Naidich DP, Megibow AJ, Hilton S, et al: Computed tomography of the diaphragm: Normal anatomy and variants. J Comput Assist Tomogr 7:633–640, 1983.

39. Naidich DP, Megibow AJ, Hilton S, et al: Computed tomography of the diaphragm: Peridiaphragmatic fluid localization. J Comput Assist Tomogr 7:641–649, 1983.

40. Somogyi J, Cohen WN, Omar MM, et al: Communication of right and left perirenal spaces demonstrated by computed tomography. J Comput Assist Tomogr 3:270–273, 1979.

41. Raptopoulos V, Kleinman P, et al: Renal fascial pathway: Posterior extension of pancreatic effusions within the anterior pararenal space. Radiology 158:367–374, 1986.

42. Hadar H, Natan G: Positional relationships of the colon and kidney determined by perirenal fat. AJR 143:773–776, 1984.

43. Sherman JL, Hopper KD, Greene AJ, Johns TT: The retrorenal colon on computed tomography: A normal variant. J Comput Assist Tomogr 9:339–341, 1985.

44. Love L, Demos TC, Posniak H: CT of retrorenal fluid collections. AJR 145:87–91, 1985.

45. Kunin, M: Bridging septa of the perinephric space: Anatomic, pathologic and diagnostic considerations. Radiology 158:361–365, 1986.

46. McClennan BL, Lee JKT, Peterson RR: Anatomy of the perirenal area. Radiology 158:555–557, 1986.

47. Donovan PJ, Zerhouni EA, Siegelman SS: CT of the psoas compartment of the retroperitoneum. Semin Roentgenol 16:241–251, 1981.

48. Vigneri P, Arger P, Pollack H, Kligerman M: Localization and protection of kidneys in radiation treatment planning using computed tomography. Int J Radiat Oncol Biol Phys 11:1209–1213, 1985.

49. Williams P, Warwick R, (eds): Gray's Anatomy, 36th British Ed, WB Saunders Company, 1980.

50. Feldberg MAM, Koehler PR, Van Waes PFGM: Psoas compartment disease studied by computed tomography: Analysis of 50 cases and subject review. Radiology 148:505–512, 1983.

51. Reynes CJ, Churchill RJ, Moncada R, Love L: Computed tomography of the adrenal glands. Rad Clin North Am 117:91–103, 1979.

52. Kneeland JB, Auh YH, Rubenstein WA, et al: Perirenal spaces: CT evidence for communication across the midline. Radiology 164:657, 1987.

53. Simpson EL, Mintz MC, Pollack HM, et al: Computed tomography in the diagnosis of renal pseudotumors. Comput Tomogr 10:341, 1986.

54. Zeman RK, Cronan JJ, Rosenfield AT, et al: Computed tomography of renal masses: Pitfalls and anatomic variants. Radiographics 6:351, 1986.

55. Hopper KD, Sherman JL, Luethke JM, Ghaed N: The retrorenal colon in the supine and prone patient. Radiology 162:443, 1987.

56. Dodds WJ, Darweesh RMA, Lawson TL, et al: The retroperitoneal spaces revisited. AJR 147:1155, 1986.

57. Rubenstein WA, Whalen JP: Extraperitoneal spaces. AJR 147:1162, 1986.

COMPUTED TOMOGRAPHY OF THE LOWER URINARY TRACT AND PELVIS

ELIAS KAZAM □ YONG HO AUH □ WILLIAM A. RUBENSTEIN □ JOHN A. MARKISZ
KENNETH ZIRINSKY

In the last decade computed tomography (CT) and ultrasonography have revolutionized imaging of the pelvis and lower urinary tract. More recently, magnetic resonance imaging (MRI) has become available, and is currently being used to supplement or occasionally replace CT and ultrasonography in pelvic imaging. With these developments, sectional anatomy, already a valuable tool for the interpretation of conventional radiographs,[1] has acquired greater significance.[2]

Anatomically, the pelvis is arbitrarily divided into two major components.[3] The greater pelvis extends from the first sacral vertebra to the level of the upper acetabula, where the iliac, pubic, and ischial bones unite. Below it, the lesser pelvis extends inferiorly to the level of the ischial tuberosities, with its floor being formed by the urogenital diaphragm.

The CT images displayed here were obtained with third-generation scanners, using 10-mm collimation and scan times of 2 to 3 seconds, or occasionally of 10 seconds. Interscan intervals were 10 to 12 mm. Intravenous and oral contrast media were administered routinely, unless contraindicated. The ultrasound images were obtained with real-time scanners using the highest frequency transducers, usually 3.5 MHz, which provided adequate penetration. The MRI scans were obtained with the Technicare 0.5 T Teslacon using spin-echo (SE) techniques. Multiple-slice, multiple-echo images were obtained routinely. These were usually in the transverse plane, with echo times (TE) of 32, 64, and 96 msec, and intersequence intervals (TR) of 1500 to 2100 msec. Additional images were usually obtained in the sagittal and/or coronal planes, using a single-echo, multiple-slice technique (TR = 500 msec/TE = 32 msec). Slice thickness was 7.5 mm for all studies. The interslice gap was 2.5 mm for single-echo images, and 5.0 mm for the multiple-echo images. Occasionally, two interleaved runs with a gap of 7.5 mm were used to image the same region. It was desirable for the patient to have a partially filled urinary bladder, in order to displace small-bowel loops that can mimic masses superiorly. An alphabetized list of anatomical abbreviations and pertinent figures is included in Table 13–2. A brief description of the major structures and organs appears below.

THE BLOOD VESSELS

Just above the inlet to the greater pelvis, the abdominal aorta divides into two common iliac arteries, which diverge as they extend inferiorly.[1] At the L4 (fourth lumbar) and upper L5 vertebrae, the common iliac arteries lie in front of the vena cava, medial to the psoas muscles (Fig. 13–29A). Below this level, they lie anterior to the common iliac veins. Between the L5 and S1 (first sacral) vertebrae, the common iliac arteries divide further into external and internal iliac (hypogastric) branches (Fig. 13–29B).

The External Iliac Branches. The external iliac arteries course forward and laterally, anterolateral to the external iliac veins, to the inguinal ligaments, where they become the femoral arteries (Figs. 13–29A–D, 13–30A,B, 13–34A). Thus, the external iliac vessels diverge progressively from their internal iliac counterparts as they course inferiorly within the pelvis, medial to the psoas muscles. The following two important external iliac branches are consistently identifiable on CT and MRI.

The *inferior epigastric vessels* arise from, or drain into, their parent external iliac vessels just above the inguinal ligament. They extend anterosuperiorly along the medial margin of the internal inguinal ring to the anterior abdominal wall, where they course behind the rectus abdominis muscles (Figs. 13–30, 13–31, 13–32A, 13–34A, 13–35, 13–36A,B, 13–37B).

The *deep circumflex iliac vessels* ascend anterolaterally from the external iliac vessels, behind the inguinal ligament and the internal inguinal ring, to the anterosuperior iliac spines (Figs. 13–30, 13–34A, 13–35, 13–36A,F).

The Internal Iliac Branches. The internal iliac arteries course posteroinferiorly, in front of the internal iliac veins (Figs. 13–39B–D, 13–31B), to the inferior margins of the sacroiliac joints, where they divide into anterior and posterior trunks.

The *anterior trunk* gives rise to vesical, prostatic, and rectal branches (Figs. 13–33A, 13–36C, 13–37). These course with their corresponding venous plexuses, lateral to the organs they supply, within the visceral layer of the pelvic fascia.[3, 4] The terminal branches of the anterior trunk are the internal pudendal and inferior gluteal arteries (Figs. 13–30, 13–37A–C, 13–38C,D and Figs. 13–30, 13–36D, 13–37D, 13–40D,E). Both exit the greater sciatic foramen below the piriformis muscle, accompanied by the internal pudendal and inferior gluteal veins, the pudendal nerve, and the sciatic nerve. The inferior gluteal vessels then continue downward, along with the sciatic nerve, into the back of the thigh, while the internal pudendal vessels and pudendal nerve curve inward through the lesser sciatic foramen, to course in the pudendal canal at the medial borders of the obturator internus muscles.

The *posterior trunk* gives rise to iliolumbar, lateral sacral, and superior gluteal branches. The iliolumbar vessels course anterior to the sacrum, behind the obturator nerve, to supply the iliacus and psoas muscles (Fig. 13–29B). The lateral sacral vessels enter the sacral foramina, while the superior gluteal vessels exit the greater sciatic foramen above the piriformis, to supply the gluteal muscles (Fig. 13–29E).

In general, the iliac vessels appear denser than muscle or isodense with muscle on contrast-enhanced CT scans. They become markedly hyperdense on dynamic CT scans.

Text continued on page 415

Table 13–2. Alphabetized List of Anatomical Abbreviations and Pertinent Figures

Abbreviation		Figures	Abbreviation		Figures
abm	adductor brevis muscle	13–38C,D, 13–39B,C	ipvs	internal pudendal vessels	13–30, 13–36D, 13–37A,D, 13–40C,D
alm	adductor longus muscle	13–38C,D, 13–39A–C	isb	ischial bone	13–36D, 13–37D, 13–39A–C
amm	adductor minimus muscle	13–39A–C	isrf	ischiorectal fossa	13–39B,C
ans	anus	13–38H, 13–39C, 13–40E	L4n	lumbar nerve #4	13–29A
arc	arcuate line	13–34A	lfcn	lateral femoral cutaneous nerve	13–29C
asis	anterosuperior iliac spine	13–29D	lsf	lesser sciatic foramen	13–36C, 13–37A
bft	biceps femoris tendon	13–36D, 13–39B,C	lsn	lumbosacral trunk	13–29B–D
blp	bulb of penis	13–39A–C, 13–39B,C	lting	lateral inguinal fossa	13–31C, 13–34, 13–35D
bspm	bulbospongiosus muscle	13–39B,C, 13–40E	ltul	lateral umbilical ligament/fold	13–31C, 13–34, 13–35B–D
ccm	coccygeus muscle	13–33C, 13–36C	lva	levator ani muscle	13–29E, 13–38A,B,E,F,H, 13–40C,D
cds	cul de sac	13–31B, 13–33A,B	mling	medial inguinal fossa	13–31C, 13–34, 13–35B,D
cec	cecum	13–29A–D, 13–31C, 13–32A, 13–34B, 13–39D	mlul	medial umbilical ligament/fold	13–30A,B, 13–31C,D, 13–32A, 13–34, 13–35, 13–36A,E,F
cia	common iliac artery	13–29A	mnul	median umbilical ligament/fold	13–30, 13–31C, 13–34A, 13–35D, 13–36E,F
civ	common iliac vein	13–29B	mrsc	median raphe of scrotum	13–40A,B
crp	crus of penis	13–39A–C, 13–40E	myo	myoma of uterus	13–32C
csp	corpus spongiosum penis	13–38H, 13–39A,D,E, 13–40C,D	obe	obturator externus muscle	13–29E, 13–37D, 13–38A,C,D, 13–40C,D
cvp	corpus cavernosum penis	13–38H, 13–39, 13–40C,D	obf	obturator foramen	13–38E,F
dc	descending colon	13–29A–D, 13–31D	obi	obturator internus muscle	13–29E, 13–30, 13–33A, 13–37A,B–F, 13–40C,D
dcivs	deep circumflex iliac vessels	13–30A,B, 13–34A, 13–35A,C,D, 13–36A,B,F	obln	obturator lymph nodes	13–30A,B, 13–36E,F, 13–37A–C
ddvp	deep dorsal vein of penis	13–38A, 13–39D,E	obn	obturator nerve	13–29A–D, 13–30A,B
eia	external iliac artery	13–29A–D, 13–30, 13–34	obt	obturator tendon	13–38B,E,F, 13–40C,D
eiln	external iliac lymph node	13–36E,F, 13–37A	obvs	obturator vessels	13–30, 13–38B
eiv	external iliac vein	13–29C,D, 13–30A,B, 13–34A,B	p	peritoneum	13–31, 13–32A, 13–34
eivs	external iliac vessels	13–29E, 13–31C,D, 13–32A,C, 13–36A,E,F	pal	pubic arcuate ligament	13–38H
ephd	epididymal head	13–40A,C,D	pdn	pudendal nerve	13–30
esm	erector spinae muscle	13–29B,D	pec	pectineus muscle	13–38A,C,D
fa	femoral artery	13–33D, 13–36C, 13–38E,F	pef	perivesical (periurachal) fat	13–35C,D
fab	fibrous adventitia of bladder	13–31B, 13–33B	pev	perivesical space	13–31A–C, 13–32B, 13–33A,B, 13–34B
fcn	femoral canal	13–33D	pir	piriformis muscle	13–30, 13–35A–C, 13–36A
fmh	femoral head	13–29E, 13–37E	pl	puboprostatic ligament	13–31
fmn	femoral nerve	13–29	pnb	perineal body	13–39B,C, 13–40E
fv	femoral vein	13–36C, 13–38E,F	pns	penis	13–29E, 13–40A
gem	gemelli muscles	13–38B,E,F, 13–40E,F	ppf	parietal pelvic fascia	13–31C, 13–32A, 13–33B
gme	gluteus medius muscle	13–29A,B,D,E, 13–30A,B, 13–38B	pr	prostate	13–29E, 13–37D, 13–38, 13–40C,D
gmi	gluteus minimus muscle	13–29D,E, 13–30A,B	prcp	prostatic capsule	13–38C
gmx	gluteus maximus muscle	13–29D, 13–30, 13–38B,E,F	prgl	glandular prostate	13–38A–F, 13–40C,D
gsf	greater sciatic foramen	13–30, 13–35A,C, 13–36A,E,F	pris	prostatic isthmus	13–38A–G, 13–40C,D
icvm	ischiocavernosus muscle	13–29E, 13–37D, 13–39B,C, 13–40E	prrf	perirectal fat	13–35A,B
			prsh	posterior rectus sheath	13–34A
ievs	inferior epigastric vessels	13–30A,B, 13–31A–D, 13–32A, 13–35, 13–36A,B, 13–37B	prv	prevesical space	13–31A–C, 13–32, 13–33, 13–34B
igvs	inferior gluteal vessels	13–30, 13–37B,C, 13–38C,D	prvf	prevesical fat	13–38E,F
iia	internal iliac artery	13–29A–D, 13–31D, 13–38C,D	prvs	prostatic vascular plexus	13–37D, 13–38E,F
iir	internal inguinal ring	13–30, 13–35A, 13–37B,C	ps	psoas muscle	13–29, 13–30A, 13–31D, 13–32A, 13–34B, 13–38E
iiv	internal iliac vein	12–29C,D	pu	pubic bone	13–31B, 13–33A, 13–36D, 13–38H
iivs	internal iliac vessels	13–29E	qfm	quadratus femoris muscle	13–29E
il	ileum	13–29A,B, 13–31C, 13–32A, 13–34B	rab	rectus abdominis muscle	13–29C,D, 13–30A,B, 13–31C,D, 13–32A, 13–34
ilb	iliac bone	13–29C	re	rectum	13–31B, 13–32B,C, 13–33, 13–35A,B, 13–37B,C, 13–38E,F, 13–40C,D
ilfs	iliac fascia	13–30A			
ilm	iliacus muscle	13–29E, 13–30A, 13–31C,D, 13–32A, 13–37B,C, 13–38E,F	rfm	rectus femoris muscle	13–29B, 13–38E,F
ilvs	ileolumbar vessels	13–29B	rvs	rectovesical septum	13–31B
imvs	inferior mesenteric vessels	13–29A	sar	sartorius muscle	13–30, 13–38B,E,F
			sb	small bowel	13–35A,C,D
ingc	inguinal canal	13–36C	scn	sciatic nerve	13–30A,B, 13–37C,D
ingl	inguinal ligament	13–30A	sdvp	superficial dorsal vein—penis	13–39E
ingn	inguinal lymph node	13–38E, 13–39E			
iob	internal oblique muscle	13–29A,C,D, 13–30A,B			

Table 13–2. Alphabetized List of Anatomical Abbreviations and Pertinent Figures *Continued*

Abbreviation		Figures	Abbreviation		Figures
sevs	superficial epigastric vessels	13–35C,D	ts	testis	13–38H, 13–39E, 13–40A–E
sgc	sigmoid colon	13–29A–D, 13–30A,B, 13–31C,D, 13–32A, 13–34B, 13–35C, 13–37D	tvs	testicular vessels	13–29A,B, 13–30, 13–35, 13–36E,F, 13–40B,C
sll	semilunar line	13–29C,D	u	umbilicus	13–31B
slp	suspensory ligament of penis	13–39D	ua	umbilical arteries	13–31A,C
			ub	urinary bladder	13–31, 13–32B,C, 13–33, 13–34, 13–35A,B, 13–36A,B, 13–38B,D, 13–39D
spc	spermatic cord	i3–36A–D, 13–39A–C,E, 13–40C,D			
spp	septum of penis	13–39B–E	ubvs	vesical vascular plexus	13–33A, 13–36C, 13–37A–C
ssl	sacrospinous ligament	13–37A	ugd	urogenital diaphragm	13–29E, 13–37D, 13–39B,C
stl	sacrotuberous ligament	13–38B–F, 13–40C,D	upv	umbilical prevesical fascia	13–31C
sv(s)	seminal vesicle(s)	13–33A, 13–35A,B, 13–36B,C,E,F, 13–37A–D, 13–38G,H	ur	ureter	13–29A–C, 13–30A,B, 13–31C,D, 13–34B, 13–35, 13–37B,C
			urc	urachus	13–31A–C, 13–35B–D
syn	sympathetic nerve trunk	13–29E	urth	urethra	13–38D–F, 13–40C,D
tab	transverse abdominis muscle	13–29A,C,D, 13–31D	ut	uterus	13–31B,C, 13–32A–C, 13–33B,D, 13–34B
tabp	tunica albuginea penis	13–38H, 13–39B–E	uv	umbilicovesical fascia	13–31A–C, 13–32, 13–33A–C, 13–34B
tabt	tunica albuginea testis	13–40C–E	vc	inferior vena cava	13–29A
tf	transversalis fascia	13–31A–C, 13–32A, 13–33B	vd	vas deferens	13–30, 13–34A, 13–35A,C, 13–36, 13–37, 13–38H
tfl	tensor fascia lata	13–30	vpf	visceral pelvic fascia	13–30, 13–32B,C, 13–33A,B, 13–35A
tpsm	transversus perinei sup muscle	13–39B,C, 13–40E	vur	vesicouterine recess	13–31C, 13–32A, 13–34B

Figure 13–29. The pelvic inlet. *A,* CT through L5 vertebra. The right common iliac artery (cia) lies anterior to the inferior vena cava (vc) and right ureter (ur). The left common iliac artery is beginning to divide into external (eia) and internal (iia) branches. Testicular vessels (tvs), inferior mesenteric vessels (imvs), cecum (cec), ileum (il), and sigmoid and descending colon (sgc, dc) are indicated. The femoral and obturator nerves (fmn, obn) have just emerged from the posteroinferior margin of the psoas muscles (ps), and the fourth lumbar nerve (L4n) is shown. The nerves are relatively prominent in this patient with neurofibromatosis. The following muscles are also indicated: external oblique (eob), internal oblique (iob), transversus abdominis (tab), gluteus medius (gme). *B,* CT through S1 vertebra, 30 mm below *A.* The left external iliac artery (eia) has moved anterolaterally and is now separated from the left internal iliac artery (iia) by the left ureter (ur). The right common iliac artery has just divided into external (eia) and internal (iia) iliac artery branches. Right ureter (ur) and common iliac veins (civ) are indicated. The obturator nerves (obn) lie at the posteromedial aspects of the psoas muscles (ps), anterior to the iliolumbar vessels (ilvs). The femoral nerves (fmn) course between the psoas and iliac muscles (ilm). Also indicated are the lumbosacral trunk (lsn), testicular vessels (tvs), and erector spinae muscle (esm). *C,* CT 30 mm below *B.* The left external iliac artery (eia) now lies just anterior to its corresponding vein (eiv), medial to the psoas muscle (ps). The left internal iliac artery (iia) is contiguous and just anterior to its corresponding vein (iiv). The right external iliac artery and vein (eia, eiv) are separated from the right internal iliac vessels (iia, iiv) by the right ureter (ur). The lateral femoral cutaneous nerve (lfcn) is visible just behind the descending colon (dc). Also indicated are the urinary bladder (ub), rectus abdominis muscle (rab), semilunar line (sll), and iliac bone (ilb). *D,* MRI (SE 500/32) of another patient at approximate level of *C.* The left external iliac artery and vein (eia, eiv) have nearly the same configuration as in *C.* The right external and internal iliac vessels (*arrows*) are not as clearly delineated from each other. Compare with *C* for visualization of nerves, muscles, and bones. (*A–D* from Kazam E, Auh YH, Rubenstein WA, et al: Normal CT anatomy of the pelvis with ultrasound and MRI correlations. *In* Putnam CE, Ravin C (eds): Textbook of Diagnostic Imaging. Philadelphia, WB Saunders, 1988.) *E,* Coronal MRI (SE 500/32) through the femoral heads (fmh). The lumbosacral trunk (lsn) lies at the medial aspect of the psoas (ps) muscle, while the femoral nerve (fmn) lies between the psoas and iliac (ilm) muscles. Also shown are the external and internal iliac vessels (eivs, iivs), superior gluteal vessels (sgvs), prostate (pr), penis (pns), sympathetic nerve trunk (syn), and the following muscles: obturator internus (obi), levator ani (lva), obturator externus (obe), quadratus femoris (qfm), ischiocavernosus (icvm), gluteus minimus (gmi), gluteus medius (gme).

See illustration on following page

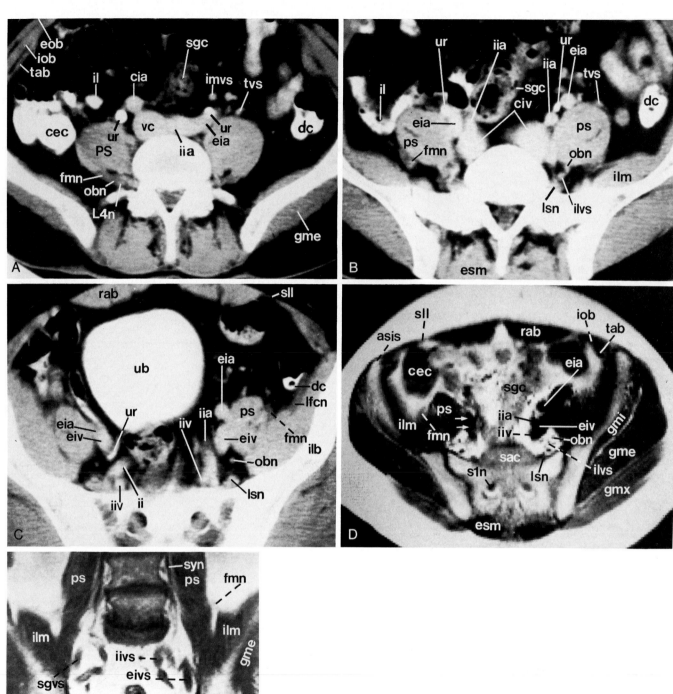

Figure 13–29 *See legend on previous page*

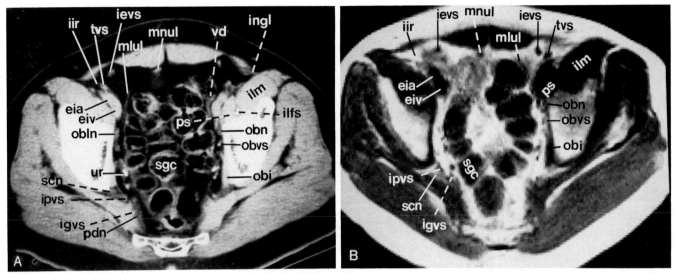

Figure 13–30. The internal inguinal ring and the greater sciatic foramen. CT scan (*A*) and MR scan (*B*, SE 500/32) of same patient show a tortuous sigmoid colon (sgc) occupying most of the pelvis at this level. Also shown are the internal inguinal ring (iir), inferior epigastric vessels (ievs), testicular vessels (tvs), and inguinal ligament (ingl). The left vas deferens (vd) courses just medial to the external iliac artery (eia) and vein (eiv) on the CT scan (*A*), analogous to the round ligament in the female, but is not as clearly delineated on MRI (*B*). The external iliac vessels (eia, eiv) blend with the isointense psoas muscle (ps) on MRI, but not on CT. Radiodense iliac fascia (ilfs), surrounded by a thin rind of fat, separates the psoas from the iliac (ilm) muscles. The obturator (obn) and sciatic (scn) nerves are well seen with both techniques. Also indicated are the obturator lymph nodes (obln), obturator vessels (obvs), obturator internus muscle (obi), pudendal nerve (pdn), median umbilical ligament (mnul), and medial umbilical fold (mlul). The ureter (ur) is indistinguishable from pelvic vessels on MR scan. (*A, B* from Kazam E, Auh YH, Rubenstein WA, et al: Normal CT anatomy of the pelvis with ultrasound and MRI correlations. *In* Putnam CE, Ravin C (eds): Textbook of Diagnostic Imaging. Philadelphia, WB Saunders, 1988.)

Figure 13–31. The urinary bladder and the extraperitoneal paravesical spaces. *A*, Schematic diagram of the extraperitoneal spaces in the ventral abdominal wall. The urinary bladder (ub), urachus (urc), and obliterated umbilical arteries (ua) lie within the perivesical space (pev), surrounded by the umbilicovesical fascia (uv). The prevesical space (prv) lies anterior to the umbilicovesical fascia and posterior to the transversalis fascia (tf). The peritoneum (p) lies behind the umbilicovesical fascia. Inferior epigastric vessels (ievs). *B*, Midsagittal view of *A*. The umbilicovesical fascia (uv) surrounds the urinary bladder (ub) and urachus (urc), which lie within the perivesical space (pev). The fibrous adventitia of the bladder (fab) is a derivative of the umbilicovesical fascia. The prevesical space (prv) is represented mainly by the darkly shaded area, anterior to the umbilicovesical fascia and posterior to the transversalis fascia (tf), but also extends into the small potential space (*small arrows*) between the umbilicovesical fascia and peritoneum (p). The pubovesical ligament (pl) forms the anteroinferior boundary of the prevesical and perivesical spaces. The rectovaginal septum (rvs) is formed by fusion of the anterior and posterior layers of peritoneum which line the cul de sac (cds). Indicated are the umbilicus (u), pubis (pu), uterus (ut), and rectum (re). Lines A, B, and C indicate the levels of the transverse sections in *C* and Figures 13–32*B, C,* and 13–33*B,* respectively.

See illustration on following page

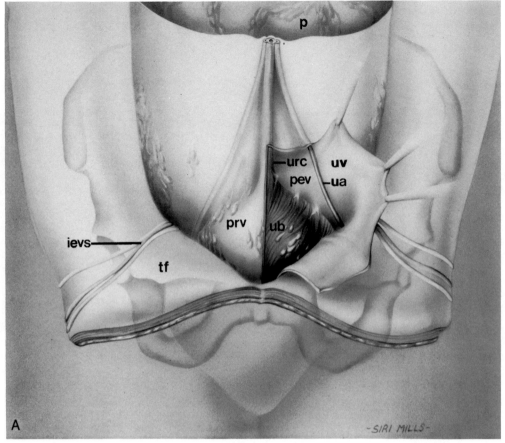

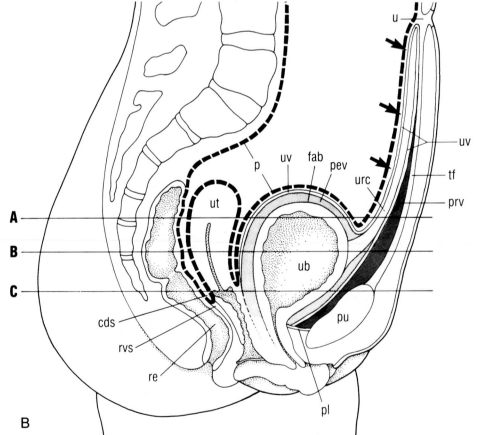

Figure 13–31 *See legend on previous and opposite pages*

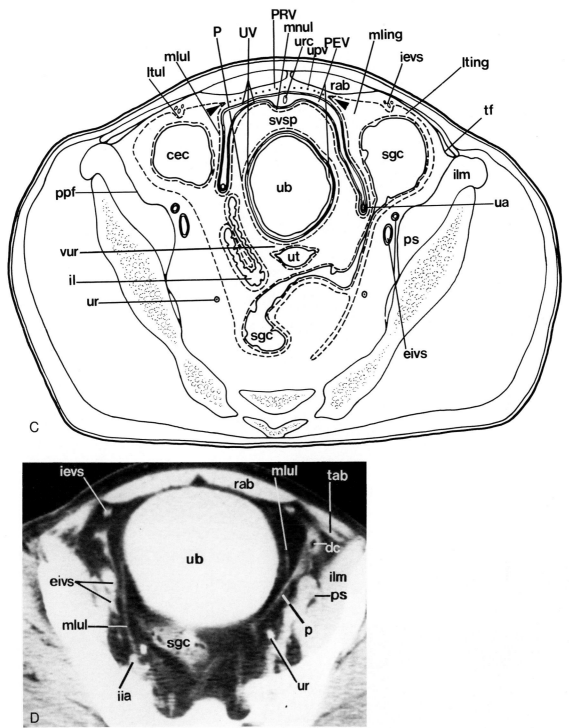

Figure 13–31 *Continued C,* Schematic drawing of a section through level A in *B.* The urachus (urc) and obliterated umbilical arteries (ua) lie within the perivesical space (pev), surrounded by umbilicovesical fascia (uv). The dome of the urinary bladder (ub) also lies within the perivesical space (pev), surrounded by umbilicovesical fascia (uv) and peritoneum (p). Prevesical space (prv) is indicated. The indentation of the peritoneum by the urachus and enveloping umbilicovesical fascia forms the median umbilical fold (mnul). The peritoneal indentations by the old umbilical arteries (umbilical ligaments) and umbilicovesical fascia form the medial umbilical folds (mlul). The inferior epigastric vessels (ievs) also indent the peritoneum, forming the lateral umbilical folds (ltul). The medial and lateral umbilical folds divide the anterior peritoneal compartment into supravesical space (svsp), medial inguinal fossa (mling), and lateral inguinal fossa (lting). The medial recesses (*large arrowheads*) of the medial inguinal fossae may extend toward the midline, anterior to the umbilicovesical fascia, and their peritoneal layers may fuse anteromedially to form the umbilical prevesical fascia (upv). Cecum (cec) and sigmoid colon (sgc) occupy the inguinal fossae. Also indicated are the ileum (il), uterus (ut), vesicouterine recess (vur), rectus abdominis muscle (rab), iliacus (ilm) and psoas (ps) muscles, external iliac vessels (eivs), ureter (ur). Transversalis fascia (tf), and parietal pelvic fascia (ppf). *D,* In vivo CT scan at approximate level of *C* shows portions of both medial umbilical ligaments or folds (mlul), with the right ligament joining the ipsilateral internal iliac artery (iia). Indicated are the external iliac vessels (eivs), parietal peritoneum (p), inferior epigastric vessels (ievs), descending (dc), and sigmoid (sgc) colons, urinary bladder (ub), ureter (ur), rectus abdominis muscle (rab), transversus abdominis (tab), iliacus (ilm) and psoas (ps) muscles. (*A–D* from Auh YH, Rubenstein WA, Schneider M, et al: Extraperitoneal paravesical spaces: CT delineation with US correlation. Radiology 159:319–328, 1986.)

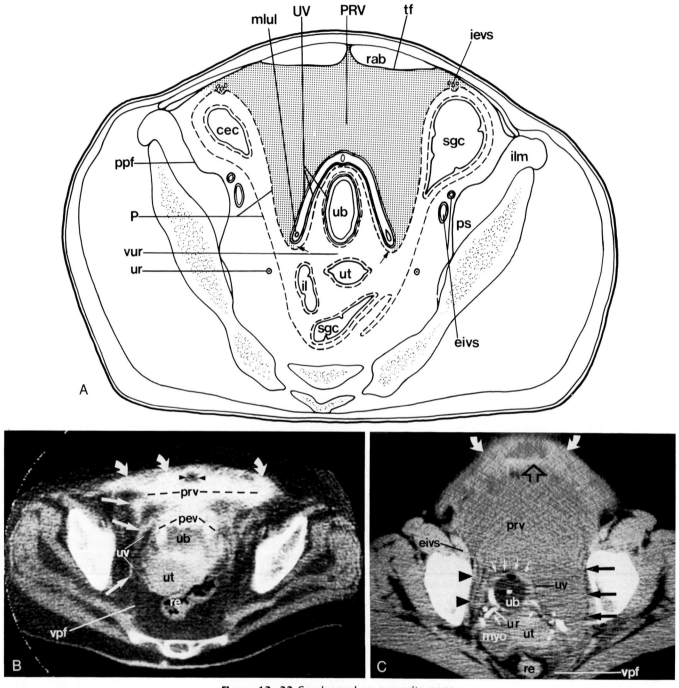

Figure 13–32 *See legend on opposite page*

They are signal poor and therefore appear black on MR scans. On sonograms, most of the internal iliac vessels are obscured by overlying bowel gas and fat. The external iliac vessels can be demonstrated as echo-poor structures, if the beam is angled laterally through the bladder.

An understanding of sectional vascular anatomy has several clinical applications. First, abnormalities of the iliac vessels, such as aneurysms or venous thrombi, which are detected with sectional imaging, may be localized correctly without having to resort to angiography. Second, the inferior epigastric and deep circumflex iliac vessels serve as important markers for the internal inguinal ring and as important collateral pathways, in case of venous or arterial obstruction. Finally, because nodes may appear isodense with vessels, even on contrast-enhanced CT, a diagnosis of pelvic lymph node enlargement should only be made after the iliac vessels are identified. At times, dynamic contrast-enhanced CT scans are required to differentiate dilated iliac vessels from lymph nodes.

THE PELVIC NODES

The pelvic nodes are grouped mainly around the common iliac, external iliac, and internal iliac vessels, with smaller groups along the sacral, inferior epigastric, deep circumflex iliac, and obturator vessels (Figs. 13–30, 13–36E,F, 13–37A–C).[3, 5] Inguinal nodes lie medial and anterior to the femoral vessels (Figs. 13–38E,F, 13–39E). Normal lymph nodes may be undetectable on CT scans, or they may appear as small structures, measuring up to 1 cm in diameter, which are either hypodense or isodense relative to muscles (Fig. 13–30A). On MR scans lymph nodes appear slightly brighter than, or occasionally as bright as, muscle (Fig. 13–37B,C, 13–38E,F). They are usually not visible with ultrasonography, unless they are enlarged.

Normal-sized nodes may be difficult to differentiate from adjacent vessels or nerves, even with the highest-quality CT scanners, but this usually has no clinical significance. Much more important is the ability to reliably differentiate enlarged pelvic nodes from adjacent blood vessels and bowel loops. This is especially important at the pelvic inlet, where the common iliac vessels are grouped together (Fig. 13–29A), and in the external iliac region, where the psoas muscle and the external iliac vessels, or adjacent bowel loops, may be confused with adenopathy on CT scans (Fig. 13–30A). Another possible source of error is the spermatic cord, which should not be mistaken for external iliac lymphadenopathy. An understanding of normal sectional anatomy helps to avoid such errors. For example, the fat that separates the psoas from the iliacus muscles is valuable for positively identifying the psoas muscle (Figs. 13–30A, 13–37B,C). Radiodense iliac fascia is often identifiable within this fat (Fig. 13–30A). This fascia appears signal poor on MRI. After positively identifying the psoas, it is important to remember that the external iliac vessels lie medial to it—with the artery anterior to the vein—and that enlarged lymph nodes generally lie medial and posterior to the external iliac vessels (Figs. 13–30A, 13–36E,F, 13–37A–C). Opacification of the blood vessels and hollow viscera with intravenous and oral contrast media is valuable for accurate CT diagnosis of pelvic lymph node enlargement.

THE PELVIC NERVES

The major pelvic nerve trunks[3, 5] can be seen well with modern CT equipment, and less well with MRI. For illustrative purposes, CT scans from a patient with neurofibromatosis and diffusely prominent nerves are included in Figure 13–29A–C. The same nerves, however, can be clearly visualized by CT and MRI in patients without neurofibromatosis (Figs. 13–29D,E, 13–30A,B, 13–37B,C).

The *femoral nerve* can be seen at the L5 level, just as

Figure 13–32. Transverse sections of extraperitoneal paravesical collections at the pelvic inlet (levels A and B in Fig. 13–31B). A, Schematic drawing of a prevesical collection at the level of 13–31C, corresponding to level A in Figure 13–31B. The collection in the prevesical space (prv) is represented by the shaded area, which has the shape of a molar tooth. The "crown" portion of the collection displaces the umbilicovesical fascia (UV) and urinary bladder posteriorly, while the "roots" extend posterolaterally, separating the peritoneal coverings (p) of the medial umbilical ligaments (mlul). The collection surrounds the inferior epigastric vessels (ievs) and is contiguous to the rectus abdominis muscles (rab), from which it is separated by only a thin and multiperforated posterior rectus sheath. Prevesical fluid may also extend into the small potential space (*small arrows*) anterior to the peritoneum and posterior to the umbilicovesical fascia. Also indicated are the uterus (ut), vesicouterine recess (vur), cecum (cec), ileum (il), sigmoid colon (sgc), iliacus (ilm) and psoas (ps) muscles, external iliac vessels (eivs), ureter (ur), transversalis fascia (tf), and parietal pelvic fascia (ppf). B, Cadaver CT scan just below the peritoneal reflection. Prevesical contrast (prv), which was injected more inferiorly (see Fig. 13–33C), displaces the urinary bladder (ub) posteriorly, and extends posterolaterally (*large arrows*) along the expected lateral contours of the umbilicovesical fascia (uv) and visceral pelvic fascia (vpf). The irregular outline of the contrast media is attributable to septations in the prevesical fat. Contrast has also extended into the rectus sheath (*curved arrows*). The relatively spared layer of prevesical fat (*arrowheads*) may be due to layering of contrast media, rather than to the presence of an umbilical prevesical fascia. Contrast within the perivesical space (pev) is confined around the anterolateral bladder contours by the umbilicovesical fascia. Uterus (ut) and rectum (re) are shown. C, CT scan of an in vivo prevesical hematoma at the level of B. The "crown" portion of the collection (prv) displaces the urinary bladder (ub) posteriorly, and extends into the rectus sheath (*curved arrows*), where it forms a blood-fluid level (*open arrow*). The larger left "root" (*large arrows*) displaces the bladder to the right, and extends posteriorly, along the expected lateral contours of the umbilicovesical fascia (uv) and visceral pelvic fascia (vpf). A smaller right "root" of the prevesical hematoma (*arrowheads*) extends posteriorly along the expected right lateral borders of the umbilicovesical and visceral pelvic fascia. Uterus (ut), uterine myoma (myo), and rectum (re) are indicated. The external iliac vessels (eivs) are contiguous to the collection. A thin layer of uninvolved perivesical fat (*small arrows*) surrounds the urinary bladder (ub) and distal ureters (ur). (A–C from Auh YH, Rubenstein WA, Schneider M, et al: Extraperitoneal paravesical spaces: CT delineation with US correlation. Radiology 159:319–328, 1986.)

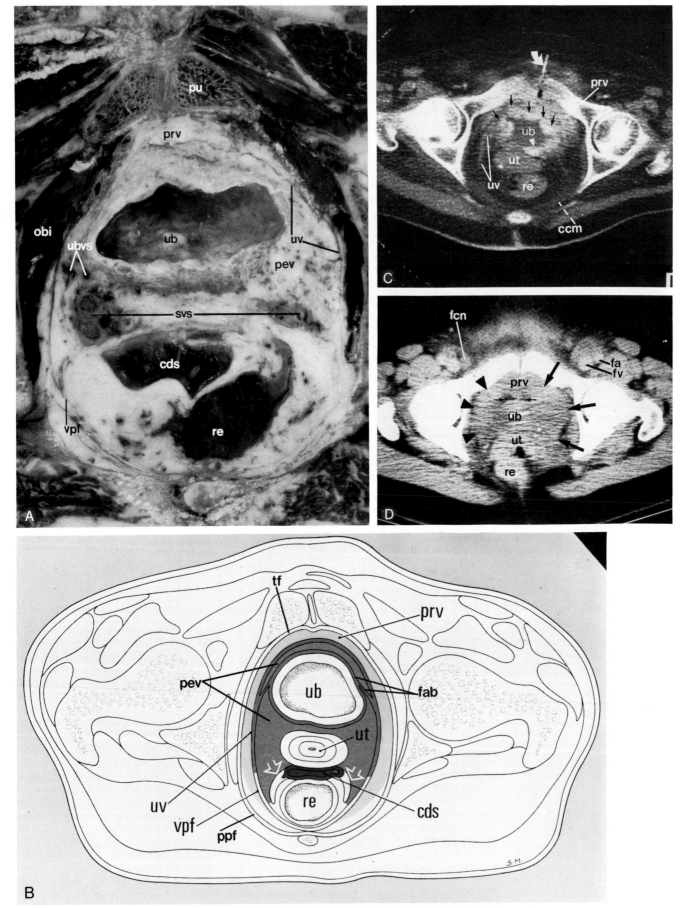

Figure 13–33 *See legend on opposite page*

it emerges from the posterior margin of the psoas muscle. At this point, it lies lateral to the obturator nerve (Fig. 13–29A). The femoral nerve then courses laterally and anteriorly between the psoas and iliacus muscles where it can occasionally be seen with CT or MRI if surrounded by sufficient fat (Fig. 13–29C,E). Just lateral to it at this level, the lateral femoral cutaneous nerve may be visible anterior to the iliacus muscle and behind the distal descending colon or cecum (Fig. 13–29C). More inferiorly, the femoral nerve continues its anterior course within the fatty groove between the psoas and iliacus muscles. In this latter location, it is usually not well seen by CT and is difficult to differentiate from radiodense iliac fascia (Fig. 13–30A), which lies anterior to the femoral nerve.

The *obturator nerve* is first visible behind the psoas muscle at the L5 level, where it lies medial to the femoral nerve, lateral to the L4 nerve, and anterior to the iliolumbar vessels (Fig. 13–29A,B). It then courses anteroinferiorly, in front of the internal iliac vessels and their obturator branches (Fig. 13–29C), and behind the external iliac lymph nodes (Fig. 13–30A). Within the obturator foramen, the obturator nerve courses laterally, adjacent to the bone, and is difficult to differentiate from the obturator vessels or nodes on CT scans (Fig. 13–38B,E,F).

The *L4 nerve* lies posteromedial to the psoas muscle at the L5 level (Fig. 13–29A). A portion of it then joins the L5 nerve below it to form the lumbosacral trunk (Fig. 13–29C,D), which continues posteroinferiorly in front of the gluteal vessels to the greater sciatic foramen, where it joins the S1–S3 nerves to form the sciatic nerve (Fig. 13–30A).

The *sacral nerves* course inferiorly from the sacral foramina into the posterior pelvis. The S1–S2 nerves are the largest of these. They are accompanied by the inferior gluteal vessels to the greater sciatic foramen, where they join the lumbosacral trunk and the S3 nerve to form the sciatic nerve (Fig. 13–30A).

The *sciatic nerve* is the largest in the body, and the most consistently visible with CT or MRI (Figs. 13–30A,B, 13–37B,C). It exits the pelvis through the greater sciatic foramen below the piriformis muscle, and descends into the posterior thigh lateral to the ischial tuberosity, with the inferior gluteal vessels and the posterior femoral cutaneous nerve at its medial aspect.

The *pudendal nerve* may be seen occasionally with CT or MRI, medial to the inferior gluteal vessels and piriformis muscle (Fig. 13–30A,B). It exits the pelvis through the inferior portion of the greater sciatic foramen, and then curves inward with the internal pudendal vessels, through the lesser sciatic foramen, to run into the pudendal canal lateral to the ischiorectal fat. Within the canal, the pudendal nerve is usually indistinguishable by CT from its accompanying vessels and the usually hyperdense fascia which surrounds them (Figs. 13–36D, 13–38E,F, 13–40C,D).

In general, nerves appear either hypodense (Figs. 13–29A and 13–30A) or isodense (Fig. 13–29A,B), relative to muscle on contrast-enhanced CT. On MRI they tend to be brighter than muscle (Fig. 13–30B) but are sometimes isointense with small vessels (Fig. 13–29D). As mentioned above, small nerves may not be differentiated reliably from contiguous small vessels and lymph nodes with either CT or MRI. Nevertheless, an understanding of the sectional anatomy of the pelvic nerves is useful. First, neural tumors, rather than enlarged lymph nodes or unspecified masses, may be diagnosed by CT and correctly localized to their nerves of origin. Second, large nerve trunks are less likely to be confused with enlarged lymph nodes, particularly in the retropsoas region at the L5–S1 levels (Fig. 13–29). Finally, nerve compression can be predicted from the CT scan when masses or fluid collections occupy the expected locations of pelvic nerves. Examples of this include compression of the retropsoas nerves by pelvic tumor, of the femoral nerve by hematoma or by an iliopsoas bursa, and of the sciatic nerve by hematoma or bone after posterior fracture-dislocation of the hip.

Figure 13–33. Transverse sections of retropubic extraperitoneal paravesical collections (at level C in Fig. 13–31B). A, Anatomical section through the pubic symphysis. Prevesical (prv) and perivesical (pev) fat are separated by the umbilicovesical fascia (uv), which is continuous posterolaterally with the visceral layer of the pelvic fascia (vpf). The urinary bladder (ub), perivesical vessels (ubvs), and seminal vesicles (svs) lie within the perivesical space. Also indicated are the cul de sac (cds), rectum (re), obturator internus muscles (obi), and pubis (pu). B, Schematic drawing of the paravesical spaces at the level of A. The prevesical space (prv) lies anterior and lateral to the umbilicovesical fascia (uv), and extends posteriorly, lateral to the visceral pelvic fascia (vpf). Large collections in this space may extend behind the rectum (re), anterior to the lower sacrum and coccyx. The perivesical space (pev) surrounds the urinary bladder (ub) and lower uterine segment (ut), but is limited posteriorly by the cul de sac (cds) and by the extraperitoneal fascia (*open arrows*), which is continuous with the peritoneal coverings of the cul de sac. The fibrous adventitia of the bladder (fab) is a derivative of the umbilicovesical fascia. Transversalis fascia (tf). Parietal pelvic fascia (ppf). C, Cadaver CT scan at the level of A and B. Contrast medium in the prevesical space (prv) extends anterior and lateral to the urinary bladder (ub) along the expected contours of the umbilicovesical fascia (uv). (Compare with A and B.) The denser contrast (*small arrows*), directly around the bladder, lies within the perivesical space. A contrast-urine level (*small arrowhead*) is visible within the urinary bladder. The 22-gauge needle (*curved arrow*) was initially introduced into the urinary bladder under CT guidance and then withdrawn gradually into the prevesical space, where contrast medium was injected. Lower uterine segment (ut), rectum (re), and coccygeus muscle (ccm) are indicated. D, In vivo CT scan, corresponding to A, B, and C, obtained 3 cm below the scan in 13–32B. The prevesical hematoma (prv) extends anterior and lateral to the urinary bladder (ub). It still resembles a tooth, with the "crown" occupying the space of Retzius, behind the pubis. The left (*large arrows*) and right (*arrowheads*) "roots" of the collection extend posteriorly along the expected lateral contours of the umbilicovesical fascia and visceral pelvic fascia. Lower uterine segment (ut) and rectum (re) are indicated. The prevesical collection has also extended into the femoral canals (fcn) and into the more lateral portions of the femoral sheaths along the femoral arteries and veins (fa, fv). A thin rim of uninvolved perivesical fat (*small arrows*) is visible. (A–D from Auh YH, Rubenstein WA, Schneider M, et al: Extraperitoneal paravesical spaces: CT delineation with US correlation. Radiology 159:319–328, 1986).

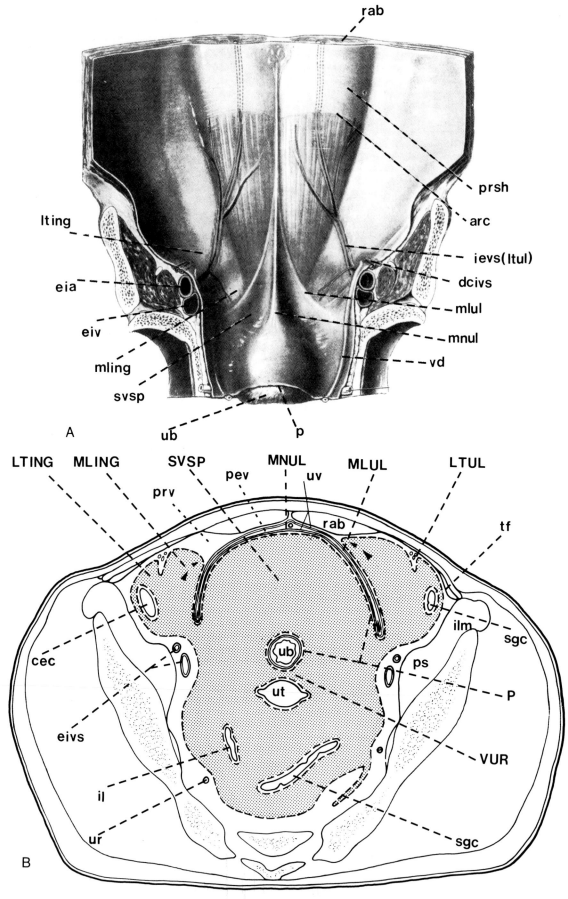

Figure 13–34 *See legend on opposite page*

THE URETERS

The ureters course anterior or lateral to the common iliac arteries at the inlet to the greater pelvis (Fig. 13–29A). As the common iliac vessels divide, the ureters may course briefly in front of the external iliac artery or vein (Fig. 13–29B), and then between the external and internal iliac vessels (Figs. 13–29C and 13–31D). They descend along the lateral aspect of the pelvis, parallel to the anterior margin of the greater sciatic foramen (Figs. 13–30A and 13–35A–D). They then turn anteromedially at the level of the ischial spines, and course anterior to the seminal vesicles (Fig. 13–37A–C) or vaginal fornices to join the urinary bladder. These anatomical markers are helpful for localizing the pelvic ureter on MRI, ultrasound, or nonenhanced CT scans, where it is not positively identified by intraluminal contrast media.

THE URINARY BLADDER

This structure lies within the extraperitoneal fat anterior to the peritoneum. Except for the bladder neck, which is fixed in position behind the pubic symphysis and in front of the prostate or upper vagina (Fig. 13–38B), the remainder of the bladder moves relatively freely within the fat around it. Its shape and position are therefore easily variable, depending on the volume of urine within it. A distended bladder is valuable for both ultrasonographic and MRI imaging of the pelvis, as it displaces potentially troublesome bowel loops superiorly.

The Bladder Wall

The bladder wall is easier to delineate by CT when the urine in its lumen is not opacified with radiopaque contrast media (Fig. 13–36B). An exception to this is the visualization of cellules and small diverticula, which is aided by positive contrast media. Gas insufflation with carbon dioxide has been used to improve CT visualization of bladder neoplasms.[6] Fatty intraluminal emulsions have also been used, in order to avoid artifacts that arise from the large differences in CT attenuation between air or positive contrast on the one hand, and bladder tumors on the other hand.[7, 8] Since contrast-laden urine is heavier than nonopacified urine, it is normal to see urine-contrast demarcation with axial images. Normally, the opacified urine constitutes the dependent layer, but in some patients the nonopacified urine may have a higher specific gravity than the opaque urine, and the layering may be reversed. An example is diabetes mellitus, in which urine containing high concentrations of glucose can be heavier than urine containing iodinated contrast material.[8a]

On MRI, the relatively long T1 and T2 relaxation times of urine provide a natural contrast for delineating the bladder wall.[9–11] On T1-weighted images (short TE and/or TR), the bladder wall appears brighter than the dark urine (Figs. 13–37B, 13–38H, and 13–39D). On T2-weighted images (longer TE and/or TR), urine becomes brighter while the bladder wall becomes relatively dark (compare Fig. 13–37B and C). Limitations of this method include the loss of spatial resolution on T2-weighted images (again, compare Fig. 13–37B and C), and the chemical shift artifact. This artifact is attributable to the chemical shift difference between the resonant frequencies of water protons and fat protons.[11] In a magnetic field of 0.5 T, the resonant frequency of fat is shifted to the down-field side of the read-out gradient (to the patient's right on transverse images, or toward the patient's head on coronal and sagittal sections) by about 4 ppm, which is approximately equal to the width of one pixel. Since localization of the signal in the read-out gradient field is dependent on the proton resonant frequencies, the down-shifted proton signal from fat is interpreted as having arisen from one pixel further down field. This leaves the pixel representing the fat that is immediately contiguous to the bladder with a significantly decreased observed intensity. The locus of all such pixels forms a dark line that may be mistaken for thickening of the bladder wall, or of a muscle (compare Fig. 13–38E and F) or cyst wall, at their interface with fat.

Because most of the bladder mucosa is loosely attached to the muscular layer, the mucosa easily becomes redundant in the partially filled bladder.[3] This may lead to the

---

Figure 13–34. The urinary bladder and the intraperitoneal paravesical spaces. A, Schematic diagram of the anterior intraperitoneal paravesical spaces. The anterior abdominal wall is viewed from behind. The urachus indents the anterior parietal peritoneum (p) in the midline, forming the *median* umbilical fold (mnul). Similarly, the medial umbilical ligaments (obliterated umbilical arteries) indent the peritoneum to form the *medial* umbilical folds (mlul). More laterally, a pair of smaller *lateral* umbilical folds (ltul) are formed by the indentations of the inferior epigastric vessels (ievs). The supravesical space (svsp) lies between the medial umbilical folds, and is bounded inferiorly by the urinary bladder (ub), as it indents the peritoneum posteriorly. The medial inguinal fossae (mling) lie between the medial and lateral umbilical folds, while the lateral inguinal fossae (lting) lie lateral to the lateral umbilical folds. Vas deferens (vd). External iliac artery (eia) and vein (eiv). Deep circumflex iliac vessels (dcivs). Rectus abdominis muscle (rab). The posterior rectus sheath (prsh) is deficient below the arcuate line (arc). (From Williams PL, Warwick R, [eds]: Gray's Anatomy, 36th Ed. Philadelphia, WB Saunders, 1980.) B, Schematic transverse section through dome of urinary bladder in the presence of a large amount of ascites. Compare with A and Figure 13–31C. The supravesical space (svsp) is now distended with ascites, which displaces the medial umbilical folds (mlul) anterolaterally. The inguinal fossae are partially subdivided by the lateral umbilical folds (ltul) into medial (mling) and lateral (lting) inguinal fossae. The extraperitoneal prevesical (prv) and perivesical (pev) spaces are compressed against the anterior abdominal wall. The bladder has been displaced inferiorly, compared with Figure 13–31C, so that only a small portion of its dome (ub) is now visible. The medial recesses (*large arrowheads*) of the medial inguinal fossae may extend further anteromedially toward the midline (*small arrowheads*), anterior to the umbilicovesical fascia (uv). Also indicated are the periotoneum (p), cecum (cec), sigmoid colon (sgc), vesicouterine recess (vur), uterus (ut), ileum (il), rectus abdominis muscle (rab), iliacus (ilm) and psoas (ps) muscles, external iliac vessels (eivs), and ureter (ur). (B from Auh YH, Rubenstein WA, Markisz JA, et al: Intraperitoneal paravesical spaces: CT delineation with US correlation. Radiology 159:311–317, 1986.)

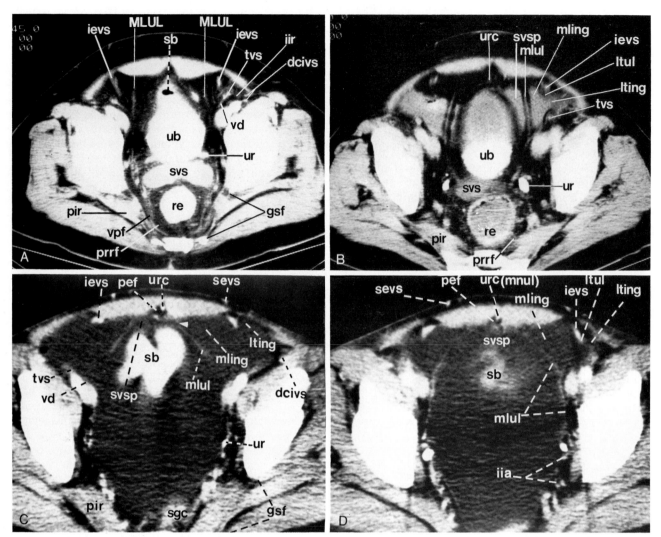

Figure 13–35. In vivo CT appearance of the intraperitoneal paravesical spaces. *A, B,* Moderate amount of ascites. *A,* CT scan through greater sciatic foramen (gsf) in a patient with lymphoma shows small bowel loops (sb) within the supravesical space anterior to the urinary bladder (ub). The medial umbilical folds (mlul) are visible on either side of the bladder. The inferior epigastric vessels (ievs) mark the location of the lateral umbilical folds. Internal inguinal ring (iir), testicular vessels (tvs), vas deferens (vd), and deep circumflex iliac vessels (dcivs) are shown. The visceral layer of the pelvic fascia (vpf) appears thickened, and the perirectal fat (prrf) has an increased density, consistent with edema or a diffuse cellular infiltrate. Seminal vesicles (svs), ureters (ur), rectum (re), and piriformis muscle (pir) are indicated. *B,* CT scan of the patient in *A,* at the same level, obtained 4 months later. Ascites is now present in the supravesical space (svsp), which is separated from the medial inguinal fossae (mling) by the medial umbilical folds (mlul). The lateral umbilical folds (ltul), subtended by the inferior epigastric vessels (ievs), partially separate the lateral (lting) from the medial inguinal fossae. Also indicated are the urachus (urc), urinary bladder (ub), seminal vesicles (svs), ureters (ur), rectum (re), infiltrated perirectal fat (prrf), piriformis muscle (pir), and testicular vessels (tvs). (*A, B* from Auh YH, Rubenstein WA, Markisz JA, et al: Intraperitoneal paravesical spaces: CT delineation with US correlation. Radiology 159:311–317, 1986.) *C,D,* Marked ascites. *C,* CT scan through greater sciatic foramen (gsf). The medial umbilical folds (mlul) are outlined by ascites in the supravesical fossa (svsp) and in the medial inguinal fossae (mling). The inferior epigastric vessels (ievs) indent the anterior parietal peritoneum, separating the fluid in the medial (mling) and lateral (lting) inguinal fossae. The medial recesses of both medial inguinal fossae are considerably deeper in their medial extent (*arrowheads*) than those in *A* and *B*. The urachus (urc) (or median umbilical ligament) is clearly outlined by perivesical fat (pef). Small bowel loops (sb) occupy most of the supravesical space. The ureters (ur) are displaced laterally by the ascites. Also indicated are the vas deferens (vd), testicular vessels (tvs), deep circumflex iliac vessels (dcivs), superficial epigastric vessels (sevs), distal sigmoid colon (sgc), and piriformis muscle (pir). *D,* CT scan 15 mm below *C.* The medial umbilical folds (mlul) are extending posteriorly toward the internal iliac arteries (iia). The supravesical fossa (svsp) contains mainly ascites, but also small bowel (sb). The lateral umbilical fold (ltul) is clearly visible on the left, separating fluid in the medial inguinal fossa (mling) from the lateral inguinal fossa (lting). Inferior epigastric vessels (ievs). The median umbilical fold (mnul) is formed by the posterior invagination of the urachus (urc) and surrounding perivesical fat (pef). Also shown are ureters (ur), testicular vessels (tvs), deep circumflex iliac vessels (dcivs), and superficial epigastric vessels (sevs).

mistaken impression of a thickened bladder wall on CT and MRI (Figs. 13–38H and 13–39D). The bladder mucosa is closely adherent to the muscularis layer over the trigone, a triangular area on the posterior wall. The base of the trigone extends between the ureteral orifices and is usually thickened by the interureteral crest, produced by intravesical extension of the longitudinal muscles of the ureters (Fig. 13–37A–C). This interureteral crest should not be mistaken for focal bladder thickening. The apex of the trigone lies at the urethral orifice, 25 to 50 mm below the ureteral orifices, depending on the degree of bladder distention.[3] Another diagnostic pitfall may arise in elderly individuals with bladder diverticula, which may mimic seminal vesical or adnexal cysts, or other extravesical pelvic masses, if their narrow communications with the bladder are not demonstrated.

Bladder volume can be estimated from sectional images by multiplying the maximal length, width, and anteroposterior dimensions with an empirically derived correction factor.[12] The standard error of such an estimate is likely to reach 20%.[12] More accurate estimates can be obtained from the sum of the areas of closely spaced (5 to 10 mm), sequential, transverse sections of the bladder.[13]

THE PARAVESICAL SPACES

The urinary bladder, urachus, and obliterated umbilical arteries, surrounded by umbilicovesical fascia, lie within a potentially large space anterior to the peritoneum. The same structures also indent the anterior parietal peritoneum to form intraperitoneal paravesical recesses. The extraperitoneal and intraperitoneal paravesical spaces are potentially large compartments, separated by only a thin layer of peritoneum, or more medially, by only peritoneum and umbilicovesical fascia.[14, 15] They are described briefly below.

The Extraperitoneal Space

Around the urinary bladder, the extraperitoneal space is lamellated by the umbilicovesical fascia, just as the retroperitoneal space around the kidneys is lamellated by the renal fascia. The bladder, urachus, and obliterated umbilical arteries lie within the perivesical space, surrounded by umbilicovesical fascia, just as the kidney lies in the perinephric space within the renal fascia (Fig. 13–31A–D). A much larger prevesical space, which, to continue the analogy with the kidney, might be compared to the anterior paranephric space, lies anterior and lateral to the umbilicovesical fascia (Figs. 13–31A,B, 13–32, and 13–33). Posterior to the urinary bladder, the seminal vesicles or lower uterine segment lies within the perivesical space, rather than in a separate compartment. Here, the analogy with the lumbar area ends, since nothing in the pelvis is comparable to the posterior paranephric space (Fig. 13–33A,B). The cul de sac and the inferolateral extension of its peritoneal layers as the rectovesical or rectovaginal septum separate the posterior perivesical space from the rectum (Fig. 13–33A,B).[14]

Near the bladder dome the course of the umbilicovesical fascia is delineated on the CT scan by the frequently visible medial umbilical folds (Figs. 13–31C,D, and 13–34A). These folds are formed by the medial umbilical ligaments (obliterated umbilical arteries), as they and their surrounding umbilicovesical fascia indent the anterior parietal peritoneum. They extend posteriorly toward the anterior trunks of the internal iliac arteries, where the medial umbilical ligaments become continuous with the superior vesical arteries (Fig. 13–31C). Thus, the linear densities visualized by CT at this level represent the medial umbilical ligaments, their surrounding umbilicovesical fascia, and the contiguous peritoneum, which they indent (compare Fig. 13–31C and D). At the same level, the obliterated urachus is often visible as the median umbilical ligament (Fig. 13–30), which slightly indents the peritoneum to form a median umbilical fold (Figs. 13–31C and 13–34A).

Occasionally, an additional linear structure, most likely representing the umbilical prevesical fascia (Fig. 13–31C), is visible on a CT scan anterior to the median and medial umbilical folds. The prevesical fascia is probably formed by apposition of the peritoneal layers that line the medial recesses of the medial inguinal fossae. These fused layers may extend anteromedially, in front of the umbilicovesical fascia, to form the umbilical prevesical fascia (Fig. 13–31C). The prevesical fascia is therefore analogous to the rectovesical septum (or the rectovaginal septum in the female), which is formed by extraperitoneal extension of the fused peritoneal layers of the cul de sac (Fig. 13–31B). Unlike the rectovesical septum, however, the umbilical prevesical fascia has not been consistently visualized on anatomical studies.

Below the peritoneal reflection, the umbilicovesical fascia extends to the pelvic floor on either side of the urinary bladder (Fig. 13–33A,B), but is too thin to visualize consistently by CT, as it is not accompanied by peritoneum. It is posteriorly continuous with the visceral pelvic fascia along the lateral aspects of the lower uterine segment, seminal vesicles, prostate, and rectum (Fig. 13–33A,B). Although the umbilicovesical fascia is not consistently seen by CT below the peritoneum, its presence is clearly indicated by extraperitoneal paravesical fluid collections.

Prevesical Collections

Because the umbilicovesical fascia lies anterior and lateral to the urinary bladder, prevesical effusions assume a "molar-tooth" configuration as they accumulate between the umbilicovesical fascia, and the transversalis fascia or parietal pelvic fascia (Fig. 13–32). The "crown" portion of the molar tooth lies anterior to the urinary bladder, between the umbilicovesical fascia and transversalis fascia of the anterior abdominal wall, and displaces the bladder posteriorly (Fig. 13–32). The "root" portion of the molar tooth extends posteriorly, between the umbilicovesical fascia and the peritoneum (Fig. 13–32A). Below the peritoneum, the "root" of the prevesical collection lies between the umbilicovesical fascia and the parietal pelvic fascia (Fig. 13–32B). The bladder is displaced medially, or away from the midline if the "roots" are asymmetrical in size (Fig. 13–32). Superiorly, prevesical collections extend up to the umbilicus (Fig. 13–31B), while inferiorly they occupy the retropubic prevesical fat, also known as the space of Retzius (Fig. 13–33B–D). The puboprostatic ligament in the male (or the pubovesical ligament in the female) forms the anteroinferior boundary of the prevesical space (Fig. 13–31B). These ligaments

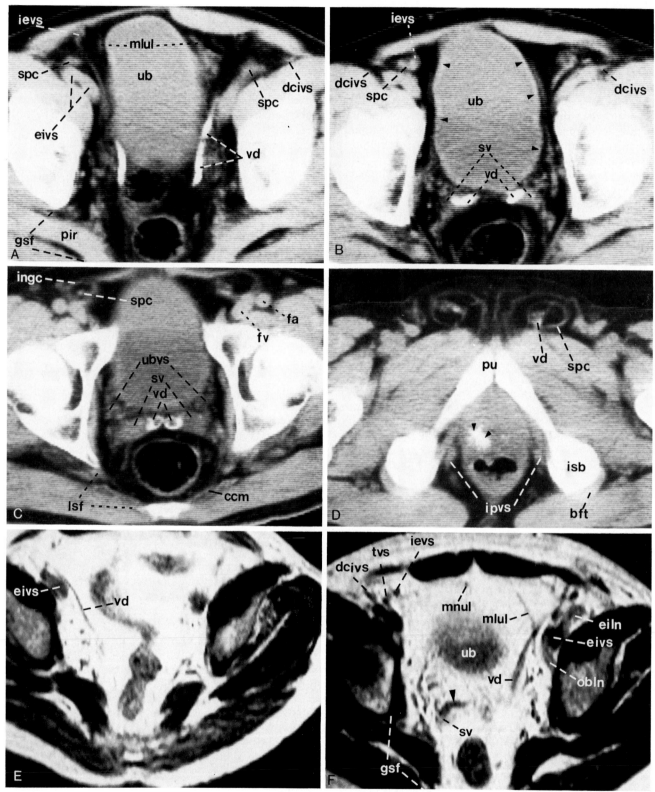

Figure 13–36 *See legend on opposite page*

are attached to the back of the pubis near the middle of the pubic symphysis. From the prevesical space, large collections may extend to the following locations.[14]

The *rectus sheath* may be involved by anterior extension of prevesical collections (Fig. 13–32*B*) through the thin transversalis fascia, which forms the only posterior lining for the rectus abdominis muscles below the arcuate line (halfway between the umbilicus and pubic symphysis, Fig. 13–34*A*). In this location, the transversalis fascia is perforated by branches of the inferior epigastric vessels. Thus, a prevesical hematoma may present clinically as a rectus sheath hematoma. Similarly rectus sheath collections may extend posteriorly into the prevesical space (Fig. 13–32*C*).

The *retroperitoneal paranephric spaces* may be reached after posterolateral extension of prevesical fluid around the parietal peritoneum, and into the properitoneal fat, which is continuous with posterior paranephric fat.

The *presacral space* may be involved by posterior extension of prevesical fluid along the lateral aspect of the visceral pelvic fascia, with which the umbilicovesical fascia is continuous, and then posterior to the pelvic fascia and rectum into the presacral fat (Fig. 13–33*B*).

The *internal inguinal ring* may be reached by anterolateral extension of prevesical fluid along the vas deferens (Fig. 13–34*A*) and spermatic cord, or along the round ligaments of the uterus. Prevesical fat accompanying the vas deferens and retroperitoneal fat accompanying the testicular vessels form the internal spermatic fascia, which is the innermost layer of the spermatic cord.[14] It follows, then, that prevesical fluid can extend along the vas deferens into the spermatic cord. After renal transplantation, prevesical fluid may traverse the inguinal canal to enter the scrotum.[14]

The *femoral sheath* may be entered after anterolateral extension of prevesical fluid along the external iliac vessels. Within the femoral sheath, the fluid collection may surround the femoral vessels or occupy the femoral canal more medially (Fig. 13–33*D*).

Perivesical Collections

These collections are confined within a relatively narrow compartment by the umbilicovesical fascia (Figs. 13–31*A–C*, 13–32*C*, and 13–33*B–D*). As a result, the perivesical space is much smaller than the prevesical space. This is not to imply that the thin umbilicovesical fascia is impregnable, as extension of prevesical contrast into the perivesical space is common in vivo, resulting in partial or complete obliteration of the perivesical fat (Fig. 13–33*D*). We have observed only one predominantly perivesical collection among 40 cases with extraperitoneal paravesical effusions. It was attributable to fluid extravasation after multiple transurethral bladder biopsies. In the remaining 39 cases, involvement of the perivesical space was seen in conjunction with larger prevesical collections.

The Intraperitoneal Paravesical Spaces[15]

The Anterior Intraperitoneal Paravesical Spaces

The urinary bladder, located within the extraperitoneal space of the anterior abdominal wall, indents the parietal peritoneum behind it, forming intraperitoneal paravesical spaces on either side of the bladder (Fig. 13–34*A*). Each paravesical space is subdivided further by the umbilical folds, which are formed by posterior indentations of the obliterated umbilical arteries (medial umbilical folds) and inferior epigastric vessels (lateral umbilical folds) (Figs. 13–34*A* and 13–31*C*). These anterior intraperitoneal paravesical spaces may be occupied by hollow viscera, ascites, abscesses, or peritoneally disseminated metastases.

The *supravesical space* extends along the bladder, and then above it, between the medial umbilical folds (Figs. 13–31*C*, 13–34, and 13–35). It is usually occupied by small-bowel loops, and by the fundus of the distended urinary bladder, which protrudes into it from the anterior extraperitoneal space (Fig. 13–34*A*). In the presence of small to moderate amounts of ascites, both the fundus of the urinary bladder and peritoneal fluid may be visualized within the supravesical space (Fig. 13–35*B*). Larger amounts of ascites, however, usually displace the bladder dome inferiorly, so that only fluid, and/or small bowel, is visible within the supravesical space (Figs. 13–34*B* and 13–35*C,D*). In such cases, the medial umbilical folds may be displaced anterolaterally, with widening of the su-

---

Figure 13–36. The spermatic cord and vas deferens. *A,* CT scan through greater sciatic foramen (gsf) shows the spermatic cords (spc) within the proximal inguinal canals, lateral to the inferior epigastric vessels (ievs), and anterolateral to the external iliac vessels (eivs). Deep circumflex iliac vessels (dcivs). The larger size of the left spermatic cord is attributable to a larger pampiniform venous plexus (small varicocele) on the left. The calcified vas deferens (vd) has already left the spermatic cord at the internal inguinal ring and courses posteriorly, medial to the external iliac vessels and lateral to the urinary bladder (ub). Medial umbilical fold (mlul) and piriformis muscle (pir) are indicated. *B,* CT scan 15 mm below *A.* The ampullary portions of each calcified vas deferens (vd) are now seen at the anteromedial aspect of the upper seminal vesicles (sv). The wall (*arrowheads*) of the urinary bladder (ub) is clearly delineated from its lumen. Also shown are the spermatic cord (spc), inferior epigastric vessels (ievs), and deep circumflex iliac vessels (dcivs). *C,* CT scan through the lesser sciatic foramen (lsf), 15 mm below *B.* The preterminal ampullary portions of the vas deferens (vd) are beginning to descend along the medial borders of the seminal vesicles (sv). Below this level the narrower terminal portion of each vas joins the seminal vesicle duct to form the ejaculatory duct (not shown here). Also indicated are the vesical venous plexus (ubvs), inguinal canals (ingc), spermatic cord (spc), femoral artery (fa) and vein (fv), and coccygeus muscle (ccm). *D,* CT scan 45 mm below *C.* The calcified vas deferens (vd) is posteriorly located within the spermatic cord (spc), which has exited the inguinal canal. Also indicated are the prostatic calcifications (*arrowheads*), internal pudendal vessels (ipvs) within the pudendal canal, inferior pubic symphysis (pu), ischial tuberosity (isb), and biceps femoris tendon (bft). *E,F,* Transverse MR scan (SE 1500/64) just above (E) and through (F) the greater sciatic foramen (gsf). The proximal intrapelvic portion of each vas deferens (vd) is visible medial to the external iliac vessels (eivs). Also indicated are the ampulla of the right vas deferens (*arrowhead*), right superior seminal vesicle (sv), dome of urinary bladder (ub), median umbilical ligament (mnul), medial umbilical fold (mlul), inferior epigastric vessels (ievs), testicular vessels (tvs), deep circumflex iliac vessels (dcivs), and mildly enlarged obturator (obln) and external iliac (eiln) lymph nodes.

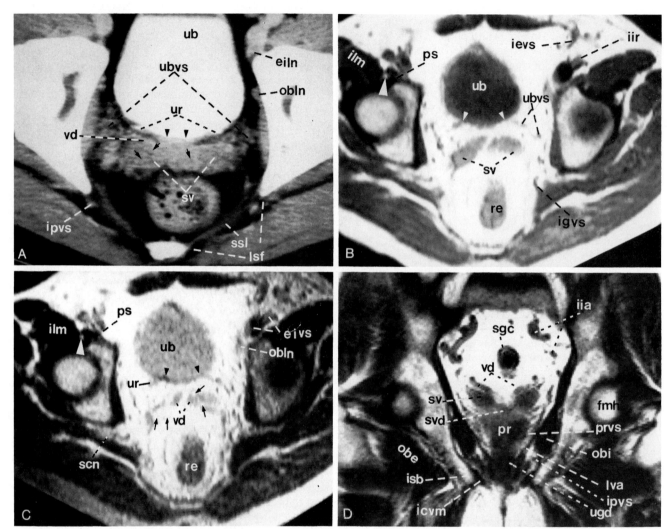

Figure 13–37. The seminal vesicles. *A,* CT scan. The seminal vesicles (sv) lie posterior to the urinary bladder (ub) at its junction with the ureters (ur). The radiolucencies (*small arrows*) within the seminal vesicles are attributable to their fluid-filled lumina. The vas deferens (vd) is considerably narrower than in Figure 13–36. The posterior thickening of the bladder wall (*arrowheads*), between the ureteral orifices, marks the interureteral ridge at the superior aspect of the trigone. Also indicated are the sacrospinous ligament (ssl), lesser sciatic foramen (lsf), internal pudendal vessels (ipvs), vesical venous plexus (ubvs), and mildly enlarged obturator (obln) and external iliac (eiln) lymph nodes. *B, C,* Transverse MR scan through the seminal vesicles (sv), obtained with a multislice, multiecho spin-echo (SE) technique. On the first-echo image (SE 1500/32) in *B,* only slight heterogeneity of the seminal vesicles (sv) is evident. On the more T2-weighted third-echo image (SE 1500/96) in *C,* fluid within the seminal vesicle lumina (*small arrows*) appears as bright as the surrounding pelvic fat. Urine within the bladder lumen (ub) shows a lesser degree of enhancement in brightness between the first-echo (*B*) and third-echo (*C*) images. The medial ampullary portions of the vas deferens (vd) remain relatively low in signal intensity on the third-echo image. The ureters (ur) are visible at their junction with the bladder. Interureteral crest (*small arrowheads*). Also indicated are the vesical venous plexus (ubvs), external iliac (eivs) and inferior epigastric (ievs) vessels, internal inguinal ring (iir), inferior gluteal vessels (igvs), sciatic nerve (scn), rectum (re), and mildly enlarged obturator (obln) lymph nodes. A fatty groove (*large arrowhead*) separates the psoas (ps) from the iliacus (ilm) muscles. *D,* Coronal MR scan (SE 500/32) through the posterior acetabula. The seminal vesicles (sv) lie above the cone-shaped prostate (pr) and inferolateral to the ampullary portions of the vas deferens (vd). Indicated are the seminal vesicle duct (svd), prostatic venous plexus (prvs), sigmoid colon (sgc), internal iliac artery and posterior ramus (iia), levator ani muscles (lva), internal pudendal vessels (ipvs), urogenital diaphragm (ugd), obturator internus (obi) and obturator externus (obe) muscles, ischiocavernosus muscle (icvm), ischium (isb), and posterior femoral head (fmh).

pravesical space at the expense of the adjacent inguinal fossae (Figs. 13–34B and 13–35C, D).

The *medial inguinal fossae* lie between the medial and lateral umbilical folds (Figs. 13–31C, 13–34, and 13–35C, D). The extent of their separation from the lateral inguinal fossae depends on the depth of the lateral inguinal folds, which varies among individuals and is most marked at the level of the proximal inferior epigastric vessels. They are usually occupied, at least partially, by cecum or ileum on the right, and by sigmoid colon on the left (Figs. 13–31C and 13–34B). However, these hollow viscera can be displaced either partially or completely by ascites. Large amounts of ascites also tend to efface the lateral inguinal folds, so that the medial and lateral inguinal fossae become continuous (Fig. 13–35C, D).

The medial recesses of the medial inguinal fossae may extend anteromedially, in front of the urachus and umbilicovesical fascia (Fig. 13–31C). The degree of medial exter ion varies among individuals, and with the amount of ascites (compare Fig. 13–35A, B and C, D). Thus, with respect to the medial extent of their medial recesses, the medial inguinal fossae resemble the paracolic gutters, pararectal fossae, and the cul de sac, which have depths that vary with the degree of posterior or inferior extension of their peritoneal lining.[16]

The femoral rings lie at the inferomedial aspects of the proximal inferior epigastric vessels[3] and therefore at the inferolateral aspects of the medial inguinal fossae. In the presence of a femoral hernia, ascites may extend into the femoral canal from the medial inguinal fossa.

The *lateral inguinal fossae* lie between the lateral umbilical folds and the lateral parietal peritoneum as it is reflected over the vas deferens or round ligament. They are the smallest of the anterior paravesical fossae (Figs. 13–31C, 13–34, and 13–35C, D). They are occupied, at least partially, by cecum or sigmoid colon but may also be filled exclusively with ascites. The internal inguinal ring lies lateral to the inferior epigastric vessels[3] at the anteromedial aspect of the lateral inguinal fossa. In the presence of an indirect inguinal hernia, ascites may extend from the lateral inguinal fossa into the inguinal canal. In contrast, direct inguinal hernias usually involve the medial inguinal fossa, or to a lesser extent, the supravesical space.[15]

The Posterior Intraperitoneal Paravesical Recesses

The peritoneum covering the posterior surface of the urinary bladder is reflected onto the rectum to form a large recess, which is the rectovesical space. In women, this space is further subdivided by the uterus into the vesicouterine recess and the cul de sac (pouch of Douglas). The pararectal fossae are posterior extensions of the rectovesical space along the lateral aspects of the rectum.[16] They are bounded laterally by peritoneal folds, the sacrogenital folds, which are reflected over the blood vessels to the bladder and the adjacent pelvic ureter.[15, 16] These folds are not consistently visible with CT, unless the peritoneum is thickened.[16]

THE MALE REPRODUCTIVE ORGANS

The normal sectional anatomy of the male reproductive organs is briefly described.

The *spermatic cord* (Figs. 13–36A–D, 13–39A–C, E, 13–40C) is formed at the internal inguinal ring by the junction of the vas deferens with the testicular, deferential, and cremasteric vessels, and with the genital, cremasteric, and testicular nerves.[2] Of these structures the vas deferens and testicular vessels are visible on CT and MR scans (Figs. 13–30, 13–35A, 13–36A–C, E–F, 13–37, and 13–38H; and Figs. 13–29A, B, 13–30, 13–35, and 13–36E, F). The fat within the internal spermatic fascia of the cord is derived in part from the retroperitoneal fat around the testicular vessels and from the prevesical fat around the vas deferens. Occasionally, it may form lipomas within the spermatic cord.

The *vas deferens* lies in the posterior part of the spermatic cord (Fig. 13–36D),[2, 4] where it is usually obscured by adjacent structures on CT or MR scans. After leaving the cord at the internal inguinal ring, the vas can be seen by CT at the anteromedial aspect of the external iliac vessels (Figs. 13–30A and 13–35A, C). It is also visible more inferiorly, as it courses medially in front of the ureter (Fig. 13–36A, E, F). It then continues its medial course between the bladder and the upper seminal vesicles, where it becomes dilated and tortuous (ampullary segment) (Figs. 13–36B, C, 13–37A, C, D, and 13–38H). The terminal portion of the vas is narrowed again. It descends vertically in the midline, where it joins the seminal vesicle duct to form the ejaculatory duct, which in turn empties into the urethra at the verumontanum. This most distal portion of the vas is obscured on sectional images by the adjacent seminal vesicles.

The *seminal vesicles* are tubular structures that lie at the superior aspect of the prostate, behind the lower urinary bladder and terminal ureters (Figs. 13–33A, 13–35A, B, 13–36B, C, F, 13–37, and 13–38G, H).[3, 5] The longest axis of each vesicle measures approximately 5 cm and consists of a coiled, compacted tube, measuring 10 to 15 cm in length and 3 to 4 mm in diameter. The saccules formed by this tube are readily apparent on cut section (Fig. 13–33A) and can be demonstrated as echo-poor structures by ultrasonography. These same saccules appear relatively bright on MRI (Fig. 13–37B) and become so bright on T2-weighted images (longer echo times or intersequence intervals) that the seminal vesicles blend with the surrounding pelvic fat (Fig. 13–37C).[17] On CT scans the saccules may appear isodense with muscle (Figs. 13–35A, B and 13–36B, C) or they may be visualized as focal lucencies (Fig. 13–37A), particularly in patients with marked prostatic hypertrophy. The seminal vesicles lie with the urinary bladder in the perivesical space. They are separated from the rectum by the cul de sac superiorly, and by the rectovesical septum (Denonvilliers' fascia) inferiorly. The seminal vesicle duct (Fig. 13–37D) joins with the ipsilateral vas deferens to form the ejaculatory duct.

The *prostate* lies behind the pubic symphysis, posteroinferior to the bladder neck, and anterior to the rectum (Figs. 13–29E, 13–37D, 13–38, and 13–40A–D).[3, 5] It is separated from the rectum by the rectovesical septum, which is formed by fusion of the peritoneal envelope of the cul de sac, analogous to the rectovaginal septum (Fig. 13–31B). The prevesical space extends downward, in front of the anterosuperior prostate (Fig. 13–38A, E, F), to the attachments of the puboprostatic ligaments, analogous to the pubovesical ligaments in the female (Fig. 13–31B), which form its floor. The prostate is shaped like

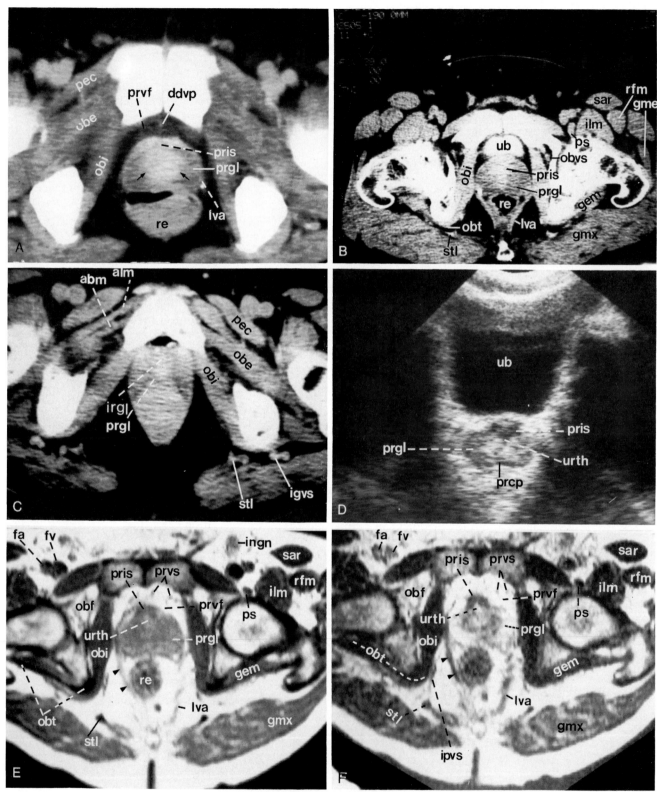

Figure 13–38 *See legend on opposite page*

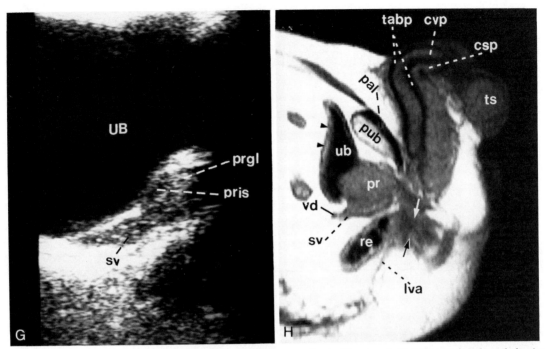

Figure 13–38. *A,* Contrast-enhanced CT scan through the pubic symphysis. The prostatic isthmus (pris) and the inner glandular tissues around the prostatic urethra (central zone) (*small arrows*) are clearly delineated from the more radiolucent peripheral zone of the prostatic glandular tissue (prgl). The central zone (*small arrows*) is mildly hyperplastic in this individual. Levator ani muscle (lva) surrounds the prostate and rectum (re). The deep dorsal vein of the penis (ddvp) is visible within the preprostatic fat in the prevesical space of Retzius (prvf). Obturator internus (obi), externus (obe), and pectineus (pec) muscles are shown. *B,* CT scan through the prostatic base in another patient. The prostatic isthmus (pris) and inner gland (central zone) have a different configuration than in *A* but are still radiodense relative to the peripheral glandular portion (prgl). Also indicated are the neck of urinary bladder (ub), levator ani muscle (lva), rectum (re), obturator internus muscle (obi) and tendon (obt), obturator vessels (obvs) within the obturator foramen, sacrotuberous ligament (stl), and the following muscles: sartorius (sar), rectus femoris (rfm), psoas (ps), iliacus (ilm), gluteus medius (gme), gluteus maximus (gmx), and gemelli (gem). *C,* CT scan through the inferior pubic symphysis. The cone-shaped prostate is narrower on this lower section, but the radiodense isthmus (irgl) and inner gland are still distinguishable from the more radiolucent peripheral gland (prgl). Obturator internus (obi), externus (obe), and pectineus (pec) muscles are shown. Also indicated are the adductor longus (alm) and adductor brevis (abm) muscles, inferior gluteal vessels (igvs), and sacrotuberous ligament (stl). *D,* Transverse abdominal sonogram of the prostate (pr). The echo-poor prostatic isthmus (pris) and periurethral tissue (urth) are clearly demarcated from the echogenic peripheral glandular portions (prgl) (compare with *A–C*). Prostatic capsule (prcp) and urinary bladder (ub) are indicated. (*B,D* from Kazam E, Auh YH, Rubenstein WA, et al: Normal CT anatomy of the pelvis with ultrasound and MRI correlations. *In* Putnam CE, Ravin C, (eds): Textbook of Diagnostic Imaging. Philadelphia, WB Saunders, 1988. *E,F,* Transverse MRI of the base of the prostate. On the first echo image (*E,* SE 1500/32) the prostatic isthmus (pris) and central zone are poorly differentiated from the peripheral glandular portion (prgl). On the third echo image (*F,* SE 1500/96), the predominantly fibromuscular isthmus (pris) remains low in signal intensity, while the peripheral zone of the glandular portion (prgl), which is rich in secretions, becomes nearly as bright as the prevesical fat (pruf). The central zone of the prostate is intermediate in intensity between the fibromuscular isthmus and the peripheral zone. Prostatic urethra (urth). The levator ani muscle (lva) appears thicker on the right (*arrowheads*) because of the chemical shift artifact. Also indicated are the rectum (re), prostatic veins (prvs), femoral artery (fa) and vein (fv), mildly enlarged left inguinal lymph node (ingn), obturator internus muscle (obi) and tendon (obt), obturator foramen (obf), sacrotuberous ligament (stl), and the following muscles: sartorius (sar), rectus femoris (rfm), psoas (ps), iliacus (ilm), gluteus maximum (gmx), and gemelli (gem). *G,* Parasagittal abdominal sonogram shows a normal-sized prostate (pris, prgl), and seminal vesical (sv). Urinary bladder (ub) is indicated. *H,* Parasagittal MR scan (SE 500/32) (patient supine). An enlarged prostate (pr) indents the base of the urinary bladder (ub). The redundant wall (*small arrowheads*) of the nearly empty bladder should not be mistaken for true bladder thickening. Indicated are the seminal vesicle (sv), vas deferens (vd), rectum (re), levator ani muscle (lva), external anal sphincter (*small arrows*), pubis (pu), pubic arcuate ligament (pal), testicle (ts), and the corpus cavernosum (cvp), corpus spongiosum (csp), and tunica albuginea (tabp) of the penis.

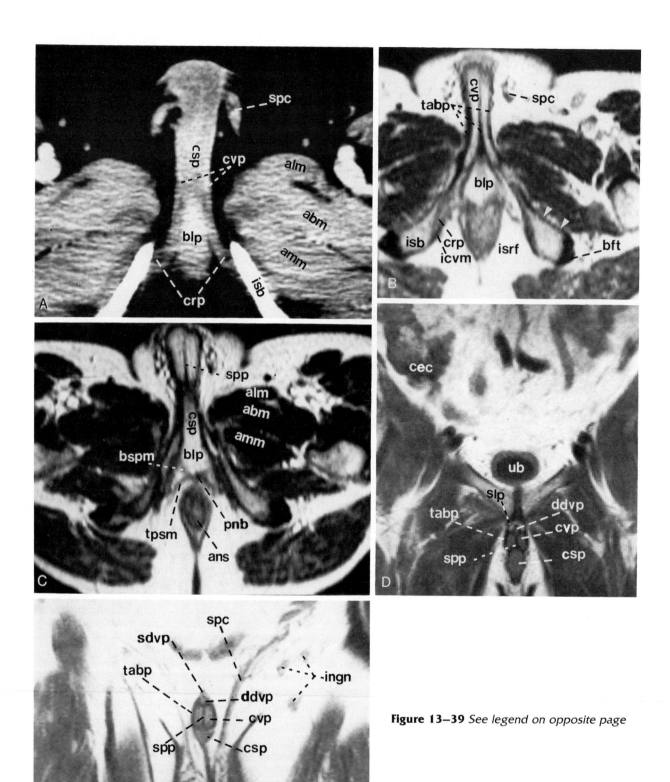

Figure 13–39 *See legend on opposite page*

an inverted cone, with its base directed superiorly toward the bladder neck, and its apex directed inferiorly toward the levator ani and transversus perinei profundi muscles (Figs. 13–29E and 13–37D). On section it consists of an anterior fibromuscular isthmus where the fibromuscular elements predominate, and a larger glandular portion, lateral and posterior to the isthmus, where the glandular elements predominate.[3] The urethra courses posterior to the isthmus, between the anterior and middle third of the glandular prostate. McNeal has further divided the glandular prostate into a smaller central zone (CZ) and a larger peripheral zone (PZ).[18] While these areas are not readily differentiable by CT, they are regularly demonstrated by MRI.

The isthmic and glandular portions of the prostate may be differentiated with sectional imaging (Figs. 13–38A–F and 13–40C,D). On contrast-enhanced CT, the isthmus usually appears radiodense, whereas the glandular portion appears relatively more lucent (Fig. 13–38A–C). The isthmus tends to appear echo poor on a sonogram (Fig. 13–38D,G) and of low signal intensity on an MR scan (Figs. 13–38E,F and 13–40C–E), while the glandular portion tends to be echogenic on a sonogram and brighter on T2-weighted MR images. Occasionally, the tissues around and behind the prostatic urethra (CZ) appear similar on CT to the more anterior isthmus (Fig. 13–38A,B), possibly because they contain mainly short glands, in contrast to the long branching glands of the PZ. In some patients, the distinction between the isthmic and glandular prostate is not possible with sectional imaging. This may be due to fibromuscular hyperplasia, or to atrophy of the long branching glands of the prostate.

The prostate is surrounded peripherally by a capsule of fibrous tissue and by a plexus of prostatic veins (Figs. 13–37D and 13–38D–F). These may account for the echo poor peripheral rim visualized by ultrasonography (Fig. 13–38D). The levator ani muscles around the inferior prostate are best delineated with MRI (Figs. 13–37D, 13–38B,E,F, and 13–40C,D).

Prostatic volume may be estimated from its longest, widest, and greatest anteroposterior dimensions by using the formula for the volume, V, of a sphere (V = 0.52 × length × width × thickness).[19] Since the prostate is not truly spherical, more accurate estimates may be obtained from the sum of the areas of the prostate on closely spaced (2.5 to 5 mm) transverse sections, multiplied by the interslice interval.[20, 21] As MRI becomes widely available, more accurate estimates may be obtainable from the areas of the cone-shaped prostate on sequential coronal sections. Prostatic weight is roughly equivalent to its volume, because the density of the prostate (mass divided by volume) is nearly one.[19]

The *penis* is relatively fixed proximally within the perineum (the penile root), and mobile distally (the penile body).[3] It is composed of three erectile bodies. Within the root of the penis there are two laterally placed crura and one central bulb of erectile tissue. The crura are firmly attached to the ischium and pubis, and covered by the ischiocavernous muscles (Figs. 13–29E, 13–39A–C, and 13–40E). They continue distally as the corpora cavernosa within the body of the penis (Figs. 13–38H, 13–39B–E, and 13–40C–D). The bulb of the penis (Figs. 13–39A–C and 13–40E) is attached to the perineal membrane, a strong fibrous layer that extends between the pubic and ischial rami, just below the external urethral sphincter. The penile bulb is covered by the bulbospongiosus muscles (Figs. 13–39B,C and 13–40E). Distally the bulb narrows to become the corpus spongiosum penis (Figs. 13–38H, 13–39D,E, and 13–40C,D), which is expanded at the penile tip to form the glans penis. Like the corpus spongiosum penis, the urethra that courses within it is also expanded proximally (intrabulbar fossa) and distally (navicular fossa).

With its excellent contrast resolution, MRI is superior to CT for differentiating the erectile tissues of the penis from their proximal muscular coverings (Figs. 13–39B,C, and 13–40E), and from their fibrous envelope, the tunica albuginea penis (Figs. 13–39B). The fibrous septum of the penis is continuous with the tunica albuginea, and separates the two corpora cavernosa (Fig. 13–39D,E). The deep, and occasionally superficial, dorsal veins of the penis may be seen within a groove indenting the dorsal surfaces of the corpora cavernosa (Fig. 13–39D,E). As surface coils become widely available, more detailed images of the penis are likely to be obtainable with MRI.

The *testes* are separated from each other by the median raphe of the scrotum (Figs. 13–39E, 13–40B).[3] Each testis is covered by a dense, fibrous tunica albuginea, which is

---

Figure 13–39. The penis. A, CT through the root of the penis. The crura of the penis (crp) are attached posteriorly to the ischium (isb), and are continuous anteriorly with the corpora cavernosa penis (cvp). The bulb of the penis (blp) is continuous anteriorly with the corpus spongiosum penis (csp). Also indicated are the spermatic cord (spc) and the adductor longus (alm), adductor brevis (abm), and adductor minimus (amm) muscles. B,C, Transverse scan (SE 1500/64) through the root of the penis. C is 10 mm below B. The crura of the penis (crp) are attached posteriorly to the ischial bones (isb) and continuous anteriorly with the corpora cavernosa penis (cvp), (B). The crura and corpora cavernosa have a bright MR signal, whereas the ischiocavernous muscle (icvm) covering them has a low MR signal. Similarly the penile bulb (blp) and its continuation as the corpus spongiosum penis (csp) appear bright, while their bulbospongious (bspm) muscular covering appears relatively dark. The fibrous tunica albuginea (tabp) surrounding the corpora cavernosa and corpus spongiosum, and the septum of the penis (spp) appear as dark as the cortex of the ischium (arrowhead) and the biceps femoris tendon (bft). Also indicated are the perineal body (pnb), transversus perinei superficialis muscle (tpsm), anus (ans), ischiorectal fat (isrf), spermatic cord (spc), and the adductor longus (alm), brevis (abm), and minimus (amm) muscles. D, Coronal MR scan (SE 500/32) through the root of the penis. The corpora cavernosa penis (cvp) are indented dorsally and superiorly by the deep dorsal vein of the penis (ddvp), and ventrally and inferiorly by the corpus spongiosum penis (csp). The fibrous tunica albuginea penis (tabp) surrounds the corpora cavernosa and corpus spongiosum and is inseparable from the fibrous fascia of the penis, which covers them anatomically. Also indicated are the penile septum (spp), suspensory ligament of the penis (slp), urinary bladder (ub), and cecum (cec). E, Coronal MR scan (SE 500/32) through the body of the penis. Shown are the corpora cavernosa penis (cvp), tunica albuginea penis (tabp), penile septum (spp), corpus spongiosum penis (csp), deep (ddvp), and superficial (sdvp) dorsal veins of penis, spermatic cord (spc), testis (ts), and mildly enlarged inguinal nodes (ingn).

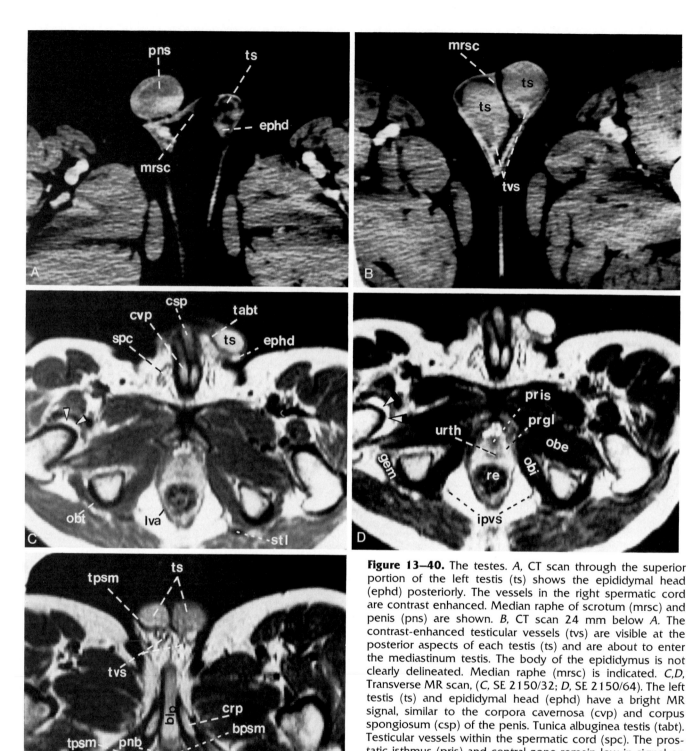

Figure 13–40. The testes. *A*, CT scan through the superior portion of the left testis (ts) shows the epididymal head (ephd) posteriorly. The vessels in the right spermatic cord are contrast enhanced. Median raphe of scrotum (mrsc) and penis (pns) are shown. *B*, CT scan 24 mm below *A*. The contrast-enhanced testicular vessels (tvs) are visible at the posterior aspects of each testis (ts) and are about to enter the mediastinum testis. The body of the epididymus is not clearly delineated. Median raphe (mrsc) is indicated. *C,D*, Transverse MR scan, (*C*, SE 2150/32; *D*, SE 2150/64). The left testis (ts) and epididymal head (ephd) have a bright MR signal, similar to the corpora cavernosa (cvp) and corpus spongiosum (csp) of the penis. Tunica albuginea testis (tabt). Testicular vessels within the spermatic cord (spc). The prostatic isthmus (pris) and central zone remain low in signal on the second echo (*E*), while the peripheral zone (prgl) becomes brighter. Indicated are the prostatic urethra (urth), levator ani muscle (lva), rectum (re), internal pudendal vessels (ipvs), obturator internus (obi) and externus (obe) muscles, obturator tendon (obt), gemelli muscles (gem), sacrotuberous ligament (stl), and effusion (*arrowheads*) within right hip joint. *E*, Transverse MR scan (SE 2150/32). Testicular vessels (tvs) are visible at the posterior aspects of each testis (ts). Indicated are the tunica albuginea testis (tabt), crura (crp) and bulb (blp) of the penis, ischiocavernous (icvm) and bulbospongious (bspm) muscles, transversus perinei superficialis muscle (tpsm), perineal body (pnb), and anus (ans).

best seen as a relatively dark envelope with MRI (Fig. 13–40C,D). The testicular contour is convex anteriorly, and relatively straight posteriorly. Internally, the testis consists of 200 to 300 cone-shaped lobules, separated from each other by incomplete fibrous septula, which radiate peripherally into the testicle from its posteriorly placed vascular hilus, the mediastinum testis. Each lobule consists of one to three coiled seminiferous tubules. At the apices of the lobules, the coiled seminiferous tubules unite to form 20 to 30 straight ducts, measuring 0.5 mm in diameter. The straight ducts enter the mediastinum testis and course superiorly within it, forming an anastomosing network, the rete testis. At the upper end of the mediastinum testis, a group of 12 to 20 efferent ductules is formed from the rete testis. These pass into the epididymal head, where they enlarge to form the lobules of the epididymis.

The vessels within the mediastinum testis can be seen by means of MRI (Fig. 13–40E), ultrasonography (Fig. 13–40B), and CT. However, the testicular septula, lobules, straight ducts, rete testis, and efferent ducts cannot be delineated with any of these methods. The epididymal head superiorly, and the epididymal body below it, lie along the posterolateral surface of the testis. The epididymal head appears isoechoic with testicular parenchyma on a sonogram and is either isointense or brighter than testicular parenchyma on an MR scan (Figs. 13–40C,D). The epididymal body also appears isoechoic with testicle on sonography although it may be difficult to delineate from the testis with any imaging method.

THE INTESTINES

The *cecum* lies in the right lower quadrant anterior to the iliacus muscle (Fig. 13–29A,D, 13–31C, 13–32A, 13–34B, and 13–39D). Although it is saccular in most patients (Figs. 13–39D), it may occasionally have a conical configuration with a narrow inferior portion. The cecum may extend into the pelvis, where it lies in the right inguinal fossa, and may herniate through the right inguinal canal. It is intraperitoneal. Ascites may be found within the retrocecal recess.

The *appendix*, not illustrated here, may be visualized as a narrow tubular structure posteromedial to the cecum. It may extend into the pelvis, between the bladder and rectum. Occasionally, it may be seen posteromedial to the psoas muscle at the L5–S1 level, in close proximity to the retropsoas nerves.

The *distal ileum* may be seen not only in the right lower quadrant, but also within the right inguinal fossa, and the cul de sac, between the bladder and rectum.

The *distal descending colon* lies in front of the iliacus muscle, just above the acetabular roof (Fig. 13–29A–C), where it curves medially to form the sigmoid colon. It may have a complete mesentery, or mesocolon, in 36% of patients.[3] In such cases, ascites may be found within its deep lateral or medial paracolic gutters.

The *sigmoid colon* forms a loop that extends anteriorly to the right, and then posteriorly on one or both sides of the midline. It may be found within the left inguinal fossa, at the pelvic inlet above the urinary bladder (Figs. 13–29B and 13–30A,B), and behind the upper urinary bladder (Figs. 13–29C and 13–31D).

The *rectum* begins at approximately the S3 vertebral level and extends inferiorly to the anus (Figs. 13–32B,C, 13–33, 13–38H, and 13–39C). The rectal columns, which are prominent longitudinal folds, may be visualized as tiny mucosal ridges on CT of the nondistended distal rectum (Fig. 13–38B). Above them, the rectum is typically dilated in its ampullary portion (Fig. 13–38A). The rectum is surrounded by perirectal fat and by the visceral layer of the pelvic fascia (Figs. 13–33A,B, and 13–35A), which may become thickened on CT in the presence of perirectal disease.

THE MUSCLES

In and around the pelvis the muscles may serve as valuable anatomical landmarks, or as pathways for extension of pelvic collections. Occasionally, they may contribute to diagnostic errors on sectional imaging.

1. The iliacus and psoas muscles course anterolaterally through the pelvis, and exit behind the inguinal ligament to insert via a common tendon onto the lesser trochanter (Figs. 13–29A–E, 13–30, 13–31D, and 13–38B,E,F). They are separated from each other by a small fatty groove (Figs. 13–37B,C) that contains iliac fascia (Fig. 13–30A) and the femoral nerve. Often, the pelvic portion of the psoas muscle is small and oval in cross section and should not be mistaken for lymphadenopathy (see earlier discussion of the pelvic nodes). A similar pitfall exists below the inguinal ligament (Figs. 13–37B–C and 13–38B), where the relatively small psoas at the medial aspect of the iliacus muscle should not be mistaken for enlarged nodes, or for a distended iliopsoas bursa.[22] Retroperitoneal collections may extend inferiorly along the iliopsoas muscle into the thigh.

2. The piriformis muscle courses from its attachments around the anterior sacral foramina, anterolaterally and inferiorly, to exit the greater sciatic foramen (Figs. 13–30A,B, and 13–35A–C). Above the piriformis the superior gluteal vessels and nerves also exit the greater sciatic foramen. Below the piriformis pass the sciatic, pudendal, and posterior femoral cutaneous nerves, and the inferior gluteal and internal pudendal vessels. The piriformis inserts onto the greater trochanter, in close proximity to the gluteus medius muscle. Collections may extend from the pelvis to the buttocks, and vice versa, along the piriformis muscle and through the greater sciatic foramen.

3. Musculus coccygeus courses from the ischial spine to the coccyx in contiguity with the sacrospinous ligament, separating the greater sciatic foramen above from the lesser sciatic foramen below (Figs. 13–33C and 13–36C). Through the lesser sciatic foramen pass the nerve and tendon of the obturator internus muscle, the pudendal nerve, and the internal pudendal vessels.

4. M. levator ani are visible, especially with MRI, in the pelvic floor along the lateral aspects of the prostate and rectum (Figs. 13–29E, 13–38A,B,E,F,H, and 13–40C,D). They are thicker than the visceral pelvic fascia directly above them (Figs. 13–30A,B, 13–33A,B, and 13–35A).

5. The urogenital diaphragm is composed of a superficial and a deep layer of perineal muscles (Fig. 13–37D). The deep layer consists of the external urethral sphincter and transversus perinei profundi muscles. These lie su-

perior to the muscles of the superficial layer, namely, the ischiocavernosus, bulbospongiosus, and transversus perinei superficialis muscles. The superficial muscles of the urogenital diaphragm are easily seen with MRI, as is the perineal body, a fibromuscular node in the midline at the convergence of the bulbospongiosus, transversus perinei superficialis, and the superficial external anal sphincter (Figs. 13–39B,C, and 13–40E).

6. The rectus abdominis muscles are separated from the internal oblique and transversus abdominis muscles by the semilunar line, which contains no muscle fibers (Figs. 13–29C,D). Spigelian hernias may occur at this point. The rectus sheath is formed by only a thin layer of transversalis fascia, below the arcuate line, which is midway between the pubis and umbilicus (Fig. 13–34A). The prevesical space and rectus sheath communicate with each other through this thin layer, along perforating inferior epigastric vessels and nerves.

THE LIGAMENTS AND TENDONS

On CT images, the ligaments and tendons may appear hyperdense because of their highly attenuating fibrous tissues. These include the sacrospinous ligament between the greater and lesser sciatic foramina, the sacrotuberous ligament which marks the posterior borders of the greater and lesser sciatic foramina (Fig. 13–38B), and the iliac fascia between the psoas and iliacus muscles (Fig. 13–30A). These same fibrous tissues are generally devoid of signal on MRI, and appear black, like blood vessels (Fig. 13–38E,F). Fibrous structures, which appear so bright on CT that they blend with adjacent bone, can be delineated with MRI. These include the tendons of the rectus femoris and biceps femoris (Fig. 13–39B,C), the iliofemoral, ischiofemoral, and pubic arcuate ligaments (Fig. 13–38H), and the lumbosacral fascia.

Acknowledgments

We are grateful to Joseph P. Whalen, M.D., Patrick T. Cahill, Ph.D., and James R. Knowles, Ph.D., without whose efforts the comparisons of CT, ultrasound, and MRI would not have been possible. We also thank Thomas Hom, R.T., R.D.M.S., Peter McCormick, R.T., and Richard Fischer, B.S., R.T., for their technical assistance. Kwan Seh Lee, M.D. (Jung Ang University Hospital, Seoul, South Korea), and Yup Yoon, M.D. (Kyung Hee University Hospital, Seoul, South Korea) lent their expertise to the preparation of the illustrations. Fereshteh Kazam assisted in manuscript preparation.

References

1. Whalen JP: Radiology of the Abdomen: An Anatomic Approach. Philadelphia, Lea & Febiger, 1976.
2. Kazam E, Auh YH, Rubenstein WA, et al: Normal CT anatomy of the pelvis with ultrasound and MRI correlations. In Putnam CE, Ravin C (eds): Textbook of Diagnostic Imaging. Philadelphia, WB Saunders Company, 1988.
3. Williams PL, Warwick R (eds): Gray's Anatomy, 36th Ed. Philadelphia, WB Saunders Company, 1980, pp 277–283, 378–385, 474–475, 593–604, 717–726, 759–763, 793–798, 1106–1117, 1352–1363, 1402–1423.
4. Hollinshead WH: Anatomy for Surgeons, 2nd Ed, Vol. 2. The Thorax, Abdomen, and Pelvis. New York, Harper & Row, 1971 pp 644–645, 731–732.
5. Eycleshymer AC, Shoemaker DM: A Cross-Section Anatomy. New York, Appleton-Century-Crofts, 1970, pp 86–101, 104–113.
6. Seidelman FE, Cohen WN, Bryan PJ, et al: Accuracy of CT staging of bladder neoplasms using the gas-filled method: Report of 21 patients with surgical confirmation. AJR 130:735–739, 1978.
7. Hildell JG, Nyman URO, Norlindh ST, et al: New intravesical contrast medium for CT: preliminary studies with Arachis (peanut) oil. AJR 137:777–780, 1981.
8. Ahlberg N-E, Berlin T, Calissendorff B, et al: Intravesical fat emulsion at computed tomography of bladder tumours. Acta Radiol (Diagn) 22:645–647, 1981.
8a. Savit RM, Udis DS: "Upside-down" contrast-urine levels in glycosuria: CT features. J Comput Assist Tomogr 11:911, 1987.
9. Fisher MR, Hricak H, Crooks LE: Urinary bladder MR imaging. Part I. Normal and benign conditions. Radiology 157:467–470, 1985.
10. Fisher MR, Hricak H, Tanagho EA: Urinary bladder MR imaging. Part II. Neoplasm. Radiology 157:471–477, 1985.
11. Soila KP, Viamonte M Jr, Starewicz PM: Chemical shift misregistration effect in magnetic resonance imaging. Radiology 153:819–820, 1984.
12. Poston GJ, Joseph AEA, Riddle PR: The accuracy of ultrasound in measuring changes in bladder volume. Br J Urol 55:361–363, 1983.
13. Beacock CJM, Roberts EE, Rees RWM, Buck AC: Ultrasound assessment of residual urine. A quantitative method. Br J Urol 57:410–413, 1985.
14. Auh YH, Rubenstein WA, Schneider M, et al: Extraperitoneal paravesical spaces: CT delineation with US correlation. Radiology 159:319–328, 1986.
15. Auh YH, Rubenstein WA, Markisz JA, et al: Intraperitoneal paravesical spaces: CT delineation with US correlation. Radiology 159:311–317, 1986.
16. Rubenstein WA, Auh YH, Zirinsky K, et al: Posterior peritoneal recesses: Assessment using CT. Radiology 156:461–468, 1985.
17. Hricak H, Williams RD, Spring DB, et al: Anatomy and pathology of the male pelvis by magnetic resonance imaging. AJR 141:1101–1110, 1983.
18. McNeal JE: The zonal anatomy of the prostate. Prostate 2:35, 1981.
19. Rifkin MD: Ultrasonography of the lower genitourinary tract. Urol Clin North Am 12:645–656, 1985.
20. Bartsch G, Egender G, Hubscher H, Rohr H: Sonometrics of the prostate. J Urol 127:1119–1121, 1982.
21. Arger PH: Computed tomography of the lower urinary tract. Urol Clin North Am 12:677–686, 1985.
22. Steinbach LS, Schneider R, Goldman AB, et al: Bursae and abscess cavities communicating with the hip: Diagnosis using arthrography and computed tomography. Radiology 156:303–307, 1985.

14 Magnetic Resonance Imaging

HERBERT Y. KRESSEL

The emergence of magnetic resonance imaging (MRI) techniques in the 1980s presents a powerful new diagnostic tool for the evaluation of the urological patient.[1-6] This new modality, which by means of magnets, radiowaves, and computers can generate medically useful images, offers several distinct advantages over existing imaging approaches. Because MRI relies on differences in the magnetic properties of tissues, which are often more pronounced than their differences in x-ray attenuation, MR images show more contrast than conventional x-ray–based images. Thus, parenchymal detail in normal tissues is usually greater, and lesions are frequently more conspicuous.

Like computed tomography (CT), MRI is a tomographic technique; images are presented as a stack of tomographic sections. In contrast to CT, however, MR images can be obtained in any plane. Thus, in addition to cross-sectional axial images, which are commonly obtained on x-ray CT, direct, nonreformatted MR images may also be obtained in the coronal and sagittal planes. Oblique imaging is also possible. This benefit markedly reduces partial volume problems that may be common on x-ray CT.

MRI appears to be a safe technique, and no ionizing radiation is required for the examination. At present, it is not necessary to use iodinated contrast materials in MRI to achieve adequate contrast for purposes of diagnosis. Thus, the examinations may be easily performed in patients with marginal renal function.

MRI techniques, as described below, are remarkably sensitive to blood flow, and excellent vascular detail may be obtained. This is useful in assessing vascular involvement of a variety of neoplasms.

Since its introduction, MRI has undergone tremendous change and development, in both technical approach and medical applications. New technical developments such as local or surface coils, new gradient-echo–based fast-scan techniques, novel approaches to reduce motion effects, and the acquisition of high-speed cine cardiac images have all resulted in new areas of application.[7-16] Although at first the primary application areas for MRI were in the central nervous system, new technical developments have improved the image quality that can be obtained in the abdomen, pelvis, and extremities. As a result, MRI is increasingly applied in these regions.

The physical basis of MR imaging is unique, and the ongoing rate of technological change in the modality is tremendous. Consequently, understanding the principles of MRI is of the utmost importance: the content of the images is more accurately interpreted, artifactual appearances are less mysterious, and new developments in the field are more easily understood.

The purpose of this chapter is to describe the physical principles of MRI and to review the current imaging approaches and contrast mechanisms as they apply to the genitourinary tract. Also discussed are the anatomical features of the genitourinary system as demonstrated by MRI.

BASICS OF MRI

Nuclei that possess an odd number of nucleons (protons and neutrons) demonstrate a property called spin. Nuclei with spin have a magnetic moment and thus generate a small magnetic field. These nuclei can be considered as tiny bar magnets whose lines of force show a definite magnitude and direction. As a result, the magnetic moment of the nuclei may be thought of as small vector quantities. In MRI, the most important nucleus is the hydrogen nucleus, owing to its great abundance in biological tissues. However, many other biologically active nuclei, such as phosphorus 31 and sodium 23, also possess nuclear spin and are potentially available for study with MR techniques.

In the absence of an externally applied magnetic field, the vectors of these magnetically sensitive nuclei have a random orientation, and there is no net magnetization in the sample. When an external magnetic field is applied to a sample of randomly oriented nuclei, they tend to align themselves along the direction of the applied magnetic field. Those aligning in the direction of the applied magnetic field (i.e., parallel) tend to be more stable (i.e., at a lower energy state) than those oriented in the opposite direction of the applied magnetic field (i.e., antiparallel). Eventually, the parallel nuclei slightly outnumber the antiparallel nuclei, and the sample has a resultant net magnetization (Fig. 14–1).

Once subject to the external magnetic field, the hydrogen nuclei exhibit a complex motion that is termed *precession*. Precession is the spinning and wobbling motion, resembling that of a spinning toy top. The rate or frequency of this nuclear precession depends on the strength of the external magnetic field and the gyromagnetic ratio. The precessional frequency of the nuclei is in the radiofrequency (RF) range. The precessional frequency of a particular nucleus can be readily determined by the Larmor equation:

$$\omega = \gamma B_0$$

This equation states that the resonance frequency (ω), or frequency of precession, for a given nucleus is equal to the gyromagnetic ratio (γ, which describes the magnetic properties of the sensitive nucleus) multiplied by the magnetic field strength (B_0). Thus, for any given nucleus and magnetic field strength, it is possible to precisely predict the precessional or resonance frequency.

Although nuclei of the same type align and precess at the same rate, they do not initially precess in phase (i.e., in synchrony) with one another. Rather, the magnetic moment vector of an individual nucleus may be thought

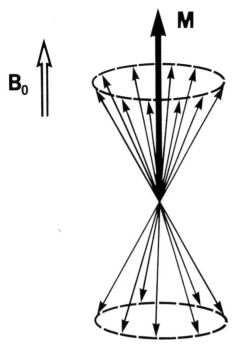

Figure 14–1. In the presence of a extrinsic magnetic field (B_0), the nuclei align either parallel or antiparallel to the main magnetic field. The slight excess of nuclei aligning parallel to the main magnetic field results in a net magnetization vector, which lies parallel to the main magnetic field. The aligned nuclei precess at a rate determined by the Larmor equation. However, they are not phase coherent. (Courtesy Felix Wehrli, Ph.D., General Electric Medical Systems.)

of as randomly distributed along its precessional path. The net magnetization vector of the entire sample may be thought of as parallel to the external magnetic field; however, the constituent spins (nuclei) are precessing at the same rate but out of phase with one another, and they may be oriented either parallel or antiparallel to the externally applied field (Fig. 14–1).

The basic MR experiment consists of adding RF energy to the sample at the resonance frequency of the nuclei to be studied, thus inducing transitions between the two potential energy states. If an RF pulse, at or near the natural Larmor frequency, is applied to the sample for a sufficient duration, the net magnetization of the sample may be deflected ("tipped") 90 or even 180 degrees. In the typical MR experiment, an RF pulse at the Larmor frequency of a duration sufficient to deflect the net magnetization vector of the sample 90 degrees is applied ("90-degree pulse") (Fig. 14–2). Immediately after the RF excitation, the excited spins are temporarily in phase, and the nuclei are precessing in synchrony. In addition, because the net magnetization of the sample is now rotated 90 degrees, it is present in the transverse plane. While the magnetization vector is in the transverse orientation, it precesses around the axis of the magnetic field, inducing a voltage in the receiver coil that is sensitive to the transverse component of the magnetization. The signal, called the *free-induction decay* (FID), decreases exponentially, as the excited spins lose their phase coherence and return to asynchronous precession.

The signal that is received by the receiver coil is then analyzed by a Fourier transform. This mathematical proc-

ess determines what RFs were present in the received signal.

Magnetic Relaxation

The return to the equilibrium state after the excitation pulse ceases is termed magnetic relaxation. Two exponential time constants describe the return to the baseline equilibrium state. The T2 relaxation time, otherwise known as the spin-spin or transverse relaxation time, is the exponential time constant that describes the irreversible decay of the transverse component of the magnetization. As the nuclei are excited and deflected 90 degrees to precess in the xy, or transverse plane, they are initially phase coherent (synchronous) with one another (Fig. 14–3C). However, soon after the excitation, relative slowing and speeding of some of the nuclei occur, because of local differences in the magnetic environment of neighboring nuclei. Phase coherence is lost as a result of these local field changes (Fig. 14–3B).

The T1 relaxation time is the exponential time constant that describes the regrowth of the longitudinal component of the magnetization following excitation. If one considers

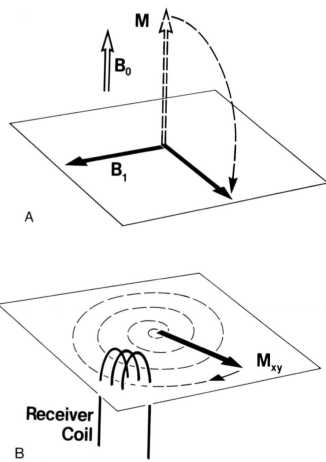

Figure 14–2. The basic MR experiment. *A,* An RF pulse at or near the Larmor frequency is applied for a duration sufficient to deflect the net magnetization (M) 90 degrees. *B,* The phase-coherent magnetization vector in the transverse plane (M_{xy}) generates a signal that is picked up by the receiver coil, which is sensitive to the transverse component of the magnetization. (Courtesy Felix Wehrli, Ph.D., General Electric Medical Systems.)

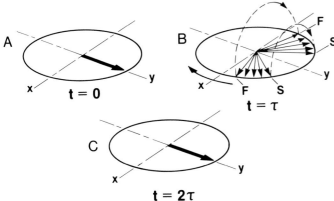

Figure 14–3. Spin-echo formation. *A*, Following the 90-degree RF excitation pulse, the net magnetization is transversely oriented, and the component nuclei are in phase with one another. *B*, Shortly after initial excitation, the excited nuclei begin to lose their phase coherence with one another, and the faster nuclei (F) separate from the slower nuclei (S). The 180-degree refocusing spin-echo pulse at time T = tau inverts the transverse magnetization. *C*, At twice the interval after the application of the 180-degree refocusing pulse, the transverse magnetization is refocused, and the nuclei are in phase once again. (Courtesy Felix Wehrli, Ph.D., General Electric Medical Systems.)

that RF excitation has resulted in an absorption of energy by some of the nuclei, which has caused a shift from the parallel to the antiparallel state, the T1 relaxation time is then the constant that describes the rate of dissipation of this excess energy to the surrounding lattice. Thus, the process is termed spin lattice relaxation. As the previously excited spins lose their additional energy, they return to the baseline equilibrium state, parallel to the main magnetic field. The T1 relaxation time then is the time required for 63% of the net magnetization to return to its original alignment with the main magnetic field. In three T1 relaxation times, 95% of the longitudinal magnetization will have recovered.

Variations in the local molecular environment clearly have a great influence on the apparent T1 and T2 of the biological tissue. In fact, the differences in the relaxation times of different tissues and of normal and pathological states are keys to ascertaining the potentially available MR contrast, and largely determine our ability to image these. The reader who is interested in a more detailed description of the physical principles of MR and MRI is referred to the standard texts in the field.[62, 63]

Chemical Shift

Differences within the local intramolecular magnetic environment may affect the Larmor frequency of a given nucleus, owing to the magnitude of magnetic shielding of the nucleus by nearby electrons. This phenomenon is termed chemical shift. The magnitude of this shift is typically quite small relative to the resonance frequency, is proportional to the magnetic field strength in which the sample is placed, and is typically described in parts per million of the resonance frequency. Thus, owing to the chemical shift phenomenon, a 3.5 parts-per-million difference is found in comparing the resonance frequency of

the hydrogen nucleus in a water molecule with that of the hydrogen nucleus in a fat molecule. At 1.5 tesla (T), this chemical shift is 220 Hz, whereas the resonance frequency of hydrogen is 64 MHz. These minute differences are the basis of differentiation of a variety of molecular compounds of a given nucleus in MR spectroscopy and form a potential source of contrast in MRI.[17–19]

Fundamentals of Magnetic Resonance Imaging

Conceptually, the key to obtaining images with MR data is the ability to localize, three-dimensionally, the received signal. By means of accurate three-dimensional localization, the signal arising from one region or organ may be distinguished from that of tissue in another organ or region sampled. In 1973, Lauterbur proposed an ingenious method of obtaining MR images, which employed magnetic field gradients to encode spatial information onto the signal.[20] Through the use of orthogonally oriented magnetic field gradients, the effective resonance frequency and phase of the MR signal may be predictably controlled. By analyzing the frequency and phase distribution of the returning signal, precise spatial localization may be obtained. This is illustrated in Figure 14–4, in which an MR experiment is performed by placing two water samples in a static magnetic field and exciting them first in a uniform magnetic field and then in a field with a linear gradient. In the first instance, when an RF pulse of a duration sufficient to deflect the net vector of the nuclei 90 degrees is applied, a simple FID signal results. Because both samples of water are in exactly the same magnetic field, all the nuclei precess at the same frequency, and the signals received from each sample of water cannot be distinguished.

In the presence of a linear gradient, the precessional frequency of the water sample in the weaker portion of the magnetic field is lower than that of the water sample in the higher portion of the magnetic field. As a result, the water in each vial produces a signal of a different frequency.

When a Fourier transform is performed on the received signal (in the experiment performed in a homogeneous magnetic field), one peak representing the resonance frequency of the water in both samples is obtained. In the presence of a magnetic field gradient, the Fourier transform yields two peaks: the one at lower frequency represents the signal derived from the sample in the weaker portion of the magnetic field; the higher-frequency peak represents the signal emitted from the vial in the stronger portion of the magnetic field. It is also apparent that the physical distance between the two peaks obtained is directly related to the physical distance of the two objects in the graded magnetic field. Thus, in the presence of a gradient, the Fourier transform yields a simple projection of the two water samples. By varying the direction of the magnetic field gradients, additional projections may be obtained. This series of projections or views may be analyzed through so-called back projection techniques, as are employed in x-ray CT to generate the image. In practice, these techniques are seldom employed in present-day imaging. Instead, simultaneous incoding of the signal in the *x* and *y* planes is performed, and a two-dimensional Fourier transform is utilized to

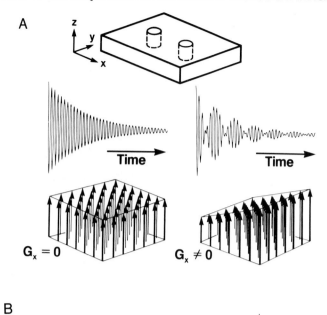

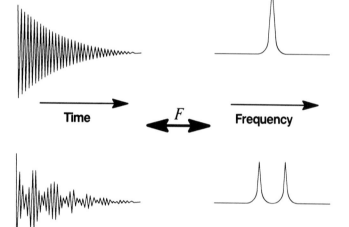

Figure 14–4. Spatial localization using gradients. *A,* A nuclear magnetic resonance (NMR) experiment performed on two vials of water and a static magnetic field ($G_x = 0$). This results in a uniform free-induction decay (FID) signal that is due to the signal contributions of the water in both vials, which are precessing at the same frequency. When the same NMR experiment is performed in a field with linear gradient ($G_x \neq 0$), the FID signal is more complex; this is because the signal is derived from the two vials precessing at different frequencies, owing to the differences in local magnetic fields. *B,* The Fourier transform performed on the signal obtained in the uniform magnetic field yields one peak corresponding to the resonance frequency of the water in both vials. When a Fourier transform is performed and the signal derived from the experiment carried out in the presence of a magnetic field gradient, two distinct peaks result, representing a simple projection of the image of the two vials. (Courtesy Felix Wehrli, Ph.D., General Electric Medical Systems.)

obtain the image.[21] This is discussed more extensively later in the chapter.

Spin Echo

Following a 90-degree RF excitation pulse, the resultant signal (the FID) decays exponentially, as the excited spins lose their phase coherence. In addition to true T2 relaxation, this exponential signal loss is also caused by spatial inhomogeneities in the magnetic field. These may be due to inhomogeneities in the magnet, as well as spatial inhomogeneities caused by the application gradients used to spatially encode the signals. These extrinsic effects serve to further accelerate the dephasing after excitation and the resultant signal loss. The exponential time constant, which describes the observed loss of transverse magnetization following an RF excitation, is termed T2*, the effective transverse relaxation time.

Once the transverse magnetization begins to decay, and if a 180-degree RF pulse is applied some time after the 90-degree pulse, phase coherence is re-established at twice the interval from the 90-degree pulse to the application of the 180-degree pulse, and the signal reappears. The refocused or returning signal is termed the spin echo. The time from the initial excitation to the peak of the spin echo is the echo time (TE). Figure 14–3 demonstrates that after the initial RF excitation, the excited spins begin to speed up or slow down, relative to one another, because of T2 effects and the other sources of spatial inhomogeneity of the magnetic field. The 180-degree RF pulse flips the partially dephased magnetization to a mirror image of itself, and the faster components now trail the slower ones. At twice the interval after the application of the 180-degree pulse, the excited spins are once again in phase and the signal reappears.

An analogy useful for understanding spin-echo formation is that of watching runners in a foot race on a video cassette recorder. Initially, all the runners are lined up along the starting line (in phase). Shortly after the starter's gun sounds, the runners begin to separate; the faster runners gain speed, and the slower runners trail behind. The effect of the spin echo may be likened to the effect of watching the race after the video reverse button has been pushed. The faster runners continue to appear to run faster, although they are moving backwards. The slower runners still appear to run slower, although backwards. All the runners appear to reach the starting line at exactly the same time, namely at twice the interval from the beginning of the race to the time the video reverse button was pushed.

Not all phase losses are refocused with a 180-degree spin echo RF pulse. Only phase losses due to extrinsic magnetic field inhomogeneities, and gradient effects are refocused by the spin-echo 180-degree RF pulse. Phase losses due to T2 relaxation are not refocused by the spin-echo RF pulse. This feature is useful in providing T2-weighted information on images, or in calculating T2 relaxation times. Spin-echoes are useful in T2-weighted imaging because, since the signal losses due to T2 relaxation are not recovered, images created at increasingly later TEs may demonstrate apparent differences in T2 as signal differences on the image. Regions with shorter T2 relaxation times lose signal earlier and are not refocused by the spin-echo pulse. They appear as darker images, whereas regions with tissues of longer T2 relaxation times continue to generate signals at increasingly longer TEs and appear brighter.

Spin echoes are also useful in calculating T2 relaxation time. This is accomplished by plotting the serial fall-off in the returning signal after a series of spin echoes have been obtained.

COMPONENTS OF THE MAGNETIC RESONANCE INSTRUMENT

Magnet

The magnet is a key component of the MR imager. It must be stable and generate a remarkably homogeneous magnetic field throughout the volume to be imaged. Clinical MRI has been performed with magnetic field strengths varying from 200 gauss (0.02 T) to fields of 20,000 gauss (2.0 T). Although the optimum magnetic field strength for imaging is controversial, there is little doubt that signal-to-noise ratios continue to increase with increasing field strength.[22] As a result, a shift to imaging at the higher field strengths has occurred over the last 5 years. At present, imagers most often operate at fields of 0.5 T to 1.5 T.

A variety of magnet designs have been employed in MRI. Resistive magnets, permanent magnets, and superconducting magnets have all been successfully utilized in MRI systems. In view of their ability to generate higher magnetic field strengths and the potential for achieving high homogeneity, superconducting magnets are the most common type found in imagers today.

Resistive Magnet

The magnetic field in resistive magnets is generated by current flowing through multiple turns of copper wire. The electrical resistance in the wires produces a significant amount of heat when ample current—sufficient to generate a strong magnetic field—flows through the magnet. The heating limits the strength of the magnetic field that can be obtained with resistive designs.[23] As a result, these magnets rarely exceed 0.04 T. In addition, they tend to be less homogeneous and require considerable power to function adequately.

Permanent Magnet

Permanent magnets are made of ferromagnetic materials, such as iron, or rare-earth alloys, such as samarium cobalt and neodynium iron. They do not require current to generate a magnetic field, and (typically) minimal fringe magnetic fields surround them. These magnets do tend to be quite heavy (as much as 100 tons) and may be difficult to site. It is also difficult to achieve a homogeneous magnetic field over a large volume with this design. In addition, requirements for temperature stability are stringent. Whole-body permanent magnets of field strengths up to 0.6 T have been produced; however, most permanent-magnet MR imagers operate at field strengths below 0.3 T.

Superconducting Magnet

The magnetic fields generated by superconducting magnets result from current flowing through turns of superconducting wire. When cooled to very low temperatures (4.2° K), these wires lose their resistance to current flow. Thus, high magnetic field strengths may be generated without significant heating problems. In addition, because of the lack of resistance in the wires, energized superconducting magnets have minimal power requirements.

To maintain the low temperatures necessary for the wires to exhibit superconductivity, the coils of wire are surrounded by liquid helium in a container, which is then surrounded by a series of containers with vacuum or liquid nitrogen. The housing that insures adequate low temperatures for the magnet coil is the cryostat. Since the liquid helium and liquid nitrogen in the cryostat tend to vaporize over time and must be replaced frequently, these magnets are associated with substantial cryogen costs. They are capable of generating very high magnetic fields (greater than 2.0 T) and of achieving the high degree of homogeneity necessary for MR applications such as spectroscopy. Superconducting magnets, particularly those operating at higher magnetic field strengths, are frequently associated with substantial fringe magnetic fields. Thus, siting in a clinical environment may be difficult or may require the installation of expensive magnetic shielding in the form of steel plates.

Gradient Coils

Gradient coils are electronic coils that lie in the bore of the magnet and produce a linear variation in magnetic field strength across a given plane, once current passes through them. Typically, three sets of gradient coils are present within the bore of the magnet. These produce gradients in the x, y, and z planes. By using combinations of gradient coils, linear gradients in oblique orientations may be produced.[24] Although the magnetic field strengths used for imaging are quite strong, the strength of the gradient used to spatially encode the signal is analyzed as rather weak—typically 1 gauss/cm or less. Thus, in a 50-cm bore magnet, a gradient of 50 gauss across the bore is sufficient for most imaging applications.

Radiofrequency Coils

Radiofrequency coils or antennae are necessary to transmit the RF energy to the sample and to receive the signal arising from the sample. For some imaging procedures, separate transmitter and receiver coils are utilized. For others, the same coil, a transceiver coil, transmits the excitation pulse and receives the resultant signal. The RF coils must be oriented at 90 degrees to the main magnetic field. Thus, the shape of the RF coils varies with the orientation and design of the magnet. Both solenoid coils and saddle-shaped coils have been utilized in MR imagers.

For high-resolution imaging applications, local or surface coils may be employed. These RF antennae are sensitive to signals arising near the surface, but are not subject to noise contribution from the deeper portions of the body.[7, 25, 26] For structures near the surface, substantial improvements in signal-to-noise can be achieved with surface coils.

The sensitive volume of a surface coil is determined by its size and shape. Circular coils with a variety of sizes are commonly employed in MRI of the spine, orbit, and shoulder. Other shapes, including rectangular surface coils or more complex coil designs, have been used. The development of local or surface coils has facilitated many emerging MR applications.

IMAGING TECHNIQUES

Spatial localization of the signal is the key requirement for MRI. We have previously described in a general fashion the use of magnetic field gradients to spatially localize the received signal.

A variety of approaches have been employed for MR imaging. The sequential point method detects signal, voxel by voxel. Sequential line acquisition techniques acquire data, simultaneously, for a row of voxels in a given plane. The sequential planar method simultaneously detects signals in an entire plane of voxels; it is the most common imaging method utilized at present and is used in essentially all the MR imagers now operating. True three-dimensional acquisition techniques have also been employed. These may be isotropic, in which case each voxel in the acquisition is a cube, or anisotropic, in which case the voxels are rectangular and resolution in plane of acquisition is improved. Although intriguing, three-dimensional acquisition techniques are time-consuming, and until recently had little clinical application. With the emergence of gradient-echo fast-scan techniques, three-dimensional acquisitions have become more feasible in the clinical setting.[11] As the multiplanar two-dimensional Fourier transform imaging approach is overwhelmingly the most commonly employed method to date, it is described below in greater detail.

Two-Dimensional Fourier Transform Multislice Imaging

The timing diagram that describes two-dimensional Fourier-transform spin-echo imaging is illustrated in Figure 14–5A. Three distinct steps are performed to localize the signal in three dimensions: (1) selective excitation, (2) phase encoding, and (3) frequency encoding. Each process employs a specific set of gradient coils oriented in a given plane. Selective excitation is the process that defines the slice to be imaged. For cross-axial imaging, selective excitation consists of applying a gradient in the craniocaudal direction (z axis) and applying an RF pulse in which frequencies are chosen to correspond precisely to a given slab of tissue in the gradient field (Fig. 14–5B). For coronal imaging, selective excitation would be performed utilizing the y gradient (AP direction), and for sagittal imaging selective excitation would be performed utilizing the x (side-to-side) gradient coils. After selective excitation, the net magnetization has been deflected 90 degrees within a given slab of tissue, but further spatial localization is required to localize the signal in the remaining two dimensions.

After selective excitation (slice selection), phase encoding follows (Fig. 14–5C). For axial body imaging, this is typically done in the y or AP dimension. A gradient of variable magnitude is briefly applied in the y direction. For each line to be ultimately reconstructed in the y dimension of the matrix, a separate excitation with a y-gradient application of a different magnitude will be applied. Thus, to acquire the information for a 256-by-

256–matrix MR image, 256 excitations—with phase encoding of a different magnitude for each—will be required. The brief application of the y gradient induces a phase shift across the sample in the y direction. This shift encodes position as a function of phase in the recovered signal. The net amount of phase shift introduced for a given magnitude of y-gradient application affects the amount of signal that is ultimately received. The sum of the phase information is then recovered by means of a Fourier transform to localize the y components of the signal. The plane used for selective excitation is fixed and determined by the desired orientation of the acquired slices. However, either of the two remaining dimensions may be used for phase encoding; typically, the narrowest remaining dimension of the image is used.

Following phase encoding, the signal refocused by a spin echo or gradient echo is read out in the presence of a gradient, which is applied in the remaining dimension (Fig. 14–5D). For axial imaging this will be the x coordinate (side-to-side). The application of the fixed gradient across the sample causes local variations in the resonance frequency that are positional; thus, according to the Fourier transform, the amount of signal at a given frequency relates to the amount of signal source per row of voxels along the x coordinate. This process is called frequency encoding.

Through selective excitation, phase encoding, and frequency encoding, localization of the MR signal in three dimensions is achieved. To acquire the information for multiple sections, this process is repeated serially across the total volume of the sample to be imaged. To improve the signal-to-noise ratio from a given voxel, repeated excitations at each y gradient step are useful. This process is termed signal averaging.

The time necessary to obtain an image is defined by the time between excitations (TR) and the number of phase-encoding steps (e.g., the size of the y dimension of the matrix multiplied by the number of excitations [NEX] or number of signal averages [NSA] obtained for each voxel).

$$\text{Acquisition time} = \text{TR} \times \text{matrix size (N)} \times \text{NEX}$$

The time between excitations (TR) greatly affects the contrast and the number of slices obtained during a given data acquisition. For a given field of view, the number of phase-encoding steps or lines on the image relates to the ultimate resolution obtained. The larger the number of phase-encoding steps, the higher the achievable resolution, assuming adequate signal-to-noise per voxel. The NEX affects the signal-to-noise per voxel. Each additional excitation provides a square-root-of-two improvement in signal-to-noise ratio.

PULSE SEQUENCES

Spin-Echo–Based Pulse Sequences

The series of RF excitations and refocusing pulses used to acquire the signal, which when analyzed generates the image, is termed a pulse sequence. Pulse sequences consist of an exciting pulse and a method of refocusing some of the acquired phase shifts, either through the use

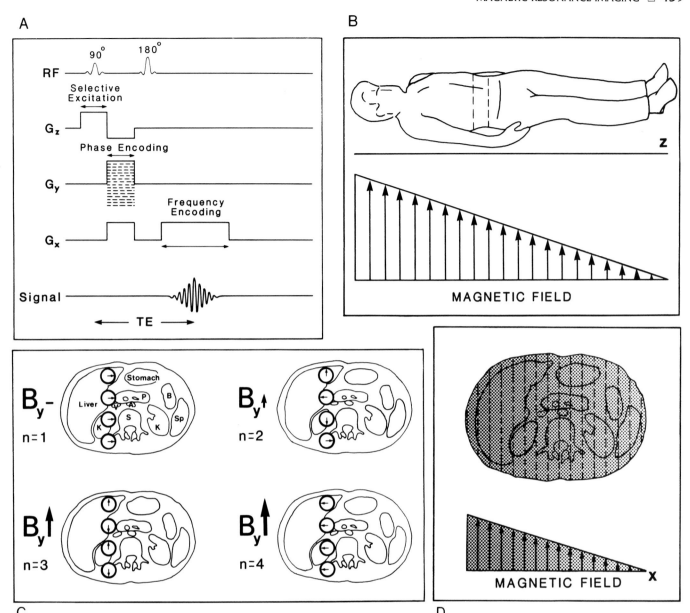

Figure 14–5. Two-dimensional Fourier transform (2DFT) imaging. *A,* Timing diagram for 2DFT imaging is shown. G_z = *z* gradient, G_y = *y* gradient, G_x = *x* gradient. This timing diagram assumes an axial slice. *B,* Selective excitation in the presence of a gradient in the z direction is illustrated. A specific range of radiofrequencies (band width) are chosen, which will excite a specific anatomical slice location. *C,* Phase encoding: With increasing values of *y*-gradient application and sequential excitations, phase shifts are induced in the *y* dimension. These phase shifts serve to encode the *y* dimension of the image. *D,* Frequency encoding: The signal is read out in the presence of a fixed magnetic gradient in the *x* direction, which alters the resonance frequency locally, as a function of position.

of spin echoes, or gradient echoes, or both. Thus, pulse sequences are commonly described in terms of the following: (1) a repetition time (TR), which is the time between the beginning of one pulse sequence and the beginning of the succeeding pulse sequence at a given tissue location, and (2) an echo time (TE), which represents the time interval between the center of a 90-degree pulse and the center of the refocused spin echo or gradient echo.

Inversion-recovery pulse sequences are also characterized by the inverting pulse time (TI), which is described below.

Most MRI currently performed utilizes spin-echo–based techniques to obtain tissue contrast that may be either T1 dependent, T2 dependent, or proton-density dependent (Table 14–1). With spin-echo–based techniques, signal intensity is dependent on proton density, T1, T2, TR, and TE, and it is expressed by the following

Table 14–1. Contrast in Spin-Echo Pulse Sequence

	TR	TE
T1 weighted	Short (0.5 × T1 tissue)	Short ($<$/$-$ 20 msec)
Proton-density weighted	Long (3 × T1 tissue)	Short ($<$/$-$ 20 msec)
T2 weighted	Long (3 × T1 tissue)	Long (e.g., 40 msec, 80 msec)

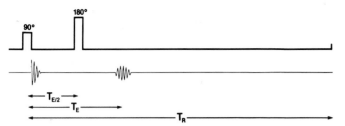

Figure 14–6. Single spin-echo pulse sequence. A 90-degree pulse is followed by a 180-degree pulse. The resultant spin-echo signal is used to generate the image. (Courtesy Felix Wehrli, Ph.D., General Electric Medical Systems.)

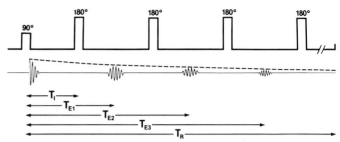

Figure 14–7. Multiple spin-echo pulse sequence. The initial 90-degree excitation pulse is followed by a series of 180-degree refocusing pulses. The signal in each of the spin echoes is used to generate a separate image. The dotted line represents the serial fall-off in the returning signal and reflects the T2. (Courtesy Felix Wehrli, Ph.D., General Electric Medical Systems.)

equation (where S = signal intensity and N(H) = proton density).

$$S = N(H)\,(1 - e^{-TR/T1})\,e^{-TE/T2}$$

T1-Weighted Images With Spin Echoes

T1-weighted imaging with spin echoes is commonly performed with a single spin-echo pulse sequence that utilizes a short TE to minimize T2 effects on the image. This pulse sequence has been referred to in the literature as a partial saturation technique.

The pulse sequence is depicted (Fig. 14–6) and consists of a 90-degree pulse, which is followed shortly thereafter by a 180-degree pulse and signal readout. The time between 90-degree pulses is the TR, whereas the time of the maximal refocusing of the echo is the TE.

To maximize T1 contrast with spin-echo techniques, the TR must be short, relative to the mean tissue T1s in the image.[27, 28] Ideally, choosing a TR that is half the mean T1 times of the two substances one wishes to contrast is ideal. In practice, the TR for T1-weighted images commonly varies between 250 and 600 msec. As the TR is increased, T1 contrast decreases. Once the TR exceeds three times the mean tissue T1 time, nearly complete T1 relaxation of all tissue in the slice has occurred between each exciting 90-degree pulse. As a result, T1 contrast is lost and, assuming that the TE remains short (less than 20 msec), the image becomes more proton-density weighted. It is important in T1-weighted or proton-density–weighted spin-echo imaging to minimize T2 effects as a contrast mechanism on the images. This is accomplished by minimizing the TE. On T1-weighted pulse sequences, tissues or substances with relatively short T1 times appear bright, whereas tissues or structures with long T1 times generate less signal and appear dark.

T2-Weighted Imaging with Spin Echoes

Obtaining T2-weighted contrast using spin echoes is facilitated by the use of long TRs (3 × T1), which minimizes the contribution of T1 differences as a source of image contrast.[27, 28] For T2-weighted imaging, longer TEs are employed, typically 40 to 100 msec. In clinical practice, T2-weighted images are commonly obtained as part of a multiple spin-echo pulse sequence (Fig. 14–7). In this sequence, the time between exciting 90-degree

pulses is referred to as the TR. The resulting TEs refer to the time of the center of the spin-echo production. Multiple spin-echo acquisitions are useful in calculating T2 values from different regions, or in tracking the apparent T2 decay from a number of different tissues or regions. On T2-weighted images, tissues or substances with short T2 times generate less signal, whereas substances with longer T2 times continue to generate signal and appear bright, even at relatively late TEs (80 to 100 msec).

Inversion Recovery

Inversion recovery is another pulse sequence that commonly employs spin echoes and is used to generate T1-weighted images. As depicted in Figure 14–8, this pulse sequence consists of an initial 180-degree pulse followed—after an interval (inverting pulse time [TI])—by a 90-degree pulse and shortly thereafter by a refocusing spin-echo 180-degree pulse. Recovery of the longitudinal magnetization in the interval between the inverting 180-degree pulse and the 90-degree pulse is the basis of the T1 contrast on these images. In general, the TE of the refocusing spin echo is kept as short as possible to minimize the effect of T2 differences on the images. Typically, TRs for inversion recovery pulse sequences are about two to three mean T1 times, and the TI is about one T1 time.

When short TIs are used, a contrast inversion results; that is, substances with long T1s generate increased signal relative to substances with shorter T1s, which may appear

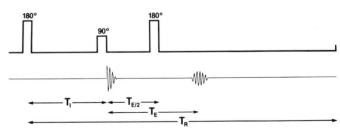

Figure 14–8. Inversion recovery pulse sequence. The initial 180-degree pulse is followed after an interval (TI) by a 90-degree pulse. The resultant signal is refocused with a spin echo. (Courtesy Felix Wehrli, Ph.D., General Electric Medical Systems.)

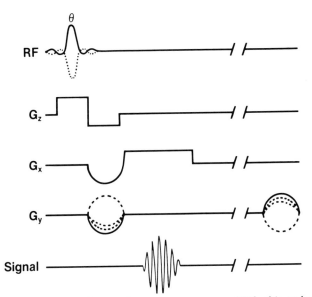

Figure 14–9. Gradient-echo pulse sequence. With this pulse sequence, refocusing is accomplished through gradient reversal. A rephasing gradient along the *y* axis is applied at the end of the pulse sequence to compensate for view-to-view phase change induced by the phase-encoding gradient (G$_y$). (Courtesy Felix Wehrli, Ph.D., General Electric Medical Systems.)

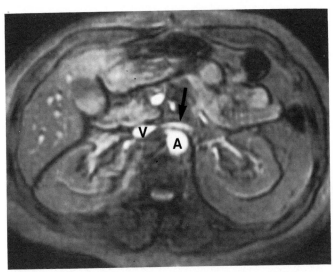

Figure 14–10. Gradient-echo scan through the midabdomen. There is little parenchymal contrast. Note the high signal in the aorta (A), inferior vena cava (V), and left renal vein (*arrow*).

dark. Thus, short TI inversion recovery (STIR) imaging has been useful in abdominal imaging by generating high-contrast images in which the signal from fat is reduced, and the associated image degradation through motion artifact is also reduced. Another benefit of STIR sequences is that, because of the contrast inversion at short inverting pulse times, the T1 and T2 contrast effects tend to be additive, and overall contrast on the image may be increased.[29]

Gradient-Echo Imaging Sequences

Recently, a number of new pulse sequences have been developed, in which the magnitude of the initial excitation pulse may be varied (5 to 90 degrees) and refocusing of the transverse component of the magnetization accomplished through gradient reversal, rather than a true 180-degree spin-echo pulse (Fig. 14–9).[10, 11] The refocusing of the transverse component of the magnetization through gradient reversal is termed a gradient echo, or field echo. For gradient-echo–based pulse sequences, flip angles of less than 90 degrees are commonly employed, and the TRs tend to be short, relative to those used in spin-echo imaging—typically less than 400 msec, and frequently less than 100 msec.

T2*-weighted, T1-weighted, and density-weighted images may be obtained by the proper selection of TR, flip angle, and TE (Table 14–2).[30] Gradient-echo images

become more T1-weighted when short TEs and larger flip angles are used. T2*-weighted images may be obtained with smaller flip angles (thereby reducing the T1 effect) and longer TEs. T2*-weighted images may also be produced in the "steady state" when very short TRs, small flip angles, and moderate TEs are used. Proton-density–weighted images are obtained when small flip angles and short TEs are used. In view of the relatively short TR, MR gradient-echo–based images may be acquired quite rapidly (in 2 to 4 seconds), depending on the parameters chosen. Clearly, when longer TRs are used, the acquisition time increases.

Gradient-echo images have properties that make them particularly useful in abdominal imaging. At the same time, certain inherent properties limit their general application. Gradient-echo images typically demonstrate marked intravascular signals attributable to flowing blood (Fig. 14–10). The increased signal results from the wash-in of previously fully relaxed spins between RF excitations, known as "flow-related enhancement." The high signal of flowing blood on gradient-echo–based pulse sequences facilitates vascular recognition and the identification of vascular obstructions or intravascular masses. Thus, these pulse sequences are particularly helpful in defining the intravascular extension of renal cell carcinoma.

Since the gradient echo is less effective than the spin echo in refocusing phase losses due to magnetic field inhomogeneities, gradient-echo–based images are markedly degraded by magnetic field inhomogeneities and are exceedingly sensitive to magnetic susceptibility differences. This latter feature may be useful in detecting hemorrhage or hemorrhagic components within a lesion,

Table 14–2. Contrast in Gradient-Echo Images

| | T1 Weighted | T2* Weighted | | Proton-Density Weighted |
		"STEADY STATE"		
TR	200–400	20–60 msec	200–400 msec	200–400 msec
TE	Short (e.g., 8–15 msec)	Short 8–15 msec	30–60 msec	Short 8–15 msec
Flip angle	45–90	30–60*	5–20	5–20

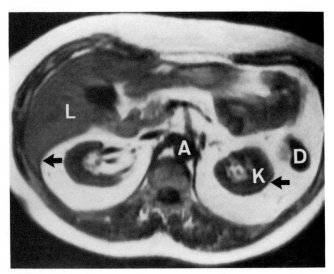

Figure 14–11. T1-weighted abdominal image, 1.5 tesla (T) field strength. Short TR/TE (TR = 400 msec, TE = 20 msec) imaged through the abdomen. Note the high signal from intra-abdominal and subcutaneous fat; this is reflective of its relatively short T1 time. The liver (L) has the highest signal intensity of the solid organs in the abdomen, in view of its shorter T1 relaxation time. The kidneys (K) are demonstrated bilaterally. Note the abundant renal sinus fat. Chemical shift artifact is also identified (*arrows*). Signal is absent in the aorta (A). This is due to the "flow void" phenomenon. There is also absent signal in the lumen of the descending colon (D). This is due to its low proton density.

but may also create problems when the decreased signal due to gas within bowel extends beyond the anatomical confines of the bowel and obscures regions of interest.

Fast acquisitions utilizing gradient-echo techniques are also of interest in the abdomen because of their potential to reduce motion artifacts caused by respiration. With the short data acquisition times, images may be acquired during breath holding, thus reducing motion-related artifacts.[31] In general, gradient-echo–based pulse sequences have been used as an adjunct in the evaluation of the genitourinary tract, particularly in the assessment of vascular structures and their relationship to masses.

CLINICAL ASPECTS OF MR IMAGING

Image Contrast

A number of intrinsic tissue parameters are potential sources of contrast in MRI. The most important contrast mechanisms are T1 and T2 relaxation time differences, proton-density differences, and blood flow. In addition, chemical shift, magnetic susceptibility, and molecular diffusion may be potential contrast sources. On T1-weighted spin-echo MR images (those with TRs that are short relative to the T1 times, and short TEs [typically 20 msec or less]), tissues or substances with short T1 relaxation times produce increased signal and appear bright on the MR images. Tissues with longer T1 times generate less signal and appear darker (Fig. 14–11).

On T2-weighted pulse sequences, tissues with short T2 relaxation times lose signal more rapidly, and appear darker at earlier echo times than tissues or substances

with long T2 times. These continue to generate signal and appear bright on the longer-echo images (Fig. 14–12).

The relative T1 and T2 times of commonly encountered tissues in the abdomen and pelvis are summarized in Table 14–3, as are their resulting signal intensities. Both a pulse sequence that emphasizes T2 differences and a second pulse sequence emphasizing T1 differences are required to adequately characterize a region or lesion. As a general rule, optimal contrast of intra-abdominal intrapelvic structures with surrounding fat is best obtained with T1-weighted images (short TR, short TE); optimal intraparenchymal contrast is commonly obtained with T2-weighted images (long TR, long TE). Although MR is capable of acquiring images in a variety of planes, axial imaging is still the dominant plane of acquisition for abdomen and pelvis. Coronal or sagittal scanning is useful as an adjunct, typically to identify the spread of a lesion to contiguous structures, a task that might be difficult by using only a series of axial images.

The differences in proton density in the organs of the abdomen and pelvis are not great. As a result, proton density is not an important source of parenchymal contrast in MR imaging. The low proton density of intraluminal gas is the source of the absent signal within the lumen of gas-containing bowel loops. Proton-density effects are also responsible for the low signal generated from cortical bone. Similarly, intraparenchymal calcification may appear as low signal because of its low proton density.

Blood flow is another major source of contrast in MRI. With spin-echo pulse sequences, blood flowing at normal velocities typically does not produce signal; therefore, the lumen of vessels with normal blood flow tends to appear low in signal intensity. Thus, vessels may be easily recognized. As discussed previously, flowing blood generates

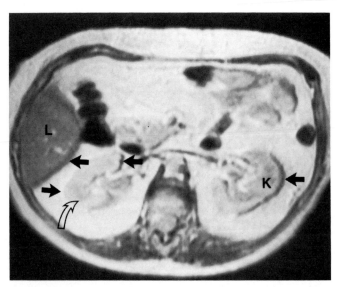

Figure 14–12. T2-weighted abdominal image (TR = 2500 msec, TE = 80 msec), 1.5 T field strength. The kidneys (K) demonstrate increased signal relative to the liver (L) in view of their longer T2 relaxation times. The renal cortex and medulla can be differentiated on the T2-weighted images (*open arrow*). Note the chemical shift artifact (*arrows*) and the decreased contrast between kidneys and fat, compared with short pulse sequence images.

Table 14–3. Relating Relaxation Times and Resultant Signal Intensities in Abdomen and Pelvis

	Relaxation Time		Signal Intensity	
	T1	T2	Short TR/TE	Long TR/TE
Water (urine)	V long	V long	V dark	V bright
Fat	V short	Long	V bright	Bright
Liver	Mod	Short	Intermediate	Dark
Renal cortex	Mod	Long	Intermediate	Bright
Renal medulla	Long	Short	Dark	Intermediate
Fibrosis	Long	Short	Dark	V dark
Tumor	Long	Long	Dark	Bright
Old hematoma	Short	Long	V bright	V bright
Fresh hematoma	Long	Short	Intermediate	Dark
Gas	—	—	Dark	Dark
Cortical bone	—	—	Dark	Dark
(Calcification)	—	—	Dark	Dark

high-signal intensities and appears bright, and the vascular structures are thereby recognized.

Paramagnetic contrast materials, such as gadolinium diethylenetriaminepenta-acetic acid (DTPA), are another potential source of contrast on the MR image. These may be administered intravenously or orally. Unlike the iodinated contrast materials used in x-ray–based techniques, paramagnetic contrast materials are not directly imaged in MRI; rather, they exert an influence on the relaxation properties of the hydrogen nuclei in their immediate environment by decreasing T1 and T2. At the lower dose ranges, the T1 shortening effects appear to predominate. As a result, T1-weighted images show signal enhancement where the contrast medium accumulates. At higher doses, the T2 effects appear to predominate, resulting in signal loss on the T2-weighted images.

At first it appears that gadolinium diethylenetriamine-penta-acetic acid (DTPA) is useful for evaluating the central nervous system. However, it (and other paramagnetic contrast agents) may prove useful in assessing renal blood flow and tubular function. This is because gadolinium DTPA is filtered by the glomerulus, concentrated in the renal tubules, and excreted into the urinary collecting system. These agents may also aid in the detection and characterization of abnormalities of the renal parenchyma and collecting system.

Safety

MRI is a safe imaging technique for which there is little documentation of biological hazard. At the magnetic field strengths currently employed, no significant bioeffects due to the static magnetic field have been noted. Similarly, the magnitude and duration of the time-varying magnetic field gradients that encode the spatial information are such that no abnormalities of ventricular rhythm or muscular contractility have been reported. The RF pulses used for excitation and refocusing may result in heating of body tissues. Typically, the heat generated is less than 1°C and of no clinical significance in patients without cardiovascular compromise or other sources of diminished capacity to dissipate heat.

Ferromagnetic materials brought into the high magnetic field strength environment can pose a health hazard. Care must be taken to secure the MRI examining room from materials that may be ferromagnetic, such as IV poles, wheelchairs, and stretchers. The examination is contraindicated in patients with cardiac pacemakers or cerebral aneurysm clips, some of which are ferromagnetic. The examination is also contraindicated in patients who may have ferromagnetic intraorbital foreign bodies. Other than cerebral aneurysm clips, surgical clips do not appear to present a hazard, and the examination may be safely performed in postoperative patients. Typically, the image distortion due to surgical clips on MRI examinations is less than is commonly encountered on x-ray CT images.

Technique Optimization

The problem of consistently acquiring high-quality MR images of the abdomen and pelvis has been a considerable technical challenge. A number of sources of image degradation and artifact can arise in the abdomen and pelvis, and these must be minimized or overcome to generate high-quality images.

Artifacts that are due to motion, namely, blurring and the periodic ghost images, serve to degrade markedly the image quality obtained in the abdomen and, to a lesser extent, the pelvis.[32–34] Respiratory motion, cardiac pulsation, peristaltic motion, and gross patient motion during the time of acquisition all contribute to possible image degradation. Vascular pulsations, and flow phenomena may also be responsible. The third major artifact source in abdominal and pelvic imaging is aliasing, namely the foldover onto the image plane, of signal from structures outside the image field of view.

Motion during acquisition is a major source of artifact on MR images. Motion may occur between RF excitation and signal readout sampling, and from view to view (between phase-encoding steps). Any repetitive or periodic motion in any direction results in ghosting, or smearing in the plane used for phase encoding. The amplitude and location of the ghosts depend partly on the rate and amplitude of the motion.[32] Probably, motion artifact is produced by both motion between RF excitations and spin-echo formation, as well as from view to view. As a result, methods that tend to reduce either of these sources of motion degradation have been partially effective.

A number of technical approaches to controlling and reducing motion-related artifacts have been employed to improve image quality in the abdomen and pelvis. These include cardiac and respiratory gating, short TR, short TE, scans with extensive signal averaging, respiratory ordered phase encoding, gradient moment mulling techniques, STIR, and gradient-echo fast-scan techniques.

Both respiratory and cardiac gating techniques have

been advocated as methods for improving upper abdominal image quality.[34-36] However, the length of time required to complete a scan may increase by a factor of two or more. Therefore, the techniques have not been widely employed on a routine basis.

By means of short TR/TE techniques and signal averaging, high-quality T1-weighted images may be obtained, with marked reduction of apparent motion artifacts.[37] Investigators working with a midfield strength system utilizing a short TR/TE pulse sequence with 16 averages have reported a marked reduction in motion-related artifacts on abdominal images. Although these reports appear to be confirmed by others working at medium field strengths,[38] they have not been widely confirmed by workers on systems of higher field strengths.[39] In addition, in view of the requirement for extensive signal averaging, these techniques are most easily applicable in short TR/TE pulse sequences and are not practical for the more time-consuming long TR/TE pulse sequences, which are diagnostically important.

The respiratory ordered phase encoding (ROPE) technique employs a respiratory monitor, such as a bellows, to assess the rate and phase of respiration. These data are then used to determine the sequence of phase-encoding steps to be employed in the two-dimensional Fourier transform imaging sequence. By ordering the steps according to the respiratory cycle, less discrete ghosts appear on the images.[12] This technique is effective on both short TR/TE and long TR/TE scans, but appears to be relatively less effective on the long TR/TE images.

Gradient moment nulling techniques attempt to reduce motion-related artifacts by shaping the rephasing lobe of the signal readout gradient, in order to compensate for velocity-dependent phase shifts acquired by nonstationary nuclei during the period of image acquisition.[14, 15] This technique is particularly effective in reducing motion effects caused by motion between the initial exciting pulse and the refocusing pulse. With gradient moment nulling, the signal-to-noise ratio improves, and motion-related artifacts decrease. In addition, the phase losses due to blood flow in the plane of acquisition are also recovered. This blood flowing in many blood vessels appears bright (Fig. 14-13D).

Another approach to reducing apparent motion-related artifacts is the STIR pulse sequence. As previously noted, contrast inversion occurs at short inverting pulse times; tissues with short T1 times (e.g., fat) appear as regions of decreased signal intensity, whereas substances with long T1 times demonstrate increased intensity. Because the high signals arising from intra-abdominal and subcutaneous fat are the major sources of the high-signal ghosts on MR images, decreasing the signal from these structures by using short inverting pulse times reduces apparent motion-related artifacts.[29]

Gradient-echo techniques are another potential method of reducing motion-related artifacts. By means of short acquisition times, scans may be obtained during breath holding.[31] In spite of excellent vascular detail and adequate tissue contrast obtained with these pulse sequences, the problems due to associated magnetic susceptibility artifacts, particularly in gas-containing structures such as bowel, have limited the widespread application of these techniques as the primary method of imaging the abdomen and pelvis.

Blood Flow Effects

On spin-echo images, blood flowing at normal velocities typically generates little or no signal (Fig. 14-11). This effect has been termed the flow void phenomenon. The signal loss commonly observed in blood vessels flowing at normal velocity has two major underlying causes: the wash-out of spins from the time of selective excitation to the time of the refocusing spin-echo pulse, and the phase shifts, which are acquired by spins moving along magnetic field gradients.[40, 41]

Although the flow void is the most common effect observed in vessels on spin-echo imaging, considerable signal is frequently found within vessels, derived from flowing blood. Potentially, this is a source of motion-related artifact or may provide confusion in image interpretation. Three major factors may result in signal from flowing blood: (1) flow-related enhancement, (2) even-echo rephasing, and (3) diastolic pseudogating.[40-42] Flow-related enhancement occurs when slowly flowing blood that has previously been unsaturated (i.e., not previously excited by the RF pulses) enters the imaging volume and replaces that blood, which was partially saturated from previous excitations. When subject to the RF excitation, the unsaturated blood is a source of relatively high signal intensity on the image. This effect is commonly observed on the "entry slices" (i.e., the most superior and inferior slices in multislice acquisition).

Just as the blood flow velocities in the arterial tree vary with the cardiac cycle, so does the relative amount of velocity-induced phase shift as a source of signal loss. Thus, rapid flow is encountered during systole, while flow may be very slow or absent during diastole. When the repetition of the pulse sequence approximates the pulse rate, it is possible to inadvertently gate the acquisition to diastole. When this occurs, the requirements for generating the flow void will not be met, and signal may increase in the arterial structures. This effect is termed diastolic pseudogating.[41]

The third source of increased signal from flowing blood is even-echo rephasing. Although the initial spin echo in a symmetrical multiecho pulse sequence refocuses the acquired phase losses of stationary spins, the phase losses due to spins moving through gradient are not recovered by the initial spin echo. With the second, or even, echoes (a series of symmetrical spin echoes) there is compensation of these phase effects. Thus, at slower velocities an intraluminal signal increase from the first to the second echo is observed.[42]

Artifacts arising from signal from within the blood vessel may be minimized through the use of spatial presaturation techniques.[43] These consist of applying 90-degree RF pulses outside the imaging volume to saturate the spins in blood vessels that enter the imaging volume during the acquisition. This spatial presaturation, in turn, reduces both the intraluminal signal that may be derived from the vessel and the ghosting that may arrive from the intravascular signal. Spatial presaturation is an effective method of reducing blood flow artifact.

Aliasing

Aliasing is the mapping of signal that arises outside the reconstructed field of view onto the image. This "wraparound" occurs when the diameter of the object to be imaged exceeds the reconstructed field of view. For abdominal or pelvic imaging, the most common source of aliased signal are the arms, which lie at the patient's sides during data acquisition. In addition, during coronal imaging, aliasing of signals that arise from the thorax or extremities may be encountered. Generally the artifact is obvious on the image; on occasion, however, it may mimic disease or obscure the identification of a lesion.

Aliasing may occur in either the phase-encoding or frequency-encoding directions. Aliasing in the frequency-encoded direction may be eliminated by RF filters, which limit the bandwidth of the analyzed signal. Aliasing may also be eliminated through the use of over-sampling techniques. By means of these techniques, the effective field of view is expanded during imaging, but only the requisite field of view is displayed. The aliased signal is on the undisplayed portion of the image.

Chemical Shift

As indicated earlier, there is a 3.5 parts-per-million shift in the resonance frequency of the hydrogen nucleus

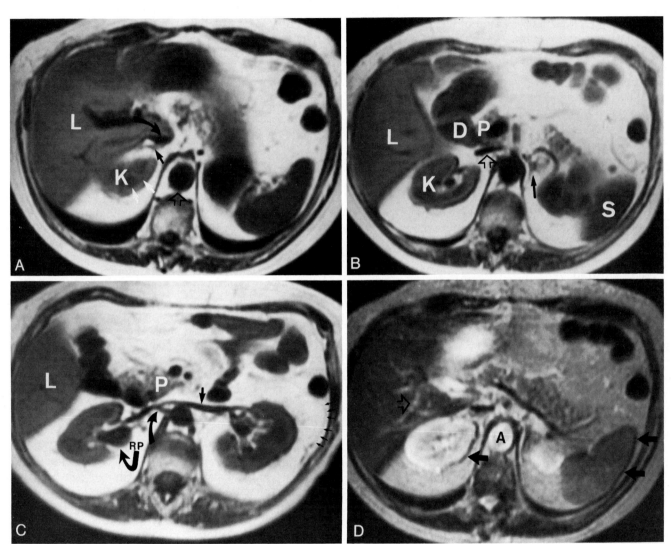

Figure 14–13. MR scan of the upper abdomen and kidneys, 1.5 T. *A*, Short TR/TE (TR = 400 msec, TE = 20 msec) axial MR image (T1 weighted) was taken through the level of the upper pole of the left kidney (K). The renal medulla is of lower signal intensity (*white arrows*) than the cortex, and it appears darker. The right adrenal gland (*arrow*) is identified with an inverted V configuration, immediately posterior to the inferior vena cava (*curved arrow*). The inferior vena cava and the aorta (*open short arrow*) demonstrate the flow void phenomenon and appear low in signal intensity. *B*, This T1-weighted, short TR/TE (TR = 400 msec, TE = 20 msec) scan was performed 1.5 cm below that seen in *A*. The left adrenal gland is now identified (*black arrow*). The liver (L), kidney (K), spleen (S), duodenum (D), pancreas (P), and inferior vena cava (*open arrow*) are also noted. *C*, T1-weighted, short TR/TE (TR = 400, TE = 20 msec) scan through the renal hila is shown. The left renal vein is identified (*short arrow*) as it traverses anterior to the aorta and enters the inferior vena cava. The right renal artery (*upper curved arrow*) is identified posterior to the inferior cava. The somewhat dilated extrarenal pelvis (RP) is identified as a structure of low signal intensity, arising in the hilus. A minimal amount of renal sinus fat is identified as a high-signal region surrounding the renal pelvis. Gerota's fascia is faintly visualized (*short arrows*) on the left. Also identified are the liver (L) and the pancreas (P). *D*, This is a T2-weighted image in the midabdomen. The kidney is of higher signal intensity than the liver or spleen. Chemical shift artifact is demonstrated (*arrows*). The aorta (A), and intrahepatic vessels (*open arrow*) are of a high signal intensity, owing to the gradient moment nulling techniques that have been employed to minimize motion artifacts in this patient.

in water, compared with fat. This difference (220 Hz in a 1.5-T system) is small enough that excitation of both water and liquid protons may occur with a single-slice selective RF pulse. However, in the presence of a relatively small readout gradient, which is applied during frequency encoding, the 3.5 parts-per-million shift is sufficient to cause spatial misregistration of the fat and water protons to an incorrect location.[18, 19]

Chemical shift misregistration artifacts are typically seen at the interface between structures that are predominantly fat containing and those that are mainly water containing (e.g., at the junction of the bladder wall and perivesical fat). Chemical shift artifact appears as a bright band of signal intensity along one side of a fat-water boundary and a symmetrical band of decreased signal at the opposite interface (Figs. 14–11 and 14–12). Chemical shift artifact occurs along the axis used for frequency encoding of the signal. This is in contrast to motion-related artifacts (ghosting), which occur along the phase-encoding direction. When chemical shift misregistration artifact occurs and mimics pathological change, altering the planes used for frequency encoding and phase encoding will shift the direction of the propagated chemical shift misregistration artifact and help to identify it. Chemical shift artifact may also be reduced by increasing the frequency-encoding gradient level or decreasing the magnitude of the main magnetic field. The latter is of course generally not practical in the clinical setting. The chemical shift artifact may actually be utilized in clinical MRI to enhance or highlight the interfaces between fat and non-fatty structures (echo-offset imaging).

MAGNETIC RESONANCE IMAGING: ANATOMY IN RETROPERITONEUM AND PELVIS

Kidneys and Retroperitoneum

The well-defined fascial compartments of the retroperitoneum[44, 45] can be demonstrated by MRI. These include the anterior paranephric space, the perinephric space, and the posterior paranephric space. The anterior paranephric space lies in direct relation to the posterior parietal peritoneum anteriorly, and the anterior layer of the perinephric (Gerota's) fascia posteriorly. This space contains the pancreas, the second portion of the duodenum, and the ascending and descending colons.

The perinephric space, which is bounded by Gerota's fascia, contains the adrenal glands, kidneys, renal vessels, and adrenal vessels, as well as lymphatic structures and perinephric fat. Although Gerota's fascia can occasionally be visualized on MRI, normal fascial compartments appear to be less constantly visualized than they are on x-ray CT.

The posterior paranephric space is bordered by the transversalis fascia posteriorly, and the perinephric fascia anteriorly. Laterally, it is bounded by the lateroconal fascia formed by the fusion of the transversalis fascia and the parietal peritoneum.

Adrenal Glands

Like the kidneys, the adrenal glands also lie within the perinephric space and are located superiorly and antero-

medially in relation to the kidneys. The right adrenal gland is situated more superiorly than the left adrenal gland. It lies dorsal to the inferior vena cava and is supported laterally by the liver and medially by the right diaphragmatic crus. The right adrenal gland typically assumes an inverted V or comma-shaped appearance on the cross-axial views (Fig. 14–13A, B).[46–48] The left adrenal gland is bounded inferolaterally by the splenic vein and tail of the pancreas, and medially by the diaphragmatic crus. On axial views, the left adrenal gland typically assumes an inverted V or Y configuration, although a triangular appearance is also common.[46] On T1-weighted spin-echo images, the adrenal glands appear to be of intermediate signal intensity and are well contrasted by surrounding fat.[49, 50] Differentiation of the adrenal cortex from the medulla is generally not possible on routine spin-echo images. On T2-weighted images, the normal adrenal glands decrease in signal intensity and appear isointense with liver.

Kidneys

The improved contrast resolution of MRI permits separate visualization of the renal cortex and medulla on both T1- and T2-weighted images.[1, 51] On the short TR/TE T1-weighted images, renal cortex appears brighter than the renal medulla because of its shorter T1 relaxation time (Fig. 14–13). Corticomedullary differentiation on T1-weighted MR spin-echo images is commonly observed, although it may be more difficult to discern in patients with poor hydration or those examined with spin-echo pulse sequences providing only minimal T1 weighting.[52] The calyces are generally not well visualized on MRI, although in some patients, particularly those with extra-renal pelves, the renal pelvis may be visualized as a low signal intensity structure on the short TR/TE images (Fig. 14–13D), and of relatively high signal on the long TR/TE images. Visualizations of the cortex, medulla, and renal pelvis are all significantly enhanced by the use of para-magnetic contrast agents such as gadolinium DTPA, which also shows promise as an indicator of renal function.[65] Fat in the renal sinus may be easily identified as regions of relatively increased signal on both T1- and T2-weighted images. The renal arteries lying posteriorly in relationship to the renal veins may be visualized, although in older individuals they are commonly tortuous and difficult to demonstrate throughout their entire course (Fig. 14–13C). The renal veins cross anteromedially and drain into the inferior vena cava. These are commonly identified on the spin-echo images as regions of decreased signal; on gradient-echo images these vascular structures commonly demonstrate high signal because of flow-related enhancement (Fig. 14–13D). The usefulness of MRI in evaluating renal disease has recently been summarized.[64]

Para-aortic lymph nodes may be visualized on MR images, particularly when they are enlarged and measure greater than 1 cm. Lymph nodes are best visualized on the short TR/TE images when they contrast easily with surrounding fat. On long TR/TE images, such contrast may be decreased and lymph nodes may be more difficult to identify. In general, the criteria most useful in assessing lymph node status are related to size. Signal intensity has not proven useful,[53] in that both reactive or inflammatory lymph nodes, as well as lymph nodes containing malignant tumor, may exhibit an overlapping range of signal intensities on the T2-weighted images.

Male Pelvis

Bladder

The bladder lies in the anterosuperior portion of the pelvic cavity. The bladder is separated anteriorly from the pubic rami by the fatty Retzius' space. Superiorly, the bladder is enveloped by peritoneum, which continues posteriorly and is then reflected onto the anterior surface of the rectum. The fatty space between the bladder and rectum is known as the rectovesical pouch. The bladder is surrounded by perivesical fat; laterally, it is bordered by the obturator internus muscles and inferiorly by the prostate gland. The bladder is best evaluated on MRI in moderate distention. Typically, the wall of the distended normal bladder is approximately 2 to 3 mm thick. On T1-weighted images, the bladder wall is of intermediate signal intensity and commonly is poorly visualized. This results from a partial volume error due to averaging with surrounding urine that has low signal intensity (Fig. 14–14A). The wall of the bladder is best visualized on T2-weighted images. There it is seen as intermediate in signal intensity, separating the surrounding perivesical fat from the urine of relatively high signal intensity on the T2-weighted images (Fig. 14–14B). Estimating bladder wall thickness may be difficult because of chemical shift effect, which exaggerates the thickness of the wall along one side of the frequency-encoding direction and minimizes it along the other side in the same plane (Fig. 14–14B). Such thickening may also be observed normally near the bladder trigone. The bladder is well visualized in all planes. Definition of tumor extent in the direction of the pelvic sidewall is best achieved on serial axial images, whereas extension to the surrounding organs is best evaluated on sagittal views.

Prostate

Caudal to the bladder, lying between the pubis and the rectum, is the prostate. The prostate is oriented as an inverted pyramid. The base is just caudal to the bladder. On short TR/TE T1-weighted images, the signal intensity of the prostate approximates that of skeletal muscle and little intraparenchymal prostatic detail is visible on the images (Figs. 14–15A and 14–16A). On these short time pulse sequences, however, the relationships of the prostate to surrounding periprostatic fat, internal obturator muscles, and levator ani muscles are well demonstrated.[4]

On the T2-weighted images, considerable intraprostatic morphological detail is discernible[54–56] (Figs. 14–15B,C and 16B). Anterior to the intraprostatic urethra lies the anterior fibromuscular stroma, which has a relatively lower signal intensity. The peripheral zone, which constitutes approximately 70% to 75% of the glandular tissue in young males, occupies the caudal, lateral, and posterior portions of the prostate gland. On T2-weighted images, the peripheral zone of the prostate is relatively high in signal intensity and can be easily discerned in all planes. It is more conspicuous in older men.[68] In the more cranial portion of the gland, lying between the anterior fibromuscular stroma and the peripheral zone, is an area of intermediate signal intensity that presumably comprises the central, periurethral, and transitional zones, as described by Sommer and colleagues.[54] Aging leads to enlargement of this central glandular region, generally caused by the development of benign prostatic hyperplasia within the transitional and periurethral zones (Fig. 14–17). As a result, the heterogeneity of signal intensity increases. At present, it is not possible to separate the zonal components in the central glandular region on the basis of signal intensity changes.

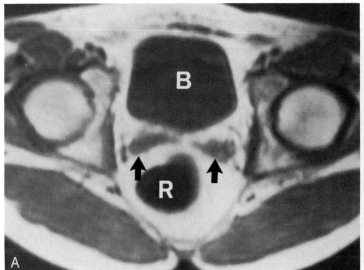
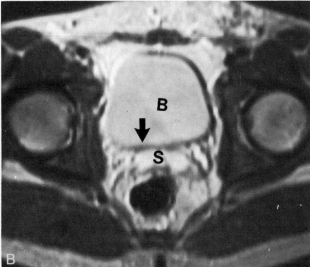

Figure 14–14. MR scan of the bladder, 1.5 T. A, T1-weighted (short TR/TE) axial scan was taken through the bladder (B). The urine in the bladder is of low signal intensity. The bladder wall is difficult to discern. The seminal vesicles (*arrows*) appear as ovoid structures of intermediate signal intensity. The rectum (R) is of low signal intensity because of the low proton density of intraluminal gas. B, Long TR/TE scan is shown. The urine in the bladder (B) is of high signal intensity because of its long T2. The seminal vesicles (S) are also of high signal intensity. The bladder wall is easily visualized posteriorly (*arrow*), although its lateral margins are difficult to discern, owing to associated chemical shift artifact.

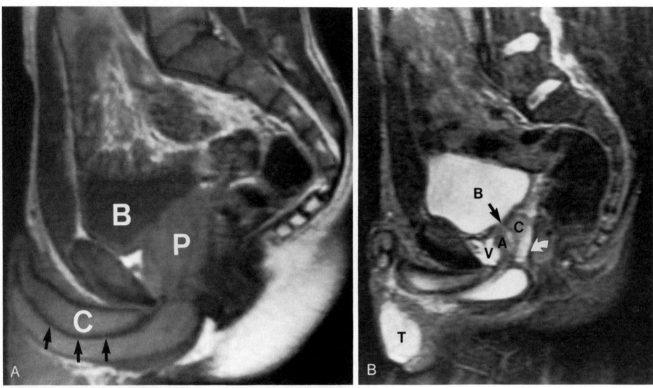

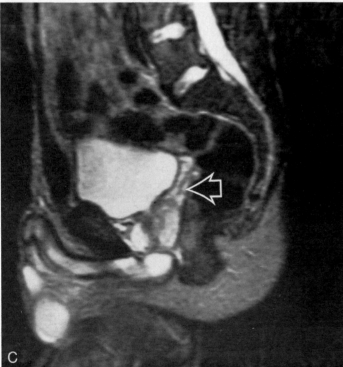

Figure 14–15. Prostatic anatomy, sagittal view, 1.5 T. *A,* T1-weighted (short TR/TE) sagittal scan through the midpelvis. The prostate (P) is an intermediate signal intensity structure identified posterior to the bladder (B). Little intraprostatic parenchymal detail is identified on this image. The corpus cavernosum (C) is of intermediate signal intensity and is surrounded by the lower-signal tunica albuginea (*arrows*). *B,* Midsagittal T2-weighted scan (long TR/TE image) shows high-signal urine in the bladder (B). The intraprostatic urethra is identified (*arrow*). Considerable intraprostatic parenchymal detail is present. The lower-signal anterior fibromuscular stroma (A) is noted anterior to the intraprostatic urethra. Posteriorly, the high-signal peripheral zone (*white arrow*) is identified. The central glandular portion (C) is posterior to the intraprostatic urethra and anterior to the peripheral zone. The anterior venous plexus (V) is noted outside the prostate margins. It is of high signal intensity in view of the slow flow in these venous structures. The normal high-signal testes (T) are also noted on the parasagittal images. The corpora cavernosa are increased in signal compared with Figure 14–15A. Note how the intervertebral discs have also become high signal intensity structures, owing to their water content. *C,* T2-weighted parasagittal scan slightly lateral to 14–15B again shows the intraprostatic detail. High signal in the seminal vesicle (*open arrow*) is readily apparent on the parasagittal view.

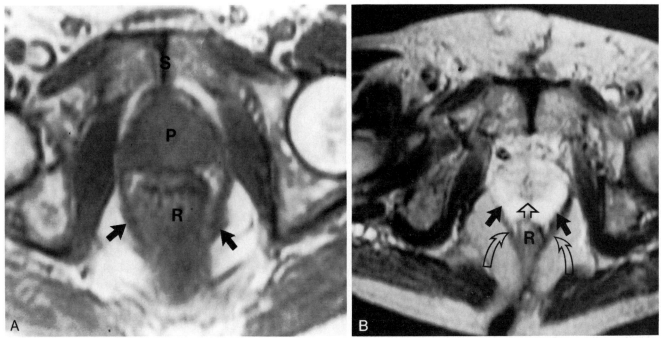

Figure 14—16. Prostatic anatomy (axial view), 1.5 T. *A*, T1-weighted image (short TR/TE) was taken at the level of the symphysis pubis (S). The prostate (P) is of intermediate signal intensity. No discernible intraprostatic detail is evident. The rectum (R) is identified immediately posterior to the rectum. The levator ani muscles are identified bilaterally (*arrows*). These are surrounded by the high-signal ischiorectal fat. *B*, T2-weighted (long TR/TE) axial scan is at the level of the symphysis pubis. The high-signal peripheral zone is identified (*short black arrows*) anterior to the rectum (R). The central gland (*open short arrow*) is heterogeneous, but of lower signal intensity. The levator ani muscles are identified bilaterally (*curved open arrows*).

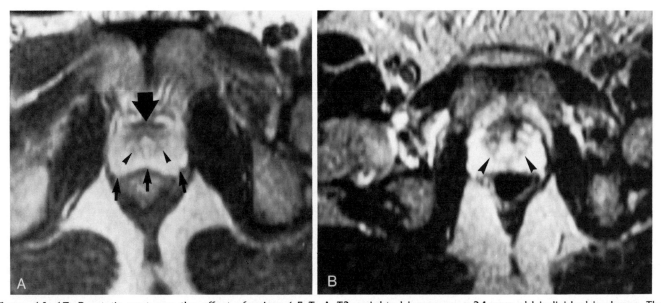

Figure 14—17. Prostatic anatomy: the effect of aging, 1.5 T. *A*, T2-weighted image on a 24-year-old individual is shown. The higher signal peripheral zone (*short arrows*) can be differentiated from the lower signal central portions of the gland (*arrowheads*). The dark fibromuscular stroma (*short fat arrow*) is identified anteriorly. *B*, In this T2-weighted image on a 65-year-old male, the gland is enlarged. There is increased heterogeneity of signal in the central gland (*arrowheads*), where round high-signal areas correspond to nodular BPH. The anterior fibromuscular stroma is thinned and is more difficult to discern.

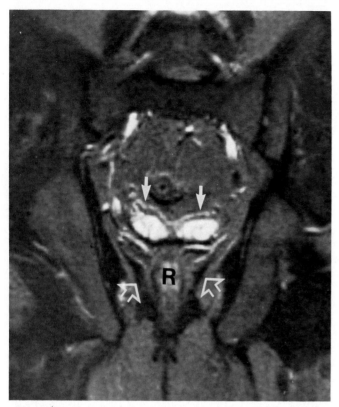

Figure 14–18. Coronal T2-weighted scan through the seminal vesicles. The paired ovoid seminal vesicles are high in signal intensity. Note the tubular convolutions within the seminal vesicles. The vasa deferentia may be identified bilaterally as intermediate signal intensity structures (*arrows*). Note the levator ani muscles (*open arrows*) and rectum (R).

The prostate is surrounded by a thin prostatic capsule that is typically not visualized by MRI. The vascular relationships about the prostate may be discerned. The neurovascular bundle is easily identified on axial views surrounding the prostate at the 5 o'clock and 7 o'clock positions.[55] Anteriorly, the anterior venous Santorini's plexus may be visualized on T2-weighted images as a region of high signal intensity due to the slow flow in the vascular plexus (see Fig. 14–15B). The axial plane clearly demonstrates the zonal architecture of the prostate and also serves to identify the relationships of the gland to surrounding fat and muscle. The relationships of the prostate to the bladder and the extension of prostatic tumors into the bladder are best demonstrated on sagittal images.

Posterior and superior to the prostate are the paired ovoid seminal vesicles. On T1-weighted images, the seminal vesicles are typically of intermediate signal intensity. They can be well differentiated from surrounding fat, from the bladder anteriorly, and from the rectum posteriorly (see Fig. 14–14A). On T2-weighted images, the seminal vesicles appear as symmetrical structures of high signal intensity. In some older individuals, the discrete convoluted tubules that constitute the seminal vesicles may be discerned (Fig. 14–18; see also Fig. 14–14B). Occasionally, the vas deferens may be identified as a structure of intermediate signal intensity on both the short TR/TE and the long TR/TE images as it traverses along the superomedial aspect of the seminal vesicles.

The penis consists of two corpora cavernosa and a single corpus spongiosum, which surround the urethra.

On short TR/TE (T1-weighted) images, the corpora are typically of the intermediate signal intensity and appear to be of somewhat higher signal intensity than skeletal muscle (Fig. 14–15C). On the T2-weighted images, both the corpora cavernosa and the corpus spongiosum demonstrate increased signal intensity, presumably because of the slow vascular flow (Fig. 14–19). Occasionally, in normal individuals, the corpora cavernosa may appear somewhat more intense than the corpus spongiosum on the T2-weighted images. The corpora are encased in a fibrous tunica albuginea, which appears as a rim of low signal intensity surrounding them. Alterations in normal corporal flow, such as that produced by cavernous thrombosis in priapism, are vividly demonstrated,[66] as are Peyronie's disease, hematomas, and tumor extension.[69]

Testes and Scrotum

The scrotum is the cutaneous pouch containing testes, portions of the vas deferens and epididymis, and the testicular vascular supply. Each ovoid testis is surrounded by fibrous capsule, the tunica albuginea. The testes are intermediate in signal intensity on the T1-weighted images and increase strikingly in signal intensity on the T2-weighted images (see Figs. 14–15 and 14–25).[57] This high-intensity signal provides a sensitive background against which testicular disorders of lower signal contrast markedly.[67] The epididymis surrounds the testis superiorly and posteriorly and contains some areolar or fatty tissue. The epididymis is intermediate on signal intensity in the T1-weighted image; however, on the T2-weighted image, it remains intermediate in signal intensity and may be readily differentiated from the testis. The vascular supply of the testes traverses the inguinal canal with the vas deferens. The testicular artery, and pampiniform venous plexus may be identified superior to the epididymis in the scrotum. Depending on the flow rates and pulse sequences used, it may appear of either low or high signal intensity.

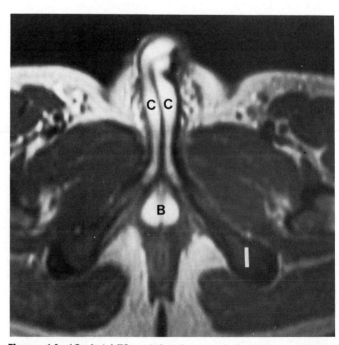

Figure 14–19. Axial T2-weighted image below the symphysis pubis. The ischium is identified (I). There is high signal intensity in the corpora cavernosa (CC) and in the bulb of the penis (B).

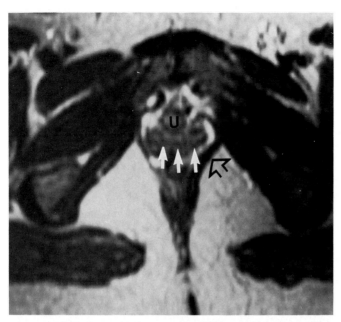

Figure 14–20. Vaginal anatomy: T2-weighted axial scan through the vagina. The intermediate signal urethra (U) is identified anteriorly. The higher-signal vaginal mucosa is surrounded by a lower-signal muscular wall (*white arrows*). High signal in the perivaginal venous plexus is also present. Note the levator ani (*open arrow*).

The vas deferens may be identified in the inguinal canal or as it enters the pelvis anteriorly to the bladder and courses across the dome of the bladder to enter the prostate. The vas deferens appears to be of low or intermediate signal intensity on both the short TR/TE and long TR/TE images.

Female Pelvis

Vagina

The vagina measures some 6 to 7 cm along its wall and approximately 9 cm along its dorsal surface.[6] It is best visualized in either the axial or sagittal planes. The vagina is commonly separated into two components: (1) the upper portion surrounding the uterine fornix, referred to as the vaginal wall, and (2) the lower portion, considered the body.

On short TR/TE pulse sequences (T1-weighted) the vagina is generally of intermediate signal intensity. Occasionally, some central increase in signal intensity is noted on the T1-weighted images, presumably as a result of proteinaceous vaginal secretions. On T2-weighted images, the vaginal mucosa and secretions appear as regions of increased signal intensity. The surrounding muscular and fibrous layers are relatively decreased in signal intensity, thereby providing a rim of decreased signal about the vagina (Fig. 14–20).

On sagittal sections, the relationship of the vagina to the anterior bladder and to the posterior rectum is easily demonstrable. The retropubic, retrovaginal, and perianal fat planes may also be demonstrated as regions of relatively high signal intensity on both short TR/TE and long TR/TE images.

On axial images below the base of the bladder, the empty vagina commonly assumes a crescentic orientation with anterior concavity. Anterior to the vagina, a round structure of intermediate signal intensity is identified on both long TR/TE and short TR/TE images. This is the urethra (Fig. 14–20). At the level of the bladder base, the vagina commonly assumes a more ovoid configuration. Axial scans above the bladder base commonly demonstrate the vagina as a crescentic structure with posterior concavity; this is caused by the posterolateral extension of the vaginal fornix. This symmetry may be distorted if a vaginal tampon has been placed to outline the anatomical confines of the vagina (Fig. 14–21).

Uterus and Uterine Cervix

The uterus is formed by the fusion of müllerian ducts and is extraperitoneal in location.[58] It is readily identified in all planes. Although often in the midline, it may be deviated to one side or the other. Normally the uterus is anterosuperior to the vagina. The uterus may assume a more anterior flexion (anteroflexion) (Fig. 14–22) or may lie posterior to the vagina (retroverted or retroflexed). In view of the variability of uterine orientation in the AP dimension, sagittal imaging is the plane most useful for its evaluation. The uterine fundus is typically superior to the bladder and is commonly seen in direct relation to the bladder wall on the sagittal views.

On the short TR/TE images (T1-weighted), the uterine signal intensity is generally equal to or slightly greater than striated muscle, and relatively little intraparenchymal detail is discernible. In approximately 50% of cases on the short TR/TE images, the endometrium can be identified as an area of slightly increased signal intensity

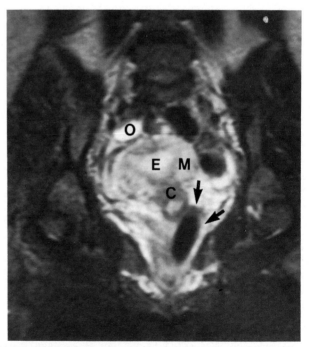

Figure 14–21. Coronal pelvic anatomy: T2-weighted image through the pelvis. A vaginal tampon has been placed and is extending into the left vaginal fornix (*arrows*). The lower signal cervix (C) is identified. The higher-signal endometrial cavity is noted (E), as is the higher signal portion of the myometrium (M), which is separated from the endometrial cavity by the lower-signal junctional zone. Also noted is the right ovary (O), which is high in signal intensity.

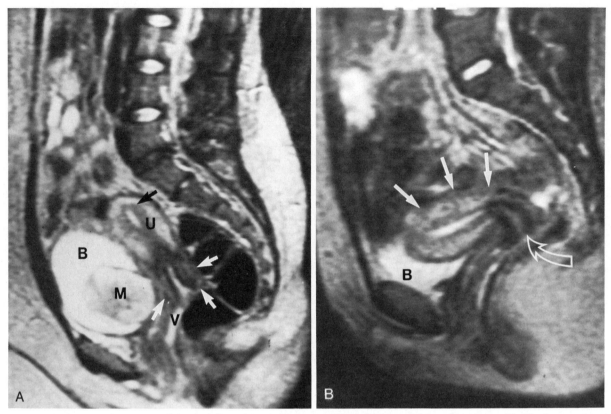

Figure 14–22. Sagittal midline scan of the female pelvis. *A,* High signal intensity is noted in the vagina (V). The lower signal cervix is readily identified (*white arrows*). The uterine zonal architecture within the uterus (U) is easily discerned. The low-signal junctional zone (*black arrow*) separates the high-signal endometrium from the more peripheral and high-signal myometrium. Also identified are the high signal in the bladder (B), and an intramural bladder mass (M), which proved to be a leiomyoma of the bladder. *B,* Anteverted uterus is seen in a T2-weighted sagittal image in a patient with an anteverted uterus. Anterior displacement of the uterine body and fundus (*white arrows*) has occurred. The uterine zonal architecture is visualized, as are the low-signal cervix and the higher-signal endocervical canal (*curved open arrow*). High signal intensity in the compressed bladder (B) is also demonstrated.

within the myometrium (Fig. 14–23). The short TR/TE images are generally most useful in ascertaining the relationships between the uterine wall and surrounding fat.

On the long TR/TE images (T2-weighted), intraparenchymal detail within the uterus is commonly discernible (Fig. 14–24; see also Figs. 14–21 and 14–22). Three distinct zones of different signal intensity are routinely identified within the uterus of women during their reproductive years. The most central is a region of high signal intensity, which represents the signal arising from the endometrium, from both the stratum basale and stratum functionale. Surrounding this area is a ring of relatively decreased signal intensity, referred to as the junctional zone. Originally believed to represent the stratum basale of the endometrium,[6] the zone has convincingly been demonstrated to represent the proximal portion of the myometrium.[59] The low signal arising within the junctional zone may be secondary to the vascularity of the proximal portion of the myometrium, or it may reflect the lower water content in the proximal myometrium.

The surrounding myometrium is homogeneous with relatively increased signal intensity, comparable to or greater than that of surrounding fat. Although skeletal muscle typically does not demonstrate increased signal on the long TR/TE images, Hricak and associates[6] have attributed this higher signal to the greater water content of smooth muscle relative to striated muscle.

The relative sizes of uterine zones on MRI images

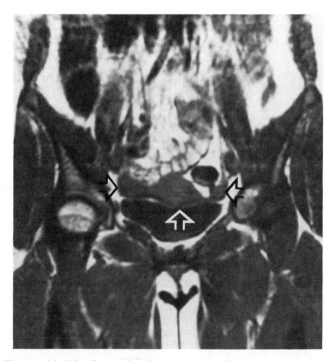

Figure 14–23. Coronal pelvic anatomy: T1-weighted image. The intermediate signal intensity uterus (*open white arrow*) is identified, immediately superior to the low-signal urine-filled bladder. Both ovaries (*open black arrows*) appear as intermediate signal intensity structures, bilaterally.

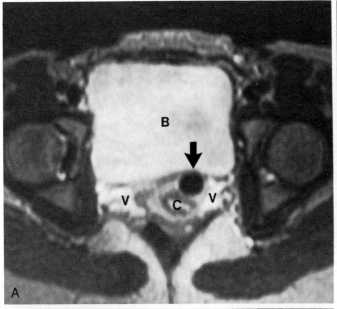

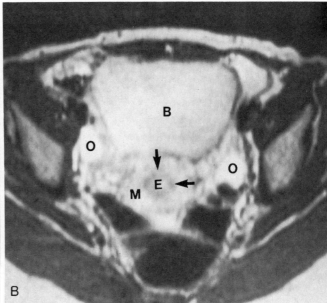

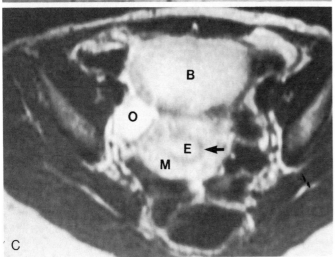

Figure 14–24. Axial T2-weighted imaging of the female pelvis. *A,* Axial T2-weighted scan at the level of the femoral heads. The high-signal bladder (B) is identified. A tampon lies in the left fornix of the vagina (*arrow*). The lower signal intensity cervix is identified and high signal is noted centrally (C). High signal in the paracervical vascular plexus is present (V). *B,* Axial scan 1 cm superior to that in *A.* High-signal ovaries (O) are noted bilaterally. The endometrium (E), peripheral myometrium (M), and lower-signal junctional zone (*arrows*) are noted. High signal is identified in the urine of the bladder (B). *C,* Axial T2-weighted scan 1 cm superior to that in *B,* scanned at the level of the uterine fundus. The high-signal endometrium is separated from the peripheral portions of the myometrium (M) by the low-signal junctional zone (*arrow*). The right ovary (O) is identified as a high signal intensity structure on the right. The bladder (B) is again noted.

depend on the patient's age, last menstrual period, and exogenous hormonal stimulation. In women of reproductive age, the high signal endometrium is 1 to 3 mm thick during the proliferative stage and increases to 5 to 7 mm thick during the midsecretory phase.[60, 61] This increase in the endometrium during the midsecretory phase is also accompanied by a slight increase in uterine volume and increased prominence in the junctional zone. Total uterine volume is greater throughout the menstrual cycle and is greatest in the midsecretory phase.

For women on oral contraceptives, the endometrium is often less than 3 mm thick or may not be visualized at all. In these women, cyclical changes are not as pronounced. Both premenarchal and postmenopausal uteri are small, typically with indistinct junctional zones and relatively thin endometrium.[60, 61]

The uterine cervix lies superiorly in relation to the vagina. On T1-weighted, short TR/TE images, the cervix is of intermediate signal intensity and can generally not be distinguished from the contiguous uterus. Occasionally, a central high-signal zone representing proteinaceous endocervical mucus may be identified.[59–61] On long TR/TE images, the anatomical confines of the cervix and its differentiation from the uterus and vagina are facilitated.

In view of its thick fibrous stroma, the cervix demonstrates a pronounced region of decreased signal immediately surrounding the central high signal of the mucosa and cervical mucus (Figs. 14–21 and 14–22).

The cervical parametrium is generally isointense with the cervix on the short TR/TE, T1-weighted images, but slow flow typically leads to the pericervical venous plexus showing relatively increased signal on the long TR/TE images (Fig. 14–24A).

The cardinal ligaments, the uterosacral ligaments, and the broad ligaments are the supporting or suspensory structures of the uterus.[58] As the cardinal and uterosacral ligaments are primarily thin condensations of extraperitoneal tissue, these are not routinely visualized. The broad ligament consists of peritoneum folding upon itself and enclosing the fallopian tubes. Adjacent to the uterine fundus, the two folds are closely opposed, whereas laterally the ligament assumes a more characteristic triangular appearance that may be visualized on parasagittal scans. The broad ligament can be generally recognized on MR images acquired in the coronal plane (Fig. 14–23). Recognition of the broad ligament facilitates the identification of the ovaries and adnexal lesions as well as their separation from uterine masses.

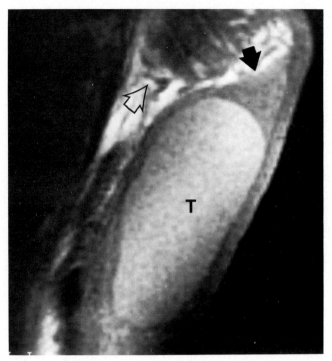

Figure 14–25. Surface coil examination of the testis: short TR/TE parasagittal scan (TR = 600 msec, TE = 20 msec), 1.5 T field strength. The testis (T) is of relatively high signal intensity. The intermediate signal intensity epididymis is identified superiorly (*closed arrow*). The pampiniform venous plexus is also identified (*open arrow*).

Ovaries

In the coronal plane it is usually possible to identify the ovaries by identifying the broad ligament and fallopian tubes and tracing these structures laterally (Fig. 14–23). As the ovaries are mobile, they may be found almost anywhere in the pelvis, including the cul-de-sac. Contiguous slice imaging may facilitate the recognition of the ovaries. In general, ovaries are most easily recognized in coronal and axial scan acquisitions. On short TR/TE images, the ovaries have a signal intensity, approximately equal to that of muscle. Typically, they are relatively homogeneous but may contain focal areas of increased or decreased signal. The areas of decreased signal may represent follicular cysts, while regions of focal increased signal on short TR/TE images may represent blood in corpus luteum cysts.[61]

On long TR/TE images, typically, the ovaries dramatically increase in signal (Fig. 14–24). They commonly have a signal intensity equal to or slightly greater than that of adjacent fat. In patients with follicular cysts, further increase in signal representing the cyst may be identified. Functional hemorrhagic cysts may demonstrate increased or decreased signal, depending on the age of the hemorrhagic collection.

The ovaries are on the posterior surface of the broad ligament; the fallopian tubes are located superiorly and somewhat medially. The ovary has two ligamentous supports. The first is the ovarian ligament, which attaches from the lower pole of the ovary to the uterine fundus and is located within the broad ligament. We have not been able to identify this structure discretely by MRI. The second attachment, the suspensory ligament, begins on the fascia overlying the external iliac vessels and psoas

muscle and attaches to the upper pole of the ovary. It is contiguous with the broad ligament and contains the ovarian vessels. On occasion this structure has been recognized on MRI images.

Vascular Relationships

The uterine artery, which arises from the internal iliac artery, is the major vascular supply of the uterus. It originates along the sidewall of the pelvis, then turns medially to cross along the cardinal ligament. It branches at the base of the broad ligament, near the cervix, and continues cephalad along the uterine body, as well as caudad toward the cervix and vagina. The uterine veins parallel the arterial structures. The ureter is medial to the internal iliac vessels. It traverses the cardinal ligament posterior and caudal to the uterine arteries. The ureter is typically of intermediate or low signal intensity on both the T1- and T2-weighted images, unless there is evidence of ureteral obstruction, in which case increased signal from the ureter may be observed on T2-weighted images. Flow effects also serve to separate the ureter from the uterine vessels on spin-echo sequences.

The ovaries receive a dual blood supply. The ovarian artery, which arises from the abdominal aorta, courses toward the ovary in the suspensory ligament. In addition, an ovarian branch of the uterine artery travels in the broad ligament from the uterus toward the ovary, as a second component of the ovarian blood supply.

The vaginal artery may arise from the uterine artery or the anterior portion of the internal iliac artery, or both. Surrounding the cervix and vagina is the uterovaginal venous plexus. These veins are the source of the serpiginous increased signal that surrounds the cervix, uterus, and vagina on long TR/TE images (Fig. 14–24).

An awareness of the vascular relationships and resulting signal intensity is useful in analyzing suspected uterine or adnexal masses.

Acknowledgment

The author acknowledges Marcy Kreamer for technical assistance in preparing the manuscript.

References

1. Hricak H, Crooks L, Sheldon P, Kaufman L: Nuclear magnetic resonance imaging of the kidney. Radiology 146:425–432, 1983.
2. Choyke PL, Kressel HY, Pollack HM, et al: Focal renal masses: Magnetic resonance imaging. Radiology 152:471–477, 1984.
3. Hricak H, Demas BE, Williams RD, et al: Magnetic resonance imaging in the diagnosis and staging of renal and perirenal neoplasms. Radiology 154:709–715, 1985.
4. Hricak H, Williams RD, Spring DB, et al: Anatomy and pathology of the male pelvis by magnetic resonance imaging. AJR 141:1101–1110, 1983.
5. Bryan PJ, Butler HE, LiPuma JP, et al: NMR scanning of the pelvis, initial experience with a 0.3 T system. AJR 141:1111–1118, 1983.
6. Hricak H, Alpers C, Crooks LE, et al: Magnetic resonance imaging of the female pelvis, initial experience. AJR 141:1119–1128, 1983.
7. Axel L: Surface coil magnetic resonance imaging. J Comput Assist Tomogr 8:381–384, 1984.
8. Schenck JF, Hart HR, Foster TH, et al: Improved MR imaging of the orbit with surface coils. AJR 144:1033, 1985.
9. Doornbos J, Grimbergen HAA, Booijen PE, et al: Application of

anatomically shaped surface coils in MRI at 0.5 T. Magn Reson Med 3:270–281, 1986.

10. Frahm J, Haase A, Matthaei D, et al: FLASH imaging rapid NMR imaging using low flip angle pulses. J Magn Res 67:258–266, 1986.

11. Frahm J, Haase A, Matthaei D: Rapid three-dimensional imaging using the FLASH technique. J Comput Assist Tomogr 10:363–368, 1986.

12. Bailes DR, Gilderdale DJ, Bydder GE, et al: Respiratory ordered phase encoding (ROPE): A method for reducing motion artifacts in MR imaging. J Comput Assist Tomogr 9:835, 1985.

13. Stark DD, Wittenberg J, Edelman RR, et al: Detection of hepatic metastases: Analysis of pulse sequence performance in MR imaging. Radiology 159:365–370, 1986.

14. Haacke EM, Lenz GW: Improving image quality in the presence of motion by using rephasing gradients. AJR 148:1251–1258, 1987.

15. Pattany PM, Phillips JJ, Chiu LC, et al: Motion artifact suppression techniques (MAST) for MR imaging. J Comput Assist Tomogr 11:369–377, 1987.

16. Glover GH, Pelc NJ: A rapid gated cine MRI technique. In Kressel HY (ed): Magnetic Resonance Annual 1988. New York, Raven Press, 1988.

17. Dixon WT: Simple proton spectroscopic imaging. Radiology 153:189–194, 1984.

18. Soila KP, Viamonte M, Starewicz PM: Chemical shift misregistration effect in magnetic resonance imaging. Radiology 153:819–820, 1987.

19. Weinreb JC, Brateman L, Babcock EE, et al: Chemical shift artifact in clinical magnetic resonance images at 0.35 T. AJR 145:183–185, 1985.

20. Lauterbur PC: Image formation of induced local interactions: Examples employing NMR. Nature 242:190–191, 1973.

21. Edelstein WA, Hutchinson JMS, Johnson G, Redpath TW: Spin warp NMR imaging and application to whole body imaging. Phys Med Biol 25:751–756, 1980.

22. Hart HR, Bottomley PA, Edelstein WA, et al: Nuclear magnetic resonance imaging: Contrast-to-noise ratio as a function of strength of the magnetic field. AJR 141:1195–1201, 1983.

23. Hanley P: Superconducting and resistive magnets in NMR scanning. In Witcofski RL, Karstaedt N, Partain CL (eds): NMR Imaging. Winston-Salem, Bowman Gray School of Medicine, 1982.

24. Dinsmore RE, Wismer GL, Levine RL, et al: Magnetic resonance imaging of the heart—positioning and gradient angle selection for optimal imaging planes. AJR 143:1135, 1984.

25. Schenck JR: High resolution imaging with surface coils. In Kressel HY (ed): Magnetic Resonance Annual 1986. New York, Raven Press, 1986.

26. Edelman RR, McFarland E, Stark DD, et al: High resolution surface coil magnetic resonance of abdominal viscera I. Theory, technique and initial results. Radiology 157:425–430, 1985.

27. Wehrli FW, MacFall JR, Glover GH, et al: The dependence of nuclear magnetic resonance (NMR) image contrast on intrinsic and pulse sequence timing parameters. Magn Res Imag 2:3–16, 1984.

28. Wehrli FW, MacFall JR, Shutts D, et al: Mechanisms of contrast in NMR imaging. J Comput Assist Tomogr 8:369–380, 1984.

29. Bydder GM, Yound IT: MRI clinical use of the inversion recovery sequence. J Comput Assist Tomogr 9:659–675, 1985.

30. Buxton RB, Edelman RR, Rosen BR, et al: Contrast in rapid MRI T1 and T2 weighted imaging. J Comput Assist Tomogr 11:7–16, 1987.

31. Edelman RR, Hahn PF, Buxton R, et al: Rapid MR imaging with suspended respiration: Clinical application in the liver. Radiology 161:125–131, 1986.

32. Axel L, Summers RM, Kressel HY, Charles C: Respiratory effects in 2DFT MR imaging. Radiology 160:795–801, 1986.

33. Schultz CL, Alfidi RJ, Nelson AD, et al: Effect of motion on two-dimensional Fourier transformation magnetic resonance images. Radiology 152:117–121, 1984.

34. Wood ML, Henkelman RM: MR imaging artifacts from periodic motion. Med Phys 12:143–151, 1985.

35. Runge VM, Clanton JA, Partain CL, James EA Jr: Respiratory gating in magnetic resonance imaging at 0.5 tesla. Radiology 151:521–523, 1984.

36. Ehman RL, McNamara MT, Pallack M, et al: Magnetic resonance imaging with gating: Techniques and advantages. AJR 143:1175–1182, 1985.

37. Stark DD, Hendrick RE, Hahn PF, et al: Motion artifact reduction with fast spin echo imaging. Radiology 164:183–191, 1987.

38. Reinig JW, Dwyer AJ, Miller DL, et al: Liver metastases detection: Comparative sensitivities of MR imaging and CT scanning. Radiology 162:43–47, 1987.

39. Spritzer CE, Baker ME, Blinder RA, et al: Comparison of short repetition time (TR)/echo time (TE) and long TR/TE spin echo pulse sequences for detecting hepatic metastases at 1.5 T. Chicago, Proc 73rd Scient Assembl Ann Meet Radiol Soc North Am, pp 202, 1987.

40. Axel L: Blood flow effects in magnetic resonance imaging. AJR 143:1157–1166, 1984.

41. Bradley WG, Waluch V: Blood flow: Magnetic resonance imaging. Radiology 154:443–450, 1985.

42. Waluch V, Bradley WG: NMR even echo rephasing in slow laminar flow. J Comput Assist Tomogr 8:594–598, 1984.

43. Felmlee JP, Ehman RL: Spatial presaturation: A method for suppressing flow artifacts and improving of vascular anatomy in MR imaging. Radiology 164:559–564, 1987.

44. Meyers MA: Dynamic radiology of the abdomen: Normal and pathologic anatomy. Berlin, Springer-Verlag, pp 113–194, 1976.

45. Raptopoulos V, Kleinman PK, Marks S, et al: Renal fascial pathways: Posterior extension of pancreatic effusions within the pararenal space. Radiology 158:367–374, 1986.

46. Montagne JP, Kressel HY, Korobkin M, Moss AA: Computed tomography of the normal adrenal glands. AJR 130:903–966, 1978.

47. Reynes CJ, Churchill R, Moncada R, Love L: Computed tomography of the adrenal glands. Radiol Clin North Am 17:91–104, 1979.

48. Karstaedt N, Sagel SS, Stanley RJ, et al: Computed tomography of the adrenal gland. Radiology 129:723–730, 1978.

49. Moon KL, Hricak H, Crooks LE, et al: Nuclear magnetic resonance imaging of the adrenal gland: A preliminary report. Radiology 147:155–160, 1983.

50. White EM, Edelman RR, Stark DD, et al: Surface coil MR imaging of abdominal viscera: Part II. The adrenal glands. Radiology 157:431–436, 1985.

51. LiPuma JP: Magnetic resonance imaging of the kidney. Radiol Clin North Am 22:925–941, 1984.

52. Demas B, Thurnher S, Hricak H: The kidney, adrenal gland and retroperitoneum. In Higgins CB, Hricak H (eds): Magnetic Resonance Imaging of the Body. New York, Raven Press, pp 373–401, 1987.

53. Lee JKT, Heiken JP, Ling D, et al: Magnetic resonance imaging of abdominal and pelvic lymphadenopathy. Radiology 153:181–188, 1984.

54. Sommer FG, McNeal JE, Carrol CL: MR depiction of zonal anatomy of the prostate at 1.5 T. J Comput Assist Tomogr 10:983–989, 1986.

55. Phillips ME, Kressel HY, Spritzer CE, et al: Normal prostate and adjacent structures: MR imaging at 1.5 T. Radiology 164:381–386, 1987.

56. Hricak H, Dooms GC, McNeal JE, et al: MR imaging of the prostate gland: Normal anatomy. AJR 248:51–58, 1987.

57. Baker LL, Hajek PC, Burkhard TK, et al: MR imaging of the scrotum: Normal anatomy. Radiology 163:89–92, 1987.

58. Hollinshead W: Anatomy for Surgeons, 2nd Ed. New York, Harper & Row, 1971, pp 788–819.

59. Lee JKT, Gersell DJ, Balfe DM, et al: The uterus: In vitro MR-anatomic correlations of normal and abnormal specimens. Radiology 157:175–179, 1985.

60. Demas BE, Hricak H, Jaffe RB: Uterine MR imaging: Effects of hormonal stimulation. Radiology 159:123–126, 1986.

61. McCarthy S, Tauber C, Gore J, et al: Female pelvic anatomy: MR assessment of variations during the menstrual cycle and with the use of oral contraceptives. Radiology 160:119–123, 1986.

62. Stark D, Bradley WG: Magnetic Resonance Imaging. St Louis, CV Mosby Company, 1987.

63. Partain CL, Price RR, Patton JA, et al: Magnetic Resonance Imaging. Philadelphia, WB Saunders Company, 1988.

64. Choyke PL, Pollack HM: The role of MRI in diseases of the kidney. Radiol Clin North Am 26:617, 1988.

65. Kikinis R, von Shulthess GK, Jäger P, et al: Normal and hydronephrotic kidney: Evaluation of renal function with contrast-enhanced MR imaging. Radiology 165:837, 1987.

66. Kimball DA, Yuh WTC, Farner RM: MR diagnosis of penile thrombosis. J Comput Assist Tomogr 12:604, 1988.

67. Thurnher S, Hricak H, Carroll PR, et al: Imaging the testis: Comparison between MR imaging and US. Radiology 167:631, 1988.

68. Allen KS, Kressel HY, Arger PH, Pollack HM: Age-related changes of the prostate: evaluation by MR imaging. AJR 152:77, 1989.

69. Hricak H, Marotti M, Gilbert TJ, et al: Normal penile anatomy and abnomal penile conditions: Evaluation with MR imaging. Radiology 169:683, 1988.

15 Angiography of the Genitourinary Tract: Techniques and Applications

JOSEPH J. BOOKSTEIN

You can't hit 'em if you can't see 'em
Attributed to various sources, originally in reference to the pitching skills of Walter Johnson, of the early 1900s.

Modern angiography may be traced back to the middle 1950s, when development of the following key techniques and devices matured within a relatively few years: image amplifiers, reliable serial changers, relatively safe contrast agents, pressure injectors, catheters, and Seldinger's technique for percutaneous catheterization.[1] The clinical value of renal angiography soon became apparent, particularly in the study of renovascular hypertension[2] or renal mass lesions.[3] In the United States at that time, most renal angiography was still performed by intravenous or translumbar techniques; quality was ludicrously poor by the standards of today, and the studies were stressful and hazardous. Since then, renal angiography has undergone remarkable improvement. High-quality arteriograms now depict arteries as small as 150μm, and images of glomeruli are usually apparent on magnification studies. Small catheters and modern contrast agents have made the technique safe enough for outpatient use.

In angiography, perfect is barely tolerable. Every compromise in performance or interpretation may carry a price of diagnostic error, incorrectly planned management, morbidity, or even mortality.

INDICATIONS

Angiography is indicated for a wide variety of diseases of the kidney and, to a lesser extent, for diseases of other genitourinary organs. Recognized indications for angiography (or catheterization) of genitourinary vessels may be classified as shown in Table 15–1.

SPACE REQUIREMENTS AND LAYOUT OF AN ANGIOGRAPHY SUITE

Recommended room sizes for an angiography suite have increased considerably in the past decade. Larger equipment, such as the new U arms (Fig. 15–1), requires more space than older equipment. More complicated procedures require larger tables for setting up, and space for accessory equipment. The angiography room itself should be at least 20 × 30 feet; in addition, a control booth (at least ~8 × 12 feet) must be attached, from which the angiography room can be broadly viewed. Immediately adjacent should be a preparation room (~8 × 12 feet), dark room (~8 × 10 feet), and reading room (at least ~10 × 12 feet). Within the angiography room, and also nearby, must be abundant storage facilities. Thus, at least 1000 square feet must be set aside for a modern angiographic facility.

Table 15–1. Classification of Indications for Angiography (or Catheterization) of Genitourinary Vessels.

Renal Arteriography

Renovascular hypertension: diagnosis, determination of cause, evaluation of hemodynamic significance, determination of suitability for surgery or transluminal angioplasty, and performance of transluminal angioplasty
Renal masses: determination of presence, differential diagnosis, evaluation of operability, transcatheter therapy
Renal donors: suitability, arterial number and anatomy
Hematuria: diagnosis and occasional treatment
Renal trauma: determination of presence and extent, possible transcatheter therapy of hemorrhage
Unexplained acute renal failure: exclude renal venous or arterial obstruction, acute tubular necrosis, DIC (disseminated intravascular coagulation)
Suspected vascular diseases of small renal vessels: i.e., polyarteritis nodosa, intravascular coagulopathy
Suspected renoparenchymal hypertension
Transplant dysfunction: exclude arterial stenosis, rejection
Unusual renal parenchymal disorders: i.e., medullary cystic disease, xanthogranulomatous pyelonephritis
Chronic renal failure: diagnosis of cause (rarely), possible transcatheter renal ablation
Miscellaneous (i.e., suspected acute arterial obstruction, arterial mapping, anomalous kidneys, intraoperative and prior to partial nephrectomy)

Renal Phlebography

Suspected renal vein thrombosis
Exclude tumor invasion of renal vein
Unexplained hematuria (search for renal and ureteral varices)
Sampling for renal vein renin concentration
Confirm diagnosis of renal agenesis
Renal vein abnormalities after transplant
Confirm patency of spleno-renal shunts; evaluate suitability

Penile Angiography (Impotence)

Pharmacoarteriography
Pharmacocavernosography
Pharmacocavernosometry

Adrenal Angiography

Phlebography (and sampling) for diagnosis of small tumor, differentiation of tumor from hyperplasia; transcatheter therapy
Arteriography: evaluation of large tumors

Testicular Angiography

Varicocele; phlebography for diagnosis and transcatheter therapy
Undescended testis: arteriography or phlebography for diagnosis of presence of testis, and localization
Suspected testicular tumor (obsolete)

Ovarian Angiography

Sampling for localization of hormonally active tumor
Pelvic congestion syndrome
Ovarian arteriography for tumor (obsolete)

Pelvic Arteriography

Localization and therapy of hemorrhage
Staging of pelvic neoplasms

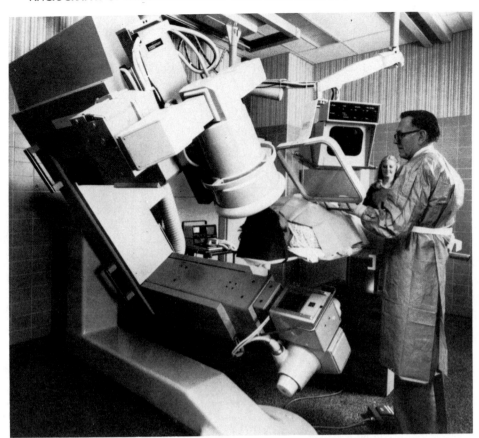

Figure 15–1. Basic angiographic assembly. One of several types of L-U carriage systems for cut-film angiography. These units allow (1) rapid exchange between image amplifier and cut-film changer, without moving the patient; (2) opportunity for complex oblique projections along any axis; (3) opportunity for installation of a second plane (not shown here). The L arm in this case pivots about a vertical axis, while the U arm pivots around a horizontal axis. (Courtesy Robert Barrazzo, General Electric Corporation.)

RADIOGRAPHIC EQUIPMENT

As of 1985, the cost of a fully equipped angiography suite was well over $1,000,000. The basic radiographic equipment required for genitourinary angiography consists of at least an 800 mA three-phase generator, a double-focus x-ray tube with a small focal spot of 0.1 to 0.3 mm and a large focal spot of about 1 mm, a single 14 × 14-inch serial cut-film changer, a 9-inch image intensifier and television chain, and a movable angiographic table. (Of course, most angiography suites are not designed exclusively for genitourinary angiography and will require other pieces of equipment, such as a long-leg changer for lower-extremity arteriography and biplane changers for neuroangiography.) Serial changers may be either the larger AOT capable of six exposures per second, or the flatter Puck or Cannon changer, capable of four frames per second.

The following list of equipment for use in the genitourinary system is presented in the order of decreasing importance. This list is necessarily subjective and based on my prejudices, developed since 1959.

1. Facilities for magnification are essential and should be a fundamental component of any angiographic facility. Direct magnification radiography markedly increases resolution (Fig. 15–2)[4] and is necessary in evaluating the following: small vessels of the kidney, penis, and other organs; small collateral vessels; renal parenchymal disorders; and disorders in children. The additional resolution is often of crucial clinical value and *in almost every case reveals some features that are not apparent on the non-magnified studies.* The x-ray tube should be specially selected to assure that the small focal spot is truly small; power capacity should be at least 4 kW for a 0.1- to 0.2-mm spot, and 11 kW for a 0.3-mm spot. Rare earth screen-film combinations are highly advantageous, and allow significant reductions in tube output. The table must be capable of elevation and/or the film changer must be capable of depression so that target–object distance and object–film distance can simultaneously be increased to at least 50 cm each. I find that a rotating grid adds appreciably to the quality of the magnified images,[5] but this item is no longer commercially available, and if desired must be custom made.

2. The newly available U-arm configurations are highly desirable (see Fig. 15–1). With the film changer mounted on one limb of the U arm, the patient need not be moved over a film changer for arteriography; rather, the position of the changer can simply and rapidly be exchanged for that of the image amplifier, and then replaced after the radiographic series has been obtained. The U-arm system, in conjunction with rotation of the apex of the U arm via an L arm, allows easy performance of multiple complicated angulated views without moving the patient. Such views are often helpful in visualizing the origins of the renal arteries (right posterior oblique [RPO] view), separating overlapping segmental branches and catheterizing smaller branches for transcatheter therapy. If multiple views of an organ are desired during a single injection, the U arm can be rotated during filming, especially in combination with recording on a 100-mm camera. U arms are also very useful during extravascular interventional procedures.

3. Methods should be available for freezing the fluoroscopic image of the opacified vascular system on the television monitor while live fluoroscopy is displayed on the same monitor (reversed densities), or on an adjacent monitor. This technique, called road mapping, facilitates

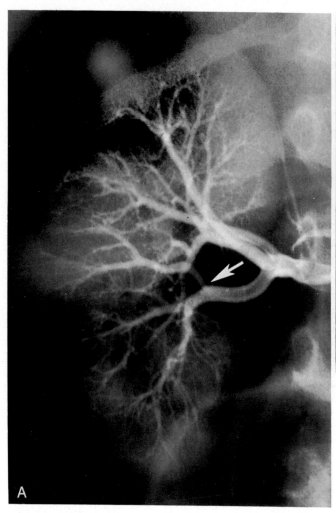

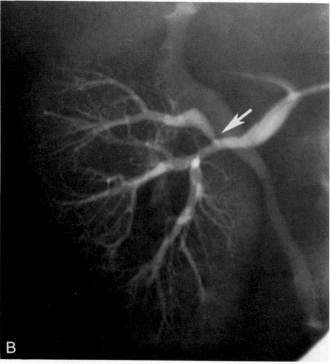

Figure 15–2. Value of selectivity, and cut-film magnification techniques. Five-year-old boy with renovascular hypertension due to segmental stenosis. The stenosis was not seen on aortography. *A*, Selective arteriogram, × 1.5 magnification. Suspected segmental stenosis at arrow. *B*, Magnification × 4 showing definite stenosis of segmental branch, with post-stenotic dilation. Patient was cured after nephrectomy.

Figure 15–3. Quality of recording obtainable with 105-mm camera. Hypertension and renal failure after renal transplantation. Transplanted kidney with anastomotic stenosis (*arrow*). Note the reasonable demonstration of the segmental branches, in comparison with the digital study of Figure 15–4*A*.

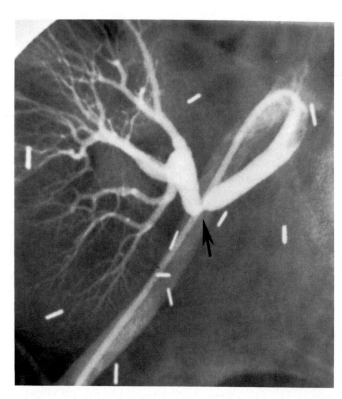

difficult catheterizations by simultaneously demonstrating the position of the catheter and the target artery during fluoroscopy.

4. A spot-film camera is often desirable. It allows quick image recording without the need for loading the large 14 × 14-inch magazines. Image quality is usually sufficient, particularly for interventional procedures, and usually it is better than that provided by digital subtraction techniques (Fig. 15–3). This equipment costs about $35,000, approximately one-seventh the cost of digital equipment.

5. High-resolution television chains are available with 1024 × 1024 matrices (rather than the conventional 525 × 525). Disadvantages include additional cost of about $25,000, and quadrupling of the required radiation. The high-resolution systems facilitate the use of fine catheters and guide wires and the catheterization of small arteries, such as the internal pudendal arteries, for penile angiography. When used with digital subtraction, these high-resolution packages may improve the quality of the final image.

6. Assuming that $250,000 in funds remain, a digital subtraction system may be added. In my opinion, vital information is usually sacrificed when film recording is replaced with digital recording systems (Fig. 15–4), and I believe such equipment will eventually be used infrequently for genitourinary angiography. Some investigators, however, do recommend digital techniques for a variety of indications in the genitourinary system, particularly in screening for renovascular hypertension. Furthermore, digital equipment is used increasingly for other purposes involving the vascular system, so that it will likely become standard equipment in most modern angiography suites.

7. Biplane filming is sometimes an advantage in renal angiography, although much less so than in neuroangiography or thoracic angiography. Nevertheless, many angiography suites are equipped in the biplane configuration, which can occasionally be exploited for renal studies. Biplane filming is commonly employed during arteriography of abdominal aortic aneurysms, in evaluating the positions of renal ostia relative to the aneurysm, and during inferior vena cavography.

In addition to radiographic equipment, the angiography suite must have a great variety of supporting facilities and equipment: outlets for oxygen and suction, space for

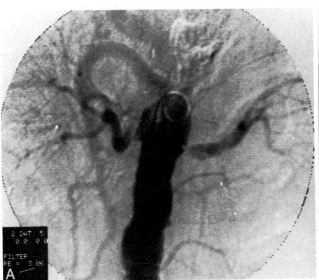

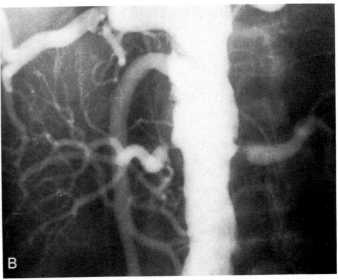

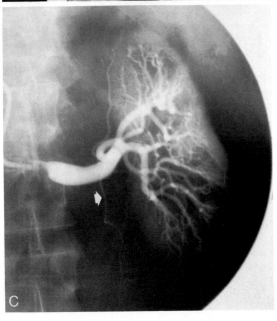

Figure 15–4. Comparison of intra-arterial digital injection with film aortography, and selective arteriography. *A,* Digital arteriogram (30 ml contrast material, 15% iodine [4.5 gm iodine]) suggests bilateral stenoses at the renal artery orifices. On the left, it is difficult to decide whether the plaque is situated within the renal artery (and is therefore more amenable to balloon angioplasty), or whether it involves the aorta at the renal origin (and is therefore less suitable for angioplasty). *B,* Conventional aortogram (30 ml contrast, 37% iodine [11.1 gm iodine]) in the same patient corroborates the digital impression. However, the following additional important information is present: (1) the stenoses can be seen to involve primarily the renal arteries, rather than the aorta, and therefore can be dilated with a better chance of success, and (2) the segmental branches are much better seen on the right, excluding coexistent segmental disease. *C,* The selective injection (6 ml contrast, 37% iodine [2.2 gm iodine]), most clearly shows the anatomy, excludes coexistent left segmental disease, and shows orthograde flow in poststenotic extraparenchymal branches (*arrow*). This branch was no longer visible after acetylcholine vasodilation, confirming the hemodynamic significance of the stenosis (see Chapter 71 for explanation).

anesthesia, facilities for physiological and ECG monitoring, surgical lamps and some surgical equipment, equipment for management of emergency conditions and reactions, and communications facilities.

CATHETER MATERIALS, GUIDE WIRES

A panoply of equipment is now available to serve the needs of angiography. Habit and experience often determine the selection of specific items, and the recommendations below reflect personal bias. I still prepare and steam shape many catheters from purchased rolls of polyethylene material; pink Formocath is still a favorite (OD 2.2 mm; ID 1.2 mm, Becton-Dickinson), offering a good combination of "shapability," visibility, and torque control. Forming one's own catheters has several advantages: Catheter shapes can be better customized, particularly after the patient's anatomy is ascertained. Cost is decreased, relative to that of preshaped catheters, and catheter inventory may be minimized. The process also promotes understanding of the relationship between arterial anatomy, proper catheter shape, and physical properties—information vital to a vascular radiology training program.

Nevertheless, the trend is certainly toward use of commercially prepared catheters, 5 F or smaller, often with wires incorporated into the wall for greater torque control. For abdominal aortography, catheters usually need be no larger than 5 F. When fabricated from thin-walled low-friction materials, such catheters can conduct warmed 76% contrast agents at flow rates up to about 25 ml/second. Pigtail configurations are acceptable (Fig. 15–5); however, the pigtail sometimes opens and deposits contrast subintimally or selectively into visceral or lumbar arteries. Consequently, I prefer straight catheters with multiple side holes.

For selective work, thin-walled small catheters facilitate catheterization of small arteries (i.e., segmental renals), or passage into distal vessels (i.e., the distal testicular vein). Thicker-walled catheters, with or without wires, augment torque control and are helpful in exerting sufficient downward traction when reversed-curve catheters (Simmons or Mikaelsson, Fig. 15–6B, E, F) are used. Catheter shapes and sizes are further selected based on the specific organ undergoing angiography.

Guide wires have improved greatly in reliability and maneuverability. During my very first percutaneous procedure, the guide wire broke secondary to repeated kinking after attempted passage through a tortuous iliac artery. At that time, the guides were constructed without the central safety wire that is now generally available. My preference is a 0.035-inch wire with a very floppy (Bentson) tip.

Deflector wires are a mandatory staple of an angiography suite (Fig. 15–5). To my knowledge, these wires are manufactured exclusively by Cook Incorporated, Bloomington, Indiana. By deflecting the guide wire within a catheter, and then feeding the catheter off the bent wire, catheters can be advanced much farther around bends than would otherwise be possible. The deflector wires are particularly useful in reforming reversed-curve catheters (i.e., the Simmons or Mikaelsson shapes).

Special torque-control guide wires are now available, composed of a relatively stiff body and a flexible, curved

distal tip. They can be obtained in sizes as small as 0.014 inch, although for conventional subselective renal work (i.e., during subselective embolization), 0.025 inch is small enough.

With regard to needles, a simple coaxial system suffices, with or without a Cournand extension. The usual needle size is 18 gauge. However, when 5-F catheter systems are used, a 19-gauge needle may reduce the frequency of paracatheter leak.

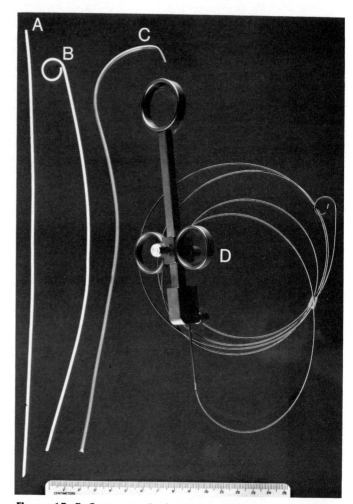

Figure 15–5. Some standard commercial equipment for basic angiography. *A*, Straight 5 F catheter with multiple small side holes near the tip (holes are invisible on this reproduction). The high-flow characteristics of these small catheters allow flow rates in the range of 24 ml/second. *B*, Pigtail catheter of same material, used for aortography. The pigtail configuration directs the contrast material more laterally than a straight catheter, often producing better opacification of the renal arteries with less obscuration by intestinal branches. These tips may straighten during injection and rarely deposit contrast subintimally or into an undesired branch. *C*, "Visceral cobra" shape, used by some for selective renal arteriography. In small calibers, these catheters have a strong tendency to recoil from the renal artery. (The author prefers to shape his own catheters for renal arteriography, as in Fig. 15–6.) *D*, A deflector guide (Cook, Inc., Bloomington, Indiana). This device is extremely helpful for reforming Simmons curves, feeding catheters out into subselective positions, passing catheters around the aortic bifurcation, and other functions. The distal tip bends variably as the finger grip is pulled (position shown), thus altering the bend on the catheter. When the handle is released, the tip will straighten.

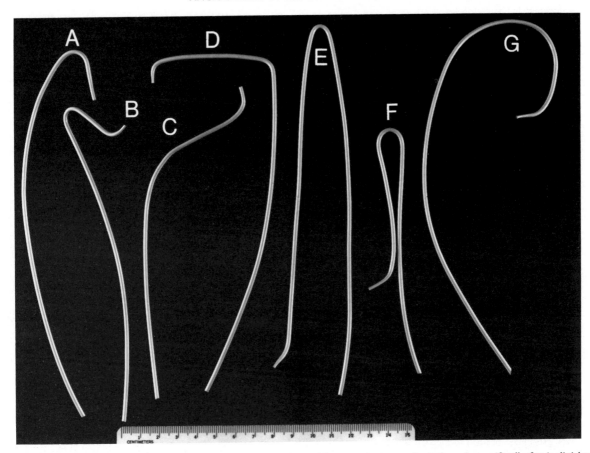

Figure 15–6. An assortment of polyethylene catheters steam shaped from catheters rolls, tailored specifically for individual arterial branch patterns. *A*, Standard J-shaped renal artery catheter. The J shape resists expulsion from the renal artery during injection. However, the catheter size must fit the aorta reasonably well. If the J is too long, catheterization of the renal artery is difficult and may produce dissection; if too short, recoil is still possible. From apex to tip is usually 2 to 2.5 cm. *B*, The short reversed curve. Basically, this is used to catheterize small branches arising from the abdominal aorta, i.e., adrenal or testicular artery. It is also useful to prevent excessive distal entry into a renal artery, as, for example, if a branch arises proximally or if one wants to remain proximal to an atherosclerotic stenosis. May be used for right adrenal phlebography. *C*, Left adrenal vein catheter. *D*, Right adrenal vein catheter. *E*, Long reversed. Used for engaging and distal passage into contralateral internal iliac, internal pudendal artery, or any other internal iliac branch, i.e., transplant arteriography, penile arteriography, transcatheter embolization for bleeding. *F*, Medium reversed. Used for engaging and distal passage into ipsilateral internal iliac, internal pudendal or other internal iliac branch. With slight anterior direction of distal tip, used for engaging the right gonadal vein from the inferior vena cava. *G*, Large cochlear. Used for entry into and passage down the left gonadal vein. Also useful for retrograde passage from one iliac around the bifurcation into the other.

EQUIPMENT FOR PEDIATRIC STUDIES

Percutaneous puncture of the femoral artery or vein can be accomplished in infants as small as 4 to 5 pounds, although such punctures are difficult. The infants should be immobilized on a board, with the pelvis extended by placing padding under the buttocks. The infants can be under light anesthesia, but sedation with one of several pharmacological mixtures is often adequate. Currently, meperidine hydrochloride (Demerol) 2mg/kg, chlorpromazine (Thorazine) 1 mg/kg, and promethazine hydrochloride (Phenergan) 1 mg/kg, mixed in one syringe, and injected intramuscularly is preferred. In my experience, the most difficult group is children 5 to 8 years of age; with such patients I generally welcome the assistance of an anesthesiologist.

Progressively smaller needles, catheters, and guide wires are now available that greatly increase the simplicity and safety of catheterization in the pediatric age group. For infants, I generally use a 20-gauge needle in conjunc-tion with a *flexible* 0.021-inch guide wire and a 3.9 or 4 F catheter. Three-French and smaller sizes are available, but these are needed only rarely, and in premature infants. Although small volumes of contrast agents are used in these small patients, a high injection rate must be maintained because of the rapid circulation. For example, in an 8-pound infant an abdominal aortogram can be performed with about 3 ml of contrast medium (Conray—28% iodine), but the injection rate should be about 6 ml/second (i.e., an injection time of only about 0.5 second). The rate of filming should also be rapid, that is, 3/second during the first 2 to 3 seconds.

In newborns, the umbilical artery often provides a convenient access route. This artery can frequently be recannulated for up to 1 week after birth, and when patent, is preferred. Using the umbilical approach, I have performed selective renal arteriograms in patients as light as 3 pounds (28 weeks premature) (Fig. 15–7). Direct magnification is indispensible in small children (Figs. 15–2 and 15–7).

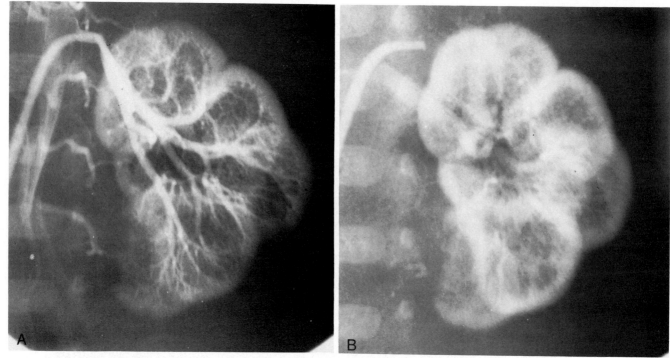

Figure 15–7. Arteriography facilitated by small catheters and magnification in a 3-lb, 29-week premature infant with suspected renal vein thrombosis. *A*, Selective catheterization with a 3.7 F catheter passed retrograde from the umbilical artery. One ml of contrast material (Conray-60) was injected in 0.5 seconds, with × 5 magnification filming. Despite some blurring, the interlobar, arcuate, and even interlobular arteries can be visualized. *B*, Nephrogram phase 1 second after *A*. Note clearly demarcated corticomedullary junction and prominent fetal lobation. (From Bookstein JJ, Clark RN: Renal Microvascular Disease: Angiographic-Micrographic Correlates. Boston, Little, Brown & Company, 1980.)

CONTRAST AGENTS

Despite continuing improvement, contrast agents remain somewhat nephrotoxic, and the desire for high contrast must always be balanced against kidney (and patient) tolerance. The incidence of significant impairment of renal function after radiographic contrast administration is between 0.6% and 1.4% among patients with normal renal function.[6-9] Pre-existing renal insufficiency is the single most important risk factor; in such patients, reversible renal failure occurred in 15% to 44% in three series.[6-8] Other risk factors include diabetes mellitus, multiple myeloma, dehydration, large doses of contrast agent, and repeated examinations within a short interval. I generally perform aortography with diatrizoate mixtures (i.e., Renografin, Angiovist) containing about 37% iodine. Renal arteriography can also be performed with this concentration of contrast medium if the volumes are moderate (i.e., ~8 ml). Alternatively, renal arteriography can be performed with media containing as little as 28% iodine (i.e., Conray-60). For abdominal aortic aneurysms, and most phlebography, the less concentrated agents are preferable. For selective internal pudendal arteriography, I use 37% iopamidol to reduce discomfort. For cavernosography, half-diluted Conray-60 is used (14% iodine).

The risk of nephrotoxicity can be reduced markedly by hydrating the patient immediately before and during angiography.[9, 10] Eisenberg and coworkers[10] hydrated their patients with normal saline before, during, and after the procedure, and reported no instances of acute renal failure in 537 patients undergoing angiography. Our hydration protocol requires that the patient drink two glasses of water orally the morning of examination. Whenever the use of more than 50 ml of contrast material is anticipated, the protocol also requires infusion of 250 ml/hour of one-half normal saline for 2 hours before and during the procedure, as well as for two hours after it.

Within the past few years, several contrast agents of low osmolality have been introduced for clinical use, including the nonionic agent iopamidol, and the dimer ioxaglate (Hexabrix). These contrast agents are less toxic, in general, than their diatrizoate or iothalamate predecessors.[11, 12] Although it seems reasonable to presume that these agents will also prove to be less nephrotoxic, reduced nephrotoxicity has to date been difficult to demonstrate.[13-16]

In patients with a history of significant prior contrast reaction, we generally pretreat with prednisone for 24 to 48 hours at a dose of 80 mg/day. Patients also receive an H_1 and H_2 blockade: hydroxyzine (Vistaril), 50 mg TID, and cimetidine, 300 mg TID, each 1 day before and the morning of the examination. The newer low-osmolality contrast agents are less allergenic than conventional contrast agents, and they can often be used without reactions in patients with a history of severe and repeated reactions to ionic contrast medium.[21, 22]

APPROACHES

The Retrograde Femoral Approach

By far, most genitourinary angiography is performed via a retrograde femoral approach. This is the simplest and safest method, and can usually be performed even when the femoral pulses are moderately reduced, or the iliac arteries are tortuous. There are many wrong ways to puncture a femoral artery, but only one or at most a few correct ways. The puncture site should be made within a few millimeters of the inguinal crease; this is usually the area of greatest palpability of the artery and where the artery generally runs a fairly straight course. I do not find fluoroscopic localization of bony landmarks to be helpful. After generous local infiltration of the superior and both lateral aspects of the artery with 2% lidocaine, a needle-cannula combination is advanced through both walls. Extreme concentration, almost to the point of self-hypnosis, is sometimes necessary in puncturing small deep arteries. The needle should enter the artery at about 45 degrees and should be imagined to be within a vertical plane that includes the course of the target artery. Two fingers mark the position and course of the artery at the anticipated point of arterial entry, cephalad to the skin puncture site. The arterial spurt is encountered upon slow withdrawal of the needle.

When the arterial flow from the needle is brisk, a guide wire, usually a very flexible (Bentson) type is advanced into the abdominal aorta. The Bentson type wire usually negotiates very tortuous iliacs; for the rare failure, a dilator with a slight bend can be advanced to a point just distal to the guide-wire tip, from which enough leverage is usually provided to facilitate passage of the guide wire into the aorta.

For aortography, I prefer a 5 or 6 F straight catheter with multiple side holes near the tip. The pigtail catheters are also acceptable; potential problems with this type are mentioned above. For renal arteriography, the catheter tip should be placed at the upper level of the most proximal renal artery. A strong Valsalva maneuver for about 8 seconds before injection decreases cardiac output to about half, and produces much denser vascular opacification.

The Axillary Approach

If the femoral approach is not feasible, one must choose from a variety of much less acceptable approaches. Trans-axillary catheterization is usually feasible, unless there is compromise of the involved axillary pulse. The left axillary approach is easier and, because it avoids the carotid system, safer than the right. However, the axillary approach is associated with a major risk of bleeding around the axillary sheath, with secondary severe chronic pain and nerve deficit.[23] Great care must be taken to properly compress the puncture site after catheter withdrawal, to apply a pressure dressing, and to keep the arm immobilized in a sling for 24 to 48 hours. The patient must be followed closely for 24 hours after angiography to detect increasing pain or sensory or motor deficits. *Should signs of nerve deficit develop, prompt exploration and decompression of the axillary sheath are mandatory.* Rarely, periaxillary hemorrhage may develop days after the procedure.

Passage of the catheter into the descending aorta from the axillary artery may sometimes be difficult. Judicious use of a sharply curved C-shaped initial catheter, flexible guide wires, deflector wires, and proper training and experience almost always lead to success.

Translumbar Aortography

The translumbar needle approach has largely been supplanted by catheter techniques—and for good reason. Translumbar aortography offers little opportunity for multiple injections or various projections; it does not allow selectivity, and the danger of serious intramural injection is always present. Femoral catheterization is faster, safer, more comfortable, and generally far preferable. In some instances in which the retrograde femoral approach is not feasible (i.e., distal aortic thrombosis), a distal translumbar aortogram is also not feasible. Although a catheter can be exchanged for the translumbar needle, by means of the Seldinger technique, such a maneuver is sometimes difficult, and is infrequently indicated. Translumbar aortography may be considered largely obsolete.

SPECIAL RADIOGRAPHIC TECHNIQUES

Digital Arteriography

Image quality of digital arteriography is inferior to conventional, selective, or magnification angiography, and represents a compromise that I find generally unacceptable for abdominal angiography. The purported cost savings frequently evaporate into costs of maintenance, costs of repeated injections, or costs of conventional arteriography that may be subsequently required. The presumed safety increment afforded by small intra-arterial doses of contrast agent becomes less important when renal protection techniques, such as hydration and non-ionic contrast agents, are used. Outpatient studies can be performed with approximately equal ease, using either film or digital recording systems.

Digital arteriography is performed by subtracting video arteriographic images from preliminary images without vascular opacification. The differences are electronically amplified and displayed as a video image of the vascular tree only (see Fig. 15–4).[24] The digital technique provides excellent contrast resolution, but spatial resolution compares unfavorably to film recording.

When contrast medium is injected from a peripheral or central vein or the right atrium (IV digital subtraction angiography [DSA]), about 40 ml of relatively concentrated agent (i.e., Renografin-76, 37% iodine) injected within about 2 seconds is required. A number of factors combine to limit the quality of IV digital renal arteriography, such as excessive contrast dilution in patients with prolonged circulation times, overlapping vessels, and patient and bowel motion. Repeat injections are often required, and the IV procedure is progressively losing favor for abdominal vascular imaging. Better quality with less contrast medium can be achieved with the intra-arterial (IA) approach. A common IA dose for renal DSA is 30 ml of contrast medium, containing only 15% iodine, injected within 2 seconds. This quantity of iodine is approximately one-third that required for conventional aortography or IV DSA.

Intra-arterial DSA, however, also has major disadvantages, primarily due to inherent limitation of the spatial resolution of ordinary video systems. *The limited resolution assumes clinical significance in the majority of cases.*

For example, fine ridges of fibromuscular dysplasia sometimes can not be resolved digitally, and the diagnosis may be missed. Visualization of the small renal vessels, which are important in evaluating parenchymal diseases, renovascular hypertension, and collateral flow, is usually inadequate on digital studies. Field sizes are often too small to allow visualization of both kidneys on one injection; larger field sizes can be obtained, but at considerable sacrifice in terms of equipment cost, resolution, and/or radiation dose.

Direct Magnification Techniques

The principles of magnification radiography are now widely appreciated.[4, 5] The image is enlarged by increasing the object–film distance relative to target–object distance. In order to reduce penumbra and geometric unsharpness, the focal spot must be very small. The lowest practical focal spot size for abdominal work is about 0.1 mm. To ascertain that a focal spot is appropriate for magnification, its behavior under simulated clinical conditions should be evaluated. The changes in focal spot size with increasing mA, variation in kV, and variations with focusing (bias) voltage are well known.[25, 26] A line pair phantom, such as the Siemens star (Fig. 15–8) makes an excellent test object for evaluating focal spot behavior. To test focal spot size, an exposure of the test pattern should be made over nonscreen film using the magnification clinically desired, and without interposition of scattering medium. The star is utilized in seeking areas of phase shift in the pattern of lines and spaces. The frequency of line pairs in the region of phase shift can be determined from the following formula:

$$\text{Line pairs/mm} = \frac{360 \times \text{magnification}}{\text{degrees of wedge} \times 2 \times 3.14 \times \text{diameter}}$$

For example, if the Siemens star has black wedges of 1.5 degrees, and the points of phase shift describe a circle of diameter 18 mm on the image, and magnification is × 3, then the line pairs/mm resolved equals

$$\text{Line pairs/mm} = \frac{360 \times 3}{1.5 \times 2 \times 3.14 \times 18 \text{ mm}}$$
$$= 6.37 \text{ line pairs/mm}$$

It is convenient to express the focal spot size in terms of its effective size, which can be evaluated by the number of line pairs resolved on magnification films, as follows:

$$\text{Effective focal spot size} = \frac{\text{magnification}}{(\text{magnification minus 1}) \times \text{line pairs/mm} \times 2}$$

A good 0.3-mm nominal focal spot should have an effective size of less than 0.15 mm by this technique. The figure obtained indicates the focal spot dimension perpendicular to the lines of the phantom.

Conventional radiography of phantoms will resolve about two line pairs/mm. With a good 0.3-mm focal spot, and using × 2 magnification, four or more line pairs/mm should be resolved. With a good 0.1-mm focal spot, low mA, proper kV, and magnification of × 3 to × 5, more than 10 line pairs/mm can be resolved (Fig. 15–8). By way of comparison, a 9-inch image amplifier in combination with a 512 × 512 matrix is theoretically capable of resolving slightly over one line pair/mm.

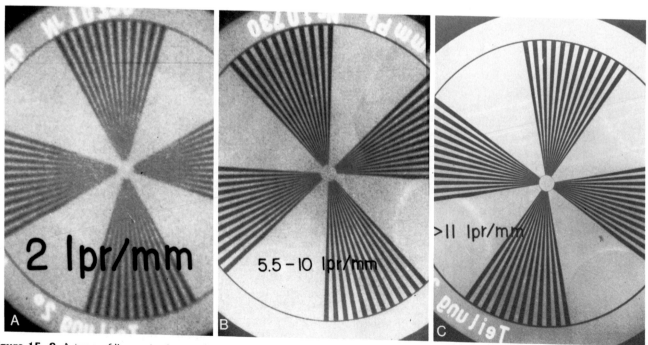

Figure 15–8. A type of line-pair phantom (the Siemen's star) useful in comparing the resolution of various radiographic recording systems and in quality-control procedures. *A,* With a conventional film system, and a 1-mm focal spot, only two line pairs per ml can be resolved in a 16-cm water phantom. *B,* Using a 0.1-mm focal spot, and ×3 magnification, 5.5 to 10 line pairs per ml can be resolved under the same conditions. *C,* Same as *B,* except the phantom is in air. Scatter is reduced, contrast is enhanced, and 11 line pairs per mm can be resolved. (*A–C* from Bookstein JJ, Clark RN: Renal Microvascular Disease: Angiographic-Micrographic Correlates. Boston, Little, Brown & Company, 1980.)

Pharmacoangiography

In conjunction with angiography, vasodilator or vaso-constrictive agents may be injected in order to alter the usual distribution of contrast flow. The most common indications for use of genitourinary *vasoconstrictor* angiography are

1. Diversion of contrast medium into a renal tumor.[27]
2. Evaluation of the hemodynamic significance of a demonstrated renal artery stenosis.[28] (See Chapter 71.)
3. Decreasing renal arterial blood flow to augment the quality of renal phlebography.[29]

The most common indications for genitourinary *vasodilator* pharmacoangiography are

1. Evaluation of the hemodynamic significance of a demonstrated renal artery stenosis.[28] (See Chapter 71.)
2. Penile arteriography, in order to overcome constriction of the penile arteries.
3. Cavernosography with papaverine and regitine, in order to activate the veno-occlusive mechanism.

The most commonly used vasoconstrictor agent for renal arteriography is epinephrine. The dose varies, depending on whether slight or major decrease in blood flow is desired. About 3 μg are used for evaluating the hemodynamic significance of stenoses, 3 to 10 μg for evaluating tumors, and about 20 μg to stop arterial flow during phlebography.[27-29] The epinephrine is usually administered as a 2- to 3-ml bolus, dissolved in saline, and followed by injection of contrast agent within about 10 seconds. Angiotensin II is the most potent vasoconstrictor agent on a weight basis, and 0.25 to 1 μg into the renal artery produces marked slowing of blood flow.[30] In my experience, angiotensin II seems to constrict only the smaller intrarenal arteries, whereas epinephrine sometimes constricts the medium or large size vessels as well. Vasopressin (0.2 to 0.3 units) is also used.[31] Despite the differences in dose, there seems to be little basic difference in the diagnostic value of these various agents.

Several vasodilator drugs have been used in the renal bed. Acetylcholine is probably the most potent.[32, 33] I use 80 μg/minute for 5 minutes in evaluating the hemodynamic significance of stenoses, and sometimes in trying to bring out small arteriovenous malformations that might be responsible for hematuria. Other agents that have been used include bradykinin and glucagon.[31-33]

PERFORMANCE OF RENAL ANGIOGRAPHY

Details of performance of renal arteriography vary somewhat, depending on the indication and renal functional status. The following describes my technique in otherwise healthy patients suspected of having renovascular hypertension.

The patients are frequently studied on an outpatient basis. After catheterization of the aorta from a femoral artery (see earlier discussion), the renal arteries are identified fluoroscopically by a small hand injection of contrast medium, and the catheter tip is placed at the upper level of the highest visualized renal artery; 40 ml of contrast (approximately 37% iodine concentration) is injected at the rate of 20 ml/second, beginning after 8 seconds of Valsalva maneuver in the inspiratory position. The filming program is two/second for 3 seconds, one/

second for 1 second, and one/3 seconds for 9 seconds. The films are examined (Fig. 15–9A).

If the aortogram is completely normal and both kidneys are very well seen, no further films are obtained. If there is any question, however, selective × 2 to × 2.5 magnification arteriograms are performed (Figs. 15–9B, C, and 15–10), commonly in contralateral oblique projection to best demonstrate the segmental branches, and in expiration to demonstrate possible respiratory changes (Fig. 15–11). The catheter configuration is usually a J shape (see Fig. 15–6A), formed from thick-walled 6 to 6.5 F material to prevent recoil. The length from apex to tip is normally a few millimeters longer than the magnified diameter of the aorta, as seen on the control aortogram. Radius of curvature is about 5 mm, and angle of curvature about 135 degrees. There are no side or top holes. Such catheters are easily passed a short distance into the renal artery, and they tend not to recoil. A dose of 7 ml of about 76% contrast agent (~37% iodine), injected at a rate of 6 ml/second, is suitable in the average case. Alternatively, 9 ml of 60% contrast (~28% iodine) is acceptable, injected at the same rate. The sequence is the same as for aortography. The less concentrated solution is used in children, and volume is reduced in proportion to weight, according to the following formula:

$$ml = \frac{Kg}{2} + 1$$

The Normal Aortogram and Renal Arteriogram

Typically a single renal artery supplies each kidney. These arteries originate from the lateral aspects of the aorta at about the lower level of the first lumbar vertebral body (see Fig. 15–9). Considerable variation exists, however, with levels of origin varying between T12 and L2.[34] The caliber of single main renal arteries varies considerably with kidney size.[34] Luminal diameter, as determined angiographically, is 6.0 to 9.5 mm (mean 7.9 mm) in men, and 5 to 8 mm (mean, 6.4 mm) in women.[35] A supplemental renal artery is present in 20% to 30% of kidneys,[34] generally arising distal to and within 3 cm of the main renal artery. In older patients, the aorta rotates so that the right renal artery often arises from the right anterolateral aspect, while the left arises from the posterolateral aspect.

The main renal artery gives rise to primary ventral and dorsal rami, which pass anterior and posterior, respectively, to the renal pelvis. The ventral ramus tends to be larger than the dorsal and often represents a continuation of the main artery (see Figs. 15–4C, 15–9, and 15–14A) Branching patterns within the kidney vary considerably, but in general the ventral artery supplies the entire ventral and some dorsal cranial aspects of the kidney, while the dorsal artery supplies the mid dorsal region and variable portions of the dorsal caudal aspects. The ventral artery can be identified angiographically by tracing back from the branches that reach the lateral margin of the kidney in its midportion (see Fig. 15–9D, E).

Branches of the primary rami pass in the renal sinus, and are termed "segmental arteries" (see Fig. 15–9). Beyond the papillae, they penetrate the parenchyma, pass between medullary pyramids, and are termed "interlobar arteries." Interlobar arteries progressively

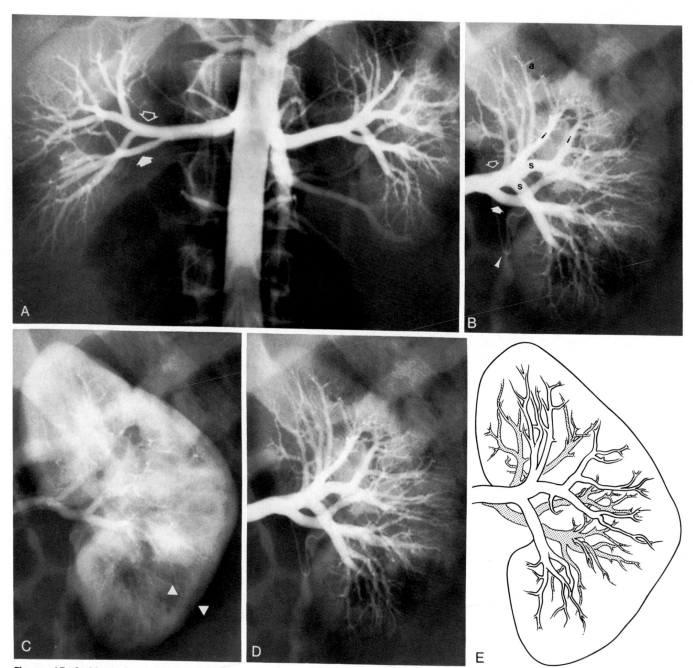

Figure 15–9. Normal donor renal arteriogram. *A*, Aortogram, using a pigtail catheter. Note limited proximal propagation of contrast medium, and preferential opacification of the renal arteries, due to the pigtail catheter configuration. A single renal artery is present bilaterally, originating at the usual level near the L1–2 interspace. The major continuation of the renal artery represents the ventral ramus (*hollow arrow*). The proximal branch (*solid arrow*) crosses branches of the ventral ramus, and therefore must represent a dorsal ramus. *B*, Selective injection with slight magnification again demonstrates on the left the ventral (*hollow arrow*) and dorsal (*solid arrow*) branches. Segmental (s), interlobar (i), and arcuate (a) branches are also indicated. A single extrarenal branch, a ureteropelvic artery (*arrowhead*) is seen. Observations regarding these extra-renal branches are very important in evaluating the hemodynamic significance of renal artery stenoses (see Chapter 71). *C*, Early nephrogram, showing smooth cortical outline, relative medullary lucency, and 8-mm cortical thickness (*between arrowheads*). *D*, Normal left renal arteriogram from another patient, AP projection. *E*, Diagrammatic representation of dorsal (*shaded*) and ventral (*unshaded*) systems. Note that ventral ramus is dominant, and sends branches to caudal, cranial, and middle poles, while the dorsal branch in this case supplies primarily cranial and middle poles. Terminal twigs of the ventral ramus reach more peripherally than do those of the dorsal.

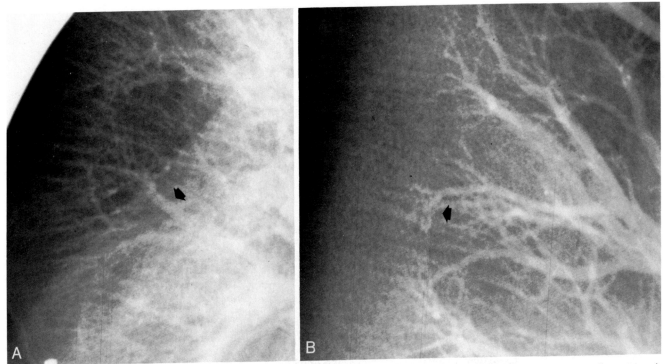

Figure 15–10. Normal cortical vascularity, transplant renal arteriogram, × 3 magnification. This patient had a transplant stenosis, and the magnification study served to exclude coexistent rejection. Slight delay in glomerular opacification, secondary to the arterial stenosis, allows better visualization of the interlobular arteries. *A,* An arcuate artery (*arrow*), and innumerable normal interlobular arteries are seen, excluding the presence of coexistent rejection. This type or resolution cannot be achieved with conventional nonmagnified arteriography, 105-mm, or digital systems. *B,* One second later, fine granularity becomes evident along the interlobular arteries, reflecting normal glomeruli. The arcuate artery (*arrow*) and dense cortical stain demarcate the cortex from medulla. (*A, B* from Bookstein JJ, Clark RN: Renal Microvascular Disease: Angiographic-Micrographic Correlates. Boston, Little, Brown & Company, 1980, pp 19–54.)

branch and taper and terminate in arcuate arteries, about 1 mm in diameter, which demarcate the corticomedullary junction. Arcuate arteries do not form a continuous subcortical arcade, and do not communicate with each other. Instead, they taper near the center of the renal pyramid, and terminate as interlobular arteries (see Fig. 15–10).

Along the course of the arcuate arteries, thousands of interlobular arteries arise, 75 to 200 μm in diameter, and pass through the cortex perpendicular to the corticomedullary junction. These arteries are sufficiently small and numerous as to be invisible on most conventional arteriograms, but they can be recognized as striae, representing overlapping arteries, on good-quality magnified arteriograms (see Fig. 15–10).[36]

The interlobular arteries give rise to about 20 afferent glomerular arterioles, each supplying one or more glomeruli. The afferent glomerular arterioles are invisible on clinical angiograms.

About 1.5 million glomeruli are in the normal kidney, distributed uniformly throught the entire cortex. Mean glomerular diameter in adults is about 300 μm, a size large enough to be visualized arteriographically. The number and cross-sectional area of glomeruli indicate approximately 10-fold overlap on two-dimensional projection. Good-quality magnified cortical images demonstrate during the late arterial phase a granular pattern that reflects, in a complicated manner, the presence of these overlapping glomeruli (see Fig. 15–10*B*).[36]

Beyond the glomeruli, efferent arterioles pursue one of two courses. Many of those originating from juxtame-

dullary glomeruli pass into the medulla and divide into bundles of vasa recta. The vasa recta are only 20 to 50 μm in diameter and cannot be discretely resolved on clinical angiograms, although they do contribute to the nephrographic density of the medulla. The efferent glomerular arterioles of the outer cortex do not contribute to the vasa recta but instead form a peritubular capillary plexus that nourishes the proximal and distal convoluted tubules.

The cortical peritubular capillaries drain via interlobular veins primarily toward the corticomedullary junction and coalesce to form arcuate veins. These smaller veins are not visible arteriographically, but may be seen on good-quality renal phlebograms (Fig. 15–12). Arcuate veins conduct flow sequentially into interlobar, segmental, and main renal veins. Numerous connections exist between interlobar veins, and between segmental veins; communications between arcuate veins are rare.[36] A single main renal vein is usually present at the upper level of L1; on the left, a second inferior, usually retroaortic, renal vein is present in about 11% of patients.[37]

The radiographic appearances secondary to selective injection of contrast medium into the renal artery have been traditionally divided into three phases: arterial, nephrographic, and venous. The arterial phase lasts about 2 seconds beyond termination of injection and demonstrates the vascular tree from the main renal artery to the interlobular arteries. Interlobular arteries usually opacify within 1 to 1.5 seconds after the onset of injection. In normals, interlobular arteries are almost immediately obscured by the granular densities of surrounding glo-

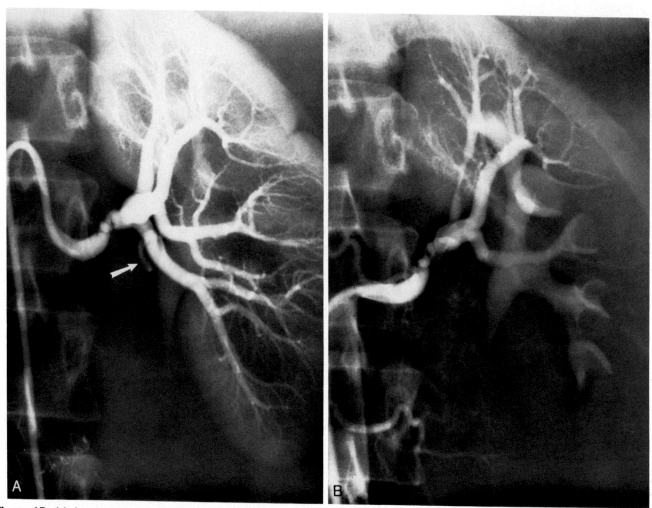

Figure 15–11. Inspiration and expiration arteriography, demonstrating changes in severity of stenosis, and changes in secondary manifestations of hemodynamic effects. *A,* Inspiratory film demonstrates moderately severe stenosis secondary to fibromuscular dysplasia. Orthograde flow is noted in a large potential collateral (*white arrow*). There is no significant retrograde flow into the aorta. *B,* Expiratory film demonstrates much more severe stenosis, with retrograde aortic flow at the same injection rate as *A.* Middle and lower pole renal arteries are no longer seen because they are being perfused entirely from collaterals, including the one indicated by the arrow in *A.* (*A, B* from Bookstein JJ, Walter JF: The role of abdominal radiography in hypertension secondary to renal or adrenal disease. Med Clin North Am 59: 169–200, 1975.)

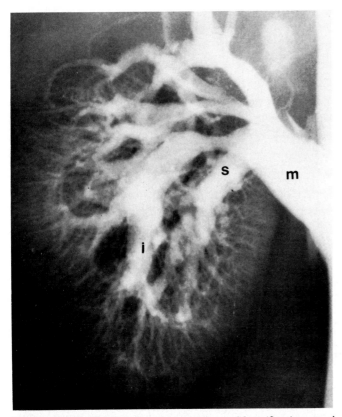

Figure 15–12. The renal venous anatomy. Magnification renal phlebogram after IA injection of epinephrine. The straight interlobular venules are seen joining arcuate veins. The appearance of arcuate venous arcades is illusory, and in the vast majority of cases represent overlap only. Progressively larger veins are termed interlobar (i), segmental (s), and main renal (m).

meruli (Fig. 15–10B). Contrast medium normally ascends in the interlobular arteries so rapidly that all levels of the cortex are opacified virtually simultaneously.

The nephrogram begins within 1.5 seconds after the onset of injection, reaches a maximum 2 seconds after termination of injection, and fades gradually over 15 or more seconds. The early nephrogram is largely attributable to opacification of microvascular structures below the resolution of the radiographic system, while the late nephrogram is increasingly attributable to contrast medium within the collecting tubules. The cortex is normally much more densely opacified than the medulla and is sharply demarcated from it. Cortical density reflects the large integrated sum of glomerular capacitance. Cortical thickness is usually approximately equal throughout both kidneys, except for some increase in the subhilar lip. Interindividual thickness in a series of normals, however, varied between 4.2 and 12 mm after correction for magnification.[36] Cortical invaginations (septa of Bertin) can be seen extending between the medullary pyramids in most cases (see Fig. 15–7). Fetal lobation may be quite prominent, but it can usually be distinguished from scar by noting that the lobation is between calyces and overlies the center of a septum of Bertin.

Renal veins are ordinarily only faintly opacified after arteriography (see Fig. 15–20B). The renal venous phase may begin as early as 4 seconds after the onset of selective injection and may persist for 6 to 10 seconds. The poor

but prolonged venous opacification partially reflects the varying rates of blood flow in the cortex, outer medulla, and inner medulla. In addition, approximately 20% of the contrast medium is filtered and therefore unavailable for venous opacification.[38]

In addition to branches to the renal parenchyma, nonparenchymal branches arise from the renal artery, including the inferior adrenal artery, multiple extrarenal capsular arteries, perforating capsular arteries that arise from the arcuates and perforate the cortex, arteries to the renal pelvis, and ureteral arteries. Noticing these arteries is important for a number of reasons, not the least of which is that they provide important collateral routes in the presence of renovascular hypertension (Figs. 15–13 to 15–15; see also Figs. 15–4C, 15–9C and 15–11A).[39] Pelvic branches course in the renal sinus and may provide collateral flow between segmental branches (Fig. 15–14C).[40] Ureteral arteries may be prominent in ureteral infections (Fig. 15–15). Capsular vessels may provide important information in perinephric infection and masses.

Principles Determining Injection Rates

Optimal demonstration of renal vascular morphology, and maximum nephrographic opacification, require an injection rate that approximates the rate of renal blood flow.[41] There is little purpose in injecting 8 ml/second into a diseased kidney that will accept only 1 ml/second. On the other hand, injection rates considerably less than the rate of blood flow result in excessive dilution and suboptimal vascular contrast. To estimate flow rate, the rapidity of passage of a small bolus of contrast medium is observed fluoroscopically, and subjectively compared with prior rates of flow in normals (~8 ml/second). Acceptable accuracy can be achieved after a little practice.

Physiological Determinations During Renal Angiography

The Spill-Over Flowmeter Technique

The rate of renal blood flow may be roughly estimated angiographically by the use of principles of the "spill-over technique."[42] A preliminary estimate of blood flow is made fluoroscopically, as above, and the injection rate is set to about this level. If the estimate has been accurate, then mild reflux into the aorta will occur during diastole, and this should be evident on the films. Reflux should disappear during systole, and this too will be manifested on films by intermittent absence of aortic reflux, and possibly by systolic dilution of injected contrast. The accuracy of this technique is reputed to be about ±25%, which seems to be acceptable for most clinical purposes.

Gross estimation of the rate of renal blood flow is of value under a variety of circumstances. Decreased renal arterial blood flow is a nonspecific manifestation of many renal parenchymal disorders. In acute tubular necrosis, for example, blood flow is commonly reduced to about 3 ml/second, and quantitation has some prognostic value. If blood flow is less than about 1 ml/second in a transplanted kidney, irreversible cortical necrosis is usually present. The corollary of these observations is also true:

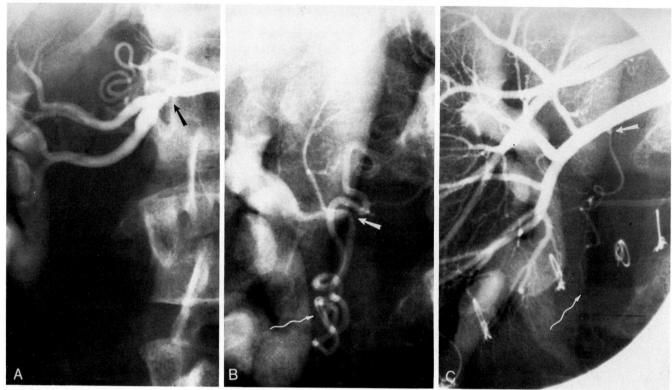

Figure 15–13. Value of observing extraparenchymal renal branches, in this case collateral arteries and preoperative collateral flow around a renal artery stenosis. *A,* The stenosis (*black arrow*) appears to be of moderate severity only, but the presence of collateral vessels *and* flow proves the hemodynamic significance of the stenosis. *B,* Conclusive demonstration of the presence of collateral *flow* requires demonstration of inflow into the renal artery beyond the stenosis (*arrow*). A dilution defect is noted in the ureteral artery (*tortuous arrow*), reflecting further collateral inflow into the ureteral collateral. *C,* Post-operative arteriogram, same magnification as *A* and *B.* The ureteral artery (*arrow*) no longer conducts collateral flow. Its caliber has decreased markedly. The branch previously conducting retrograde flow, and indicated by the tortuous arrow here and in *B,* now conducts contrast (and blood) in orthograde direction. (*A–C* from Bookstein JJ, Walter JF: The role of abdominal radiography in hypertension secondary to renal or adrenal disease. Med Clin North Am 59:169–200, 1975.)

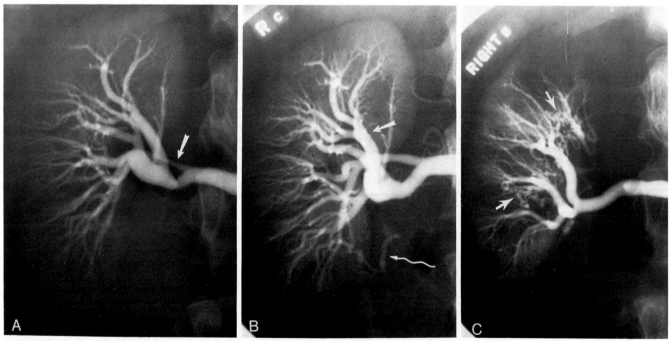

Figure 15–14. Demonstration of sinusoidal collateral vessels, and differentiation from tumor vessels. *A,* Segmental arterial stenosis (*arrow*), as commonly seen in the presence of parahilar renal pheochromocytoma. *B,* Repeat arteriogram after alpha-blockade with phenoxybenzamine demonstrates relief of vasospasm of the segmental branch and appearance of arterial flow (*tortuous arrow*) into the pheochromocytoma. The tumor vessels can be distinguished from collaterals by the fact that they carry blood away from the renal branches, rather than toward them, and by their inappropriate caliber. *C,* A segmental branch was unavoidably ligated during resection of the tumor (*arrow in B*). Now, a few months postoperatively, sinusoidal collaterals have developed (*small arrows*), conducting blood between segmental branches. (*A–C* from Velick WF, Bookstein JJ: Pheochromocytoma with reversible renal artery stenosis. AJR 132(6):294–296, 1978, © Am Roentgen Ray Soc., 1978.)

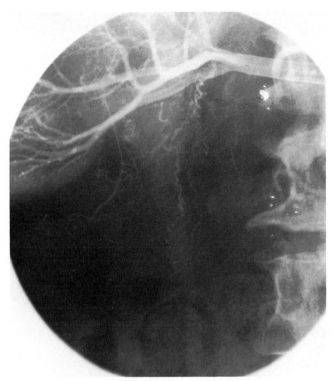

Figure 15–15. Prominent ureteral arteries in a patient with hematuria. Hypervascularity of the ureteropelvic junction was due to chronic inflammation. A faint calculus was visible at the ureteropelvic junction on the plain radiograph.

Preservation of renal blood flow can serve to exclude significant degrees of various parenchymal disorders. Decreased flow is a nonspecific response and may also be evident in conditions other than parenchymal disease, such as apprehension, hypotension, vasoconstrictive pharmacoangiography, and severe renal artery stenosis. Flow is occasionally increased, as in hypervascular tumor, large arteriovenous fistula or malformation, and after vasodilatory pharmacoangiography. By matching injection rate to estimated rate of blood flow, maximum angiographic quality can be derived from a given quantity of contrast agent. Estimations of renal blood flow are also helpful in determining amounts and rate of injection of embolic materials or alcohol.

I have found the accuracy of the spill-over technique sufficient for most clinical angiography. However, angiographic techniques are available that are reputed to provide more precise estimates, such as videodensitometry[43] and digital arteriography.[44, 45] Basically, these modalities may be used (1) to determine the linear velocity of the blood–bolus interface or (2) to calculate concentration curves after intravascular injection of known concentrations.[46] The most commonly used methods depend on determination of the linear velocity of advance of the blood–bolus interface within the renal artery, following aortic injection. Theoretically, the linear velocity of flow multiplied by the cross-sectional area of the artery will equal the volume of renal blood flow. The techniques, however, are fraught with pitfalls. First of all, the linear velocity of blood flow varies markedly between systole and diastole, so that the phase of the cardiac cycle during which the single measurement can be made is critical. Second, the renal artery may not be visualized orthogonally, so that actual linear progression may be greater than projected progression. Third, accurate determination of blood flow will depend on accurate determination of renal artery cross-sectional area throughout the length of observed bolus passage. Such an assessment is very difficult and assumes a nearly uniform caliber and circular cross-sectional contour. For all these reasons, precise angiographic measurement of renal blood flow by these methods is virtually impossible. In my own prior laboratory experience, the range of error was great. Although estimates were often within 10% of true flow rates, unpredictable errors of up to 100% were not uncommon. I have not yet found a simple clinical method that promises significantly greater reliability than the spill-over technique.

Pressure Determinations

Pressure gradients are routinely obtained across renal artery stenoses before and after transluminal angioplasty. I avoid such measurements in the usual diagnostic situation, because of the need for full heparinization before, and the risks of dissection or thrombosis during, catheter passage across an atherosclerotic stenosis. It must be recalled that pressure determinations under circumstances of antegrade trans-stenotic catheter passage may be grossly inaccurate. A catheter that occupies more than about 25% of the residual lumen will significantly exaggerate a pre-existing gradient or will be totally responsible for a measured gradient.[47] However, if one uses a catheter of 1-mm diameter (usually coaxial) for determining pressure gradient in a standard-sized (5 to 6 mm) renal artery, the presence of a measured gradient of over 25 mmHg usually means that a significant pre-existing gradient was present. In other words, with a small catheter, a large gradient should not be attributed entirely to the trans-stenotic position of the catheter.

Modifications of Angiographic Routines by Indications and Circumstances

Suspected Renovascular Hypertension

If a stenosis of possible hemodynamic significance is found, then pharmacoangiography is performed.[48] This important technique is described under Renovascular Hypertension, Chapter 71. A renal vein renin assay may also be performed at the same sitting. If a stenosis was evident on the inspiratory aortogram, then the selective study is performed in the expiratory phase, because stenoses may occasionally fluctuate markedly in severity between inspiration and expiration (see Fig. 15–10).

Suspected Renal Mass

Ultrasonography, CT, radionuclide imaging, MRI, and percutaneous puncture with aspiration biopsy are usually adequate to prove the presence of suspected renal mass and to differentiate renal cyst from tumor. Nevertheless, in a significant minority of lesions such information cannot be reliably obtained with the above methods, and for these arteriography is indicated. Examples include difficulty in differentiating scar and hypertrophy from renal tumor, differentiating tumor from complex cyst, or evaluating retroperitoneal or hepatic metastases. Because of its usual characteristic hypervascularity, arteriography is quite reliable in diagnosis of renal cell cancer, evaluation of its extent, and differentiation from other mass lesions. Angiography is often indicated primarily for preoperative or palliative ablation, using injection of particles or alcohol.

In nephrectomy candidates, diagnostic accuracy may be enhanced by using unusually large doses of contrast medium (approximately 25 ml), thus improving demonstration of tumor vessels, the extent of tumor, and the possibility of invasion of the renal vein.[49] In the past, pharmacoangiography was frequently employed to augment tumor demonstration. The technique was based on the observation that tumor vessels constricted less after epinephrine than did normal arteries, owing to the deficiency of musculature in newly formed pathological vessels.[27] Thus, contrast injected shortly after intra-arterial injection of 5 to 20 μg of epinephrine was often diverted into the renal tumor. Other vasoconstrictor agents (angiotensin, vasopressin)[50, 51] had similar effects (Fig. 15–16). My experience over many years, however, has indicated that the technique almost never demonstrated a tumor that was not visible to some extent on a good-quality conventional study. Others describe occasional tumors that were visible only after pharmacoarteriography.[52] Acccurate estimation of the proper dose of vasoconstrictor is difficult, and the degree of vascular obstruction after injection of vasoconstrictor is sometimes so severe as to prevent all flow, thus nullifying the value of

the examination. The advent of CT, ultrasonography, and percutaneous puncture have further restricted indications for pharmacoangiography in renal mass.

Inferior vena cavography and selective renal venography are sometimes also indicated in order to assess intravenous tumor extension. Again, CT, ultrasonography and MRI have reduced the need for this step.

Hematuria

Angiography is frequently indicated in patients with gross or unilateral hematuria, generally in the setting of negative urography, CT, and ultrasonography, and non-localization by endoscopy. Although it only rarely provides definitive diagnosis, endoscopy is often valuable in lateralization. The angiogram is specifically targeted at demonstrating small arteriovenous malformations (Fig. 15–17), although occult tumor or other abnormality is also possible.

The study is initiated with aortography in order to detect possible ureteral abnormality. Selective magnification renal arteriography usually follows, beginning on the side of endoscopic lateralization when appropriate. If selective magnification arteriography is negative, I continue to employ vasoconstrictive (epinephrine) pharmacoarteriography in the hope of demonstrating a small otherwise occult malformation. In my experience, this technique still has to demonstrate its first abnormality when the conventional selective study is negative. If the arteriogram remains negative, bilateral renal phlebography is performed in order to demonstrate possible renal

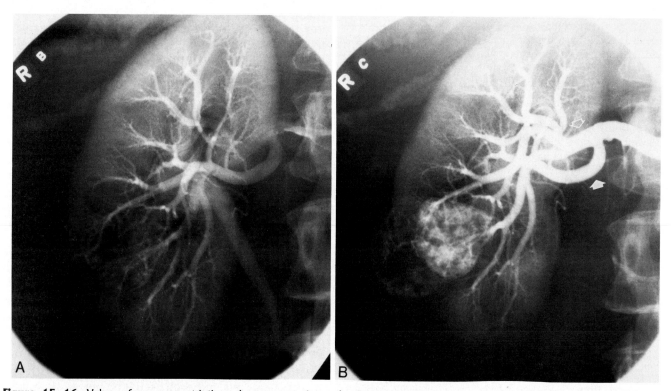

Figure 15–16. Value of vasoconstrictive pharmacoarteriography in augmenting demonstration of renal tumor. *A,* Control arteriogram barely demonstrates abnormal vessels in the lower portion of the right kidney. *B,* Arteriography after injection of a vasoconstrictor agent (0.5 μg angiotensin in this case) shows diversion of contrast material into the tumor. Epinephrine (3 to 10 μg) would probably have accomplished the same purpose. This case also serves to demonstrate some features of an otherwise normal arterial tree. The main renal artery divides into a dorsal (*solid arrowhead*) and ventral ramus (*hollow arrowhead*). The ventral ramus, as usual, represents the continuation of the main renal artery. In *A* the arcuates and corticomedullary demarcation are well shown.

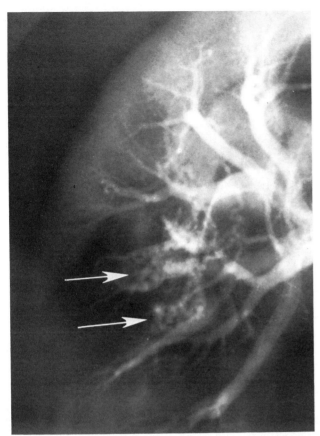

Figure 15–17. Abnormal vessels visible on magnification arteriography, representing a small arteriovenous malformation (*arrows*).

vein varices, even though such demonstration would not prove an etiological relationship to the hematuria.

Renal Parenchymal Diseases

If the indication for arteriography is unexplained acute or chronic renal failure, aortography is frequently omitted, in order to reduce contrast load. In evaluating parenchymal disease, it is of crucial importance to maximize nephrographic density by observing the principles of "flow-dependent injection rates," described above. The nephrographic phase is often critical in diagnosis. Although arteriography provides useful information in most renal parenchymal diseases (Fig. 15–18),[53] it may be diagnostic and specifically indicated when renal arterial occlusion, intravascular coagulopathy, arteritis, or renal vein thrombosis is suspected. Renal phlebography is also indicated for the latter condition.

Transplant Dysfunction

Transplant dysfunction can be evaluated by various imaging modalities, particularly ultrasonography for urinary extravasation, and isotopic methods to determine renal blood flow and excretion. Angiography is most frequently indicated for renal failure and marked hypertension, when other features of rejection are absent, that is, in circumstances that suggest the possibility of stenosis of the transplant artery. Assuming pelvic transplantation, the examination begins with an ipsilateral iliac arteriogram in the frontal projection. Various oblique projec-

tions, and/or the lateral projection, may be necessary to adequately demonstrate the status of the arterial anastomosis. Subsequently, the transplanted artery is selectively catheterized, pressures are obtained within the renal artery and across the anastomosis, the volume of renal blood flow is estimated fluoroscopically and by the spillover technique, and a selective magnification arteriogram is performed, centering on portions of the kidney projected free of bone. The magnification arteriogram is very useful in demonstrating signs of rejection (Fig. 15–19).[54] If a significant stenosis is identified, dilation is usually performed at a subsequent sitting.

Donor Arteriograms (Fig. 15–20)

The study is often limited to a simple aortogram. If there is any question about the number of renal arteries, a selective arteriogram is performed, with examination of the nephrogram for completeness (Fig. 15–20C). If the potential donor kidney has multiple arteries, then selective arteriograms are performed in search of a ureteral artery (see Fig. 15–15), the origin of which should be preserved.

Intraoperative Arteriography

Intraoperative arteriography is occasionally performed in conjunction with renal revascularization or bench sur-

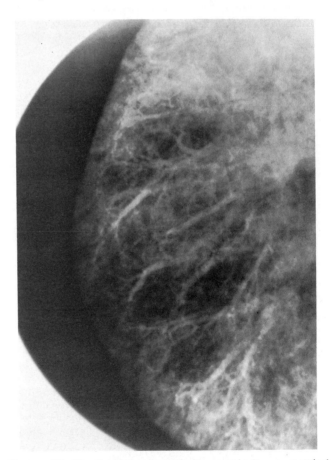

Figure 15–18. Cortical microinfarcts, producing a mottled nephrogram, characteristic of occlusive disease of the interlobular arteries. In this case, scleroderma was the underlying cause. (From Bookstein JJ, Clark RN: Renal Microvascular Disease: Angiographic-Micrographic Correlates. Boston, Little, Brown & Company, 1980, pp 121–166.)

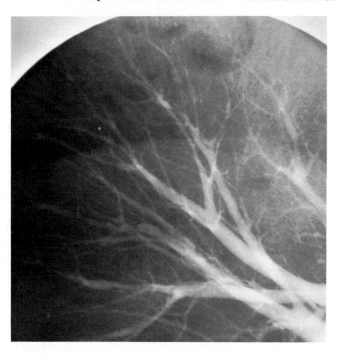

Figure 15–19. Value of magnification arteriography in evaluating renal rejection. In this patient with mild stenosis of the transplant artery, × 2 magnification studies demonstrate distal interlobar stenoses characteristic of rejection. (From Bookstein JJ, Clark RN: Renal Microvascular Disease: Angiographic-Micrographic Correlates. Boston, Little, Brown & Company, 1980, pp 351–382.)

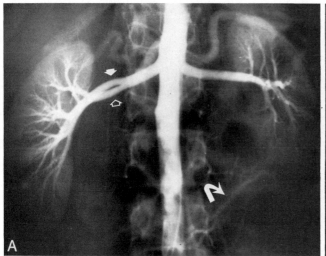

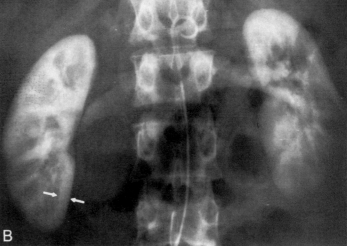

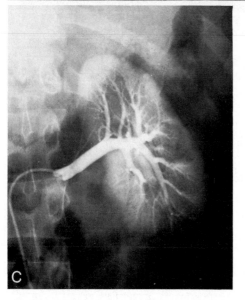

Figure 15–20. Donor arteriogram demonstrating normal features on the right and an accessory artery on the left. *A*, Aortogram shows the usual origin of a single artery on the right from the L1–2 level. Notice how the interlobar branches of the dorsal (*solid arrow*) and ventral (*hollow arrow*) rami cross, indicating that representative vessels from both the dorsal and ventral rami are present on this side. On the left, branches do not cross, suggesting the presence of a second artery. As is not infrequently the case, this second artery is difficult to visualize (*curved arrow*) and could easily have been missed. *B*, The renal veins are faintly opacified. A complete nephrogram is present bilaterally, and shows the normal cortical accentuation (*between arrows*) and the relative medullary lucency, especially on the right. *C*, Selective left renal arteriogram was performed to confirm the presence of a second artery. Note the characteristic large nephrographic defect, in contrast to the complete nephrogram in *B*, proving the presence of a second artery.

gery when some question exists regarding persistent or new arterial compromise. One technique is to clamp the aorta immediately above and below the renal arteries, insert a 20-gauge needle into the aorta (not into the renal artery), and obtain a single film after contrast injection. Image quality is just sufficient to recognize severe obstructions of major renal arteries that may require immediate repair.

Technique of Cavography and Renal Phlebography

Inferior vena cavography may be indicated in the investigation of suspected caval or renal vein thrombosis or obstruction, caval extension of renal tumor, retroperitoneal mass, anomalies, and before caval filter placement. A straight catheter with multiple side holes is passed percutaneously from a femoral vein into the lower cava. Contrast medium 20 ml/second for 2 seconds is injected, followed by serial (usually biplane) filming at the rate of one and one-half or two/second, for 3 seconds.

Renal venous catheterization is most commonly performed for selective renal vein renin assay, though in this instance usually without phlebography. Renal phlebography is most commonly performed for suspected renal vein thrombosis, suspected tumor invasion of the renal vein, or in patients with hematuria to exclude ureteral varices (Fig. 15–21A, B).[37] A gently curved 7 F catheter is passed from a femoral vein into the distal portion of the renal vein. Passage may be facilitated by gentle use of flexible guide wires to pass renal vein valves,[55] or by deflecting the catheter over a deflector wire.

Better demonstration of the renal veins, particularly the small intracortical branches, can be achieved by slowing renal arterial flow before the injection. Arterial flow can be easily stopped with an injection of 20 μg of epinephrine into the renal artery immediately beforehand.[29] Balloon occlusion of the renal artery is also feasible but is less simple than the epinephrine injection.

An injection of 20 ml/second of ~30% iodinated contrast material for 1.5 to 2 seconds, followed by serial films at the rate of two/second for 3 seconds, and one/second for 3 seconds. Multiple side holes are essential to minimize recoil during the rapid injection.

COMPLICATIONS OF RENAL ARTERIOGRAPHY

Nephrotoxic and allergic contrast complications are described earlier in this chapter. Although transient proteinuria and mild, self-limited reduction in renal blood flow are seen following selective renal arteriography, renal function is not permanently affected, and the incidence of nephrotoxicity does not appear to be greater than the incidence after injection of contrast material into other arteries, or intravenously.[56] Nonionic contrast agents produce less proteinuria than do ionic agents.[56a] Allergic reactions are thought to be less frequent after intra-arterial than after intravenous injections.[57]

Renal arteriography is associated with the usual remote mechanical complications of catheterization: femoral

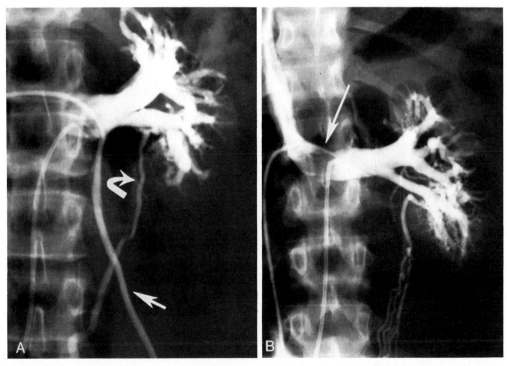

Figure 15–21. Renal phlebography. *A,* Left renal phlebogram. A catheter is within the renal artery, through which 10 μg of epinephrine had been injected to temporarily stop renal blood flow. Twenty ml/second of contrast medium was then injected into the renal vein for 1.5 seconds, producing reasonably effective retrograde flow. Testicular (*straight arrow*) and ureteral (*curved arrow*) veins are also shown. The dilated distal ureteral vein could conceivably be related to the patient's hematuria. *B,* In this patient with hematuria, lucency of the renal vein is seen (*arrow*), owing to compression between the aorta and superior mesenteric artery, a frequent anatomical variant. A 4-mmHg pressure gradient existed across this stenosis. Ureteral veins are somewhat enlarged, raising the question of bleeding from ureteral varices. However, proof of this association was lacking.

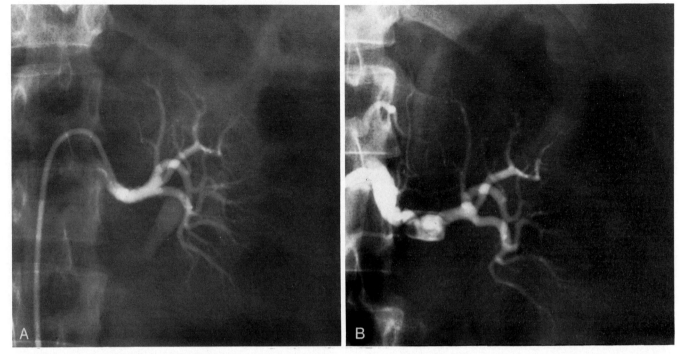

Figure 15–22. Complication of arteriography: renal artery dissection. *A,* Control arteriogram, showing fibromuscular dysplasia of little or no hemodynamic significance. The catheter curve is too long, and passes too far distally into the renal artery in a direction that does not conform well to the course of the artery. Shortly afterward, during preparation for pharmacoangiography, a minimal dissection was noted fluoroscopically, and the procedure was abandoned. Hypertension progressed markedly to 180/110, and could not be well controlled with drugs. *B,* Repeat arteriography 2 weeks later demonstrates a large dissecting aneurysm, markedly narrowing the true renal lumen. The kidney length had decreased by 1 cm. (From Talner LB, McLaughlin AP, Bookstein JJ: Renal artery dissection: A complication of catheter arteriography. Radiology, 117:291–295, 1975.)

thrombosis, hematoma, arteriovenous fistula, embolization, guide-wire perforation, and others. Clinically significant local complications are now quite uncommon, occurring at our institution in about 0.2% of cases after retrograde femoral catheterization. As already stated, the complications of transaxillary catheterization are much more frequent.[23] Unlike ionic contrast agents, which are weak anticoagulants, ionic media do not affect the coagulation process. Blood clot formation in angiographic syringes containing nonionic contrast media has been reported.[57a] As a basic principle, therefore, nonionic contrast media should not be allowed to mix with blood prior to injection, and they should be flushed from the catheter immediately after injection.

Local mechanical complications can also occur from selective renal catheterization. The renal artery can be dissected, with secondary hypertension (Fig. 15–22).[58] Frequency of this complication can be minimized by avoiding forceful advance of catheters with excessively long or insufficiently curved limbs into the renal artery. Emboli are occasionally injected, which can be treated immediately by local infusion of streptokinase or urokinase, if large or symptomatic.

PENILE ANGIOGRAPHY

Penile angiography is primarily indicated for the evaluation of suspected vasculogenic impotence. Erection is largely a circulatory phenomenon, and angiography would seem to be an effective method for study of the process of erection, as well as the causes of impotence. My early experience, however, convincingly demonstrated that conventional methods of arteriography and cavernosography were completely unreliable in the evaluation of the penile circulatory anatomy and function. The development of special angiographic methods was required.

The erectile process is initiated by neurogenic and psychogenic stimuli.[59, 60] Coincident with the onset of erection, arterial flow increases markedly.[61–63] The augmented arterial flow, supposedly mediated via precapillary shunting into the corpora cavernosa, was thought to be the major, if not the only, immediate cause of erection.[64] The error of this concept has clearly been demonstrated through the recent discovery of the erectogenicity of intracavernosal injection of papaverine and other smooth muscle relaxants.[61, 65, 66] This discovery abruptly shifted to emphasize relaxation of smooth muscle in the walls of cavernosal sinusoids as the initiating process of cavernosal erection.[66] As sinusoidal muscle tone diminishes and the sinusoids begin to distend with blood, the small peripheral venous tributaries become compressed between the peripheral sinusoids and the unyielding tunica albuginea. Thus, activation of a veno-occlusive mechanism is an intrinsic sequela of cavernosal muscular relaxation.

Besides activating the veno-occlusive mechanism, relaxation of cavernosal smooth muscle inherently reduces resistance to cavernosal arterial inflow. Thus, intracavernosal injection of papaverine markedly augments cavernosal arterial flow and arterial diameter, and greatly facilitates both visualization of the small penile arteries and evaluation of penile arterial physiology.[67, 68]

PENILE VASCULAR CATHETERIZATION IN THE EVALUATION OF IMPOTENCE

With the advent of intracavernosal injection of smooth muscle relaxants, penile angiography has become a highly reliable and informative diagnostic study, comparable in many respects to catheterization of the heart. Like cardiac catheterization, the catheter study now enables precise evaluation of the morphologic and physiologic nature of both the arterial and venous (right and left) components of the penile vasculature, during both relaxed and flaccid states. I prefer to emphasize the comprehensive morphologic and physiologic nature of the examination by the term *penile vascular catheterization,* rather than arteriography or cavernosography.

The primary prerequisite for penile vascular catheterization is impotence for 3 months or more in an individual who, for one of several reasons, wants to know with certainty whether or not he has vasculogenic impotence. Usually, some other objective criterion of organic vasculogenic impotence is present, such as a decreased penile blood pressure or an abnormal rigidity test, although these noninvasive studies have not proven highly reliable to date. The study is performed on an outpatient basis, under mild sedation and local anesthesia, and requires about 1.25 hours.

Arteriography

An adequate arteriogram must demonstrate the arterial pathways from the aorta to at least one distal cavernosal artery. One groin is anesthetized locally in preparation for arterial catheterization, and the root of the penis is locally anesthetized in preparation for later cavernosal needle punctures. A 5 F catheter is percutaneously passed from the femoral artery to the aortic bifurcation, and pelvic arteriography is obtained in both 25-degree posterior oblique projections, using a small amount of contrast medium. These films adequately demonstrate the larger arteries only, and serve as a road map for selective catheterization of the internal pudendal artery.

Presuming the pelvic arteriogram demonstrates patency of the internal iliac arteries, a long reversed high-torque catheter is manipulated into the ipsilateral (most often) internal pudendal artery, the usual major source of cavernosal blood flow. Proper placement in the internal pudendal artery can be best confirmed by observing the course of the artery near the inferior ischial ramus; the patient is in the anterior oblique projection. A preliminary film is then obtained, in 30-degree anterior oblique projection, using × 2 direct magnification technique. In younger men, the testicles are shielded.

Before arteriography, however, the penile arterial vasculature must be dilated; otherwise little or no opacification of penile arteries can be obtained, and even normal patients may appear to have organic arterial occlusion. In my early experience, I obtained moderate arterial dilation by injecting a mixture of nitroglycerin (300 μg) and papaverine (30 mg) directly into the internal pudendal artery.[67] Others have obtained penile vasodilation by using spinal or general anesthesia.[69] Over the past 2 years,

however, it has become evident that intracavernosal (IC) injection of a mixture of papaverine (60 mg) and phentolamine (1 mg) in about 10 ml of nonheparinized saline is a preferred method of obtaining dilation of the cavernosal arteries. This injection is made via a 21-gauge needle while the preliminary arteriographic film is being developed. A tourniquet is placed around the base of the penis for 2 minutes to prolong intracavernosal drug retention. The needle is left in place for later cavernosal studies.

Arteriography is then performed within about 5 minutes of the IC papaverine-phentolamine injection. Concentrated nonionic media are used, for example, iopamidol containing 37% iodine; 3 ml/second are injected for 6 seconds. Two films per second are obtained for 3 seconds, then one film every 2 seconds for seven more films. The arteriogram is inspected, and if complete patency is evident to the distal cavernosal artery, the arteriographic portion of the procedure is terminated. If cavernosal arterial patency is not clearly visible throughout, or if contralateral collateral flow is suspected, then an additional ipsilateral projection, or a contralateral injection, is obtained.

It has been argued that a more proximal site of injection (i.e., the anterior division of the internal iliac artery) is preferable to injection from the internal pudendal artery because of the frequency of supplemental penile arteries that arise from the anterior division or other branches. These arguments, however, are invalidated by the rich system of inosculations (precapillary arterial-arterial communications) around the root of the penis, which allow good and consistent opacification of any existing supplemental pudendal or cavernosal arteries after selective internal pudendal injection. They also frequently enable visualization of the contralateral dorsal penile and cavernosal arteries. Injections from the internal pudendal arteries result in significantly better opacification of small penile and collateral branches and, in addition, are much less painful than more proximal injections.

Cavernosometry and Cavernosography

Following the arteriogram, and within 20 to 30 minutes of the intracavernosal injection of the papaverine-phentolamine mix, pharmacocavernosometry is performed. The primary purpose of pharmacocavernosometry is to quantify the volume of cavernosal leak during full relaxation of cavernosal smooth musculature. A second 21-gauge needle is placed in the opposite corpus cavernosum, and connected to a recording manometer. (Proper placement should always be confirmed fluoroscopically by a small test injection of contrast agent.) Using one of several types of infusion pumps, saline is infused into the corpus cavernosum at a rate that raises cavernosal pressure to about 150 mmHg. The flow required to maintain this pressure is termed the pharmacological maintenance erectile flow (PMEF).[70] At a pressure of 150 mmHg, no significant arterial flow enters the corpus cavernosum, so that the PMEF is, in effect, the rate of cavernosal leakage at that pressure. In a few patients the veno-occlusive insufficiency is severe enough to preclude raising cavernosal pressures to 150 mmHg.

The normal PMEF varies from about 2 to 12 ml/minute. I have had a few patients develop normal erections despite PMEF as high as 30 ml/minute. However, PMEF of 45 ml/minute or more has always been associated with erectile failure, and I consider this figure to be the lower limit of venogenic impotence.

There are other methods of quantifying cavernosal leakage. Goldstein and colleagues[71] observe the rate of fall of the cavernosal pressure after discontinuing the infusion at a level of 150 mmHg cavernosal pressure (see Chapter 78). Normally the rate of fall is less than 1 mmHg/second over a range of 50 mmHg; faster rates reflect excessive venous leak. In my experience, this method does not allow a determination of venous leak as precise as does the PMEF method.

Cavernosometry also enables determination of several other useful parameters of erectile physiology. After IC injection of papaverine-phentolamine, pulsations are normally evident in the cavernosal pressure trace. These pulsations probably reflect systolic inflow via the helicine arteries. Normally the pulse amplitude is greater than 2 mmHg; a lower amplitude of pulsations is found in about 80% of patients with an arteriographic diagnosis of arteriogenic impotence. Systolic cavernosal arterial occlusion pressure can also be obtained. A Doppler flow probe is placed on the lateral aspect of the penis and oriented to detect the flow pulse within the cavernosal artery. As the cavernosal pressure is raised by IC infusion of saline at a rate equal to or greater than the PMEF, the Doppler signal will disappear. The level at which disappearance occurs is called the systolic cavernosal occlusion pressure and normally is 20 to 30 mmHg below the peak systemic systolic pressure.[71] In my experience, decreased systolic occlusion pressures are found in about 80% of patients with arteriographic diagnosis of arteriogenic impotence.

Cavernosography is performed only if cavernosometry indicates excessive leakage. The cavernosogram is designed to indicate the sites of leakage, in which case the possibility of operative[72] or transluminal therapy is considered.[73] Dilute contrast material (~14% iodine) is infused at or just above the PMEF rate, and films are exposed in oblique projection at IC pressures of 75, 100, 125, and 150 mmHg.

Complications

Dissection, thrombosis, or embolization are theoretical complications of selective pudendal arteriography, but they have not occurred in my experience (175 examinations to date). Aside from transient hypotension, no untoward sequelae have followed the IC injection of vasodilators. Likewise, there have been no major complications of cavernosography or cavernosometry. In several patients studied early in this series, contrast material extravasated from the corpus cavernosum during infusion, leading to penile edema that subsided within 1 or 2 days. One patient developed an area of skin slough from the extravasation, emphasizing the importance of immediately stopping the injection if extravasation is observed. About 3% of these patients developed prolonged erection. This must be treated within 4 hours, usually by repeat cavernous puncture with an 18-gauge needle, aspiration of about 20 ml of blood, and IC injection of 12 μg of norepinephrine.[74]

Normal Arterial Anatomy

The arterial supply to the penis is derived almost entirely from the two internal pudendal arteries, which typically arise as independent branches of the anterior division of the internal iliac artery (Fig. 15–23A).[69, 75, 76] The internal pudendal artery sweeps around the inner aspect of the pelvis: beyond the origin of a scrotal branch it is termed the penile artery. Typically, the penile artery then gives rise to an artery to the urethral bulb, one or more branches to the ipsilateral corpus cavernosum (called deep or cavernosal arteries), and the deep dorsal artery of the penis (Figs. 15–23 and 15–24). Common variants include a supplemental cavernosal artery, or the origin of both cavernosal arteries from one side.[68]

The arteriogram is considered inadequate unless the arterial tree is visualized as far as the distal cavernosal artery on at least one side. If the cavernosal artery is not visualized on a pharmacoarteriographic study (i.e., after IC injection of a vasodilator), and technical deficiency is excluded, then it is likely that the cavernosal arteries arise entirely from the opposite side and will be demonstrated by the contralateral injection. On the other hand, when a cavernosal artery is obstructed by organic disease, distal reconstitution via collaterals is usually visible. Such collateral flow commonly arises from the obturator artery, the dorsal penile artery, spongiosal branches, or the external pudendal artery and will be demonstrated through the inosculations discussed above.

Although visualization of the cavernosal artery is the primary aim of the arteriogram, all the other terminal branches of the internal pudendal artery are also demonstrated: the dorsal penile artery, cavernosal branches arising from the dorsal penile, the artery to the bulb, and communicating branches to the opposite side. The spongiosum, particularly the bulb, may stain densely. The corpus cavernosum also stains to some degree, but the degree of stain shows no correlation with the presence or absence of arteriogenic impotence.

In the past, arteriography was performed without vasodilation. Such studies rarely demonstrated flow beyond the origin of the penile arteries, reflecting either spasm at this level or more distal vasoconstriction preventing distal flow (Figs. 15–24 and 15–25). Such nonvasodilated arteriograms were frequently misinterpreted as indicative of organic occlusive arterial disease.

Arteriographic Features of Arteriogenic Impotence

Of 175 patients in our series of penile vascular catheterizations, approximately 30% had normal studies, 23% had pure arteriogenic impotence, 24% had venogenic impotence, and 23% had both arteriogenic and venogenic impotence. Arteriogenic impotence is diagnosed arteriographically in the presence of bilateral hemodynamically significant obstructions of flow proximal to the midcavernosal arteries. Hemodynamic significance is inferred from the anatomical severity of obstruction and/or the demonstration of collateral circulation. Venogenic impotence indicates a PMEF greater than 45 ml/minute.

In patients with arteriogenic impotence, the usual site of the most distal significant disease is the distal internal

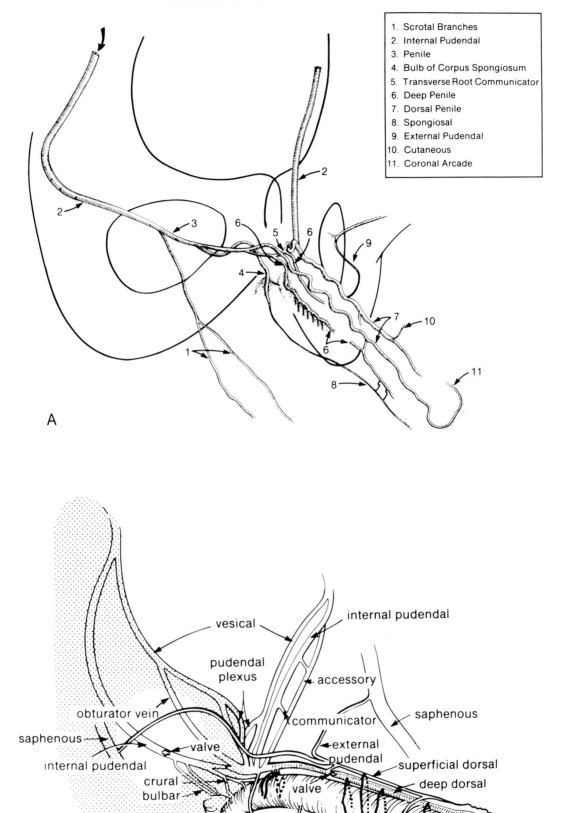

1. Scrotal Branches
2. Internal Pudendal
3. Penile
4. Bulb of Corpus Spongiosum
5. Transverse Root Communicator
6. Deep Penile
7. Dorsal Penile
8. Spongiosal
9. External Pudendal
10. Cutaneous
11. Coronal Arcade

Figure 15–23. Artist's depiction of the normal penile vascular anatomy, in oblique projection. *A*, Arterial anatomy. *B*, Venous drainage of the corpus cavernosum.

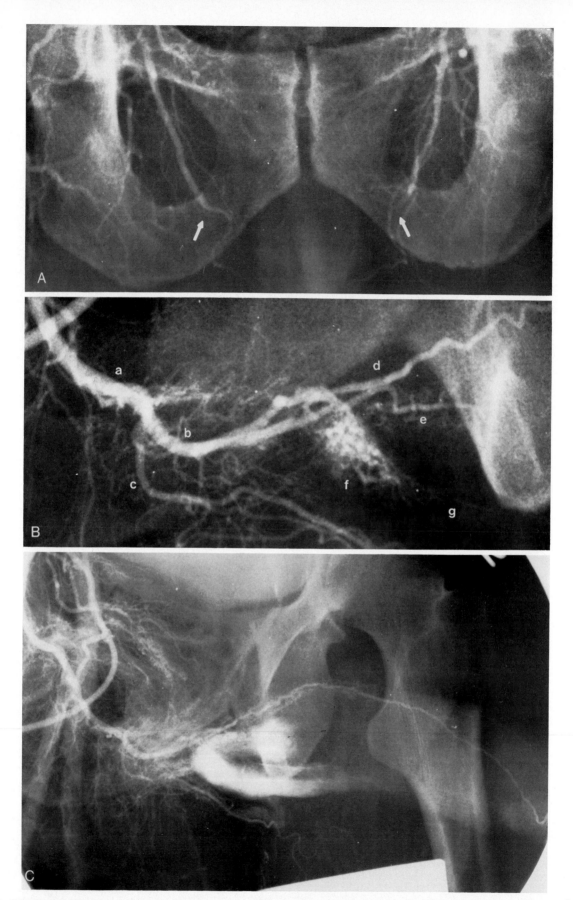

Figure 15—24. Normal internal pudendal arteriogram in 45-year-old impotent male. *A,* After aortography, the penile arteries appear to be occluded as they approach the root of the penis (*arrows*). The small branch continuing from each pudenal artery is a scrotal branch. *B,* Same patient as in *A.* Magnification selective oblique arteriogram of the root of the penis, after intrapudendal arterial injection of a mixture of 200 μg of nitroglycerin and 30 mg of papaverine. The constriction of the pudendal artery, shown in *A,* has been relieved. Key to arteries: a = distal pudendal; b = penile; c = scrotal; d = dorsal penile; e = deep penile with branches (cavernosal); f = stain of bulb; g = spongiosal. *C,* Same case, 6 seconds later. The dorsal penile is visualized to the glans and the glans stains. Cutaneous branches are also seen. There is dense stain of the bulb of the corpus spongiosum (lower region), and moderate stain of the right corpus cavernosum (upper stain).

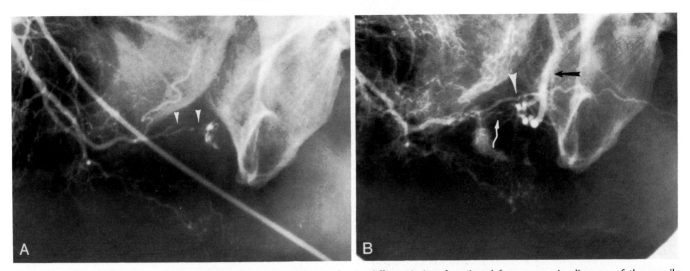

Figure 15–25. Importance of vasodilator pharmacoangiography in differentiating functional from organic disease of the penile vasculature. *A,* Control pudendal arteriogram demonstrating irregularity and occlusion of the dorsal penile artery, strongly suggesting organic atherosclerotic disease (*arrowheads*). *B,* After intra-arterial injection of 300 μg of nitroglycerin, and 30 mg papaverine, the apparent disease has disappeared, and the dorsal penile artery is opacified (*arrowhead*). An anterior communicating branch is also seen (*tortuous arrow*), which conducts contrast into the contralateral internal pudendal artery (*black arrow*).

pudendal artery (Fig. 15–26), the penile artery, or the origins of the cavernosal arteries (Fig. 15–27). Obstructive arterial disease is usually remarkably symmetrical bilaterally.

Cavernosal Studies

Normal (Fig. 15–28) and abnormal (Fig. 15–29) cavernosometry have been described above.

Anatomical studies indicate that cavernosal effluent flows predominantly via circumflex veins into the deep dorsal penile vein (see Fig. 15–23*B*). The deep dorsal vein then passes below the symphysis pubis and drains via 4 to 8 large preprostatic veins that in turn join vesical veins.[77] The deep dorsal vein can drain laterally via communication with one or two internal pudendal veins on each side. Crural veins arise from the crura and drain into the internal pudendal veins, providing a second major route of cavernosal drainage. From the internal pudendal

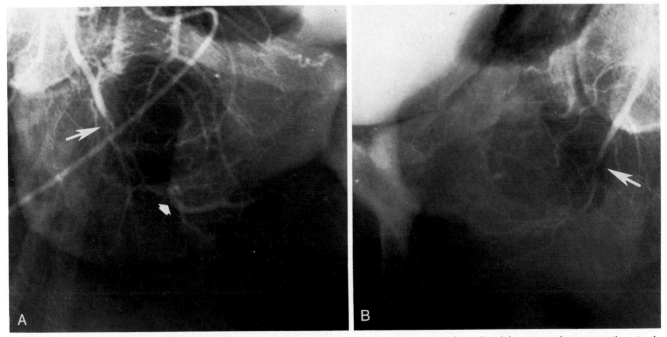

Figure 15–26. Arteriogenic impotence, with true organic obstruction of the internal pudendal artery, demonstrating typical bilateral symmetry. The almost invariably bilateral and symmetrical nature of penile arterial disease generally obviates the need for bilateral arteriography, if the initial side injected is normal. *A,* Right internal pudendal arteriogram demonstrating obstruction. The organic nature of the obstruction is indicated by its persistence, despite administration of 300 μg nitroglycerin and 30 mg papaverine (*white arrow*). Collateral circulation reopacified the internal pudendal after 2 cm (*arrowhead*). *B,* Identical findings on the left.

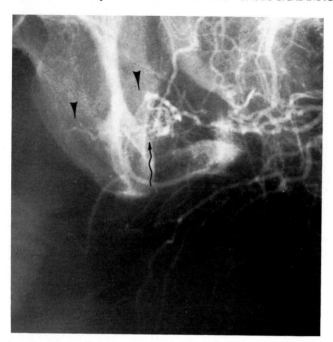

Figure 15–27. Arteriogenic impotence, due to small artery disease. The dorsal penile artery is irregularly narrowed until it becomes occluded (*proximal arrowhead*). Collateral flow then occurs via small cavernosal collaterals (*tortuous arrow*), to opacify the distal cavernous artery or the dorsal penile artery by collateral flow (*distal arrowhead*).

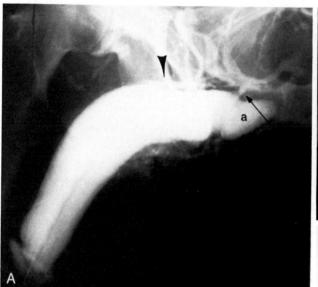

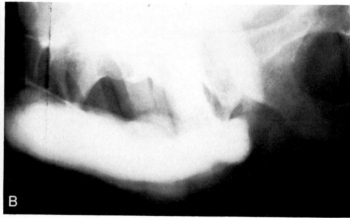

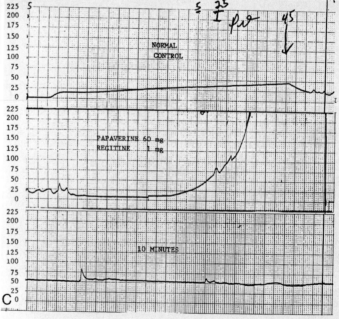

Figure 15–28. Normal cavernosography, pharmacocavernosography, and cavernosometry. Sexually normal 57-year-old volunteer. *A*, 100 ml of diluted contrast medium was injected at the rate of 1 ml/second into one corpus cavernosum, with filming in oblique projection. Note abundant flow into the deep dorsal penile vein (*arrowhead*) and deep penile veins (*narrow arrow*). The crus of the corpus cavernosum (a) opacifies well because of drainage from the crus via the deep penile veins. *B*, After intracavernosal infusion of papaverine 60 mg and phentolamine 1 mg, cavernosography demonstrates occlusion of all veins. The corpora are somewhat larger and are erect. The crura are not opacified because complete occlusion of deep penile veins converts each crus into a blind sac; thus, the corpus cavernosum appears to be displaced from the ischial ramus, simulating avulsion. *C*, Cavernosometry before and after pharmacological veno-occlusion. During the control infusion of 100 ml of dilute contrast, cavernosal pressure rose to 45 mmHg. After pharmacological veno-occlusion, pressure rose off-scale to over 300 mmHg. (Infusion should be terminated if pressures rise to over 200 mmHg.) After 10 minutes, pressures returned to 50 mmHg. Erection then returned and gradually abated over a 6-hour period. If erection had persisted beyond this point, pharmacological detumescence with IC epinephrine would have been performed.

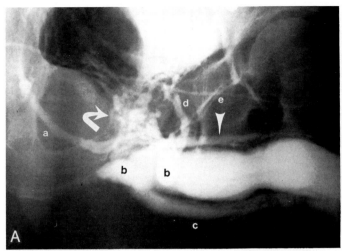

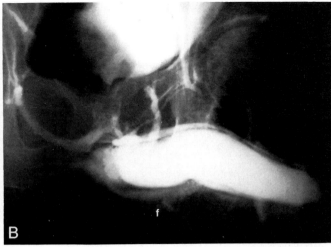

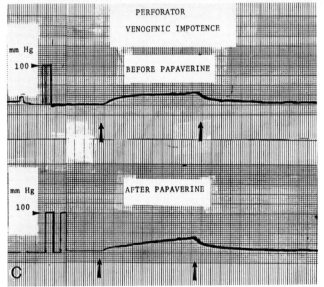

Figure 15–29. Sixty-six-year-old man, impotent on the basis of incompetence of the veno-occlusive mechanism of the deep dorsal penile venous system. *A,* Control cavernosography demonstrates free flow via the deep dorsal vein (*arrowhead*), and via deep penile veins into the pudendal plexus (*curved arrow*) and internal pudendal veins. Abundant flow into the corpus spongiosum is observed as well. Key to venous structures: a = right internal pudendal; b = crura; c = corpus spongiosum; d = left internal pudendal; e = external pudendal. *B,* After intracavernosal administration of papaverine only, the deep penile flow into the pudendal plexus has stopped, while flow continues into the deep dorsal and internal pudendal veins. With closure of the deep penile veins, the crus is now poorly opacified (f = corpus spongiosum). *C,* Cavernosometry demonstrates insignificant pressure increment during postpapaverine infusion.

veins, flow may proceed centrally or peripherally. Abundant venous communications also exist between the corpora cavernosa and the body and glans of the corpus spongiosum. There are no central intracavernosal veins. The superficial dorsal penile vein primarily drains the skin and conducts flow into the external pudendal veins.

Cavernosography performed without IC injection of a smooth muscle relaxant will opacify all of the above-named venous pathways (see Fig. 15–28).[78] After IC injection of papaverine, all venous pathways will be almost completely closed in normal men. Thus, cavernosography after IC injection of papaverine-phentolamine should normally demonstrate cavernosal erection and little or no opacification of draining veins. If, however, the injection of contrast medium is maintained for a considerable period of time (i.e., 1 to 2 minutes) at the approximate PMEF, the veins draining the cavernosa will eventually opacify. The amount of venous leak cannot be judged accurately by the density or size of opacified veins.

In patients with venogenic impotence, leakage can occur via any combination of routes of cavernosal venous drainage. Most patients leak via the deep dorsal penile vein alone or in combination (Fig. 15–29), but almost as many also drain via the crural perforators (Fig. 15–30).

A few may drain predominantly via the spongiosum or the superficial venous network.

ADRENAL ANGIOGRAPHY

Most diseases of the adrenal gland are associated with endocrine dysfunction and produce relatively characteristic clinical and biochemical abnormalities. Diagnosis of the basic disease process, therefore, is usually accomplished clinically, and imaging modalities, including angiography, are reserved for localization of an adrenal or extra-adrenal tumor, or for differentiating adrenal tumor from hyperplasia. For most adrenal mass lesions CT has superseded other modalities to become the imaging procedure of first choice. Adrenal venous sampling and phlebography remain useful procedures in occasional patients, particularly in localizing small hormonally active tumors such as aldosteronomas, and for differentiating bilateral tumors from bilateral nodular hyperplasia. Arteriography is useful in evaluating larger tumors such as pheochromocytomas, or carcinomas, and despite the advent of CT is still occasionally indicated. (Fig. 15–31 shows a diagram of normal adrenal vascularity.)

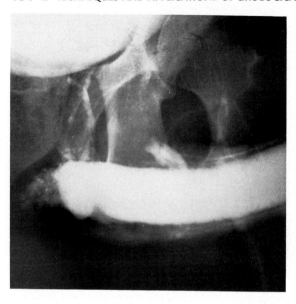

Figure 15–30. Male in his forties, with cavernosal venous leak via a single perforator. This perforator was surgically ligated, with immediate intraoperative improvement in the postpapaverine pressure response to infusion.

PHLEBOGRAPHY AND VENOUS ANATOMY

Technique of Adrenal Phlebography

The catheter material may be the same as that described for arteriography; the shapes are as indicated in Fig. 15–6B to D. A tiny side hole is punched on the under surface of the distal portion of the right adrenal vein catheter, within 5 mm of the tip, to facilitate aspiration of blood for biochemical assay. I prefer to catheterize the right adrenal vein first. Search begins on the posterior aspect of the inferior vena cava, at the anticipated level of the center of the gland, that is, just above the upper pole of the kidney. When minor advances and withdrawals of the catheter shaft do not produce corresponding motions at the tip, a test injection is performed to determine whether the adrenal vein has been engaged. Considerable experience is required to recognize the characteristic patterns of the right adrenal veins. One looks for the typical stellate appearance, produced by two or three central tributaries opacifying from the short main trunk (Fig. 15–33). Small accessory hepatic veins are often encountered in the same region; a hepatic vein may be differentiated from adrenal by the following:

1. Injection into the adrenal vein is usually somewhat painful, whereas injection into a hepatic vein is painless.

2. Injection into a hepatic vein often produces a homogeneous persistent blush, whereas a blush does not usually occur after adrenal venous injection.

3. Downward-coursing adrenal and renal capsular veins are often opacified after adrenal injections, as opposed to the upward-curving hepatic veins visualized after hepatic vein injections.

In experienced hands, the right adrenal vein can be successfully catheterized in about 95% of cases.[78] Difficulty is sometimes due to the adrenal vein joining a hepatic vein immediately proximal to the inferior vena cava. This problem can be overcome by elongating the distal tip so that it will reach through the hepatic vein to the adrenal vein.

If adrenal venous sampling is to be performed, it must be done before definitive injections of contrast medium, since such injections may markedly increase the concentration of adrenal hormones (J.J.B. unreported observations).

In order to minimize the incidence of intra-adrenal rupture and hemorrhage, gentle technique is required. The amount of contrast to be injected varies greatly and is best determined by noting the point at which the patient experiences the pain of glandular distention. I perform the injections by hand and generally load about 6 ml of contrast (~28% iodine) into the syringe. The patient is asked to clench his fist in a visible position, usually near his ear, and to extend one finger when discomfort is noted. The injection is then begun slowly, during filming, and the injection rate gradually increases until the finger snaps open. At this point, the injection is stopped. In most patients, about 3 or 4 ml will have been injected, with the final injection rate often being about 1.5 ml/second. Sometimes, however, a much greater or lesser volume or rate is required. Filming is at the rate of two films/second for 3 seconds, and one/second for 3 seconds. Anteroposterior projections are used, usually with magnification. Repeat injections or projections are performed infrequently, in order to minimize the incidence of extravasation.

Following completion of right adrenal catheterization, the right adrenal catheter is passed into the left renal vein. A guide wire is advanced far into the peripheral renal venous bed, and a catheter shaped as in Fig. 15–6C is exchanged. The catheter is then slowly withdrawn while the tip is directed superiorly, until a sudden visible cephalad motion indicates entrance into the phrenicoadrenal trunk, usually within 1 cm of either side of the left lateral vertebral margin. After engagement of the trunk, a test injection should show most of the contrast ascending into the central vein; if toward the phrenic vein, adjustment of catheter shape or position may be necessary. Blood samples are then withdrawn, and phlebography is

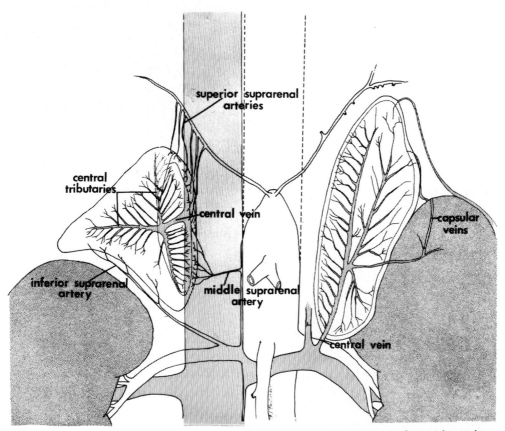

Figure 15–31. Diagrammatic representation of normal adrenal vascularity. Note three sets of arterial supply to each adrenal, but only a single central vein. (From Bookstein JJ: The roles of angiography in adrenal disease. *In* Abrams HL (ed): Abrams Angiography. Boston, Little, Brown & Company, 1983.)

performed in a manner comparable to that already described. The dose of contrast medium is often 1 ml greater on the left than right.

Technique of Venous Sampling

Despite a catheter position satisfactory for phlebography, aspiration of amounts sufficient for radioimmunoassay (about 5 ml at our institution) from the right gland may be difficult and time consuming. As described, a small hole on the under surface of the curve, along with minor changes in position or respiration, usually suffices. If all else fails, the adrenal vein wall can be displaced from the catheter tip by passing a narrow guide wire with a blunt distal bead (Cook, Inc.) just beyond the catheter tip, and then aspirating through a gasketed side arm.

Normal Phlebographic Anatomy

On the left side the venous anatomy is relatively constant. The central vein is valveless, usually solitary, and passes down the entire long axis of the gland (Fig. 15–32). It generally meets an inferior phrenic vein just above the left renal vein, and joins the left renal vein as a phrenicoadrenal trunk. The junction of phrenicoadrenal trunk and renal vein usually occurs within 1 cm of a parasagittal plane passing through the left lateral aspect of the vertebral column. The phrenic vein is medial to

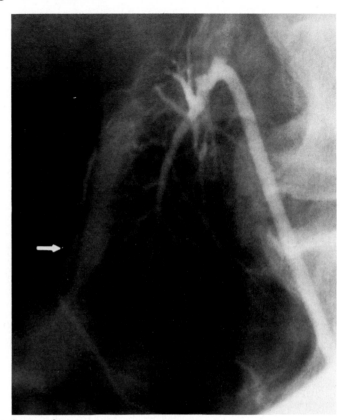

Figure 15–33. Normal right adrenal phlebogram. The central vein arises from the posterior aspect of the inferior vena cava near the anticipated center of the adrenal gland. In this case, one main and one small trunk join the central vein; in other cases, three trunks join to form the central vein. The capsular vein courses distally over the kidney (*arrow*), helping to differentiate the injected vein from a hepatic vein.

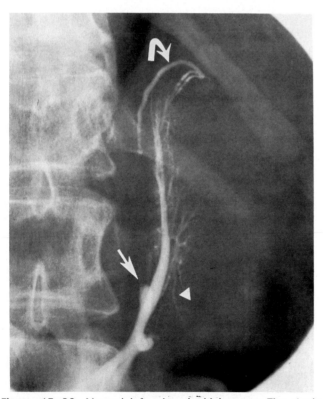

Figure 15–32. Normal left adrenal phlebogram. The single central vein is typical. Note the apical capsular perforator (*curved arrow*), valve of the inferior phrenic vein (*straight arrow*), and normal lower-pole recurrent vein (*arrowhead*). (From Bookstein JJ: The roles of angiography in adrenal disease. *In* Abrams HL (ed): Abrams Angiography. Boston, Little, Brown & Company, 1983.)

the adrenal vein and generally contains a competent terminal valve. During left adrenal phlebography and sampling, special manipulations or catheter shapes are sometimes necessary to direct the catheter from the inferior phrenic vein toward the central adrenal vein.

The central vein of each gland usually communicates via perforator veins with an adenal capsular vein (Figs. 15–32 to 15–35), particularly at the apex of the gland. The adrenal capsular veins in turn communicate with renal capsular veins. Observation of these communications during right adrenal phlebography is helpful in distinguishing an adrenal from a hepatic vein.

On the right, two or three central tributaries are generally present, from superior, inferior, and posterior aspects of the gland. These tributaries join to form a short central trunk, which passes forward to enter the right posterior aspect of the inferior vena cava. In about 10% of individuals, the right adrenal vein joins the posterior aspect of a hepatic vein near the inferior vena cava, rather than directly joining the inferior vena cava. Successful catheterization is still possible, despite this anatomical arrangement. Rarely, the right adrenal vein drains into the right renal vein.

A normal right adrenal phlebogram is illustrated in Fig. 15–33. Note two or three diverging branches from the short central vein. The pinnate branching pattern of the central venous tributaries is evident.

Figure 15–32 illustrates the normal left adrenal phlebogram. Note the single central venule and the clear

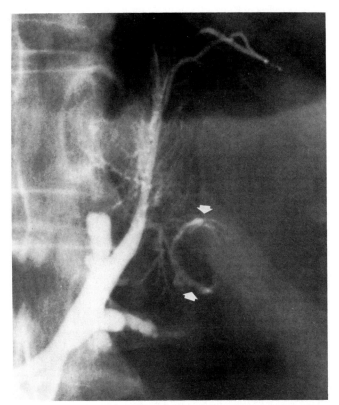

Figure 15–34. Left adrenal phlebogram, aldosteronoma. Note the typical arcuate displacement of small veins around the tumor (*arrowheads*). (From Bookstein JJ: The Roles of Angiography in Adrenal Disease. *In* Abrams HL (ed): Abrams Angiography. Boston, Little, Brown & Company, 1983.)

demonstration of the normal size, contour, and position of the gland. The pinnate branching pattern of the central vein is particularly evident. The phrenic vein is seen medial to the adrenal vein. Because the venules lie within the medulla, the cortex is infrequently opacified. Communications with adrenal and renal capsular venules are noted.

Small adrenal tumors produce characteristic convex displacements of intra-adrenal venules (Figs. 15–34 and 15–35). Large tumors are rarely studied now, but they may produce spectacular venous patterns (Fig. 15–36).

Arterial Anatomy and Arteriography

Classically, each adrenal gland has three sources of arterial supply: a superior adrenal artery originating from the inferior phrenic artery, a middle adrenal artery that arises from the lateral aspect of the aorta between the renal and celiac arteries, and an inferior adrenal artery arising from the superior aspect of the renal artery (Fig. 15–31). Each arterial trunk then breaks up into 10 to 20 smaller twigs that ramify and intercommunicate over the outer aspect of the gland. The twigs terminate as perforating branches that pass perpendicularly through the cortex into the medulla. No direct arterial supply to the adrenal medulla seems to be present.

The perforating arteries gradually assume the histological characteristics of veins as they pass centripetally into the medulla, and no other direct cortical venous supply

is present. Upon reaching the central medulla, these venules join the central vein at right angles. The junction of perforating and central veins is deficient in medial musculature[79] and probably constitutes a site of predilection for rupture during adrenal phlebography.[80]

Adrenal arteriography is generally initiated with an aortogram, for two reasons: (1) to possibly localize an adrenal or extra-adrenal mass, and (2) to facilitate localization of the major adrenal arteries prior to selective catheterization. In searching for masses such as pheochromocytoma, two injections are often necessary, one centered for the upper abdomen, a second for the lower. For large hypervascular tumors, aortography alone may provide sufficient information (see Fig. 15–40). Subtraction films should be obtained, which occasionally demonstrate tumors, particularly pheochromocytomas, that are invisible on conventional films (see Fig. 15–40C).

If selective arteriography is necessary, the aortogram catheter is replaced with a "shepherd's crook" (see Fig. 15–6B), using catheter material with good torque characteristics. The tip should be narrow to facilitate entry into the small adrenal arteries; that is, it should be tapered tightly over a 0.028-inch guide wire. I still prefer to shape my own from pink Formocath material (Becton-Dickinson), with OD 2.2 mm, ID 1.3 mm; preformed wire-ensheathed No. 5 catheters are also excellent (Cook, Inc.).

Complete selective arteriography of both adrenal

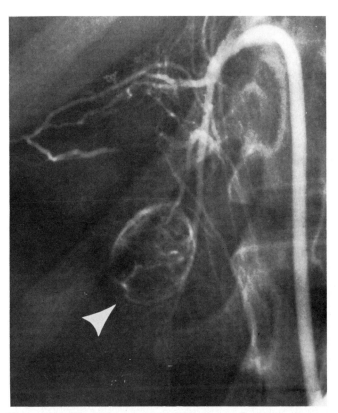

Figure 15–35. Right adrenal phlebogram, Cushings disease due to bilateral neoplasms. Typical arcuate displacement of intra-adrenal veins is again noted (*arrowhead*). This patient had bilateral adenomas, and does not demonstrate the atrophy of the remaining gland that is usually seen in cortisol-producing adenomas. (From Bookstein JJ: The roles of angiography in adrenal disease. *In* Abrams HL (ed): Abrams Angiography. Boston, Little, Brown & Company, 1983.)

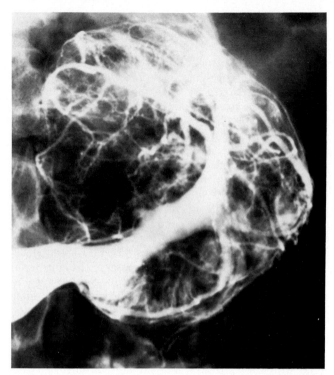

Figure 15–36. Pheochromocytomas tend to be much larger and more vascular than aldosteronomas; this is an extreme example of the venous circulation of a pheochromocytoma. (From Bookstein JJ: The roles of angiography in adrenal disease. *In* Abrams HL (ed): Abrams Angiography. Boston, Little, Brown & Company, 1983.)

glands would usually require selective injection of six arteries. The small interarterial communications over the surface of the gland usually do not permit visualization of an entire gland from one injection (Figs. 15–37 and 15–38). To visualize the superior adrenal artery, the catheter is initially passed above the celiac artery, and the correct reversed configuration within the aorta is obtained. The anterior aorta, just above the origin of the celiac artery, and/or the proximal celiac artery is then explored, and the inferior phrenic arteries (from which the superior adrenal arteries arise) are engaged (Fig. 15–37). From 4 to 6 ml of ~28% iodinated contrast medium is injected in 3 seconds, and serial films are obtained at diminishing frequency for about 9 seconds. The discomfort of injection can be reduced by using low-osmolality contrast agents, or admixing lidocaine with contrast material to a final concentration of 0.2% lidocaine.

The middle adrenal artery can be found by exploring the lateral aspect of the aorta above the renal arteries with the same catheter. Once engaged, filming is performed as above, with reduction in the rate and amount of injection in proportion to the size of the artery.

In order to catheterize the inferior adrenal artery, the catheter is passed into the renal artery. Continued withdrawal directs the tip superiorly. As the tip retreats medially, small injections of contrast medium indicate the point at which the inferior adrenal artery is encountered. The tip may have to be shortened, or the upward angulation increased, to achieve successful engagement.

At times, selective adrenal arteriography may not be possible. In such cases, selective renal arteriography after 3 to 5 μg epinephrine may provide an acceptable alternative (Fig. 15–39). The epinephrine causes a dispropor-

tionate constriction of renal microvasculature, diverting contrast medium into the inferior adrenal artery.

Normal adrenal arteriograms are demonstrated in Figs. 15–37 and 15–38. Note that the gland is not usually entirely opacified after injection of any one artery. The parallel folds of the cortex produce a characteristic double density resembling railroad tracks (Fig. 15–37). Each cortical track measures about 2 mm in thickness. The medulla is not distinctly opacified. Because only a portion of the gland is visualized after each selective injection, the overall appearance of the gland can be appreciated only by mental integration of separate injections, or sophisticated summation of photographic images.

Complications

Two potential complications are somewhat more frequent after adrenal arteriography than after other types of arteriography. Hypertensive reaction to the injection of contrast medium is an expected sequela in patients with pheochromocytoma (Fig. 15–40),[81] especially after selective injection. For this reason, premedication with an α blocker (phenoxybenzamine hydrochloride [Dibenzyline]), and also a β blocker (propranolol) in the presence of tachycardia, are necessary before arteriography (or phlebography) when pheochromocytoma is suspected.

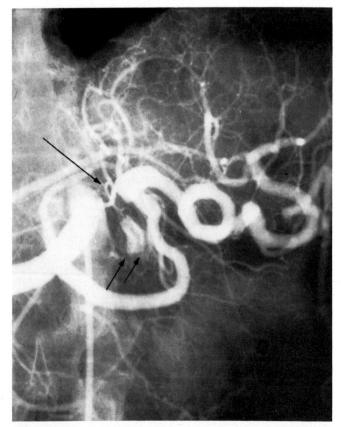

Figure 15–37. Celiac arteriogram, resulting in marked opacification of the upper portion of the left adrenal gland via the superior adrenal artery (*arrow*) branch of the inferior phrenic. Note the parallel stain of both cortices (*parallel arrows*) and the segmental nature of opacification limited to the area of supply of the superior adrenal artery. (From Bookstein JJ: The roles of angiography in adrenal disease. *In* Abrams HL (ed): Abrams Angiography. Boston, Little, Brown & Company, 1983.)

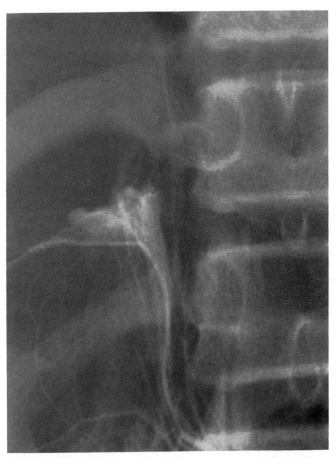

Figure 15–38. Right inferior adrenal arteriogram. The inferior adrenal artery arose in typical manner from the superior aspect of the proximal renal artery. Injection into this artery stained most of the gland, except for the apex. The entire gland does not ordinarily stain from injection of only one of the three sets of arteries that supply the adrenal gland. Thus, arteriography is not usually practical if the entire gland is to be visualized. Arteriography is more useful for demonstration of large hypervascular masses, such as an adrenal carcinoma, in which case tumors can be defined and attributed to the adrenal gland, without the necessity for selective injection of all adrenal arteries. (From Bookstein JJ: The roles of angiography in adrenal disease. *In* Abrams HL (ed): Abrams Angiography. Boston, Little, Brown & Company, 1983.)

The search for adrenal arteries may be difficult and tedious. In patients with extensive atherosclerosis, cholesterol embolism may be the result of excessive persistence in seeking the adrenal arteries.

The most common complication of adrenal phlebography is intra-adrenal extravasation of contrast medium or blood.[82] In experienced hands, this complication develops in about 4% of cases. It is more frequent in patients with aldosteronism or Cushing's disease, in whom the adrenal veins, as well as other systemic veins, are relatively fragile. Radiographic demonstration of extravasated contrast occurs in the minority of cases. More frequently the films are normal, but the patient will complain of progressive postinjection pain, which becomes excruciating within 1 or 2 hours and requires large doses of a narcotic for control. The pain, along with mild fever, usually persists for 24 to 36 hours, and then subsides.

Such a sequence of events indicates intra-adrenal hemorrhage, and is almost invariably associated with complete and permanent destruction of ipsilateral glandular function. Hormonally active tumors within these injured glands may be temporarily or permanently ablated, either accidentally[83–86] or by primary intent.[87, 88] Radionuclide adrenal scans obtained days or months later demonstrate total lack of uptake. If extravasation is bilateral, Addison's disease develops.[82] Thus extravasation recognized after the first adrenal catheterization usually contraindicates a contralateral study, unless total ablation of adrenal function is the intent of the procedure. Clinicians must be prepared to recognize and manage an acute Addisonian crisis in any patient who has undergone adrenal vein catheterization.

Extravasation of contrast medium from extra-adrenal venules is not infrequently observed during the course of the study. This complication is of little clinical significance and is accompanied by only minimal transient discomfort. Adrenal dysfunction does not occur. Differentiation from intra-adrenal extravasation is easily accomplished by noting the extra-adrenal location of contrast deposition.

MISCELLANEOUS VASCULAR PROCEDURES

Gonadal Angiography

Gonadal vasculature can be studied via phlebography or arteriography. Indications for gonadal angiography are considerably impacted by the inherent radiation exposure to the gonads, or, in pregnant women, irradiation of the

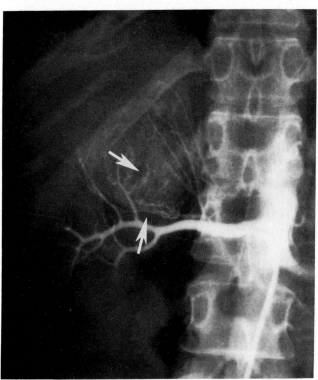

Figure 15–39. Adrenal pharmacoangiography. Control renal arteriography failed to demonstrate a pheochromocytoma. This arteriogram, after 8 μg of epinephrine, results in marked vasoconstriction of renal artery branches, and diversion of flow toward the adrenal gland. The adrenal tumor is now faintly stained (*arrows*). (From Schteingart DE, Conn JW, Orth DN, et al: Secretion of ACTH and B-MSH by an adrenal medullary paraganglioma. J Clin Endocrinol Metab 34:676–683, 1972, © by The Endocrine Soc.)

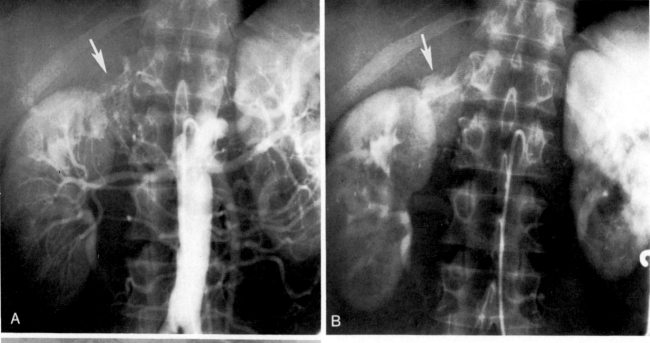

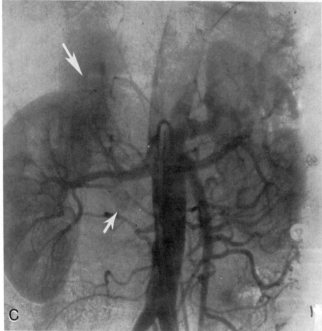

Figure 15–40. Value of subtraction arteriography in demonstrating pheochromocytoma. *A*, Aortogram demonstrates tumor vessels in the region of the right adrenal gland (*arrow*). *B*, Parenchymal phase demonstrates tumor stain in the region of the right adrenal gland (*arrow*). *C*, Subtraction film demonstrates additional unsuspected pheochromocytoma below the renal hilus (*small arrow*), as well as the right adrenal tumor (*large arrow*). (*A–C* from Reuter SR, Talner LB, Arkin T: The importance of subtraction in the angiographic evaluation of extra-adrenal pheochromocytoma. AJR 117(3):128–131, 1973, © Am Roentgen Ray Soc.)

fetus, as well as the availability and flexibility of ultrasonographic imaging, and the efficacy of CT. Current indications for catheterization of ovarian or testicular veins include the following:

1. Demonstration of incompetence of testicular veins in patients with varicocele and infertility, especially in preparation for transcatheter occlusion.[90–94]

2. Demonstration of position of pampiniform plexus in patients with undescended testicles, in order to locate the testicle before orchiopexy or before orchiectomy,[95, 96] in order to eliminate the risk of malignant degeneration.

3. Sampling from ovarian veins (along with adrenal veins), in patients with suspected hormone-producing tumors of either the ovary or adrenal glands.[97, 98]

4. Demonstration of the ovarian vein in suspected so-called right or left ovarian vein syndrome,[99–101] ovarian

vein thrombosis,[102] or a series of ill-defined and perhaps nonexistent "pelvic congestion" syndromes.[103, 104]

Gonadal phlebography for demonstration of displacement by metastatic neoplasm[105] has virtually been completely displaced by CT and other imaging modalities.

Currently, the ovarian or testicular arteries are rarely catheterized. Possible indications might include

1. Identification of location of undescended testicle.[106–109]

2. Study of testicular tumors.[108]

3. Uterine and adnexal masses.[109]

The ovarian and testicular veins arise correspondingly. On the left, the gonadal vein usually arises from the inferior aspect of the left renal vein, within several centimeters of the vertebral margin (Figs. 15–15*A* and 15–40). A valve at the origin and several valves more distally are usually present. Ahlberg and coworkers[110] noted an absence of valves in 40% of left and 23% of right testicular veins. In addition, 36% of males had incompetent valves on one side, but no men had bilaterally incompetent valves. In the presence of an accessory left renal vein, the testicular vein usually arises from the more caudal vein.[96] At autopsy Ahlberg and colleagues[110] found the veins to be slightly larger in women (circumference of about 8.5 mm in men and 10.2 mm in women). Keeping in mind the effects of 20% magnification and possible flattening in the AP dimension, these autopsy measurements are consistent with the angiographically observed diameters of 3 to 4 mm. Multiple veins, which intercommunicate, are common through at least part of the course. The gonadal veins usually also communicate with other retroperitoneal veins, such as the capsuloadipose vein of the kidney and the lumbar veins.

The testicular veins terminate in a profusion of six to 12 small tortuous veins distributed over the upper surface of the testicle, known as the pampiniform plexus (Figs. 15–42 and 15–43).[93] Phlebographic visualization of the pampiniform plexus proves the presence, and marks the site, of testicular tissue in patients with cryptorchism.[96] Abnormal dilation of these veins is the sine qua non of varicocele. The ovarian veins terminate over the ovary and communicate within the broad ligament with uterine veins (Fig. 15–41).

The left gonadal vein can usualy be easily catheterized from the femoral venous approach, using a configuration as shown in Figure 15–6G. The initial phlebogram can be performed with the catheter tip near the renal vein; distal passage is desirable if transcatheter therapeutic obstruction is to be performed for varicocele, or if the pampiniform plexus is to be consistently opacified in cryptorchidism. Valves are negotiated by a judicious combination of flexible guide wires, and trial and error. Venospasm is a problem that may be minimized, but not completely avoided, with IV vasodilators such as nitroglycerin. Depending on the relative vein and catheter sizes, a catheter can usually be advanced well into the pelvis in varicocele patients. In order to reduce radiation to the testis in younger patients, filming below the inguinal ligament is discouraged, and the testes are protected with lead.

The right gonadal vein arises from the right anterolateral aspect of the inferior vena cava in about 90% of patients,[106] just below the origin of the right renal vein. Uncommonly, it originates from the inferior aspect of the renal vein near its junction with the inferior vena cava.

The right gonadal vein, when it arises in the usual manner from the inferior vena cava, can be easily catheterized using a shepherd's crook configuration (Fig. 15–6B, F), with a slight anterior direction being imparted to the distal tip. If repeated efforts fail, a renal vein origin may be suspected. A gonadal vein arising from the right renal can be catheterized by using a shape similar to that for the left. Alternatively, if the shepherd's crook catheter is fairly long, the catheter can be rotated 180 degrees with its tip trapped in the right renal vein. This directs the tip inferiorly, and allows catheterization of the right gonadal vein from the renal vein. If distal passage into the vein is desired, as for treatment of varicocele, then a long redundant loop is needed (Fig. 15–6E). Another option is to catheterize one or both gonadal veins via a percutaneous jugular approach.[92]

The volume of contrast medium to be injected varies with the size of the veins and the need to visualize distally. Ordinarily, I would use a moderately rapid long injection to encourage distal flow. If this is insufficient to demonstrate distal portions, phlebography with the patient upright is very effective; in men, it commonly allows contrast medium to flow into the lower pelvis, even if the testicular vein is normal. The Valsalva maneuver may also promote the distal passage of contrast medium.

In keeping with the frequent judgment of incompetent valves at autopsy,[106] valvular incompetence demonstrated on injection of contrast medium can frequently be elicited

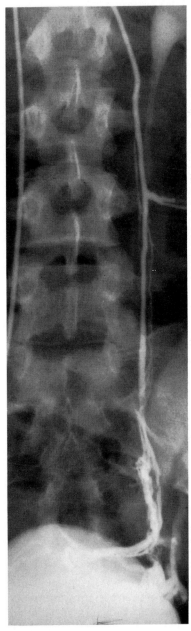

Figure 15–41. Gonadal phlebography. Ovarian phlebogram performed to document proper catheter position during adrenal and ovarian sampling for androgens. This young hirsute woman had a suspected ovarian or adrenal tumor. High concentrations of andronesteone, androstenodione, testosterone, and other hormones were found from the left ovarian vein, and a left ovarian tumor was found at laparotomy.

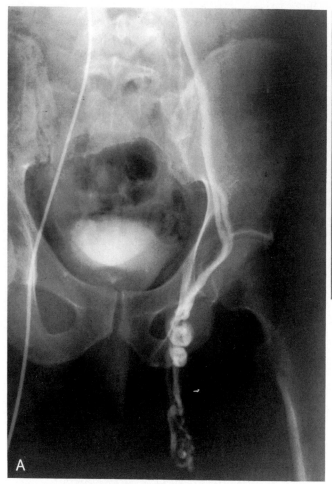

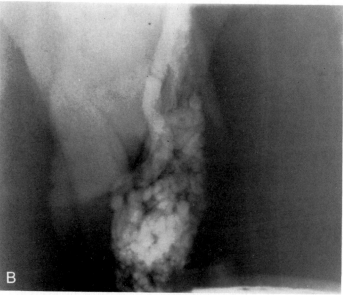

Figure 15–42. Infertility secondary to varicocele. *A*, The testicular vein was dilated, and contrast medium flowed freely in a retrograde direction. *B*, With the patient upright, contrast flowed further, outlining the dilated veins of the varicocele within the scrotum. (From Bookstein JJ: Angiographic technique. Radiology 147:583–584, 1983.)

in the upper pelvis of otherwise normal individuals, particularly if the patient is in the upright position.[111] Formanek and coworkers[92] found insufficiency of the right testicular vein in almost all patients with palpable left-sided varicocele. Marsman[112] and Slot and Miejenhorst[94] consider moderate insufficiency, in the absence of palpable varicocele, to represent a pathological entity termed "subclinical varicocele," which they suggest can be etiologically related to male hypofertility. In my opinion, moderate insufficiency in the upright position, on injection of contrast medium, may be normal.

Varicocele. Diagnosis and therapy of varicocele has assumed importance recently in view of its presumed relationship to male hypofertility. While much more frequent on the left, Chatel and coworkers[113] found palpable right-sided varicocele in 20%, and right testicular vein insufficiency in 80%, of patients with left varicocele.

The major phlebographic sign of varicocele is free retrograde flow of contrast medium into a dilated pampiniform plexus (Fig. 15–42). Patients with frank varicocele will commonly also demonstrate mild or moderate increase in caliber of the testicular vein. In planning for surgical or transcatheter therapy, it is important to note all the testicular vena comitantes, and their sites of intercommunication with the testicular vein, in order to properly plan the site(s) of surgical or transcatheter therapy.

Testicular phlebography is not infrequently indicated for recurrent varicocele, after prior surgical or transcath-

eter therapy.[114] In such cases, one of three patterns can be seen: (1) collateral veins around the site of occlusion, (2) large pre-existing branches around the obstruction, or (3) accessory testicular veins.

Cryptorchism. Testicular localization is desirable because of the risk of malignant degeneration of intra-abdominal testes, and because of the possibility of orchiopexy for inguinal testes (Fig. 15–43). Retrograde phlebography enables testicular localization through demonstration of the position of the pampiniform plexus. In a recent review of 77 phlebographic studies in impalpable testes,[95] the pampiniform plexus was visualized in about one-third, and in 95% of these a testis was present at this site. Of those in whom the testicular vein appeared to end blindly, testicular tissue was absent in 95%. Of those in whom the testicular vein could not be catheterized at all, the testis was surgically absent in 75%.[96]

Ovarian Vein Syndromes. Although of controversial reality, the ovarian vein syndrome is supposedly characterized by acute pain in pregnant women, or chronic pelvic distress in nonpregnant women, secondary to, or associated with, ureteral compression at the pelvic inlet by a dilated ovarian vein.[99–101] Although most frequent on the right, the syndrome may also occur on the left, or may be found bilaterally. The condition is commonly diagnosed on the basis of urography, when the ureter appears to be partially obstructed by extrinsic pressure at the pelvic inlet, even though such features are far from diagnostic. If the syndrome is suspected, ovarian phle-

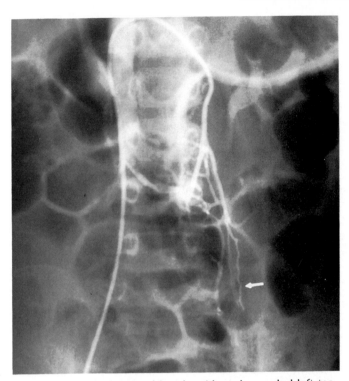

Figure 15–43. Five-year-old male with undescended left testicle. Left testicular phlebogram was performed to locate the level of the testicle, prior to replacement within the scrotum, which would be attempted, if feasible. The testicular vein terminates too high in the pelvis (*arrow*), and the left testicle was removed.

bography might be helpful in demonstrating dilation of the ovarian vein, or conceivably compression as it crosses the pelvic inlet.

Ovarian and Testicular Arteriography

These studies were occasionally performed during the late 1960s.[108, 115] Since then, most of the indications have been assumed by gonadal phlebography, ultrasonography, CT, or laparoscopy.

An initial aortogram is probably advisable, because of frequent anatomical variations. Most commonly, a single gonadal artery is present on each side, arising from the anterior aspect of the abdominal aorta. In about 25% of cases, at least one gonadal artery originates from a renal artery.[111] In 20% of cases, more than two gonadal arteries are present.

If the gonadal arteries are evident on aortography, they can almost always be catheterized. If not, failures sometimes occur. The expected site of origin, usually the anterior and anterolateral aorta just below the renal artery origins, should be explored with a well-taped shepherd's crook catheter (Fig. 15–6*B*). Once the source is found, about 1 to 2 ml/second of contrast is injected for 4 to 6 seconds, in the usual case. The injection is painful, and the newer low-osmolality agents should be used.

The normal gonadal artery is 1 to 1.5 mm in diameter[108, 109] and pursues a tortuous course to the inguinal canal and testicle in males, or to the region of the adnexae

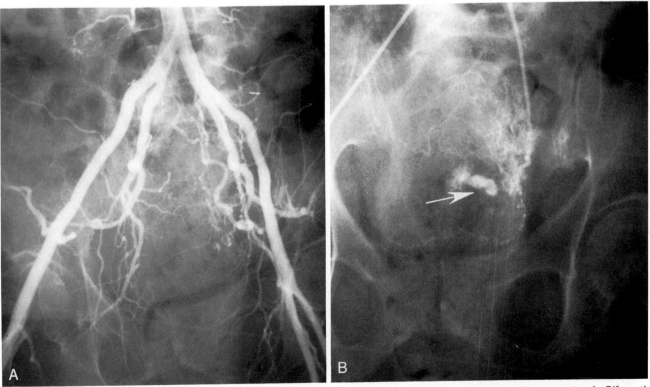

Figure 15–44. Uterine arteriography in a patient with bleeding from postirradiated carcinoma of the cervix. *A,* Bifurcation aortogram demonstrated irregular arteries in the left hemipelvis. Hemorrhage is not evident. *B,* Selective injection of the uterine artery shows hemorrhagic extravasation (*arrow*), plus pathologic vessels secondary to carcinoma and/or irradiation. Subsequently, the uterine artery was occluded with polyvinyl alcohol sponge, and the hemorrhage was permanently stopped.

in females. Gonadal arteries of greater caliber than 1.5 to 2 mm suggest the possibility of a gonadal tumor, or other pelvic tumor in females. Gonadal tumors demonstrate pathological vascularity, often sparse, in about 90% of cases.[108, 116, 117] Uterine tumors may also receive blood supply from the ovarian artery and can be visualized after ovarian arteriography.[109]

Genitourinary Arteriography in Diagnosis and Therapy of Pelvic Bleeding

Arteriography and transcatheter embolization have proven very useful, often life saving, in the localization and treatment of pelvic bleeding. Such bleeding has been attributable to a variety of causes, including trauma (foremost in our experience), cervical and bladder carcinoma before or after irradiation or surgery,[118] prostatic surgery, and obstetrical delivery.[119] Although both internal iliac arteries usually require study, I prefer a unilateral approach with a long reversed-curve catheter (see Fig. 15–6E), sequentially catheterizing and opacifying the ipsilateral side and then the contralateral side (Fig. 15–44).

Once the site of bleeding is identified, selective branch catheterization and embolization with a gelatin sponge, polyvinyl alcohol sponge, or other materials can be accomplished rapidly. Sometimes the bleeding rate is so slow as to be invisible angiographically, a common situation in postirradiation vaginal bleeding from carcinoma of the cervix. In such cases, the uterine arteries are embolized on the basis of the history and clinical findings, usually with gratifying results.[118]

Arteriographic Staging in Neoplasms of the Bladder, Prostate, and Urethra

Therapy of pelvic neoplasms is often dependent on stage. Staging on the basis of clinical examination is notably unreliable,[116] and a variety of imaging modalities may be applied for greater accuracy. In the past, arteriography was utilized to a considerable extent, particularly by Lang.[120, 121] CT, dynamic CT, and CT-guided needle biopsy have now largely displaced angiography as a staging procedure.

Uterine Phlebography

Transmyometrial injection of contrast medium has been used in the past to visualize the uterine, pelvic, and ovarian veins.[100, 101] Contrast is injected via a long needle that is passed through the vaginal canal into the apex of the uterus. The examination was supposed to have been useful in the diagnosis of a variety of uterine and pelvic masses, as well as in the ovarian vein syndrome.[103, 104] Most of the indications seem to have been replaced by uterine ultrasonography or CT, and suspected pathology of the ovarian vein can be more easily evaluated with ovarian phlebography. The paucity of current articles on the subject suggests that the technique has been generally abandoned.

References

1. Seldinger SI: Catheter replacement of the needle in percutaneous arteriography. A new technique. Acta Radiol 39:368–376, 1953.
2. Bookstein JJ, Abrams HL: Surgically correctable renal hypertension. Radiology 75:207–214, 1960.
3. Boijsen E, Folin J: Angiography in the diagnosis of renal carcinoma. Radiole 1:173–191, 1961.
4. Bookstein JJ, Voegeli E: A critical analysis of magnification radiography. Radiology 98:23–30, 1971.
5. Bookstein JJ, Powell TJ: Short target–film rotating–grid magnification. Comparison with air-gap magnification. Radiology 104:399–402, 1972.
6. D'Elia JA, Gleason RE, Alday M, et al: Nephrotoxicity from angiographic contrast material. Am J Med 72:719–725, 1982.
7. Harkonen S, Kjellstrand CM: Exacerbation of diabetic renal failure following intravenous pyelography. Am J Med 63:939–946, 1977.
8. Mason RA, Arbeit LA, Giron F: Renal dysfunction after arteriography. JAMA 253:1001–1004, 1985.
9. Berkseth RO, Kjellstrand CM: Radiologic contrast-induced nephropathy. Med Clin North Am 68:351–370, 1984.
10. Eisenberg RL, Bank WO, Hedgock MW: Renal failure after major angiography can be avoided with hydration. AJR 136:859–861, 1981.
11. Drayer BP (ed): Iopamidol. Invest Radiol 19(Suppl 5):S157–S286, 1984.
12. McClennan BL (ed): Ioxaglic acid: A new low-osmolality contrast medium. Invest Radiol 19(Suppl 6):S6–S392, 1984.
13. Khoury GA, Hopper JC, Varghese Z, et al: Nephrotoxicity of ionic and nonionic contrast material in digital vascular imaging and selective renal arteriography. Br J Radiol 56:631–635, 1983.
14. Gale ME, Robbins AH, Hamburger RV, Widrich WL: Renal toxicity of contrast agents: Iopamidol, iothalamate, and diatrizoate. AJR 142:333–335, 1985.
15. Ford KK, Newman GE, Dunnick NR: The optimal contrast material for digital subtraction angiography of the renal arteries: Ionic or nonionic. Invest Radiol 19(Suppl 5):S244–S246, 1984.
16. Barth K, Mertens MA: A double-blind comparative study of Hexabrix and Renograffin-76 in aortography and visceral arteriography. Invest Radiol 19(Suppl 6):S323–S325, 1984.
17. Shehadi WH, Toniolo G: Adverse reactions to contrast media. Radiology 137:299–302, 1980.
18. Lasser E: Adverse reactions to intravascular administration of contrast media. Allergy 36:369–373, 1981.
19. Witten DH, Hirsch FD, Hartman GW: Acute reactions to urographic contrast medium. Incidence, clinical characteristics, and relationship to history of hypersensitivity. AJR 119:832–840, 1973.
20. Ansell G, Tweedie MCK, West CR, et al: The current status of reactions to contrast media. Invest Radiol (Suppl)15:S32–S39, 1980.
21. Rapoport S, Bookstein JJ, Higgins C, et al: Experience with metrizamide in patients with previous severe anaphylactoid reactions to ionic contrast agents. Radiology 143:321–325, 1982.
22. Lasser E, Simon R, Long J, et al: Contrast media reactions: Idiosyncratic or anaphylactic. Invest Radiol 19(Suppl 4):S103, 1984.
23. Molnar W, Paul DJ: Complications of axillary arteriotomies: An analysis of 1762 consecutive studies. Radiology 104:269–276, 1972.
24. Kruger RA, Mistretta CA, Houk TL, et al: Computerized fluoroscopy in real time for noninvasive visualization of the cardiovascular system. Radiology 130:49, 1979.
25. Bookstein JJ, Steck W: Effective focal spot size. Radiology 98:31–33, 1971.
26. Mattson O: Focal spot variations with exposure data. Acta Radiol 7:161–169, 1968.
27. Abrams HL: The response of neoplastic renal vessels to epinephrine in man. Radiology 82:217–224, 1964.
28. Bookstein JJ, Ernst C: Vasodilatory and vasoconstrictive pharmacoangiographic manipulation of renal collateral flow. Radiology 108:55–59, 1973.
29. Olin TB, Reuter SR: Pharmacoangiographic method for improving nephrophlebography. Radiology 85:1036–1042, 1965.
30. Ekelund L, Gothlin J: Effect of angiotensin on normal renal circulation determined by angiography and a dye dilution technique. Acta Radiol 18:39–48, 1977.
31. Carlsson B, Erickson U: Renal angiography under the influence of vasopressin and bradykinin. AJR 109:161–166, 1970.
32. Abrams HL, Obrez I, Hollenberg NK, Adams DF: Pharmacoangiography of the renal vascular bed. Curr Prob Radiol 1:1–50, 1971.
33. Ozer H, Hollenberg NK: Renal angiographic and hemodynamic responses to vasodilators. Invest Radiol 9:473–478, 1974.

34. Boijsen E: Angiographic studies of the anatomy of single and multiple renal arteries. Acta Radiol (Suppl)183:1, 1959.

35. Edsman G: Angionephrography and suprarenal angiography. Acta Radiol (Suppl)155:1–141, 1957.

36. Bookstein JJ, Clark RN: Renal Microvascular Disease: Angiographic-Micrographic Correlates. Boston, Little, Brown & Company, 1980, pp 19–54.

37. Abrams HL: Renal venography. In Abrams HL (ed): Abrams Angiography. Boston, Little, Brown & Company, 1983.

38. Josephson B: Mechanisms of excretion of renal contrast substances. Acta Radiol 38:299–306, 1952.

39. Abrams HL, Cornell S: Patterns of collateral flow in renal ischemia. Radiology 84:1001–1012, 1965.

40. Bookstein JJ: Segmental renal artery stenosis in renovascular hypertension: Morphologic and hemodynamic considerations. Radiology 90:1073–1083, 1965.

41. Bookstein JJ, Clark RN: Renal Microvascular Disease: Angiographic-Microangiographic Correlates. Boston, Little, Brown & Company, 1980, p 6.

42. Olin T, Redman H: Spillover flowmeter. A preliminary report. Acta Radiol 4:217–222, 1966.

43. Silverman NR, Intaglietta M, Tompkins WR: A videodensitometer for blood flow measurement. Br J Radiol 46:594–598, 1973.

44. Bursch JH, Hahne HJ, Brennecke R, et al: Assessment of arterial blood flow measurements by digital angiography. Radiology 141:39–41, 1981.

45. Kruger RA, Bateman W, Liu PY, Nelson JA: Blood flow determination, using recursive processing: A digital radiographic method. Radiology 149:293–298, 1983.

46. Lantz B, Foerster JM, Link DP, Holcroft JW: Determination of relative blood flow in single arteries: A new video dilution technique. AJR 134:1161–1168, 1980.

47. Leiboff R, Bren G, Katz R, et al: Determinants of transstenotic gradients observed during angioplasty: An experimental model. Am J Cardiol 52:1311–1317, 1983.

48. Bookstein JJ, Walter JF: Pharmacoangiographic manipulation of renal collateral blood flow. Circulation 53:328–334, 1976.

49. Chang V, Fried AM: High-dose renal pharmacoangiography in the assessment of hypovascular renal neoplasms. AJR 131:807–811, 1978.

50. Ekelund L, Lunderquist A: Pharmacoangiography with angiotensin. Radiology 110:533–540, 1974.

51. Gothlin J, Sakuma S, Ishigaki T: Effects of vasopressin in experimental nephroangiography. Acta Radiol 16:609–617, 1975.

52. Bosniak MA, Maydayag MA, Ambos MA, et al: Epinephrine-enhanced renal angiography in renal mass lesions: Is it worth performing? AJR 129:647–651, 1977.

53. Bookstein JJ, Clark RN: Renal Microvascular Disease: Angiographic-Micrographic Correlates. Boston, Little, Brown & Company, 1980.

54. Bookstein JJ, Clark RN: Renal Microvascular Disease: Angiographic-Micrographic Correlates. Boston, Little, Brown & Company, 1980, pp 351–382.

55. Beckman CF, Abrams HL: Renal vein valves; incidence and significance. Radiology 127:351–356, 1978.

56. Moreau JF, Droz D, Abto J: Osmotic nephrosis induced by water soluble tri-iodinated contrast media in man. Radiology 115:329–336, 1975.

56a. Holtás S, Tejler L: Proteinuria following nephroangiography IV: Comparison in dogs between ionic and non-ionic contrast media. Acta Radiol (Diagn) 20:13–18, 1979.

57. Lang EK: Clinical evaluation of side-effects of radiopaque contrast medium administered via intravenous and intra-arterial routes in the same patient. Radiology 85:666–669, 1965.

57a. Robertson HJF: Blood clot formation in angiographic syringes containing nonionic contrast media. Radiology 163:621, 1987.

58. Talner LB, McLaughlin AP, Bookstein JJ: Renal artery dissection: A complication of catheter arteriography. Radiology 117:291–295, 1975.

59. Krane RJ, Sirosky MB: Neurophysiology of erection. Urol Clin North Am 1:350, 1981.

60. Benson GS, McConnell J, Lipschultz LI, et al: Neuromorphology and neuropharmacology of the human penis. J Clin Invest 65:506–513, 1980.

61. Lue TF, Takamura T, Schmidt RA, et al: Hemodynamics of erection in the monkey. J Urol 130:1237–1241, 1983.

62. Dorr LD, Brody MJ: Hemodynamic mechanisms of erection in the canine penis. Am J Physiol 213:1526–1531, 1967.

63. Andersson PO, Bloom SR, Mellander S: Haemodynamics of pelvic nerve induced penile erection in the dog: Possible mediation by vasoactive intestinal polypeptide. J Physiol 350:209–224, 1984.

64. Conti G: L'erection du penis human et ses bases morphologico-vasculaires. Acta Anat 14:217–262, 1952.

65. Valji K, Bookstein JJ: The veno-occlusive mechanism of the canine corpus cavernosum: Angiographic and pharmacologic studies. J Urol 138:1467–1470, 1987.

66. Fournier GR, Juenemann KP, Lue TF, Tanagho EA: Mechanisms of venous occlusion during canine penile erection: An anatomic demonstration. J Urol 137:163–167, 1987.

67. Bookstein JJ, Valji K, Parsons L, Kessler W: Pharmacoarteriography in the evaluation of impotence. J Urol 137:333–337, 1987.

68. Bookstein JJ, Lang E: Penile magnification pharmacoarteriography: Details of intrapenile arterial anatomy. AJR 148:883–888, 1987.

69. Ginestie JF, Romieu A: Radiologic exploration of impotence. The Hague, Martinus-Nijhoff, 1978.

70. Bookstein JJ: Cavernosal venoocclusive insufficiency in male impotence: Evaluation of degree and location. Radiology 164:175–178, 1987.

71. Goldstein I, Payton T, Padma-Nathan H: Diagnostic roles of intracavernosal papaverine. J Cardiovasc Intervent Radiol (in press).

72. Wespes E, Schulman CC: Venous leakage: Surgical treatment of a curable cause of impotence. J Urol 133:796–798, 1985.

73. Bookstein JJ, Lurie AL: Transluminal penile venoablation for impotence. A progress report. J Cardiovasc Intervent Radiol (in press).

74. Virag G: About pharmacologically prolonged erection. Lancet 2:519–520, 1985.

75. Warwick R, Williams PL (eds): Gray's Anatomy, 35th British Ed. Philadelphia, WB Saunders, 1973, pp 669–672, 1346–1348.

76. Merland J-J, Chiras J: Arteriography of the pelvis. Berlin, Springer-Verlag, 1981.

77. Bookstein JJ, Lurie AL: Selective penile venography: Anatomical and hemodynamic observations. J Urol 140:55–60, 1988.

77a. Bookstein JJ, Valji K, Parsons L, Kessler W: Penile pharmaco-cavernosography and cavernosometry in the evaluation of impotence. J Urol 137:772–776, 1987.

78. Horton R, Finck E: Diagnosis and localization in primary aldosteronism. Ann Intern Med 76:885–890, 1972.

79. Dobbie JW, Symington T: The human adrenal gland with special reference to the vasculature. J Endocrinol 34:479–490, 1966.

80. Mikaelsson CG: The adrenal glands after epinephrophlebography. Acta Radiol (Diagn) 11:65–77, 1970.

81. Meaney TF, Buonocore E: Selective arteriography as a localizing and provocative test in the diagnosis of pheochromocytoma. Radiology 87:309–314, 1966.

82. Bookstein JJ, Conn J, Reuter SR: Intra-adrenal hemorrhage as a complication of adrenal venography in primary aldosteronism. Radiology 90:778–779, 1968.

83. Eagan RT, Page MI: Adrenal insufficiency following bilateral adrenal venography. JAMA 215:115–116, 1971.

84. Fisher CE, Turner FA, Horton R: Remission of primary hyperaldosteronism after adrenal venography. N Engl J Med 285:334–336, 1971.

85. Kahn PC, Kelleher MD, Egdahl RH, Belby JC: Adrenal arteriography and venography in primary aldosteronism. Radiology 101:71–78, 1971.

86. Taylor HC, Sachs CR, Bravo EL: Primary aldosteronism: Remission and development of adrenal insufficiency after adrenal venography. Ann Intern Med 85:207–209, 1976.

87. Teixeira PE, Dwyer DE, Voil GW: Remission of primary hyperaldosteronism consequent on adrenal venography. Can Med Assoc J 117:789–790, 1977.

88. Jablonski RD, Meaney TF, Schumacher OP: Transcatheter adrenal ablation for metastatic carcinoma of the breast. Cleve Clin Q 44:57–63, 1977.

89. Zimmerman CE, Eisenberg H, Rosoff CB: Transvenous adrenal destruction: Clinical trials in patients with metastatic malignancy. Surgery 75:550–556, 1974.

90. Seyforth W, Jecht E, Zeitler E: Percutaneous sclerotherapy of varicocele. Radiology 139:335–340, 1981.

91. White RI, Kaufman SL, Barth KH: Occlusion of varicoceles with detachable balloons. Radiology 139:327–334, 1981.

92. Formanek A, Rusnak B, Zollikofer C, et al: Embolization of the spermatic vein for treatment of infertility: A new approach. Radiology 139:315–321, 1981.

93. Tjia TT, Rumping WJM, Landman GHM, Cobben JJ: Phlebog-

raphy of the internal spermatic vein (and the ovarian vein). Diag Imag 51:8–18, 1982.

94. Slot B, Miejenhorst GCH: Venography of the left internal spermatic vein in patients with fertility problems. Diag Imag 51:214–223, 1982.

95. Khan O, Krausz G: Testicular venography in impalpable testis. Eur Urol 9:341–342, 1983.

96. Weiss RM, Glickman MG: Venography of the undescended testis. Urol Clin North Am 9:387–395, 1982.

97. Weiland AJ, Bookstein JJ, Cleary RE, Judd HL: Pre-operative localization of virilizing tumors by selective venous sampling. Am J Obstet Gynecol 131:797–802, 1978.

98. Moltz L, Pickartz H, Sorensen R, et al: Ovarian and adrenal vein steroids in seven patients with androgen-secreting ovarian neoplasms: Selective catheterization. Fertil Steril 42:585–593, 1984.

99. Clark JC: The ovarian vein syndrome. *In* Witten DM, Myers GH, Utz DC (eds): Clinical Urography. Philadelphia, WB Saunders, 1964, pp 2149–2155.

100. Rundqvist E, Sandholm L-E, Larsson G: Treatment of pelvic varicosities causing lower abdominal pain with extraperitoneal resection of the left ovarian vein. Ann Chir Gynecol 73:339–341, 1984.

101. Frea B, Tizzani A, Cicigoi A, et al: Sindrome della vena ovarica. Min Urol Nefrol 36:349–352, 1984.

102. Adachi A, Segren J, Li JKH: Ovarian vein thrombosis mimicking ectopic pregnancy. N Y State J Med 84:567–568, 1985.

103. Bellina JH, Dougherty CM, Mickal A: Transmyometrial pelvic venography. Obstet Gynecol 34:194–199, 1969.

104. Murray E, Comparato MR: Uterine phlebography. Am J Obstet Gynecol 102:1088–1093, 1968.

105. Lien HH, Kolbenstvedt A, Talle K, et al: Comparison of computed tomography, lymphography, and phlebography in 200 consecutive patients with regard to retroperitoneal metastases from testicular tumor. Radiology 144:129–132, 1983.

106. Nordmark L: Angiography of the testicular artery. I. Method of examination. Acta Radiol (Diagn) 18:25–32, 1977.

107. Nordmark L, Bjiersing L, Domellof L, et al: Angiography of the testicular artery. II. Cryptorchism and testicular agenesis. Acta Radiol (Diagn) 18:167–176, 1977.

108. Kahn PC, Fratas RE: The value of angiography of the small branches of the abdominal aorta. AJR 102:407–417, 1968.

109. Karlsson S, Persson PH: Angiography in uterine and adnexal tumors. Acta Radiol (Diagn) 20:11–20, 1980.

110. Ahlberg NE, Bartley O, Chidekel N: Right and left gonadal veins:

111. Bookstein JJ: Angiographic technique. Radiology 147:583–584, 1983.

112. Marsman JWP: Clinical versus subclinical varicocele: Venographic findings and improvement of fertility after embolization. Radiology 155:635–638, 1985.

113. Chatel A, Bigot JM, Dectot H: Anatomie radiologique des veins spermatiques. J Chirurg 115:443–450, 1978.

114. Morag B, Rubinstein ZJ, Madgar I, Lunnenfeld B: The role of spermatic venography after surgical high ligation of the left spermatic veins: Diagnosis and percutaneous occlusion. Urol Radiol 7:32–34, 1985.

115. Fratas RE: Selective angiography of the ovarian artery. Radiology 92:1014–1019, 1969.

116. Eliska O: Venae et arteriae spermaticae a jejich variabilita. Morfologie 9:200–208, 1961.

117. Ichijo S: Vascular patterns of testicular tumors: A microangiographic study. J Urol 113:360–363, 1975.

118. Higgins CB, Bookstein JJ, Davis GB, et al: Therapeutic embolization for intractable chronic bleeding. Radiology 122:473–478, 1977.

119. Pais SO, Glickman M, Schwartz P, et al: Embolization of pelvic arteries for control of postpartum hemorrhage. Obstet Gynecol 55:754–758, 1980.

120. Lang EK: Neoplasms of the bladder, prostate, and urethra. Semin Roentgenol 18:288–297, 1983.

121. Lang EK: Angiography in the diagnosis and staging of pelvic neoplasms. Radiology 134:353–358, 1980.

122. Velick WF, Bookstein JJ: Pheochromocytoma with reversible renal artery stenosis. AJR 132:294–296, 1978.

123. Bookstein JJ: The roles of angiography in adrenal disease. *In* Abrams HL (ed): Abrams Angiography. Boston, Little, Brown & Company, 1983, pp 1395–1426.

124. Reuter SR, Talner LB, Arkin T: The importance of subtraction in the angiographic evaluation of extra-adrenal pheochromocytoma. AJR 117:128, 1973.

125. Bookstein JJ, Walter JF: The role of abdominal radiography in hypertension secondary to renal or adrenal disease. Med Clin North Am 59:169–200, 1975.

126. Schteingart DE, Conn JW, Orth DN, et al: Secretion of ACTH and B-MSH by an adrenal medullary paraganglioma. J Clin Endocrinol Metab 34:676–683, 1972.

An anatomical and statistical study. Acta Radiol (Diagn) 4:593–601, 1966.

16

Digital Subtraction Angiography

BRUCE J. HILLMAN

Digital subtraction angiography (DSA) is a relatively new technologic development that takes advantage of the greater dynamic range of using an image intensifier, rather than film, as the x-ray receptor.[1] DSA may be performed using either intravenous (IV-DSA) or intra-arterial (IA-DSA) administration of contrast material. The advantages of DSA relate to the high contrast sensitivity of image intensification and the ability to manipulate or to post-process digital images. They include (1) performance of angiography with reduced concentration and total dose of contrast material; (2) reduced time for procedures because viewing of images is instantaneous, (3) improved safety related to shortened procedure times and use of venous or smaller arterial catheters, (4) reduced cost related to shortened time of procedure and enhanced capacity for performing outpatient angiography.

Simply described, a DSA system consists of the following: an image intensifier–video chain; a means of converting pictorial (analogue) data into computerized (digital) information; a computer; and a storage, retrieval, and viewing system. The image intensifier transmits the image via a high signal-to-noise video camera to an analogue-to-digital (A/D) converter. The A/D converter changes the image information from pictorial to computerized form, and the data are stored on a digital disc. Following an angiographic run, the radiologist—using an interactive keyboard—electronically subtracts an image exposed prior to the administration of contrast material from one exposed after the circulation of interest has been opacified. The result is a subtraction image that the radiologist views on a video (CRT) screen. The radiologist can postprocess the images to alter brightness and contrast, improve the registration of precontrast and postcontrast images, and filter the final diagnostic images that will be used for interpretation (Fig. 16–1). Desired raw data and subtraction images can be transferred to film or stored on tape.

INTRAVENOUS DIGITAL SUBTRACTION ANGIOGRAPHY

Although IV-DSA was the first technique used in the development of DSA, it is generally out of vogue in the United States, where IA-DSA is preferred. Nonetheless, IV-DSA is still a commonly performed procedure in Europe, where it is favored as a minimally invasive technique for depicting the arterial circulation.

Renal IV-DSA depends on administering a venous bolus of contrast material and waiting for transit of the material to the renal arterial circulation. An optimal IV-DSA technique is predicated on the principle that the bolus of contrast must be administered in a form as compact as possible and in a quantity sufficient to achieve diagnostically adequate opacification of the renal arteries. Digital technology requires only about one-tenth the intra-arterial concentration of contrast material needed to depict arteries of the same size by conventional angiography.[2] However, the smaller the vessel that must be seen, the higher the concentration of contrast material needed for diagnostic opacification. Because arterial contrast concentration with IV-DSA is limited by the dose deliverable to the right atrium and by dilutional effects incurred in contrast reaching the renal arteries, the technique is reliably applicable only to diagnosis of main arterial lesions. A further limitation is that spatial resolution is poorer with digital than with conventional radiography.

Optimal contrast administration dictates that the site of administration should be central, preferably in the right atrium. Both laboratory and clinical data support that this approach will produce superior arterial opacification relative to peripheral vein or even superior vena cava catheterization.[3] Central catheterization is performed by the Seldinger technique, via an antecubital or groin puncture, with a pigtail catheter. The curl of the catheter and its multiple side holes reduce the risk of a subendocardial or intramural injection. Prior to injection, abdominal compression should be applied to displace bowel gas from the region of interest; additionally, 1 mg of intravenous glucagon may help to reduce subtraction misregistration artifact related to bowel peristalsis. Depending on the patient, 25 to 35 cc of 76% contrast material will be required for each injection-exposure sequence. This is best administered at a rate of 20 to 35 cc/second. A slower injection rate results in lower peak opacification of the renal arteries; a faster injection rate may cause wasteful reflux of contrast material into the superior vena cava.[3] Several precontrast images should be exposed immediately following injection to serve as masks for subtraction. One image/second is exposed during renal arterial opacification.

Several problems with IV-DSA have led to United States practitioners' disenchantment with the technique. Much disappointment was related to the primitive state of early commercial systems and the tendency of many to purchase "add-on," rather than dedicated, units. However, as noted, the resolution of IV-DSA, particularly for smaller vessels, is not up to the standard of conventional angiography. Patient respiratory and body motion obviate subtraction and make uninterpretable a small but significant percentage of studies. Therefore, uncooperative patients cannot be imaged by the technique. IV-DSA is nonselective angiography; repeat injection-exposure sequences must be performed in varying obliquities and angulations to depict all the relevant circulation. As a result, total patient contrast dose may be quite high, even exceeding that required for conventional arteriography. Finally, patients with diminished cardiac output will have greater dilutional compromise of renal artery contrast concentration. Consequently, many examinations on such patients will be suboptimal.

497

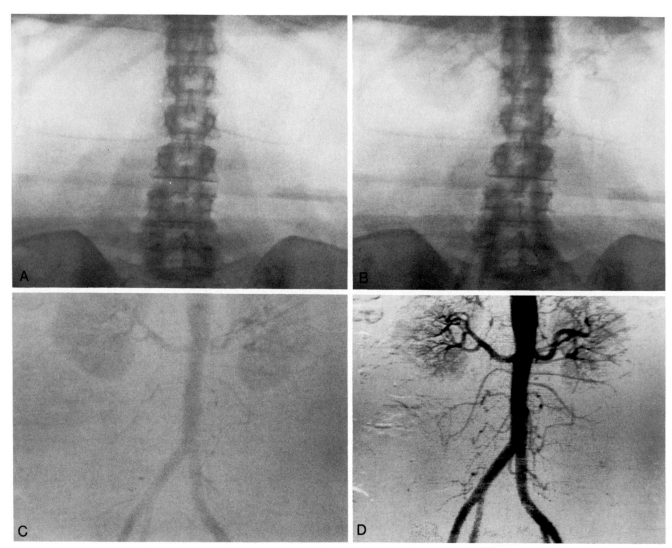

Figure 16–1. Digital intravenous angiogram of the normal abdominal circulation. *A,* The mask, or precontrast, images are exposed shortly after contrast administration, prior to contrast reaching the abdominal circulation. *B,* The postcontrast images are exposed during contrast transit through the renal circulation. *C,* Subtraction image. The mask image is subtracted from the postcontrast image, leaving only a depiction of the renal circulation. *D,* Diagnostic image. Brightness and contrast of the subtraction image are manipulated by the radiologist in order to produce an image of diagnostic quality.

INTRA-ARTERIAL DIGITAL SUBTRACTION ANGIOGRAPHY

For renal arteriography, IA-DSA overcomes a number of the problems cited for IV-DSA while retaining many of the advantages of digital technology. Because contrast material is injected intra-aortically or selectively into the renal arteries, there is no practical limit to intra-arterial contrast concentration. Indeed, the 10-fold contrast resolution of digital radiography permits reduced contrast material concentration and total dose with IA-DSA relative to conventional angiography. Since patients do not have to hold still for the period of cardiac and pulmonary contrast transit, immobility requirements are greatly reduced; nearly all patients can be imaged by this technique. Obviously, no limitation is imposed by the patient's cardiac status. There is dispute over whether the performance of IA-DSA is sufficient for evaluating very small vessels, such as those affected by the renal arteritides, which may be better depicted by magnification film-screen examination.

Following conventional femoral or axillary puncture and Seldinger catheterization of the aorta, an aortogram is usually performed to evaluate the anatomy of the renal circulation. Abdominal compression and or glucagon is again helpful in reducing bowel motion artifact. The injection technique for the aorta follows the same general rules as for selective injection: contrast volume should be maintained similar to conventional arteriography to avoid mixing and layering artifacts, but the concentration of contrast material should be reduced. For the aorta, 25% to 40% contrast material is sufficient for good aortic and branch vessel opacification. Selective renal artery injection with good branch vessel depiction can be achieved by administering 30% to 40% contrast material. Mask exposures are obtained prior to injection. During contrast transit through the renal arteries, images are exposed at a rate of three/second (Fig. 16–2). Postprocessing and

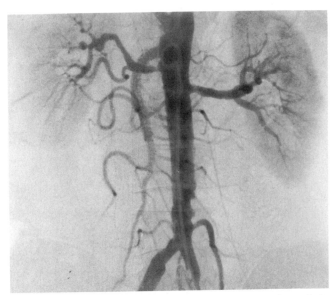

Figure 16–2. Digital arterial aortogram. A pigtail catheter is in the suprarenal aorta. There is aortic irregularity reflective of atherosclerosis. There is also a severe proximal right renal artery stenosis.

interpretation are carried out as with IV-DSA. Patients are held several hours following angiography for observation and to avoid hemorrhage related to activity too soon after the procedure.

References

1. Hillman BJ: Digital radiology. Rad Clin North Am 23:211, 1985.
2. Verhoeven LAJ: Comparison of enhancement capabilities of film subtraction and digital subtraction methods. Pro SPIE 314:114, 1981.
3. Saddekni S, Sos TA, Srur M, Cohn DJ: Contrast administration and techniques of digital subtraction angiography performance. Rad Clin North Am 23:275–291, 1985.

17

Lymphography

RONALD A. CASTELLINO

Lymphography is the radiographic technique whereby lymphatic channels and lymph nodes are opacified by the introduction of radiopaque contrast material. The terms *lymphangiography* and *lymphadenography* are more precisely applied to the radiographic study of the opacified lymphatic channels and of the lymph nodes, respectively. The vast majority of lymphographic studies are performed by infusing oily contrast media into cannulated lymphatic channels on the dorsum of the foot, with subsequent opacification of lymph nodes in the pelvis and retroperitoneum, groups that are of importance in evaluating patients with genitourinary tract malignancies. Cannulation of lymphatics on the dorsum of the hand, spermatic cord, and neck, although technically feasible, is rarely performed in clinical practice.

HISTORY AND DEVELOPMENT

Lymphography was introduced as a clinically useful tool in the middle 1950s as an outgrowth of studies by Kinmonth and associates in their evaluation of patients with lymphedema.[15] They subcutaneously injected vital blue dyes, which were then absorbed by the lymphatics after which they could be visualized in the skin or subcutaneous tissues. This was followed by the surgical cannulation of the visualized subcutaneous lymphatic channels and the introduction of radiopaque contrast media. Initially, aqueous contrast media were utilized, and although the lymphatic channels were well delineated, there was poor spatial resolution of the opacified nodes. The use of an iodinated poppy seed oil (Ethiodol, Savage Laboratories, Melville, New York) provided markedly improved radiographic spatial resolution of the opacified lymph nodes, with the added advantage of sustained opacification for many months.

In the early 1960s, lymphography was widely employed as the definitive test for studying the pelvic and retroperitoneal lymph nodes. Early enthusiasm for the spectacular radiographic images of the opacified lymph nodes was dampened significantly when meaningful radiological-histological correlative studies developed data regarding false-positive and false-negative interpretations. During the latter 1960s and 1970s, further studies provided data leading to refinement in radiographic interpretation and a more realistic assessment of the advantages and disadvantages of lymphography. Its contribution to the management of patients with Hodgkin's disease and the non-Hodgkin's lymphomas was clearly established, and its usefulness in patients with a variety of pelvic tumors was defined.

The introduction of computed tomographic (CT) scanning (and, to a lesser extent, diagnostic ultrasound) provided an alternate means of directly identifying lymph nodes without having to perform the lymphatic cannulation required for lymphography. As occurred with lymphography, early enthusiasm for CT as a means to evaluate lymph nodes was tempered when more carefully performed clinical correlative studies were completed. Currently, the utilization of lymphography has decreased, owing to the contribution to patient management from the less invasive and more readily performed CT examination. Lymphography does possess the advantages of increased spatial resolution and the ability to evaluate internal architectural changes within each lymph node. The advantages of CT are that it is not invasive, it can potentially evaluate lymph node groups not opacified by lymphography, and it provides assessment of the primary tumor as well as of other organs. Magnetic resonance imaging (MRI), which has recently been introduced, is the object of yet another cycle of early enthusiasm. One hopes that careful clinical studies will critically define the advantages and limitations of this diagnostic modality for assessing pelvic and abdominal lymph nodes for metastases. In this chapter, the technique of lymphography is presented, with an evaluation of the advantages and limitations of this procedure. The intent is not to provide guidelines or conclusions regarding preferred imaging modalities or sequencing of lymph node imaging studies in clinical management; that is more properly discussed in chapters about specific disease entities.

TECHNIQUE

The basic technique of lymphography consists of the (1) identification of a lymphatic channel, (2) cannulation of the surgically exposed lymphatic channel, (3) infusion of radiopaque contrast medium, and (4) radiographic documentation of the opacified lymphatic channels (initial films) and lymph nodes (delayed or 24-hour films). With experience, the procedure is frequently completed within 1 hour although at times difficulty in successfully cannulating a lymphatic channel is encountered.

Patient Preparation

The patients are interviewed by the radiologist to assess respiratory status and allergy history, to answer questions, and to obtain an informed consent. No patient preparation or premedication is required in adults. Since patient cooperation is necessary to keep the foot relatively motionless, children may require sedation or a general anesthesia. Studies are routinely performed on an outpatient basis, unless the patient is in the hospital for other reasons. Patients are therefore asked to bring slippers, which they can use comfortably over the small bandage following the procedure. The feet, ankles, and lower legs are thoroughly scrubbed and draped to provide a sterile field for the subsequent lymphatic identification and cannulation.

Lymphatic Channel Identification

Traditionally, a vital blue or green dye is injected intradermally and subcutaneously, usually mixed in a one-to-one solution with a local anesthetic, into the webs between the first three toes. Within minutes, lymphatics over the dorsum of the foot are selectively stained, which facilitates lymphatic channel identification. With experience, lymphatic channels in subcutaneous tissues can be identified without the use of these vital dyes. This avoids the discomfort of the injection, the potential risks from allergic reaction to these substances, and the temporary discoloration of the tissues over the foot and lower legs.

The skin and subcutaneous tissue over the middle third of the dorsum of the foot is infiltrated with a local anesthetic, which also serves to separate the tissues. A small, usually 1-cm, incision is made through the superficial layers of the skin, and the remainder of the exposure is performed by blunt dissection so that the lymphatic channels are not inadvertently injured. If a vital dye has been used, the lymphatic channel is appropriately stained. Differentiation from a small vein can be made by stripping the channel, which refills with blood if it is a vein.

Lymphatic Cannulation

The lymphatic channel is carefully cleaned of surrounding tissues to enable maximum distention, and is isolated in preparation for needle cannulation. Various technical modifications and cannulating aids have been proposed to facilitate successful lymphatic channel puncture. Some distention of the channel can be accomplished by temporary proximal obstruction with forward milking distal to the incision site. Care should be taken to puncture only the anterior wall of the lymphatic channel. Careful antegrade threading of the needle shaft follows. The shaft is then stabilized by a previously placed loose suture or other device. Intralymphatic injection of a small amount of saline confirms successful cannulation if slight distention of the channel without leakage is observed.

Infusion of Contrast Medium

Although infusion pumps can be used, a simple mechanical system consisting of varying weights applied to the plunger of a syringe is adequate for controlled infusion of the viscous oily contrast material. Following 0.5 to 1.0 cc of contrast medium infusion, intralymphatic infusion should be radiographically confirmed, either by fluoroscopy or radiographs. Lymphatic infusion results in opacification of one or more branching, fine, continuously opacified structures of approximate unchanging caliber. Intravenous infusion produces discontinuous collections of contrast medium, usually in droplet form.

Sufficient contrast medium should be infused to obtain diagnostic opacification of the pelvic and retroperitoneal lymph nodes. This is accomplished by periodic fluoroscopic or radiographic monitoring of the ascent of contrast medium (Ethiodol). The volume infused for each extremity depends on the size, number, and status of the patient's lymph nodes. Small individuals (and certainly children) require less contrast medium than the average

adult. Lymphatic infusion can be discontinued when the opacified channels reach the level of L4 (Fig. 17–1), because sufficient contrast medium will be in the lymphatic channels of the lower extremity to subsequently flood the middle and upper retroperitoneal lymph nodes. (This approach is altered if the primary purpose of the study is to identify the thoracic duct.) If the visualized lymph nodes appear to be massively enlarged, then the infusion can be cautiously continued to more completely opacify the more cephalad lymph node groups. It is important to determine the amount of contrast medium infused by careful monitoring, rather than by a predefined dose schedule.

After withdrawal of the needle, the small incision is approximated with either a few fine sutures or tape, and is then covered by a sterile gauze bandage. Patients are instructed that they should not wet their feet for several days and that they should keep the area clean. If sutures are used, they are removed 7 to 10 days later.

Radiographs

In order to adequately evaluate the fine internal architectural detail of the opacified lymph nodes, every effort

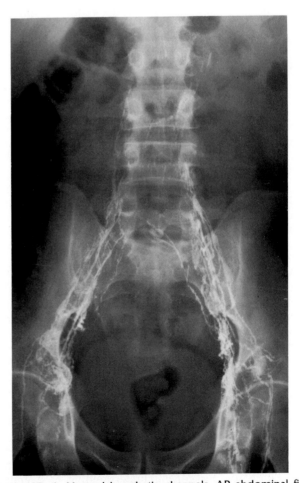

Figure 17–1. Normal lymphatic channels. AP abdominal film shows opacification of normal lymphatic channels in the pelvis and retroperitoneum. Note that they accompany the blood vessels, that is, the aorta, inferior vena cava, and common and external iliac arteries and veins.

must be made to obtain films with excellent spatial resolution. Careful patient positioning, coning of the roentgen beam, utilization of a fine focal spot, and short exposure times to decrease lymph node motion from adjacent pulsating vessels are critical. A technically successful cannulation can be negated by suboptimal radiographs that fail to provide diagnostic images. Low kilovoltage exposure enhances contrast and therefore detail of the infused contrast material.

Preliminary Films. Recent frontal and lateral chest radiographs should be obtained to assess for underlying pulmonary disease, either intrinsic or extrinsic, which might affect the decision as to whether the lymphogram will be performed. An abdominal radiograph (KUB) records the status of the abdomen prior to infusion of contrast medium.

Initial (Lymphangiogram) Films. A frontal abdominal film will document opacification of lymphatic channels in the pelvis and retroperitoneum. Additional films are taken if the clinical question is one of lymphatic channel/lymphodynamic evaluation. Although some authors have found an analysis of the channels helpful in subsequently interpreting the appearance of the opacified lymph node (thus requiring oblique and lateral views), we and others have not found this to be contributory.[16]

Twenty-Four Hour (Lymphadenogram) Films. In most patients, the contrast material has left the lymphatic channels within 24 hours, so that the nodes are optimally visualized the day after the procedure. Routine films include coned AP, both posterior oblique, and lateral views of the opacified retroperitoneal and pelvic lymph nodes. The oblique views are most helpful in projecting the opacified retroperitoneal lymph nodes away from the underlying lumbar spine as well as in displaying the pelvic lymph nodes, which are oriented in a posterior-to-anterior sweep. Suspicious or poorly visualized areas can often be better visualized by obtaining detailed views in various projections limited to a specific lymph node group.

Supplemental techniques, although rarely needed, include conventional linear or complex motion tomography and direct magnification radiography. Tomography particularly helps to eliminate confusing overlying shadows as well as to more convincingly demonstrate abnormalities seen on the conventional studies. Magnification radiography has a more limited use.

Abdominal Surveillance Films. The residually opacified lymph nodes, which retain sufficient contrast media to evaluate lymph node size and position for over 1 year in most patients (an average of 18 months in two-thirds of patients), can be conveniently monitored with serial abdominal radiographs.[6]

LYMPHATIC DRAINAGE

Knowledge of the normal lymphatic drainage of the organ containing the primary tumor is essential for interpretation of imaging studies related to lymph node metastases. The excellent book by H. Rouviere[23] serves as a foundation for our current understanding of lymphatic drainage, and is the basis for the following information. A diagram of the major pelvic and retroperitoneal lymph nodes pertinent to the urinary tract is shown in Figure 17–2.

Testis

The rich lymphatic network of the testis is drained by 4 to 8 lymphatic vessels that ascend along the vessels of the spermatic cord. (The lymphatic drainage of the epididymis likewise runs adjacent to the testicular lymphatics and considerable anastomosis is normally found between these lymphatic channels.) Some of the channels drain into the same nodes that receive lymphatic trunks from the kidney and adrenal, or may directly anastomose with these lymphatic vessels prior to piercing the substance of the node.

The first lymphoid echelon from the testis and epididymis is (1) on the right side, to nodes adjacent to the aorta and inferior vena cava, from the renal vein to the aortic bifurcation—several precaval nodes always receive several lymphatic vessels, and the lowermost precaval node lying adjacent to the aortic bifurcation usually receives a lymphatic channel as well; (2) on the left side, to the left para-aortic nodes adjacent to the renal vascular pedicle, although some may end in nodes closer to the aortic bifurcation; and (3) on both sides, a lymphatic channel draining the testis, as well as channels draining the epididymis (tail), to the external iliac nodes. (Invasion of the scrotum by a testis tumor, or alteration of the usual lymphatic drainage by prior inguinal or scrotal operations, can lead to metastases to the inguinal nodes.)

Prostate

The periprostatic subcapsular lymphatic network drains into four major trunks, which accompany the arterial supply of this organ. A number of intercalating lymph nodules (rather than true lymph nodes), which are retroprostatic, are present. If these are excluded from consideration, the first echelon of lymph nodes collecting these lymph pedicles are as follows: (1) external iliac nodes (to which the surgical obturator nodes belong); (2) an internal iliac node along the branches of the middle hemorrhoidal artery; (3) a node medial to the second sacral foramen, and other nodes of the sacral promontory; and (4) an internal iliac node near the origin of the internal pudendal artery.

Bladder

The lymphatic network in the mucosa and muscular layers of the bladder drains into a superficial lymphatic plexus, from which three major lymphatic trunks drain the bladder. They are known as the collecting trunks of the trigone, posterior wall, and anterior wall. Excluding the interposed intercalating lymph nodules, the first echelon of nodes draining the bladder are the external iliac lymph nodes, particularly the medial and middle groups. Only rarely are lymph nodes in the internal iliac or common iliac region the first lymphoid echelon for the lymphatics of the bladder.

Kidney

Three major collecting trunks drain the kidneys. These are the anterior, middle, and posterior groups, which exit

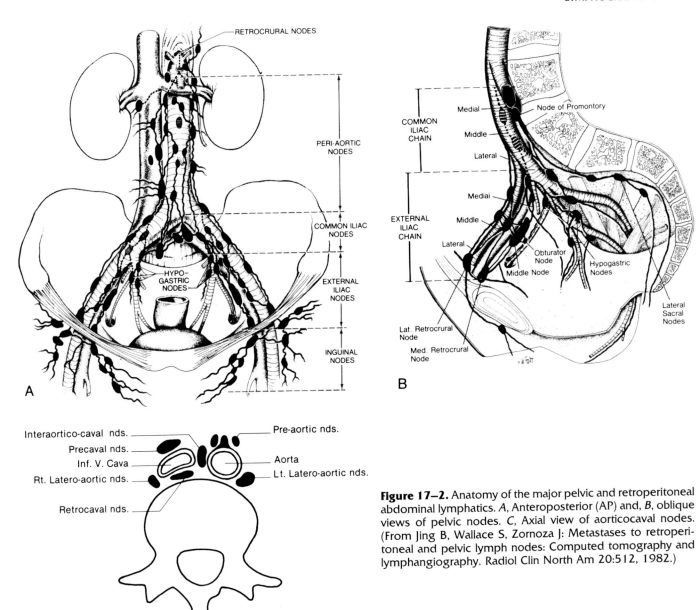

Figure 17–2. Anatomy of the major pelvic and retroperitoneal abdominal lymphatics. *A*, Anteroposterior (AP) and, *B*, oblique views of pelvic nodes. *C*, Axial view of aorticocaval nodes. (From Jing B, Wallace S, Zornoza J: Metastases to retroperitoneal and pelvic lymph nodes: Computed tomography and lymphangiography. Radiol Clin North Am 20:512, 1982.)

the renal hilus and accompany the vessels medially. The first echelon of lymph nodes for the drainage of the kidney consists of (1) para-aortic nodes between the origins of the renal and inferior mesenteric arteries; (2) from the left kidney, the nodes along the left renal vein near the termination of the left adrenal and gonadal veins; and (3) from the right kidney, the paracaval nodes near the termination of the right renal vein.

Renal Pelvis and Ureter

A network of lymphatics drains the renal collecting system and ureter into adjacent lymph nodes. The first echelon of lymph nodes are: (1) from the renal pelvis, to the para-aortic nodes situated near the origin of the ipsilateral renal artery; (2) from the upper ureter, to the para-aortic nodes from near the origin of the renal artery

to the aortic bifurcation; and (3) from the lower ureter, to the common iliac, external iliac, and internal iliac nodes. The intravesical portion of the ureter has the same lymphatic drainage as the bladder trigone.

Urethra

In the male, four collecting groups of lymphatics drain as follows: (1) in the region of the glans, to the superficial or deep inguinal nodes, and occasionally the external iliac, or even internal iliac, nodes; (2) from the penile urethra, to the same location; (3) from the bulbomembranous urethra, to the retrofemoral and medial external iliac nodes; and (4) from the prostatic urethra, to the lymphatic drainage of the prostate. In the female, the lymphatic drainage is similar to that of the prostatic and membranous portions of the male urethra.

Penis

The first lymph node echelons for various portions of the penis are as follows: (1) from the integument of the penis, to the superficial inguinal nodes; (2) from the glans penis, to the superficial and deep inguinal nodes, and occasionally external or internal iliac nodes; and (3) from the erectile bodies, to the superficial inguinal nodes, and occasionally to the deep inguinal and retrofemoral external iliac nodes.

Seminal Vesicles

The first lymphoid echelon is the external iliac nodes. Drainage to an internal iliac node probably occurs as well.

Adrenal Glands

The first lymphoid echelon of the adrenal gland is primarily the adjacent para-aortic lymph nodes, from the celiac axis to the renal vascular pedicles. A few collecting trunks occasionally drain into intrathoracic prevertebral and posterior mediastinal lymph nodes.

LYMPHOGRAPHIC INTERPRETATION

Lymphographic interpretation is based on an understanding of normal lymph node anatomy and its variations, and a knowledge of the normal lymphatic drainage of the organ that is the primary site of the tumor under evaluation (because patterns of lymph node metastases are quite predictable). Consideration must always be given to various nonmalignant processes that can affect gross lymph morphology, such as various types of hyperplasia and replacement of lymph node tissue by fat or fibrosis.

Anatomy

Lymph nodes are ovoid structures surrounded by a capsule from which trabeculae penetrate into the substance of the gland. The afferent lymphatic channels enter the gland at various points along its periphery. The efferent lymphatic channels, together with blood vessels, exit at the hilus of the node.

The lymph node parenchyma is composed of two histological and functional entities. The dense aggregates of cells situated in the cortex and medulla are the lymphoid follicles and medullary cords, respectively. These vary in size, averaging 1 mm in diameter, and play a role in immune surveillance and antibody production. In comparison, the interconnecting sinusoidal system is relatively acellular and is honeycombed by reticular fibers, the main function of which is filtration and macrophage activity. The sinusoidal system conducts the flow of lymph from the peripheral afferent lymphatics to the draining efferent channels.

The Normal Lymphogram

The infused droplets of oily contrast medium follow the flow of lymph fluid and become trapped in the sinusoidal system. Very little contrast medium enters the lymphoid follicles and cords. Therefore, the normal radiographic appearance is that of numerous droplets of contrast medium homogeneously distributed throughout the lymph node (in the sinusoids), in which the nonopacified areas represent the lymphoid tissue (follicles) (see Fig. 17–3A).[26] This normal lymphographic pattern can be altered by changes in the lymphoid follicles, sinusoidal system, or both, with or without a concomitant change in lymph node size. The lymphogram therefore presents a detailed rendition of the macroscopic appearance of the lymph node.

In pedal lymphography, the inguinal/femoral, the external and common iliac, and the para-aortic and para-caval lymph nodes are routinely opacified to the level of the renal vascular pedicles. Cephalad to this level, the contrast material passes through the thoracic duct to the venous system, although nodes in the retrocrural, supraclavicular, and other sites may be opacified.

Because the inguinal/femoral (and lowest, superficial external iliac) nodes frequently contain hyperplastic/inflammatory changes, their appearance is disregarded, unless markedly abnormal. Note that the *surgical* obturator nodes are in fact part of the external iliac lymph node group, and are thus *always* opacified (see page 511) during routine lymphography.

The Abnormal Lymphogram

Compression and/or obliteration of the sinusoidal system, either by benign or malignant enlargement of the follicular tissue (e.g., reactive follicular hyperplasia and malignant lymphoma, respectively) or destruction/replacement of portions of the lymph node (e.g., fatty or fibrous infiltration, metastases, microabscesses) will produce an inhomogeneous radiographic appearance. When occurring as more focal, relatively sharply marginated processes, these changes are often referred to as "filling defects," which are seen most typically with metastases from solid, epithelial tumors (Figs. 17–3B, 17–4A, and 17–5). When diffusely scattered throughout the lymph node the appearance is often termed "foamy" and is the classic appearance of malignant lymphomas. However, malignant lymphomas can also produce focal filling defects (Fig. 17–4B), and solid tumors can produce diffuse foamy patterns (Fig. 17–4B and 17–6). These architectural changes are usually accompanied by enlargement of the node, although perhaps only focally at the site of the internal architectural abnormality. However, the degree of nodal enlargement may be insufficient to be detected with confidence on cross-sectional imaging studies. Therefore, the major diagnostic advantage of lymphography over other lymph node imaging techniques is the ability to detect internal architectural abnormalities in nodes that have not enlarged sufficiently to permit diagnosis on CT, ultrasound, or MRI studies (Figs. 17–7 and 17–8).

Filling defects caused by metastases from epithelial (solid) tumors typically produce relatively well-circum-

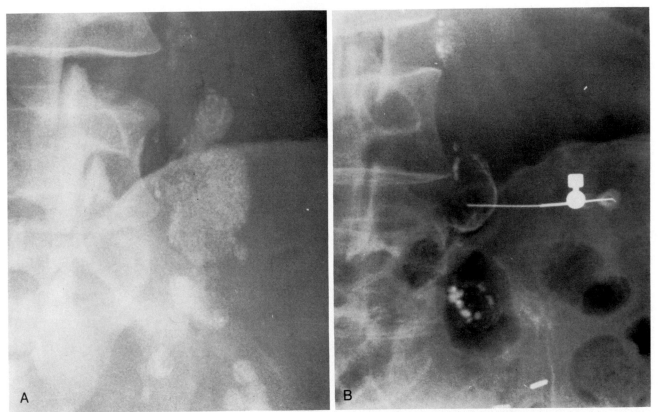

Figure 17-3. Importance of internal architecture in lymphography. Lymphograms from two different patients, left posterior oblique (LPO) projections, demonstrate a large lymph node at the junction of the aorta and left common iliac artery. *A,* Normal internal architecture characterized by homogeneously distributed fine, punctate droplets of contrast medium, indicating that the large size of this node was not related to replacement by tumor. This node was excised and was histologically normal. (*A,* Reproduced by permission from Castellino RA: Relative Merits. *In* Margulis A, Burhenne J [eds]: Alimentary Tract Radiology. St Louis, 1979, The CV Mosby Co.) *B,* Classic filling defect with a "rim sign," interpreted as metastases from this patient's prostate carcinoma. Percutaneous needle aspiration yielded malignant cells. (*B,* from Castellino, RA: Lymphography. *In* Moss A, Goldberg H [eds]: Computed Tomography, Ultrasound and X-ray: An Integrated Approach. Chicago, Masson, 1979. © Masson Publishing USA, Inc.)

scribed lesions with focal enlargement of the lymph node (Fig. 17-9; see also Figs. 17-3*A,* 17-4*A,* 17-5, and 17-8). In general, partial replacement of nodes by fat and fibrous tissue often produces defects with ill-defined margins and without focal lymph node enlargement. This is helpful in distinguishing malignant from benign filling defects, a relatively frequent problem in the pelvic lymph nodes in the older age group who develop pelvic genitourinary tract malignancies.

The diffusely granular or foamy internal architectural changes, typically seen with the malignant lymphomas and nonspecific reactive (follicular) hyperplasia, frequently cause modest to moderate lymph node enlargement. A helpful distinguishing feature is that nonspecific hyperplasia tends to involve all lymph node groups relatively equally and symmetrically, whereas involvement by metastases spares certain lymph node groups or, if all are involved, some groups demonstrate alterations more pronounced than others. Diffuse hyperplasia is also more commonly seen in children and young adults.

Complete replacement of lymph nodes results in failure of the involved nodes to opacify. This is frequently accompanied by the visualization of fine, meandering lymphatic collaterals, indicative of lymphatic obstruction (Fig. 17-10).

Careful comparison of serial abdominal films provides important information in assessing the effects of therapy, thus providing important information for patient management. Detection of disease relapse by interval increase in lymph node size or definite change in lymph node position may be the first, or confirmatory, evidence of relapse (Figs. 17-11 and 17-12). Since the droplets of contrast medium (Ethiodol) are lost in a random fashion, the residually opacified lymph nodes normally in time, develop internal architectural appearances that might be categorized as foamy or containing filling defects. Thus, when surveillance abdominal radiographs are evaluated, the changes in size and/or position, and not the internal architectural patterns, are the basis of interpretation.

Interpretation

Knowledge of the primary site and histological subtype of the tumor under study, the lymphatic drainage of the organ harboring the tumor, and any prior intervention or treatment, will enhance diagnostic confidence and accuracy. Lymph node metastases occur in a predictable fashion. For example, in patients with bladder or prostate cancer, worrisome abnormalities in the para-aortic region with normal-appearing opacified pelvic lymph nodes warrants a diagnosis of negative for metastases from the primary tumor, with the possibility of a second disease process. This is based on multiple surgical studies showing

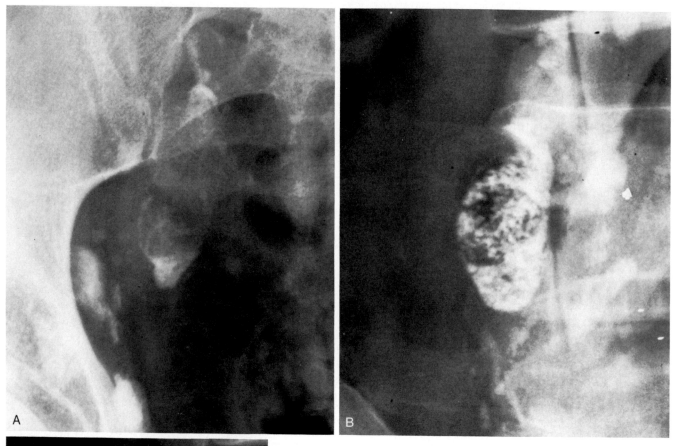

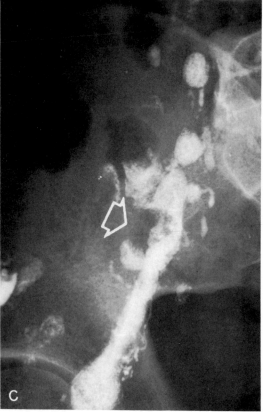

Figure 17–4. Abnormal lymphographic patterns. *A*, Filling defect with a rim sign, causing focal bulging of node from solid tumor metastases (prostate carcinoma). *B*, Foamy node that, although typical for lymphoma, is also compatible with metastases from a solid tumor (prostate carcinoma). *C*, Filling defect with focal node enlargement (*arrow*) that, although typical for a solid tumor, is also compatible with malignant lymphoma (Hodgkin's disease).

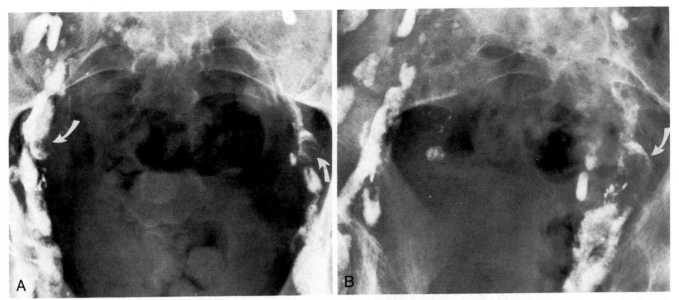

Figure 17–5. Filling defects in normal-size nodes. *A*, AP, and *B*, right posterior oblique (RPO) projections demonstrate sharply marginated, discrete filling defects, with focal bulging of lymph node contours, (*arrows*) typical for metastases from solid tumors (confirmed at surgical staging of this patient's prostate carcinoma). These nodes are in a typical location for the "surgical obturator" nodes. (From Spellman MC, Castellino RA, Ray GR, et al: An evaluation of lymphography in localized carcinoma of the prostate. Radiology 125:637–644, 1977.)

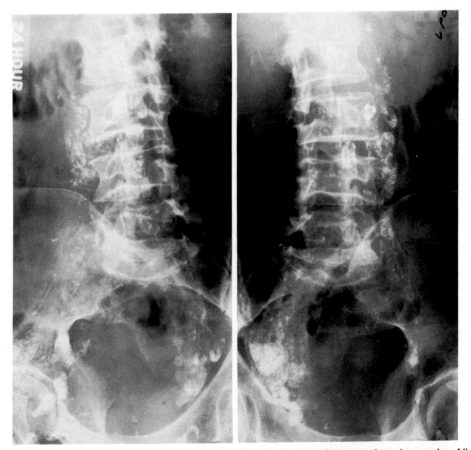

Figure 17–6. Widespread nodal metastases from prostate cancer simulating lymphoma on lymphography. All nodes are enlarged and demonstrate marked architectural derangement, reminiscent of the "foamy" appearance usually associated with malignant lymphoma. Note the greater involvement of the pelvic, as compared with retroperitoneal, lymph nodes. The lymphographic pattern is quite compatible with widespread lymph node metastases in a patient with a known pelvic solid tumor (biopsy proven). (From Spellman MC, Castellino RA, Ray GR, et al: An evaluation of lymphography in localized carcinoma of the prostate. Radiology 125:637–644, 1977.)

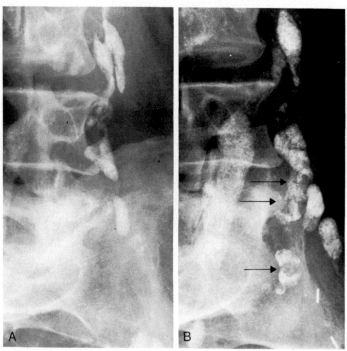
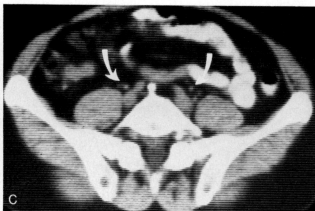

Figure 17–7. Repeat lymphography demonstrating development of lymph node metastases. The initial staging lymphogram (*A*) in a patient with prostate carcinoma was interpreted as negative, which was subsequently confirmed at staging laparatomy. A repeat lymphogram (*B*) several years later demonstrated interval appearance of multiple filling defects (*arrows*) with slight increase in nodal size, interpreted as representing metastases (proven with percutaneous needle aspiration). A computed tomographic (CT) scan (*C*) obtained just prior to the repeat lymphogram was unremarkable, even in retrospect, because the lymph nodes with metastases (*arrows*), although architecturally abnormal, were not enlarged sufficiently to warrant concern on the CT study. (From Castellino RA, Marglin SI, Carroll BA, et al: The radiographic evaluation of abdominal and pelvic lymph nodes in oncologic practice. Cancer Treat Rev 7:153–160, 1980.)

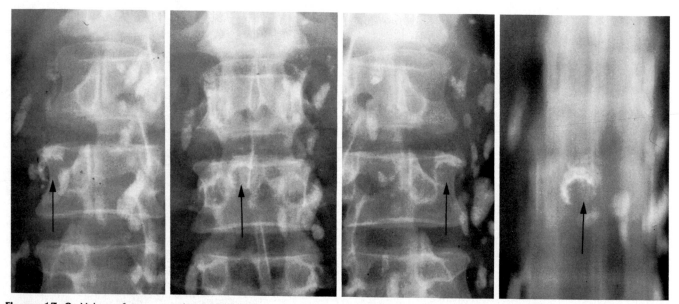

Figure 17–8. Value of tomography to delineate focal lesions. RPO, AP, and LPO views of opacified retroperitoneal nodes demonstrate a normal-size node that is almost completely replaced, creating a sharply demarcated filling defect and rim sign (*arrows*). AP tomogram convincingly demonstrates this abnormality. It is the evaluation of internal architecture, and not lymph node size, shape, or position, that provides unique information in lymphography. (Reproduced by permission from Castellino RA: Lymphangiography. *In* Margulis A, Burhenne J [eds]: Alimentary Tract Radiology. St Louis, 1979, The CV Mosby Co.)

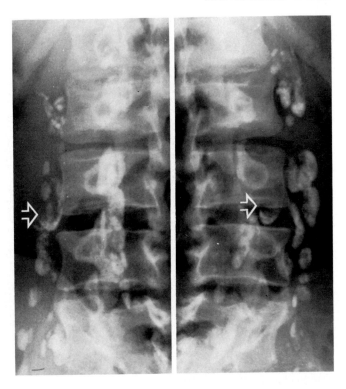

Figure 17–9. Focal filling defect with moderate node enlargement from metastases from a right testicular tumor. The RPO and LPO projections demonstrate an almost completely replaced paracaval lymph node, just above the vena cava bifurcation (*open arrows*). This is a common site for lymph node metastases from right testicular tumors (biopsy proven). (Reproduced by permission from Castellino RA: Lymphangiography. *In* Margulis A, Burhenne J [eds]: Alimentary Tract Radiology. St Louis, 1979, The CV Mosby Co.)

that the para-aortic lymph nodes are rarely, if ever, involved without concomitant pelvic node metastasis.[8, 19] If both lymph node groups are involved, then the degree of pelvic nodal involvement is greater than in more cephalad nodes (Figs. 17–13 and 17–14).

If the patient is having a repeat lymphogram (Figs. 17–15 and 17–16), careful comparison with the initial study is very helpful in assessing stability of unusual-appearing nodes or development of disease based on subtle architectural changes. In this clinical setting, careful attention to prior treatment is important, as surgery, radiotherapy, or chemotherapy can cause lymph node alterations.

False-Negative Lymphographic Interpretations. These are primarily the result of the inability of this imaging

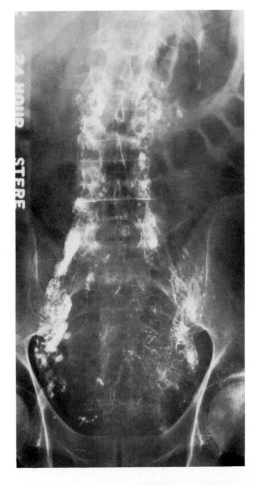

Figure 17–10. Abnormal lymphatic channels. AP abdominal film shows opacification of multiple fine meandering channels in the pelvis, characteristic of collateral filling secondary to obstruction. At times, these collateral channels will decompress to the abdominal, pleural, or pericardial spaces, producing effusions.

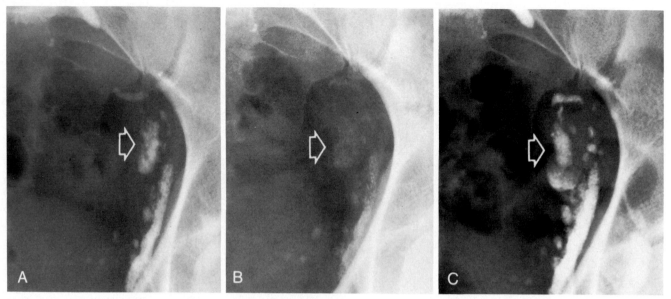

Figure 17–11. Detection of unsuspected relapse with routine surveillance abdominal films. *A,* Initial staging lymphogram for a right testicular seminoma was interpreted as normal. Patient received "hockey stick" (ipsilateral pelvic and para-aortic/caval lymph node) radiotherapy. *B,* Periodic routine surveillance films were negative until this study was obtained 6 months after *A,* which demonstrated interval increase in size of the residually opacified lymph nodes (*arrow*). *C,* To confirm this observation, a repeat lymphogram was performed, clearly demonstrating interval enlargement of nodes, which were interpreted as representing metastases (biopsy proven). (Reproduced by permission from Castellino RA: Lymphangiography. *In* Margulis A, Burhenne J [eds]: Alimentary Tract Radiology. St Louis, 1979, The CV Mosby Co.)

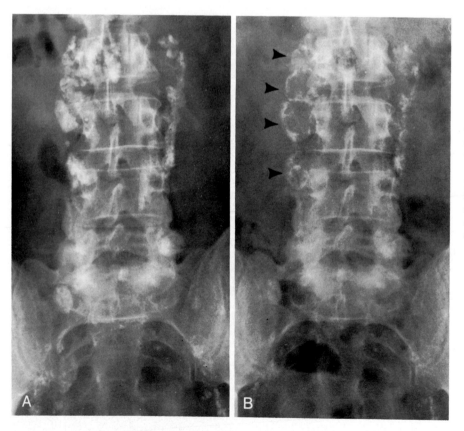

Figure 17–12. Detection of unsuspected relapse on surveillance films. *A,* Initial lymphogram for staging newly diagnosed prostate cancer was interpreted as normal. The patient was treated with radiation therapy to the prostate and pelvic lymph nodes to the level of L4–L5. *B,* Three months later, an abdominal radiograph demonstrated marked enlargement, with development of multiple large filling defects (*arrowheads*), in the right retroperitoneal nodes immediately cephalad to the previous radiation therapy port. (From Spellman MC, Castellino RA, Ray GR, et al: An evaluation of lymphography in localized carcinoma of the prostate. Radiology 125:637–644, 1977.)

It should be noted, however, that the so-called "surgical obturator" nodes, which are frequent sites of lymph node metastases from pelvic tumors, are part of the external iliac group just distal to the bifurcation of the common iliac artery and are, in fact, routinely opacified during foot lymphography. Merrin and coworkers and Zoretic and coworkers have convincingly shown that the nodes excised and called "obturator nodes" by the surgeon contain lymphographic contrast medium.[20, 28]

False-Positive Lymphographic Interpretations. These interpretations result from benign reactive changes, such as fat, fibrosis, and hyperplasia, which cause macroscopic alterations in the lymph node internal architecture that can mimic metastases (Fig. 17–17). This can be a particularly difficult problem in the older group affected by genitourinary malignancies, in whom the middle and lower pelvic lymph nodes frequently display nonuniform opacification due to fatty and fibrous replacement, presumably the result of normal lymph node involution and/or prior inflammatory changes.

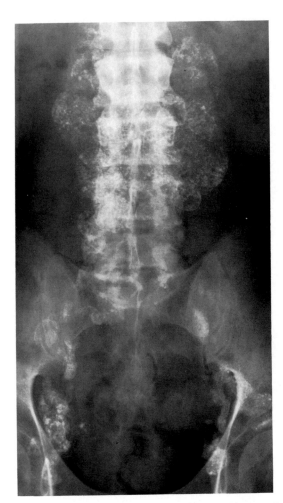

Figure 17–13. Lymphogram for staging prostate carcinoma demonstrates markedly enlarged and foamy retroperitoneal nodes with similar, but less striking findings, in the right pelvic nodes. The foamy pattern, although more typical of lymphoma, is still compatible with prostate carcinoma. However, the anatomical distribution of the most abnormal nodes being in the paraortic rather than pelvic region is not consistent with the lymphatic drainage of the prostate. Therefore, the lymphographic interpretation suggested the possibility of an additional disease entity, which was confirmed at laparotomy where multiple para-aortic lymph node biopsies revealed non-Hodgkin's lymphoma.

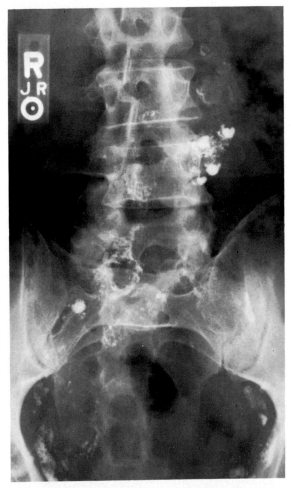

Figure 17–14. Lymphogram in a patient with previously treated non-Hodgkin's lymphoma and newly diagnosed prostatic carcinoma. The opacified nodes are markedly abnormal, with multiple filling defects as well as some foamy nodes. Major abnormalities are present in the right iliac nodes with similar, but less striking findings, more cephalad. Although this could represent the patient's non-Hodgkin's lymphoma, the anatomical distribution is also compatible with prostate cancer. Percutaneous needle aspiration of pelvic and para-aortic lymph nodes revealed prostatic carcinoma. (Courtesy W. Rogaway, M. D.)

technique to display "micrometastases," that is, isolated metastatic deposits of less than to 0.3 to 0.5 cm that do not significantly alter the internal architecture or contour of the opacified node. Should a lymph node contain several deposits of this size, the result may be a detectable foamy-appearing lymph node. Occasionally, false-negative studies are the result of the inability to adequately evaluate opacified lymph nodes due to overlying structures. In this setting, tomography can be quite useful. False-negative diagnoses can also result when lymphographic abnormalities are incorrectly interpreted as benign reactive changes (such as fat or fibrous replacement), when in fact they represent nodal metastases. Finally, false-negative studies are encountered when lymph nodes involved with tumor are not opacified during lymphography. Because the internal iliac lymph nodes are almost never opacified during bipedal lymphography, metastasis to these nodes by pelvic tumors will go undetected.

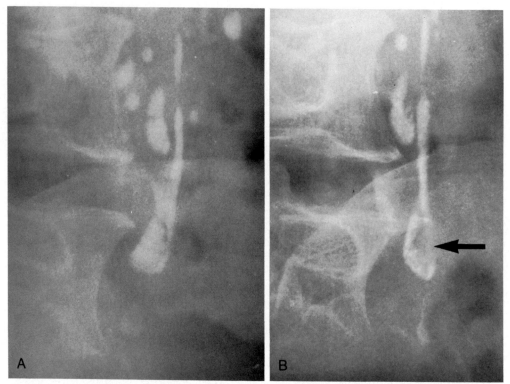

Figure 17–15. Detection of unsuspected relapse by repeat lymphography. *A*, Staging lymphogram for prostate cancer was interpreted as normal, following which the patient received pelvic radiotherapy. *B*, Repeat lymphogram 4 years later demonstrated development of a prominent filling defect in one lymph node (*arrow*) that had not increased in size. Since this node had previously been homogeneously opacified, a diagnosis of metastases was made (biopsy confirmed). (Reproduced by permission from Castellino RA: Lymphangiography. *In* Margulis A, Burhenne J [eds]: Alimentary Tract Radiology. St Louis, 1979, The CV Mosby Co.)

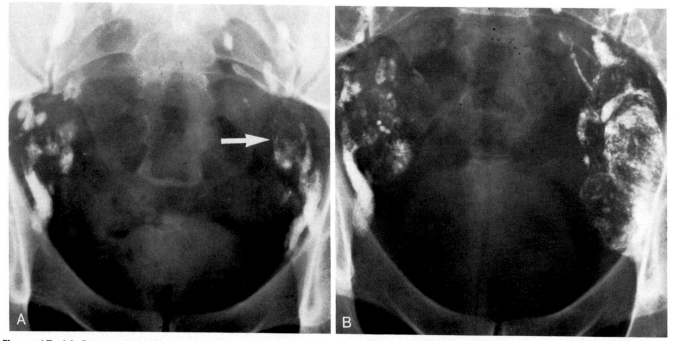

Figure 17–16. Progression of lymph node metastases from prostate cancer. *A*, Staging lymphogram, performed elsewhere, was incorrectly interpreted as negative. Nodes in the left pelvis, at the site of the "surgical obturator nodes," demonstrate distorted internal architecture (*arrow*). This can be more readily appreciated by comparing these nodes with other, more cephalad, opacified nodes. *B*, Repeat lymphogram obtained 4 years later demonstrated interval marked enlargement of all left pelvic nodes, which now contain a striking foamy internal architecture. Although this appearance is more typical for lymphoma, it is also quite compatible with carcinoma. Note also interval change of several right pelvic nodes.

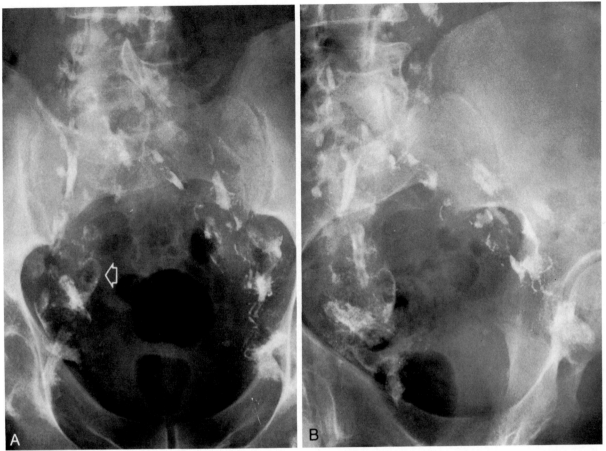

Figure 17–17. False-positive lymphogram caused by extensive fatty replacement of pelvic lymph nodes. Bilateral pelvic nodes are enlarged and demonstrate multiple filling defects (*open arrow*) interpreted as representing metastases in this patient with newly diagnosed Stage C prostate adenocarcinoma. At staging laparotomy, pelvic nodes were palpably enlarged and believed to be positive for metastases; however, multiple excised nodes showed only marked fatty replacement at microscopy, without evidence of tumor. (Reproduced by permission from Castellino RA: Lymphangiography. *In* Margulis A, Burhenne J [eds]: Alimentary Tract Radiology. St Louis, 1979, The CV Mosby Co.)

Sensitivity, Specificity, and Accuracy. Various studies have addressed lymphographic accuracy in patients with cancer of the prostate[7, 11, 14, 18, 22, 24, 25, 30] and testis,[3, 5, 10, 17, 21, 27] with lesser experience for other genitourinary tract primary carcinomas.[13, 25, 27] Such data are limited, owing to difficulty in obtaining histological verification of the lymphographic interpretation and patient selection in various studies.

On balance, when evaluating patients with newly diagnosed, previously untreated solid tumors, the ability to detect the presence of lymph node metastases (sensitivity) ranges between 50% and 75%, whereas the ability to correctly predict the absence of lymph node metastases (specificity) is higher.[1, 4, 12] Overall accuracy is around 70% to 80%. In practical terms, therefore, a positive lymphographic diagnosis has a very high likelihood of correctly indicating lymph node metastases; whereas, a negative lymphographic diagnosis does not exclude this possibility. Percutaneous neeedle aspiration of suspicious or presumptively positive lymphographic abnormalities, performed under fluoroscopic guidance, will further increase diagnostic certainty and accuracy.[7, 9, 14, 24, 29] A positive study is very useful in this clinical setting. Negative studies provide less meaningful information, since small deposits of tumor may not have seen sampled.

INDICATIONS

Initial Staging of Malignant Tumor

The lymphogram assesses the pelvic and retroperitoneal lymph nodes for metastases. As stated above, studies with typical findings for metastases from solid tumors have a high degree of accuracy. Urological malignancies most commonly evaluated with lymphography include those involving the testis, prostate, bladder, and urethra, whereas the primary nonurological indication is in the assessment of Hodgkin's disease and non-Hodgkin's lymphomas.

Lymph Node Biopsy/Dissection Guidance

The opacified nodes are readily accessible to fluoroscopically guided percutaneous needle aspiration (see Figs. 17–3B, 17–7B, and 17–14). Should the patient undergo a surgical staging procedure, the opacified nodes serve as an important guide to surgical exploration. If the patient has a therapeutic lymph node dissection, an intraoperative film assesses the completeness of this procedure.

Radiotherapy Treatment Planning

The opacified nodes serve as important landmarks for defining radiation treatment fields. As bulky lymph node metastases respond to treatment as assessed on surveillance abdominal films, radiotherapy ports can be appropriately decreased to reduce the dose to adjacent, uninvolved tissues and organs.

Evaluating Therapeutic Response

Serial abdominal radiographs monitor decrease in size of abnormal nodes following radiotherapy or chemotherapy. Not infrequently, such changes in the opacified lymph nodes will be the only objective evidence of treatment response, an assessment facilitated by the simplicity of obtaining an abdominal radiograph.

Detection of Relapse

The surveillance abdominal radiograph can depict an increase in the size or a change in the position of the residually opacified lymph nodes, which may indicate metastases. At times, such findings are the only evidence of relapse in otherwise asymptomatic and apparently disease-free patients. In patients with suspected or known relapse, such findings can provide strong confirmatory or contributory evidence, respectively.

Repeat Lymphography

If necessary, the study can be repeated as the residual contrast medium becomes insufficient to provide adequate monitoring. Performance of the repeat lymphogram is technically similar to the initial study and is accomplished with the same success rates. Repeat lymphography for genitourinary tumors has largely been replaced by reliance on CT scanning, although at times the improved evaluation of lymph nodes based on architectural abnormalities prompts performance of a repeat lymphogram.

COMPLICATIONS

Complications encountered relate to the surgical incision and adverse reactions to the local anesthetic, vital dye, or lymphographic contrast media. Currently, lymphography is a procedure with an extremely low rate of significant complication. Data on complications from the 1960s do not translate into current practice, since the earlier studies were performed with larger volumes of contrast material (Ethiodol).

Allergic Reactions

Such reactions can result from the local anesthetic, vital dye, or iodinated oily contrast media. Since they are all administered within a short time of each other, it may be difficult to determine which produced the allergic reaction. It does appear, however, that most major allergic complications, such as cardiovascular and respiratory compromise, were related to the vital dye. To date, we have had no major allergic complications with Evans blue dye (Harvey Labs, Inc., Philadelphia, PA).

Pulmonary Oil Embolization

All patients will have some contrast medium trapped within their pulmonary capillary bed, although the amount is small when the infusion is carefully monitored, as previously described. The fine dispersion of oily droplets may be noted on a chest radiograph. Most patients are asymptomatic; however, when questioned some note an occasional cough and low-grade fever. Pulmonary function studies, if performed, demonstrate diminished function, particularly in the carbon monoxide diffusing capacity. Clinically important pulmonary compromise is rare and is associated with excessive amounts of contrast material entering the venous system, such as occurs with unintentional cannulation of a small vein, rather than a lymphatic channel, or with lymphaticovenous communications. An intense pulmonary inflammatory response, representing perhaps a chemical pneumonitis or a hypersensitivity reaction to the contrast medium, is a rare event, occurring several days to 1 week after the study. This can be associated with significant hemoptysis.

Systemic Oil Embolization

Clinically apparent systemic embolization is very rare, and very few cases of documented cerebral embolization have been reported. The presence of right-to-left cardiac shunting permits access of the oily contrast media to the systemic circulation.

Local Complications

Local infection or lymphangitis following lymphography is unusual. Significant infections must be rare indeed. A peculiar dermatitis, usually in the distribution of the opacified lymphatic channels, is occasionally seen 5 to 15 days following the procedure, is of unknown etiology, and regresses spontaneously.

CONTRAINDICATIONS

Right-to-Left Shunts

A known right-to-left shunt is an absolute contraindication to lymphography, because it permits bypass of the filtering mechanism of the pulmonary capillary bed and allows embolization of the oily droplets into the systemic circulation. Patients with known left-to-right intracardiac shunts should be assessed for possible bidirectional shunting due to pulmonary arterial hypertension.

Impaired Pulmonary Function

Reviewing the preliminary chest radiographs and taking a short respiratory history from the patient in most instances serves as an adequate screen to evaluate pulmonary function and reserve. Radiographic or clinical evidence of significant pulmonary compromise should be carefully evaluated. Pulmonary function studies may be of help in deciding whether to proceed. At times, the cause of the pulmonary impairment can be reversed, for example, by treating congestive failure or by tapping large pleural effusions that compromise pulmonary volume, so that the study can be safely performed.

Allergic History

Known hypersensitivity to the local anesthetic can be addressed by utilizing another agent that has no known cross reactivity. Most patients have no known exposure to vital dyes, although many such dyes are apparently ubiquitous, perhaps accounting for the occasional allergic reactions encountered with these substances. Most patients will not have previously received Ethiodol, although many will have had aqueous iodinated contrast media during urography or CT. The molecular structure for the latter is considerably different from Ethiodol, and there appears to be little cross reactivity. If necessary, premedication with adrenal corticosteroids might be used.

Patients who have severe allergic histories, and particularly those who have had allergy-induced cardiovascular and respiratory compromise, presumably represent increased risks for similar major allergic complications from a variety of substances. Such patients are difficult clinical problems for whom the advantages of obtaining the lymphogram must be carefully assessed against the potential risks. Alternate means of obtaining similar information should be considered.

MISCELLANEOUS CONDITIONS

Chyluria

Intestinal chyle appears in the urine (chyluria) when abnormal fistulous communications exist between the lymphatics containing chyle and the urinary collecting system. Lymphatic obstruction due to lymphangitis and lymphadenitis from parasites, usually filaria, can result in so-called tropical chyluria. Nontropical causes are usually secondary to lymphatic obstruction due to malignancy or chronic inflammatory disease.

Lymphangiography demonstrates opacification of abnormal channels in the region of the kidneys (as well as elsewhere) and subsequent entrance of contrast material into the renal collecting system (Fig. 17–18; see also Figs. 30–21 and 30–22). Abnormal lymphaticorenal communications can also be suspected when profuse pyelolymphatic backflow occurs during retrograde pyelography performed at relatively low pressures.

Retroperitoneal Fibrosis

Retroperitoneal fibrosis may be an idiopathic process, although there appears to be some relationship to adjacent arterial (aneurysm, aortitis) vascular disease. This inflammatory process, associated with scarring, can cause partial to complete obstruction of lymphatics as well as of the ureter, the latter bringing the patient to the urologist's attention.

Lymphographic findings are those of distorted lymphatic channels with evidence of collateral filling. The opacified nodes are often difficult to evaluate, owing to the persistently opacified channels caused by stasis, but may contain irregular nonspecific defects. Lymphaticovenous communications have been reported.

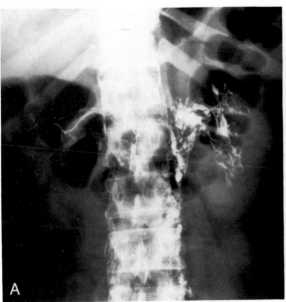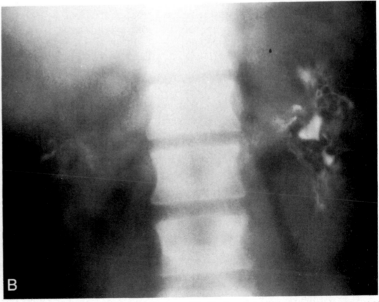

Figure 17–18. Chyluria due to filariasis. A 34 year-old Samoan woman with painless "milky" urine. The lymphogram (A) demonstrates an abnormal collection of lymphatic channels at both renal hila, left more extensive than right, extending into the kidney. AP tomogram (B) confirms the intrarenal location of the lymphographic contrast and opacification of a part of the renal collecting system on the left. (Courtesy Ronald Becker, M. D.)

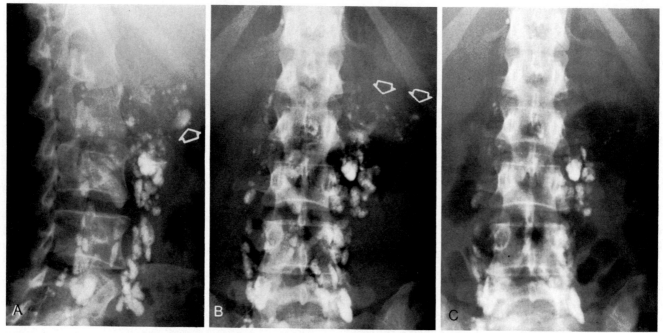

Figure 17–19. Retroperitoneal lymphangioma. Following lymphography, globular collections of contrast material (*arrows*) are seen in the left upper para-aortic region in the LPO (*A*) and AP (*B*) views. Three days later, AP view (*C*) shows disappearance of most of these globules, which were in the dilated spaces of a subsequently resected retroperitoneal multiloculated lymphangioma. (From Castellino RA, Finkelstein S: Lymphographic demonstration of a retroperitoneal lymphangioma. Radiology 115:355–366, 1975.)

Retroperitoneal Lymphangioma

These rare, benign tumors of the lymphatic system are classified as simple, cavernous, or cystic. Presumably congenital, they are single or multiple, unilocular or multilocular, and contain clear or chylous fluid. Lymphangiectasis, which consists of masses of lymphatic cysts, is similar to the spectrum of lymphangiomas.

Lymphangiomas that communicate with the opacified lymphatic system can be visualized with lymphography.[2] One or more irregular dilated lymphatic spaces are opacified, often with disappearance of the contrast material within several days (Fig. 17–19).

References

1. Castellino RA, Marglin SI: Imaging of abdominal and pelvic lymph nodes: Lymphography or computed tomography? Invest Radiol 17:433–443, 1982.
2. Castellino RA, Finkelstein S: Lymphographic demonstration of a retroperitoneal lymphangioma. Radiology 115:355–356, 1975.
3. Chassard JL, Papillon J, Serin D, et al: La lymphographie dans les dysembryomes malins dut testicule. Confrontation radio-anatomique a propos de quarante curages ganglionnaires. (Lymphography in malignant dysembryomas of the testis. Radioanatomical comparison based on 40 lymph node dissections.) Ann Radiol 22:29–38, 1979.
4. Dooms GC, Hricak H: Radiologic imaging modalities, including magnetic resonance, for evaluating lymph nodes. West J Med 144:49–57, 1986.
5. Dunnick NR, Javodpour N: Value of CT and lymphography: Distinguishing retroperitoneal metastases from nonseminomatous testicular tumors. AJR 136:1093–1099, 1981.
6. Fabian CE, Nudelman EJ, Abrams HL: Post-lymphangiogram films as an indication of tumor activity in lymphoma. Invest Radiol 1:386, 1966.
7. Flanigan RC, Mohler JL, King CT, et al: Preoperative lymph node evaluation in prostatic cancer patients who are surgical candidates: The role of lymphangiography and computerized tomography scanning with directed fine needle aspiration. J Urol 134:84–87, 1985.
8. Flocks RH, Culp D, Porto R: Lymphatic spread from prostatic cancer. J Urol 81:194–196, 1959.
9. Gothlin JH: Post-lymphographic percutaneous fine needle biopsy of lymph nodes guided by fluoroscopy. Radiology 120:205–207, 1976.
10. Heiken JP, Balfe DM, McClennan BL: Testicular tumors: Oncologic imaging and diagnosis. Int J Radiat Oncol Biol Phys 10:275–287, 1984.
11. Hoekstra WJ, Schroeder FH: The role of lymphangiography in the staging of prostatic cancer. Prostate 2:433–440, 1981.
12. Jing B-J, Wallace S: Lymphatic imaging of solid tumors. *In* Clouse ME, Wallace S (eds): Lymphatic Imaging. Baltimore, Williams & Wilkins, 1985.
13. Juimo AG, Masselot J, Markovits P, et al: Interet de la lymphographie dans le bilan pre-therapeutique des cancers vesicaux de l'adulte. (Lymphography as an investigation method for bladder cancer in adults.) J Radiol 63:415–421, 1982.
14. Kidd R, Crane RD, Dail DH: Lymphangiography and fine-needle aspiration biopsy: Ineffective for staging early prostate cancer. AJR 141:1007–1012, 1984.
15. Kinmonth JB: Lymphangiography in clinical surgery and particularly in the treatment of lymphoedema. R Coll Surg 15:300–315, 1954.
16. Kolbenstvedt A: Lymphography in the diagnosis of metastases from carcinoma of the uterine cervix stages I and II. Acta Radiologica 16:81–97, 1975.
17. Lackner K, et al: Computertomographischer nachweis von lymphknotenmetastasen bei malignen hodentumoren, ein vergleich der ergebnisse von lymphographie und computertomographic. (Computer tomographic demonstration of lymph-node metastases from malignant testicular tumors. A comparison of lymphography in computer tomography.) Fortschr Rontgenstr (Rofo) 130:636, 1979.
18. Liebner EJ, Stefani S, et al: An evaluation of lymphography with nodal biopsy in localized carcinoma of the prostate. Cancer 45:728–734, 1980.
19. McLaughlin AP, Saltzstein SL, McCullough DL, Gittes RF: Pros-

tatic carcinoma: Incidence and location of unsuspected lymphatic metastases. J Urol 115:89–94, 1976.

20. Merrin C, Wajsman Z, Baumgartner G, Jennings E: The clinical value of lymphangiography: Are the nodes surrounding the obturator nerve visualized? J Urol 117:762–764, 1977.

21. Musumeci R, Tesoro-Tess JD, Milani A, et al: Tumors of the testis: Lymphography and other imaging techniques. Ettore Majorana Int Sci Ser Life Sci 18:99–107, 1985.

22. Prando A, Wallace S, von Eschenbach AC, Jing B-S, Rosengren J-E, Hussey DH: Lymphangiography in staging of carcinoma of the prostate. Radiology 131:641–645, 1979.

23. Rouviere H: Anatomy of the Human Lymphatic System. Compendium. Tobias MJ (translator). Ann Arbor, Edwards Brothers, 1938.

24. Spellman MC, Castellino RA, Ray GR, et al: An evaluation of lymphography in localized carcinoma of the prostate. Radiology 125:637–644, 1977.

25. Taddei L, Fuochi C, Menichelli E, Luciani L: Accuracy of lym-
phography in staging of prostatic and bladder carcinoma: 88 cases with aspirative cytological and postlymphadenectomy histological verification. Diagn Imag Clin Med 53:91–98, 1984.

26. Tjernberg B: Lymphography: An animal study in the diagnosis of V × 2 carcinoma and inflammation. Acta Radiol (Suppl)214:1–184, 1962.

27. Vinje B, Skjennald A, Fryjordet A: Lymphography in the evaluation of urinary bladder carcinoma. Clin Radiol 31:551–553, 1980.

28. Zoretic SN, Wajsman Z, Beckley SA, Pontes JE: Filling of the obturator nodes in pedal lymphangiography: Fact or fiction? J Urol 129:533–535, 1983.

29. Zornoza J, Wallace S, Goldstein HM, et al: Transperitoneal percutaneous retroperitoneal lymph node aspiration biopsy. Radiology 122:111–115, 1977.

30. Castellino, RA: Lymphography in clinically localized prostate cancer. In NCI Monograph #7: Management of Clinically Localized Prostate Cancer, 1988, pp 37–39.

18 Urological Applications of Radionuclides

EUGENE J. FINE □ M. DONALD BLAUFOX

Diagnostic genitourinary (GU) evaluation with radiotracers remains an area of underutilized potential for urologists, radiologists, nephrologists, and internists.[1] Reasons for this suboptimal utilization include confusion on the part of many physicians with respect to (1) the relative diagnostic roles and values of a profusion of renal radiotracers and (2) inadequate recognition of renal physiological principles and their integration with anatomical findings (for example the widespread confusion of hydronephrosis, an anatomical diagnosis, with outflow obstruction, a functional disorder). The advantages of using radiotracers in evaluating the GU tract are so powerful that every effort should be made to understand their unique diagnostic role. The proper choice of a radionuclide tracer examination provides useful and often invaluable functional information that may not be easily obtained by other methods. Additionally, it offers the advantages of substantially lower patient absorbed radiation dose, and a significantly lower morbidity (virtually zero) than do contrast radiographic procedures. Ultrasonography is limited to the depiction of anatomical information with poor functional correlates. Nuclear magnetic resonance imaging (MRI) is an exciting and powerful, but expensive tool. Its use in clinical practice remains to be determined. Radionuclide studies, however, combine anatomical and functional information, have a proven record of clinical utility, and can be provided at relatively low cost.

RADIOTRACER EVALUATION OF THE KIDNEY: TRACER PRINCIPLES AND HISTORY

A biological tracer may be defined as a very small quantity of a substance that can be used to explore the function of an organ or system without disturbing the normal physiological and metabolic processes. Radioactive isotopes of elements that can be incorporated into biologically important molecules were recognized as ideal tracers by investigators as early as the 1920s.[2] It was appreciated that such substances (1) could be administered in quantities that had no discernible biological effect; (2) were nonetheless easily and accurately measurable; and (3) could be detected externally.

Hevesy[2] demonstrated the biological distribution of a naturally occurring radioisotope of lead after absorption by plants. Radiotracers for practical use in humans, however, needed to be further developed.

Nuclear fission was first demonstrated in Germany in 1938.[3] The reaction uranium-235 + n → uranium-236 fission → iodine-131 + yttrium-101 + 4n was discovered to be one of many possible fission reactions, with many other daughter products possible, most of them radioactive. This discovery, preceded by the invention of the cyclotron by Lawrence and Sloan in 1931[4] opened the way toward the widespread availability of radioactive isotopes of many common nuclides.

Radioactive isotopes of iodine were employed in the 1940s in the first practical clinical use of radiotracers, which was directed toward the evaluation of thyroid function.[5, 6] Radioactivity was detected externally over the thyroid with probes (such as the Geiger-Müller tube) to provide information on the rate of accumulation of iodine-131 (I-131) in the gland. Blood and urine samples at various times after ingestion of I-131 also provided information concerning the kinetics of iodide disappearance from plasma.

During the 1950s, the same principles were directed toward the evaluation of the kidney and GU tract. Initial studies were performed with iodopyracet (Diodrast), a urographic contrast medium in wide use at that time. Diodrast is both filtered by the glomerulus and secreted by the proximal renal tubule. Its radiopacity is due to its content of high-molecular-weight nonradioactive iodine. When nonradioactive iodine in the iodopyracet molecule was substituted with I-131, iodopyracet could be detected after intravenous administration of tracer quantities with none of the ill effects sometimes associated with its use as a radiographic contrast agent. Dual crystal-detector measurements over the kidneys produced the first curves of renal uptake and excretion of a radiotracer, which were called renograms.[7] Unfortunately, a significant degree of hepatic uptake interfered with measurement from the right kidney, and extensive protein binding rendered this agent less useful than was originally hoped.

In 1960, I-131 orthoiodohippurate (OIH), a chemical analogue of para-aminohippurate (PAH), was first used in an attempt to surpass the limitations of iodopyracet in measuring the kinetics of renal tubular function.[8, 9] During the next 5 years, the biological properties of I-131 OIH were found to differ somewhat from PAH,[10, 11] but OIH, labeled with I-131, or more recently I-123, remains the best radiotracer available to reflect renal tubular function.

The invention of the rectilinear scanner by Cassen and coworkers in the 1950s[12] and proliferation of this device in the 1960s made possible the imaging of radiotracers. Radioactive agents that bind to renal parenchyma were explored for morphological evaluation of the kidney. Radiotracers such as chlormerodrin[13] labeled with mercury-203 or mercury-197 were utilized for this purpose. In Europe, Hg-197 chloride[14] was used for morphological and functional renal evaluation with excellent results. The radiation dose to the kidney was considered to be too high for use in the United States, and this agent was never approved for routine application. The rectilinear scanner was limited in its resolution capabilities, and its low sensitivity made it incapable of imaging quickly; hence, dynamic sequence imaging was not possible.

The gamma scintillation camera invented by Anger in the 1950s,[15] which did not come into widespread use until the late 1960s, has now replaced the rectilinear scanner for nearly all nuclear medicine imaging applications. Its superior sensitivity and resolution characteristics allow both dynamic and improved static imaging. The nearly simultaneous availability of tracers labeled with technetium-99m (Tc-99m)[16] allowed nuclear physicians to exploit the superior properties of the gamma camera; whereas I-131 has a half-life of 8 days and emits beta radiation, Tc-99m decays by isomeric transition with a half-life of only 6 hours. As a consequence, Tc-99m may be administered in much higher amounts. A large number of Tc-99m–labeled tracers have been developed since that time, including diethylenetriaminepentaacetic acid (DTPA),[17] dimercaptosuccinic acid (DMSA),[18] glucoheptonate (GHA),[19] iron ascorbate,[20] among many others. The principle agents in clinical use in this category are discussed in the next section.

The multiple crystal autofluoroscope was developed by Bender and Blau[21] at about the time the gamma camera was becoming popular. This device has extremely high count rate capabilities. It has achieved limited use in high photon flux dynamic studies only, due to its low resolution of photon detection.

Interfacing the gamma camera with digital computers facilitated ready quantification of renal studies and rendered probe renograms obsolete by the middle 1970s. It is possible, using I-131-OIH or I-123-OIH[22] to measure effective renal plasma flow by either in vitro blood sampling techniques[23, 24] or by computerized gamma camera techniques, which do not require blood sampling.[25] Similarly Tc-99m-DTPA may be used to measure the glomerular filtration rate by either in vitro procedures[26–29] or computerized gamma camera methods.[30] Other parameters of renal function, such as filtration fraction,[31] and parenchymal transit times[32] of physiological tracers can be measured. Investigators continue to report new clinical applications for such measurements.

Combining angiography with radiotracer techniques permits additional functional information to be obtained: the rate of wash-out of xenon-133 (Xe-133) from the kidneys can be measured by external detector probes after bolus injection into the renal artery.[33–35] The information thus obtained allows a measurement of flow per gram of renal tissue, as well as information on the distribution of intrarenal blood flow.

The power of the tracer concept allows for exploration of fundamental biochemical processes by other techniques as well: incorporation of radiotracers in molecularly intact biochemicals such as carbon-11–labeled glucose, fatty acids, nucleotides, and neurotransmitters permits evaluation of fundamental metabolic processes. Incorporation of such metabolic substrates into their biological milieu can be detected invasively by biopsy followed by autoradiography, or noninvasively by positron-emission tomographic (PET) imaging. These last applications have not yet been widely applied to the clinical or physiological evaluation of the GU tract. An exciting arena of physiological investigation has accompanied the development of monoclonal antibodies. Theoretically, this technique may permit differentiation of various immunological diseases of the kidney, including glomerulonephritis, transplant rejection, Goodpasture's syndrome, and others. It has also been used to image neuroblastomas.[35a]

RADIOTRACERS, PHARMACOLOGY AND DOSIMETRY, AND PROCEDURES

The radioactive tracers most commonly used to evaluate the GU tract clinically are compounds labeled with Tc-99m, I-131, or I-123. The physical properties of these radionuclides as well as the administered doses and radiation absorbed doses are indicated in Table 18–1. It should be noted that an ideal agent for imaging with modern scintillation cameras should emit a photon in the range of 100 to 200 KeV. To minimize the radiobiological hazards, the emissions should contain no particulate radiation (e.g., beta particles) and should have the shortest possible half-life compatible with performing a diagnostic examination. Tc-99m is ideal in every regard; I-123 is nearly so, except for a longer than needed half-life. I-131 is really a vestige of an earlier era; with a photopeak of 364 KeV, it is far too penetrating to be imaged sensitively by modern scintillation cameras. Furthermore, its beta radiation and 8-day half-life are radiobiologically undesirable, especially because of potential damage to the thyroid gland. These factors contribute to a relatively higher absorbed radiation dose, making this a less optimal radionuclide for patient studies than Tc-99m, or I-123. The main attribute of I-131-OIH is its extremely rapid elimination from the body, rendering the physical half-life relatively unimportant. In renal failure, I-131-OIH is excreted much more slowly than normally and consequently delivers a higher radiation burden to the patient's thyroid gland due to dissociation of I-131 from the OIH molecule. The dosage, however, does not constitute a contraindication to its use, since the absolute amount of radioactivity administered is quite low.

The alternative to I-131–labeled OIH is I-123–labeled OIH,[22] but its expense has limited its use in the United States. I-123 has a half-life of 13 hours and no particulate emissions. Recent changes in pricing by several companies have made its use more attractive.

Technetium-99m–labeled agents include DTPA,[17] DMSA,[18] and GHA;[19] the first is commonly used for both imaging and renal functional assessment, the latter two for morphological evaluation of the kidneys and, to a lesser degree, functional assessment. Tc-99m bone-seeking agents, such as methylene diphosphonate (MDP) often yield serendipitous information about the kidneys because of their high renal uptake. Simple sodium Tc-99m pertechnetate may be used in rapid-sequence images to assess renal perfusion. A number of Tc-99m–labeled tubular agents are under investigation as potential alternatives to OIH. The advantages of such an agent are numerous. It is not possible at this time, however, to determine which, if any, of these agents will prove superior for clinical use. Data from Europe and preliminary data from the U.S. suggest that Tc-99m MAG$_3$ may be the first agent to seriously challenge the use of Radiohippuran. It is expected to be approved for use in the United States in the near future.

Gallium-67 (Ga-67) in citrate form has a role in the evaluation of renal infections, inflammatory conditions and tumors. Other agents, such as indium-111 (In-111)–labeled leukocytes, In-111–labeled platelets, and Tc-99m sulfur colloid have a limited role in the evaluation of renal infection and transplant function.

OIH

This agent, which was described in 1960,[8, 9, 36, 37] is structurally related to PAH (Fig. 18–1). PAH is extracted

Table 18–1. Renal Radiotracers

Labeled Tracer	Physical Characteristics				Uses and Advantages	Disadvantages	Administered Activity	Rads/mCi			Refs
	Decay Mode	Photon Energy	T½	Renal Handling				Kidney	Bladder	Whole Body	
Tc-99m-DTPA	Isomeric Transition	140 keV	6 hr	GFR	Assess perfusion Individual and total GFR, transit, excretion, leaks, obstruction	Less useful in renal failure	5–15 mCi	0.042	0.55	0.016	177
Tc-99m-GHA				Complex; GFR and tubular secretion with binding to parenchymal tissues	Assess perfusion Individual renal function Morphology, localization Pathological significance of suspected mass	Less useful in renal failure, hepatic excretion	5–10 mCi	0.17	0.80	.007	178, 181
Tc-99m-DMSA				Complex; GFR and tubular secretion with binding to parenchymal tissues	Individual renal function or mass Morphology Pathological significance of suspected mass	Less useful in renal failure High radiation absorbed to kidney makes flow study impractical	2–3 mCi	0.62	0.28	0.016	177, 180
Tc-99m-MDP				Complex	Incidental information provided on bone scan	Major uptake by bone	15–20 mCi	—	0.34	0.013	177
Tc-99m-TcO$_4^-$				Complex	Assess perfusion	Poor renal images	10–20 mCi	—	0.053	0.014	177, 178
I-131-OIH	Beta decay	364 keV	8 days	80% tubular secretion 20% GFR	Individual and total ERPF, transit, excretion, leaks, obstruction	Radiation dose limits administered activity Not imaged well on modern gamma cameras	200–400 μCi	0.11	4.12	0.024	179, 180
I-123-OIH	Electron capture	159 keV	13 hr	80% tubular secretion 20% GFR	Individual and total ERPF transit, excretion, leaks obstruction Imaged well on modern gamma cameras	Expensive	200–400 μCi	0.025	0.86	0.010	179, 180
Ga-67 citrate	Electron capture	Multiple 90 190 300 390	78 hr	Complex	Renal inflammation and/or infection or neoplasm	Nonspecific uptake	3–5 mCi	0.41	—	0.26	182

from renal arterial plasma virtually completely in a single transit through the kidneys; hence, it may be used to measure the effective renal plasma flow (ERPF). A small quantity of PAH within renal venous blood is attributable to shunting of blood through physiologically inactive regions of the kidney, or ineffective plasma flow; thus, the term *effective* is used to describe the renal plasma flow as measured with this substance. The structural similarity of OIH to PAH is not a guarantee of identical physiological behavior. In fact, OIH does behave qualitatively in a manner similar to PAH, but differs quantitatively. Approximately 70% to 80% of OIH is extracted from renal arterial blood in one pass through the kidney; most of the clearance is due to proximal tubular secretion, but about 20% of its total excretion is from glomerular filtration.[10, 11] (After blocking tubular secretion of OIH with probenecid, some investigators have used OIH to measure the glomerular filtration rate.[29]) In tracer quantities, after intravenous administration, approximately 70% of OIH is weakly protein bound in the serum,[38] in contrast to only a few per cent of PAH (when administered in macroscopic quantities). However, protein binding appears to be quite reversible in vivo. The binding of

I-131 or I-123 to OIH is greater than 99% in vitro and is quite stable; however a small amount of free I-131 or I-123 does appear in the circulation.[11] In commercial preparations, the maximum amount of free I-131 is limited to 2%. This can expose a patient to significant thyroidal irradiation, especially from I-131, although the risk can be reduced significantly by blocking thyroid uptake with Lugol's solution before the tracer injection. Good correlations between total ERPF from PAH measurements and from various measures of OIH clearance have been reported.[10, 11, 39] Liver excretion is quite low,[38] an advantage for quantitative renal function evaluation and for imaging in advanced renal insufficiency.

Scintigraphy and Renography

The major uses of scintirenography using OIH include evaluation of total and individual renal function (either qualitatively or quantitatively), parenchymal transit, and renal excretion. Only 25 to 50 μCi of I-131-OIH need be administered for nonimaging probe studies of renal function.[11, 36, 40] Such studies are now primarily of historical interest, since the vast majority of dual crystal detector

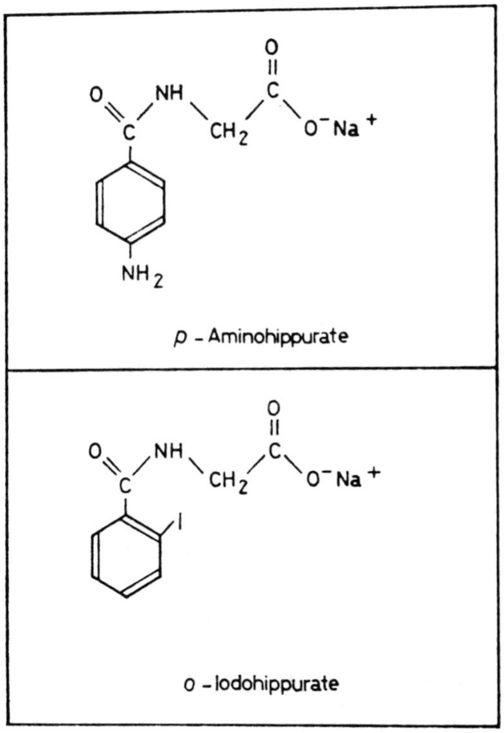

Figure 18–1. The structural formula for para-aminohippurate (PAH) (top) and for orthoiodohippurate (OIH) (bottom). (From Mailloux L, Gagnon JA: Measurement of effective renal plasma flow. *In* Blaufox MD: Evaluation of renal function and disease with radionuclides. Baltimore, S. Karger AG, Basel/University Park Press, 1972, pp 54–70.)

units have been retired in favor of the gamma scintillation camera because of the added imaging capabilities of the latter. The acquisition of reasonable images with minimally acceptable counting statistics requires 200 to 300 μCi of tracer. A major limitation on the amount of tracer administered is the thyroid uptake of free I-131. In the case of I-123-OIH, free I-123 also is present but poses a lower risk to the thyroid because of its shorter half-life and the absence of particulate radiation. However, the expense of I-123-OIH limits its practical use to about 300 μCi as well.

A medium-energy parallel-hole collimator is required for I-131-OIH, whereas a low-energy all-purpose collimator is used with I-123-OIH. A standard scintillation camera with a 12-inch crystal diameter usually encompasses both kidneys within the field of view. The patient should be normally hydrated, as dehydration or overhydration may affect the appearance of the renal uptake.[41] It should be noted that the question of how to deal with uncertainties of hydration remains an unsolved technical problem of renal scintigraphy. Three to five drops of Lugol's iodine in orange juice prior to radiotracer injection is advisable to block thyroidal uptake of free radioiodine. Studies are done with the patient usually prone under the gamma camera after 150 μCi of OIH is injected for each kidney. Alternatively, the patient may be in the sitting or supine position. Sequential posterior-projection 3-minute images are obtained during the first 20 to 30 minutes. It is particularly useful to acquire the images simultaneously on a computer where sequential 15-second 32 × 32–byte matrix images offer adequate temporal resolution for most quantitative applications. A bladder (and/or urine collection bag) image should be obtained

at the end of the 30-minute examination to evaluate for excretion. A large-field-of-view gamma camera might allow the bladder to be included with the kidneys, but standard cameras generally do not permit this. Delayed images of the kidneys are frequently helpful in the evaluation of ureteral obstruction, particularly after ambulation or voiding.[42] Other specialized views may be useful as well; for example, post-void bladder images may be used to quantify residual urine.[43, 44]

The normal appearance of the OIH scintirenogram appears in Figure 18–2. Normally, there should be bilaterally symmetric uptake of tracer in the first 3-minute image with a high kidney-to-background ratio. The intensity of renal visualization on this first image in comparison to background activity is a qualitative index of renal function. (More precise quantification of the kidney uptake using the computerized images allows one to measure total and individual effective renal plasma flow. This is described later in greater detail.) Since the normal transit time of OIH through the kidney is from 3 to 5 minutes,[45] the renal pelves usually can be identified on the second frame (3- to 6-minute) image. Progressive cortical and pelvic emptying occurs through the remainder of the normal examination. The computerized acquisition of these images makes possible the placement of regions of interest around the kidneys and the generation of the time-activity histograms known as renograms. The normal renogram appearance is shown and described in Figure 18–3*B*.

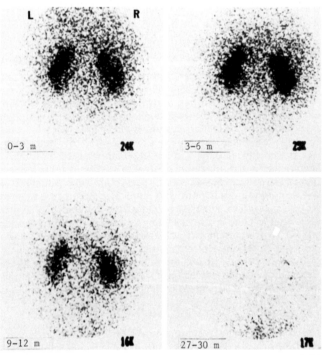

Figure 18–2. Normal scintirenogram with iodine-131 OIH. Four frames are demonstrated from a normal OIH study performed in the posterior projection. During the first 3 minutes of acquisition, activity accumulates symmetrically within the renal cortex. The renal collecting systems are not seen until the 3- to 6-minute image, where they appear as medial prominences. Excretion proceeds rapidly so that less activity is noted within the kidneys on the 9- to 12-minute image, and virtually none remains on the 27- to 30-minute image shown. (See Figure 18–3*B* for another normal OIH study with accompanying renogram curves and their description.)

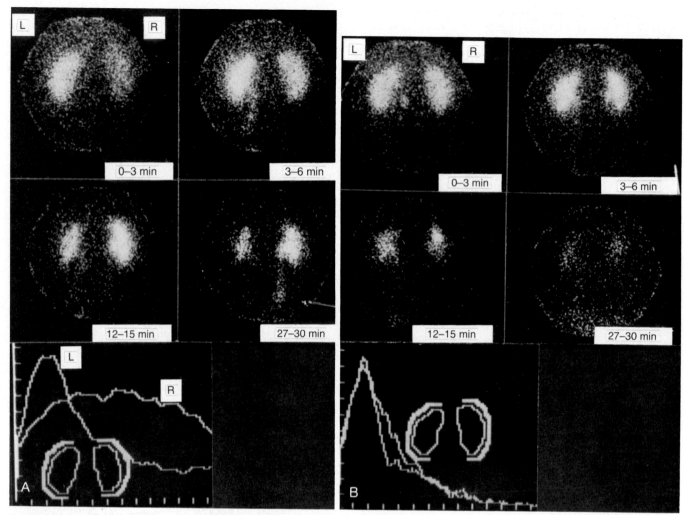

Figure 18–3. Distal ureteral stone, before and after passage. *A,* A 32-year-old woman presented with right flank pain and evidence, on abdominal plain film, of a distal right ureteral stone. The scintirenogram shows normal left kidney uptake on the 0- to 3-minute image, normal transit into the collecting system and ureter on the 3- to 6-minute image, and subsequent normal excretion. However, the right kidney demonstrates less initial uptake, corresponding to decreased renal function. In addition, transit into the collecting system is not clearly noted on the 3- to 6-minute image, indicating a delay. The medial collecting system prominence is noted on the 12- to 15-minute image. On the 27- to 30-minute image there is still substantial activity within the right kidney, and the right ureter is also visualized. A normal left renogram curve is shown. The progressive initial accumulation with markedly delayed excretion is reflected in the right renogram curve by a prolonged plateau. The renal regions of interest and the areas used for background correction are also shown. *B,* After the stone passed, a repeat study was performed. The scintirenogram is normal. It should be noted that right renal function has returned to normal, as have transit and excretion. Normal renogram curves show a rapid initial uptake phase and a peak between 3 and 4 minutes. This corresponds to arrival of radiolabeled urine in the collecting system and subsequent excretion from the kidney. The decrement in renal activity seen in the images is reflected in a rapidly falling curve after the peak. The curves are derived by simultaneously obtaining the imaging data on a computer and determining the time course of radioactivity within a region of interest surrounding the kidney. The regions of interest for the kidneys are superimposed on the image with the renogram curves. Background regions of interest are also shown, but not the curves appropriate to them. (From Fine EJ, Scharf SC, Blaufox MD: The role of nuclear medicine in evaluating the hypertensive patient. *In* Freeman, LM, Weissmann HS (eds): Nuclear Medicine Annual 1984. New York, Raven Press, 1984.)

Abnormalities detectable by OIH scintirenography include ureteral obstruction, acute tubular necrosis, extravasation of urine, renal artery stenosis, and chronic renal failure. Other purposes to which this examination is applicable include detection of a kidney nonvisualized by intravenous urogram (IVU); monitoring of qualitative or quantitative (see Clinical Applications) individual and/or total renal functional changes following interventional procedures (e.g., nephrostomy, angioplasty, lithotripsy, and antibiotic therapy for pyelonephritis); and determination of renal salvageability.

Diuretic Scintirenography

Dilatation of the renal pelvis and ureter (hydroureteronephrosis) is an anatomical diagnosis that, in adults, correlates well with the functional diagnosis of renal outlet obstruction. In the appropriate clinical setting, the scintirenographic diagnosis of obstruction is obvious (Fig. 18–3A). Dilatation, however, may be present without obstruction. This is frequently true in infants and young children with reflux nephropathy, "prune-belly" syndrome, primary megaureter, and other congenital condi-

renal pelvis is prominent at 30 minutes after OIH injection, suggesting obstruction, Rosenthall and coworkers[42] suggest ambulating the patient and obtaining delayed images. They argue that pelvic retention indicates obstruction (Fig. 18–7) and that drainage rules it out, with an accuracy comparable to that of diuretic renography (Fig. 18–8). However, it is difficult to standardize such an examination with respect to hydration, which in turn affects urine flow rate. One may anticipate slow drainage from a minimally dilated, nonobstructed system in the face of dehydration, leading to an erroneous diagnosis of obstruction. Similarly, a partially obstructed system may drain sufficiently to be misdiagnosed as normal. These studies need further confirmation, as Figure 18–9 illustrates. Clearly, long-term follow-up is necessary to clarify the roles of different approaches to the evaluation of hydroureteronephrosis.

Measurement of Renal Function: Effective Renal Plasma Flow (ERPF)[191]

Total ERPF. The classic measurement of ERPF utilizes the constant infusion of para-aminohippurate (PAH),[57] which is cumbersome for both patient and physician. The examination requires a constant intravenous infusion of PAH and multiple venipunctures for sampling of blood to ensure a constant serum PAH concentration. Once this state of equilibrium has been achieved, the rate of influx must equal the rate of efflux (excretion by the kidneys) and is measured by carefully timed urine collections:

$$PAH \text{ clearance} = ERPF \text{ (ml/min)} = \text{(mg/min PAH excreted in urine)}/\text{(PAH concentration in serum)}.$$

Theoretically, the rate of disappearance of PAH from the plasma after bolus injection can provide the same information. In practice, however, a bolus of PAH in amounts sufficient for chemical analysis of delayed blood samples produces early plasma concentrations that may exceed the tubular maximum for PAH secretion by the kidneys.[58] Alternatively, a small bolus of PAH, initially, would lead to serum concentrations of PAH in delayed blood samples that would be too low for accurate chemical measurement. OIH may be used as a reasonable analogue of PAH[10, 11] and has none of the above problems. On the other hand, in the face of marked ERPF reductions, tracer doses of OIH may not be extracted as efficiently as macroscopic quantities of PAH. The typical disappearance of I-131-OIH from the plasma is shown in Figure 18–10.[190] Evaluation of a complete curve in a given subject requires multiple blood sample determinations, but various compartmental analyses[59–61] of this type of disappearance curve have led to simplified methods requiring fewer blood specimens.

An open two-compartment model requires, minimally, four to six blood specimens for measurement of OIH activity. Two slopes and two intercepts may be obtained

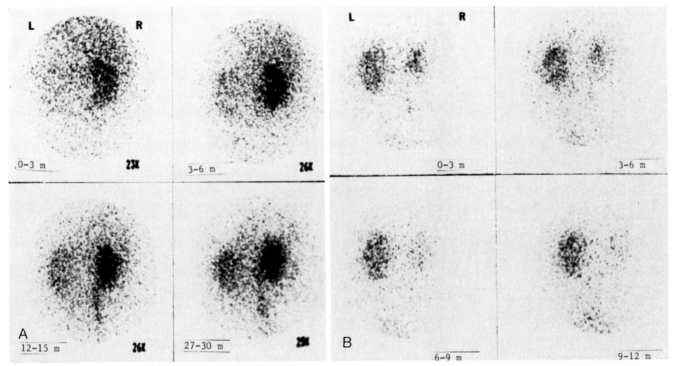

Figure 18–6. Effect of poor renal function on furosemide study. *A,* Furosemide may not distinguish between obstructive and nonobstructive disease. There is bilaterally decreased renal function, more severe on the left. The right kidney demonstrates a dilated collecting system and ureter in the 27- to 30-minute image, while the left kidney has accumulated relatively little activity. *B,* Furosemide was administered, and images were subsequently obtained. The right kidney responded by washing out its activity from the collecting system and ureter; its obstruction is therefore excluded. The left kidney, however, progressively accumulates activity. One cannot state with certainty that the left side is obstructed, because its function may be too poor to respond to furosemide. The study must be considered nondiagnostic for the left kidney. Renogram curves, which are not displayed for this study, did not alter the stated conclusions.

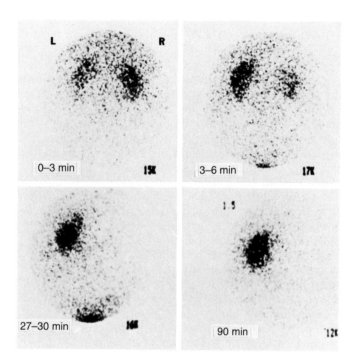

Figure 18–7. Furosemide wash-out with ambulation. This posterior-view OIH study demonstrates normal right-sided function, transit, and excretion. However, the left side demonstrates diminished uptake and therefore decreased function, as seen on the initial 0- to 3-minute image. In addition, transit into the collecting system and subsequent excretion are delayed, as is indicated by progressive accumulation through the 27- to 30-minute image. The patient was asked to ambulate and void, and a repeat image was obtained 90 minutes after injection of the radiotracer. The image shows no significant change in the amount of tracer activity in the left kidney. This pattern has been reported to be highly suggestive of obstruction of the left kidney.

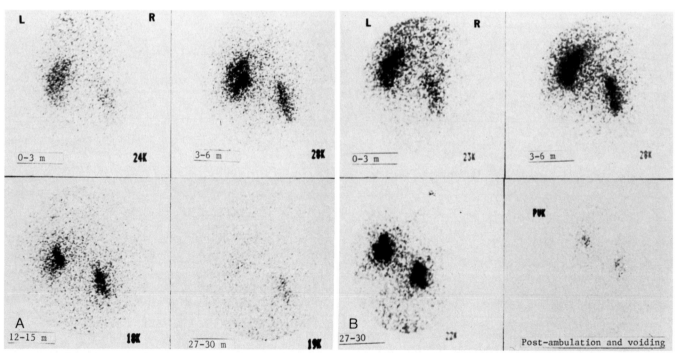

Figure 18–8. Dehydration simulating obstruction. A, This patient was being evaluated for flank pain, and the initial image of an OIH study in the posterior view demonstrates asymmetry of uptake between the kidneys. This may reflect decreased function on the right side. However, normal transit to the collecting systems is indicated on the 3- to 6-minute image and by subsequent excretion, which is nearly complete in the 27- to 30-minute image. B, A repeat study performed approximately 18 months later, again for flank pain, demonstrates the same asymmetry of initial uptake. This time, however, by 27 to 30 minutes there is marked retention of radiolabeled urine within both collecting systems, which appear dilated. The last frame shows normal excretion from both kidneys, after ambulation and voiding. This indicates the value of ambulation and voiding in excluding obstruction. The patient was somewhat dehydrated on this second scan, which accounts for the delay in excretion and the appearance of a dilated collecting system.

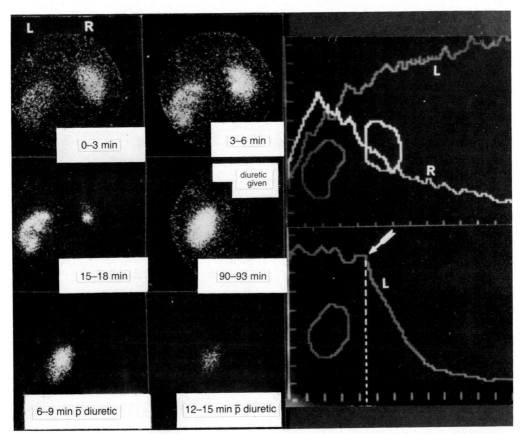

Figure 18–9. Discordance between furosemide and ambulation studies. A discrepancy is demonstrated between the technique of ambulating the patient and the diuresis scintirenogram. A large and relatively poorly functioning left kidney has a dilated collecting system that shows no activity through the initial 18 minutes of images. After ambulation and voiding, a huge collecting system is filled. Evidence at this point suggests obstruction of the left kidney. However, after intravenous furosemide was administered, the dilated left collecting system emptied rapidly. This is also demonstrated by the renogram curve (*arrow*). Such discrepancies are occasionally seen in the diagnosis of obstruction by diuretic scintirenography versus delayed imaging after ambulation and voiding. It is probably more difficult to standardize the latter procedure for states of hydration.

by curve stripping.[59–61] ERPF may be calculated as follows:

$$ERPF = (dose \times b_1 b_2)/(Ab_2 + Bb_1)$$

where A and B are intercepts and b_1 and b_2 are slopes of the fast and slow compartments, respectively (Fig. 18–10).

Further simplification into a one-compartment model requires only two blood specimens.[39] Specimens obtained at 20 and 30 minutes after OIH injection are used to calculate ERPF as follows:[39]

$$ERPF = -dose \times slope/intercept$$

Only one slope and one intercept can be derived from two blood specimens. This introduces a potential loss of accuracy in exchange for the greater simplicity and convenience of a reduced number of blood samples. Nonetheless, good correlations with PAH clearances are obtained with this method as well. Although it has excellent precision, it tends to overestimate the true clearance by about 10%.

Even further simplifications have been attempted. A single sample technique attributable to Tauxe and colleagues[24, 62] has surprising accuracy, nearly comparable to the two-sample method. Another technique described

by Schlegel and Hamway[25] requires no blood samples, as it utilizes the gamma camera–derived renal uptake from computerized images. This, however, appears to be less accurate than the blood-sampling in vitro procedures.[63]

Individual Renal Function. Divided renal function may be derived from computerized gamma camera data. After the OIH injection, computer matrix images are obtained (usually at 15-second intervals). After the first 3 minutes, the likelihood of pelvic accumulation and excretion becomes high.[64] Therefore, only data obtained during the first 3 minutes may be used for evaluation of split renal function. For individual renal function measurements, the relative function is determined quite simply by the relative activity accumulated in one kidney compared with the other, usually in the first- to second-minute interval after injection. The major problems are twofold: (1) selecting appropriate background regions to approximate nonrenal activity measured within the renal region of interest, and (2) correcting for renal depth. To date, no consensus has been reached about how to choose renal background.[25, 65–68] Renal depth correction has also been attempted by a variety of means, including formulas based on height and weight,[25] ultrasonography,[69] and single[70] and double isotope[71] depth-finding techniques. Formulas based on height and weight are not sufficiently reliable to recommend their general use.[63]

Quantitative total and split renal function measure-

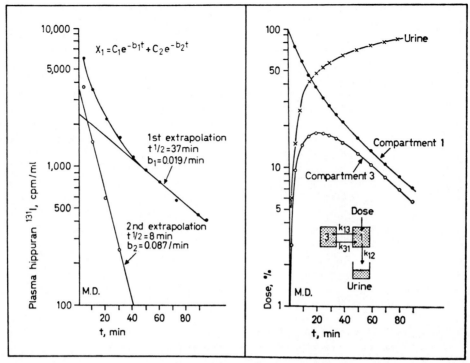

Figure 18–10. Disappearance curve and two-compartment model. On the left, the curve fitted to the black dots indicates the disappearance of OIH from the plasma after a bolus intravenous injection. The equation, with two exponential terms, indicates effectively a two-compartment model for the disappearance of OIH; the fast component is indicated by the sharply falling line with slope b_2 and the slow component is indicated by the line with a shallower slope with value b_1. On the right is an attempt to demonstrate the distribution of the OIH between the plasma compartment (Compartment 1) as well as a somewhat ill-defined compartment that represents all that is not plasma, noted as Compartment 3. (From Blaufox MD: A compartmental analysis of the radiorenogram and kinetics of ^{131}I Hippuran. *In* Blaufox MD: Evaluation of renal function and disease with radionuclides. Baltimore, S. Karger AG, Basel/University Park Press, 1972, pp 107–146.)

ments enable clinicians to follow the progress of a patient's renal function objectively and noninvasively. The utility of this method of studying renal pathophysiology is only beginning to show its promise. Other agents used to measure individual renal function include Tc-99m-DTPA, DMSA, and GHA (see later discussion).

Transit Time Estimates

The transit time of OIH through the renal parenchyma varies according to the length of the nephron being traversed. Juxtaglomerular nephrons extend more deeply into the renal medulla than do cortical nephrons and require a correspondingly longer time for transit of OIH to the collecting system. Because 90% of renal blood flow normally is to the renal cortex, the normal transit of OIH predominantly reflects cortical transit. In normal patients, the mean transit time of OIH ranges from about 3 to 5 minutes.[45, 64] This is reflected in the scintigram by the appearance of the renal collecting system on the 3- to 6-minute image. The renogram curve correspondingly shows its peak at that time, after which OIH begins to leave the kidney. The actual calculation of the mean transit time is performed from data obtained during a standard scintirenogram acquired on computer matrix. Any alteration in intrarenal blood flow distribution increases the mean transit time, because blood flow will be redirected toward the longer juxtaglomerular nephrons. This is reflected in the scintigram by a delay in the appearance of the collecting system, and in the renogram

by a delayed peak. Unfortunately, these patterns of delayed or prolonged transit appear to be nonspecific. Britton and colleagues and Gruenewald and coworkers have attempted to examine the mean transit time as well as the distribution of transit times within the kidney by the technique of deconvolution analysis.[72–74] Deconvolution analysis mathematically reconstructs the passage of activity through the kidney as if a simple compact bolus of OIH had entered the renal artery. The division of this bolus into many segments, each with different transit times through the kidney, allows determination of the distribution of individual transit times. Britton and coworkers have obtained interesting correlations with obstructive uropathies. In particular, they have found prolonged parenchymal transit in patients with obstruction, but no such prolongation in nonobstructed dilated systems.[74a]

Tc-99m–Labeled Agents

Sodium Tc-99m Pertechnetate (Na Tc-99m-TcO₄⁻)

Sodium Tc-99m pertechnetate is the chemical form in which Tc-99m is eluted from commercial molybdenum-99 generators. Wide availability and inexpensiveness are its major advantages. The chemical form of pertechnetate is similar to perchlorate and other iodide-like monovalent anions. Pertechnetate, too, concentrates in tissues with an affinity for such anions, including as the thyroid gland, salivary glands, gastric mucosa, and choroid plexus. Renal handling of Tc-99m-TcO$_4^-$ is complex, involving GFR and net tubular reabsorption. Because of its slow renal clearance and complex handling, this agent is a poor choice in renal imaging or the evaluation of renal function. However, virtually any Tc-99m–labeled tracer, including simple pertechnetate may be administered as an intravenous bolus, for a rapid-sequence renal scintiangiogram. Choice of the appropriate form of Tc-99m usually depends on the clinical context. If only perfusion information is required, 10 to 15 mCi of Tc-99m-TcO$_4^-$ may be used. The major advantage of this agent is its low cost. If information about renal function, transit, and/or excretion is desired, Tc-99m-DTPA would be far more valuable (see section, Radionuclide Angiography and Transit Times). If morphologic information is needed Tc-99m GHA could be used (see discussion, Tc-99m-GHA and DMSA).

Tc-99m DTPA

This chelate, available since 1970, is excreted by glomerular filtration, as are most chelates, and may be used to measure the glomerular filtration rate.[17, 29] Its clearance usually is a few per cent lower than inulin,[69] the physiological standard for this measurement. The reason for this is not entirely clear, although the presence of a small amount of excess tin in the preparation appears to cause approximately 3% to 5% of the DTPA to be protein bound in the serum. In addition, some renal parenchymal binding of Tc-99m-DTPA may occur, since it is not uncommon to be able to image the kidney at 24 hours, when all activity theoretically should be gone. The favorable imaging and dosimetric properties of Tc-99m compared with I-131 would appear to make the Tc-99m-DTPA superior to I-131-OIH for scintigraphic evaluation of qualitative renal function (see Table 18–1). In fact, significantly higher background activity is noted with Tc-99m-DTPA, owing to the much lower extraction efficiency for the glomerular agent compared with a tubular agent, such as OIH.[75] In recent years, scintillation cameras have become more sophisticated electronically. The modifications have included increasing the number of photomultiplier tubes to improve spatial resolution; decreasing crystal detector thickness for the same purpose; and decreasing electronic "dead time" between scintillations to improve detector sensitivity at high count rates. Collimators have been changed as well. The net result has been a dramatic improvement in the imaging of Tc-99m–labeled agents. Unfortunately, the image quality for agents labeled with I-131 has deteriorated.[76] Many institutions with modern scintillation cameras will find Tc-99m-DTPA to be their agent of choice for renal functional imaging. Although this may be justified for technical reasons, a tubular agent provides significant advantages. For the reliable evaluation of tubular function with modern detectors, one must use I-123-OIH.[77] Such a tubular agent provides greater renal concentration than a glomerular agent such as DTPA, and this is an advantage in the evaluation of renal failure. Validation, approval, and commercial availability of a Tc-99m–labeled tubular agent is therefore anxiously awaited. Tc-99m MAG$_3$ appears to have many of the desired characteristics of a Tc-99m–labeled tubular agent.[195]

SCINTIGRAPHY AND RENOGRAPHY

The use of Tc-99m-DTPA may be quite similar to that of OIH, although, of course, Lugol's solution is not administered. Modern gamma scintillation cameras produce high-quality images with Tc-99m-DTPA when fitted with a parallel-hole all-purpose low-energy collimator. Image quality is usually quite a bit better than with OIH.[78] Technical factors aside, the amount of administered activity alone (10 mCi of Tc-99m-DTPA) usually provides improved images for scintirenography, compared with only 300 µCi of I-131 or I-123–labeled OIH. The renal transit time of DTPA is approximately 3 to 5 minutes, as it is for OIH, so that the renal pelvis is visualized during that time interval in the normal study. Figure 18–11 demonstrates images from a normal subject. Higher tissue and liver background may cause difficulty in interpreting renal images and renal function in the presence of renal insufficiency (Fig. 18–12). As with OIH, an interface with a computer is a valuable adjunct for simultaneous computer matrix images and allows for generation of a renogram.

DIURETIC SCINTIRENOGRAPHY

The procedures for evaluating obstruction using diuretics and DTPA, described by Thrall and colleagues and Koff and coworkers[50, 79] are virtually identical to those described for OIH. However, the slower renal clearance of DTPA (compared with a tubular agent) leads to a lower kidney-to-background ratio and a protracted period of continued DTPA extraction, which introduces potential problems of interpretation. An example of hydronephrosis (not challenged for obstruction by a diuretic) is shown in Figure 18–13.

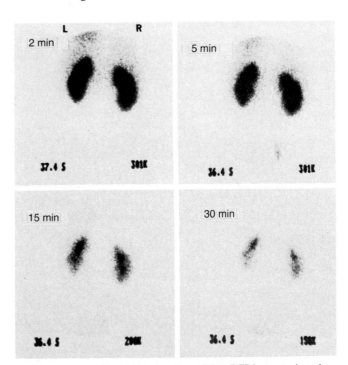

Figure 18–11. Normal technetium-99m DTPA posterior-view scintirenogram. On the 2-minute image, there is normal and symmetric uptake of radiotracer bilaterally within the kidneys. By the 5-minute image, activity has moved into both collecting systems and is seen within the ureters. Activity subsequently decreases in both kidneys, and is much less at 30 minutes.

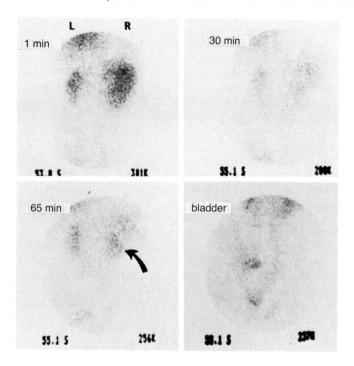

Figure 18–12. Tc-99m-DTPA scintirenogram in renal failure. This procedure is less satisfactory for functional imaging of the kidneys. On the 1-minute image the left kidney is small. It is not clear whether the right kidney is very large or whether activity of the liver is superimposed. By 65 minutes, the right kidney is more distinct (*arrow*). The delayed bladder image shows minimal accumulation of radiolabeled urine.

Measurement of Renal Function: Glomerular Filtration Rate (GFR)

Total GFR. The same general techniques for measuring the clearance of PAH apply to the use of inulin for the determination of total GFR.[80] Like the PAH clearance, the inulin clearance procedure has inherited the distinction of standard use and the inconvenience of the constant infusion procedure. Unlike PAH, single-injection clearances can be performed accurately using inulin and chemical analysis,[76] since GFR is independent of plasma concentration.

The radionuclide used clinically to measure GFR is DTPA.[29] The plasma disappearance rate after a single injection may be used to determine the GFR in ways completely analogous to ERPF determinations described earlier. Multicompartmental models of the disappearance curve require multiple blood samples for analysis,[26, 29] and simplified compartmental models exist, using fewer samples.[27, 30] The equations for calculating GFR are similar

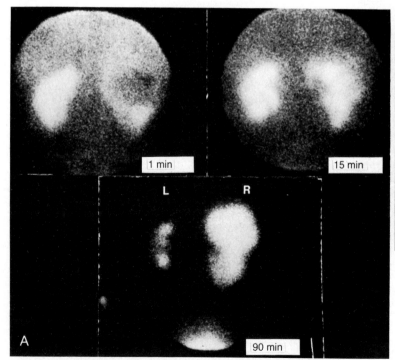

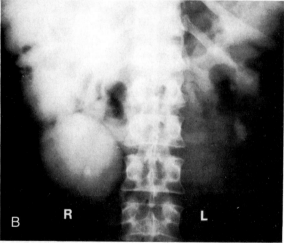

Figure 18–13. *A,* Hydronephrosis with delayed imaging. This posterior-view Tc-99m-DTPA study demonstrates normal left-sided function and excretion. The right kidney, however, is enlarged and has a sizable upper-pole defect on the 1-minute image. This region begins to fill with radiolabeled urine, as seen on the 15-minute image. By 90 minutes, marked hydronephrosis of both upper and lower poles is observed. *B,* The intravenous urogram demonstrates the radiologic correlate of the 90-minute view seen in *A.* Again, the hydronephrosis in both upper and lower poles is seen. (From Fine EJ, Scharf SC, Blaufox MD: The role of nuclear medicine in evaluating the hypertensive patient. *In* Freeman LM, Weissmann HS (eds): Nuclear Medicine Annual 1984. New York, Raven Press, 1984, p 23.)

to those for ERPF. The only significant difference is related to the time of blood sample collection. Because the GFR is approximately 20% of the ERPF, the rate of Tc-99m-DTPA disappearance from plasma is correspondingly much slower than that of OIH. Sampling must be carried out for a longer period of time to derive the GFR accurately. A two-sample method analogous to that applied to OIH requires samples at approximately 2 and 4 hours after injection, instead of 20- and 30-minute measurements for OIH (see earlier discussion). One-sample methods[27, 82] can be performed as well, analogous to the Tauxe method for ERPF. An in vivo method requiring no samples has been described by Gates and colleagues[30] and is completely analogous to the comparable method of Schlegel and Hamway[25] for ERPF (see earlier discussion). Higher tissue background activity may produce greater problems quantifying renal function by the in vivo procedure for this glomerular agent, when compared with OIH.

Individual Renal Function. Computer interfacing allows determination of relative renal uptake of DTPA, and therefore the assessment of relative renal function.[192] Again, this is analogous to the procedures described earlier for OIH and suffers from the same problems regarding proper background determination[83] and accurate depth correction.[84] Other tracers used to determine relative renal function are Tc-99m-DMSA and GHA (see later discussion).

FILTRATION FRACTION (FF)

The ratio of GFR to ERPF is known as the filtration fraction. Therefore, it is a derived and not an independent parameter of renal function. The radiotracer methods used to determine this parameter have already been described. The FF is not used widely in current clinical practice, but there is greater interest in it as a tool for physiological research. Certain pathological states appear to selectively affect GFR or ERPF disproportionately. Recently, this has been described as an effect of angiotensin converting enzyme inhibitors such as captopril, particularly in renal artery stenosis.[85, 86] Whether the FF will become a clinically useful marker of disease awaits further investigation.

RADIONUCLIDE ANGIOGRAPHY AND TRANSIT TIMES

Rapid-sequence imaging in the posterior projection, after bolus Tc-99m-DTPA administration in amounts exceeding 10 mCi, yields qualitative information about relative arterial flow to the kidneys.[87] In principle, virtually any Tc-99m–labeled tracer may be used for this evaluation, including Tc-99m-TcO$_4^-$, Tc-99m-MDP, Tc-99m-GHA, and others (see discussion, Sodium Tc-99m Pertechnate NaTc-99m-TcO$_4^-$). Images obtained at intervals of 1 or 2 seconds usually are used. The resultant radionuclide angiogram may be stored in a computer for generation of time-activity histograms derived from renal regions of interest. Actually, any Tc-99m agent may be used, but DTPA is preferred because its rapid excretion causes lower absorbed radiation doses per mCi administered. Tc-99m-DMSA should not be used for perfusion studies because of the high renal dose (see Table 18–1); nor is it feasible to obtain perfusion studies using OIH.

I-131-OIH in mCi amounts would provide an excessive dose to the kidneys, bladder, and thyroid. I-123-OIH, although dosimetrically safe in mCi amounts and technically acceptable, is prohibitively expensive.

Figure 18–14 shows a normal "flow study" performed with Tc-99m-DTPA. This type of examination provides crude visual information about the symmetry and existence of renal flow. Asymmetry of flow is a rather nonspecific finding; consequently, the imaging portion of a radionuclide angiogram has rather limited utility. However, interest in the procedure has been revived, because the transit time of the bolus (which can be derived by deconvolution analysis from the computerized study only) may have interesting properties more specific to different disease states.[88] This is currently under investigation.

Tc-99m-GHA and Tc-99m-DMSA

These agents are handled by the kidneys in a complex manner, being both filtered and concentrated by the tubules to differing degrees. Approximately 80% to 90% of the administered GHA is excreted by filtration, with the remaining 10% to 20% concentrated in the renal tubular cells,[19] where it remains in the cytosol. This probably takes place in the proximal tubule, since its uptake is inhibited by PAH and by probenecid, both of which act there.[89] The path of the subsequent elimination of this portion of the dose from the body has not been defined. DMSA is both filtered at the glomerulus and concentrated by the renal tubular cells. The filtered portion of the dose is excreted from the body, 16% of

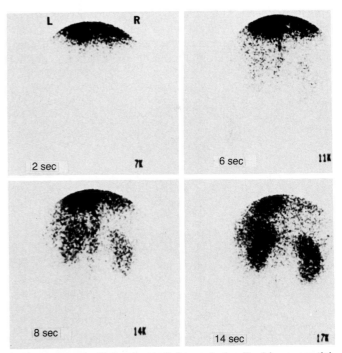

Figure 18–14. Normal renal flow study. Rapid sequential images obtained after intravenous injection of 15 mCi of ^{99m}Tc may be used to obtain a radionuclide angiogram or "flow study." In this instance the radiotracer was labeled with DTPA. Selected 2-second interval frames obtained in the posterior projection demonstrate nearly simultaneous visualization of the aorta and kidneys on the 6-second image, with symmetrical and progressive accumulation of radiotracer on subsequent images.

the total dose by 2 hours. The portion of the dose concentrated by the tubular cells remains predominantly bound (up to 50% of the total dose bound to cortical nephrons by 24 hours),[90] probably by disulfide binding to intracellular mercapto groups. In the rat kidney, 54% is localized in the kidney within 1 hour; 5% is in the liver and spleen and 19% remains in the blood.[18] Its uptake is presumed to occur largely in the distal tubule, since its uptake is inhibited by acidification of the urine.[89]

Both agents are used primarily to elucidate renal morphology.[91, 92] Since neither is excreted by simple mechanisms, they cannot easily be used to measure total ERPF or GFR. However, both have been employed more commonly to measure individual renal function (as a percentage of total function).[93, 94] In renal failure, hepatic uptake limits the utility of GHA to a greater degree than DMSA, both in the measurement of individual renal function and in the evaluation of morphology. The advantage of DMSA can be accounted for, in part, by its more extensive tubular extraction, compared with the predominant glomerular filtration of GHA.

IMAGING

Either of the agents may be used as renal imaging agents. Posterior projection images are obtained 1 to 2 hours after injection of 5 mCi GHA or 1 to 3 mCi of DMSA. Because both tracers are excreted to a degree, it is necessary to wait this long to be certain that collecting system activity has cleared. It should be noted that in the presence of urinary tract obstruction renal pelvic activity obscures the parenchyma, rendering the agents less useful. Parallel-hole, low-energy collimation, or pinhole collimation should be used when higher-resolution images are desired. Despite the relatively high-resolution renal images that can be obtained with these tracers, neither

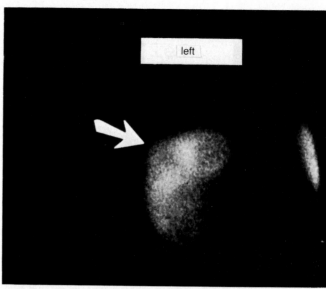

Figure 18–16. Fetal lobation, Tc-99m-DMSA scan. An intravenous urogram (not shown) demonstrated a questionable left upper-pole mass. Further evaluation with Tc-99m-DMSA demonstrates a fetal lobation in the region of the suspicious mass (*arrow*). The concentration of DMSA in this region indicates normal-functioning parenchymal renal tissue. Malignant neoplasms will not concentrate DMSA, DTPA, or GHA, any of which may be used.

provides the anatomical resolution (available with CT or ultrasonography) necessary to recommend it as a primary diagnostic tool to evaluate renal morphology or size. A possible exception is for study in the case of acute trauma or in patients with contrast-media sensitivity. Another situation in which nuclear studies are preferable to radiological studies employing contrast is in diabetic patients with renal insufficiency. Ultrasonography, IVU, or CT scanning usually is performed first in most evaluations of renal size and morphology or in tumor detection. Radiotracer procedures are useful in evaluating the function, and hence the pathological significance, of questionable masses seen on the other studies.[92] A fetal lobation may be identified and distinguished from a solid tumor. The functional status of the connecting tissue in a horseshoe kidney may also be evaluated with these radiotracers.

A normal GHA imaging study is shown in Figure 18–15. Figure 18–16 demonstrates a lobulated but otherwise normal kidney, in which the lobations function as normal renal tissue. The accompanying IVU could not distinguish these normal variants from abnormal masses. Kidney location and orientation may vary with the patient's position. Such "floating kidneys" may produce pain and obstruction, but even when asymptomatic should not be confused with a renal mass (Fig. 18–17).

Severe parenchymal renal dysfunction causes poor background clearance and enhances alternate routes of GHA excretion (namely gastrointestinal and biliary) (Fig. 18–18). Poor images result.

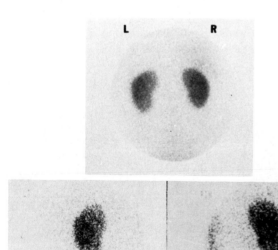

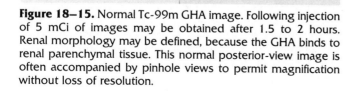

Figure 18–15. Normal Tc-99m GHA image. Following injection of 5 mCi of images may be obtained after 1.5 to 2 hours. Renal morphology may be defined, because the GHA binds to renal parenchymal tissue. This normal posterior-view image is often accompanied by pinhole views to permit magnification without loss of resolution.

RELATIVE RENAL FUNCTION

When static images are obtained on a computer matrix, relative renal function can be determined. At 2 hours after injection of radiotracer, the renal pelves are usually free of activity. The relative counts in one kidney com-

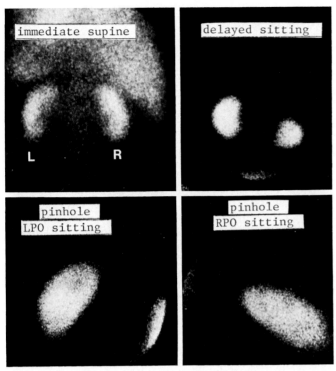

Figure 18–17. Renal pseudotumor, secondary to sitting position. In this woman with flank pain and hematuria, immediate blood pool images were obtained after a Tc-99m-GHA injection. In the supine position, the kidneys appeared normal. Delayed images would have suggested a mass in the upper pole of the right kidney on the posterior sitting views. Further clarification is obtained using pinhole views from oblique projections. The kidney rotates in the sitting position. No mass is seen in the upper pole of the right kidney; this pitfall can be avoided by obtaining additional views in the appropriate projections as displayed.

pared with the other provide the relative function. Although GHA has been used for this purpose[94, 94a] DMSA has been studied more extensively.[93, 95–97] The measurement of relative renal function becomes important in following the results of interventions, whether medical or surgical. In some cases, the decision to perform an indicated nephrectomy may depend on the proportion of total renal function provided by the contralateral kidney. Figure 18–19 demonstrates the use of Tc-99m-GHA to measure relative renal function.

Tc-99m–labeled Tubular Agents

Radiopharmacists and synthetic chemists have worked for years to develop a Tc-99m–labeled agent with excretory properties based predominantly on tubular secretion. Most such agents have been disappointing when used in humans, despite promise shown in animal models. Two recent families of compounds (one group is related to N,N′-bis(S-benzoylmercaptoacetyl)ethylenediamine with a Tc-99m core, known as Tc-99m-DADS[98]: the other similar to [Tc-99m]mercaptoacetylglycylglycine or Tc-99m-MAG[99]) appear to demonstrate excellent properties as tubular agents in humans, although problems remain with respect to purification procedures. Tc-99m MAG$_3$ is rapidly emerging as a practical clinically useful agent.[195]

Tc-99m Phosphates and Phosphonates

Popularly used as bone scanning agents, this class of compounds is recognized to be valuable because of coincidental information about the kidneys, which may be derived during the course of a bone scan. After intravenous injection, these agents gradually accumulate in metabolically active bone, by unresolved mechanisms (possibly by adsorption to hydroxyapatite crystals).[100, 101] The portion not taken up by bone is excreted predominantly by the kidneys. The entire family of compounds demonstrates renal excretion, although in differing degrees depending on the specific agent. Among the more commonly used agents, pyrophosphate (PYP) demonstrates better renal visualization than does MDP. Approximately 60% of MDP is excreted, normally within 3 hours of injection.[102] While the "poor man's renal scan" can deliver useful results, one should not depend on the bone scan for definitive information about the kidneys. An abnormality detected on bone scan should be pursued by another, more specific modality. Figures 18–20 to 18–24 demonstrate the variety of abnormalities related to the urinary tract that may be seen on bone scans.

Ga-67 Citrate

Radiogallium in tracer doses acts as an iron analogue, reversibly binding in the Ga^{+++} form to transferrin, after intravenous administration.[103] The half-life of Ga-67 is 78 hours. Consequently, it is less than ideal, from the radiobiological perspective. Fortunately, it does not produce particulate radiation. From an imaging perspective Ga-67

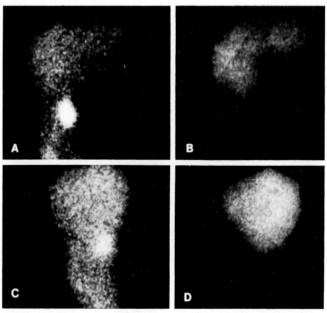

Figure 18–18. Tc-99m-GHA imaging in renal failure. This procedure is not useful in patients with severe renal dysfunction. Alternate routes of excretion are usually found and most commonly involve the hepatobiliary system. Twenty-four hours after injection of Tc-99m-GHA, images A and C demonstrated hepatic and biliary concentration of the radiotracer. B and D demonstrate the corresponding images obtained in this patient, using Tc-99m-sulfur colloid to localize the liver precisely in the corresponding projections.

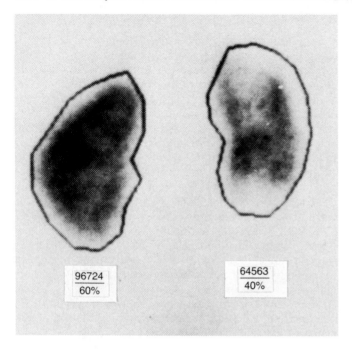

96724
60%

64563
40%

Figure 18–19. Use of Tc-99m DMSA for split renal function determination. Tc-99m-DMSA may be used for assessing relative renal mass. Two hours after injection of the radiotracer, images acquired on computer matrix are usually free of collecting system activity. Sometimes further delay helps to improve collecting system drainage and to decrease background activity. Here, regions of interest are drawn around the kidneys to determine relative renal counts, which reflect relative function and/or mass. As indicated the left kidney accounts for 60% of total function, the right for 40%. (From Handmaker H: Nuclear renal imaging in acute pyelonephritis. Semin Nucl Med 12:246, 1982.)

is not ideal either, with four photopeaks at 90, 190, 300, and 390 keV.

In the first 24 hours after injection Ga-67 is excreted, predominantly by the kidneys. From 24 hours on, Ga-67 is excreted primarily in the colon. Currently, however, it is considered acceptable to visualize kidneys faintly with modern scintillation cameras, even on 48 hour images.[104] Faint kidney visualization and nonvisualization by scintigraphy during this period are therefore both considered normal findings. Intense or focal accumulation at 48 hours or on subsequent images is abnormal.[104, 105] Ga-67 is known to accumulate in areas of inflammation as well as

in certain tumors by uncertain mechanisms, perhaps by binding to lactoferrin (present in granulocytes and certain tumors) in preference to transferrin. As a result, Ga-67 may be used in the evaluation of suspected pyelonephritis, renal or perinephric abscess, interstitial nephritis, and renal tumors.

Xe-133

Radioactive forms of inert xenon gas have been used for invasive measurement of renal perfusion.[32-34] Selective catheterization of the renal artery with a subsequent bolus

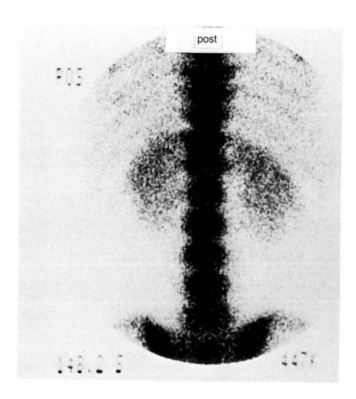

post

Figure 18–20. Normal Tc-99m-methylene diphosphonate (MDP) bone scan showing normal renal excretion. This posterior projection was obtained during a Tc-99m-MDP bone scan. This image was taken 3 hours after injection of 15 mCi of the radiotracer.

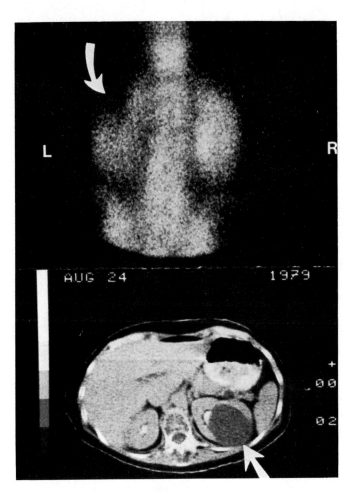

Figure 18–21. Incidental finding of renal cyst on Tc-99m-MDP bone scan. Renal masses may be identified on bone scans, usually as serendipitous findings. In this case, a posterior-view Tc-99m-MDP bone scan demonstrates a defect in the left upper pole (*arrow*). The accompanying CT study demonstrates a cyst in this region (*arrow*).

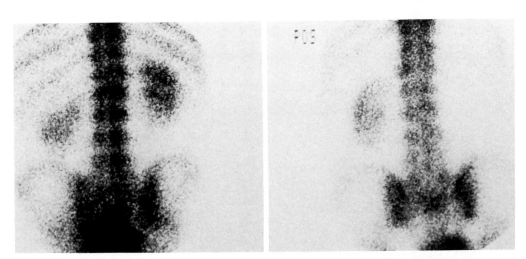

Figure 18–22. Incidental renal abnormalities detected on Tc-99m-MDP bone scan. Left, is the posterior projection of a bone scan on a 70-year-old woman with metastatic breast carcinoma. The upper pole of the left kidney is not well defined on the study. Right, is the bone scan from a 57-year-old man with congestive heart failure, hypertension, diabetes mellitus, and lung carcinoma. The right kidney is not visualized. In both circumstances, follow-up was initially suggested but was not pursued, because the clinical condition of the patients did not warrant further intervention.

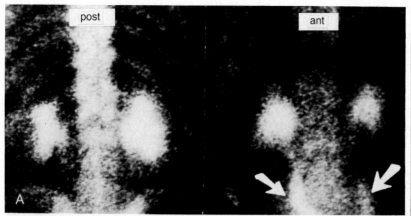

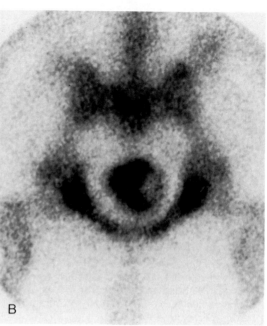

Figure 18–23. Incidental pathology on Tc-99m-MDP bone scan (bladder tumor). *A,* Posterior and anterior views of this bone scan demonstrate marked dilatation within both renal collecting systems. Bilateral ureterovesical junction obstructions are strongly suggested on the basis of the bone scan finding in this patient with carcinoma of the bladder. Dilated ureters are indicated by the arrows. *B,* Technetium-99m MDP bone scan with markedly increased bone uptake. Bladder tumor detected on bone scan in patient with osteoarthritis reveals photon-deficient area in urinary bladder. Asymptomatic transitional cell carcinoma is present.

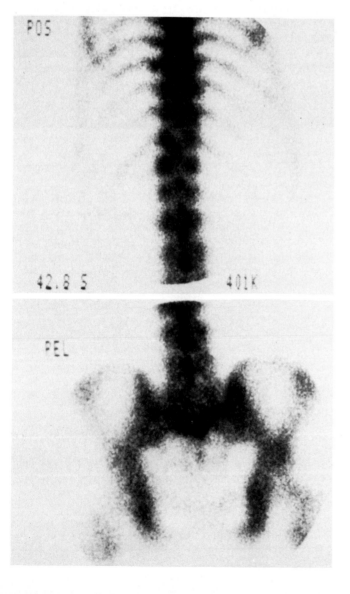

Figure 18–24. "Superscan" of prostate cancer with confluent metastases and obstruction with renal failure. The "superscan" may be misinterpreted as a normal bone scan. Key distinguishing characteristics are higher-than-normal bony uptake compared with background soft tissue and absent kidney and bladder visualization. The common underlying diseases that give rise to this pattern include renal failure with secondary or tertiary hyperparathyroidism and diffuse confluent osteoblastic metastases, usually from prostate carcinoma. Primary hyperparathyroidism and hematologic diseases with marrow expansion can cause diffuse increased osteoblastosis, resulting in increased bony uptake, but absence of urinary tract uptake in such patients is a less reliable distinguishing sign. This patient had prostatic carcinoma with diffuse confluent metastatic disease to spine and pelvis, as well as obstructive uropathy with resultant renal failure. Both factors undoubtedly contributed to the superscan pattern.

injection of dissolved Xe-133 is performed. The rate of Xe-133 wash-out is recorded with external detectors and is related to renal blood flow.

This procedure has achieved utility in the physiology lab but has not had widespread clinical application.

Chromium-51 (Cr-51)-EDTA (edetic acid), Ytterbium-169 (Yb-169)-DTPA, Cobalt-57 (Co-57)-Cyanocobalamin and Other Chelates

Most chelates are excreted by glomerular filtration. Many have been tagged with radioactive tracer labels for the purpose of exploring renal physiology. Radioactive Co-57 and Co-58 labeled Vit B-12 (cyanocobalamin)[106, 107] are, in fact, biochemically identical to their nonradioactive molecules, and therefore share physiological behavior. The Cr-51 and Yb-169 tags (on EDTA and DTPA, respectively) do not appear to alter the physiological behavior of these molecules significantly, and they too can be used to measure GFR by in vitro blood sampling procedures. None of these agents has emission suitable for imaging studies. Many other nonimaging radiotracers have been employed successfully in measuring the glomerular filtration rate as well, including I-131 iothalamate and I-125 iothalamate.[108] Although the iothalamates have been used in humans,[108] they are used primarily in animal investigations. Chelates of DTPA include In-111-DTPA[109] and In-113m-DTPA.[110, 111] The most popular chelates in use are Cr-51-EDTA[112, 113] and Yb-169-DTPA,[111] which have become standards in the measurement of GFR, nearly to the extent of inulin.

CLINICAL APPLICATIONS

The nuclear medicine approach to the patient depends on the details of the case and the overall experience of the attending physician. As a result, a flow-sheet approach cannot be expected to describe all situations. The following examples, therefore, are illustrative of a general approach to several specific problems. Renal failure, both acute and chronic, as well as problems of patients with renal transplants are presented in detail in Chapters 102 and 108 respectively.

Obstruction (See discussion, Diuretic Scintirenography, Chapter 55.)

Suspected Renovascular Hypertension (RVH)

The first major application of nuclear medicine in urology/nephrology was in patients with hypertension. Although at present this application is considered to be less useful than that in many other diseases of the GU tract such as obstructive uropathy, the high worldwide prevalence of hypertension and the many misconceptions of the role of nuclear medicine in its management justify a detailed discussion. (See also Chapter 71.)

Untreated elevations of blood pressure are responsible for damage of several organ systems, probably as a result of direct damage to small blood vessels. These complications include stroke due to associated cerebrovascular disease, renal failure as a consequence of nephrosclerosis,

claudication from peripheral vascular disease, heart failure as a result of left ventricular hypertrophy, and coronary artery disease as the result of direct damage to the coronary arteries.

In the vast majority of hypertensive patients, the disease has no identifiable cause. Table 18–2 lists the major causes of secondary or correctable hypertension. The clinical dilemma is to identify these patients and separate them from the vastly larger number of essential hypertensive patients. Essential hypertension is not usually associated with symptoms. Therefore symptomatic disease should alert the physician to the possibility of secondary hypertension or the development of end-organ damage. It is often difficult to determine whether end-organ damage is the consequence or the cause of hypertension. For this reason, the interpretation of renal radionuclide studies in hypertensive patients presents a considerable problem.

Stenosis of the renal artery is a cause of decreased perfusion to the involved kidney. Baroceptors within the afferent arterioles sense the lower perfusion pressure and trigger the release of renin from cells within the juxtaglomerular apparatus. Consequent increases in circulating angiotensin II produce generalized arteriolar vasoconstriction, and increased aldosterone secretion by the adrenal cortex. The resultant increase in peripheral vascular resistance and fluid and sodium retention causes sustained hypertension. Once the physiological variables are stabilized, peripheral plasma renin activity is frequently elevated, although it can be normal. The usual screening tests for RVH are listed in Table 18–3. Their complex interrelationship is a major problem in interpreting such tests.

In RVH virtually any pattern may be observed on an excretion study performed with OIH. The most useful pattern, however, is decreased and delayed accumulation and excretion of radiotracer seen on the affected side (Figs. 18–25 and 18–26). Much has been published in the attempt to quantify the delay necessary to invoke a diagnosis of renal artery stenosis. Normal values of "time to peak" and "time to half-peak" have been devised, but they have little meaning in view of wide variations due to hydration factors. Prolonged transit time may be seen as a result of decreased urine flow secondary to increased water reabsorption on the affected side. Bilateral ureteral

Table 18–2. Causes of Secondary Hypertension

Endocrine	Vascular
Cushing's syndrome	Coarctation of the aorta
Conn's syndrome	Renal ischemia
Pheochromocytoma	
Hyperthyroidism	Renal
Drugs	Chronic pyelonephritis
Amphetamines	Congenital renal disease
Estrogens and oral contraceptives	Diabetes
Steroids	Glomerulonephritis
Miscellaneous	Gout
Increased intracranial pressure	Interstitial nephritis
Licorice	Obstructive uropathy
Toxemia of pregnancy	Polycystic kidney disease
Lead poisoning	Renin-secreting neoplasms
	Vasculitis

From Fine EJ, Scharf SC, Blaufox MD: The role of nuclear medicine in evaluating the hypertensive patient. *In* Freeman LM, Weissmann HS (eds): Nuclear Medicine Annual 1984. New York, Raven Press, 1984.

Table 18–3. Screening Tests for Renovascular Hypertension

Test	Comments	References
Peripheral plasma renin activity	Helpful if very high	183
Intravenous urography	Rapid sequence films obtained every minute for 5 minutes	184
Renography and renal scintigraphy	Convenient and useful screening test	185
Renal vein renin	Helpful in lateralization of lesion and predicting response to surgery	134
Angiography	Required for definitive diagnosis and surgery	186
	Digital intravenous angiography may simplify the procedure and reduce morbidity	
Blood pressure response to angiotensin competitor	Has not gained widespread clinical utility	187
Blood pressure response converting enzyme inhibition	Has not gained widespread clinical utility	188

From Fine EJ, Scharf SC, Blaufox MD: The role of nuclear medicine in evaluating the hypertensive patient. *In* Freeman LM, Weissmann HS (eds): Nuclear Medicine Annual 1984. New York, Raven Press, 1984.

catheterization for split renal function evaluation (Stamey-Howard test) may demonstrate decreased urine volume with decreased sodium concentration of the affected side.[114] If it is chronically diseased, the involved kidney may be small with reduced blood flow. Unfortunately, the scintigraphic pattern described is not specific for RVH. Chronic pyelonephritis or unilateral obstruction (when the collecting system is not clearly dilated) may produce similar patterns on OIH scintirenograms, falsely suggesting RVH. Even essential hypertension cannot necessarily be distinguished, as asymmetrical renal function is more common in patients with essential hypertension than in normal subjects. Even more complicating is the fact that chronic renal diseases may cause secondary hypertension. False-negative examinations may also be seen. Most series report sensitivities of approximately 80% to 85% and specificities in the same range for the diagnosis of RVH.[115–121] Although false-positive rates of 10% to 15% are usually reported, this is a reflection of the lack of specificity of the test more than of its inaccuracy. That is, although these 10% to 15% of patients do not have RVH, they do have an asymmetry of renal function that is accurately documented by the OIH excretion study, indicating the presence of one of the other numerous conditions that result in unilateral renal disease.

The Tc-99m-DTPA radionuclide angiogram was also greeted enthusiastically when first proposed as a diagnostic test for RVH. Unfortunately, it is influenced by asymmetrical renal disease of any etiology, and therefore suffers from the same lack of specificity (Fig. 18–27)[122] associated with its predecessor, the radiohippurate renogram.

There is growing interest in the use of angiotensin-converting enzyme inhibitors (ACEI) to enhance the sensitivity, and perhaps specificity, of radionuclide studies

in the diagnosis of renal artery stenosis.[85, 86, 123] In normal subjects these agents cause peripheral arterial vasodilation and lower peripheral vascular resistance. In patients with essential hypertension ERPF may increase, whereas the GFR does not change after administration of ACEI. In patients with RVH the effects may be more complex. Some investigators report a marked decrease in GFR of the affected kidney after ACEI administration, and an increase in the ERPF of the contralateral kidney.[86] These changes may enhance the functional differences between a normal and abnormal kidney caused by renal artery stenosis. Both OIH and DTPA scintirenograms may more sensitively detect RVH using ACEI. A carefully designed investigation is necessary to clarify the role of this class of compounds in the diagnosis of RVH.

It is important to consider the prevalence of the disease before adopting a diagnostic algorithm for RVH, so that the expensive and/or invasive tests from Table 18–3 can be used in an efficient and productive manner.

RVH is the most common form of secondary hypertension. The prevalence of secondary hypertension is variously reported as less than 1%, to 30% and depends not only on the source of the study population but also on the definition of hypertension in that population and on its severity.[124–130] Recent studies have demonstrated a substantial benefit from treating patients with mild diastolic blood pressure elevation.[131] The prevalence of renovascular disease in this group is probably well below 1%.

Population-based studies typically have found a low prevalence of secondary hypertension. In the Hypertension Detection and Follow-up Program,[128] 9.1% of patients with severe hypertension (diastolic blood pressure greater than 115 mmHg) may have had renovascular hypertension. However, the apparent prevalence in the entire group, including mild and moderate hypertensive patients, was only 0.13%. Recent data demonstrate a higher prevalence of RVH in patients with severe disease. In one study, 31% of all patients presenting with a diastolic blood pressure greater than 125 mmHg or Grade 3 or 4 hypertensive retinopathy were discovered to have renovascular hypertension. When white patients were analyzed separately from blacks (in whom severe hypertension is common), the figure was over 40%.[129] In general it may be assumed that for not more than 5% to 10% of hypertensive patients in a hospital-based population have identifiable causes for the disease been found, and even fewer in a general hypertensive population. An identifiable cause, in a patient, signals the potential for cure to the referring physician. Unfortunately, often this possibility cannot be realized. Diagnostic tests are more valuable if they can prognosticate the likelihood of curing hypertension with further intervention—and if they provide information about the level of function of the involved kidney.

From a selected patient sample, with characteristics indicating a higher likelihood of secondary hypertension, it is possible to devise an algorithm to search for the cause.[132] If the patient's clinical characteristics are more suggestive of RVH, one may proceed with either an OIH scintirenogram or a digital intravenous subtraction angiogram (IV-DSA) also (see Chapter 71). The best available data do not distinguish clearly among these examinations on the basis of sensitivity or specificity. Clearly, one

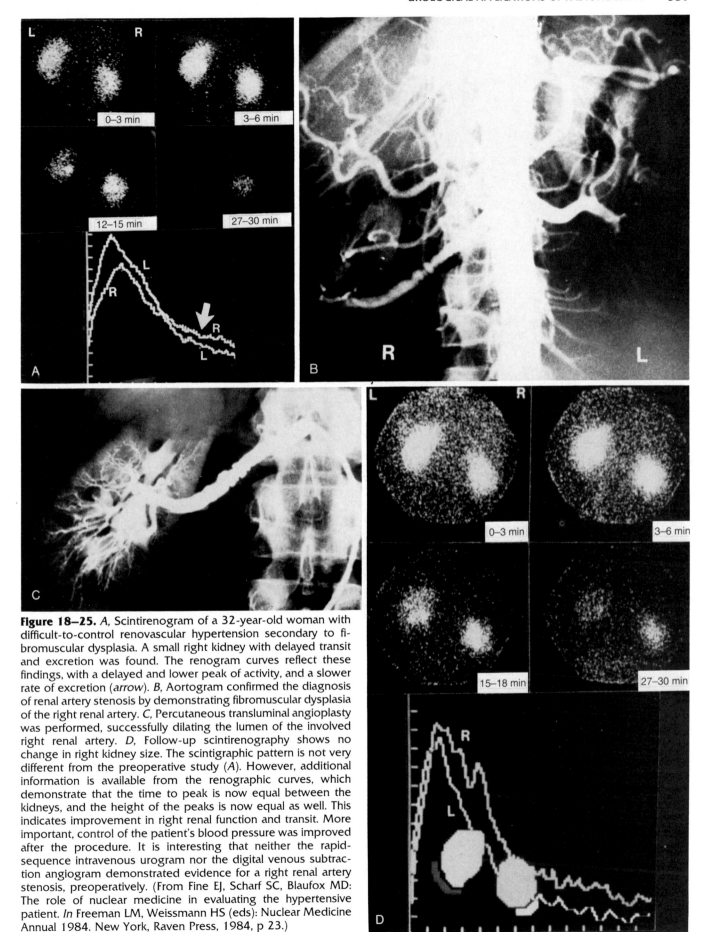

Figure 18–25. *A,* Scintirenogram of a 32-year-old woman with difficult-to-control renovascular hypertension secondary to fibromuscular dysplasia. A small right kidney with delayed transit and excretion was found. The renogram curves reflect these findings, with a delayed and lower peak of activity, and a slower rate of excretion (*arrow*). *B,* Aortogram confirmed the diagnosis of renal artery stenosis by demonstrating fibromuscular dysplasia of the right renal artery. *C,* Percutaneous transluminal angioplasty was performed, successfully dilating the lumen of the involved right renal artery. *D,* Follow-up scintirenography shows no change in right kidney size. The scintigraphic pattern is not very different from the preoperative study (*A*). However, additional information is available from the renographic curves, which demonstrate that the time to peak is now equal between the kidneys, and the height of the peaks is now equal as well. This indicates improvement in right renal function and transit. More important, control of the patient's blood pressure was improved after the procedure. It is interesting that neither the rapid-sequence intravenous urogram nor the digital venous subtraction angiogram demonstrated evidence for a right renal artery stenosis, preoperatively. (From Fine EJ, Scharf SC, Blaufox MD: The role of nuclear medicine in evaluating the hypertensive patient. *In* Freeman LM, Weissmann HS (eds): Nuclear Medicine Annual 1984. New York, Raven Press, 1984, p 23.)

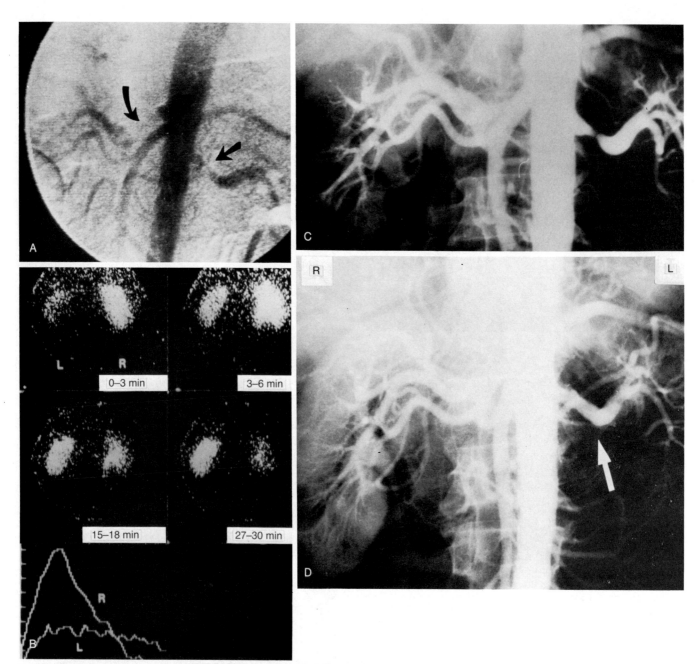

Figure 18–26. Right ventricular hypertrophy in a 55-year-old man, secondary to atherosclerosis. *A,* A man with peripheral vascular disease as well as severe hypertension refractory to medical management had an intravenous digital subtraction angiogram, as shown. It was interpreted as a tight left-sided renal artery stenosis (*short arrow*). In addition, a near-complete right-sided renal artery stenosis was believed to be in the region of the long arrow. *B,* An OIH scintirenogram was performed, which demonstrates normal right-sided renal function, transit and excretion, confirmed on the renogram curve. The left kidney, however, is small and demonstrates decreased uptake indicating decreased function, as well as delayed transit and delayed excretion without evidence of a dilated collecting system. The pattern is that of left-sided renal artery stenosis. *C,* A midstream aortogram confirms the left-sided renal artery stenosis seen on the scintirenographic study. The digital venous subtraction angiogram was falsely positive on the right side, owing to identification of the splenic artery as the origin of the right renal artery. In addition, there was oversubtraction of vessels in the region of the duplicated right renal artery that is more clearly seen on the direct-contrast angiogram. *D,* Percutaneous transluminal angioplasty was performed, restoring toward normal the caliber of the left renal artery.

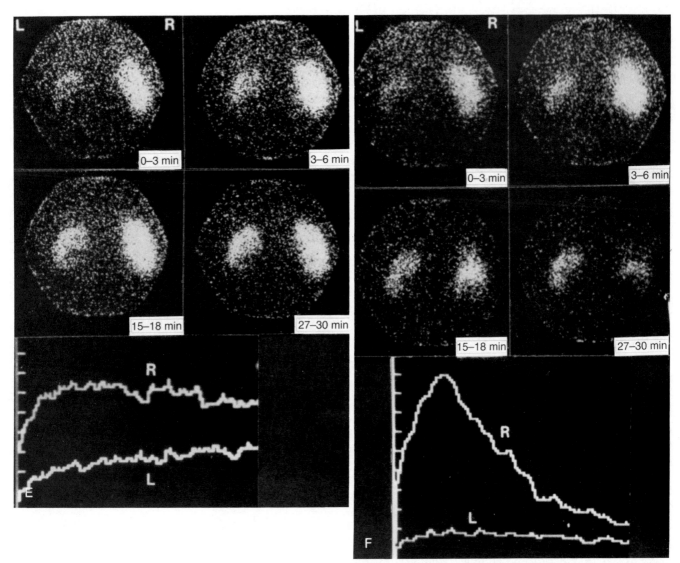

Figure 18–26 *Continued E,* The immediate (1 day later) postoperative scintirenogram demonstrates progressive accumulation of radiotracer on both sides. This is the pattern of acute tubular necrosis, which in this instance is likely to be a reaction to intra-arterial contrast material administered at the time of arteriography. An infarct appears to be in the left lower pole. *F,* Two months later a repeat scintirenogram is changed little from the initial scintirenogram seen in *B.* (From Fine EJ, Scharf SC, Blaufox MD: The role of nuclear medicine in evaluating the hypertensive patient. *In* Freeman LM, Weissman HS (eds): Nuclear Medicine Annual 1984. New York, Raven Press, 1984.)

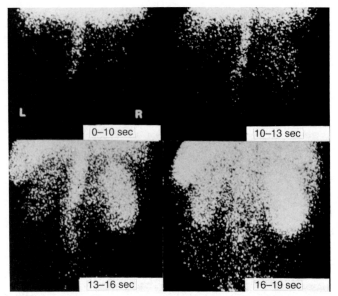

Figure 18–27. The nonspecific appearance of a small kidney. Asymmetry of flow is demonstrated on this radionuclide scintiangiogram, and the left kidney is smaller than the right. Although the findings are compatible with renal artery stenosis on the left, they are not specific. In this instance, the patient had chronic pyelonephritis on the left. (From Fine EJ, Scharf SC, Blaufox MD: The role of nuclear medicine in evaluating the hypertensive patient. *In* Freeman LM, Weissman HS (eds): Nuclear Medicine Annual 1984. New York, Raven Press, 1984.)

advantage of the radionuclide study is its noninvasive nature. Another is its relatively low cost.[133] A positive study implies a post-test likelihood of RVH of about 70%, while a negative study suggests a likelihood of RVH of about 7%.[132] Although both IV-DSA and radiorenography have proponents of their use as screening tests for RVH, we prefer the latter, for reasons already stated, reserving IV-DSA for those with negative or equivocal results who are still suspected of having RVH.[133] The case for IV-DSA as a primary screen for RVH is well presented in Chapter 71.

One may obtain renal vein renins at the time of the IV-DSA study; this provides physiological data about the likelihood that a stenotic renal artery is the cause of the patient's hypertension; it also provides some prognostic information[134, 135] about the probability that vascular surgery or percutaneous transluminal angioplasty will improve the hypertension.

Regardless of the work-up chosen, radionuclides are extremely valuable for follow-up. All patients submitted to surgery of RVH or angioplasty should have renal scintirenograms, preoperatively for baseline evaluation, followed by post-treatment studies. This is especially important in patients undergoing angioplasty, in whom several procedures may be necessary before success is achieved (see Figs. 18–25 and 18–26).

Masses

These present most often as hematuria, or as abdominal or flank masses or pain. Ultrasonography, CT scanning, or an IVU is then usually performed. Nuclear medicine has a limited primary role in this evaluation, but is invaluable if a questionable mass is found (see Fig. 18–16). Fetal lobations, columns of Bertin, dromedary

humps, and other pseudotumors can be identified positively by following the initial radiographic or sonographic examination with Tc-99m-GHA[92] or DMSA[91] scintigraphy. A pathological mass will not function normally and its lack of radioactive uptake will be apparent as a photopenic renal defect (see Fig. 18–28). Similar information, but at greater cost, can be obtained by dynamic CT or MRI.

Trauma

Prevailing opinion favors the use of CT (or in less severe injuries, IVU) in the event of abdominal trauma, to document the nature and extent of traumatic damage. However, once renal trauma has been established, there is evidence to support the use of the radionuclide procedures as important adjuncts.[136] CT provides limited information on the extent of renal functional damage, and this information is both vital and easily obtainable by radio-

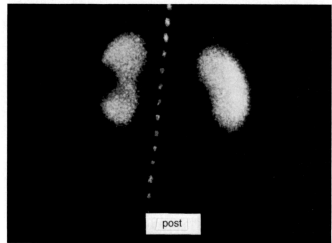

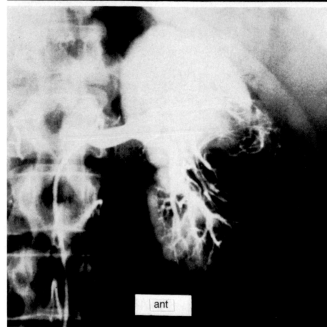

Figure 18–28. Renal parenchymal defect secondary to renal cell carcinoma. The posterior view from a Tc-99m-GHA renal morphology study reveals a clear-cut defect in the lateral margin of the left kidney. The arteriogram is shown for comparison in this patient with renal cell carcinoma.

Tc-99m angiogram

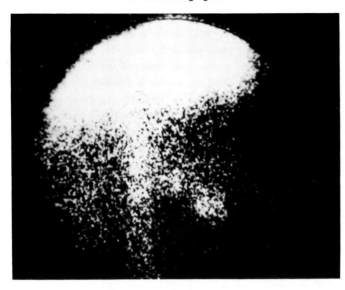

0–10 sec

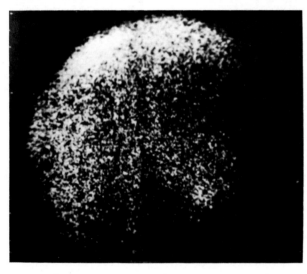

10–14 sec

Figure 18–29. Renal AV fistula. This patient had a renal biopsy followed by persistent hematuria. On this Tc-99m-TcO$_4^-$ angiogram, there is evidence of a traumatic arteriovenous fistula. In the first image, there is pooling of radioactivity within the kidney. The inferior vena cava is seen.

nuclide imaging. The addition of vitally important perfusion information can be achieved with many of the Tc-99m agents (DTPA, GHA, TcO$_4^-$). A post-traumatic arteriovenous fistula is demonstrated in Figure 18–29. DTPA, GHA, and DMSA produce high-quality anatomical images of renal trauma (Fig. 18–30). I-131-OIH produces images of poorer spatial resolution, although urinary extravasation may sensitively be detected. DTPA can be used for this purpose as well and has the advantage of photon flux higher than that of OIH in the doses used (Fig. 18–31). In the event of sensitivity to contrast material, excretory urography and contrast-enhanced CT may not be feasible. Here the radionuclide procedures assume a role even more important in documenting the

nature and extent of renal anatomical and functional damage. In severe renal insufficiency, I-131-OIH or I-123-OIH may be the only agents capable of visualizing the kidneys.

The importance of documenting the extent of renal damage with a radiotracer study, independent of obtaining a CT scan or IVU deserves additional emphasis. It is only the radionuclide study that allows multiple noninvasive follow-up examinations to be performed with the disclosure of anatomical, perfusion, and functional information.

Infarcts

The demonstration of renal infarcts can be achieved easily and noninvasively with a Tc-99m-GHA or DMSA morphology scintiscan. The nuclear procedure has some distinct advantages over morphologic imaging by IVU, ultrasonography, or CT. In particular, the typical wedge-shaped peripheral defect in the renal cortex is quite easy to demonstrate by this procedure, and additional perfusion information is quite important (Fig. 18–32). In contrast, CT exposes the patient to more radiation as well as the possibility of radiographic contrast material, as does the IVU. Ultrasonography may show no abnormality in an acute renal infarct.

Congenital and Pediatric Conditions

Tc-99m DTPA is useful in most situations requiring evaluation of the kidneys in the pediatric age group. The agent is used in a manner similar to that used in adults, except that the administered activity is lower in proportion to body surface area. Special considerations in this group include the need for sedation. I-131-OIH is used much less frequently. The higher absorbed radiation dose to the kidneys from this agent in comparison with Tc-99m-DTPA cause this agent to be less attractive in this age group. On the other hand, I-123-OIH is important in the evaluation of children.

Evaluation of hydronephrosis and megaureter to rule out obstruction is a common indication for pediatric renal scintigraphy. The IVU often is obtained first, although in many instances it provides no diagnostic information that is not obtainable by the Tc-99m-DTPA scintirenogram and a sonogram (a less invasive combination with less radiation absorbed by the child). In any event, at least a concurrent Tc-99m-DTPA scintirenogram is suggested, to allow for noninvasive follow-up of the patient. The examination using Tc-99m-DTPA must sometimes be carried out for several hours, to follow the slow course of radioactive urine into a dilated renal pelvis (Fig. 18–33). The use of IV furosemide (1 mg/kg) just as in adults, helps to distinguish true obstruction from nonobstructed hydronephrotic kidneys.[79, 137–139] Renal function, both total and individual, may be quantified by means similar to those used in adults. This is useful in following the progress of disease, especially before and after corrective surgery.

Also common in the pediatric group is vesicoureteral reflux. Patients presenting with multiple urinary tract infections usually will have a voiding cystourethrogram

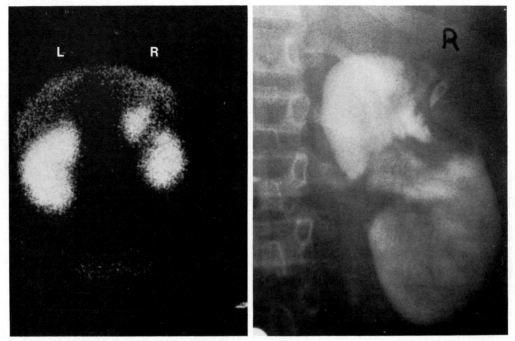

Figure 18–30. Fracture of the kidney. Many technetium-labeled agents may be used in the evaluation of renal trauma. On the left is a posterior view of a blood pool image of a Tc-99m-DTPA study. A clear fracture line passes through the upper pole of the right kidney. A film from this patient's intravenous urogram is shown for comparison. The urogram is from the posterior projection. Correlation of the images is excellent.

performed at some phase of their evaluation. The radionuclide cystogram[140, 141] is more sensitive in detecting reflux with a substantially lower absorbed radiation burden to the child than the contrast radiographic study. Its primary drawback, however, is that it does not provide anatomical information about the bladder neck or urethra. Again, we recommend the scintigraphic technique, regardless of whether the contrast examination is performed (Fig. 18–34). This allows for sequential follow-up using the lower-radiation-dose radionuclide procedure.

Most renal morphological studies are often performed with CT, ultrasonography, or IVU. However, in small

children the resolution of renal studies performed with radionuclides is quite high, particularly with DMSA. Renal scars are reported to be detectable with a 94% sensitivity in children, using DMSA.[142] In patients showing a questionable mass, the level of function of the mass can be seen using Tc-99m-GHA or DMSA, as with adults. Nonfunctioning tissue indicates disease, whereas functioning tissue, that is, tissue that concentrates Tc-99m-GHA or DMSA, does not.

Patients with a horseshoe kidney may profit from radionuclide evaluation. The problem that often needs to be addressed is the degree of function of the isthmus or

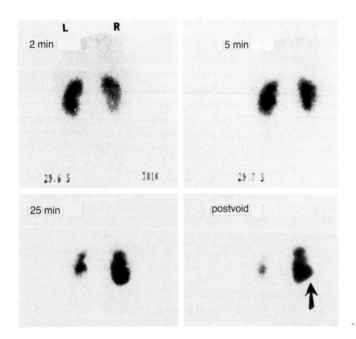

Figure 18–31. Renal trauma with extravasation. Urinary extravasation may be evaluated with radionuclides in renal trauma. This Tc-99m-DTPA study was performed with 8 mCi in a 10-year-old boy who had sustained abdominal trauma. The right kidney is not functioning as well as the left, which is shown by a decreased level of uptake on the 2-minute image, compared with the left kidney. The left kidney demonstrates normal transit and excretion, but the right progressively accumulates activity, particularly in a misshapen lower pole. The activity exceeds the boundaries of a normal renal contour and indicates urinary extravasation on the 25-minute image and especially in the postvoid image (arrow). Equally important is the reduced renal function already described. A follow-up study is necessary to insure return of function on the affected side.

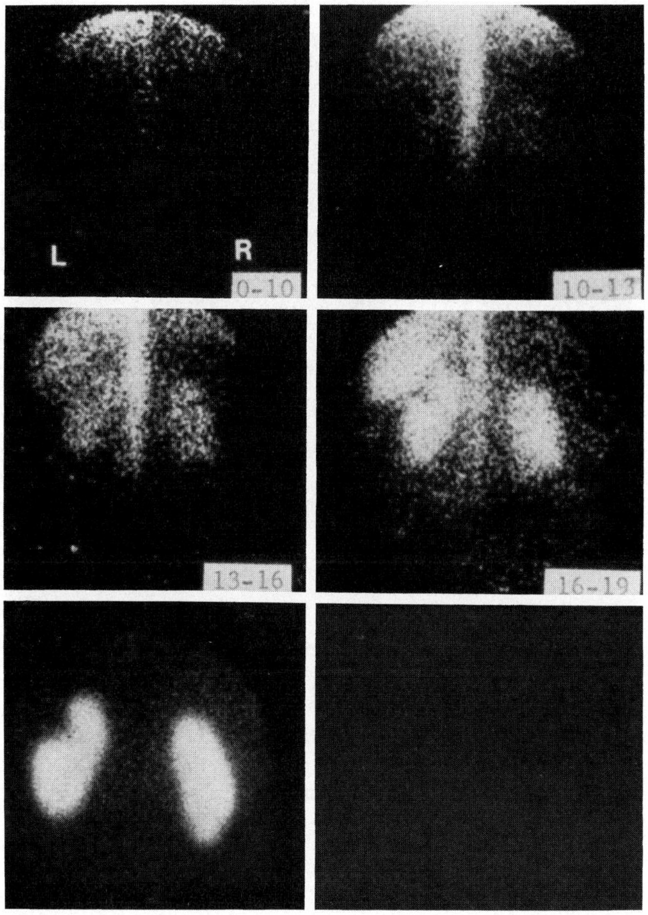

Figure 18–32. Renal infarct. In this Tc-99m-GHA flow study, a defect in the left upper pole is noted, which becomes more clearly defined on the delayed morphology image. This wedge-shaped peripheral defect is typical for a renal infarct, which was confirmed by angiography (not shown). (Labels denote seconds.)

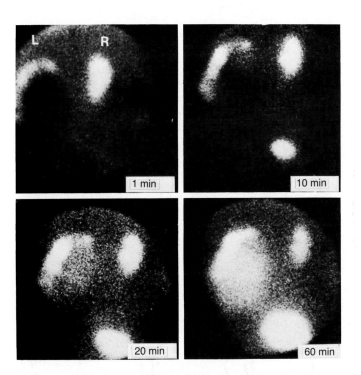

Figure 18–33. Hydronephrosis. A huge hydronephrosis sac is demonstrated on the left in these Tc-99m-DTPA scintireno-grams obtained in a 10-month-old boy. Sixty minutes of delayed imaging are required to demonstrate the extent of the sac. Prior to this it appears merely as a photon-deficient area. Renal function is also evident in a rim of cortex around the dilated renal pelvis.

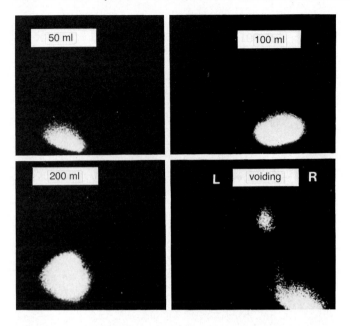

Figure 18–34. Radionuclide VCU—recurrent left pyelonephritis in a child. 500 μCi of Tc-99m-TcO$_4$⁻ were administered via a urethral catheter. Subsequent filling of the bladder with sterile saline indicated no reflux. However, during voiding, reflux up the left ureter and into the left renal pelvis is noted.

connecting segment. Particularly if there is evidence of obstruction (which may be evaluated with Tc-99m diuretic scintirenography), it may be desirable to separate surgically the left and right portions to free the ureters. Again, a Tc-99m-GHA scintiscan, performed from the anterior projection, can determine the degree of function of the interconnecting segment (Fig. 18–35). Functioning tissue will show concentration of the radiotracer, whereas fibrous nonfunctioning tissue will not.

Renal agenesis, when suspected clinically (usually by incidental nonvisualization on IVU performed for another purpose) can easily be confirmed or refuted using radiotracers. One may use Tc-99m-GHA or DMSA with delayed images as well as Tc-99m-DTPA or I-123-OIH to locate a kidney. The last agent has particular value if the differential diagnosis includes severe renal dysfunction within a chronically diseased, atrophic kidney. When searching for a "missing kidney," it is essential to image the pelvic region as well as the abdomen, since pelvic kidneys may be described as missing kidneys by other procedures. This is not a problem in the young pediatric patient in whom the entire abdomen and pelvis will fit on a large-field-of-view scintillation camera. In an adult with recent suspicion of renal agenesis, however, it is necessary to remind oneself to obtain a pelvic image. The bladder must be emptied and shielded to complete the examination.

Polycystic and multicystic kidneys may be detected serendipitously in a renal scan evaluation, but the multiple defects seen within a large kidney are certainly suggestive of the former (see Fig. 18–36). Multiple defects, however, may be caused by other renal masses, or large calculi and therefore ultrasonography is mandatory to confirm the cystic or calcareous nature of the lesions. Generally, the

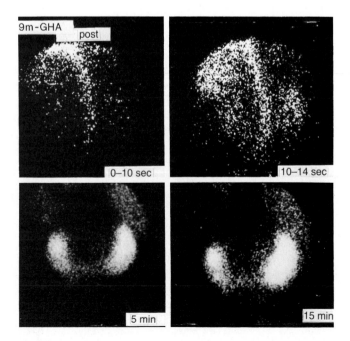

Figure 18–35. Horseshoe kidney. Two frames from a Tc-99m-GHA flow study are demonstrated along with delayed images obtained at 5 minutes and 15 minutes after injection of the tracer. The axis of each kidney points medially and an interconnecting segment of tissue is noted in this typical example of horseshoe kidney with apparent thin parenchymal isthmus. An anterior view might have shown more impressive uptake in the connecting segment.

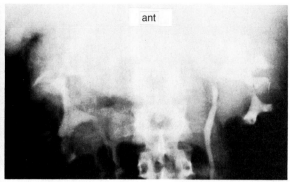

Figure 18–36. Autosomal dominant polycystic kidney disease. In this patient with polycystic kidneys, the posterior view Tc-99m-DTPA image demonstrates defects in the region of the dilated pyelocalyceal systems. Right-sided defects are more subtle.

distinction between a hydronephrotic and a multicystic kidney is possible with radionuclides. In hydronephrosis, the renal parenchyma is seen as a shell-like structure surrounding a photopenic dilated renal pelvis and calyceal system. Delayed images usually provide a morphological representation of a distended collecting system in even the most severely damaged kidneys, if properly delayed images are obtained. With multicystic dysplastic kidneys, however, there may be no visible excretion of radionuclide. If excretion does occur, its distribution will not conform to a recognizable renal pelvis or collecting system, but rather will be spotty and heterogeneous. Whatever kidney tissue is present will not be reniform in outline, but will be irregular and amorphous in its appearance.[143]

Duplication of the renal collecting systems is more common in females and is often bilateral. This condition may produce no symptoms or signs throughout life, in which case it would have to be considered a normal variant. However, in general, patients with this anatomical curiosity have a substantially higher incidence of GU disorders including obstruction, reflux, and infection. Scinti-imaging procedures with Tc-99m-DTPA, I-123-OIH, Tc-99m-DMSA, or Tc-99m-GHA are of value in demonstrating this condition, particularly to assess function of the upper versus lower pole.[144, 145] Persistent pain, obstruction, or infection may require surgery. The decision to perform heminephrectomy of a nonfunctioning upper or lower pole can be assisted by a radionuclide assessment of regional renal function.

The use of Ga-67 citrate in the evaluation of pediatric tumors has not been widespread. In a small series[146] Ga-67 did not appear sensitive in detecting primary or metastatic disease in either Wilms' tumors or neuroblastomas. Chest and abdominal radiographs, ultrasonograms, and IVUs appear to be superior in the definition of these tumors.

Splenic-gonadal fusion is an unusual congenital anomaly representing fusion of splenic and gonadal anlagen during early fetal development and most frequently associated with cryptorchism. It may be detected by Tc-99m sulfur colloid imaging.[147]

Infection and Inflammation

The symptom complex of fever, dysuria, and flank or back pain suggests infection of the kidneys, but on occasion lower urinary tract infections produce these same symptoms.

In cases where kidney infection is suspected, but cannot be proven by conventional or simpler means, other diagnostic tools may be employed, including the IVU, CT scan, sonogram, and Ga-67-citrate and Tc-99m-DMSA scintiscans. Features that dictate the order of these examinations usually include the familiarity and preferences of the referring physician, and the availability of the given examination. In general, the IVU and sonogram are of limited value in the setting of acute pyelonephritis. On the other hand, Ga-67 citrate imaging has been reported to be 85% accurate in distinguishing upper from lower GU infections.[148] Intrarenal parenchymal infection is not readily distinguishable from renal or perinephric abscess (Fig. 18–37); therefore ultrasonography or CT should follow a positive study to establish the possibility of abscess. Handmaker reports 100% sensitivity in one series for Tc-99m-DMSA scintiscanning in acute pyelonephritis.[149] These results suggest that these procedures may be of great value in cases of suspected pyelonephritis that cannot be proved by other noninvasive means.

Patients with spinal cord injury are often young and must be followed for many years to observe the complications of their trauma. They run the risk of recurrent GU tract infection, with concomittent loss of renal function. The IVU has been used for many years by urologists to follow renal function in such patients. However, a growing body of investigation[150, 151] has demonstrated the utility of OIH scintigraphy with ERPF measurements to screen these patients sensitively for loss of renal function. The IVU, with its superior anatomical resolution, may be reserved, then, to evaluate patients who have demonstrated decreased renal function by OIH scintigraphy.

Ga-67 has been useful in cases of interstitial nephritis in demonstrating bilaterally diffuse, often markedly increased uptake (Fig. 18–38).[152]

Determination of Recoverability of Renal Function

The need to determine the salvageability of a kidney is closely related to the determination of individual renal function. As such, any of the agents and procedures described above can be utilized for this purpose. The specific agent chosen, depends on the particulars of the clinical situation. Although a badly damaged kidney may

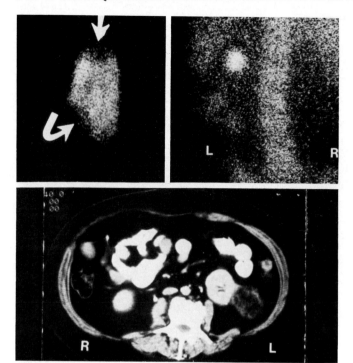

Figure 18–37. Renal abscess coexistent with angiomyolipoma. In this patient with fever, left flank pain and pyuria, a Tc-99m-GHA study (upper left) revealed a defect in the left upper pole (*short arrow*) and in the left lower pole (*curved arrow*). A Ga-67-citrate study (upper right) performed in the posterior projection 48 hours after injection of radiotracer showed striking focal accumulation of radiogallium in the left upper-pole region and more diffuse and hazy uptake in the left lower-pole region. The right kidney demonstrated no appreciable uptake, a normal finding. A CT scan of the abdomen demonstrates the left lower-pole finding, which was determined by angiography to be an angiomyolipoma. The left upper pole finding was found to be a left renal abscess. Ga-67 is known to concentrate avidly in neutrophils, and therefore the intense uptake seen in the left upper pole is both consistent with and suggestive of an abscess in this region. Gallium uptake in tumors is variable, and depends on the affinity of the individual tumor for this radiotracer.

require nephrectomy, preservation of, for example, upper-pole renal function may allow partial nephrectomy to be a viable option. Finally, the degree of contralateral renal function must be sufficient to justify a nephrectomy. In many situations of this kind a Tc-99m-GHA or DMSA study would probably provide the most information, since what is requested requires a combination of regional morphologic and functional information. Attempts to predict the degree of renal viability remaining in a chronically obstructed kidney have largely been disappointing. Except for the most far-advanced cases, it is all but impossible to determine by radionuclide methods which kidneys are worth "saving" and which are best removed forthwith. All things being equal, and assuming no contraindications, it is often worthwhile to defer such decisions until after an 8- to 10-week period of trial nephrostomy.[193] By this time, renal function will usually have returned maximally, and a more reasoned clinical decision can be made. The results are often surprising.

In acute renal failure the questions asked about salvageability include the prognosis for the return of renal function. The agent of choice for renal evaluation in such a case is OIH. The intensity of kidney visualization during the first 30-minute scinti-images correlates with the prognosis for the spontaneous return. In acute obstruction, however, renal nonvisualization may occur more rarely without necessarily implying a poor prognosis (Figure 18–39).[154, 155] On the other hand, in the setting of acute nonobstructive renal failure, nonvisualization almost invariably implies end-stage disease.[153]

Renal Localization

Tc-99m-DMSA or GHA can be used in a simple fashion to localize the kidneys prior to radiotherapy or biopsy. Oncologists and radiation therapists need to identify the kidney locations in order to avoid the kidneys in their selection of radiation portals. Renal localization may be performed by a routine morphology scan with DMSA or GHA, with the aid of lead strips or small sources of radioactivity. Either the nonradioactive lead strips or the small radioactive sources can be visualized on the imaging oscilloscope screen simultaneously with the kidneys. Outlining the kidneys is a simple matter, and the outlines can be traced onto the patients back. A long-lasting ink should be used to account for an extended course of radiotherapy (Fig. 18–40).

OTHER GENITOURINARY TRACT APPLICATIONS

Urinary Conduit Evaluation

The urinary conduit, a "bladder equivalent," usually is formed of a loop of ileum, into which the ureters are implanted in patients who have had cystectomies. This

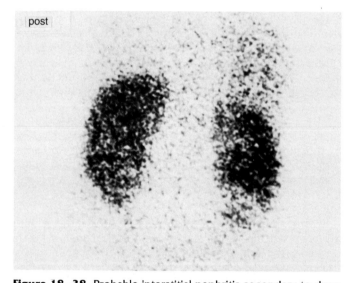

Figure 18–38. Probable interstitial nephritis secondary to drug abuse. A Ga-67 study was performed in this posterior projection with 3 mCi of the tracer. Striking diffuse accumulation of the radiogallium is noted bilaterally. The patient was an intravenous drug abuser on multiple antibiotic therapy for *Escherichia coli* endocarditis. The pattern on the gallium study is suggestive of diffuse interstitial nephritis. The defect in the lower pole of the right kidney is unexplained.

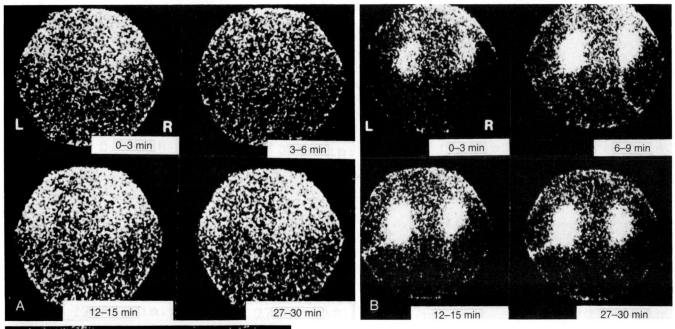

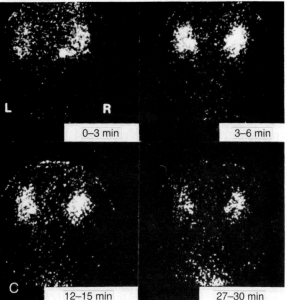

Figure 18–39. Improved renal function after relief of obstruction. *A,* A 65-year-old man presented in renal failure and was demonstrated to have bilateral hydronephrosis upon ultrasonography. Staghorn calculi obstructed both kidneys. A scintirenogram performed with OIH shows no significant renal accumulation on either side, consistent with severe renal failure. *B,* Bilateral nephrostomies were placed. After 2 weeks, recovery of renal function occurred, as demonstrated by the scintirenogram. Delayed excretion is commonly seen from nephrostomy tubes. *C,* After improvement in the patient's clinical condition, the staghorn calculi were removed. Following removal of the nephrostomies, a scintigraphic study performed 6 months later revealed satisfactory renal function, transit, and excretion. The importance of this example is that renal function can recover in patients with obstruction, even if renal failure is severe. (From Fine EJ, Scharf SC, Blaufox MD: The role of nuclear medicine in evaluating the hypertensive patient. *In* Freeman LM, Weissmann HS (eds): Nuclear Medicine Annual 1984. New York, Raven Press, 1984.)

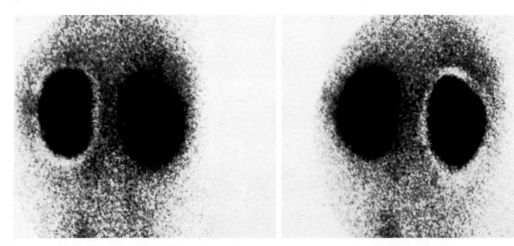

Figure 18–40. Renal scintigraphy in radiation treatment planning. This 65-year-old woman with non-Hodgkin's lymphoma was administered 3 mCi of Tc-99m-GHA to localize her kidneys for renal portals prior to radiotherapy. Lead markers were placed around the kidneys with the aid of the persistence oscilloscope, as the accompanying images demonstrate. By marking the patient's back with indelible ink in the region of the lead markers, radiation portals can be defined.

reanastamoses of ureters may function suboptimally; reflux, infection, and obstruction may ensue. To test the patency of the ureteral-conduit anastamoses, Tc-99m-DTPA or OIH scintirenography with or without a diuretic are useful to evaluate the dilatation commonly seen. The technique is similar to that described previously on diuretic scintirenography. Evaluation for the possibility of ureteral reflux is accomplished in more or less the same fashion as that employed for evaluating reflux in the intact bladder (see section Vesicoureteral Reflux).

Residual Urine Determination

Little or no urine remains in the normal bladder following physiological voiding. A persistent residual urine reflects urinary stasis and may predispose a patient to urinary tract infection. The condition may be seen in cases of neuropathic bladder (e.g., due to spinal cord injury, transverse myelopathy, poliomyelitis, diabetes mellitus) as well as bladder outlet obstruction. An extremely simple, accurate, noninvasive means of measuring residual urine is with radiotracers.

Originally described as an adjunct to dual crystal detector "probe" renography,[156, 157] the procedure now is usually the final step in gamma camera scintirenography[158] with OIH or Tc-99m-DTPA. The dose administered is by intravenous injection exactly as for an excretion study. OIH is preferable in some respects, since excretion into the bladder is completed more quickly. By 45 minutes, with OIH, a bladder image may be obtained by means of a computer matrix. Using regions of interest to surround the bladder and define a background region, total net bladder counts per minute (CPM) may be obtained, before and after voiding. Voided volume can be directly determined, and the difference in net bladder CPM can be obtained from the computer. Residual urine is calculated as follows:

Voided volume = K × difference in net bladder CPM,

where K = constant of proportionality relating urine volume to CPM.

Therefore K = voided volume (ml)/difference in bladder CPM.

Finally, we can determine that

Residual volume = K × net residual bladder CPM.

Thereby, residual volume is determined from residual bladder counts. Strauss and Blaufox[157] report the correlation between the radionuclide determination and catheterization in 20 patients to be y = 0.085x + 9.9 ml, where x is the catheter-determined volume and y represents the uncorrected radionuclide-determined volume. The correlation coefficient, r = 0.966, indicates outstanding correspondance between the techniques. The average catheter-determined volume in this study was 80 ± 18 ml, whereas by radionuclide techniques the average was 77 ± 17 ml.

Vesicoureteral Reflux

The detection of vesicoureteral reflux may be performed sensitively using radiotracer imaging techniques. Direct and indirect procedures have been devised. The indirect technique involves the latter phase of an excretion study performed with OIH. Detection of activity in the ureter of kidney in the late phase of this examination is a finding so common that false-positive studies recommend against the indirect procedure. (See discussion, Infection and Inflammation.)

Far superior is the direct procedure, in which the patient is first asked to void, after which Tc-99m-TcO$_4^-$ is instilled into the bladder via urethral catheter. Sterile saline then is instilled gradually through the catheter into the bladder by gravity infusion. (Simply hanging a bottle of saline above the level of the bladder is sufficient.) Scinti-images in anterior and/or posterior projections, with the patient sitting in front of the gamma camera usually are obtained at sequentially noted intervals of filling (e.g., 50 ml, 100 ml, 150 ml) until the patient expresses a desire to void, indicating bladder fullness. Images are obtained during voiding as well. Reflux may be demonstrated either during filling or voiding or both, the determinant apparently relating to the vesicoureteral pressure gradient during the respective phase of the examination. Indwelling ureteral stents will, of course, produce vesicoureteral reflux.[196]

Scrotal Imaging

Testicular Torsion versus Epididymitis

In several conditions of excessive testicular motility, the testis may twist on its pedicle, causing occlusion of the arterial blood supply (internal and external spermatic arteries and deferential artery) arriving via the spermatic cord.[159] The incidence of testicular torsion has a bimodal distribution with peaks occurring between ages 0 and 5 and again between 12 and 15 years. This condition constitutes a surgical emergency. Detorsion must be accomplished as quickly as possible or testicular viability will be lost. After 10 hours of torsion, the rate of salvage may be as low as 20%.[160]

Acute epididymo-orchitis is an inflammatory disease, usually seen in adults, and in most cases it is treated medically rather than surgically. In any individual patient, the differentiation between torsion and epididymo-orchitis may be difficult. In such individuals scrotal scinti-imaging is extremely helpful to distinguish the two conditions.

It is imperative that scinti-imaging be performed

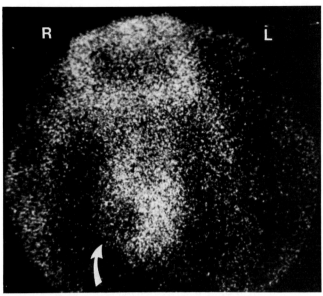

Figure 18–42. Acute torsion of testis. A classic example of acute torsion is demonstrated with a photon deficiency involving the right hemiscrotal contents on this delayed blood pool image performed with Tc-99m-TcO$_4^-$ (*arrow*).

promptly: time is of the essence should acute torsion prove to be the diagnosis. If imaging cannot be started promptly, for whatever reason, one must question its utility in a given patient, and surgery may have to be considered without the imaging study.

The study may be performed with any Tc-99m agent that remains in the blood pool. Tc-99m pertechnetate or DTPA are commonly used, although Tc-99m–labeled human serum albumin (HSA) is a reasonable choice also. Rapid sequential images (each 2 to 5 seconds) are obtained over the scrotal region and an immediate blood pool image also is obtained. A lead marker to separate and distinguish the left and right hemiscrotal regions is helpful. Symmetrical appearance of tracer on the flow study and on the delayed image constitute a normal study (Fig. 18–41). Use of a pinhole collimator improves resolution of anatomical detail and is an important adjunct for this purpose.

Acute torsion is characterized by an activity deficiency on the symptomatic side on both "flow" and blood pool images (Fig. 18–42). Epididymo-orchitis does not have this scintigraphic appearance and demonstrates either normal or increased activity on the painful side (Fig. 18–43). Increased activity is thought to reflect the increased vascularity due to inflammatory vasodilatation.

When torsion has been present long enough to cause infarction, the devitalized testis cannot be salvaged. Scintigraphically, such a structure appears as an activity deficiency surrounded by a "vascular" rim, representing scrotal hyperemia (Fig. 18–44).[161] The scrotum, as distinct from its contents, is supplied by branches of the internal and external pudendal arteries, which do not arrive via the spermatic cord, and is therefore spared during testicular torsion. An inflammatory response to the infarcted testis causes vasodilatation of the scrotal blood vessels, accounting for the scintigraphic appearance of the "missed torsion." This pattern is important to recognize from a prognostic point of view, since it indicates a tendency toward torsion in that individual. Although the infarcted testis cannot be saved, the surgeon, in all

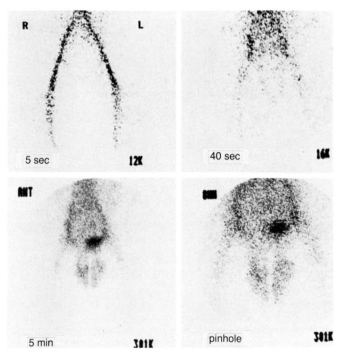

Figure 18–41. Normal scrotal scan in a 13-year-old. Representative images are obtained in this scintigraphic scrotal study. Two images from the angiogram demonstrate the iliac vessels and faint tracer accumulation in the scrotal region on the 2-second image obtained at 40 seconds after injection. The 5-minute blood pool image demonstrates homogeneous and symmetric accumulation of tracer as does the pinhole magnified view. This is a normal study in a 13-year-old boy with right-sided testicular pain. The delayed blood pool images often provide substantially more information than do the initial blood flow images.

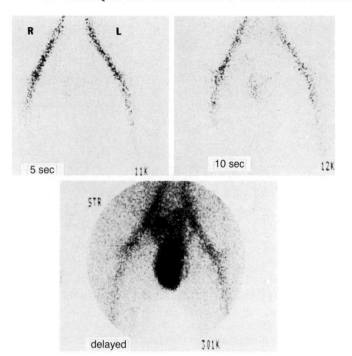

Figure 18–43. Right epididymitis—scrotal scan. In this 14-year-old boy with right scrotal pain and swelling, the flow study suggests increased activity on the right side compared with the left. The delayed static image shows markedly increased right-sided blood pool activity, compared with the left. This pattern indicates inflammatory disease on the right side, rather than torsion.

likelihood, will want to perform an orchiopexy on the contralateral, viable testis at a later time.

Tumors, abscesses, cysts, hydroceles, and hematomas may demonstrate deficiencies of radioactivity on scrotal scinti-images, mimicking torsion or missed torsion.[161] In other words, these diagnostic patterns are not specific for torsion. However, the typical pattern of acute torsion in the appropriate clinical setting is extremely helpful in mandating a surgical approach for an individual. A normal-appearing scan rules out torsion with a nearly 100% predictive value.[162]

Blood pool imaging of the scrotum is not indicated, in general, for evaluation of scrotal masses when the clinical context is not that of acute disease. Ultrasonography is better able to characterize scrotal masses. Blood pool imaging has been successfully employed for the demonstration of varicoceles.[163]

Penile Vascularity and Impotency Evaluation[164]

Blood pool labeling is performed easily with a wide variety of Tc-99m–labeled tracers, just as for scrotal imaging procedures. Any of these agents in amounts of 10 to 15 mCi may be used for blood pool evaluation of the penis as well. After ordinary IV injection of these agents, the penis may be visualized on delayed blood pool images. It is essential to shield surrounding blood pool activity with lead aprons so that the penis alone is imaged by the gamma camera, using parallel-hole, low-energy, or pinhole collimation.

The value of the procedure is in distinguishing organic

disease with decreased penile vascularity (diabetes mellitus, sickle cell anemia) from nonvascular causes of impotency, including psychogenic causes. Similar information has been obtained by Nseyo and colleagues, employing Xe-133 wash-out techniques.[165]

Prostatic Lymphoscintigraphy

Tc-99m antimony sulfide (not approved for general use) can be produced in colloidal particles of 100 μm. Colloidal particles of this size are trapped and phagocy-

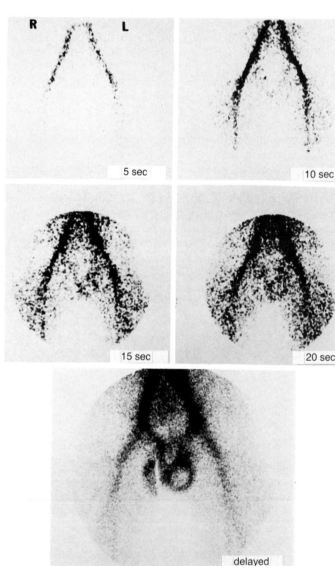

Figure 18–44. Missed testicular torsion. This 9-year-old boy with 2 days of left-sided scrotal pain demonstrates a rounded activity deficiency surrounded by a radioactive rim. This is seen on the flow study but is better demonstrated on the delayed image. The pattern is consistent with a missed torsion in which the central photon deficiency represents an avascular, nonviable, necrotic testis. The radioactive blood pool in the rim is the result of inflammatory changes in the surrounding scrotum, which is supplied by pudendal vessels—and not by arterial flow—through the spermatic cord. In the appropriate clinical setting, this pattern is very helpful in identifying a missed torsion, although it is not specific for it. This pattern may also indicate an abscess or a necrotic or hypovascular tumor with surrounding inflammation.

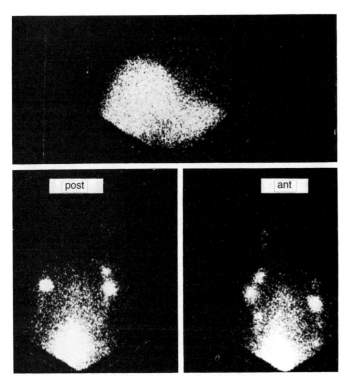

Figure 18–45. Prostatic lymphoscintigraphy. 250 mCi of Tc-99m antimony sulfide colloid was administered by direct injection into each prostatic lobe. Anterior and posterior images of the pelvis and lower abdomen are obtained and reveal focal accumulation in the draining lymphatics of the prostate. Some activity that has escaped into the blood stream accumulates in the liver, as demonstrated in the scintigram. Phagocytosis by reticuloendothelial cells confirms the colloidal nature of this agent (similar to Tc-99m-sulfur colloid). The small particulate size explains the absence of spleen visualization. This study demonstrates normal lymphatic drainage from the prostate. The clinical role of this agent has not yet been clearly defined.

tized in regional lymph nodes after subcutaneous or intramuscular injection. Direct injection into the lobes of the prostate gland allow for visualization of regional lymph node drainage (Fig. 18–45). This procedure is under investigation for its potential role in the preoperative staging of prostatic carcinoma.[166, 167] Pedal lymphoscintigraphy has been used in evaluating patients with chyluria.[194]

Evaluation of the Pregnant Patient

Scant data are available about the use of renal radiotracers in pregnancy. Wax and Rudolph, in 1967,[168, 169] examined seven women undergoing therapeutic abortion between 10 and 26 weeks of pregnancy with I-131-OIH renograms performed 6 to 24 hours prior to operation. OIH was not detected in fetal kidney or gonads in any trimester of fetal life. We may conclude that fetal kidneys between 10 and 26 weeks gestational age cannot be evaluated using OIH. However, free I-131 did cross the placenta, as evidenced by uptake in the thyroid of two fetuses, a potential hazard during the second and third trimesters. In six pregnant women at term, premedicated with Lugol's iodine, OIH renograms were followed by delivery within 4 to 24 hours. In these infants, thyroid activity was not detected.

On the other hand, I-123-OIH produces the lowest absorbed radiation of all renal excretory agents (see Table 18–1). In doses of 300 μCi, the mother's whole-body dose would be about 10 mrad. Since first- and second-trimester fetuses do not appear to accumulate OIH, the fetal absorbed dose would be predictably lower. An IVU would produce substantially higher absorbed doses of radiation to both mother and fetus. OIH, therefore, would be a reasonable choice for evaluating the mother, should the clinical need arise. Premedication with Lugol's solution would be appropriate. However, further information is required before OIH scintirenography can be recommended in a more general context for pregnant women.

ADRENAL IMAGING

Huge adrenal tumors have been detected serendipitously during radionuclide imaging (Fig. 18–46). Several cholesterol analogues labeled with I-131 have been utilized in attempts to image the adrenal cortex more specifically. These agents depend on uptake and storage of cholesterol and its analogues by the adrenal cortex. Most bodily tissues contain cholesterol, but only the adrenal cortex, ovary (corpora luteal cells), and testes (Sertoli's cell) normally store it, to any degree, by esterification. Historically, 19-iodocholesterol was used first in 1970.[170]

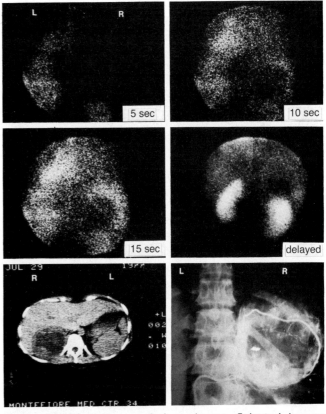

Figure 18–46. Adrenocortical carcinoma. Selected images from a flow study and a delayed blood pool image performed with Tc-99m-DTPA reveal an activity deficiency superior to the right kidney surrounded by a vascular rim. A hypodense lesion is noted superior to the right kidney on the CT study, and the angiogram demonstrates a large tumor. This represents a surgically proven right adrenocortical carcinoma.

However, the most successful adrenocortical agent to date has been I-131-6-beta-iodomethyl-19-norcholest-5-(10)-ene-3-beta-ol, known as NP-59.[171]

At room temperature, NP-59 may degrade from 95% bound radioactivity to as low as 70% within 6 days. It is best stored in a cold, dark environment.[172] The recommended shelf life is no more than 2 weeks,[173] and greater than 10% free iodide is unacceptable for use. Patients should be prepared with 1 and preferably 2 days of pretreatment with Logol's iodine—3 drops, twice daily—to protect their thyroid glands. This should be continued for 2 weeks after the examination. The patient is given 1 to 2 mCi/1.7 m² body surface area of high specific activity NP-59 by slow intravenous injection (over 1 to 2 minutes).[174] Imaging should be performed with a gamma camera using a medium-energy parallel-hole collimator and interfaced with a computer; it should begin at least 4 to 5 days after tracer injection to allow background to clear. The gamma camera should be "peaked" for the 364-keV photopeak of I-131 with a ±40 keV window. Positioning is done posteriorly at the T12-L1 level. A minimum of 50,000 counts is obtained. Absorbed radiation to the adrenal is higher than to any other organ evaluated with current diagnostic nuclear studies. This is a potential limitation in using this procedure.

Quantification of adrenal uptake, analogous to thyroid uptake, may be performed, and is most conveniently done with the computer matrix images. A lateral view should also be obtained to allow depth calibration of the adrenals. Uptake percentage of the initial dose may then be calculated after correcting for depth attenuation. Normal uptake ranges have been determined for NP-59[175] as well as for I-131-19-iodocholesterol.[176] High values have been reported to be associated with adrenocortical hypersecretion. More recently, agents for adrenal medullary imaging, such as meta-iodo-benzyl guanidine (MIBG) have been developed and applied successfully in a clinical setting. A complete discussion of the clinical applications of radionuclide adrenal imaging in the various forms of hyperadrenalism and in pheochromocytoma appears in Chapter 90.

Acknowledgments

The authors wish to thank Dr. L. M. Freeman for much of the illustrative material, and Joyce Rush for patience and superior secretarial support.

References

1. Blaufox MD, Fine E, Lee H-B, Scharf S: The role of nuclear medicine in clinical urology and nephrology. J Nucl Med 25:619, 1984.
2. Hevesy G: The absorption and translocation of lead by plants, a contribution to the application of the method of radioactive indicators in the investigation of changes of substances in plants. Biochem J 17:439, 1923.
3. Hahn O, Strassman F: Uber den nachweis und das verhalten der beider bestrahlung des urans mittels neutronen entstehenden Erdalkalimetalle. (Covering the detection and behavior of alkaline earths resulting from the irradiation of uranium with neutrons.) Naturwissenschaften 27:11, 1939.
4. Lawrence EO, Sloan DH: The production of high speed canal rays without the use of high voltages. Proc Natl Acad Sci 17:64, 1931.
5. Livingood JT, Seaborg GT: Radioactive isotopes of iodine. Physiol Rev 54:775, 1938.
6. Hamilton JF, Soley MH: Studies in iodine metabolism by the use of a new radioactive isotope of iodine. Am J Physiol 127:557, 1939.
7. Taplin GV, Meredith OM, Kade H, Winter CC: The radioisotope renogram. An external test for individual kidney function and upper urinary tract patency. J Lab Clin Med 48:886, 1956.
8. Nordyke RA, Tubis M, Blahd WH: Use of radioiodinated hippuran for individual kidney function tests. J Lab Clin Med 56:438, 1960.
9. Tubis M, Posnick E, Nordyke RA: Preparation and use of ¹³¹I labelled sodium iodohippurate in kidney function tests. Proc Soc Exp Biol Med 109:497, 1960.
10. Schwartz FD, Madeloff MS: Simultaneous renal clearances of radiohippuran and para-aminohippurate in man. Clin Res 9:208, 1961.
11. Burbank MK, Tauxe WN, Maher FT, Hunt JC: Evaluation of radioiodohippuran for the estimation of renal plasma flow. Proc Staff Meet Mayo Clin 36:372, 1961.
12. Cassen B, Curtis L, Reed C, et al: Instrumentation for ¹³¹I use in medical studies. Nucleonics 9:46, 1951.
13. McAfee JG, Wagner HN Jr: Visualization of renal parenchyma. Scintiscanning with ²⁰³Hg neohydrin. Radiology 75:820, 1960.
14. Raynaud C, Desgrez A, Kellershohn C: Measurement of renal mercury uptake by external counting. Separate functional testing of each kidney. J Urol 99:248, 1968.
15. Anger HO: Scintillation camera: Rev Sci Instrum 29:27, 1958.
16. Harper PV, Lathrop KA, McCardle RJ, Andros G: The use of ⁹⁹ᵐTc as pertechnetate for thyroid, liver and brain scanning. In Medical Radioisotope Scanning. International Atomic Energy Agency, Vienna, IAEA, 1964.
17. Hauser W, Atkins HL, Nelson KG: ⁹⁹ᵐTc-DTPA—a new radiopharmaceutical for brain and kidney imaging. Radiology 94:679, 1970.
18. Lin TH, Khentigan A, Winchell HS: A ⁹⁹ᵐTc chelate substitute for organoradiomercurial renal agents. J Nucl Med 11:34, 1974.
19. Charamaza O, Budikova M: Method of preparation of a ⁹⁹ᵐTc-complex for renal scintigraphy. Nucl Med (Stuttgart) 8:301, 1969.
20. Harper PV, Lathrop KA, Hinn GM, et al: Technetium-99m iron complex, In Andrews Kniseley RM, Wagner HN Jr (eds): Radioactive Pharmaceuticals. Conf 651111, USAEC, 1966.
21. Bender MA, Blau M: Autofluoroscopy—the use of a nonscanning device for tumor localization with radioisotopes (abstr). J Nucl Med 1:105, 1960.
22. Stadalnik RC, Vogel JM, Jansholt A-L, et al: Renal clearance and extraction parameters of ortho-iodohippurate (I-123) compared with OIH (I-131) and PAH. J Nucl Med 21:168, 1980.
23. Blaufox MD, Merrill JP: Simplified hippuran clearance. Measurement of renal function in man with simplified hippuran clearance. Nephron 3:274, 1966.
24. Tauxe WN, Dubovsky EV, Kidd T Jr, et al: New formulas for the calculation of effective renal plasma flow. Eur J Nucl Med 7:51, 1982.
25. Schlegel JU, Hamway SA: Individual renal plasma flow determination in 2 minutes. J Urol 116:282, 1976.
26. Braren V, Versage PN, Touya JJ, et al: Radioisotopic determination of glomerular filtration rate. J Urol 121:145, 1979.
27. Piepsz A, Denis R, Ham HR, et al: A simple method for measuring separate glomerular filtrate rate using a single injection of ⁹⁹ᵐTc-DTPA and the scintillation camera. J Pediatr 93:769, 1978.
28. Carlsen JE, Møller ML, Lund JO, Trap-Jensen J: Comparison of four commercial Tc-99m (Sn) DTPA preparations used for the measurement of glomerular filtration rate: Concise communication. J Nucl Med 21:126, 1980.
29. Klopper JF, Hauser W, Atkins HL, et al: Evaluation of ⁹⁹ᵐTc-DTPA for the measurement of glomerular filtrate rate. J Nucl Med 13:107, 1971.
30. Gates GF: Glomerular filtration rate: Estimation from fractional renal accumulation of ⁹⁹ᵐTc-DTPA (stannous). Am J Radiol 138:565, 1982.
31. Donadio C, Tramenti G, Cotronei T, et al: Filtration fraction in unilateral hypertensive renal disease and a new non-invasive method for its measurement. Contrib Nephron 11:29, 1978.
32. Coe FL, Burke G: Renal transit time: Its measurement by the I-131-Hippuran renogram. J Nucl Med 6:269, 1965.
33. Rosen SM, Hollenberg NK, Dealy JB Jr, Merrill JP: Measurement of the distribution of blood flow in the human kidney using the

intraarterial injection of ^{133}Xe: Relationship to function in the normal and transplanted kidney. Clin Sci 34:287, 1968.

34. Ladefoged J: Measurements of the renal blood flow in man with the ^{133}Xe wash-out technique. Scand J Clin Lab Invest 18:299, 1966.

35. Blaufox MD, Fromowitz A, Gruskin A, Meng C-H, and Elkin M: Validation of the use of xenon-133 to measure intrarenal distribution of blood flow. Amer J Physiol 219:440, 1970.

35a. Miraldi FD, Nelson AD, Kraly C, et al: Diagnostic imaging of human neuroblastoma with radiolabelled antibody. Radiology 161:413, 1986.

36. Scheer KE, Meier-Borst W: Die darstellung von ^{131}I-orthoiodohippuran ourch Austauchmarkierung. Nuklearmedizin 2:193, 1961.

37. Mitta AEA, Fraga A, Veall N: A simplified method for preparing ^{131}I-labelled hippuran. Int J Appl Radiol 12:146, 1961.

38. Smith WW, Smith HW: Protein binding of phenol red, diodrast, and other substances in plasma. J Biol Chem 124:107, 1938.

39. Blaufox MD, Merrill JP: Simplified Hippuran clearance: Measurement of renal function in man with simplified Hippuran clearances. Nephron 3:274, 1966.

40. Taplin GV, Dore EK, Johnson DE: The quantitative radiorenogram for total and differential renal blood flow measurement. J Nucl Med 4:409, 1963.

41. Wedeen RP, Goldstein MH, Levitt MF: The radioisotope renogram in normal subjects. Am J Med 34:765, 1963.

42. Rosenthall L, Tyler JL, Arzoumanian A: A cross-over study comparing delayed radiohippurate images with furosemide renograms. Diagn Imag 52:267, 1983.

43. Strauss BS, Blaufox MK: Estimation of residual urine and urine flow rates without urethral catheterization. J Nucl Med 11:81, 1970.

44. Rosenthall L: Residual urine determination by roentgenographic and isotopic means. Radiology 80:454, 1963.

45. Dore EK, Taplin GV, Johnson DE: Current interpretation of the sodium iodohippurate I-131 renocystogram. JAMA 185:925, 1963.

46. Lundstam S, Wihed S, Suurkula M, et al: Acute radiorenography during attacks of renal colic. J Urol 130:855, 1983.

47. Bueschen AJ, Witten DM: Radionuclide evaluation of renal function. Urol Clin N Am 6:307, 1979.

48. Belis JA, Belis TE, Lai JCW, et al: Radionuclide determination of individual kidney function in the treatment of chronic renal obstruction. J Urol 127:636, 1982.

49. Whitaker RH: Methods of assessing obstruction in dilated ureters. Br J Urol 45:15, 1973.

50. Thrall JH, Koff SA, Keyes JW Jr: Diuretic radionuclide renography and scintigraphy in the differential diagnosis of hydroureteronephrosis. Semin Nucl Med 11:89, 1981.

51. O'Reilly PH, Testa HJ, Lawson RS, et al: Diuresis renography in equivocal urinary tract obstruction. Br J Urol 50:76, 1978.

52. O'Reilly PH, Lawson RS, Shields RA, et al: Idiopathic hydronephrosis—the diuresis renogram: A new non-invasive method of assessing equivocal pelvi-ureteral junction obstruction. J Urol 121:153, 1979.

53. O'Reilly PH, Lupton EW, Testa HJ, et al: The dilated nonobstructed renal pelves. Br J Urol 53:205, 1981.

54. Lupton EW, Richards P, Testa HJ, et al: A comparison of diuresis renography: The Whitaker test and renal pelvic morphology in idiopathic hydronephrosis. Br J Urol 57:119, 1985.

55. Koff SA: Experimental validation of diagnostic methods in idiopathic hydronephrosis. In O'Reilly PH, Gosling JA (eds): Idiopathic Hydronephrosis. New York, Springer-Verlag, 1982.

56. O'Reilly PH: Diuresis renography 8 years later: An update. J Urol 136:993, 1986.

57. Smith HW, Finkelstein N, Aliminosa, et al: The renal clearance of substituted hippuric acid derivatives and other aromatic acids in dog and man. J Clin Invest 24:388, 1945.

58. Landowne M, Alving A: A method of determining the specific renal functions of glomerular filtration, maximum tubular excretion (or reabsorption) and "effective blood flow" using a single injection of a single substance. J Lab Clin Med 32:931, 1947.

59. Blaufox MD: A compartmental analysis of the radiorenogram and uretics of ^{131}I-Hippuran. In Blaufox MD (ed): Evaluation of Renal Function and Disease with Radionuclides. Baltimore, Karger, 1972, p. 107.

60. Blaufox MD, Orvis A, and Owen CA Jr: Compartmental analysis of the radiorenogram and distribution of Hippuran ^{131}I in dogs. Am J Physiol 204:1059, 1963.

61. Blaufox MD, Merrill JP: Compartmental analysis of the Hippuran I-131 renogram in man. Fed Proc 24:405, 1965.

62. Tauxe WN, Maher FT, Taylor WF: Effective renal plasma flow: Estimation from theoretical volumes of distribution of intravenously injected ^{131}I-ortho-iodohippurate. Mayo Clin Proc 46:524, 1971.

63. Fine EJ, Axelrod M, Gorkin J, et al: Measurement of effective renal plasma flow: A comparison of methods. J Nucl Med 28:1393, 1987.

64. Kenny RW, Ackery DM, Fleming JS, et al: Deconvolution analysis of the scintillation camera renogram. Br J Radiol 48:481, 1975.

65. Britton KE, Brown NJ: The clinical use of CABBS renography. Investigation of the "non-functioning" kidney and renal artery stenosis by the use of ^{131}I-Hippuran renography by computer assisted blood background subtraction (CABBS). Br J Radiol 41:570, 1968.

66. Farmelant MH, Sachs CE, Burrows BA: The influence of tissue background activity on the apparent renal accumulation of radioactive compounds. J Nucl Med 11:112, 1970.

67. Rosenthall L, Damtew B, Kloiber R: Selection of renal background for quantitative ^{131}I-hippurate relative renal function studies. Diagn Imaging 50:159, 1981.

68. Mlodkowska E, Liniecki B, Surma M: A method for subtraction of the extrarenal "background" in dynamic ^{131}I-hippurate renoscintigraphy. Nucl Med (Stuttgart) 18:36, 1979.

69. Tonnesen KH, Munck O, Haid T, et al: Influence on the radiorenogram of variation in skin to kidney distance and the clinical importance thereof. In zum Winkel K, Blaufox MD, Bretano JLF (eds): Radionuclides in Nephrology. Stuttgart, Georg Thieme, 1975, p. 79.

70. Piepsz A, Denis R, Ham HR, et al: A simple method for measuring separate glomerular filtration rate using a single injection of ^{99m}Tc-DTPA and the scintillation camera. J Pediatr 93:769, 1978.

71. Ostrowski ST, Tothill P: Kidney depth measurements using a double isotope technique. Br J Radiol 48:291, 1975.

72. Britton KE, Whitfield HN, Nimmon CC, et al: Obstructive nephropathy: Successful evaluation with radionuclides. Lancet 1:905, 1979.

73. Whitfield HN, Britton KE, Nimmon CC, et al: Renal transit time measurements in the diagnosis of ureteric obstruction. Br J Urol 53:500, 1979.

74. Gruenewald SM, Nimmon CC, Nawaz MK, and Britton KE: A non-invasive gamma camera technique for the measurement of intrarenal flow distribution in man. Clin Sci 61:385, 1981.

74a. Britton KE, Nawaz MK, Whitfield HN, et al: Obstructive Nephropathy: Comparison between parenchymal transit time index and furosemide diuresis. Br J Urol 59:127, 1987.

75. Kempi V, Persson BRR: Evaluation of renal function parameters with simultaneously administered ^{99m}Tc-DTPA and ^{131}I-Hippuran. Eur J Nucl Med 8:65, 1983.

76. Zuckier LS, Axelrod MS, Wexler JP, et al: The implications of decreased performance of new generation gamma-cameras on the interpretation of ^{131}I-Hippuran renal images. Nucl Med Commun 8:49, 1987.

77. Jewkes RF, Jayasingh K: Comparison of ^{123}I-Hippuran and ^{99m}Tc-DTPA. Nucl Med Commun 2:278, 1981.

78. Buck AC, Macleod MA, Blacklock NJ: The advantages of ^{99m}Tc-DTPA (Sn) in dynamic renal scintigraphy and measurement of renal function. Br J Urol 52:174, 1980.

79. Koff SA, Thrall JH, Keyes JW: Assessment of hydro-ureteronephrosis in children using radionuclide urography. J Urol 123:531, 1980.

80. Shannon JA, Smith HW: The excretion of inulin, xylose and urea by normal and phlorinized man. J Clin Invest 14:393, 1935.

81. Alving A, Miller B: A practical method for the measurement of the GFR (inulin clearance). Arch Intern Med 66:306, 1940.

82. Fisher M, Veall N: Glomerular filtration rate based on a single blood sample. Br Med J 2:542, 1975.

83. Harris CC, Ford KK, Coleman RE, Dunnick NR: Effect of region assignment on relative renal blood flow estimates using radionuclides. Radiology 151:791, 1984.

84. Gruenewald SM, Collins LT, Fawdry RM: Kidney depth measurement and its influence on quantitation of function from gamma camera renography. Clin Nucl Med 10:338, 1984.

85. Nally JV, Clarke HS Jr, Grecos GP, et al: Effect of captopril on ^{99m}Tc-diethylenetriaminepentaacetic acid renograms in two kidney, one clip hypertension. Hypertension 8:685, 1986.

86. Blythe WB: Captopril and renal autoregulation. N Engl J Med 308:390, 1983.

87. Koenigsberg M, Novich I, Lory M, Blaufox MD: Limits of sensitivity of radio-pertechnetate flow studies in the detection of asymmetrical renal perfusion. *In* Berlyne GM et al (eds): Contributions to Nephrology. Basel, S. Karger, 1978, p. 73.

88. Conrad GR, Wesolowski C, Kirchner PT: Intrarenal blood flow distributions from first transit recording of Tc-99m radiochelates (abstr). J Nucl Med 26:132, 1985.

89. Lee H-B, Blaufox MD: Mechanism of renal concentration of technetium-99m glucoheptonate. J Nucl Med 26:1308, 1985.

90. Enlander D, Weber PM, dos Remedios LV: Renal cortical imaging in 35 patients: Superior quality with ^{99m}Tc-DMSA. J Nucl Med 15:743, 1974.

91. Bingham JB, Maisey MN: An evaluation of the use of ^{99m}Tc-dimercaptosuccinic acid (DMSA) as a static renal imaging agent. Br J Radiol 51:599, 1972.

92. Older RA, Korobkin M, Workman J, et al: Accuracy of radionuclide imaging in distinguishing renal masses from normal variants. Radiology 136:443, 1981.

93. Kawamura J, Hosokawa S, Yoshid O, et al: Validity of ^{99m}Tc-DMSA renal uptake for an assessment of residual kidney function. J Urol 119:305, 1978.

94. Pieretti R, Gilday D, Jeffs R: Differential kidney scan in pediatric urology. Urology 4:665, 1974.

94a. Zeissman HA, Balsiero J, Fahey FH, et al: ^{99m}Tc-glucoheptonate for quantitation of differential renal function. Am J Roentgenol 148:899, 1987.

95. Daly J, Jones W, Rudd TG, et al: Differential renal function using technetium-99m dimercaptosuccinic acid (DMSA): In vitro correlation. J Nucl Med 20:63, 1979.

96. Kawamura J, Hosokawa S, Yoshida A, et al: Renal function studies using ^{99m}Tc-dimercaptosuccinic acid. Clin Nucl Med 4:39, 1979.

97. Price RR, Born ML, Jones JP, et al: Comparison of differential renal function by Tc-99m DMSA, Tc-99m DTPA, I-131 Hippuran and ureteral catheterization (abstr). J Nucl Med 20:631, 1979.

98. McAfee JG, Subramanian G, Schneider RF, et al: Technetium-99m DADS complexes as renal function and imaging agents: II. Biological comparison with iodine-131 Hippuran. J Nucl Med 26:375, 1985.

99. Taylor A Jr, Eshima D, Fritzberg AR, et al: Comparison of iodine-131 OIH and technetium-99m MAG3 renal imaging in volunteers. J Nucl Med 27:795, 1986.

100. Rosenthall L, Kaye M: Observations on the mechanism of ^{99m}Tc-labelled phosphate complex uptake in metabolic bone disease. Semin Nucl Med 6:59, 1976.

101. Jones AG, Francis MD, Davis MA: Bone scanning—radionuclide reaction mechanisms. Semin Nucl Med 6:3, 1976.

102. Subramanian G, McAfee JG, Blair R, et al: ^{99m}Tc methylenediphosphonate—a superior agent for skeletal imaging: Comparison with other technetium complexes. J Nucl Med 16:744, 1975.

103. Larson SM: Mechanisms of localization of gallium-67 in tumor. Semin Nucl Med 8:193, 1978.

104. Hauser MF, Alderson PO: Gallium imaging in abdominal disease. Semin Nucl Med 8:251, 1978.

105. Staab EV, McCartney WH: Role of gallium-67 in inflammatory disease. Semin Nucl Med 8:219, 1978.

106. Weeke E: ^{57}Co-cyanocobalamin in the detection of the glomerular filtration rate. Scan J Clin Lab Invest 21:139, 1968.

107. Cutler RE, Glatte H: Simultaneous measurement of glomerular filtration and effective renal plasma flow with ^{57}Co-cyano-cobalamin and ^{125}I-Hippuran. J Lab Clin Med 65:1041, 1965.

108. Sigman EM, Elwood CM, Knox F: The measurement of glomerular filtration rate in man with sodium iothalamate ^{131}I (Conroy). J Nucl Med 7:60, 1967.

109. McAfee JG, Gagne G, Atkins HL, et al: Biological distribution and excretion of DTPA labelled with Tc-99m and In-111. J Nucl Med 20:1273, 1979.

110. Reba RC, Hosain F, Wagner HN: Indium-113m diethylenetriaminepentaacetic acid (DTPA): A new radiopharmaceutical for study of the kidneys. Radiology 90:147, 1968.

111. Sziklas JJ, Hosain F, Reba RC, Wagner HN Jr: Comparison of ^{169}Yb-DTPA, ^{113m}In-DTPA, ^{14}C-inulin and endogenous creatinine to estimate glomerular filtration. J Nucl Biol Med 15:122, 1971.

112. Stacy BD, Thorburn GD: Chromium-51 ethylenediaminetetraacetate for estimation of glomerular filtrate rate. Science 152:1076, 1966.

113. Garnett ES, Parsons V, Veall N: Measurement of glomerular filtration rate in man using a ^{51}Cr/Edetic acid complex. Lancet i:818, 1967.

114. Connor TB, Thomas WC Jr, Haddock L, Howard JE: Unilateral renal disease and its detection by ureteral catheterization studies. Ann Intern Med 52:544, 1960.

115. Maxwell MH, Lupu AN, Taplin GV: Radioisotope renogram in renal arterial hypertension. J Urol 100:376, 1968.

116. Nordyke RA, Gilbert FI Jr, Simmons EL: Screening for kidney disease with radioisotopes. JAMA 208:493, 1969.

117. Wall CA, Hilario EM, Whalen TJ: An orderly search for a vascular lesion producing hypertension. J Urol 108:511, 1972.

118. Keane JM, Schlegel JU: The use of a scintillation camera system for scanning of hypertensive patients. J Urol 108:12, 1972.

119. Maxwell MH: Cooperative study of renovascular hypertension. Kidney Int 8:S153, 1975.

120. Secker-Walker RH, Sheperd EP, Cassell KJ: Clinical applications of computer assisted renography. J Nucl Med 13:235, 1975.

121. Farmelant MH, Sachs SE, Burrows BA: Prognostic value of radioisotope renal function studies for selecting patients with renal arterial stenosis for surgery. J Nucl Med 11:743, 1970.

122. Keim HJ, Johnson PM, Vaughan D Jr, et al: Computer assisted static/dynamic renal imaging. A screening test for renovascular hypertension. J Nucl Med 20:11, 1979.

123. Drew H, LaFrance N, Bender W, et al: Renal function in patients with renovascular hypertension following inhibition of angiotensin converting enzyme (abstr). J Nucl Med 25:836, 1984.

124. Gifford RW: Evaluation of the hypertensive patient with emphasis on detecting curable causes. Milbank Mem Fund Q 47:170, 1969.

125. Iimura O: Actual incidence of secondary hypertension. Jpn Circ J 37:1040, 1973.

126. Rudnick KV, Sackett DL, Hirst S, Holmes C: Hypertension in a family practice. Can Med Assoc J 117:492, 1977.

127. Burglund C, Andersson O, Wilhelmsen L: Prevalence of primary and secondary hypertension. Studies in a random population sample. Br Med J 2:554, 1976.

128. Lewin A, Blaufox MD, Castle H, et al: Apparent prevalence of curable hypertension in the Hypertension Detection and Follow-Up Program. Arch Intern Med 145–424, 1985.

129. Davis BA, Crook JE, Vestal RE, et al: Prevalence of renovascular hypertension in patients with grade III or IV hypertensive retinopathy. N Engl J Med 301:1273, 1979.

130. Simon N, Franklin SS, Bleifer KH, Maxwell MH: Clinical characteristics of renovascular hypertension. JAMA 220:1209, 1972.

131. Hypertension Detection and Follow-Up Program Cooperative Group: Five-year findings of the Hypertension Detection and Follow-Up Program: I. Reduction in mortality of persons with high blood pressure, including mild hypertension. JAMA 242:2562, 1979.

132. Fine EJ, Scharf SC, Blaufox MD: The role of nuclear medicine in evaluating the hypertensive patient. *In* Freeman LM, Weissmann HS (eds): Nuclear Medicine Annual 1984. New York, Raven Press, 1984, p. 23.

133. McNeil BJ, Varady PD, Burrows BA, et al: Measures of clinical efficacy. Cost-effectiveness calculation in the diagnosis and treatment of hypertensive renovascular disease. N Engl J Med 293:216, 1975.

134. Mark LS, Maxwell MH: Renal vein renin. Value and limitations in the prediction of operative results. Urol Clin North Am 4:155, 1975.

135. Tucker RM, Strong CG, Brennan LA, et al: Renovascular hypertension. Relationship of surgical curability to renin-angiotensin activity. Mayo Clin Proc 53:373, 1978.

136. Chopp RT, Hekmat-Raven H, Mendez R: Technetium-99m glucoheptonate renal scan in diagnosis of acute renal injury. Urology 15:201, 1980.

137. English PJ, Testa HJ, Gosling JA, Cohen SJ: Idiopathic hydronephrosis in childhood—a comparison between diuresis renography and upper tract morphology. Br J Urol 54:603, 1982.

138. Gonzales R, Chiou R-K: The diagnosis of upper urinary tract obstruction in children. Comparison of diuresis renography and pressure flow studies. J Urol 133:646, 1985.

139. Senac MO Jr, Miller JH, Stanley P: Evaluation of obstructive uropathy in children. Radionuclide renography vs. the Whitaker test. AJR 143:11, 1984.

140. Maizels M, Weiss S, Conway JJ, Firlit CF: The cystometric nuclear cystogram. J Urol 121:203, 1979.

141. Blaufox MD, Gruskin A, Sandler P, et al: Scintigraphy for

detection of vesico-ureteral reflux in children. J Pediatr 79:239, 1971.

142. Merrick MV, Uttley WS, Wild SR: The detection of pyelonephritis scarring in children by radioisotope imaging. Br J Radiol 53:544, 1980.

143. Ash JM, Antico VF, Gilday DL, Houle S: Special considerations in the pediatric use of radionuclides for kidney studies. Semin Nucl Med 12:345, 1982.

144. O'Reilly PJ, Lawson RS, Shields RA, et al: A radioisotope method of assessing uretero-ureteric reflux. Br J Urol 50:164, 1978.

145. Meller ST, Eckstein HB: The value of renal scintigraphy in reduplication, In Joekes AM, Constable AR, Brown JG, Tauxe WN (eds): Radionuclides in Nephrology. London, Academic Press, 1982, p 229.

146. LePanto PB, Rosenstock J, Littman P: Gallium-67 scans in children with solid tumors. Am J Roentgenol Rad Ther Nucl Med 126:179, 1976.

147. McLean GK, Alavi A, Ziegler MM, et al: Splenic-gonadal fusion: Identification by radionuclide scanning. J Pediatr Surg 16(Suppl). 1:649, 1981.

148. Hurwitz SR, Kessler WO, Alazraki NP, et al: Gallium-67 to localize urinary tract infection. Br J Radiol 49:156, 1975.

149. Handmaker H: Nuclear renal imaging in acute pyelonephritis. Semin Nucl Med 12:246, 1982.

150. Lloyd LK, Dubovsky EV, Bueschen AJ, et al: Comprehensive renal scintillation procedures in spinal cord injury: Comparison with excretory urography. J Urol 126:19, 1981.

151. Kuhlemeier KV, Huang CT, Lloyd LK, et al: Effective renal plasma flow: Clinical significance after spinal cord injury. J Urol 133:758, 1985.

152. Wood BC, Sharma JN, Germann DR, et al: Gallium citrate 67Ga imaging in non-infectious interstitial nephritis. Arch Intern Med 138:1665, 1978.

153. Sherman RA, Blaufox MD: Clinical significance of nonvisualization with 131I-Hippuran renal scan. In Hollenberg NK, Large S (eds): Radionuclides in Nephrology. Thieme, Stuttgart, 1980, p 235.

154. Kalika V, Bard RH, Iloreta A, et al: Prediction of renal functional recovery after relief of upper urinary tract obstruction. J Urol 126:301, 1981.

155. Sherman RA, Blaufox MD: Obstructive uropathy in patients with nonvisualization on renal scan. Nephron 25:82, 1980.

156. Rosenthall L: Residual urine determination by roentgenographic isotopic means. Radiology 80:454, 1963.

157. Strauss BS, Blaufox MD: Estimation of residual urine and urine flow rates without urethral catheterization. J Nucl Med 11:81, 1970.

158. O'Reilly PJ, Lawson RS, Shields RA, et al: Radionuclide studies of the lower urinary tract. Br J Urol 53:266, 1981.

159. Holder LE, Melloul M, Chen D: Current status of radionuclide scrotal imaging. Semin Nucl Med 11:232, 1981.

160. Skoglund RW, McRoberts JW, Ragde H: Torsion of the spermatic cord: A review of the literature and an analysis of 70 new cases. J Urol 104:604, 1970.

161. Vieras F, Kuhn CR: Nonspecificity of the "rim sign" in the scintigraphic diagnosis of missed testicular torsion. Radiology 146:519, 1983.

162. Levy OM, Gittleman MC, Strashun AM, et al: Diagnosis of acute testicular torsion using radionuclide scanning. J Urol 129:975, 1983.

163. Marmar JL, Zeiger LS, DeBenedictis TJ, Praiss DE: Comprehensive scrotal flow and scan technique for detection of varicoceles. Urology 25:505, 1985.

164. Fanous FN, Jevitch MJ, Chen DCP, et al: Radioisotope penogram in diagnosis of vasculogenic impotence. Urology 20:499, 1982.

165. Nseyo UO, Wilbur HJ, Kang SA, et al: Penile xenon (133Xe) washout: A rapid method of screening for vasculogenic impotence. Urology 23:31, 1984.

166. Stone AR, Merrick MV, Chisholm GD: Prostatic lymphoscintigraphy. Br J Urol 51:556, 1979.

167. Whitmore WF III, Blute RD, Jr, Kaplan WD, Gittes RF: Radiocolloid scintigraphic mapping of the lymphatic drainage of the prostate. J Urol 124:62, 1980.

168. Wax SH, Rudolph JH: The 131I renogram in pregnancy. I. Safety. Obstet Gynecol 30:381, 1967.

169. Rudolph JH, Wax SH: The 131I renogram in pregnancy. II. Normal pregnancy. Obstet Gynecol 30:386, 1967.

170. Beierwaltes WH, Lieberman LM, Ansari AN, et al: Visualization of human adrenal glands in vivo by scintillation scanning. JAMA 216:275, 1971.

171. Sarkar SD, Cohen EL, Beierwaltes WH, et al: A new and superior adrenal imaging agent, 131I-6 iodomethyl-19-norcholesterol (NP-59): Evaluation in humans. J Clin Endocrinol Metab 45:333, 1974.

172. Hotte CE, Ice RD: Thermal and radiolytic decomposition of 131I-19 iodocholesterol. J Nucl Med 15:38, 1974.

173. Beierwaltes WH, Wieland DM, Yu T, et al: Adrenal imaging agents: Rationale, synthesis, formulation and metabolism. Semin Nucl Med 8:5, 1978.

174. Thrall JH, Freitas JE, Beierwaltes WH: Adrenal scintigraphy. Semin Nucl Med 8:23, 1978.

175. Freitas JE, Thrall JH, Swanson DP, et al: Normal adrenal imaging (abstr). J Nucl Med 18:599, 1977.

176. Moses DC, Schteingart DE, Sturman MF, et al: Efficacy of radiocholesterol imaging of the adrenal glands in Cushing's syndrome. Surg Gynecol Obstet 139:201, 1974.

177. Kereiakes JG, Rosenstein M: Handbook of radiation dose in nuclear medicine and diagnostic x-ray. Boca Raton, CRC Press, 1980.

178. MIRD Dose Estimate Report No 8: Summary of current radiation dose estimates to normal humans from 99mTc as sodium pertechnetate. J Nucl Med 17:74, 1976.

179. zum Winkel K, Hermann H-J, Eisenhut M, et al: Renal imaging and diagnostic studies, radiation dose and labelling procedure using 123I-hippurate. In Hollenberg NK, Large S (eds): Radionuclides in Nephrology. Proc 6th International Symposium. New York, Thieme-Stratton, 1980, p. 31.

180. Roedler HD, Kaul A, Hine GJ: Internal radiation dose in diagnostic nuclear medicine. Berlin, Verlag H. Hoffman, 1978.

181. Arnold RW, Subramanian G, McAfee JG, et al: Comparison of 99mTc complexes for renal imaging. J Nucl Med 16:357, 1975.

182. MIRD Dose Estimate Report No 2: Summary of current radiation dose estimates to humans from 66Ga-, 67Ga-, 68Ga-, and 72Ga-citrate. J Nucl Med 14:755, 1973.

183. Wallach L, Nyarai I, Dawson KG: Stimulated renin: A screening test for hypertension. Ann Intern Med 82:27, 1975.

184. Bookstein JJ, Abrams HL, Buenger RE, et al: The role of urography in unilateral renovascular disease. JAMA 220:1225, 1972.

185. Blaufox MD, Kalika V, Scharf S, Milstein D: Applications of nuclear medicine in genitourinary imaging. Urol Radiol 4:155, 1982.

186. Buonocore E, Meaney TF, Borkowski GP, et al: Digital subtraction angiography of the abdominal aorta and renal arteries: Comparison with conventional angiography. Radiology 139:281, 1981.

187. Brunner RR, Garvas H, Laragh JH, et al: Angiotensin II blockade in man by Sar-ala8-angiotensin II for understanding and treatment of high blood pressure. Lancet 2:1045, 1973.

188. Case D, Wallace JM, Keim HJ, et al: Possible role of renin in hypertension as suggested by renin-sodium profiling and inhibition of converting enzyme. N Engl J Med 296:641, 1977.

189. Eshghi M, Silver L, Smith AD: Technetium-99m scan in acute scrotal lesions. Urology 30:586, 1987.

190. Blaufox MD: A compartmental analysis of the radiorenogram and kinetics of 131I Hippuran. In Blaufox MD: Evaluation of Renal Function and Disease with Radionuclides. Baltimore, S. Karger/University Park Press, 1972, pp 107–146.

191. Mailloux L, Gagnon JA: Measurement of effective renal plasma flow. In Blaufox MD: Evaluation of Renal Function and Disease with Radionuclides. Baltimore, S. Karger/University Park Press, 1972, pp 54–70.

192. Heyman S, Duckett JW: The extraction factor: An estimate of single renal function in children during routine radionuclide renography with 99mtechnetium diethylene triaminepentactetic acid. J Urol 140:780, 1988.

193. Taha SA, Al-Mohaya S, Abdulkader A, et al: Prognosis of radiologically non-functioning obstructed kidneys. Br J Urol 62:209, 1988.

194. Pettit J, Sawczuk IS: Use of lymphoscintigraphy in chyluria. Urology 32:367, 1988.

195. Taylor A Jr, Ziffer JA, Steves A, et al: Clinical comparison of I-131 orthoiodohippurate and the Kit formulation of Tc-99m mercaptoacetyltriglycine. Radiology 170:721, 1989.

196. Greenstein A, Chen J, Matzkin H, et al: Potential pitfalls in obstructive renal scan in patients with double-pigtail ureteral catheters. J Urol 141:283, 1989.

III SPECIFIC DISORDERS OF THE URINARY TRACT

SECTION 1 Developmental and Congenital Disorders

GERALD W. FRIEDLAND
Editor

---

19 Congenital Anomalies of the Urinary Tract

GERALD W. FRIEDLAND □ PIETER A. DEVRIES
MATILDE NINO-MURCIA □ RONALD COHEN □ MATTHEW D. RIFKIN

INTRODUCTION

Congenital anomalies of the urinary tract are both important and common—so common that about 10% of infants and children in an autopsy series were found to have such disorders.[1] The anomalies can be dangerous. They may, in fact, be responsible for some stillbirths and for other kinds of problems (discussed later in greater detail).

A significant feature of congenital anomalies of the urinary tract, however, is that they often do not occur in isolation. The same factors that produce these disorders may also produce anomalies elsewhere in the body; these can be equally important, equally common, and equally dangerous. If we focus exclusively on the urinary tract, we run a great risk of failing to think about the body as a system in which underlying etiological factors affect the whole as well as the parts.

Therefore, in order to understand the larger significance of congenital anomalies of the urinary tract, we begin by discussing the embryological basis of multiple associated congenital anomalies.

Some of the material on scintigraphy and ultrasound in this chapter was provided by Massoud Majd, M.D., Barry Potter, M.D., and Bruce Markle, M.D., courtesy of the Children's Hospital, National Medical Center, Washington, D.C.

EMBRYOLOGICAL BASIS OF MULTIPLE ASSOCIATED CONGENITAL ANOMALIES: IMPORTANCE OF STAGING OF HUMAN EMBRYOS

For almost 100 years it has been accepted that congenital anomalies result from the fact that an organ (the site of the anomaly) temporarily stopped growing during the embryonic period.[2, 3] This arrest might affect one organ, an organ system, or several systems, all at the same stage of development.[4]

To ascertain when a particular defect occurred, modern embryologists use a staging system, which is useful for deducing the exact day during which the malformation may have come about.

The identification of the approximate age of embryos, or of their stages of development, is based on the classic work of Streeter[5-8] and others.[9-13] They have collectively shown that embryonic length alone cannot be statistically correlated with development. Streeter divided human embryos into *developmental horizons* or *age groups* based on certain features (internal and external form) common to the group. Using these features, estimations of post-ovulation age were made and then checked against macaque embryos of known gestational age. As a result, Streeter divided the embryonic period into 23 horizons, beginning with the fertilized ovum on the first day and ending, somewhat arbitrarily, 56 to 60 days later with the onset of marrow formation in the humerus (Fig. 19–1). Organogenesis is largely complete by this period, and the prenatal period that follows is designated the fetal period.

Despite the appeal of the term *horizon,* which combines the concepts of continuity and advancement, O'Rahilly[9] later substituted the term *stage* and modified some of the embryonic groupings. Additional modifications were contributed by Jirasek,[11] whose staging will be followed here. Since fetal length is directly related to age in the fetal period, no classification system has proved necessary, and developmental changes of interest are discussed in terms of fetal age and fetal length alone.

One problem is that the time at which various urogenital and associated anomalies in other organs develop is not known. The procedure, therefore, is as follows: look at a normal embryo; determine what is abnormal in cases of congenital anomalies; and deduce when the appropriate growth arrest must have occurred.[4, 14, 15]

Another means to understanding the development of congenital anomalies is to study the embryology of experimental animals and relate the exact stage in animals to that in humans. This is accomplished either by denying the animal mother essential nutrients, thereby temporarily arresting growth in the organ or organ system under study,[16] or by giving the animal an appropriate teratogenic agent to accomplish the same purpose.[17] The examiner can then observe congenital anomalies that develop, and try to draw a relationship between the times of the occurrence of the same anomaly in an experimental animal and humans. Typically, rats are the experimental animals used in this work.

It has also been found that the study of rat embryology can help refine early human embryology. DeVries and Saunders[18] were not able to distinguish the heart from surrounding structures in very early human embryos; a study of a large number of early rat embryos, however, combined with special histological techniques, enabled them to distinguish the heart from surrounding structures in the rat—and subsequently in the human—at an earlier date. As a result, they found it possible to study associated anomalies, such as those in the urinary tract, earlier and with more definitive findings.[18, 19]

We turn now to a discussion of the chief associated congenital anomalies that the practicing physician may find. A number of tables follow in the sections to come. We suggest that they be used as convenient references.

MULTIPLE ASSOCIATED CONGENITAL ANOMALIES: CLASSIFICATION AND DIAGNOSTIC IMAGING

A mnemonic device has been developed for remembering the most common multiple associated congenital anomalies. This is the acronym VATER: *vertebral, anorectal, tracheoesophageal, radial and renal.*[20] Associated cardiovascular anomalies have led to the related acronym VACTERL, which stands for *vertebral, anorectal, cardiovascular, tracheoesophageal, renal, and limb* (Fig. 19–2).[21]

In addition, renal agenesis, agenesis or hypoplasia of the müllerian ducts, and cervicothoracic spine anomalies are frequently associated. This has given rise to the acronym MURCS, which stands for *müllerian ducts, renal, cervicothoracic spine.*[22, 23]

The most serious and life-threatening of the associated anomalies are esophageal atresia, anorectal malformations, and cardiac anomalies. About 10% of patients with esophageal atresia,[24] and 10% (range of 4% to 17%) of patients with congenital cardiac anomalies[25] also have urinary tract anomalies. The most common cardiac malformations associated with urinary tract anomalies are (in descending order of frequency) atrial septal defect (secundum), tetralogy of Fallot, ventricular septal and other defects, isolated ventricular septal defect, tricuspid atresia, pulmonic stenosis, mitral atresia, aortic stenosis, patent ductus arteriosus, partial anomalous pulmonary venous return, hypoplastic left heart, and truncus arteriosus.[25] Associated skeletal anomalies are also common,[26] especially vertebral anomalies. About 40% of patients with congenital scoliosis, for example, have urinary tract anomalies.[27] The most common anomaly of the bones of the extremities is absence of a bone (especially the radius), but anomalies of the metacarpals and phalanges also occur, including duplicated phalanges (Fig. 19–2*B*), cone epiphyses, and short metacarpals or phalanges. Anomalies of the central nervous system also occur, especially neural tube defects.[28]

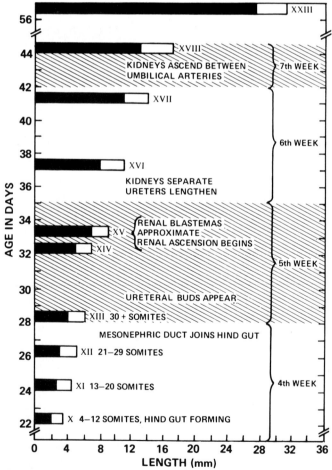

Figure 19–1. The relationship between the age of the embryo in days, the length of the embryo in millimeters, and the stage of development (Roman numerals). (From Friedland GW, deVries PA: Renal ectopia and fusion. Embryologic basis. Urology 5:698–706, 1975.)

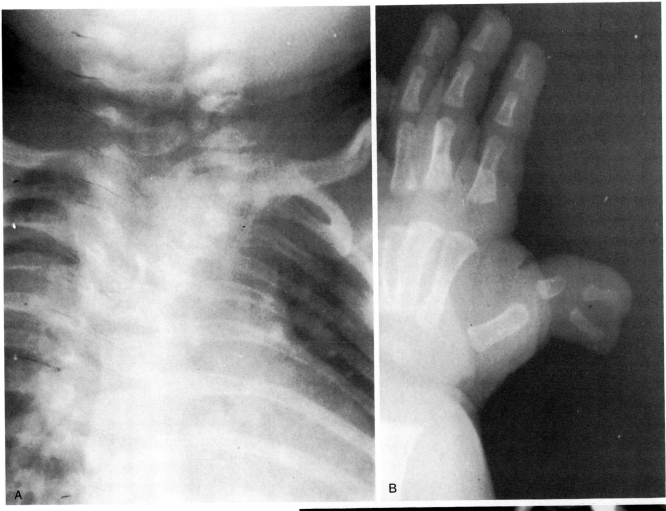

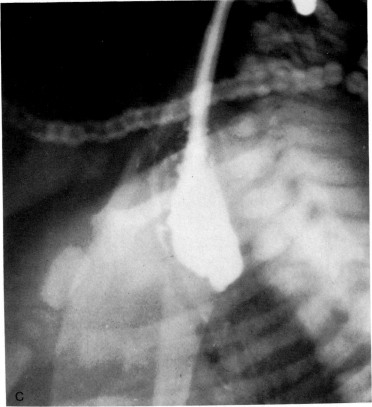

Figure 19–2. Multiple associated congenital anomalies. Neonate with crossed fused ectopia who has multiple thoracic hemivertebrae *(A)*, duplication of the terminal phalanx of the thumb *(B)*, and esophageal atresia *(C)*. (From Friedland GW, Filly R, Goris ML, et al: Uroradiology: An Integrated Approach. New York, Churchill Livingstone, 1983, p 1366. By permission.)

Table 19–1. Genetic Diseases with Autosomal Recessive Inheritance Associated with Urogenital Abnormalities

Condition No.—Syndrome	Urogenital Abnormalities	Other Major Abnormalities	Reference
1—Acrocephalopolysyndactyly Type II (Carpenter's) syndrome	Hypogenitalism	Acrocephaly, polydactyly, syndactyly of feet, lateral displacement of inner canthi	Temtamy, S. A.: J. Ped., 69:111, 1966
2—Bird-headed dwarfism (Seckel's) syndrome	Cryptorchidism, hypogenitalism	Small head, large eyes, beaklike nose, narrow face	Harper, R. G., Orti, E. and Baker, R. K.: J. Ped., 70:799, 1967
3—Cerebrohepatorenal (Zellweger) syndrome	Hypospadias, hydroureter, cryptorchidism, clitoromegaly	Hypotonia, high forehead, flat facies, hepatomegaly	Opitz, J. M., ZuRhein, G. M., Vitale, L., Shahidi, N. T., Howe, J. J., Chou, S. M., Shanklin, D. R., Sybers, H. D., Dood, A. R. and Gerritsen, T.: Birth Defects, part II, 5:114, 1969
4—Cerebro-oculofacioskeletal syndrome	Cryptorchidism, enlarged genitalia, absent ureter, and absent bladder	Neurogenic arthrogryposis, microcephaly, microphthalmia, cataract	Preus, M., Kaplan, P. and Kirkham, T. H.: Amer. J. Dis. Child., 131:62, 1977
5—Chondroectodermal dysplasia	Cryptorchidism, epispadias	Short distal extremities, polydactyly, nail hypoplasia	McKusick, V. A., Egeland, J. A., Eldridge, R. and Krusen, D. E.: Bull. Johns Hopkins Hosp., 115:306, 1964
6—Cockayne's syndrome	Cryptorchidism	Senile appearance, retinal degeneration, impaired hearing, thin skin	Macdonald, W. B., Fitch, K. D. and Lewis, I. C.: Pediatrics, 25:997, 1960
7—Cryptophthalmos (Fraser) syndrome	Cryptorchidism, clitoromegaly, penile chordee, hypospadias, vaginal atresia, urethral meatal stenosis	Cryptophthalmos, cupped ears	Fraser, G. R.: Ann. Hum. Genet., 25:387, 1962; Gupta, S. P. and Saxena, R. C.: Brit. J. Ophthalmol., 46:629, 1962, and Azevedo, E. S., Biondi, J. and Ramalho, L. M.: Brazil. J. Med. Genet., 10:389, 1973
8—De Sanctis-Cacchione syndrome	Hypogenitalism, small testes	Xeroderma pigmentosum, mental retardation, microcephaly	Smith, D. W. and Jones, K. L.: Recognizable Patterns of Human Malformation: Genetic, Embryologic and Clinical Aspects, 3rd ed. Philadelphia: W. B. Saunders Co., 1982
9—Diastrophic dysplasia syndrome	Cryptorchidism	Short tubular bones, joint limitation, hypertrophied auricular cartilage	Walker, B. A., Scott, C. I., Hall, J. G., Murdoch, J. L. and McKusick, V. A.: Medicine, 51:41, 1972
10—Dubowitz syndrome	Cryptorchidism, hypospadias	Peculiar facies, eczema, small stature, mild microcephaly	Wilroy, R. S., Jr., Tipton, R. E. and Summitt, R. L.: Amer. J. Med. Genet., 2:275, 1978
11—Dyskeratosis congenita syndrome*	Testicular hypoplasia	Skin hyperpigmentation, leukoplakia, nail dystrophy, pancytopenia	Smith, D. W. and Jones, K. L.: Recognizable Patterns of Human Malformation: Genetic, Embryologic and Clinical Aspects, 3rd ed. Philadelphia: W. B. Saunders Co., 1982
12—Ehlers-Danlos syndrome†	Bladder neck obstruction, ureteropelvic junction obstruction	Hyperextensibility of skin and joints, poor wound healing	Eadie, D. G. A. and Wilkins, J. L.: Brit. J. Urol., 39:353, 1967
13—Escobar (multiple pterygia) syndrome	Cryptorchidism, absence of labia majora	Multiple pterygia, camptodactyly, syndactyly	Escobar, V., Bixler, D., Gleiser, S., Weaver, D. D. and Gibbs, T.: Amer. J. Dis. Child., 132:609, 1978
14—Fanconi's pancytopenia	Cryptorchidism, horseshoe kidney, duplication of ureter, hypogenitalism, hypospadias	Radial hypoplasia, hyperpigmentation, pancytopenia	Nilsson, L. R.: Acta Paed., 49:518, 1960
15—Johanson-Blizzard syndrome	Double or septate vagina, clitoromegaly, rectovaginal fistula, single urogenital orifice	Hypoplastic alae nasi, hypothyroidism, deafness	Johanson, A. and Blizzard, R.: J. Ped., 79:982, 1971, and Mardini, M. K., Ghandour, M., Sakati, N. A. and Nyhan, W. L.: Clin. Genet., 14:247, 1978
16—Laurence-Moon-Biedl syndrome (Bardet-Biedl syndrome)	Bifid scrotum, cryptorchidism, hypogenitalism, micropenis, calyceal clubbing, diverticula, marked fetal lobation, diffuse parenchymal loss, horseshoe kidney	Retinal pigmentation, obesity, polydactyly	Harnett, J. D., Green, J. S., Cramer, B. C., et al.: N. Engl. J. Med., 319:615, 1988; Urol. Radiol., 10:176, 1988.
17—Lipodystrophy, congenital generalized (Seip) syndrome	Hydroureter, enlarged genitalia	Lipodystrophy, hepatomegaly, hyperlipemia	Seip, M.: Acta Paed., 48:555, 1959
18—Lissencephaly (Miller-Dieker) syndrome	Cryptorchidism	Microcephaly, incomplete brain development, vertical ridge in forehead	Azevêdo, E. S., Biondi, J. and Ramalho, L. M.: Brazil. J. Med. Genet., 10:389, 1973, and Dieker, H., Edwards, R. H., ZuRhein, G., Chou, S. M., Hartman, H. A. and Opitz, J. M.: Birth Defects, part II, 5:53, 1969

Table 19–1. Genetic Diseases with Autosomal Recessive Inheritance Associated with Urogenital Abnormalities *Continued*

Condition No.—Syndrome	Urogenital Abnormalities	Other Major Abnormalities	Reference
19—Meckel-Gruber syndrome	Cryptorchidism, incomplete external and internal genitalia	Encephalocele, polydactyly	Opitz, J. M. and Howe, J. J.: Birth Defects, part II, 5:167, 1969
20—Opitz's syndrome	Cryptorchidism, hypospadias	Hypertelorism, moderate mental retardation	Michaelis, E. and Mortier, W.: Helv. Paed. Acta, 27:575, 1972
21—Pena-Shokfir I syndrome	Cryptorchidism	Neurogenic arthrogryposis, pulmonary hypoplasia, hypertelorism	Azevêdo, E. S., Biondi, J. and Ramalho, L. M.: Brazil. J. Med. Genet., 10:389, 1973
22—Polycystic kidney disease, infantile	Duplication of urinary tract, ureteral atresia or stenosis, urethral valves, hypospadias, hypoplastic bladder	Polydactyly, chrondrodystrophy	Lieberman, E., Salinas-Madrigal, L., Gwinn, J. L., Brennan, L. P., Fine, R. N. and Landing, B. H.: Medicine, 50:277, 1971
23—Polydactyly with neonatal chondrodystrophy*	Ambiguous genitalia, cystic or hypoplastic ureters, double or small uterus, microphallus, small or absent urogenital opening	—	Majewski, F., Pfeiffer, R. A., Lenz, W., Müller, R., Feil, G. and Seiler, R.: Z. Kinderheilkd., 111:118, 1971
24—Male pseudohermaphroditism (owing to defect in androgen synthesis, four types)	Hypospadias, ambiguous genitalia, complete feminization	—	Grumbach, M. M. and Conte, F. A.: In: Textbook of Endocrinology, 6th ed. Edited by R. H. Williams. Philadelphia: W. B. Saunders Co., chapt. 9, pp. 423–514, 1981
25—Male pseudohermaphroditism, (owing to 5-α-reductase deficiency)	Ambiguous genitalia, hypospadias	—	Grumbach, M. M. and Conte, F. A.: In: Textbook of Endocrinology, 6th ed. Edited by R. H. Williams. Philadelphia: W. B. Saunders Co., chapt. 9, pp. 423–514, 1981
26—Renal-genital-middle ear syndrome*	Hemiatrophy of bladder, vaginal atresia	—	Turner, G.: J. Ped., 76:641, 1970
27—Robert's syndrome	Cryptorchidism, ureteral stenosis, hypospadias, bicornuate uterus, vaginal septum, clitoral and penile enlargement	Hypomelia, midfacial defects, severe growth retardation	Winter, J. S. D., Kohn, G., Mellman, W. J. and Wagner, S.: J. Ped., 72:88, 1968
28—Rokitansky-Küster-Hauser syndrome*	Renal agenesis, double ureter, vaginal atresia, cryptorchidism	Vertebral and rib anomalies	Anger, D., Hemet, J. and Ensel, J.: Bull. Fed. Soc. Gynec. Obst., 1:18, 1949
29—Rothmund-Thomson syndrome	Cryptorchidism, hypogenitalism	Poikiloderma, cataract, ectodermal dysplasia	Silver, H. K.: Amer. J. Dis. Child., 111:182, 1966, and Hall, J. G., Pagon, R. A. and Wilson, K. M.: Amer. J. Dis. Child., 134:165, 1980
30—Rubinstein-Taybi syndrome*	Cryptorchidism, angulated penis, posterior urethral valves, hypospadias, abnormal bladder shape	Broad thumbs and toes, hypoplastic maxilla, slanted palpebral fissure	Simpson, N. E. and Brissenden, J. E.: Amer. J. Hum. Genet., 25:225, 1973
31—Rudiger syndrome*	Bicornuate uterus, microphallus, ureterovesical stenosis	Coarse facies, flat nasal bridge, stubby nose, hoarse voice, hypoplastic fingernails	Rudiger, R. A., Schmidt, W., Loose, D. A. and Passarge, E.: J. Ped., 79:977, 1971
32—Schinzel-Giedion midface retraction syndrome*	Hypospadias, short penis	Severe midface retraction, skull anomalies, congenital heart disease, hypertrichosis	Kelley, R. I., Zackai, E. H. and Charney, E. B.: J. Ped., 100:943, 1982
33—Schwartz-Jampel-Aberfeld syndrome	Hypoplastic testes	Myotonia, blepharophimosis, joint limitation	Aberfeld, D. C., Hinterbuchner, L. P. and Schneider, M.: Brain, 88:313, 1965
34—Selective intestinal malabsorption of vitamin B$_{12}$ with proteinuria (Imerslund-Graesbeck syndrome)	Duplication of renal pelvis and ureter	Proteinuria, pernicious anemia	Imerslund, O.: Acta Paed., suppl. 119, 49:1, 1960
35—Smith-Lemli-Opitz syndrome	Cryptorchidism, hypospadias, microphallus	Anteverted nostrils, ptosis of eyelids, syndactyly of toes	Smith, D. W., Lemi, L. and Opitz, J. M.: J. Ped., 64:210, 1964
36—Wolfram (Didmoad) syndrome	Atony of urinary tract, sclerosis of bladder neck, hydroureter	Diabetes insipidus, diabetes mellitus, sensory deafness, optic atrophy	Najjar, S. S., Seikaly, M. G. and Abdelnoor, A.: Arch. Dis. Child., 60:823, 1985

*Mode of inheritance probably autosomal recessive.

†Types IVB, VI, VIIA and IX are inherited as autosomal recessive; types I, II, III, VIA and VIII as autosomal dominant; types VA and VB are X-linked, and types IVC and VIIB are uncertain.

From Barakat AY, Seikaly MG, Der Kaloustian VM: Urogenital abnormalities in genetic disease. J Urol 136(4):778–785, © by Williams & Wilkins, 1986.

A number of syndromes with associated urinary tract anomalies have been mentioned in the literature.[68, 70] Barakat and colleagues[29] have tabulated these syndromes for urinary tract anomalies according to the terminology used by McKusick,[30] and their tables are reproduced here (Tables 19–1 to 19–5). They also presented a cross referenced table of genetic conditions associated with each urogenital abnormality (Table 19–6) and listed the nine anomalies for which a locus is assigned on the human chromosome (Table 19–7). Although the tables are provided for ease of reference, they also stress that multiple associated congenital anomalies do often occur.

A relatively detailed discussion of anorectal malformations follows. We cover these malformations in detail because (1) they are one of the most common types of anomalies associated with urinary tract anomalies (26% of patients with anorectal malformations have urinary tract anomalies),[31] and (2) at one point in their embryological development, the urinary tract and hindgut were interconnected via the cloaca. This ancestral connection may persist in high anorectal anomalies. Their embryological basis is discussed in the fourth section of this chapter.

Uroradiological Aspects of Anorectal Malformations

Disagreement has long existed concerning how best to classify anorectal malformations. The suggested International Classification,[32] based primarily on the work of Browne[33] and Stephens,[34–36] represents a compromise of various views held by the participants at a conference on anorectal anomalies held in Melbourne, Australia, in 1970. That classification is outlined in Table 19–8. It is explained and correlated with Stephens' pioneering work and is based on the site of termination of the colon (Fig. 19–3).

The disorders known as high (supralevator) anorectal malformations according to the International Classification—those called rectal agenesis by Stephens—have been derived as follows. Stephens[34–36] correlated his anatomical and radiological studies by drawing a line, called the pubococcygeal (PC) line, between the top of the symphysis pubis and the sacrococcygeal junction. This line has been seen as more or less indicating the level of the bladder neck, the peritoneal pouch, the external orifice of the cervix, and the third fold of Houston of the rectum.

Stephens obtained the necessary radiograph by suspending the infant upside-down and centering the x-ray beam on the greater trochanter of the femur. A lateral radiograph was obtained, on which a line was drawn from the top of the pubic ossification site to just below the S5 vertebra. He then defined rectal agenesis, or imperforate rectum (high malformations according to the International Classification), as an anomaly in which the last part of the gas-filled bowel ends just above the pubococcygeal line (anatomically just above the levator ani muscle).

According to that definition of rectal agenesis, fistulas extending from the terminal colonic pouch are common; in the male, they are usually found in the prostatic urethra, most often just below the verumontanum, although they may extend into the bladder. Such fistulas may lead to recurrent urinary tract infections, chronic pyelonephritis, hyperchloremic acidosis, epididymitis, or seminal vesiculitis.[37] In the female, the fistulas open into the vagina or into the urogenital sinus.

An intermediate anomaly in the International Classification occurs when gas extends below the PC line, but not below a line drawn parallel to it, at the lowest level of the ossified ischial bone. Stephens called this the "ischial line," which corresponds to the most proximal level of the bulbous urethra. If fistulas occur, they open in the bulbous urethra in the male, or into the vestibule or lower vagina in the female. Stephens' third line, the pit line, marks the posteroinferior part of the bulbocavernosus muscle and is parallel to the ischial line, but 1 to 2 cm caudal to it. If bowel gas ended in this area, Stephens called the anomaly imperforate anal membrane; in the International Classification it is called a low or translevator anomaly.

Unfortunately, Shopfner and others have demonstrated that these inverted films usually fail to show fistulas, and they may distort the location of the bowel gas 40% of the time. Shopfner[38, 39] pointed out some of the pitfalls (Table 19–9). In summary, Shopfner found the entire situation far more dynamic than allowed by Stephens or the International Classification.

Shopfner[38, 39] attempted to overcome the difficulties associated with inverted plain film with the so-called flushing technique or "genitography" (Fig. 19–4). The perineum is first examined for an ectopic opening; if it is found, a blunt-nosed syringe filled with contrast material is inserted, under fluoroscopic control, just inside the opening. The barrel is pressed tightly against the skin to prevent leaks. Contrast material is injected to see what is outlined. If the opening is too small, a catheter or cannula may be inserted. The tract itself is filled, but not the rectum, so as not to obscure the available anatomy.

If there is no perineal opening, Shopfner examines the vagina in the female and the urethra in the male. In the female, vaginography is performed by pressing the syringe tightly against the skin to prevent leaks. In the male, urethrography is performed using a similar technique. If the fistula is still not filled in the male, a Foley catheter is inserted into the bladder with the balloon pressed tightly against the bladder neck, and another injection is made.

Peck and Poznanski[40] described a simple device for performing fistulography, vaginography, and retrograde urethrography, which they claim offers several advantages over the blunt-nosed syringe. A 3.5-, 5-, or 8-F feeding tube with side holes is pulled with a small hemostat through a sterile single-hole disposable nipple. To increase the firmness of the nipple, small pieces of cotton are placed inside it. The radiologist holds the device in place with a lead gloved hand or tapes it to the soft tissues. A syringe filled with contrast material is attached to the device, the contrast material is injected under fluoroscopic control, and appropriate radiographs are taken. The same can be accomplished with a small Foley catheter.

In the male or female, these radiographs are followed by routine films of the chest, abdomen, spine, and intravenous urography, to check for associated anomalies. Ultrasonography, scintigraphy, and other appropriate studies are performed as indicated.

Text continued on page 570

Table 19—2. Genetic Diseases with Autosomal Dominant Inheritance Associated with Urogenital Abnormalities

Condition No.—Syndrome	Urogenital Abnormalities	Other Major Abnormalities	Reference
37—Acrocephalosyndactyly Type III (Saethre-Chotzen) syndrome	Cryptorchidism, double collecting system	Brachycephaly, maxillary hypoplasia, syndactyly	Bartsocas, C. S., Weber, A. L. and Crawford, J. D.: J. Ped., 77:267, 1970
38—Basal cell nevus (Gorlin's) syndrome	Hypogenitalism, cryptorchidism	Basal cell nevi, broad shoulders, rib abnormalities	Gorlin, R. J., Vickers, R. A., Kellin, E. and Williamson, J. J.: Cancer, 18:89, 1965, and Gorlin, R. J., Chaudhury, A. P. and Moss, M. L.: J. Ped., 56:778, 1960
39—Ectodermal dysplasia, anhidrotic, with cleft lip and palate (Rapp-Hodgkin) syndrome?	Hypospadias	Defect in sweating, alopecia, hypodontia	Rapp, R. S. and Hodgkin, W. E.: J. Med. Genet., 5:269, 1968
40—Exomphalos-macroglossia-gigantism syndrome	Cryptorchidism, hydroureter, hypospadias	Macroglossia, omphalocele, macrosomia	Combs, J. T., Grunt, J. A. and Brandt, I. K.: New Engl. J. Med., 275:236, 1966
41—Fibrodysplasia ossificans congenita syndrome	Hypogenitalism	Fibrous dysplasia leading to ossification in muscles and subcutaneous tissue	Tünte, W., Becker, P. E. and Knorre, G. v.: Humangenetik, 4:320, 1967
42—Fifth digit (Coffin-Siris) syndrome?	Cryptorchidism	Hypoplastic or absent fifth finger and toenail, coarse facies	Weiswasser, W. H., Hall, B. D., Delavan, G. W. and Smith, D. W.: Amer. J. Dis. Child., 125:838, 1973
43—Frontometaphyseal dysplasia syndrome?	Cryptorchidism	Prominent supraorbital ridge, joint limitation, splayed metaphyses	Danks, D. M., Mayne, V., Hall, R. K. and McKinnon, M. C.: Amer. J. Dis. Child., 123:254, 1972
44—Hereditary arthro-onychodysplasia (nail-patella) syndrome	Duplication of collecting system	Nail dysplasia, patella hypoplasia, iliac spurs	Bennett, W. M., Musgrave, J. E., Campbell, R. A., Elliot, D., Cox, R., Brooks, R. E., Lovrien, E. W., Beals, R. K. and Porter, G. A.: Amer. J. Med., 54:304, 1973
45—Hydronephrosis with peculiar facial expression (Ochoa)	Hydroureter, urethral valves, cryptorchidism	Peculiar facies when smiling or crying	Elejalde, B. R.: Amer. J. Med. Genet., 3:97, 1979
46—Hypertelorism with esophageal abnormality (G or Opitz-Frias) syndrome*	Hypospadias, bifid scrotum, duplication of ureters, vesicoureteral reflux	Stridor, swallowing difficulty, hypertelorism	Opitz, J. M., Frias, J. L., Gutenberger, J. E. and Pellett, J. R.: Birth Defects, part II, 5:95, 1969
47—Hypospadias, familial*	Hypospadias	—	Perlmutter, A. D.: In: Campbell's Urology, 4th ed. Edited by J. H. Harrison, R. F. Gittes, A. D. Perlmutter, T. A. Stamey and P. C. Walsh. Philadelphia: W. B. Saunders Co., vol. 2, sect. XII, chapt. 43, p. 1535, 1979
48—Intestinal polyposis (Peutz-Jeghers syndrome)	Ureteral polyposis, bladder papillomas	Mucocutaneous pigmentation, intestinal polyposis	Dormandy, T. L.: New Engl. J. Med., 256:1093, 1957
49—Mandibulofacial dysostosis (Treacher Collins-Franceschetti) syndrome	Cryptorchidism	Malar hypoplasia, down-slanting of palpebral fissure, defect of lower lid, malformation of external ear	Stovin, J. J., Lyon, J. A., Jr. and Clemmens, R. L.: Radiology, 74:225, 1960
50—Marfan's syndrome	Hydroureter, ureteral stenosis, double ureter, hypogenitalism, cryptorchidism	Arachnodactyly, lens subluxation, aortic dilatation	Booth, C. C., Loughridge, L. W. and Turner, M. D.: Brit. Med. J., 2:80, 1957
51—Multiple lentigines	Hypogenitalism, cryptorchidism, hypospadias	Multiple lentigines, pulmonary stenosis, deafness	Moynahan, E. J.: Proc. Roy. Soc. Med., 55:959, 1962, and Swanson, S. L., Santen, R. J. and Smith, D. W.: J. Ped., 78:1037, 1971
52—Myotonic dystrophy (Steinert's disease)	Cryptorchidism, testicular atrophy	Myotonia, muscle atrophy, cataract, premature frontal baldness in males pts.	Pruzanski, W.: Brain, 89:563, 1966

Table continued on following page

Table 19–2. Genetic Diseases with Autosomal Dominant Inheritance Associated with Urogenital Abnormalities *Continued*

Condition No.—Syndrome	Urogenital Abnormalities	Other Major Abnormalities	Reference
53—Neurofibromatosis (von Recklinghausen's disease)	Neurofibromatosis of lower urinary tract	Café-au-lait spots, neurofibromas of skin and gastrointestinal tract, central nervous system involvement	Gonzalez-Angulo, A. and Reyes, H. A.: J. Urol., 89:804, 1963
54—Multiple noduli cutanei with urinary tract abnormalities*	Duplication of the collecting system	Multiple skin nodules	Selmanowitz, V. J., Lerer, W. N. and Orentreich, N.: Cancer, 26:1256, 1970
55—Noonan's syndrome	Microphallus, cryptorchidism	Webbed neck, pectus excavatum, pulmonary stenosis	Smith, D. W.: J. Ped., 70:463, 1967
56—Rieger's syndrome	Hypospadias	Iris dysplasia, hypodontia	Smith, D. W. and Jones, K. L.: Recognizable Patterns of Human Malformation: Genetic, Embryologic and Clinical Aspects, 3rd ed. Philadelphia: W. B. Saunders Co., 1982
57—Robinow's syndrome	Cryptorchidism, hypogenitalism	Flat facial profile, short forearms	Wadlington, W. B., Tucker, V. L. and Schimke, R. N.: Amer. J. Dis. Child., 126:202, 1973
58—Russell-Silver syndrome*	Hypospadias, cryptorchidism, microphallus	Short stature, skeletal asymmetry, small incurved fifth finger	Silver, H. K.: Amer. J. Dis. Child., 107:495, 1964
59—Shprintzen syndrome?	Cryptorchidism, hypospadias	Cardiac defects, craniofacial defects, short stature, deafness	Smith, D. W. and Jones, K. L.: Recognizable Patterns of Human Malformation: Genetic, Embryologic and Clinical Aspects, 3rd ed. Philadelphia: W. B. Saunders Co., 1982
60—Telangiectasia, hereditary	Telangiectasia of bladder, vagina, and uterus	Multiple telangiectasis, epistases	Bird, R. M., Hammarsten, J. F., Marshall, R. A. and Robinson, R. R.: New Engl. J. Med., 257:105, 1957
61—von Hippel-Lindau disease	Ureterocele	Retinal angiomas, cerebellar hemangioblastoma	Grossman, M. and Melmon, K. L.: In: Handbook of Clinical Neurology: The Phakomatoses. Edited by P. J. Vincken and G. W. Bruyn. Amsterdam: North-Holland Publishing Co., vol. 14, chapt. 8, pp. 241–259, 1972

*Mode of inheritance probably autosomal dominant.
From Barakat AY, Seikaly MG, Der Kaloustian VM: Urogenital abnormalities in genetic disease. J Urol 136(4):778–785, © by Williams & Wilkins, 1986.

Table 19–3. Genetic Diseases with X-Linked Inheritance Associated with Urogenital Abnormalities

Condition No.—Syndrome	Urogenital Abnormalities	Other Major Abnormalities	Reference
62—Anorchia, familial (embryonic testicular regression) syndrome	Anorchia, cryptorchidism, ambiguous genitalia	—	Perlmutter, A. D.: In: Campbell's Urology, 4th ed. Edited by J. H. Harrison, R. F. Gittes, A. D. Perlmutter, T. A. Stamey and P. C. Walsh. Philadelphia: W. B. Saunders Co., vol. 2, sect. XII, chapt. 43, p. 1535, 1979, and Josso, N. and Briard, M. L.: J. Ped., 97:200, 1980
63—Arthrogryposis multiplex congenita, distal	Microphallus, cryptorchidism	Extended arms, flexion of hands, and wrists, decreased muscle mass, major joint contractures	Hall, J. G., Reed, S. D., Scott, C. I., Rogers, J. G., Jones, K. L. and Camarano, A.: Clin. Genet., 21:81, 1982
64—Cerebellar ataxia with hypogonadism, familial	Hypogenitalism	—	Matthews, W. B. and Rundle, A. T.: Brain, 87:463, 1964
65—Faciogenital dysplasia (Aarskog-Scott) syndrome*	Cryptorchidism, cleft and "shawl" scrotum, phimosis	Ocular hypertelorism, anteverted nostrils, broad upper lip	Berry, C., Cree, J. and Mann, T.: Arch. Dis. Child., 55:706, 1980
66—Kallmann's syndrome*	Cryptorchidism, hypogenitalism	Anosmia, color blindness	De Morsier, G.: Schweiz. Arch. Neurol. Psychiatr., 74:309, 1954
67—Lenz's microphthalmia	Cryptorchidism, hydroureter, hypospadias	Narrow shoulders, double thumbs, anophthalmos, cardiovascular anomalies	Herrmann, J. and Opitz, J. M.: Birth Defects, part II, 5:138, 1969
68—Mental retardation, growth retardation, deafness, microgenitalism	Cryptorchidism, rudimentary scrotum	Growth and mental retardation, deafness, flat nasal bridge	Juberg, R. C. and Marsidi, I.: Amer. J. Hum. Genet., 32:714, 1980
69—Mental retardation with macro-orchidism, familial	Macro-orchidism	—	Bowen, P., Biederman, B. and Swallow, K. A.: Amer. J. Med. Genet., 2:409, 1978
70—Mental retardation, male hypogonadism and skeletal anomalies	Hypogenitalism, rudimentary scrotum, cryptorchidism	—	Sohval, A. R. and Soffer, L. J.: Amer. J. Med., 14:328, 1953
71—Oculo-cerebro-renal (Lowe) syndrome	Cryptorchidism	Hypotonia, cataract, renal tubular dysfunction	McCance, R. A., Matheson, W. J., Gresham, G. A. and Elkinton, J. R.: Arch. Dis. Child., 35:240, 1960
72—Male pseudohermaphroditism (owing to 17,20-desmolase deficiency)	Hypospadias, ambiguous genitalia, complete feminization	—	Grumbach, M. M. and Conte, F. A.: In: Textbook of Endocrinology, 6th ed. Edited by R. H. Williams. Philadelphia: W. B. Saunders Co., chapt. 9, pp. 423–514, 1981
73—Male pseudohermaphroditism (owing to defect in androgenation)—including testicular feminization, partial testicular feminization, and incomplete male pseudohermaphroditism (4 forms)	Hypospadias, ambiguous genitalia, complete feminization, blind vagina, absent uterus, sexual infantilism	—	Opitz, J. and Groose, F. R.: In: The Year Book of Pediatrics. Edited by S. S. Gellis. Chicago: Year Book Medical Publishers, pp. 486–491, 1971

*Mode of inheritance probably X-linked.
From Barakat AY, Seikaly MG, Der Kaloustian VM: Urogenital abnormalities in genetic disease. J Urol 136(4):778–785, © by Williams & Wilkins, 1986.

Table 19–4. Genetic Diseases with Uncertain Mode of Inheritance Associated with Urogenital Abnormalities

Condition No.—Syndrome	Urogenital Abnormalities	Other Major Abnormalities	Reference
74—Acrodysostosis syndrome	Hypogenitalism	Dwarfism, short limbs, rudimentary fibula, micrognathia	Robinow, M., Pfeiffer, R. A., Gorlin, R. J., McKusick, V. A., Renuart, A. W., Johnson, G. F. and Summitt, R. L.: Amer. J. Dis. Child., 121:195, 1971
75—Acrorenal syndrome	Ureteral hypoplasia, trigone deformity, bladder neck obstruction, hypospadias, cryptorchidism	Limb abnormalities	Curan, A. S. and Curran J. P.: Pediatrics, 49:716, 1972
76—Aniridia-Wilms tumor	Cryptorchidism, hypospadias, microphallus, ambiguous genitalia, gonadoblastoma	Mental and growth retardation, aniridia, micrognathia	Riccardi, V. M., Sujansky, E., Smith, A. C. and Francke, U.: Pediatrics, 61:604, 1978
77—Biliary atresia, extrahepatic	Atresia of ureter, megaloureter	—	Moore, T. C.: Surg., Gynec. & Obst., 96:215, 1953
78—CHARGE association	Genital hypoplasia in male pts.	Coloboma, heart defect, coanal atresia, ear anomalies	Smith, D. W. and Jones, K. L.: Recognizable Patterns of Human Malformation: Genetic, Embryologic and Clinical Aspects, 3rd ed. Philadelphia: W. B. Saunders Co., 1982
79—Cornelia de Lange's syndrome	Cryptorchidism, hypogenitalism	Mental retardation, bush eyebrows, micromelia	Opitz, J. and Groose, F. R.: In: The Year Book of Pediatrics. Edited by S. S. Gellis. Chicago: Year Book Medical Publishers, pp. 486–491, 1971, and Ptacek, L. J., Opitz, J. M., Smith, D. W., Gerritsen, T. and Waisman, H. A.: J. Ped., 63:1000, 1963
80—Femoral-facial syndrome	Hemangioma of urinary tract	Femoral hypoplasia, short nose, cleft palate	Daentl, D. L., Smith, D. W., Scott, C. I., Hall, B. D. and Gooding, C. A.: J. Ped., 86:107, 1975
81—Genital anomaly with cardiomyopathy	Hypoplastic genitalia	—	Najjar, S. S., Der Kaloustian, V. M. and Ardati, K. O.: Clin. Genet., 26:371, 1984
82—Hallermann-Streiff syndrome	Cryptorchidism, hypogenitalism	Microphthalmia, small pinched nose, hypotrichosis	Hoefnagel, D. and Benirschke, K.: Arch. Dis. Child., 40:57, 1965
83—Klippel-Trenaunay-Weber syndrome	Hemangioma of urinary tract, enlarged genitalia	Asymmetric limb hypertrophy, hemangiomas	Stephan, M. J., Hall, B. D., Smith, D. W. and Cohen, M. M., Jr.: J. Ped., 87:353, 1975
84—MURCS association	Absence of vagina and uterus	Short stature, cervical defects, renal anomalies	Duncan, P. A., Shapiro, L. R., Stangel, J. J., Klein, R. M. and Addonizio, J. C.: J. Ped., 95:399, 1979
85—N syndrome	Cryptorchidism, hypospadias	Spasticity, mental retardation, visual impairment, deafness	Hess, R. O., Kaveggia, E. G. and Opitz, J. M.: Clin. Genet., 6:237, 1974
86—Popliteal web (faciogenitopopliteal syndrome)	Cryptorchidism, bifid scrotum, hypoplastic labia majora, ambiguous genitalia	Popliteal web, cleft palate, lower lip pits	Bartsocas, C. S. and Papas, C. V.: J. Med. Genet., 9:222, 1972
87—Prader-Willi syndrome	Cryptorchidism, hypogonadism	Hypotonia, obesity, small hands and feet	Hamilton, C. R., Jr., Scully, R. E. and Kliman, B.: Amer. J. Med., 52:322, 1972, and Gabilan, J.-C. and Royer, P.: Arch. Fr. Ped., 25:121, 1968
88—Prune-belly syndrome	Cryptorchidism, large trabeculated bladder, bladder neck obstruction, hypoplastic or absent urethra, megaloureter, urethral diverticulum, posterior urethral valve	Absent abdominal muscles	Pagon, R. A., Smith, D. W. and Shepard, T. H.: J. Ped., 94:900, 1979
89—Renal agenesis, bilateral (Potter's syndrome) (see also Table 19–15)	Hypospadias, absent vas deferens, absent penis, cryptorchidism, agenesis, or hypoplasia of müllerian ducts	Pulmonary hypoplasia, limb positioning defect	Potter, E. L.: Obst. Gynec., 25:3, 1965
90—Senter syndrome	Cryptorchidism	Ichthyosiform erythroderma, sensory deafness	Smith, D. W. and Jones, K. L.: Recognizable Patterns of Human Malformation: Genetic, Embryologic and Clinical Aspects, 3rd ed. Philadelphia: W. B. Saunders Co., 1982
91—VATER association	Hypospadias, rectourethral, rectovaginal, and rectovesical fistulas; renal ectopia and fusion	Vertebral anomalies, ventricular septal defect, anal atresia, tracheoesophageal fistula, radial dysplasia	Temtamy, S. A. and Miller, J. D.: J. Ped., 85:345, 1974, and Mehrizi, A.: J. Ped., 61:582, 1962

From Barakat AY, Seikaly MG, Der Kaloustian VM: Urogenital abnormalities in genetic disease. J Urol 136(4):778–785, © by Williams & Wilkins, 1986.

Table 19–5. A Representative List of Chromosomal Aberrations Associated with Urogenital Abnormalities
(All of These Conditions May Be Diagnosed Antenatally)

Condition No.—Syndrome	Urogenital Abnormalities	Reference
	Klinefelter's syndrome	
92—XX	Small firm testes, hypogenitalism	Yunis, J. J.: Molecular Structure of Human Chromosomes. New York: Academic Press, Inc., 1977
93—XXY	Small firm testes, short penis, hydroureter, ureterocele, cryptorchidism	Yunis, J. J.: Molecular Structure of Human Chromosomes. New York: Academic Press, Inc., 1977; Caldwell, P. D. and Smith, D. W.: J. Ped., 80:250, 1972
94—XXYY	Small firm testes	Yunis, J. J.: Molecular Structure of Human Chromosomes. New York: Academic Press, Inc., 1977
95—XXXY	Small firm testes, microphallus	
96—XXXXY	Cryptorchidism, hypospadias, microphallus, bifid scrotum	Zalestki, W. A., Houston, C. S., Pozsonyi, J. and Ying, K. L.: Canad. Med. Ass. J., 94:1143, 1966
97—Mosaic	Small firm testes	Yunis, J. J.: Molecular Structure of Human Chromosomes. New York: Academic Press, Inc., 1977
98—XYY	Cryptorchidism, microphallus, hypospadias	Bergsma, D.: Birth Defects Compendium, 2nd ed. New York: Alan R. Liss, Inc., 1979
99—XXYY	Cryptorchidism	Yunis, J. J.: Molecular Structure of Human Chromosomes. New York: Academic Press, Inc., 1977
100—XYYYY	Cryptorchidism	Bergsma, D.: Birth Defects Compendium, 2nd ed. New York: Alan R. Liss, Inc., 1979
101—Turner (XO) syndrome	Meatal stenosis, ureteropelvic obstruction, double collecting system, hypoplastic uterus, hypogenitalism, horseshoe kidney	Hortling, H.: Acta Endocr., 18:548, 1955
102—Triploidy	Cryptorchidism, bifid scrotum, hypospadias, microphallus	Walker, S., Andrews, J., Gregson, N. M. and Gault, W.: J. Med. Genet., 10:135, 1973
	Trisomy	
103—4p	Cryptorchidism, hypospadias, microphallus, prolapsed bladder	Yunis, J. J.: Molecular Structure of Human Chromosomes. New York: Academic Press, Inc., 1977
104—8	Cryptorchidism, hypogenitalism, vesicoureteral reflux	Yunis, J. J.: Molecular Structure of Human Chromosomes. New York: Academic Press, Inc., 1977; Riccardi, V. M., Atkins, L. and Holmes, L. B.: J. Ped., 77:664, 1970
105—9	Cryptorchidism, microphallus	Yunis, J. J.: Molecular Structure of Human Chromosomes. New York: Academic Press, Inc., 1977
106—9p	Microphallus	Yunis, J. J.: Molecular Structure of Human Chromosomes. New York: Academic Press, Inc., 1977
107—9 mosaic	Micropenis, cryptorchidism	Smith, D. W. and Jones, K. L.: Recognizable Patterns of Human Malformation: Genetic, Embryologic and Clinical Aspects, 3rd ed. Philadelphia: W. B. Saunders Co., 1982
108—Partial trisomy 10q syndrome	Cryptorchidism, hypospadias	Smith, D. W. and Jones, K. L.: Recognizable Patterns of Human Malformation: Genetic, Embryologic and Clinical Aspects, 3rd ed. Philadelphia: W. B. Saunders Co., 1982
109—13 (Patau)	Cryptorchidism, abnormal scrotum, hypospadias, large bladder, stenosis of prostatic urethra, bladder neck stenosis, vesicoureteral obstruction, uterine cysts, bicornuate and double uterus	Patau, K., Smith, D. W., Therman, E., Inhorn, S. L. and Wagner, H. P.: Lancet, 1:790, 1960
110—18	Cryptorchidism, double collecting system, horseshoe kidney, microphallus, vaginal atresia, hypoplasia of labia majora, prominent clitoris, bicornuate uterus	Warkany, J., Passarge, E. and Smith, L. B.: Amer. J. Dis. Child., 112:502, 1966, and Egli, F. and Stalder, G.: Humangenetik, 18:1, 1973
111—20p	Genital hypoplasia, cryptorchidism	Smith, D. W. and Jones, K. L.: Recognizable Patterns of Human Malformation: Genetic, Embryologic and Clinical Aspects, 3rd ed. Philadelphia: W. B. Saunders Co., 1982
112—21	Cryptorchidism, microphallus, hypoplastic uterus, bicornuate uterus, ureteral stenosis	Egli, F. and Stalder, G.: Humangenetik, 18:1, 1973
113—22	Cryptorchidism, microphallus	Yunis, J. J.: Molecular Structure of Human Chromosomes. New York: Academic Press, Inc., 1977
114—Cri-du-chat (5p-)	Cryptorchidism, hypospadias, hypoplasia of penis and vulva, hyperplastic clitoris	Egli, F. and Stalder, G.: Humangenetik, 18:1, 1973
115—18p- syndrome	Cryptorchidism, hypoplastic testes, and external genitalia	Egli, F. and Stalder, G.: Humangenetik, 18:1, 1973
116—18q- syndrome	Hypospadias, cryptorchidism, hypoplastic penis and scrotum, unilateral anorchidism, aplasia of labia	Egli, F. and Stalder, G.: Humangenetik, 18:1, 1973
117—18 ring chromosome	Megaureter, hypospadias, bifid scrotum, cryptorchidism	Egli, F. and Stalder, G.: Humangenetik, 18:1, 1973
118—5p- syndrome	Cryptorchidism	Smith, D. W. and Jones, K. L.: Recognizable Patterns of Human Malformation: Genetic, Embryologic and Clinical Aspects, 3rd ed. Philadelphia: W. B. Saunders Co., 1982
119—4p- syndrome	Hypospadias, cryptorchidism, vesicoureteral reflux	Guthrie, R. D., Aase, J. M., Asper, A. C. and Smith, D. W.: Amer. J. Dis. Child., 122:421, 1971
120—9p- syndrome	Micropenis, cryptorchidism, hypoplastic labia majora	Smith, D. W. and Jones, K. L.: Recognizable Patterns of Human Malformation: Genetic, Embryologic and Clinical Aspects, 3rd ed. Philadelphia: W. B. Saunders Co., 1982
121—13q- syndrome	Hypospadias, epispadias, cryptorchidism, ambiguous genitalia, hydroureter	Allderdice, P. W., Davis, J. G., Miller, O. J., Klinger, H. P., Warburton, D., Miller, D. A., Allen, F. H., Jr., Abrams, C. A. L. and McGilvray, E.: Amer. J. Human. Genet., 21:499, 1969
122—13 ring syndrome	Cryptorchidism, hypospadias, epispadias	Egli, F. and Stalder, G.: Humangenetik, 18:1, 1973
123—21q- syndrome	Hypospadias, cryptorchidism	Egli, F. and Stalder, G.: Humangenetik, 18:1, 1973

From Barakat AY. Seikaly MG, Der Kaloustian VM: Urogenital abnormalities in genetic disease. J Urol 136(4):778–785, © by Williams & Wilkins, 1986.

Table 19–6. Genetic Conditions Associated with Different Urogenital Abnormalities

Urogenital Abnormality	Associated Genetic Condition
Anorchism	62, 116
Bladder abnormality	4, 12, 22, 26, 30, 36, 48, 60, 61, 75, 88, 91, 93, 103, 109
Clitoromegaly	3, 7, 15, 27, 110, 114
Collecting system, double	14, 22, 34, 37, 44, 46, 50, 54, 101, 110
Cryptorchidism	2–7, 9, 10, 13, 14, 16, 18–21, 27–30, 35, 37, 38, 40, 42, 43, 45, 49–52, 55, 57–59, 62, 63, 65–68, 70, 71, 75, 76, 79, 82, 85–90, 93, 96, 98–100, 102–105, 107–123
Epispadias	5, 121, 122
Feminization, complete	24, 72, 73
Genitalia:	
Ambiguous	15, 19, 23–25, 62, 72, 73, 76, 86, 121, 122
Enlarged	4, 17, 83
Gonadoblastoma	76
Hemangioma of urinary tract	80, 83
Hypogenitalism	1, 2, 8, 14, 16, 29, 38, 41, 50, 51, 57, 64, 66, 70, 74, 78, 79, 81, 82, 92, 101, 104, 111, 115
Hypogonadism	87
Hypospadias	3, 7, 10, 14, 20, 22, 24, 25, 27, 30, 32, 35, 39, 40, 45, 47, 51, 56, 58, 59, 67, 72, 73, 75, 76, 85, 89, 91, 96, 98, 102, 103, 108, 109, 114, 116, 117, 119, 121–123
Labia majora, aplasia or hypoplasia	13, 86, 110, 116, 120
Macro-orchidism	69
Microphallus	16, 23, 31, 35, 55, 58, 63, 76, 95, 96, 98, 102, 103, 105–107, 110, 112, 113, 116, 120
Neurofibroma of urinary tract	53
Penile abnormality	7, 27, 30, 32, 89, 93, 114
Scrotum, bifid or rudimentary	16, 45, 65, 68, 70, 86, 96, 102, 109, 116, 117
Sexual infantilism	73
Testes, hypoplastic or small	8, 11, 33, 52, 92–95, 97, 115
Ureteral abnormalities	4, 12, 22, 23, 27, 28, 31, 48, 50, 75, 77, 101, 109, 112
Hydroureter or megaureter	3, 17, 36, 40, 45, 50, 67, 77, 88, 93, 117, 121
Urethral abnormality	7, 88, 91, 101, 109
Urethral valves, posterior	22, 30, 45, 88
Uterine abnormality	23, 27, 31, 60, 73, 84, 101, 109, 110, 112
Vaginal abnormality	7, 15, 26–28, 60, 73, 84, 91, 110
Vesicoureteral reflux	46, 104, 119

Numbers refer to genetic conditions listed in Tables 19–1 to 19–5.
From Barakat AY, Seikaly MG, Der Kaloustian VM: Urogenital abnormalities in genetic disease. J Urol 136(4):778–785, © by Williams & Wilkins, 1986.

Fistulas can also be demonstrated by injecting contrast material through a diverting colostomy (Fig. 19–5). Associated urinary tract anomalies (Table 19–10) should be diagnosed before rectal surgery in order to prevent complications that might arise as a result of the associated anomaly and to differentiate between complications arising as a result of surgery and pre-existing complications.[41–44]

Congenital H-Type Fistulas

The term congenital H-type anourethral fistula was suggested by Stephens and colleagues[45] to describe a congenital fistula between the posterior urethra and an-

Table 19–7. Chromosomal Mapping of Syndromes Associated with Urogenital Abnormalities

Syndrome	Gene Locus
Aniridia-Wilms tumor	11p13
Cat eye	22pter-22q11
Ehlers-Danlos:	
Type IV	7p11?
Type VII	8p12?
Mental retardation with macro-orchidism (familial)	Xq28-Xq27
Myotonic dystrophy	19pter-19q13
Nail-patella	9q34
Prader-Willi	15q11-15q12
Testicular feminization	Near centromere X chromosome (p11-q13)
21-Hydroxylase deficiency	Near HLA-D/DR chromosome 6

From Barakat AY, Seikaly MG, Der Kaloustian VM: Urogenital abnormalities in genetic disease. J Urol 136(4):778–785, © by Williams & Wilkins, 1986.

orectal junction in patients with no evidence of anorectal atresia (Fig. 19–6). They used the term because the situation seemed somewhat analogous to that in the esophagus, in which an H-type tracheoesophageal fistula can occur without evidence of esophageal atresia.

Congenital H-type anourethral fistulas can present clinically in two age groups. Most commonly it presents during infancy, because of an associated anterior urethral stricture.[46] In cases presenting in adulthood, the anterior urethra is normal.[47, 49]

Because congenital anomalies develop in the embryo, we have taken the time earlier in this chapter to look briefly at the embryology. There is, of course, another

Table 19–8. Classification of Anorectal Malformations*

Male	Female
A. Low (translevator)	
1. At normal anal site	1. Same
a. Anal stenosis	a. Same
b. Covered anus—complete	b. Same
2. At perineal site	2. Same
a. Anocutaneous fistula (covered anus—incomplete)	a. Same
b. Anterior perineal anus	b. Same
	3. At vulvar site
	a. Anovulvar fistula
	b. Anovestibular fistula
	c. Vestibular anus
B. Intermediate	
1. Anal agenesis	1. Same
a. Without fistula	a. Same
b. With fistula	b. With fistula
i. Rectobulbar	i. Rectovestibular
	ii. Rectovaginal—low
2. Anorectal stenosis	2. Same
C. High (supralevator)	
1. Anorectal agenesis	1. Same
a. Without fistula	a. Same
b. With fistula	b. With fistula
i. Rectourethral	i. Rectovaginal—high
ii. Rectovesical	ii. Rectocloacal
	iii. Rectovesical
2. Rectal atresia	2. Same
D. Miscellaneous	
1. Imperforate anal membrane	
2. Cloacal exstrophy	
3. Others	

*See also Figure 19–3.

MALE

FEMALE

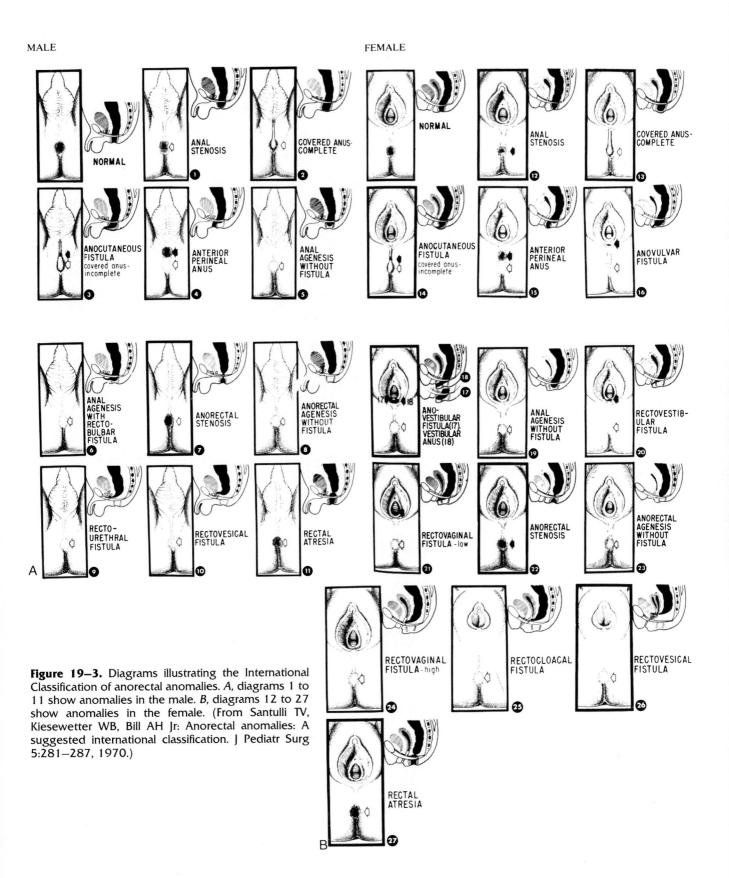

Figure 19–3. Diagrams illustrating the International Classification of anorectal anomalies. *A,* diagrams 1 to 11 show anomalies in the male. *B,* diagrams 12 to 27 show anomalies in the female. (From Santulli TV, Kiesewetter WB, Bill AH Jr: Anorectal anomalies: A suggested international classification. J Pediatr Surg 5:281–287, 1970.)

Table 19–9. Pitfalls Associated with Inverted Films

1. Meconium may be impacted in the blind part of the bowel.
2. The anal marker may be in the wrong place.
3. Gas in the vagina or small bowel may be mistaken for gas in the rectum.
4. Radiological magnification or distortion may occur.
5. The levator ani muscle may contract, making a low lesion look like a high lesion.
6. Air in the gastrointestinal tract may not have reached the distal blind segment.
7. It is sometimes difficult to draw the pubococcygeal line with accuracy.
8. The levator ani muscle ascends and descends with crying and straining, so that the gas in the terminal part of the bowel ascends and descends as well.

From Schopfner CE: Roentgenologic evaluation of imperforate anus. Reprinted by permission from the SOUTHERN MEDICAL JOURNAL 58:712–719, 1965.

point of view, which focuses on the living human being. Modern imaging techniques can provide a great deal of information to help determine whether interventional techniques or therapeutic abortion might become an option. It is important to look at the developing embryo or fetus as a living and growing organism, upon which the physician can act, should circumstances warrant intervention.

PRENATAL DIAGNOSIS OF URINARY TRACT ANOMALIES

Many genitourinary anomalies can be accurately diagnosed by prenatal ultrasonography.[50, 51, 67] Some can be identified in the early second trimester so that therapeutic intervention is possible, if it is clinically warranted. The subject has been covered in detail earlier (Chapter 12), but is presented here in a supplementary mode, and from a slightly different perspective.

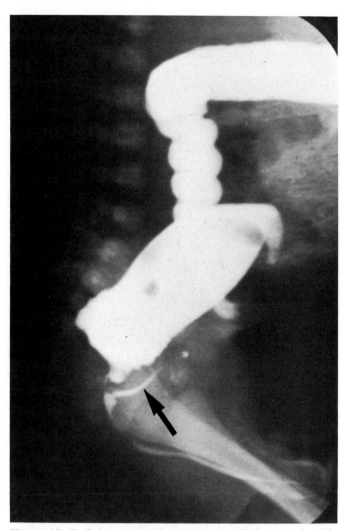

Figure 19–5. Colostogram demonstrates a high anomaly with an associated fistula to the prostatic urethra (*arrow*).

In the normal developing fetus, the kidneys can be identified in the early second trimester. They have a classic reniform appearance, and are positioned lateral to either side of the spine, immediately inferior to the stomach and liver.

There are three distinct sonographic appearances; all correlate with gestational age. Pattern one, most often seen in the second trimester, demonstrates kidneys that are poorly differentiated from the surrounding structures; in addition, the renal sinus is of low-level echogenicity. Pattern two, most frequently noted close to the third

Table 19–10. Urinary Tract Anomalies Associated with Anorectal Malformations

1. Unilateral or bilateral renal agenesis
2. Renal hypoplasia/dysplasia (multicystic)
3. Renal ectopia and/or fusion
4. Megaureter (ureterovesical junction obstruction)
5. Hydronephrosis (ureteropelvic junction obstruction)
6. Vesicoureteral reflux
7. Bladder diverticula
8. Posterior urethral valves
9. Urethral duplication
10. Congenital urethral diverticula
11. Hypospadias
12. Epispadias
13. Prune-belly syndrome

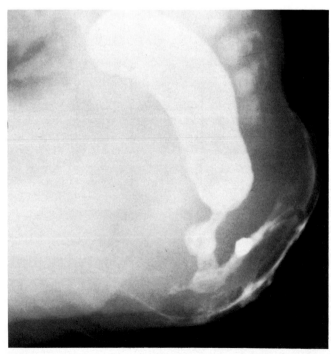

Figure 19–4. Flushing technique for evaluating anorectal anomalies. Low anorectal malformation with anterior perineal anus is shown.

CONGENITAL "H"-TYPE
ANOURETHRAL FISTULA

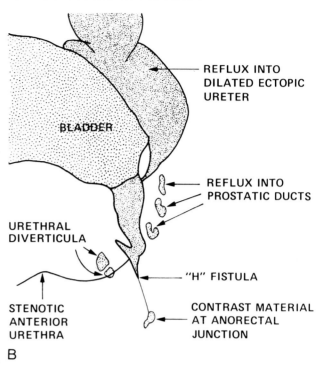

REFLUX INTO
DILATED ECTOPIC
URETER

BLADDER

REFLUX INTO
PROSTATIC DUCTS

URETHRAL
DIVERTICULA

"H" FISTULA

STENOTIC
ANTERIOR
URETHRA

CONTRAST MATERIAL
AT ANORECTAL
JUNCTION

Figure 19–6. Congenital H-type anourethral fistula is shown: *A*, voiding cystourethrogram; *B*, diagram of *A*. (From deVries PA, Friedland GW: Congenital "H-type" anourethral fistula. Radiology 113:397–407, 1974.)

trimester, has either an acoustically reflective renal margin or a renal sinus. Pattern three, seen in the late third trimester, has both an echogenic renal margin and central sinus with less reflective parenchyma (Fig. 19–7).[52]

The normal fetal kidney enlarges during gestation.[53] Formulas have been developed to measure and quantify renal volume with gestational age (Table 19–11).[54]

The fetal urinary bladder can be identified by as early as 13 weeks as a fluid-filled structure within the fetal pelvis (Fig. 19–8). It distends and empties periodically during the period of 1 hour with changes discernible in as little as 20 minutes.

When evaluating for fetal renal abnormalities, it is essential to identify the kidneys or the urinary bladder,

Figure 19–7. Normal fetal kidney. *A,* Transverse and, *B,* longitudinal images in the third trimester demonstrate a typical reniform appearance of the kidneys. Both kidneys are seen in the transverse image. In the longitudinal view, the cephalocaudal length of the kidney is noted *(arrows)* adjacent to the liver. The echogenic renal sinus echoes and renal borders are identified, as is the less echogenic renal parenchyma. (RK = right kidney, LK = left kidney, Sp = spine.)

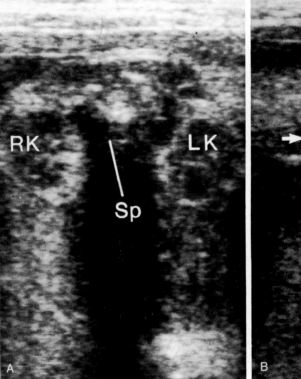

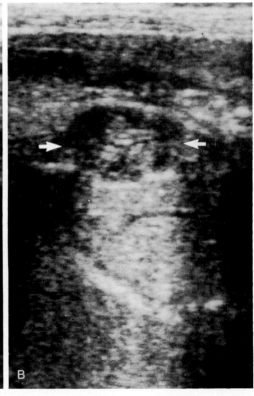

Table 19–11. Polynomial Regressions of Fetal Renal Measurements* (Also see Table 12–4)

Kidney length	0.610 W + 16.190
	0.353 BPD + 7.109
Kidney width	0.422 W + 6.592
	0.246 BPD + 0.206
	0.330 W + 7.20
Kidney thickness	0.183 BPD + 2.982
Kidney volume	0.385 W − 5.543
	0.191 BPD − 8.747

*W = weeks. BPD = biparietal diameter in millimeters.
From Jeanty P, Dramaix-Wilmet M, Elkhazen N, et al: Measurement of fetal kidney growth on ultrasound. Radiology 144:159–162, 1982.

or both, as well as the amount of amniotic fluid. Fetal urine accumulation is responsible for a large proportion of amniotic fluid from at least 18 to 20 weeks gestation until term.[55, 56]

Decreased amniotic fluid production is in part due to bilateral renal dysfunction and a lack of normal fetal urination. If one kidney functions normally and urinary bladder outflow is not obstructed, a normal amount of amniotic fluid will be present. Early diagnosis of bilateral renal dysfunction is essential because the condition is fatal after birth.

If the urinary bladder is not identified during the initial examination, the fetal pelvis should be re-examined at periodic intervals, particularly if renal abnormalities are suspected. If an observed large fluid-filled area is thought to represent the urinary bladder, it should be evaluated for normal emptying. Cystic masses in the pelvis (i.e., urachal cysts) may be mistaken for the bladder in fetuses without functioning renal tissue. The delineation of a cystic mass from the bladder is highly important, since some renal anomalies are fatal after birth.

Other causes of oligohydramnios include (1) fetal demise, (2) ruptured amniotic membranes, (3) intrauterine growth retardation, or (4) a postmature gestation.

Renal Agenesis

In renal agenesis, the fetal kidneys cannot be defined,[57, 71] and in early pregnancy, they may be difficult to identify. Thus, in the presence of oligohydramnios, the failure to identify a fluid-filled bladder may suggest bilateral renal agenesis (Fig. 19–9). The appearance of fetal adrenals may simulate that of fetal kidneys; therefore, if oligohydramnios is present and reniform structures are identified, it is important to identify a fluid-filled bladder to confirm that functioning kidneys exist. If the diagnosis is in doubt, a furosemide stimulation test should be performed. The technique for performing this examination is described in detail in Chapter 12.

Because furosemide crosses the placental membrane, it exerts a diuretic effect on both the mother and the fetus. Even if furosemide is administered, the kidneys may not be identified in the normal fetus; however, if the fetus is carefully monitored, a fluid-filled urinary bladder should become evident within 2 hours in the case of normally functioning renal tissues. If a fluid-filled urinary bladder is seen, functioning renal tissue is assumed and the study can be terminated immediately.

The furosemide test is not specific for renal agenesis, however. Fetuses severely compromised by other problems (e.g., intrauterine growth retardation) may not produce enough urine during the examination to enable the sonographer to identify a urinary bladder.[58, 59] It is important in this connection to remember that a fluid-filled loop of bowel can resemble a fluid-filled urinary bladder.

Hydronephrosis

The most common renal anomaly in the fetus is hydronephrosis. However, a transient fluid-filled renal pelvis may be seen as a result of fetal urinary bladder overdistention (Fig. 19–10).[60] The pathophysiology is unclear but is not due to maternal hydration.[61] To differentiate a clinically insignificant minimally distended renal pelvis from a possible important ureteropelvic junction obstruction, or other causes of hydronephrosis, it is important to examine the fetus over a period of time to discern whether, following fetal voiding, the dilated renal pelvis improves or worsens. Postnatal sonograms and serial studies carried out over the first few months of life are sometimes necessary to definitely establish the presence of obstruction.

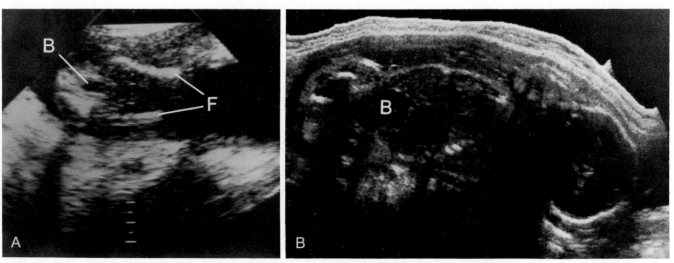

Figure 19–8. Urinary bladder. Images of the fetus in *A*, the second trimester, and *B*, the late third trimester, demonstrate the fluid-filled urinary bladder (B) in two subjects. Note that in the late third-trimester pregnancy, despite a paucity of amniotic fluid, normal renal function can be ascertained because of demonstration of the fluid-filled urinary bladder. (F = femurs.)

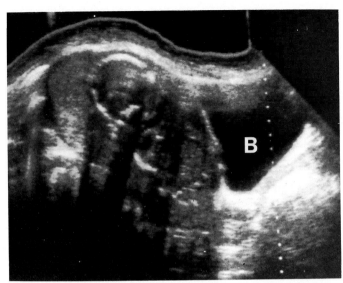

Figure 19–9. Renal agenesis. A longitudinally oriented image of the fetus in the early third trimester demonstrates a marked decrease in the amount of amniotic fluid. This finding, in conjunction with the absence of a defined urinary bladder or kidneys, is highly suggestive of renal agenesis. (B = mother's bladder.)

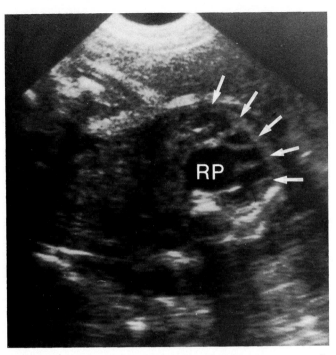

Figure 19–11. Fetal hydronephrosis secondary to ureteropelvic junction obstruction. Real-time sonographic image demonstrates a dilated renal pelvis (RP) and dilated calyces *(arrows)* in this fetus with mild obstructive changes.

Unilateral obstruction is most frequently due to a ureteropelvic junction obstruction. This diagnosis can be made with a high degree of accuracy by ultrasonography.[62, 63] Sonographically, multiple fluid-filled spaces within the kidney are seen, the renal pelvis being the largest and located medially. The smaller fluid-filled structures, the dilated calyces, extend from the dilated renal pelvis in a ringlike fashion (Fig. 19–11).

Communication of the dilated calyces with the renal pelvis should be identifiable, particularly if careful technique is used during the sonographic examination (Fig.

19–12). Frequently, a dilated renal pelvis from a ureteropelvic junction obstruction can be differentiated from a lower urinary tract obstruction, because in the former the renal pelvis appears more rounded. The normal ureter usually cannot be identified. If a unilateral dilated renal pelvis is identified, a dilated ureter (often due to ectopic ureterocele or megaureter) must be excluded. Although a dilated ureter in utero suggests the diagnosis (Fig. 19–13), exact visualization may not be possible. Subtle renal pelvic dilatation may also evade sonographic detection in utero. If a unilateral obstruction is present, and if one

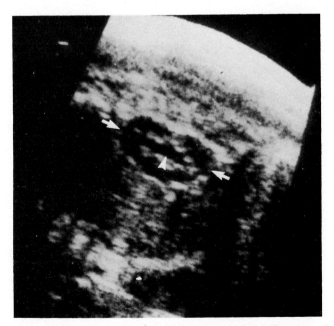

Figure 19–10. Physiological fetal renal pelvic dilatation. A longitudinal image of the fetal kidney *(arrows)* demonstrates a clinically insignificant, physiologically normal, minimally fluid-filled renal pelvis *(arrowhead)*. Sequential studies demonstrated no progression of this finding.

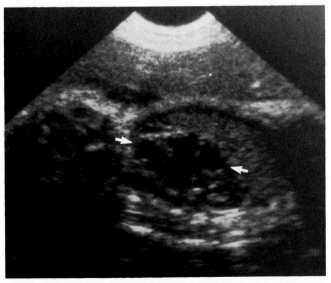

Figure 19–12. Fetal hydronephrosis. Dilated infundibula and calyces *(arrows)* are noted to be connected to a dilated renal pelvis in this fetus with moderate to severe hydronephrosis. A relatively normal quantity of residual renal parenchyma remains.

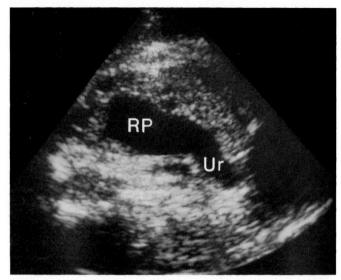

Figure 19–13. Fetal hydronephrosis secondary to distal ureteral obstruction. An enlarged real-time sonographic image of the fetus demonstrates a markedly dilated renal pelvis (RP) connected to a dilated ureter (Ur). Both are obstructed, owing to an ectopic ureterocele (not shown).

kidney functions normally, the amount of amniotic fluid will be normal.

Bilateral hydronephrosis may be due to a number of causes, the most common being posterior urethral valves.[69] In these cases, the hydronephrotic changes are due to bladder outlet obstruction. The urinary bladder is also seen as a dilated structure in the fetal pelvis (Fig. 19–14). A lack of emptying during the sonographic evaluation, even if the study is prolonged, is observed.

Oligohydramnios is usually present in cases of bilateral hydronephrosis, because of failure of fetal urination. In severe cases, pulmonary hypoplasia may also occur.

The presence of bilateral hydronephrosis with polyhydramnios may suggest the Eagle-Barrett (prune-belly) syndrome.[64] (See page 771 in this chapter for details.)

In fetuses with duplicated systems, a unilateral obstruction involving only one of the duplicated systems may be observed. This is most often due to a duplicated system with ectopic insertion of one of the ureters, usually involving the upper-pole system.

Renal Dysplasia

Where renal dysplasia is concerned, a number of sonographic images may occur.[65] The least severe, and believed to be due to focal cystic dysplasia, is the single cyst. When identified, it is almost pathognomonic of cystic dysplasia (Fig. 19–15).[66] A portion of the kidney may be involved, resulting from infundibular stenosis or atresia that is localized to a single segment.

The diagnosis of multicystic kidney is determined by demonstrating multiple small and large cystic spaces (Fig. 19–16). These are of varying sizes and are scattered throughout the kidney. However, the absence of cysts does not exclude the disease. Analysis of renal echogenicity may be helpful. Greatly increased echogenicity is highly suggestive of dysplasia, but echogenicity may be normal with the disorder. In certain cases, there may be no definable renal tissue other than cysts.

Concurrent hydronephrosis can be seen with dysplasias, but its presence is not specific. Renal pelvis dilatation may be due to other causes. When it is present unilaterally, and if no second abnormality affects the other kidney, a normal amount of amniotic fluid and a clearly defined urinary bladder are seen.

One functioning kidney is compatible with normal fetal and postnatal development. When dysplasia is bilateral, the process is incompatible with life.

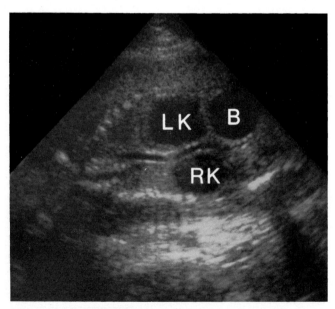

Figure 19–14. Posterior urethral valves. A longitudinally oriented image of the fetus demonstrates dilated upper collecting systems in both the left kidney (LK) and right kidney (RK) as well as a persistent fluid-filled distended urinary bladder (B). The ureters are not visualized in these images.

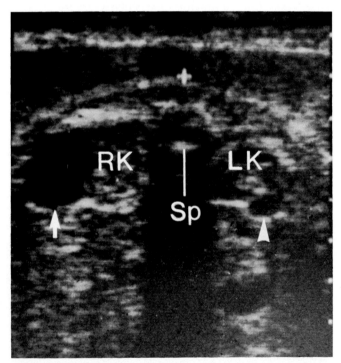

Figure 19–15. Fetal renal dysplasia. A transverse sonogram of the fetus demonstrates a small cyst (arrowhead) in the left kidney (LK). The right kidney (RK) demonstrates a single simple-appearing cyst extending off the lateral margin (arrow). These findings are pathognomonic of renal dysplasia in this fetus. (Sp = spine.)

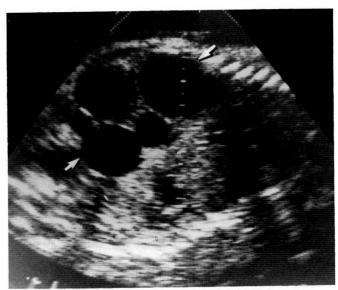

Figure 19–16. Fetal renal dysplasia. A longitudinal image of the fetus demonstrates one kidney *(arrows)* to be totally replaced by multiple simple-appearing cysts. The cysts are not connected and are of varying sizes, and the largest ones appear to be situated in the periphery. When the largest cysts are centrally placed, obstruction, as opposed to dysplasia, would be suggested.

References

1. Rubenstein M, Meyer R, Bernstein J: Congenital abnormalities of the urinary system. I. A postmortem survey of developmental anomalies and acquired congenital lesions in a children's hospital. J Pediatr 58:356–366, 1961.
2. Dareste C: Recherches sur la Production Artificielle des Monstruosities ou Essais de Teratogenie Experimentale, 2nd Ed. Paris, Reinwald, 1891.
3. Stockhard CR: Development rate and structural expression: An experimental study of twins, "double monsters," and single deformities, and the interaction among embryonic organs during their origin and development. Am J Anat 28:115–227, 1921.
4. deVries PA: Embryology of multiple congenital anomalies. *In* El Shafie M, Klippel CH (eds): Associated Congenital Anomalies. Baltimore, Williams & Wilkins Company, 1981, pp 17–20.
5. Streeter GL: Developmental horizons in human embryos. Description of age group XI, 13 to 20 somites, and age group XII, 21 to 29 somites. Carnegie Inst Wash Publ 541, Contrib Embryol 30:211–245, 1942.
6. Streeter GL: Developmental horizons in human embryos. Description of age group XIII, embryos about 4 or 5 millimeters long, and age group XIV, period of indentation of the lens vesicle. Carnegie Inst Wash Publ 557, Contrib Embryol 31:27–63, 1945.
7. Streeter GL: Developmental horizons in human embryos. Description of age groups XV, XVI, XVII and XVIII, being the third issue of a survey of the Carnegie Collection. Carnegie Inst Wash Publ 575, Contrib Embryol 32:133–203, 1948.
8. Streeter GL: Developmental horizons in human embryos. Description of age groups XIX, XX, XXI, XXII, and XXIII, being the fifth issue in a survey of the Carnegie Collection. Carnegie Inst Wash Publ 592, Contrib Embryol 34:165–169, 1951.
9. O'Rahilly R: Developmental stages in human embryos. Including a survey of the Carnegie Collection. Part A: Embryos of the first three weeks (Stages 1 to 9). Carnegie Inst Wash Publ 631, pp 1–165, 1973.
10. Oliver G, Peneau H: Horizons de Streeter et age embryonnaire. Bull Ass Anat 47:573–576, 1962.
11. Jirasek JE: Development of the Genital System and Male Pseudohermaphroditism. Baltimore, Johns Hopkins Press, 1971.
12. Iffy L, Chatterton RT, Jakobovits A: The "high weight for dates" fetus. Am J Obstet Gynecol 115:238–247, 1973.
13. Drumm JE, O'Rahilly R: The assessment of prenatal age from crown-rump length determined ultrasonically. Am J Anat 148:555–560, 1977.
14. deVries PA, Friedland GW: The staged, sequential development of the anus and rectum in human embryos and fetuses. J Pediatr Surg 9:755–796, 1974.
15. Friedland GW, deVries PA: Renal ectopia and fusion. Embryologic basis. Urology 5:698–706, 1975.
16. Warkany J, Nelson RC: Appearance of skeletal anomalies in the offspring of rats reared on a deficient diet. Science 92:383–384, 1940.
17. Fraser FC: The use of teratogens in the analysis of abnormal developmental mechanisms. *In* Fishbein M (ed): First International Conference on Congenital Malformations. Philadelphia, JB Lippincott, 1961.
18. deVries PA, Saunders JB: Development of the ventricles and spiral outflow tract of the human heart. Carnegie Inst Wash Publ 621, Contrib Embryol 256:87–114, 1962.
19. deVries PA: Evolution of precardiac and splanchnic mesoderm in relation to the infundibulum and truncus. *In:* Workshop of Mechanisms of Cardiac Morphogenesis and Teratogenesis. Institute d'Histologie et Embryologie, Paris. New York, Raven Press, 1979.
20. Quan L, Smith DW: The VATER association: Vertebral defects, anal atresia, TE fistula with esophageal atresia, radial and renal dysplasia. A spectrum of associated defects. J Pediatr 82:104–107, 1973.
21. Creizel A, Ludanyi I: An etiological study of the VACTERL association. Eur J Pediatr 144:331–337, 1985.
22. Green RA, Bloch MJ, Huff DS, Iozzo RV: MURCS association with additional congenital anomalies. Human Pathol 17:88–91, 1986.
23. Calavita N, Orazi C, Logroscino C, et al: Does MURCS association represent an actual nonrandom complex of malformations? Diagn Imag Clin Med 55:172–176, 1986.
24. Holder TM, Cloud DT, Lewis JE Jr, Pilling GP IV: Esophageal atresia and tracheo-esophageal fistula. A survey of its members by the Surgical Section of the American Academy of Pediatrics. Pediatrics 34:542, 1964.
25. Engle MA: Association urologic anomalies in infants and children with congenital heart disease. *In* El Shafie M, Klippel CH (eds): Associated Congenital Anomalies. Baltimore, Williams & Wilkins, 1981, pp 137–142.
26. Gupta NP, Gill IB: Skeletal anomalies associated with unilateral renal agenesis. Br J Urol 59:15–16, 1987.
27. Crvaric DM, Ruderman RJ, Conrad RW, et al: Congenital scoliosis and urinary tract abnormalities: Are intravenous pyelograms necessary? J Pediatr Orthop 7:441–443, 1987.
28. Hunt GM, Whitaker RH: The pattern of congenital renal anomalies associated with neural tube defects. Dev Med Child Neurol 29:91–95, 1987.
29. Barakat AY, Seikaly MG, Der Kaloustian VM: Urogenital abnormalities in genetic disease. J Urol 136:778–785, 1986.
30. McKusick VA: Mendelian Inheritance in Man: Catalogs of Autosomal Dominant, Autosomal Recessive and X-linked Phenotypes, 6th Ed. Baltimore, Johns Hopkins University Press, 1983.
31. Santulli TV, Schullinger TV, Kieswetter WB, Bill AH Jr: Imperforate anus: A survey from the members of the Surgical Section of the American Academy of Pediatrics. J Pediatr Surg 6:484–487, 1971.
32. Santulli TV, Kieswetter WB, Bill AH: Anorectal anomalies: A suggested international classification. J Pediatr Surg 5:281, 1970.
33. Browne D: Some congenital deformities of the rectum, anus, vagina and urethra. Ann Roy Coll Surg Engl 8:173.
34. Stephens FD: Congenital imperforate rectum, recto-urethral and recto-vaginal abnormalities. Aust NZ J Surg 22:161, 1953.
35. Stephens FD: Malformations of the anus. Aust NZ J Surg 23:9, 1953.
36. Stephens FD: Congenital rectal fistulae and their sphincters. Aust Pediatr 1:107, 1965.
37. deVries PA: Complications of surgery for congenital anomalies of the anorectum. *In* deVries PA, Shapiro SR (eds): Complications of Pediatric Surgery. New York, John Wiley & Sons, 1982, pp 233–262.
38. Shopfner CE: Roentgenologic evaluation of imperforate anus. South MJ 58:712–719, 1965.
39. Shopfner CE: Urologic aspects of ectopic anus (imperforate anus; anal atresia). *In* Witten DM, Myers GH, Utz DC (eds): Clinical Urography, 4th Ed. Philadelphia, WB Saunders Company, 1977, pp 791–801.
40. Peck AG, Poznanski AK: A simple device for genitography. Radiology 103:212, 1972.

41. Swenson O, Sherman JO, Fisher JH, et al: Diagnosis of congenital megacolon: An analysis of 501 patients. J Pediatr Surg 8:587, 1973.
42. Persky L: Urologic complications of surgery for imperforate anus. In deVries PA, Shapiro SR (eds): Complications of Pediatric Surgery. New York, John Wiley & Sons, 1982, pp 263–268.
43. Adkins JC, Klesewetter WB: Imperforate anus. Surg Clin North Am 56:379, 1976.
44. Smith ED: Urinary anomalies and complications in imperforate anus and rectum. J Pediatr Surg 3:337, 1968.
45. Stephens FD, Donnellan WL: "H-type" urethro-anal fistula. J Pediatr Surg 12:95–102, 1977.
46. deVries PA, Friedland GW: Congenital "H-type" anourethral fistula. Radiology 113:397–407, 1974.
47. Magee RK: Recto-urethral fistula. Report of a case. Lancet 1:140, 1948.
48. Le Duc E: Congenital rectourethral fistula: Report of a case without rectal anomaly. J Urol 93:272–275, 1965.
49. Nino-Murcia M, Friedland GW: Unusual fistulae between the rectum and the lower urinary tract: Simple techniques for diagnosis. Urol Radiol 9:240–242, 1988.
50. Rouse GA, Kaminsky CK, Saaty HP, et al: Current concepts in sonographic diagnosis of fetal renal disease. Radiographics 8:119–132, 1988.
51. Hill MC, Lande IM, Larsen JW: Prenatal diagnosis of fetal anomalies using ultrasound and MRI. Radiol Clin North Am 26:287–307, 1988.
52. Bowie JD, Rosenberg ER, Andreotti RF, Fields SI: The changing sonographic appearance of fetal kidneys during pregnancy. J Ultrasound Med 2:505–507, 1983.
53. Crannum P, Bracken M, Silverman R, Hobbins JC: Assessment of fetal kidney size in normal gestation by comparison of ratio of kidney circumference to abdominal circumference. Am J Obstet Gynecol 136:249–254, 1980.
54. Jeanty P, Dramaix-Wilmet M, Elkhazen N, et al: Measurement of fetal kidney growth on ultrasound. Radiology 144:159–162, 1982.
55. Smith FG, Adams FH, Borden M, et al: Fetus and newborn: Studies of renal function in the intact fetal lamb. Am J Obstet Gynecol 96:240–246, 1966.
56. Harrison MR, Nakayama DK, Noall R, et al: Correction of congenital hydronephrosis in utero. II: Decompression reverses the effects of obstruction on the fetal lung and urinary tract. J Pediatr Surg 17:965–974, 1982.
57. Allen RW, Rehm NE, Scott JR, et al: Antepartum diagnosis and intrapartum management of lethal renal defects. Obstet Gynecol 58:379–382, 1981.
58. Harman CR: Maternal furosemide may not provoke urine production in the compromised fetus. Am J Obstet Gynecol 140:322–323, 1984.
59. Raghavendra BN, Young BK, Greco MA, et al: Use of furosemide in pregnancies complicated by oligohydramnios. Radiology 165:455–458, 1987.
60. Hoddick WK, Filly RA, Mahony BS, Callen CW: Minimal fetal renal pyelectasis. J Ultrasound Med 4:85–89, 1985.
61. Allen KS, Arger PH, Mennuti M, et al: Effects of maternal hydration on fetal renal pyelectasis. Radiology 163:807–809, 1987.
62. Kleiner B, Callen PW, Filly R: Sonographic analysis of the fetus with ureteropelvic junction obstruction. AJR 148:359, 1987.
63. Brown T, Mandell J, Lebowitz RL: Neonatal hydronephrosis in the era of sonography. AJR 148:959, 1987.
64. Glazer GM, Filly RA, Callen PW: The varied sonographic appearance of the urinary tract in the fetus and newborn with urethral obstruction. Radiology 144:563–568, 1982.
65. Fong KW, Rahmani MR, Rose TH, et al: Fetal renal cystic disease: Sonographic-pathologic correlation. AJR 146:767, 1986.
66. Mahony BS, Filly RA, Callen PW, et al: Fetal renal dysplasia: Sonographic evaluation. Radiology 152:143–146, 1984.
67. Ahmed S, Le Quesne GW: Urological anomalies detected on antenatal ultrasound: A 9-year review. Aust Paediatr J 24:178–183, 1988.
68. Harnett JD, Green JS, Cramer BC, et al: The spectrum of renal disease in Laurence-Moon-Biedl syndrome. N Engl J Med 319:615–618, 1988.
69. Hayden SA, Russ PD, Pretorius DH, et al: Posterior urethral obstruction. Prenatal sonographic findings and clinical outcome in fourteen cases. J Ultrasound Med 7:371–375, 1988.
70. Boechat MI, Kangarloo H: MR imaging in Drash syndrome. J Comput Assist Tomogr 12:405–408, 1988.
71. Cardwell MS: Bilateral renal agenesis: Clinical implications. South Med J 81:327–328, 1988.

CONGENITAL ANOMALIES OF THE KIDNEY

NORMAL DEVELOPMENT

The permanent kidney—the metanephros—develops sequentially within the intermediate mesoderm from nephric tissue called the pronephros and mesonephros. A knowledge of the sequential development of these tissues is necessary to understand both normal and pathological renal organogenesis.

Intermediate Mesoderm

The very earliest stages in the development of the kidneys can be traced at a remarkably early stage of embryonic development: specifically, to Stage 6 (see page 559 for a discussion of stages). At this point, the future embryonic body is a flat disc, appropriately called the germ disc (embryonic disc).

The amniotic cavity is on one side of the germ disc; this side is covered with a single layer of cells, called the epiblastic layer. On the other side is another cavity, the yolk sac; this side is also coated by a single layer of cells, called the hypoblastic layer (Fig. 19–17).

The epiblastic layer becomes the ectoderm, and the hypoblastic layer becomes the endoderm. The hypoblastic layer is continuous with a layer of cells that line the yolk sac; the epiblastic layer is continuous with the ectoderm lining the amniotic cavity (Fig. 19–17).

Nephric cells are derived from specific cells of the epiblastic layer. They migrate to the primitive streak in the midline in the caudal portion of the embryonic disc. They evaginate into the primitive streak and are then distributed between the epiblastic and hypoblastic layers (Fig. 19–18).[1, 2]

These cells then become the intermediate mesoderm, so called because it lies between two other mesodermal components, the paraxial somites and the lateral plate (Fig. 19–19). The portion of the intermediate mesoderm connecting the most cranial 10 somites with the lateral plate is partially divided into 10 segments. Caudal to the 10th somite, however, the intermediate mesoderm is not segmented and forms a continuous cord. Because of its cordlike shape, and because it is the primordium of the lower pronephros and the mesonephros, this structure is called the nephrogenic cord (nephric cord).

The lateral plates and the most cranial portion of the intermediate mesoderm soon split into two layers. The

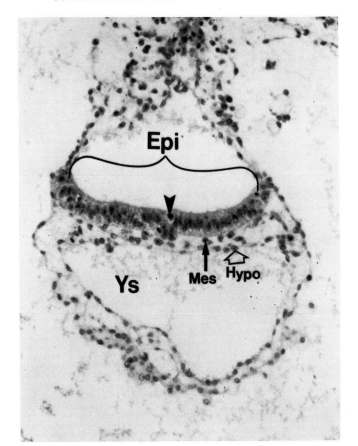

Figure 19–17. Transverse section through the primitive streak area of a Stage-7 embryo. Within the amniotic cavity is a bracket over the embryonic disc or epiblastic layer. The arrowhead points to the primitive streak, which is giving off cells into the space between the epiblast and hypoblast. These cells (*black arrow, Mes*) are the mesoblastic cells. The hypoblast (*open arrow, hypo*) is the primordium of the endoderm and is continuous with the more peripheral layer of cells surrounding the remainder of the yolk sac (Ys), just as the amniotic ectoderm is continuous with the epiblast around the amniotic cavity. (Embryo 7802, Carnegie Collection.)

AGE GROUPS 8–10
18–24 Days
Middle of 3rd to Middle of 4th Week

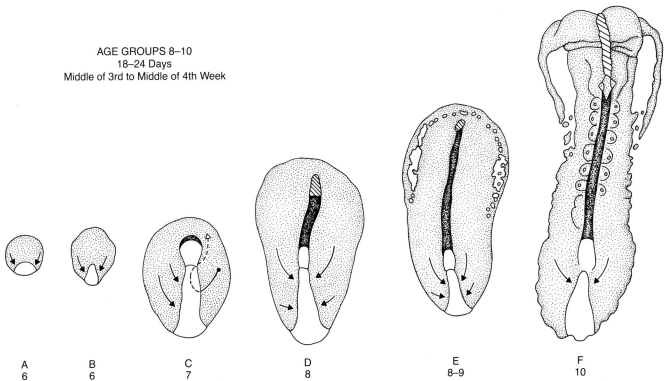

| A | B | C | D | E | F |
| 6 | 6 | 7 | 8 | 8–9 | 10 |

Figure 19–18. Illustrations of embryos during early stages of development show relative changes in size and configuration as viewed from above. Arrows show the direction of cell migration toward the caudosagittal primitive streak. Dotted and open arrow in C, Stage 7, shows the direction of migration of mesoblastic cells, which is craniolateral, following invagination at the primitive streak. Stages are as follows: A, Stage 6A; B, Stage 6B, appearance of primitive streak, Day 14; C, Stage 7, formation of notochordal process, Days 15 to 17; D, Stage 8, notochordal and neurenteric, Days 17–19; E, Stage 9, beginning of somites, Days 19 to 21; F, Stage 10, 4 to 12 somites, Days 22 to 23. (Modified from Streeter GL: Development of the mesoblast and notochord in pig embryos. Carnegie Inst Wash Publ 380, Contrib Embryol 19:73–92, 1927.)

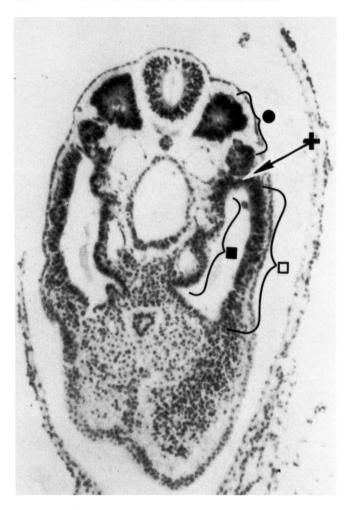

Figure 19–19. Cross section of a late Stage-10 embryo (Carnegie Collection) showing the three primary components of the embryonic mesoblast: somites (on the left side, *bracket and solid circle*); intermediate mesoblast *(solid arrow and cross)*; splanchnic layer of the lateral plate *(medial bracket and solid square)*; lateral to the coelomic cavity, somatic layer of the lateral plage *(bracket and open square)*.

outermost is called the somatic mesoderm; the inner, the splanchnic mesoderm. As a result of this split, a cavity called the coelom is formed between the layers (Fig. 19–19).

Three pairs of excretory organs develop sequentially in the intermediate mesoderm: the pronephros, mesonephros, and metanephros. It should be remembered, however, that these divisions are somewhat arbitrary; the evolving tissue is much more homogeneous than these terms might indicate.

Staged Sequential Development of the Pronephros and Primary Nephric Duct in Human Embryos

The pronephros is an incomplete abbreviated organ. It is so rudimentary and transient that some investigators argue that this most cranial portion of the intermediate mesoderm does not properly deserve this phylogenetic name.[3, 4] Its importance, however, lies in the fact that it establishes the primary nephric duct (Fig. 19–20). This event occurs in Stage-10 embryos (about 22 to 23 days, with eight to 10 somites), during which time the pronephric tubules appear.

Two theories exist regarding the formation of the primary nephric duct. The first is that it is the result of fusion of the segment tubules of the pronephros;[5] the second is that it is formed in situ by the delamination of epithelial cells of the coelomic cavity.

The more cranially located tubules of the pronephros degenerate as the caudal tubules develop. The pronephros reaches its greatest length in Stage-11 embryos (23 to 26 days with 14 somites), at which time it extends from the

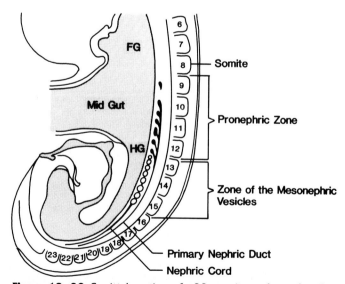

Figure 19–20. Sagittal section of a 23-somite embryo showing the developing pronephros, primary nephric duct, mesonephros, and nephric cord. (Modified from Felix W: The development of the urogenital organs. *In* Keibel F, Mall FP (eds): Manual of Human Embryology, Vol 2. Philadelphia, JB Lippincott Company, 1912.)

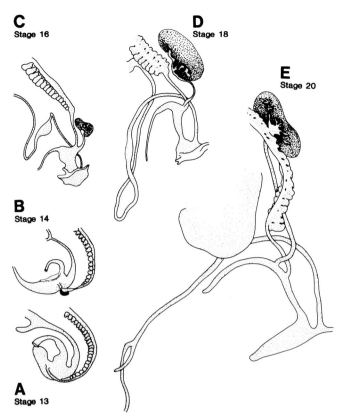

C
Stage 16

D
Stage 18

E
Stage 20

B
Stage 14

A
Stage 13

Figure 19–21. Sagittal view of the cloaca, hindgut, mesonephros, developing metanephros, primary nephric duct, ureter, and anorectum from Stages 13 through 20, all at the same magnification. (Modified from Shikinami J: Detailed form of the wolffian body in human embryos of the first 8 weeks. Carnegie Inst Publ 363, Contrib Embryol 18:49–61, 1926.)

tubules develop, extends down to about the level of the 26th somite (L3) by the beginning of Stage 13 (about 28 days). By this time each mesonephros contains 33 to 34 tubules, but the number per primary segment (somite) varies (Fig. 19–21A). By this stage the cranial growth of mesonephric tubules has ceased, and craniocaudal degeneration begins, but caudal tubular growth and differentiation continue. This results in a remarkably stable number of tubules through Stage 20 (51 to 52 days) (Fig. 19–21E).

During this period of longitudinal growth, which began at Stage 11 (about 24 days), the mesonephros expands. As a result, the secondary and collecting ducts are larger than those of the pronephros, and the malpighian corpuscles are considerably larger than those subsequently formed in the metanephros. The first result is a widening of the middle plate and the establishment of the dorsal coelomic wall on either side of the gut. This is followed by bilateral protrusions into the coelomic cavity along the length of the mesonephroi (Fig. 19–22A to C). These are the urogenital folds, into which the genital organs grow (Fig. 19–22D). After involution of the rostral portion of the mesonephroi in Stage 22 (embryonic length of 23 to 28 mm, 54 to 56 days) the folds are limited to the lumbar region. It is believed that the human mesonephros may transiently excrete prior to involution.

Some mesonephric tubules in the lumbar area play an important role in the development of the male reproductive system; others account for the development of some nonfunctional structures. Some 30 mesonephric arteries on each side originally supply the mesonephros only; however, those in the lower thoracic and lumbar regions are more numerous (like the nephric ducts) and will persist, eventually supplying the metanephros as well as the reproductive glands, suprarenal glands, and diaphragm (Fig. 19–23).

Staged Sequential Development of the Metanephros in Human Embryos and Fetuses

The first sign of the developing permanent kidneys (metanephroi) is the appearance of fusiform dilatations of the primary nephric ducts in embryos of Stage 13 (28 to 32 days) at the angulation, caudal to the mesonephroi, where they cross the nephrogenic cord ventrally, from a lateral to medial direction, to join the cloaca. The dorsomedial hemicircumference of each dilated segment is surrounded by condensations of mesenchymal cells, the metanephrogenic blastema (Fig. 19–24).

It is important for the metanephrogenic blastema to be in close contact with the primary nephric duct, in order that the ureteral bud can develop.[9] The metanephrogenic blastema secretes an inductor substance,[9] which induces the bud to grow out of the primary nephric duct. The ureteral bud, in turn, secretes inductor substances[9] that later induce the secretory tubules within the metanephrogenic blastema. This is a classic example of mutual induction.

During Stage 14 (32 to 35 days), the bilateral dilatations are transformed into dorsally protruding hollow ureteral buds of single-layered columnar epithelium that become enveloped by the multilayered blastema. This metanephrogenic tissue additionally extends cranially, between the

7th somite (3rd cervical segment) to the 14th somite (2nd thoracic segment).

By the end of Stage 12 (26 to 30 days), the pronephros, the cells of which are disappearing into the mesenchyme, has degenerated.[6] The free-growing ends of the primary nephric ducts below the 14th somite, however, have continued their growth down between the ectoderm and the nephrogenic cord. At the level of the 27th or 28th somite (L4 or L5), they angle ventromedially to reach the cloaca. By Stage 13 (28 to 32 days), when embryos are 4 to 5 mm long, the partially canalized primary nephric ducts open into the cloaca (Fig. 19–21A).

Staged Sequential Development of the Mesonephros in Human Embryos

The mesonephros develops below the pronephros in the caudal extensions of the nephrogenic cord. The mesonephros slightly overlaps the pronephros owing to rostral mesonephric growth. The developed primary nephric duct (see above) induces the mesonephric tubules.[1]

The mesonephric tubules differ from the pronephric tubules in at least two respects: (1) Bowman's capsule is vascularized by an artery arising from the aorta and a vein arising from the posterior cardinal vein to form a glomerulus, and (2) the mesonephric tubules are unambiguously united with the primary nephric ducts.

Each nephrogenic cord, within which the mesonephric

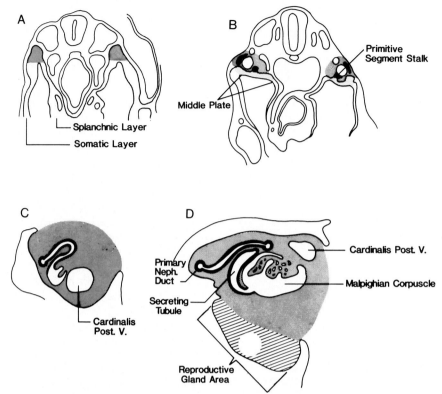

Figure 19–22. During Stages 11 through 16, the intermediate mesoderm broadens with the development of the mesonephroi and their relatively large malpighian corpuscles. *A,* Cross section through a Stage-11 embryo shows virtually no dorsal wall to the coelomic cavities between the splanchnic and somatic layers of the mesoderm *(light stipple).* Cross-hatched areas show the nephrogenic cords, the site of future mesonephroi at this level. *B,* Cross section through Stage-12 embryo shows widening of the posterior coelomic wall with the development of bilateral middle plates as a result of growth and development of the mesonephroi. *C,* Further developmental stage of mesonephros shows the urogenital fold now protruding into the coelomic cavity. *D,* Cross section through the right urogenital fold of a Stage-16 embryo shows the mature secreting tubule and the developing reproductive gland area of the urogenital fold. (Modified from Felix W: The development of the urogenital organs. *In* Keibel F, Mall FP (eds): Manual of Human Embryology, Vol 2. Philadelphia, JB Lippincott Company, 1912.)

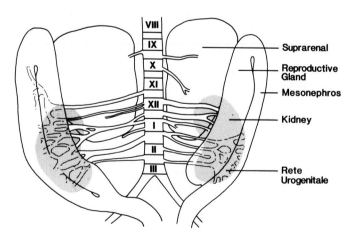

Figure 19–23. Semidiagrammatic illustration of the blood supply to the mesonephros, kidney, and suprarenal and reproductive glands, showing arteries arising from the aorta between the T9 and L3 segments. (Modified from Felix W: The development of the urogenital organs. *In* Keibel F, Mall FP (eds): Manual of Human Embryology. Philadelphia, JB Lippincott Company, 1912.)

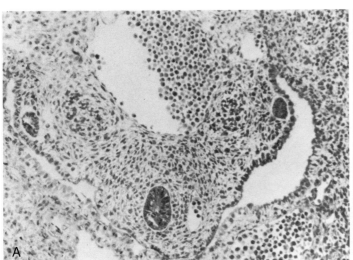

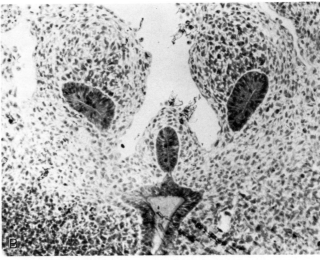

Figure 19–24. Cross sections of a Stage-13 embryo in three regions of the developing metanephros. *A,* At the cranial pole of the metanephrogenic blastema, each primary nephric duct can be seen just beneath the coelomic epithelium. The most cephalic portion of the metanephrogenic blastema lies on either side, just ventrolateral to the aorta. The hindgut is ventral and in the midline. *B,* The expanded primary nephric duct is on either side at the site of the future ureteral bud. The metanephrogenic blastema lies dorsal and medial to the expanded ducts. The hindgut joins the ventrally placed cloaca. *C,* The caudal level of the metanephrogenic blastema is shown, with the dilated primary nephric ducts inducing an orientation of the blastema. The terminal primary nephric duct is joining the cloaca, as is the hindgut. (From the Carnegie Collection.)

ureteral bud and the lower mesonephric tubules. During the next three stages, the metanephrogenic tissue is comet-shaped (Fig. 19–25).

In Stage 15 (35 to 37 days), the growing tips of the two ureteral buds become the bulbous ampullas; the relatively narrow stems from each primary duct become the ureters.

Surrounding the ampullas are two layers of cells: (1) an inner, dense metanephric blastema, the epithelial cells of which have radially oriented oval nuclei, and (2) a surrounding zwischenblastem, the cells of which have round nuclei and no detectable orientation. This outer, less dense mesenchymal tissue is pseudolamellar, and it becomes the capsule and the interstial tissue of the kidneys (Fig. 19–26). At this stage, the cells of the dorsomedial metanephrogenic blastema proliferate, causing the two metanephrogenic blastemas to grow together, and almost touch at the midline.

Simultaneously, the ureters lengthen and the angle between each lengthening ureter and the proximal primary nephric duct becomes progressively more acute. This progressive change in the angle can make it appear that the kidneys are ascending, although this is not the case; at this stage the metanephroi remain in the same position relative to the mesonephroi. A genuine ascent follows; the kidneys migrate cranially, dorsal to the mesonephroi, and ascend relative to the somites lying dorsally in the longitudinal axis and relative to the urogenital folds. This ascent is due in part to the straightening of the embryo, since the ventral side of the embryo is growing faster than the dorsal side, as well as to the increased length of the kidneys and the ureters themselves during Stages 16 through 23.

After the ampullas are formed by the expansion of the terminal ends of the ureteral buds and their tubular derivatives, they progressively divide into two. In Stage 16 (37 to 42 days), the first such dichotomous budding has led to the formation of a "primary renal pelvis" with both cranial and caudal poles (Fig. 19–27).

The kidneys, once almost touching, have been separating since the latter part of Stage 15; they now begin their ascent, passing between the two umbilical arteries, which appear to form a kind of girdle surrounding them.

Three Periods of Nephron and Tubular Development

There are three periods of nephron and tubular development within the embryonic kidney.

First Period

During Stage 17 (42 to 44 days), second- and third-generation buds develop from the ampullas at the poles

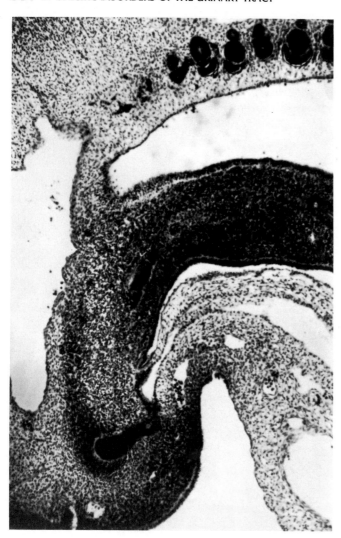

Figure 19–25. Sagittal section through Stage-14 embryo shows the developing ureteral bud surrounded by the metanephrogenic blastema, which extends cranially toward the mesonephroi and is known as the *zwischenblastem*. (From the Carnegie Collection.)

Figure 19–26. Sagittal section of a Stage-15 embryo shows the thick-walled cloaca continuous with both the allantois, which extends into the body stalk, and the primary nephric duct entering the cloaca. The ureter is longer than in Stage 14 and now extends dorsocranially to its ampullary dilatation, which is surrounded by metanephrogenic blastema, the cells of which are oriented radially. The zwischenblastem extends cranially and has an appearance like the tail of a comet. (From the Carnegie Collection.)

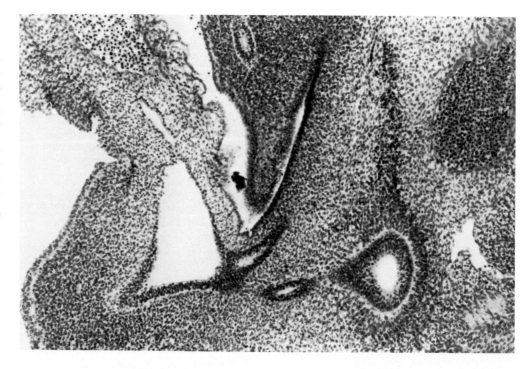

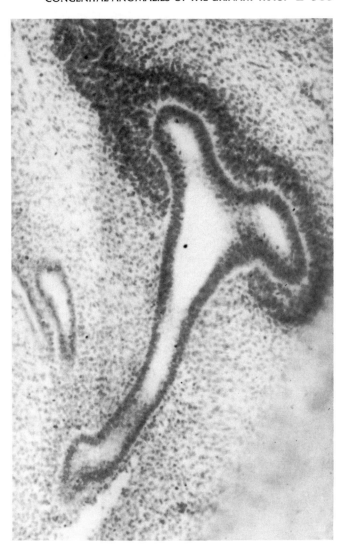

Figure 19–27. The first dichotomous budding of the ureteral ampulla is apparent as cranial and caudal diverticula. They are surrounded by metanephrogenic blastema, which extends cranially into the zwischenblastem. Note the greater area of blastema cranially. (From the Carnegie Collection.)

of the developing kidney (Fig. 19–28B–C). The metanephrogenic mantle divides as these buds develop. This budding is dichotomous and can be symmetrical or asymmetrical;[14] the developing branches tend to be longer at the poles and shorter in the interpolar area. At the poles the tubules divide faster. Consequently, the number of buds in the polar regions is almost twice that of the interpolar areas (Fig. 19–28E).

By Stage 18 (44 to 48 days), the kidneys have ascended above the umbilical arteries (Fig. 19–29); by Stage 19 (48 to 51 days), five generations branch at the poles of the kidneys, and three in the interpolar areas. At this point, 15 to 20 renal vesicles appear simultaneously, adjacent to the ampullas that induce them (Figs. 19–30[1] and 31). These are the primordial nephrons; in rapid succession they become ovoid, and then S-shaped by Stage 20 (51

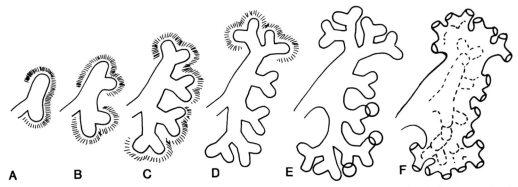

Figure 19–28. Development of the renal pelvis showing the renal blastema orienting around the dichotomously dividing ampulla. A shows the first dichotomous branching. B shows the second, C, the third, D, the fourth, and E, the fifth. The circles in E indicate the possible location of minor calyces at the level of the third-, fourth-, or fifth-generation branches. F indicates the ureteral bud branches that may dilate to form the renal pelvis. (Modified from Osathanondh V, Potter EL: Development of human kidney as shown by microdissection. Arch Pathol 76:271–302, 1963. Copyright 1963, American Medical Association.)

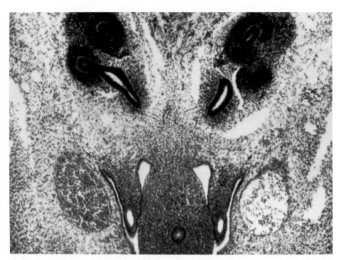

Figure 19–29. Frontal section through a Stage-18 embryo shows first-generation ampullary and ductal portions of the metanephros' collecting system on each side. Below are the primary nephric (wolffian) ducts, medial to the umbilical arteries and flanking the hindgut. (From the Carnegie Collection.)

to 53 days). Finally, the lower limb of the nephron expands and becomes Bowman's capsule (Figs. 19–30[3] and 19–32).

By Stages 21 and 22, the nephrons become attached to the ampullas; the glomerular vessels grow into an expanded, spoon-shaped capsule (Fig. 19–30[4]).

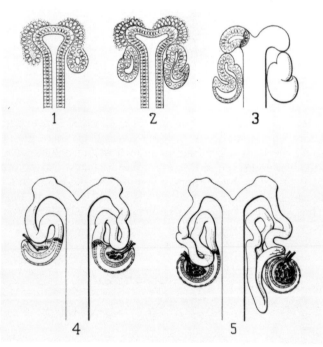

Figure 19–30. Semidiagrammatic figures of the primordia and differentiation of renal vesicles, and early developmental stages of the uriniferous tubules. *1*, Metanephrogenic blastema surrounding the ampullary expansion of the duct and early appearance of a renal vesicle are shown. *2*, Early vesicles develops adjacent to and below the dichotomously dividing ampulla. *3* Beginning of the S-shaped stage of tubular development is shown, just before fusion with the collecting tubule. *4* and *5*, Successive stages in the development of the tubule, Bowman's capsule, and glomerulus are shown. (From Huber CC: On the development and shape of uriniferous tubules of certain of the higher mammals. Am J Anat 4:1–98, 1905.)

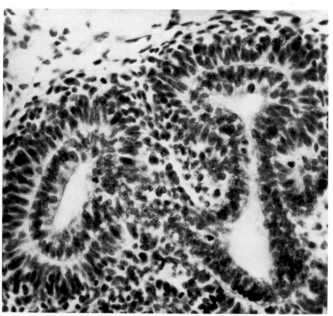

Figure 19–31. Section through the metanephros of a Stage-19 embryo showing the two branches of a dichotomous division. The one on the right has an early renal vesicle. (Embryo 4501, Carnegie Collection.)

In the same developing kidney, it is possible to see different stages; the first generation of nephrons continues to develop, but new nephrons are continuously being added at the periphery. The ampullas continue to grow and split and to induce the metanephrogenic mantle. By Stage 23 (56 to 60 days), the end of the embryonic period, large glomeruli appear and the secretory tubules have lengthened (Fig. 19–30[5]) and dilated to become 10 to 20 minor calyces (Fig. 19–28E). The proximal ends have dilated to become 4 to 10 major calyces (Fig. 19–28F). By 63 to 64 days, urine excretion may actually begin.

The whole process of dichotomous branching lasts until

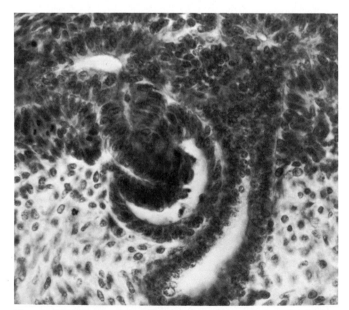

Figure 19–32. Section through the metanephros of a Stage-20 embryo, showing a significant advance over Stage 19 in the development of the nephron. It now has an S-shaped expansion of the lower limb which is destined to become Bowman's capsule. (Embryo 5537, Carnegie Collection.)

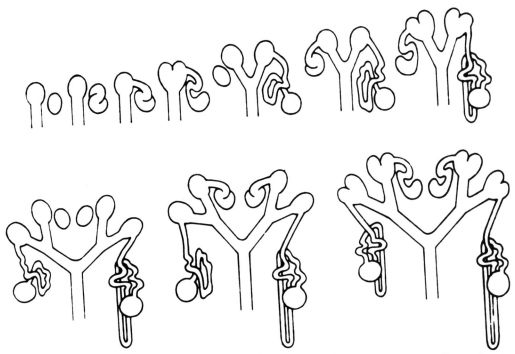

Figure 19–33. Kidney development during the first period. In dichotomous branching of the ampullas, a developing nephron is carried peripherally by continued growth of the tubule, ampulla formation, and division. (From Osathanondh V, Potter EL: Development of human kidney as shown by microdissection. Arch Pathol 76:277–289, 1963. Copyright 1963, American Medical Association.)

the 14th to the 15th week,[10] but only the ampullas not attached to a nephron can induce new ones. The nephron attached to the ampulla is carried to the periphery of the developing kidney, because the terminal end of the tubule continues to grow, to form new ampullas, and to divide (Fig. 19–33).

Second Period

During the second period of growth, which may occur from the 14th or 15th week to the 20th to 22nd week, the ampulla continues to grow but does not divide. Instead, it induces multiple (up to 14) new nephrons in series (Fig. 19–34). Each nephron, in turn, shifts its connection from the ampulla to the connecting tubule below it, so that by

the end of the second period a nephronic arcade appears with a single long main connecting tubule (Fig. 19–34).

Third Period

During the third period of growth, between 32 and 36 weeks, any remaining unbranched ampullas induce new nephrons, provided that no nephron was previously attached. Each new nephron attaches to the collecting tubule just proximal to the ampullas and differentiates serially. This is repeated four to seven times and finally leads to a terminal unbranched collecting tubule. The glomeruli belonging to the serial nephrons form the outer portion of the cortex (Fig. 19–35). Figure 19–36 illustrates the relationship of the uriniferous tubules to the collecting ducts.

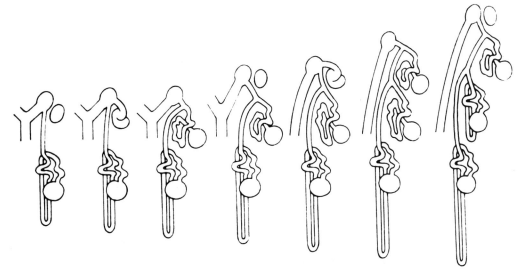

Figure 19–34. In the second period of kidney development, nondividing ampullas induce nephrons in the form of an arcade. (From Osathanondh V, Potter EL: Development of the human kidney as shown by microdissection. Arch Pathol 76:277–289, 1963. Copyright 1963, American Medical Association.)

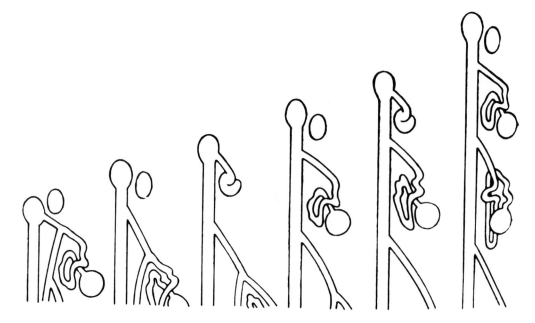

Figure 19–35. In the third period of kidney development, nonbranching ampullas induce new nephrons after each preceding nephron has been left behind on the duct. (From Osathanondh V, Potter EL: Development of the human kidney as shown by microdissection. Arch Pathol 76:277–289, 1963. Copyright 1963, American Medical Association.)

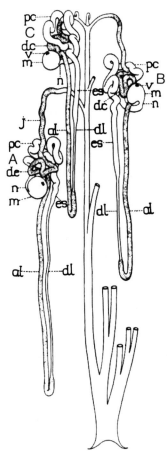

Figure 19–36. Diagram illustrates three uriniferous tubules and their relation to a collecting tubule: *A,* A tubule, the malpighian corpuscle of which is situated in the lowermost portion of the cortex; *B,* the approximate middle of the cortex; *C,* the outer portion of the cortex. (m = Malpighi's corpuscle, v = vessel porta, n = neck, pc = proximal convoluted portion, es = end segment, dl = descending limb, al = ascending limb of Henle's loop, dc = distal convoluted portion, j = junctional tubule, c = collecting tubule.) (From Huber CC: On the development and shape of uriniferous tubules of certain of the higher mammals. Am J Anat 4:1–98, 1905.)

CLASSIFICATION OF CONGENITAL ANOMALIES OF THE KIDNEY

Table 19–12 shows the classification of the major congenital anomalies of the kidney. (See Section 3, Chapters 34 to 42, for further information on congenital cystic disease of the kidney.)

Anomalies in Number

Supernumerary Kidneys

Supernumerary kidneys are present when the total number of kidneys exceeds two.[15–18] This can refer to more than two separate kidneys, or to a horseshoe kidney with an additional kidney (or kidneys). One individual may have as many as five supernumerary kidneys. A supernumerary kidney is functioning and kidney-shaped, completely surrounded by a capsule, and either not attached or attached very loosely to the usual kidney. It may be found above, below, in front of, or behind the usual kidney. It is nearly always smaller than normal or in an abnormal position, or both. Rarely, however, it may be the same size or larger than a normal kidney. It may be associated with cloacal exstrophy.

EMBRYOLOGY OF SUPERNUMERARY KIDNEYS

The earliest evidence of supernumerary kidneys in human embryos seen thus far is in Stage 16 (Fig. 19–37). Because this is long after primary induction, which occurs in Stage 13, no one has seen the true early development of the supernumerary kidney. Consequently, at this point we can only form hypotheses.

DeVries Hypothesis. In order to understand this hypothesis, as well as others, it might be helpful to review the relevant embryology. The primary nephric duct angles ventromedially immediately before it enters the cloaca; at the point of angulation, in Stage 13, the dorsomedial aspect dilates. The metanephrogenic blastema surrounds

Table 19–12. Classification of the Major Congenital Anomalies of the Kidney

A. Anomalies in number
  1. Supernumerary kidneys
  2. Renal agenesis
B. Anomalies in size
  1. Renal hypoplasia
    a. Dwarf kidney
    b. Thin kidney
    c. Oligomeganephronia
    d. The Ask-Upmark kidney
  2. Renal dysplasia
  3. Compensatory hypertrophy
C. Anomalies in position
  1. Anomalies of rotation
  2. Renal ectopia
    a. Ipsilateral ectopia
    b. Crossed renal ectopia
D. Anomalies in form: Renal fusion
  1. Horseshoe kidney
  2. Disc kidney
  3. Crossed fused ectopia
E. Anomalies in structure
  1. Large septa of Bertin (cloisons)
  2. Fetal lobation
  3. Congenital polar enlargement
  4. Other congenital masses composed of normal renal parenchyma ("pseudotumors")
  5. Congenital indentation of the left kidney
  6. Cystic diseases

blastema caudally than cranially. This is the case because the metanephrogenic blastema is delimited more sharply caudally than cranially, because cranially an additional comet-shaped tail of blastema could contribute to the renal parenchyma (Fig. 19–26).

Pohlman Hypothesis. Although it is less well developed, the Pohlman hypothesis is very similar to the deVries hypothesis.[19] The bifurcation of the ureteral bud, for example, takes place near the wolffian duct.

Geisinger Hypothesis. This hypothesis suggests either that the ureteral bud divides prematurely or that two buds come off the wolffian duct.[20] Geisinger proposes that the metanephrogenic blastema also divides. Thus, in the case of a bifurcated ureter, each limb has an independent mass of metanephrogenic blastema around it, or if two ureteral buds are present, a mass of metanephrogenic blastema develops independently around each.

Felix Hypothesis. According to this hypothesis, a phylogenetic "reversion" has occurred, such that one or more cephalically placed mesonephric ureters are present, in addition to a single caudal metanephric ureter.[5]

N'Guessan and Stephens Hypothesis.[16] This hypothesis states that separate twin metanephroi lie one behind the other. Each is induced by a branch of a bifid ureteral bud or by one or two separate ureteral buds.

this eccentric dilatation, and in Stage 14 this dilatation becomes the ureteral bud, which protrudes into the metanephrogenic blastema. In Stage 15, this bud develops a bulbous termination (the ampulla) and a narrow stem.

The metanephrogenic blastema forms a cap around this single ampulla, through Stages 13, 14, and 15. During these stages, the incipient ureter lengthens because of tubular interstitial growth. At Stage 16, the ampulla divides dichotomously. This first generation of ampullary buds is usually referred to as the cephalic and caudal poles of the primary renal pelvis.

If the first generation of ampullary buds come off the incipient ureter in late Stage 13, before the ureter has lengthened appreciably, and assuming that they do so in the usual manner (i.e., cranially and caudally at 180 degrees), then the metanephrogenic blastema would aggregate around and be induced by these widely separated ampullas. The result eventually would be two separate kidneys.

According to this hypothesis, whether the supernumerary kidney had a separate ureter or bifid ureters would depend on whether interstial growth of the incipient ureter had occurred during Stages 13 and 14.

Thus, the deVries hypothesis does not postulate any abnormality of the metanephrogenic blastema. It is consistent with the fact that either the cranial or the caudal kidney is called supernumerary, depending on which is the smaller on that side.

This hypothesis explains the hypoplasia without dysplasia, which is characteristic of the supernumerary kidney, as follows: If the inducing ampulla happens to be near either end of the metanephrogenic blastema, the amount of parenchyma the developed kidney will possess is determined by the fact that there is less blastema near the ends than elsewhere, meaning the developed kidney will be hypoplastic. The location of the supernumerary kidney is usually caudal, because there is less metanephrogenic

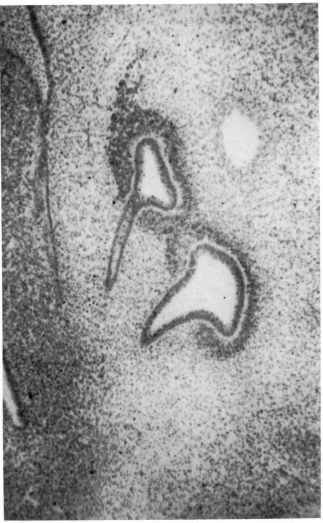

Figure 19–37. Section through duplicate ureteral buds and their surrounding metanephrogenic blastema in a Stage-16 embryo. (Embryo 6516, Carnegie Collection.)

Table 19–13. Difference Between a Duplex and a Supernumerary Kidney

Structure	Supernumerary Kidney	Duplex Kidney
Parenchyma	Completely separate	Both poles firmly attached to each other
Capsule	Completely separate	A single continuous capsule surrounds both poles
Number of calyces	Greater	Does not exceed number on opposite side

DIFFERENCE BETWEEN DUPLEX AND SUPERNUMERARY KIDNEYS

A supernumerary kidney may be confused with one pole of a duplex kidney. However, a clear distinction can be made between the two (Table 19–13).

INCIDENCE

Supernumerary kidneys are rare. About 60 cases have been described in the world literature.[16] Males and females are equally affected, and the average age at time of discovery is 36 years.* One patient with bilateral supernumerary kidneys has been reported.[16]

CLASSIFICATION AND ANATOMY

Two types of supernumerary kidney exist: (1) that drained by a bifid ureter, and (2) that drained by a separate ureter. The supernumerary ureter lies either behind or in front of the usual ureter.

When the ureters draining the usual and the supernumerary kidney are bifid, the supernumerary kidney nearly always lies below the usual kidney (Figs. 19–37 and 19–38). The junction of the two ureters in such cases is Y-shaped, although occasionally it has an inverted Y shape, because the supernumerary kidney may be located below the junction of the two ureters.

When separate ureters drain both the supernumerary and the usual kidney, the supernumerary kidney nearly always lies cranial to the usual kidney. In addition, the orifice of the ureter draining it, consistent with the Weigert-R Meyer rule, usually inserts distal to the orifice of the ureter draining the usual kidney (Fig. 19–39). Occasional exceptions occur.

If both a horseshoe and a supernumerary kidney are present, the half of the horseshoe kidney on the side of the body containing the supernumerary kidney is always small. The ureter draining the supernumerary kidney can be bifid or separate.

COMPLICATIONS

Complications vary, according to whether a bifid or separate ureter is present (Table 19–14).

IMAGING OF SUPERNUMERARY KIDNEYS

The intravenous urogram sometimes shows a complete additional kidney, nearly always smaller than usual; on rare occasions it may be normal or larger (Figs. 19–40 to

*Begg's report of a patient with "six kidneys" is intriguing, as several of the renal units appeared primordial. However, the report was not surgically confirmed, and the case must be viewed as one of bilateral triplex ureters, rather than as true supernumerary kidneys.[216]

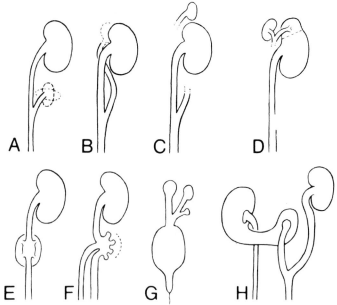

Figure 19–38. Diagram illustrates the various patterns of urinary drainage when the ureters draining the usual and the supernumerary kidney are bifid. (From N'Guessan G, Stephens FD: Supernumerary kidney. J Urol 130(4):649–653, © by Williams & Wilkins, 1983.)

19–42). It is nearly always above the usual kidney when there is a separate ureter, and usually below when there is a bifid ureter. In either case it may be in front of or

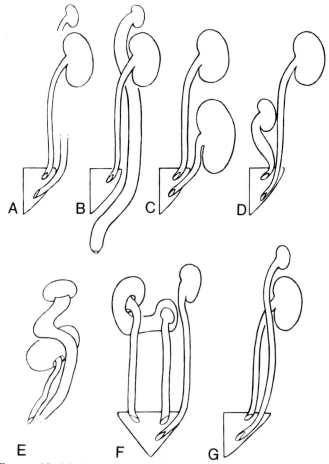

Figure 19–39. Diagram illustrates the various patterns of urinary drainage of supernumerary and ipsilateral kidneys when separate ureters drain both the supernumerary and the usual kidney. (From N'Guessan G, Stephens FD: Supernumerary kidney. J Urol 130(4):649–653, © by Williams & Wilkins, 1983.)

Table 19–14. Complications of Supernumerary Kidneys

I. Supernumerary kidney with bifid or single ureter: increased incidence of renal malignancy
II. Supernumerary kidney with bifid ureter
A. Stones—50%
B. Hydronephrosis—50%

behind the usual kidney. The side of a horseshoe kidney on side of the body containing the supernumerary kidney is always smaller.

Because the function of a small or diseased supernumerary kidney may be impaired, opacification of the collecting system is often poor, and it easy to overlook an additional renal unit. It may be impossible by urography alone to determine whether the kidneys are separate or fused, but this determination can usually be made by scintigraphy (Fig. 19–43), arteriography, ultrasonography (Fig. 19–44), or computed tomography (CT) (Fig. 19–45).

Renal Agenesis

The term agenesis of the kidney refers to a kidney that fails to develop.

INCIDENCE AND PATHOGENESIS

Bilateral agenesis is rare. Unilateral agenesis occurs in about 1 in 1000 of the general population.[21]

One recent series showed that, of patients having angiograms performed for hypertension, 3.2% have unilateral renal agenesis.[22] Another report,[23] however, suggests that all patients with hypertension and apparent

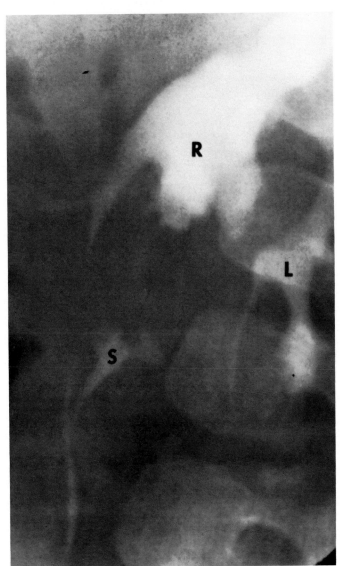

Figure 19–41. Excretory urogram, right posterior oblique view, showing the calyces and pelves of the normal right (R) and left (L) kidneys. The calyces and pelvis of the small supernumerary kidney (S) lie caudal to the right kidney, and the two share a bifid ureter that joins just above the bladder. (From McPherson RI: Supernumerary kidney: Typical and atypical features. J Can Assoc Radiol 38:116–119, 1987.)

unilateral renal agenesis must be investigated aggressively, because the kidney may be present but so dysgenetic and tiny or so diseased that imaging studies cannot always detect it, although hypertension in such patients may be cured when the affected kidney is removed.

Information is conflicting in regard to whether renal agenesis is hereditary or occurs spontaneously. The issue is obviously important with regard to bilateral agenesis, which is lethal. Thus, for a pregnant woman who has already given birth to one infant with bilateral renal agenesis, the question arises: is prenatal ultrasonography, perhaps leading to a therapeutic abortion, desirable?

Some anecdotal reports describe the recurrence of bilateral renal agenesis within the same family;[24, 25] one mother gave birth to more than one infant with bilateral agenesis. Same-sex twins have also been concordantly affected with bilateral renal agenesis.[26] The problem has recently been examined in more depth, and currently it is suggested that renal agenesis is truly hereditary.

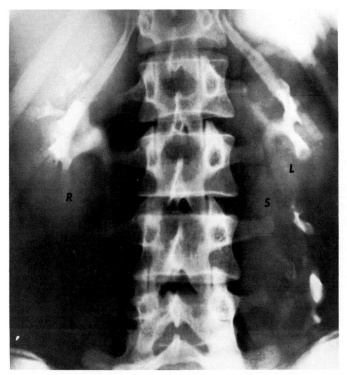

Figure 19–40. Supernumerary kidney on the left. Excretory urogram shows the normal right kidney (R), the undersized but otherwise normal left kidney (L), and the malrotated but clearly separate supernumerary kidney (S) lying caudal to the left kidney. (From McPherson RI: Supernumerary kidney: Typical and atypical features. J Can Assoc Radiol 38:116–119, 1987.)

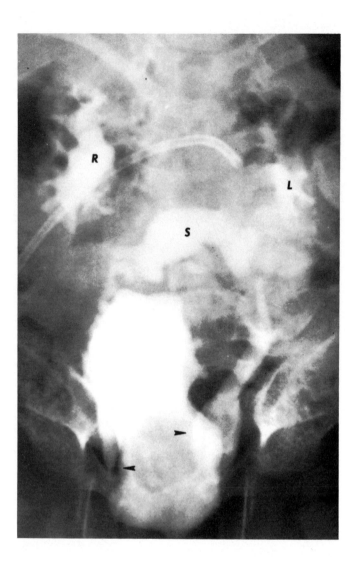

Figure 19–42. Excretory urogram in a 3-year-old child, showing the skeletal deformities and neurogenic bladder secondary to meningomyelocele. Right (R) and left (L) kidneys have a normal position, rotation, and longitudinal axis. The supernumerary kidney (S) is oriented transversely between the lower poles of the other two kidneys. Its ureter accompanies the left ureter (arrowheads) to the bladder. (From McPherson RI: Supernumerary kidney: Typical and atypical features. J Can Assoc Radiol 38:116–119, 1987.)

Figure 19–43. Tc-99m-DTPA renal scan showing a supernumerary kidney. A, Early image shows the right (R) and left (L) kidneys and their ureters (arrowheads), with the predominantly photopenic supernumerary kidney (S) between them. B, A 5-hour image shows the delayed function of the supernumerary kidney and its separate dilated ureter at the left (arrowhead). The collecting system did not wash out upon induced diuresis, indicating obstruction. (From McPherson RI: Supernumerary kidney: Typical and atypical features. J Can Assoc Radiol 38:116–119, 1987.)

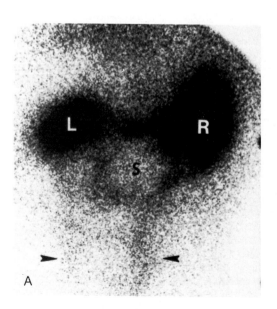

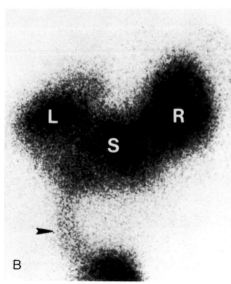

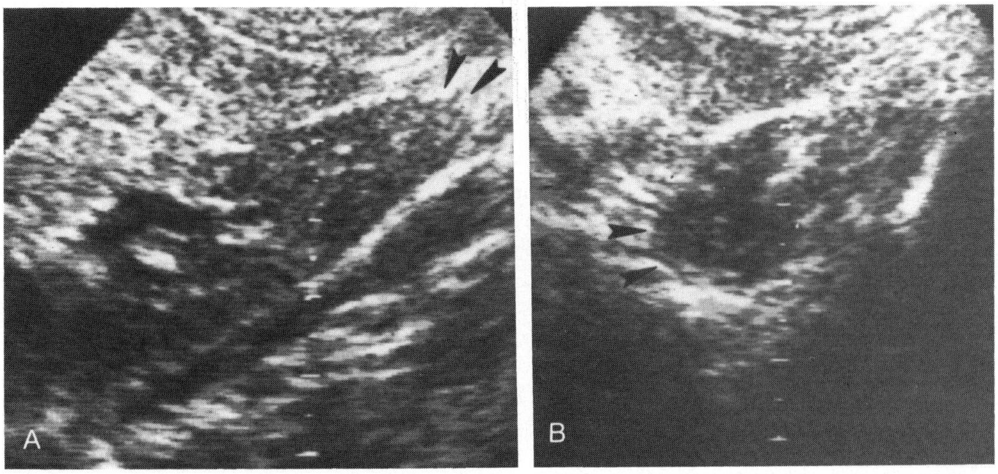

Figure 19–44. Renal ultrasonography, longitudinal scans. *A* shows the lower pole of a normal right kidney (*arrowheads*). *B* shows the upper pole of the supernumerary kidney (*arrowheads*). (From McPherson RI: Supernumerary kidney: Typical and atypical features. J Can Assoc Radiol 38:116–119, 1987.)

Unilateral or bilateral agenesis, or severe dysplasia, is now called hereditary renal adysplasia (HRA); the condition of bilateral renal agenesis or severe dysplasia is called perinatally lethal renal disease (PLRD). Two recent papers show that the overall empirical risk of recurrence in families with one child with PLRD is 3.5% to 5% in one series,[27] but 15% to 20% in another series.[28] Therefore, the current recommendation is that when an infant is born with bilateral renal agenesis, ultrasonography should be performed on subsequent fetuses in the second trimester, when therapeutic abortion is still a possibility.[29] Further routine sonographic scans should be obtained for all first-degree relatives of infants born with PLRD, in order to ascertain whether they have unilateral renal agenesis.

It is the current opinion that most cases of renal agenesis are hereditary and are transmitted as autosomal dominant traits.[28]

EMBRYOLOGY OF RENAL AGENESIS

The formation of the mesonephros is absolutely dependent on direct contact with the primary nephric duct. The proper formation of the metanephros depends on direct contact with the ureteral bud.[9, 19, 30–36] In kidney agenesis, an inhibition of growth involving either the nephric duct or the ureteral bud must have occurred. Either kind of problem may be hereditary.

If the nephric duct is deficient, the following three possibilities exist, depending on the stage of growth inhibition:

1. If inhibition occurs at the stage when the duct is at the level of pronephros, the kidney, ureter, and other structures will be absent, depending on whether the developing embryo is male or female. In the male, the epididymis, vas, and seminal vesicle—and perhaps the testis—will be absent. In the female, half the uterus will be absent (a unicornuate uterus), as will the vagina and perhaps the ovary.

2. If inhibition occurs when the duct extends half the length of the mesonephros, the gonad and the upper fallopian tube may be present in the female.

3. If inhibition occurs when the duct develops to below the urogenital fold, but above the ureteral bud segment, the seminal vesicle and the kidney will be absent in the male, but the gonad, the epididymis, and the vas will be present. In the female, the uterus and the vagina will be deficient.

Figure 19–45. Abdominal CT scans in a patient with a supernumerary kidney. *A,* Section through the middle of mildly hydronephrotic right (R) and left (L) kidneys are shown. *B,* Lower section shows the intimate relationship of the hydronephrotic supernumerary kidney (S) to the lower poles of the right (R) and left (L) kidneys. *C,* Further caudad, a section through the hydronephrotic supernumerary kidney shows its relationship to the ureters *(arrowhead). D,* Section just above the bladder shows right and left ureters *(arrowheads)* and the dilated supernumerary ureter (S) posterior to the left ureter. (From McPherson RI: Supernumerary kidney: Typical and atypical features. J Can Assoc Radiol 38:116–119, 1987.)

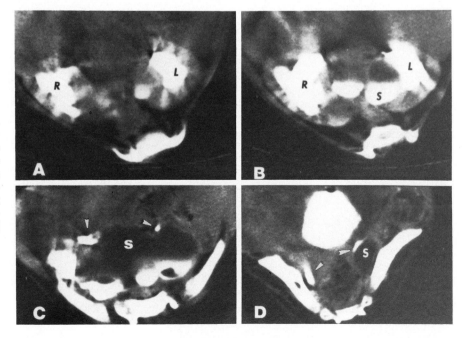

For cases in which the inhibition involves a delay in the development of the ureteral bud, or in which the metanephrogenic blastema is displaced relative to the nephric duct angle from which the ureteral bud develops, the kidney may be absent, but a ureter may well be present.[32]

A dysgenetic kidney may be resorbed. However, it may also remain, unnoticed, because it is tiny and lacks function. Such a kidney could cause hypertension.[23]

CLINICAL FEATURES

Bilateral Renal Agenesis. Bilateral renal agenesis (BRA) usually reveals itself in the antenatal period because it causes maternal oligohydramnios.[37] Because fetal urine constitutes the major part of the amniotic fluid, it will be deficient if the fetus has no kidneys. In cases of oligohydramnios the mother should undergo antenatal ultrasonography.

In the postnatal period, such infants will have the so-called Potter's facies (Fig. 19–46), bilateral pulmonary hypoplasia, and bilateral pneumothoraces. Nothing can be done for infants with bilateral renal agenesis. Rather than devote precious therapeutic resources to them, it will be more useful to establish the diagnosis by performing renal ultrasonography and, if necessary, scintigraphy.

Unilateral Renal Agenesis. Although unilateral renal agenesis (URA) is often discovered coincidentally in the asymptomatic patient, it may be suspected because one or more associated anomalies are present. Agenesis is frequently discovered when patients present with an abnormality of the one remaining kidney, in which case it becomes important to know if there is a contralateral renal unit. This can happen under the following circumstances: when a patient has had an abdominal injury and the solitary kidney is damaged; when the patient becomes acutely anuric because of acute pyelonephritis involving the solitary kidney or an acute ureteral obstruction by a

stone in the solitary ureter; when a pathological kidney spontaneously ruptures;[39] or when there is disease in the solitary kidney and a complete or partial nephrectomy is being considered, as might occur in a patient with a renal cell carcinoma.

ASSOCIATED ANOMALIES

Genitourinary Anomalies (Table 19–15). Associated genital anomalies can present as cystic pelvic masses in both sexes, although their causes differ with sex. In the female, for example, ureterovaginal atresia, especially unilateral vaginal atresia in one half of a duplicated genital tract, can produce an unusual mass.[43, 51–61] This is usually not detected until puberty, at which point menstrual blood accumulates continuously in the obstructed half, producing hydrometrocolpos. As a result, a large pelvic mass develops over time, the nature of which can be masked by a history of normal menstruation that occurs in the normal half of the uterus and the vagina (see Fig. 19–52). About 20% of women with ureterovaginal atresia (Mayer-Rokitansky-Küster-Hauser syndrome) have only one kidney,[52–55] but the incidence may be higher when there is duplication of müllerian derivatives (see Fig. 19–51).[43, 58–61] However, most women with duplication of the müllerian derivatives have a normal upper urinary tract.[64]

This anomaly is significant because an accurate diagnosis can prevent the unnecessary surgical removal of both uteri, which is clearly radical and irreversible. Such patients require only vaginal drainage and vaginoplasty. Thus women with pelvic masses should routinely undergo ultrasonography[64] or magnetic resonance imaging (MRI)[58, 217] of the pelvis and kidneys, which is an excellent means of establishing the diagnosis.

Renal agenesis with uterovaginal atresia or uterine duplication results from simultaneously faulty müllerian and primary nephric ducts.[65]

In the male, absence of the seminal vesicle or a seminal

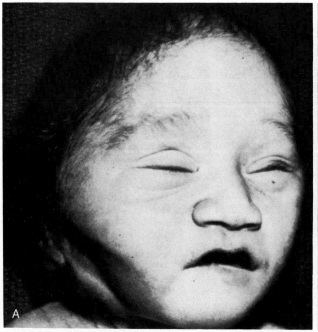
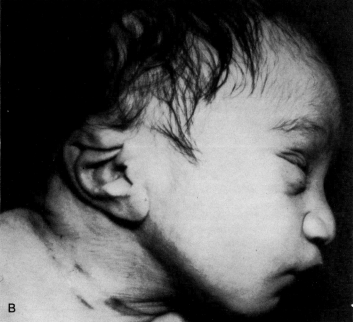

Figure 19–46. *A* and *B,* Neonate with typical Potter facies; Note the low-set flaccid ears, the prominent suborbital skinfolds, and the broad flat nose. (Courtesy Bruce Tune, M.D., Division of Pediatric Nephrology, Stanford University.)

Table 19–15. Genitourinary Anomalies Associated with Renal Agenesis*

Structure	Anomaly
Male genitalia (anomalies in 20%)[41, 42]	Absent ipsilateral epididymis, vas, and seminal vesicle (33%) (see Fig. 19–47), perhaps with absent testis[41-44]
	Isolated absence of ipsilateral seminal vesicle[41-43]
	Ipsilateral seminal vesicle cyst (see Figs. 19–48 to 19–50)[43, 45, 46]
	Ectasia of rete testis[47]
	Suprainguinal scrotum[48]
	Dermoid cyst of prostate[49]
Female genitalia (anomalies in 70%)[41, 42, 50, 51]	Absent or atretic uterus and vagina[50, 52-55]
	Unicornous uterus with absent or atretic vagina and ovary[56]
	Duplicated genital tract (see Figs. 19–51 and 19–52) with or without absence or atresia of ipsilateral vagina[43, 58-61]
	Gartner's duct cyst[62, 63]
Ipsilateral adrenal gland	Absent in 8% to 17%[42, 43, 66, 67]
Ipsilateral Gerota's fascia and perinephric fat	Absent in 100%[68]
Ipsilateral renal artery and vein	Right renal agenesis: both absent in 100%[42]
	Left renal agenesis: artery absent in 100%;[42] a vein exists that receives only left adrenal and gonadal tributaries[69]
Ipsilateral ureter	Agenesis (80%)[42]
	Blind-ending stump (20%)[42]
Contralateral ureter	Congenital ureteral valve[70]
	Ectopic insertion into Gartner's duct cyst[63]
	Hypoplasia[71]
Bladder	Bilateral renal agenesis
	Vesical agenesis (20%)[42]
	Vesical hypoplasia (30%)[42]
	Unilateral renal agenesis
	Absent ipsilateral hemitrigone (80%)[42]
	Absent ipsilateral ureteral orifice (80%)[42]

*See also Embryology.

vesicle cyst can occur on the same side as the absent kidney (Figs. 19–47 to 19–50), which may be large and may present as a large palpable pelvic mass (Fig. 19–48).[43-46, 226] It may protrude into the bladder, simulating a ureterocele, or it may prolapse through the bladder neck.

The two ways of suggesting the diagnosis,[43, 45, 46] are imaging the pelvis and kidneys by ultrasonography (Fig. 19–50) or CT (Figs. 19–47 and 19–48), but the diagnosis can be made definitively only through vasovesiculography or cyst puncture with a needle, and the subsequent instillation of contrast material (Fig. 19–49).[43, 219] These interesting lesions need be treated, however, only if they become symptomatic.[220]

Anomalies Elsewhere in the Body. The three acronyms VATER, VACTERL, and MURCS assist in remembering those regions of the body where additional associated anomalies may occur (see page 560). The most common associated anomalies located elsewhere in the body include anorectal malformations and skeletal anomalies,[72] especially anomalies of the phalanges and metacarpals.[73] One characteristic finding is brachymesophalangy in the second through the fifth digits; in addition, a small distal phalanx may be found in the first digit. These anomalies occur in 56% of patients. In addition, 48% of patients have a long proximal phalanx in the third and fourth digits; 51% have long first through fourth metacarpals.[73]

There is some disagreement regarding sacral agenesis and small pelvic outlet. Some authors have postulated an association,[74, 75] but Fellows and colleagues[76] found that renal agenesis was not associated with either of these findings.

Rare but interesting associated anomalies include total intestinal aganglionosis,[77] meningocerebral angiodysplasia,[78] and the BOR syndrome.[225]

IMAGING STUDIES

Ultrasonography. This study usually shows a normally located adrenal gland but no kidney, although in 8% to 17% of cases the adrenal gland is absent, as is the kidney.[66, 67] In such cases it is important to search in the pelvis on the same side, and to search the opposite side, to be certain that an ectopic kidney is not present.

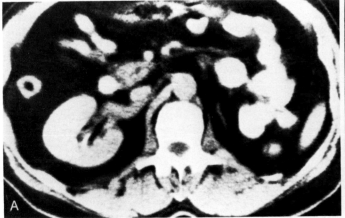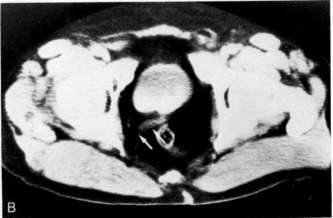

Figure 19–47. Absent left kidney and left seminal vesicle in a 63-year-old man with scrotal pain and impalpable left spermatic cord. *A,* CT scan shows absence of left kidney. *B,* CT shows absence of left seminal vesicle. Arrows indicate normal right seminal vesicle. (From Kenney PJ, Spirt BA, Leeson MD: Genitourinary anomalies: Radiologic-anatomic correlations. Radiographics 4:233–260, 1984.)

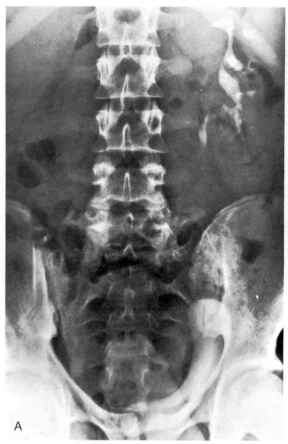

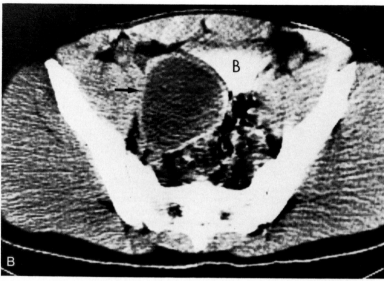

Figure 19–48. Right renal agenesis and right seminal vesicle cyst in an 18-year-old man who complained of persistent right scrotal pain, urinary frequency, and dysuria. He had a right lower quadrant mass. *A,* Intravenous urogram shows absent right kidney, hypertrophied left kidney, and mass extrinsic to bladder. *B,* CT scan shows thick-walled cyst *(arrow)* arising from right seminal vesicle displacing bladder (B). (From Kenney PJ, Spirt BA, Leeson MD: Genitourinary anomalies: Radiologic-anatomic correlations. Radiographics 4:233–260, 1984.)

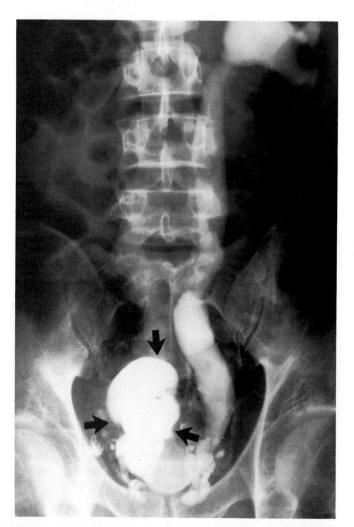

Figure 19–49. Seminal vesicle cyst *(arrows).* The radiograph was taken after bilateral seminal vesiculograms, a left retrograde pyelogram, and transrectal puncture of the right seminal vesicle cyst were performed. The right hemitrigone and right ureteral orifice were absent at cystoscopy (surgical proof).

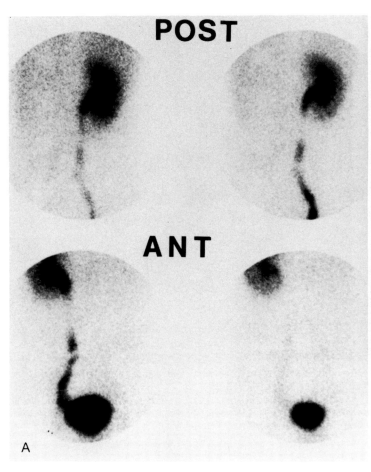

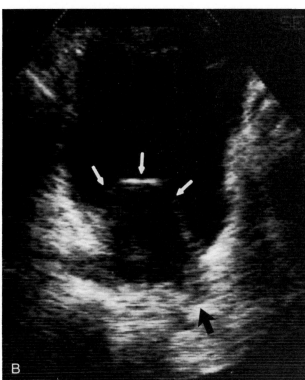

Figure 19–50. Left renal agenesis and seminal vesicle cyst. *A,* Scintigraphy demonstrates left renal agenesis. *B,* Transverse bladder sonogram shows a cystic mass *(white arrows)* at the left bladder base, distorting the seminal vesicle *(black arrow)* (surgical proof).

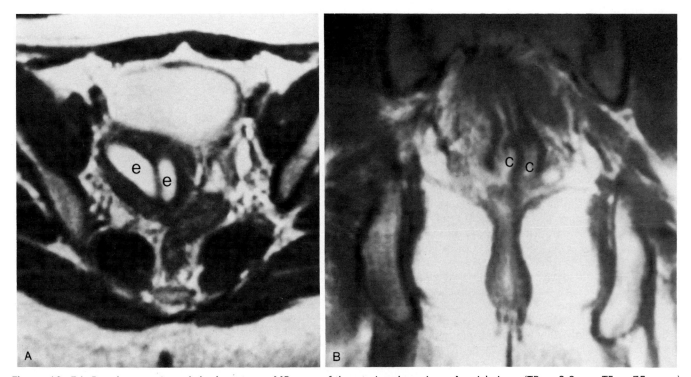

Figure 19–51. Renal agenesis and duplex uterus. MR scan of the uteri and cervices. *A,* axial views (TR = 2.0 sec; TE = 75 msec) progressing cephalad. There is an endometrial cavity (e *to* e); *B,* two cervical canals (c) are shown. (Courtesy Leroy Heinrichs, M.D., Department of Obstetrics and Gynecology, Stanford University.)

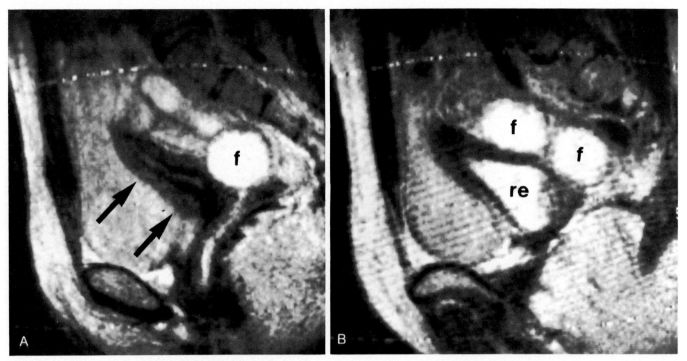

Figure 19–52. Duplex uterus with right vaginal atresia causing a right hematometrosalpinx. The patient also had a right renal agenesis. MR scan of uteri and right fallopian tubes. *A* and *B* are sagittal views (TR = 2.05 secs, TE = 75 msec). *A* demonstrates the left uterus *(arrows)*, which has a normal-appearing endometrial cavity. The right fallopian tube (F), which is distended with blood, lies posterior to the left uterus. *B* shows the right endometrial cavity (re) and the right fallopian tube (f), both of which are distended with blood. (Courtesy of Leroy Heinrichs, M.D., Department of Obstetrics and Gynecology, Stanford University.)

The adrenal hypertrophies in fetuses and neonates with renal agenesis or ectopia.[79, 80] The average length of the right adrenal in such patients is 3.4 cm, but on the left it is 2.9 cm. On both sides, the average thickness is 5 mm.[80]

The adrenal also loses its characteristic V or Y shape, and becomes elliptical, such that it can resemble a kidney.[80] However, its echogenicity, differs; the cortex is anechoic and the medulla is echogenic.[80] In BRA, the adrenal glands may be fused.

Patients of either sex can have cystic or complex masses in the pelvis, as described above. In the female these may be due to hydrometrocolpos (Fig. 19–53), and in the male to a seminal vesicle cyst (Fig. 19–50A). Problems can arise in distinguishing renal agenesis from a small hypoplastic or dysplastic kidney, because the latter can have an echogenicity similar to that of retroperitoneal fat. Furthermore, it may be obscured by gas, making the kidney difficult to find. In addition, fluid-filled bowel loops in the renal fossa, where the kidney is absent, can simulate hydronephrosis. It would be important to garner sufficient real-time ultrasonography to determine whether persistalsis is present. Sonograms would obviously indicate bowel in the presence of peristalsis, and hydronephrosis in its absence.

Scintigraphy. This study will demonstrate unilateral renal uptake and excretion (Fig. 19–50).[80] In the differential diagnosis should be included unilateral nonfunctioning kidney. In some cases, the renal fossa appears photopenic, but, as there is a long list of renal lesions which can cause photopenic renal fossae, the finding is nonspecific.[82]

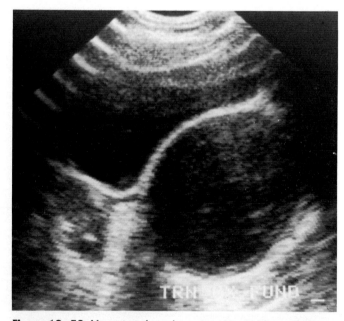

Figure 19–53. Hematocolpos-hematometra in Mayer-Rokitansky-Küster-Hauser syndrome. A transverse sonogram through the pelvis demonstrates a large complex mass behind the left side of the urinary bladder. Although the mass appears to contain considerable fluid, numerous extraneous echoes within it are attributable to blood clots and debris. This 15-year-old girl had left renal agensis, complete duplication of the uterus and vagina, and atresia of the distal left vagina resulting in unilateral hematocolpos and hematometra. (Courtesy Dr. Darrel Cannon.)

Abdominal Radiography (KUB). The plain film of the abdomen may supply the first clue to the diagnosis of agenesis. It can be a cheap and easy way to help distinguish this entity from nonfunction. Crucial for making the diagnosis are the distribution of the colon gas, the appearance of the psoas shadow, the lack of a kidney shadow on one side, and an abnormally large kidney representing a hypertrophied solitary kidney on the opposite side.

Colon Gas. The appearance of the colon gas shadows varies according to whether the absent kidney is on the left or the right side.

There are two splenic flexures: the anatomical and the radiological. The anatomical splenic flexure is the point where the colon is fixed by the phrenocolic ligament. It is the most posterior part of the colon and the point at which it becomes extraperitoneal. The radiological splenic flexure is the distal transverse colon, lying within the peritoneal cavity and attached to the transverse mesocolon.

In *left* renal agenesis, both Gerota's fascia and the phrenocolic ligament are absent, resulting in the anatomical splenic flexure occupying the left renal fossa in the left paraspinal area, posterior and medial to the stomach.

On a plain film of the normal abdomen, the gas in the anatomical splenic flexure lies lateral to the gas in the stomach. With left renal agenesis, the gas in the anatomical splenic flexure is either medial to or superimposed upon the stomach gas.[83, 84]

The diagnosis can be difficult or impossible to establish in the neonate, because it is not always possible to distinguish colon gas from small bowel gas on an abdominal radiograph. If no gas is in the anatomical splenic flexure, the diagnosis is impossible. Because the anatomical splenic flexure is the most posterior part of the colon, a prone or erect film of the abdomen may be helpful.

An identical appearance on the plain radiograph of the abdomen can occur when the patient has had an anterior (abdominal, but not flank) nephrectomy; it may also be seen with left renal ectopia and with the rare congenital absence of the phrenocolic ligament. The most common problem with the diagnosis lies in misinterpreting the unusual appearance of the colon gas as an internal hernia or malrotation, instead of recognizing it as renal agenesis.

The real value of the plain film in diagnosis of left renal agenesis is that if the anatomical splenic flexure lies in the normal location, the patient does not have left renal agenesis. Therefore, it is an easy way to distinguish agenesis from nonfunction. If the patient's hemitrigone is absent, a normal anatomical splenic flexure will further help to distinguish left renal agenesis from left multicystic renal dysplasia, in which the ipsilateral hemitrigone is often absent but the colon gas is in the normal position.

In *right* renal agenesis, the posterior part of the hepatic flexure occupies the right renal fossa. The distal part of the ascending colon and the posterior part of the hepatic flexure lie medial to the anterior part of the hepatic flexure and proximal transverse colon. This is just the opposite of what would be expected. As with left renal agenesis, erect and prone films are more useful for producing the characteristic appearance of the colon gas.

Patients with right renal agenesis may have malposition of the duodenum, visible on an upper gastrointestinal series.

The identical appearance of the colon gas can occur with right renal ectopia or after a right anterior nephrectomy. As with left renal agenesis, the abnormal colon gas shadow in patients with right renal agenesis may incorrectly be attributed to an internal hernia, malrotation, or displacement of the colon by a large mass or large organs.

If the plain abdominal radiograph is equivocal or if it suggests that the splenic flexure lies in an abnormal position, a barium enema is helpful in more precisely depicting the anatomy.

Psoas Shadow. The psoas shadow bows outward on the affected side; normally it is almost straight. Unfortunately, this sign occurs only infrequently.[21]

Kidney Shadow on the Affected Side. The soft-tissue shadow of the kidney on the affected side will be missing on the plain radiograph of the abdomen. However, it may be simulated by overlying soft tissues.

Compensatory Hypertrophy of the Solitary Kidney. An enlarged kidney due to compensatory hypertrophy of the solitary kidney will be present in all cases.[21]

Barium Enema. The barium enema is a simple and rapid way to confirm the abnormal position of either the splenic or the hepatic flexure of the colon. If left renal agenesis is suspected, the patient should be examined in the supine position.[83]

In the normal colon, as the barium flows into the patient it runs in a counterclockwise direction from the anatomical to the radiological splenic flexure. With left renal agenesis, the barium flows in a clockwise direction, because the radiological splenic flexure lies superior and lateral to the anatomical splenic flexure (Fig. 19–54).

In right agenesis, the distal ascending colon and the posterior part of the hepatic flexure lie medial to the anterior part of the hepatic flexure and the proximal transverse colon, which is just the opposite of the normal situation.[85]

Excretory Urography. This will show one kidney which is usually in the normal position (see Fig. 19–48), although it may be ectopic. In most cases the solitary kidney is huge, owing to compensatory hypertrophy, although this usually occurs only if it is in normal position.

The ureter of the remaining kidney is usually normal, although there may be ureteral valves, or an ectopic insertion into the vagina via a Gartner's duct cyst.

Retrograde Pyelography. The retrograde pyelogram can sometimes be valuable in a difficult case. If, for example, the urologist finds two ureteral orifices, and if the retrograde pyelogram shows two pyelocalyceal systems and ureters, then the patient does not have renal agenesis.

If the urologist sees two ureteral orifices, however, this does not in itself exclude renal agenesis. The patient may have a blind-ending ureter on one side with renal agenesis. Unfortunately, however, an absent ureteral orifice at cystoscopy is still not diagnostic of renal agenesis. If the kidney fails to excrete for any reason, the ureteral orifice can become very small and difficult to find over a period of time. Moreover, one-third of patients with congenital cystic dysplasia have an absent ureteral orifice, and the orifice may also be absent if it is ectopic—if, for example, the ureter is inserted into the seminal vesicle in the male. Nor is an absent hemitrigone diagnostic; it can be seen in one-third of patients with multicystic renal dysplasia and in patients with ectopic ureters.

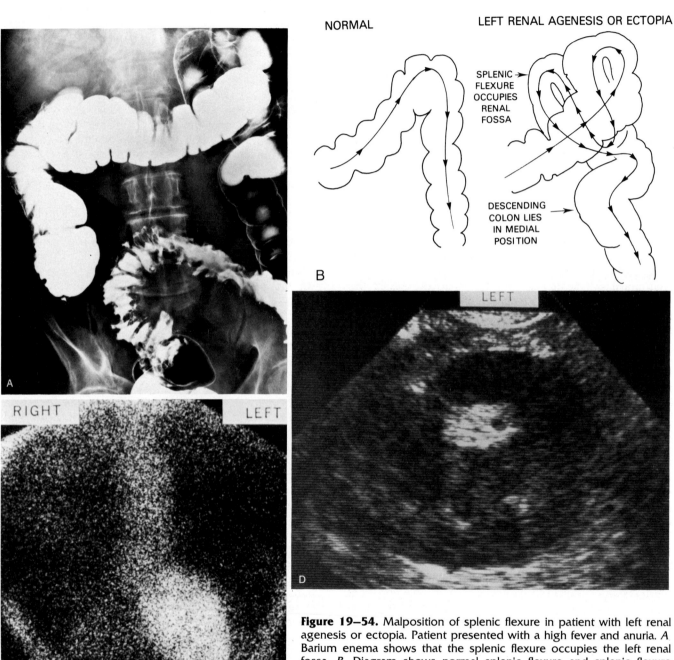

Figure 19–54. Malposition of splenic flexure in patient with left renal agenesis or ectopia. Patient presented with a high fever and anuria. *A,* Barium enema shows that the splenic flexure occupies the left renal fossa. *B,* Diagram shows normal splenic flexure and splenic flexure occupying left renal fossa. *C,* In-111–labeled white-cell scan (anterior view) shows uptake in an ectopic left kidney; this indicates acute pyelonephritis. *D,* Sonogram shows edema of the ectopic kidney.

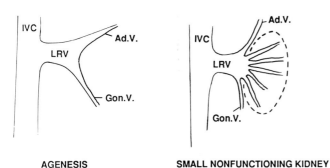

Figure 19–55. Diagram illustrating the difference between left renal agenesis and a small left nonfunctioning kidney on renal phlebography. (Ad V = adrenal vein, Gon V = gonadal vein.)

Aortography. If the patient has Potter's syndrome or bilateral pneumothoraces, a flush aortogram may be used in the isolette and performed via the umbilical artery. It will show no renal arteries if both kidneys are absent. One cannot depend on arteriography to confirm a diagnosis of unilateral renal agenesis, however, since with long-standing renal atrophy, the renal artery will be so small as to be angiographically undetectable, or the renal artery may have been occluded at its origin.

Renal Phlebography. Although in right renal agenesis the renal vein is absent, in left renal agenesis a vein exists that receives only left adrenal and left gonadal tributaries but that is otherwise surprisingly similar in appearance to a normal left renal vein (Fig. 19–55).[69] The absence of small renal tributaries may be used to differentiate small from absent kidneys if this determination cannot be made more simply (e.g., by ultrasonography or CT).[69]

Computed Tomography and Magnetic Resonance Imaging. CT[43, 86, 87] and MRI,[58] which should include the entire abdomen, will show only one kidney in patients with renal agenesis.[218, 219] The adrenals have an abnormal elliptical shape and appear linear on CT.[86, 87] In contrast to patients with agenesis, the adrenals retain their normal shape in patients with acquired renal atrophy, or in patients who have had a kidney surgically removed.[87] In addition, the colonic flexures, loops of small bowel, the duodenum, the spleen, and the tail of the pancreas may all be in an abnormal position in patients with renal agenesis.[86] None of these findings, however, is diagnostic, because they can occur as well in caudal or crossed ectopy, or following nephrectomy.[86, 87] If there are cystic masses in the pelvis, they will be visible as well (see Figs. 19–48 and 19–52). MRI, with its extreme sensitivity in detecting blood, is excellent for disclosing hematocolpos-hematometra (see Fig. 19–52).[217]

Choosing an Imaging Technique for Renal Agenesis.[218, 219] In the neonate, lesions from which renal agenesis must be differentiated are usually congenital. Combined scintigraphy and ultrasonography are needed to make the diagnosis, because one technique alone could miss the relevant findings (see Fig. 19–50). Ultrasonography, for example, might show that a nonexcreting kidney on scintigraphy is actually present but abnormal. Conversely, scintigraphy might reveal a small unilateral dysplastic or hypoplastic kidney that was difficult to find by ultrasonography, but which is nonetheless present and retains some function.

In older infants, children, or adults, a kidney may be nonvisualizing but present, if it has been destroyed by a pathological process or has been rendered temporarily nonfunctioning because of an acute process, such as acute bacterial nephritis.

Unfortunately, a high percentage of patients do not remember having the disease process that has destroyed the kidney, or even that the kidney had been removed. Thus, the radiologist should always examine the patient for a surgical scar.

It is sometimes vitally important to determine whether a kidney is absent or if it is present but nonfunctioning. Figure 19–54 depicts one such situation. Many others are possible, such as a patient having an acute trauma. Unfortunately, no imaging technique is infallible. The most accurate are CT and renal phlebography, provided the angiographer is aware of the pitfalls on the left side, as described above. The retrograde urogram can exclude renal agenesis if it shows the pyelocalyceal system and a ureter on the suspect side, but if the urologist finds an absent orifice with or without an absent hemitrigone, that is not diagnostic. Because of the pitfalls that can occur with arteriography, ultrasonography, and scintigraphy, the radiologist must diagnose by exclusion and with great caution.

Anomalies in Size

Renal Dysgenesis

Renal dysgenesis is defined as defective renal parenchymal development. Two groups exist: hypoplasia and dysplasia.[88]

RENAL HYPOPLASIA

Renal hypoplasia signifies a congenital renal parenchymal anomaly in which there are too few nephrons. The term oligonephronia (literally, "too few nephrons") is a more accurate term than renal hypoplasia.[88] To establish the diagnosis, it is necessary to obtain an accurate nephron count.[89]

Embryology of Renal Hypoplasia. The caudal portion of the metanephrogenic blastema is sharply limited, unlike its more cranial aspect, which is shaped like a comet tail. Therefore, if the ureteral bud makes contact only with the most caudal portion of the metanephrogenic blastema, that bud will be surrounded by very little blastema, and the resulting kidney will be hypoplastic. This may occur because of delayed development of the bud itself, or because of delayed contact with the blastema, which is migrating cranially.

Classification. Four types of renal hypoplasia exist (Table 19–16).

Hypoplastic Kidney with Orthotopically Draining Ureter (Miniature Kidney; Dwarf Kidney). A hypoplastic kidney drained by a ureter in which the orifice inserts orthotopically appears grossly like a normal kidney and

Table 19–16. Types of Renal Hypoplasia

Ureter draining the kidney, inserting in a normal location (orthotopic)
Ureter draining the kidney, inserting in an abnormal location (ectopic)
Oligomeganephronia: too few nephrons, all enlarged
Ask-Upmark kidney

has normal-appearing calyces, although there are fewer than usual. The ureter appears normal and the ureteral orifice opens in the normal place.[88]

A dwarf kidney can be unilateral or bilateral. The unilateral type is uncommon, although its true prevalence is difficult to estimate, because it is often impossible to differentiate the hypoplastic from the atrophic kidney. It occurs sporadically, and it affects an equal number of males and females.[88] It does not affect total kidney function unless the opposite kidney is diseased or absent, but on rare occasions it may cause severe hypertension in the neonate.[90, 91]

The bilateral form is a type of oligomeganephronia, in which there are too few nephrons. However, those present are enlarged because of compensatory hypertrophy, and renal failure results. Of these patients, 80% also have congenital central nervous system lesions.[88]

Hypoplastic Kidney with Ectopically Inserting Ureter (Thin Kidneys). Abnormal locations in which the ureter can insert are discussed on page 603.

In these kidneys, the renal parenchyma is usually thin, the calyces are clubbed, the ureteral caliber is wide, and vesicoureteral reflux is usual.[92]

Thin kidneys fall into two common subgroups:[88] (1) Kidneys with a single ureter and lateral ectopia. This occurs primarily in females; it can be inherited as an autosomal dominant with variable penetrance or as an autosomal recessive. (2) Kidneys with double ureters with vesicoureteral reflux, usually into the ureter draining the lower pole of the kidney.

Debate continues regarding the causes of thin kidney. It could arise due to high-grade or high-pressure vesicoureteral reflux, and represent one form of reflux nephropathy. Indeed, reflux nephropathy can develop in the fetus or the neonate, may often be fully developed by the age of 2 years, and is fully developed in nearly all cases by the age of 4 years. On the other hand, the defects present in infants or young children could be congenital. The question of whether or not the ureter in one of these patients should be reimplanted to prevent further deterioration of renal function is a matter of current debate.

Oligomeganephronia. Oligomeganephronia (OMN) denotes bilateral renal hypoplasia in which there are too few nephrons (hence *oligo*-nephronia), and all are enlarged (hence *mega*-nephronia).[93, 94] Because the kidneys are hypoplastic, they are small. Most contain fewer than seven renal segments instead of the normal eight; only one renal segment and one papilla may be present, this being known as the unipapillary kidney. The calyces and ureters usually appear normal, although occasionally mild hydronephrosis may occur.[95]

Oligomeganephronia is usually not familial[93] (although familial cases can occur[96]) and is not associated with other congenital anomalies. It is three times more common in boys than in girls.[93] The mother was 35 years of age or older at conception for one-third of patients with oligomeganephronia; one-third of all such patients weigh less than 2.5 kg at birth.[93]

Progressive renal failure occurs during infancy. These infants are unable to concentrate their urine, and have polyuria and polydypsia. After infancy often comes a period of no further deterioration of renal function until puberty, after which additional relative loss of renal function usually occurs.

Ask-Upmark Kidney. The Ask-Upmark kidney consists of a segmental renal scar and usually presents with hypertension, usually in girls and young women.

PATHOLOGY. Renal hypoplasia has a number of characteristic features.[97] (1) The arterioles in the affected area of the kidney are thick-walled, lie abnormally close to one another, and are very tortuous. (2) It usually affects only one kidney, which tends to be small. (3) Deep, narrow, segmental scars are usually found in the midzone of the kidney (so-called slit scars). (4) The calyces underlying these scars are usually clubbed. (5) Often, the number of calyces is less than usual. (6) Within the scarred area itself, the glomeruli are usually entirely absent, although a few fibrotic or hyalinized ones may be present. (7) The tubules have usually atrophied, and are small or distended with colloid. (8) Inflammatory cells are few or absent. (9) The renal parenchyma in the unaffected area of the kidney is histologically normal.

ETIOLOGY. Although some Ask-Upmark kidneys are congenital,[98] many—perhaps even most—are acquired.[99–103] The embryogenesis of the congenital form will have to await further study. Several cases are documented in which children with an entirely normal-appearing kidney subsequently developed all the radiological and histological features of the Ask-Upmark kidney, as a result of vesicoureteral reflux and acute focal bacterial nephritis. All the associated symptoms, including hypertension, were present.[103–105]

On pathological grounds, the Ask-Upmark kidney usually appears acquired and not congenital.[102, 103] The renal arterioles, for example, might be expected to kink and appear closer together when the destruction of renal parenchyma associated with high-pressure vesicoureteral reflux and acute focal bacterial nephritis has occurred.[97] Finally, the Ask-Upmark deformity has been produced in pigs by obstructing the urethra and slitting one of the ureteral orifices, producing high-pressure vesicoureteral reflux.[97]

RENAL DYSPLASIA

Renal dysplasia is a congenital renal parenchymal malformation in which abnormal nephrons and mesenchymal stroma are found.[89] Because these features can also arise from neoplasm or infection, however, it is necessary to first specify that both occur in the kidney in the absence of either of the above.[89]

Embryology of Renal Dysplasia. Renal dysplasia may be related to the position of the ureteral orifice in the bladder and in the urethra (Fig. 19–56).[106] This, in turn, may be related to the point at which the ureteral bud arises in the wolffian duct (Fig. 19–56).[106] Some cases of dysplasia may also result from acute in utero obstruction, in which there is secondary pyelocalyceal rupture.[107] Sanders believes that renal dysplasia is almost invariably associated with in utero obstruction.[224] He postulates that the appearance of the kidney correlates with the level of the obstruction, with more proximal obstructions producing predominantly cystic dysplastic kidneys.[224] Vesicoureteral reflux may also produce dysplasia. However, Stephens believes that the key factor in dysplasia is the position of ureteral orifice.[108]

Pathology. Histologically, the dysplastic kidney has four characteristic features: in decreasing order of impor-

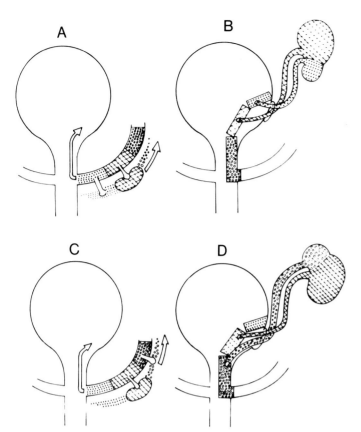

Figure 19–56. Mackie's and Stephens's correlation between the site of origin of the ureteral bud, the quality of the kidney, and the location of the ureteral orifices in duplex kidneys. *A,* Presumed orthotopic bud arises from the normal zone, while ecoptic bud arises distally. *B,* The consequences of *A* are shown. Ectopic bud has a normal site of ureteral orifice. The orthotopic bud is abnormally placed craniolaterally and is hypodysplastic. *C,* The orthotopic bud arises from the normal site, and the ectopic bud arises proximally. *D,* The results of *C* are shown: normal placement of the orthotopic ureteral orifice; ectopic, caudally displaced orifice of the ectopic bud; and a hypodysplastic segment. (From Mackie CG, Stephens FD: Duplex kidneys: A correlation of renal dysplasia with position of the ureteral orifice. J Urol 114(2):274–280, © by Williams & Wilkins, 1975.)

tance,[89] (1) primitive ducts; (2) low cuboidal epithelium lining the ductules, and mesenchymal collars surrounding them; (3) cartilage; (4) areas of loose mesenchymal fibrous tissue.

Two other findings, cysts and heterotopic erythropoiesis, often lumped together as the fifth feature, may be associated with dysplastic kidneys, but are not regarded as being particularly diagnostic. Some authors classify multicystic kidney as a separate form of renal dysplasia. This subject is considered in detail in Chapter 39.

Dysplasia is often seen in hypoplastic kidneys. The relative importance of each can be accurately determined by discovering the ratio of nephrons to dysplastic structures, by grading dysplastic structures using the five features described previously, or by a combination of these methods.

Associated Anomalies. A number of anomalies may be associated with renal dysplasia.

Ectopic Ureter. The degree of ectopia and the severity of the dysplasia are somewhat correlated.[108, 109] The more medial, caudal, or lateral the ureteral orifice, the more dysplastic the kidney usually is. When the ureteral orifice

opens caudally, the presence of a single or double ureter or an ectopic ureterocele is a factor less important to the degree of dysplasia than how caudally the ureter opens. The most severe dysplasia usually occurs when the ureter opens into the urethra, the vas, or seminal vesicle.

Posterior Urethral Valves. When a patient has posterior urethral valves and a lateral ectopic ureter, the more lateral the ectopy, the more likely is the kidney to be dysplastic.[110, 111] Others strongly dispute these data, claiming that the changes are acquired.[112]

Absent Abdominal Muscles (Prune-Belly Syndrome). In the prune-belly syndrome, the ureters are often wide and tortuous because of a lack of muscle in their walls. Often the ureteral orifices are wide and inserted ectopically in a lateral position. When these malformations occur, renal dysplasia is often associated, although the degree of the disorder may vary widely.

Dwarf Kidneys. Such kidneys can occasionally exhibit hypodysplasia.

IMAGING OF RENAL DYSGENESIS

Renal dysgenesis may be unilateral or bilateral. All such kidneys are small.

Unilateral Renal Dysgenesis. Kidneys in this category include the hypoplastic kidneys (dwarf, thin, or Ask-Upmark kidneys), and dysplastic kidneys.

Intravenous Urography. The true *dwarf kidney* looks like a miniature version of a normal kidney: it is small, usually excretes contrast material well, is smooth in outline, has normal calyces (although fewer than seven), and a normal ureter (Figs. 19–57 and 19–58). The opposite kidney is usually large, owing to compensatory hypertrophy (Fig. 19–58). If the opposite kidney is congenitally absent, or acquires intercurrent disease, the patient may present with renal failure.

Diagnosis is by exclusion. The identical appearance may present in the following entities:

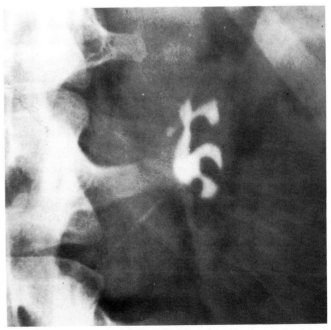

Figure 19–57. Intravenous urogram showing a left dwarf kidney. (From Friedland GW, Goris ML, Gross D, et al: Urodiology: An Integrated Approach. New York, Churchill Livingstone, 1983, p 1652. By permission.)

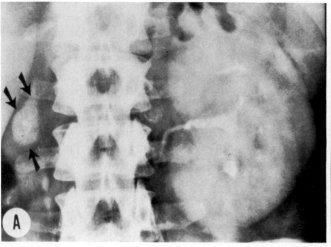

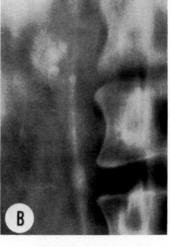

Figure 19–58. Intravenous urogram *(A)* and nephroto-mogram *(B)* showing a dwarf right kidney *(arrows)*. Note the contralateral renal hypertrophy. (From Friedland GW, Goris ML, Gross D, et al: Uroradiology: An Integrated Approach. New York, Churchill Livingstone, 1983, p 1489. By permission.)

1. Postobstructive atrophy, commonly caused by ureteral obstruction of several weeks' duration by a stone, which then passes or is removed. The usual result is backpressure atrophy with calyceal clubbing. Occasionally, however, the kidney simply shrinks, whereas the calyces retain their normal cupping, causing the kidney to resemble a dwarf kidney.[113] In such cases, the differential diagnosis cannot be made by imaging studies alone, and a careful history becomes critical.

2. High-grade renal artery stenosis, or occlusion, secondary to embolism, thrombosis, or post-traumatic intimal tear. The history is vital to the diagnosis. The affected kidney would usually have a delayed calyceal appearance time, but this finding is unreliable.

3. Postinflammatory changes. In some instances after an acute pyelonephritis in infants, the kidney does not grow, although the calyces are normal.[114] This leads to a dwarflike appearance.[114] The history is crucial for the diagnosis.

4. Sterile vesicoureteral reflux. Some claim that the only effect of sterile vesicoureteral reflux on the kidney is that it does not grow.[115] If infection supervenes, the appearance usually can no longer be confused with simple hypoplasia.

5. After radiation therapy, if the kidney has been in the treatment field. The history is essential.

6. After a heminephrectomy, especially after the upper pole of a duplex kidney has been removed. The infundibulum of the calyx draining the apparent upper pole will look too short, and it is often possible to see surgical deformity of the rib. There will be a corresponding history and a surgical scar.

7. Renal vein occlusion.[116]

The *thin kidney* resembles a small hydronephrotic kidney. It usually excretes contrast material well, is smooth in outline, possesses a thin parenchyma, and has clubbed calyces, usually fewer than seven in number.

An identical appearance can be seen in reflux nephropathy due to high-pressure vesicoureteral reflux, and backpressure atrophy. In both cases, the history and other findings are important for the differential diagnosis.

The *Ask-Upmark kidney* is small, usually excretes contrast material well, usually has fewer than seven calyces, and has a slitlike scar, usually in the midzone. The calyces under the scar usually appear clubbed.

Because in *dysplastic and hypodysplastic kidneys* the dysplastic elements do not function, these kidneys may excrete contrast material poorly or not at all, depending on the ratio of dysplastic elements to nephrons. In more severe forms, the renal outline may appear lobulated, and the calyces may be severely clubbed and fewer than seven in number. The calyces may have an odd appearance, sometimes being vertically oriented; the renal pelvis may appear more vertical than is normal. An infant's kidney that does not excrete will be shown on an intravenous urogram only if the infant fortuitously voids and refluxes.

However, some very bizarre-appearing calyces and a vertical renal pelvis can be acquired, owing to reflux nephropathy with infection.[117]

Voiding Cystourethrography. This may show vesicoureteral reflux, especially if the ureteral opening is ectopic, but reflux is unpredictable. Sometimes, if both vesicoureteral reflux and intrarenal reflux occur, the primitive ducts, the tubules, and cysts may fill with contrast material, leading to a characteristic radiological appearance (Fig. 19–59).[118]

Angiography. Angiography is infrequently employed for the investigation of renal dysgenesis. It has been alleged that the angiographic appearance can differentiate a hypoplastic or dysplastic kidney from an acquired renal lesion on the following grounds: If the orifice of the artery is wide and the proximal segment of the artery tapers rapidly, then the lesion is acquired, because a wide orifice must formerly have supplied more renal tissue. If, on the other hand, the orifice is in proportion to the rest of the renal artery, the lesion is congenital. A few cases have been reported in which the pathologic findings support this theory.[119] It has been suggested that the capsular vessels surrounding the kidney become abnormally distant from it as the shrunken kidney retracts from them. In congenital hypoplasia, however, these vessels maintain their usual close proximity to the renal capsule.[120]

However, no available data examine the crucial case of a lesion acquired during early infancy, suggesting that this theory be applied cautiously.

Ultrasonography. On sonograms the hypoplastic kidney is small but otherwise normal (Fig. 19–60). The Ask-Upmark kidney shows an area of parenchymal thinning in which corticomedullary differentiation is absent (Fig. 19–61). The dysplastic kidney is also small, but is poorly defined and hyperechoic. Like other forms of chronic

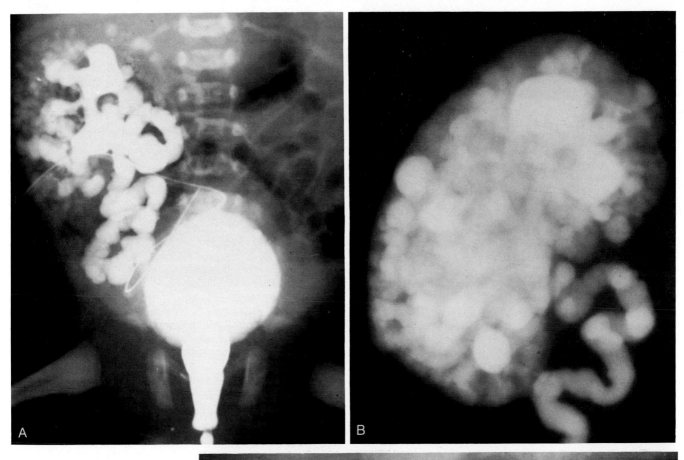

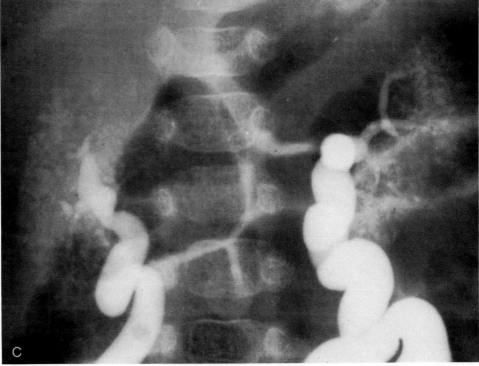

Figure 19–59. *A* to *C*, Examples of parenchymal reflux in renal dysplasia, filling the primitive ducts, the tubules and cysts. (From Pinckney LE, Currarino G, Weinberg WG: Parenchymal reflux in renal dysplasia. Radiology 141:681–686, 1981.)

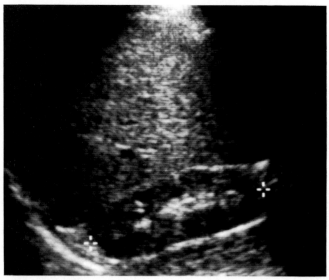

Figure 19–60. Hypoplastic kidney in a 12-year-old boy. Sonogram shows the right kidney, which measures only 5.6 cm in length. This is several standard deviations below normal for the patient's age. The kidney is otherwise normal in appearance.

renal parenchymal disease, it is not possible to differentiate cortex and medulla. In some cases there may be cortical cysts.

Scintigraphy. On scintigrams the hypoplastic kidney is small and smooth in outline, with an effective renal plasma flow less than that found on the normal opposite side. If the kidney is dysplastic, however, scintigraphy reveals a small poorly functioning or nonfunctioning kidney. A nonfunctioning dysplastic kidney may be filled via vesicoureteral reflux (Fig. 19–62).

Bilateral Renal Dysgenesis

Bilateral renal dysgenesis can occur in the following two forms: bilateral hypoplasia and bilateral dysplasia.

One of the best-known examples of bilateral hypoplasia is oligomeganephronia. Although contrast excretion is often suboptimal, both kidneys in patients with oligomeganephronia usually excrete enough contrast material to

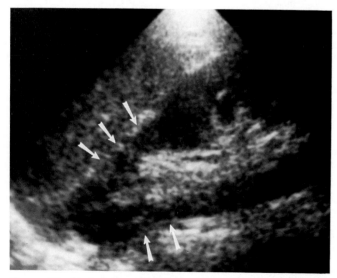

Figure 19–61. Ask-Upmark kidney. A coronal sonogram shows a generalized thinning of the parenchyma of the upper pole (*arrows*). No corticomedullary differentiation is apparent.

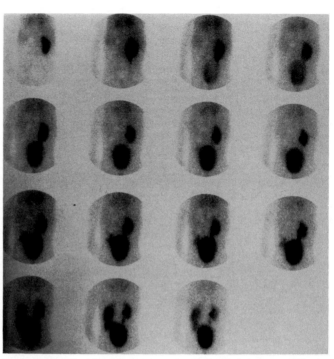

Figure 19–62. Nonfunctioning dysplastic left kidney, filled by reflux, shown in Tc-99m-DTPA scan. Sequential posterior images were taken at 2-minute intervals, from 2 to 24 minutes. In the scans taken between 2 and 14 minutes, activity is absent in the left flank. Between 14 and 20 minutes, tracer appears in the distal left ureter, indicating reflux. On the 22- and 24-minute scans, the dilated left pyelocalyceal system fills. (Courtesy of Barry Potter, M.D., and Bruce Markle, M.D.)

produce a nephrogram and a pyelogram revealing that they are both small and smooth in outline. The renal pelvis and calyces may appear relatively normal for the small-sized kidneys, but in some cases they reflect the underlying shortage of renal lobes (Fig. 19–63).

Oligomeganephronia is most often confused with nephronophthisis (medullary cystic disease). In most cases, the latter is inherited as an autosomal dominant trait with variable penetrance, although it may occur sporadically. Its characteristic feature is salt-losing nephropathy. It has been suggested that angiography is useful for differentiating oligomeganephronia from nephronophthisis; in the latter case, multiple radiolucent spaces are seen in a thin renal cortex that is poorly delineated from the medulla. However, ultrasonography and CT appear more reliable in making this distinction, because medullary cysts may be shown clearly by both modalities.

Prune-belly syndrome is another well-known example of bilateral dysplasia (Figs. 19–64 and 19–65). In severe cases, the kidneys are tiny, and there is marked fetal lobation. One kidney is often much smaller than the other. Some calyces are clubbed; others often appear normal, although they are asymmetrically distributed. The ureters show areas of dilatation and others of relative narrowing. They are very tortuous.

On sonograms, both kidneys are small, poorly defined, and hyperechoic. Some may show cortical cysts. In such cases the parenchyma is unevenly hyperechoic, and small scattered, round, sonolucent areas represent the cysts. The cortex and the medulla cannot be differentiated (Fig. 19–65A).

Scintigraphy usually shows high background activity and photopenic renal fossae (Fig. 19–65B).

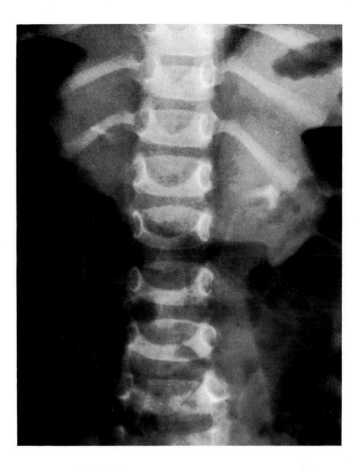

Figure 19–63. Oligomeganephronia. Intravenous urogram in a 3-year-old boy with oligomeganephronia demonstrates the typical findings of bilateral severe hypoplastic kidneys with attenuated collecting systems. The number of calyces seems less than that of a normal kidney. Creatinine was mildly elevated, but the excretion of contrast material was prompt and in good concentration. (Courtesy Massoud Majd, M.D.)

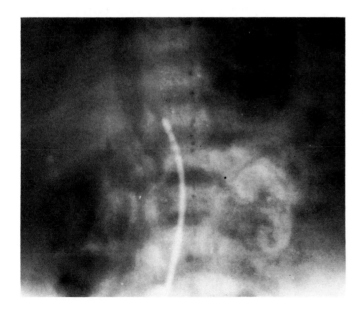

Figure 19–64. Bilateral renal dysplasia in a neonate with the prune-belly syndrome. The nephrogram phase of an arteriogram performed through an umbilical artery catheter shows two tiny kidneys. (From Friedland GW: Hydronephrosis in infants and children, Parts I and II. *In* Moseley RD Jr, (ed): Current Problems in Diagnostic Radiology. Chicago, Year Book Medical Publishers, 1978. Copyright © 1978 by Year Book Medical Publishers.)

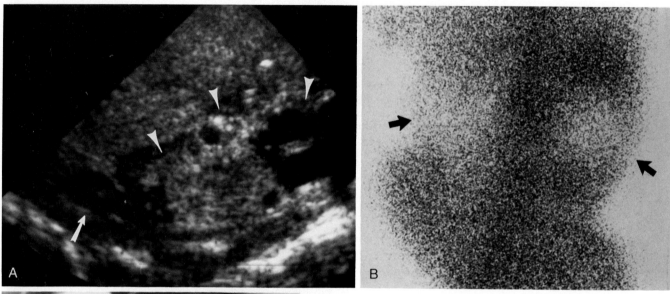

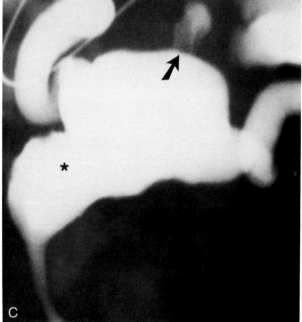

Figure 19–65. Prune-belly syndrome with severe renal dysplasia. *A,* Longitudinal right upper-quadrant sonogram shows a poorly defined, hyperechoic kidney *(arrowheads).* No recognizable corticomedullary differentiation is present; the parenchyma is unevenly hyperechoic, with scattered cortical cysts. Note the normal sonolucent adrenal gland *(arrow).* Scintigraphy *(B)* shows high background activity and photopenic renal fossae *(arrows). C,* Voiding cystourethrogram shows bilateral vesicoureteral reflux, dilated posterior urethra *(asterisk),* and a small urachal diverticulum *(arrow).* (Courtesy Massoud Majd, M.D., Barry Potter, M.D.)

Compensatory Hypertrophy

Compensatory renal hypertrophy is an acquired condition that results when one kidney is called upon to perform the work of two. Two forms of hypertrophy are recognized: diffuse and focal. The diffuse form is typically seen following nephrectomy, renal agenesis, hypoplasia, or atrophy, when the remaining kidney is healthy. The focal form occurs when the remaining kidney (or sometimes both kidneys) is diseased, as in reflux nephropathy, allowing only the remaining islands of normal renal tissue to participate in the compensatory process.

The stimulus for compensatory hypertrophy is poorly understood. Many theories have been advanced. Histologically, compensatory enlargement is seen to be mainly the result of the enlargement of existing nephrons (hypertrophy), rather than an increased mitotic cellular replication (hyperplasia).[121] Following nephrectomy in healthy kidney donors, overall renal function gradually increases, with the glomerular filtration rate (GFR) reaching 70% to 80% of the total for both kidneys within 1 year.[122]

The degree to which the normal human kidney can undergo compensatory hypertrophy is age-related, most marked in infants and young children and less marked in young adults, and it decreases with age. Some degree of hypertrophy is still possible as late as the 6th and 7th decades of life,[123–126] however, in spite of earlier reports[127] to the contrary. Compensatory hypertrophy does not occur in utero, because maternal renal function masks any fetal renal deficiency.[128] At birth, therefore, the size of a single functioning kidney is normal. It enlarges rapidly, however, reaching a volume roughly equivalent to that of two normal kidneys by 1 year of age.[128]

DIAGNOSTIC IMAGING

Compensatory hypertrophy can be detected because of changes on the intravenous urogram, sonogram, CT scan, or scintigram.

Intravenous Urography. The increase in size of the diffusely hypertrophied kidney is manifested urographically by an enlarged normal outline and an increased fullness of the collecting system and ureters (Fig. 19–66).[121]

In nodular compensatory hypertrophy, the intravenous urogram shows areas of scarring and intervening renal masses (sometimes quite large), which take up contrast material like normal renal parenchyma (Fig. 19–67).

Ultrasonography. In diffuse compensatory hypertrophy, the kidney appears enlarged but otherwise normal. In nodular compensatory hypertrophy, there are parenchymal scars, between which are areas of large mass resembling normal-appearing kidney tissue.

Computed Tomography with Contrast Enhancement. The kidney is enlarged but otherwise normal in diffuse compensatory hypertrophy. In nodular compensatory hypertrophy, scars are seen within the renal parenchyma, with masses between the scars. The masses have a normal cortex and medulla. In order to visualize this area properly, it is necessary to obtain the early vascular phase of the nephrogram.

Angiography. The renal artery of the hypertrophied kidney is usually noticeably increased in diameter. Because flow through an artery varies with the fourth power of the diameter, even slight increases are hemodynamically significant.

Scintigraphy (DMSA or Glucoheptonate Scan). Diffuse hypertrophy is revealed by scintigraphy as an enlarged

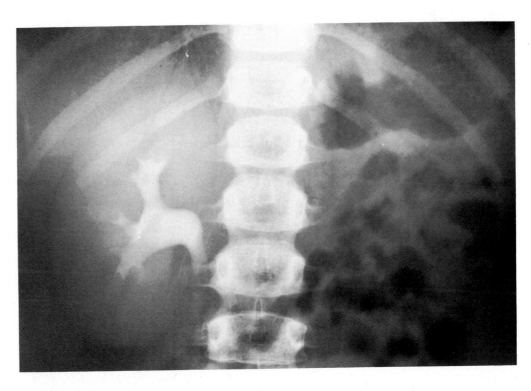

Figure 19–66. Compensatory hypertrophy of the right kidney in a child following left nephrectomy for Wilms' tumor. The intravenous urogram shows a large but otherwise normal-appearing right kidney and an absent left kidney.

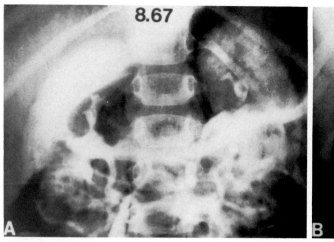
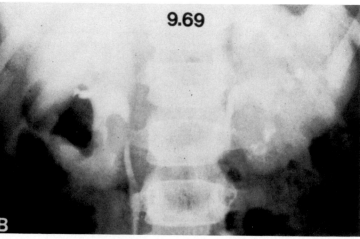

Figure 19–67. Nodular compensatory hypertrophy. *A,* Intravenous urogram performed in this child shows that the upper pole of the left kidney is normal. Between that time and 2 years later, when a second intravenous urogram *(B)* was obtained, the child had multiple episodes of acute left pyelonephritis. *B* shows clubbing of the upper pole calyces with overlying parenchymal scarring. Immediately below, in the midzone, a focal mass protrudes from the outline of the left kidney. This proved to be an area of nodular compensatory hypertrophy. The lower pole of the kidney also shows marked clubbing and scarring.

but otherwise normal-appearing kidney. With nodular hypertrophy, uptake in the large hypertrophied masses is normal. Therefore, scintigraphy is by far the best method of showing that these masses are normally functioning hypertrophied tissue.

Anomalies in Position

Anomalies of Rotation

In the supine position, the medial border of the normal kidney is much more anterior than the lateral border, so that the kidney lies at an angle of about 30 degrees from the horizontal.[129] Thus, the normal renal pelvis is anterior as well as medial to the kidney.

The following five types of rotational anomalies have been delineated (Figs. 19–68 and 19–69):[130, 131]

1. Nonrotation. The renal pelvis lies directly anterior to the kidney; the kidneys lie at an angle of about 90 degrees from the horizontal.

2. Incomplete rotation. The renal pelvis lies between 30 and 90 degrees from the horizontal.

3. Reverse rotation. The renal pelvis lies somewhere between the lateral side of the kidney and the direct anterior position. Characteristically, the renal vessels are twisted around the anterior surface of the kidney.

4. Excessive rotation. This may superficially resemble reverse rotation, except that the renal vessels are twisted around the posterior surface of the kidney, and the renal pelvis faces posteriorly or posteromedially.

5. Transverse rotation. The calyces point superiorly or inferiorly, or in some intermediate direction.

Nonrotation and incomplete rotation are the most common rotational anomalies. These may be unilateral or bilateral, and often accompany ectopia or fusion anomalies.

Malrotation has no specific complications, but affected kidneys are prone to the same diseases that affect a normal kidney.

EMBRYOLOGY OF ROTATIONAL ANOMALIES

Normally, the developing metanephros rotates from a dorsomedial position to a more lateral one relative to the collecting system. This process occurs during the "ascent" of the kidney, which occurs between Stage 16 (about 38

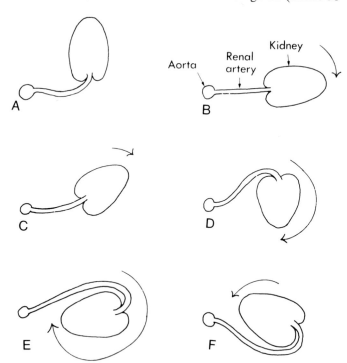

Figure 19–68. Diagram shows the following anomalies of renal rotation: *A,* nonrotation—the renal pelvis lies directly anterior to the kidney; *B,* the normal position of the adult kidney, with the hilus facing medially; *C,* incomplete rotation; *D,* excessive rotation—the renal pelvis faces posteriorly; *E,* excessive rotation—the renal pelvis lies laterally; *F,* reverse rotation—the renal pelvis lies laterally. (From Gray SW, Skandalakis JE: Embryology for Surgeons: The Embryological Basis for the Treatment of Congenital Defects. Philadelphia, WB Saunders Company, 1972, p 479.)

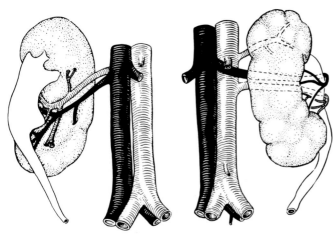

Figure 19–69. Diagram illustrates reverse rotation *(left)* and excessive rotation *(right)*. (From Weyrach HM: Anomalies of renal rotation. Surg Gynecol Obstet 69:183–199, 1939. By permission of SURGERY, GYNECOLOGY & OBSTETRICS.)

days) and Stage 19 (about 49 days) (Fig. 19–70).[132] Renal rotation occurs before definitive renal vascularization takes place.[133] Although a number of theories have been offered to explain anomalies of rotation,[131, 134, 135] at the moment they are purely speculative. The embryological basis of anomalies of rotation, therefore, is still unknown.

DIAGNOSTIC IMAGING

Intravenous Urography. Rotational anomalies are important because they are frequently mistaken for some more serious condition on an intravenous or retrograde urogram study. This mistake can happen for the following reasons:

1. The malrotation may erroneously be attributed to displacement by a paravertebral mass.

2. In nonrotation, the renal pelvis and calyces are seen on end; consequently they appear peculiar (Fig. 19–71).

3. In other types of malrotation, the calyces at first seem clubbed. The infundibula may look elongated and deformed, not unlike crab's legs. The renal pelvis can appear unusual, lying at an abnormal angle relative to the calyces (Fig. 19–71). In reverse rotation, it may even be lateral to them, as the calyces point toward the midline (Fig. 19–72). In malrotation, the ureter must always cross the lower pole of the kidney.

4. Commonly, the lower pole causes deviation in the course of the crossing ureter. Usually such deviation is anterior and lateral, sometimes creating the impression that a lower pole mass is present (Fig. 19–73).

Oblique views are of great help in establishing that the malrotated kidney is otherwise normal. In this projection the malrotated kidney resembles a normal kidney much more than on a straight anteroposterior view. It is also helpful to examine carefully the calyces and the parenchymal thickness. For this purpose, it is important to draw the interpapillary line of Hodson, connecting the tips of the papillae, and to measure the parenchymal thickness from this line to the border of the kidney at multiple points. If the problem is simply malrotation, this thickness should be normal everywhere. Focal thickness would suggest a mass; focal thinness would suggest a scar, just as with any other kidney.

Finally, the calyces of a malrotated kidney, although seen head-on or at an unusual angle, will still be cupped and the fornices will still be sharp.

When apparent malrotation is observed, it is important to be sure that the patient has not had prior surgery, since postoperative repositioning may be responsible for the abnormal orientation of the kidney. For the same reason, disease in the subcapsular, perinephric, anterior paranephric, and posterior paranephric spaces must also be excluded.

Other Studies. Neoplasms, abscesses, hematomas, uriniferous pseudocysts, or accumulations of normal extraperitoneal fat in any of these spaces can all rotate the kidney (Fig. 19–74). Thus, it is sometimes necessary to examine these other spaces by means of ultrasonography or CT to be certain that the renal malposition is not a manifestation of extrarenal disease.

Ultrasonography reveals that the nonrotated renal pelvic is directly anterior to the calyces and the renal parenchyma (Fig. 19–75). If reverse rotation has occurred, the renal pelvis is seen lateral to the kidney, instead of medial to it.

Scintigraphy shows nonrotation or other types of malrotation very well (Fig. 19–76).

Renal Ectopia

Renal ectopia describes a kidney congenitally in an abnormal location.

Figure 19–70. Diagram illustrates rotation and ascent of the kidneys: Stage 16 *(left)*; Stage 17 *(middle)*; Stage 19 *(right)*. (From Kelly HA, Burnam CF: Diseases of the Kidneys, Ureters, and Bladder, Vol 1. New York, D Appleton and Co, 1914, p 92.)

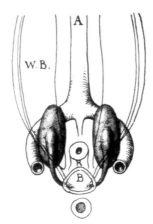
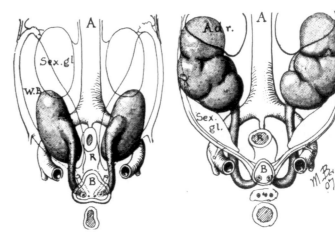

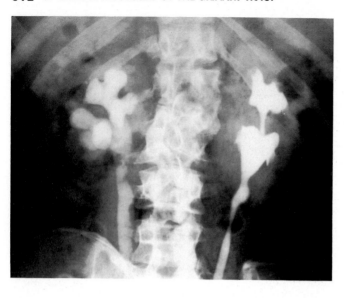

Figure 19–71. Intravenous urogram showing nonrotation of the left kidney. The renal pelvis and calyces are seen on end. Also seen are congenital anomalies of the first three lumbar vertebrae, and a congenital right ureterovesical junction obstruction accounts for the right hydronephrosis.

Figure 19–72. Excretory urogram shows reverse rotation of the right kidney. The right renal pelvis lies lateral to the calyces and infundibula.

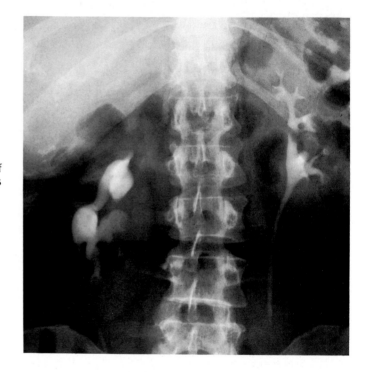

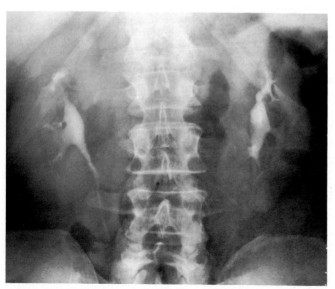

Figure 19–73. Intravenous urogram shows nonrotation of the left kidney. The lower pole of the left kidney deviates the crossing left ureter laterally.

Figure 19–74. Rotary displacement of the left kidney simulating malrotation: lymphoma. Excretory urography shows the left kidney slightly displaced laterally and the renal pelvis anteriorly rotated. Although this appearance simulates that seen in congenital malrotation, the findings in this case were produced by a paravertebral lymphoma, which rotated the left kidney on a craniaocaudal axis as it displaced the kidney laterally. Care must be taken not to overlook paravertebral masses as a cause of apparent malrotation.

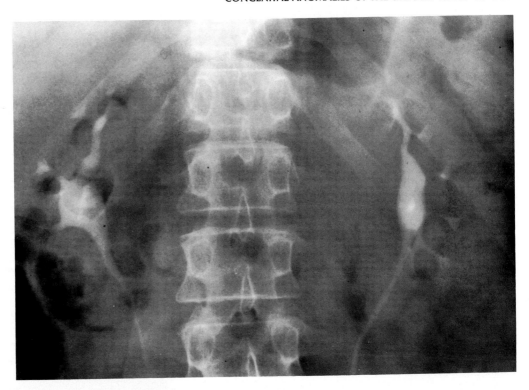

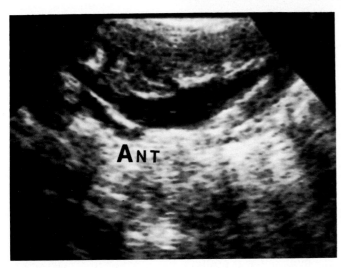

Figure 19–75. Nonrotated kidney. A prone longitudinal sonogram shows an elongated dilated renal pelvis lying directly anterior to the calyces and renal parenchyma.

Figure 19–76. Reverse rotation of the left kidney. Tc-99m-DTPA scan, posterior view, demonstrates the reverse rotation.

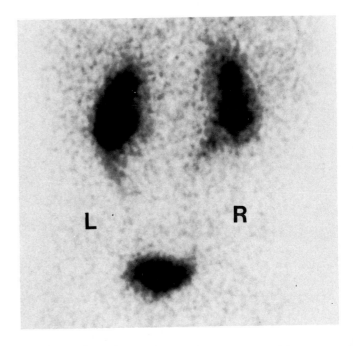

The arterial blood supply to an ectopic kidney also arises ectopically, usually from a major artery in the immediate vicinity of the malpositioned kidney. The length of the attendant ureter must adjust itself to the position of the kidney; therefore, intrathoracic kidneys have ureters that are longer than normal, whereas pelvic kidneys have shorter ones.

It is important not to confuse renal ectopia with renal ptosis, which refers to an abnormally mobile kidney that drops further down in the abdomen, especially when the patient is in the upright position. In the latter case, the attendant ureter is of normal length (although it may be quite redundant when the patient stands), and the renal arteries arise from their normal sites.

EMBRYOLOGY OF RENAL ASCENT

The kidney initially develops opposite the future S2 vertebra, but eventually comes to rest opposite the L1 or L2 vertebra (Fig. 19–70). However, in order to understand the factors leading to renal ectopy (discussed later in this section) it is helpful to review the theories that attempt to explain how the kidney reaches its normal position.

1. The ureter grows so that its tip presses against the surrounding developing kidney, forcing the kidney in a cranial direction. In fact, it is probable that diminished ureteral growth is one of the factors leading to caudal ectopy.[5]

2. Renal "ascent" is partly the result of straightening of the developing vertebral column, which tends to force the kidney cranially.[136]

3. Some investigators maintain that the kidney does not "ascend" at all, but that the caudal part of the embryo grows away from the renal blastema, and the ureters lengthen as it grows away. This caudal growth takes place both dorsally and ventrally, but it is greater in the ventral direction. It results in the spinal curvature being flattened. This flattening proceeds progressively caudally as the embryo grows.[12] A recent paper[40] disagrees with this thesis, however, arguing that the kidney really does ascend.

CLASSIFICATION

Ipsilateral Ectopia. Renal ectopia can be *ipsilateral,* meaning that the kidney is on the same side of the body as the orifice of its attendant ureter. The ureter is usually, but not always, orthotopic.

Renal ectopias may further be divided into *cranial ectopias* and *caudal ectopias,* according to whether they are above or below the normal position.[137] Cranial renal ectopias are usually *intrathoracic,* in which case the kidney lies partially or completely in the thorax.

Caudal ipsilateral ectopia, also known as *simple ectopia,* is generally classified as follows (Fig. 19–77).[138]

1. Abdominal. The kidney lies above the iliac crest, but below the level of L2.

2. Iliac. The kidney is located opposite the iliac crest or in the iliac fossa.

3. Pelvic (sacral). The kidney is located in the true pelvis.

Any of these caudal ectopias can involve one or both kidneys, although unilateral involvement is much more

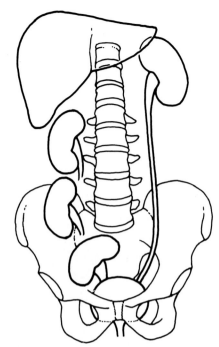

Figure 19–77. Diagram illustrates the three types of caudal ipsilateral ectopia (abdominal, iliac, and pelvic).

common. Caudal ectopias involving both kidneys are rare, but the least common form occurs in a solitary kidney.

Crossed Renal Ectopia. Also known as *contralateral renal ectopia,* this disorder occurs when the kidney is located on the side of the body opposite the orifice of its attendant ureter. In decreasing order of frequency, this may occur with fusion, without fusion, or in a solitary kidney.

COMPLICATIONS

Ectopic kidneys may develop any of the diseases that normally located kidneys may develop, but they are more prone to certain complications than are normally located kidneys.

1. Abdominal and iliac ectopic kidneys are more injury-prone, because they are unprotected by ribs and lie in a more anterior position. Participation in contact sports should therefore be carried out with great circumspection, if at all.

2. About 50% of pelvic kidneys have decreased function.

3. Ureteropelvic junction obstruction and renal stones are more common in patients with ectopic kidneys.

4. Pelvic kidneys may obstruct labor,[139, 140] although their surprising degree of mobility often allows them to be displaced into the lower abdomen, permitting normal vaginal delivery.[141]

HEREDITARY FACTORS

Only one study in the literature screened families for ectopia and malrotation. The results showed that ectopia was inherited as an autosomal recessive trait.[142] Ectopic kidneys have also been reported in monozygotic twins, which again indicates a hereditary factor;[143] a more definitive statement regarding the possible hereditary basis of renal ectopy must await further investigation.

Table 19–17. Congenital Anomalies Commonly Associated with Renal Ectopia

System	Incidence	Anomaly
Genitourinary tract[144, 145]	50%	Renal malrotation Hypospadias High ureteral insertion into renal pelvis Ectopic ureter Extrarenal calyces Calyceal diverticula Bladder exstrophy
Skeleton[144, 145]	50%	Rib anomalies Assymetrical skull Vertebral body anomalies Absence of a bone (commonly the radius)
Cardiovascular[144, 145]	40%	Valvular defects Septal defects
Gastrointestinal[144–147]	33%	Anorectal malformations Malrotations Malposition of ipsilateral colonic flexure
Ears, lips, palate[144, 145]	33%	Lowset ears Absent ears Hare lip Cleft palate
Hemopoietic[148]	7%	Fanconi's anemia

ASSOCIATED CONGENITAL ANOMALIES (Table 19–17)

Cranial Ectopia (Superior Ectopia). This kidney, also called an *intrathoracic kidney,* has partially or completely herniated into the thorax through the lumbocostal triangle or the foramen of Bochdalek.[149, 150] It is radiologically similar to another form of superior ectopy, in which the kidney is not actually intrathoracic but lies below a localized eventration of the membranous part of the diaphragm. The kidneys in 46% of patients who have an omphalocele lie in an abnormally cranial position (Fig. 19–78);[151] in 43% of these patients, the anomaly is on the right side only, and in 57% it is bilateral. If the omphalocele includes the liver, the kidney is always abnormally cranial.[151] The adrenal gland may lie above, behind, or below the ectopic kidney.[150]

This congenital anomaly is rare, occurring in approximately 1 in 15,000 autopsies performed in children,[145] and is more common in males.

In order of decreasing frequency, superior ectopic kidneys may occur with the left kidney only, the right kidney only (the liver presents some barrier to excessive right-sided ascent), or both kidneys.

Embryology of Cranial Ectopia. In the absence of restraint by any diaphragmatic structures, the kidney continues to ascend through the foramen of Bochdalek in the loose mesenchymal zone known as the sliding plane. This plane is bounded ventrally by the mesonephros, dorsally and laterally by the body wall, and medially by the mesentery or mediastinum.

Diagnostic Imaging. A superior ectopic kidney is often first seen on a chest radiograph, as a well-defined posteroinferior mediastinal mass (Fig. 19–79) that can be mistaken for other posteroinferior mediastinal masses (neurogenic neoplasms, neuroenteric cysts, meningoceles, pericardial cysts, and other hernias through the foramen of Bochdalek). The kidney may appear to be normally located at birth, with the typical radiological appearance delayed for several months.[227]

An intravenous urogram with tomograms is helpful, because it shows a nephrogram and pyelogram and helps to identify the mass as an intrathoracic kidney (Fig. 19–79C) or, if a pneumoperitoneum is performed, as a kidney lying below a diaphragmatic eventration (Fig. 19–80). CT can show the kidney residing in the thorax. An aortogram, rarely performed for this purpose, shows an elongated renal artery, usually arising from the aorta at the normal level; occasionally, an accessory renal artery arises from the thoracic aorta.[150] Either a technetium-99m (Tc-99m) DMSA or glucoheptonate scan can prove that a posterior mediastinal mass is kidney. Ultrasonography can be very helpful in showing whether a kidney is below the diaphragm. Ultrasonography can also show the diaphragm very well; it can show whether, for example, a kidney lies just below an eventrated diaphragm or is passing through a defect in the diaphragm.

Abdominal and Iliac Ectopia. Abdominal and iliac ectopia can be simple (unilateral, bilateral, or solitary) or crossed.

The incidence of simple abdominal and iliac ectopia on intravenous urography is estimated at approximately 1 in 600.[137] The adrenal gland is characteristically in the normal place, despite the malposition of the kidney. The adrenal hypertrophies in fetuses and neonates with renal agenesis or ectopia.[79, 80] The average length of the right adrenal in such patients is 3.4 cm, but on the left it is 2.9 cm. On both sides, the average thickness is 5 mm.[80]

As in renal agenesis, the adrenal also loses its characteristic V or Y shape, and becomes elliptical, such that it can resemble a kidney.[80]

Embryology of Caudal Ectopia. Several hypotheses regarding the origins of caudal ectopia are as follows:

1. Diminished ureteral growth is one factor leading to caudal ectopia.[5]

2. The umbilical arteries can block the cranial ascent of the kidney.[152, 153]

3. There is a consistent asymmetry in the level of development of the two kidneys in luxate mice; this probably occurs in humans with unilateral renal ectopia.[154]

Diagnostic Imaging. An abdominal radiograph, a barium enema, or a small-bowel series may show malposition of the colon identical to that which occurs in renal agenesis (see Fig. 19–54) and is discussed on page 599.

Intravenous urography shows that the kidney is in an abnormal position, in either the abdominal or iliac areas (Figs. 19–81 and 19–82). The kidney is usually smaller, and the ureter shorter, than normal. There is always a rotational anomaly—incomplete rotation, nonrotation, or reverse rotation. The calyces sometimes have a very bizarre appearance when the kidney is in the abdominal or iliac areas (Fig. 19–81). Extrarenal calyces are common.

Angiography is not often called for, but if performed it will show the renal arteries arising from lower in the aorta than is normal. Multiple renal arteries are common.

CT with contrast material shows the kidney and its abnormal relationship very clearly. The adrenals appear linear on CT.[86, 87] In addition, CT may reveal that the colonic flexures, duodenum, loops of small bowel, spleen, and tail of the pancreas are in an abnormal position.[86]

Both scintigraphy (with Tc-99m DMSA, glucoheptonate, or DTPA) and ultrasonography can demonstrate

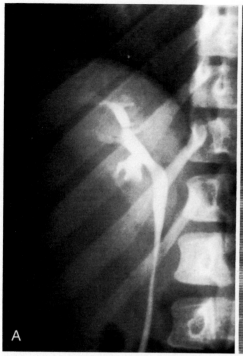
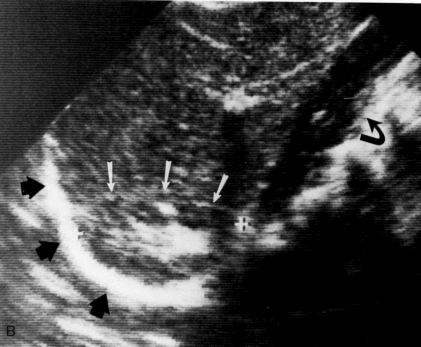

Figure 19–78. Cranial ectopia in an infant with omphalocele. *A,* An intravenous urogram, RPO view, shows cranial ectopia of the right kidney. *B,* Sonography demonstrates that the right kidney *(white arrows)* lies immediately beneath the echoic diaphragm *(large black arrows).* The kidney is displaced superiorly relative to the sonolucent psoas muscle *(curved black arrow).*

whether the kidney is in an abnormal position. In the neonate, the large and abnormally shaped adrenal can resemble a kidney. However, its echogenicity differs; the cortex is anechoic, and the medulla is echogenic.[80]

Pelvic (Sacral) Ectopia. A pelvic kidney exists when the kidney lies in the true pelvis below the terminal line, which proceeds from the superior margin of the sacral promontory to the superior margin of the symphysis pubis.[155]

Pelvic kidneys may be unilateral, bilateral crossed, or solitary. The left kidney is involved in about 70% of patients; if the congenital anomaly is bilateral, the left kidney is usually lower than the right, and the kidneys are usually fused.

Pelvic kidney occurred in 22 of 15,919 autopsies performed in children, or 1 in 724 cases; it also, however, occurred 21 times in 260,888 new pediatric admissions to the Mayo Clinic, or 1 in 12,423 cases.[145] This latter figure is probably far too low, because most patients do not have imaging studies for pelvic kidneys. The autopsy evidence is probably closer to the true prevalence. Solitary pelvic kidney is rare, being estimated to occur in 1 in 22,000 individuals.[131]

Associated Urinary Tract Anomalies. Four other anomalies are commonly associated with pelvic kidneys (Table 19–18). Other less common associations include

Table 19–18. Urinary Tract Anomalies Commonly Associated with Pelvic Kidneys

Anomalies of rotation
Ureter that is frequently too high as it exits the renal pelvis ("high insertion")
Ectopic ureter
Extrarenal calyces[140]

calyceal diverticula, absent uterus,[158] and absent or hypoplastic vagina.[159]

Diagnostic Imaging. On the abdominal radiograph, it may be possible to observe malposition of the colon. The renal outline is not visible in the expected place. Sometimes the soft-tissue outline of the kidney is visible in the true pelvis.

For the intravenous urogram, if an ectopic kidney is suspected from the preliminary abdominal radiograph, a 14- by 17-inch film, substituted for the usual coned film obtained during the nephrogram phase, is more likely to record the nephrogram of an ectopic kidney (Fig. 19–83). If a pelvic kidney has not been suspected from the preliminary abdominal radiograph, and only one kidney is visible on the intravenous urogram, a kidney may still be somewhere in the pelvis. The pelvis must be scrutinized very carefully, because pelvic kidneys can be difficult to locate, for the following reasons:

1. Sacral superimposition makes it easy to mistake the collecting system for the struts of bone between the sacral foramina (Fig. 19–84).

2. The pelvis is a common area for bowel gas and stool to collect; if the patient is not well prepared, the kidney can be obscured.

3. The collecting system of a pelvic kidney frequently empties rapidly, and hence may not be well filled with contrast material (Fig. 19–85).

4. It is impossible to apply compression to the ureter of a pelvic kidney.

Often, a clue to a pelvic kidney is the ureter itself, which can be visible even if the collecting system and the kidney are not. Even this finding must be interpreted carefully, because it is easy to mistake bowel wall for the ureter. When doubt exists, oblique views and tomograms

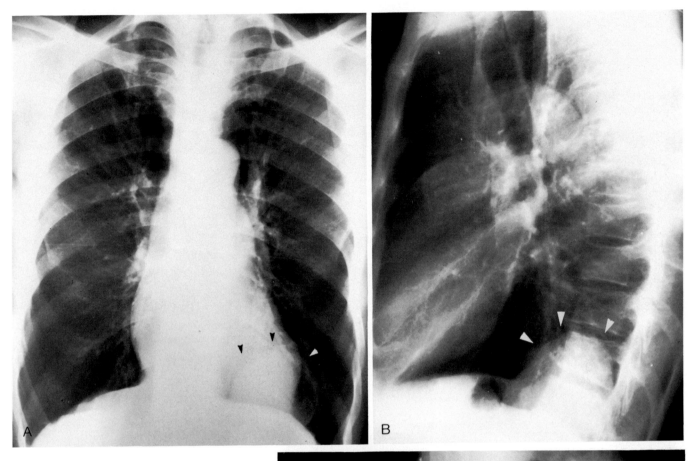

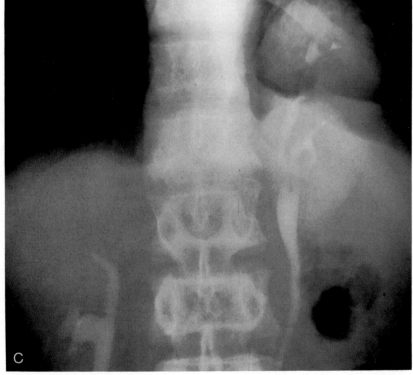

Figure 19–79. Intrathoracic kidney. *A* and *B*, Chest radiographs demonstrate a well-defined posterior inferior mediastinal mass *(arrowheads)*. *C*, An excretory urogram shows that the mass is an intrathoracic kidney.

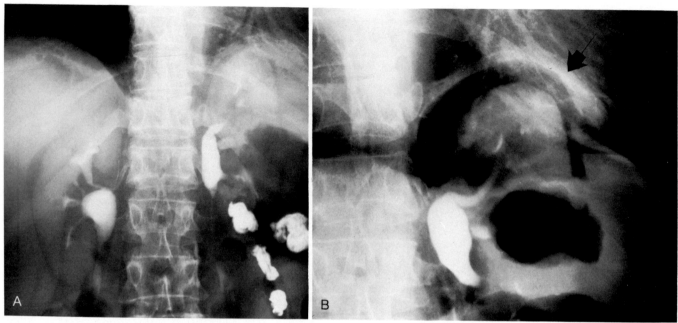

Figure 19–80. Cranial ectopia in which the kidney lies beneath the dome of the diaphragm. *A,* Excretory urogram shows cranial ectopia. *B,* A pneumoperitoneum was induced, and shows that the kidney lies below the eventrated hemidiaphragm (*arrows*).

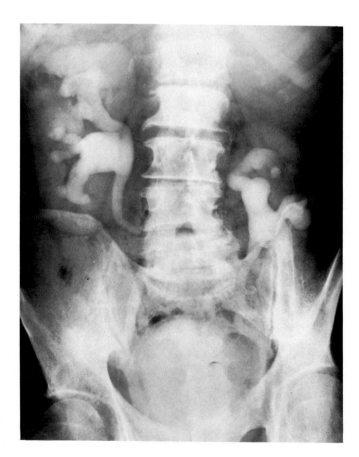

Figure 19–81. Intravenous urogram showing left caudal ectopia. A rotational anomaly is seen, and the calyces have a very bizarre appearance.

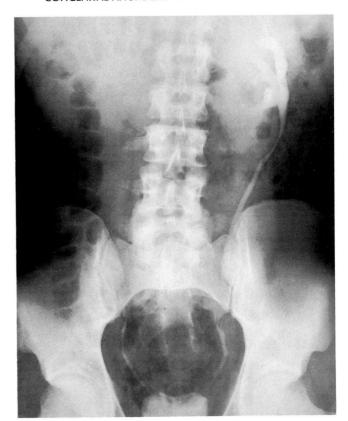

Figure 19–82. Intravenous urogram shows right caudal ectopia and left reversed rotation. The right kidney overlies the sacrum.

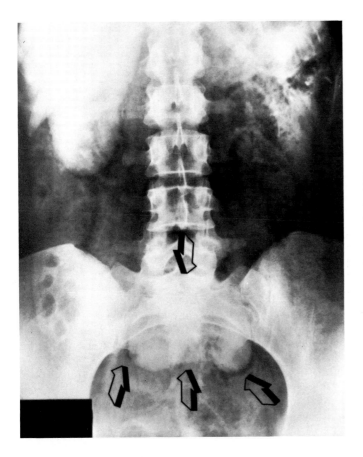

Figure 19–83. Intravenous urogram showing a presacral left kidney *(arrows)*. A presacral kidney was suspected from the preliminary abdominal radiograph, so a 14- by 17-inch film was substituted for the usual coned film obtained during the nephrogram phase. This procedure is more likely to record the nephrogram of an ectopic kidney. (From Friedland GW, Goris ML, Gross D, et al: Uroradiology: An Integrated Approach. New York, Churchill Livingstone, 1983, p 1642. By permission.)

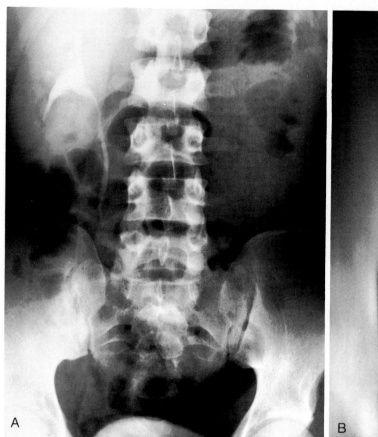
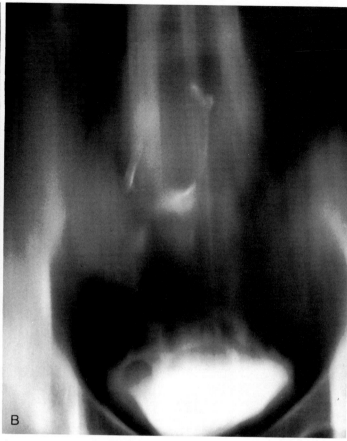

Figure 19–84. Presacral kidney. *A,* An intravenous urogram shows a right kidney. The left kidney is invisible, because sacral superimposition makes it easy to mistake the collecting for the struts of bone between the sacral foramina. *B,* Tomograms reveal the presacral kidney.

prove useful (Fig. 19–84). A retrograde pyelogram (Fig. 19–86) is rarely necessary.

When CT is used for evaluating pelvic kidneys, intravenous contrast material should always be used to avoid the chance of mistaking them for various pelvic masses. In this way, it is possible to visualize the nephrogram as well as the collecting system (Fig. 19–87).

The renal arteries, which are often multiple, usually arise from the distal aorta or the bifurcation of the aorta.

Scintigraphy (Fig. 19–88) and MRI (Fig. 19–89) can also clearly demonstrate a pelvic kidney.

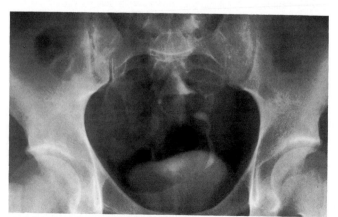

Figure 19–85. Intravenous urogram showing left pelvic kidney. A normal right kidney and ureter were present.

Crossed Renal Ectopia. Crossed renal ectopia with fusion is discussed in the renal fusion section, page 636. Crossed ectopia without fusion (Fig. 19–90) is rare,[160–162] accounting for only 10% to 15% of all crossed ectopic kidneys.

Embryology. Many hypotheses suggest possible origins of crossed renal ectopia, but ample evidence suggests that both the mesonephric ducts and the ureteral buds may stray from the normal course, giving rise to crossed ectopia.

Diagnostic Imaging. A plain abdominal radiograph shows malposition of the colon, and can indicate that the kidney is not in its normal place.

On an intravenous urogram, it is sometimes obvious that there are two kidneys clearly separated from one another. If they are not widely separated, the fact that they are separate structures may not be discernible by excretory urography. Usually this question is academic, unless one kidney is diseased and requires surgery, especially nephrectomy. Under these circumstances, or any in which the information may be useful, CT with closely spaced (4- to 5-mm) cuts can show the degree of separation of the kidneys. Angiography may be useful before any contemplated surgery, as it can provide a "road map" of the arteries.[165]

A solitary crossed ectopic kidney (Fig. 19–91) is even less common than crossed ectopia without fusion.[167–171] It may occur at the normal level, although on the wrong side of the body.[170] CT, a technetium-99m DMSA scan,

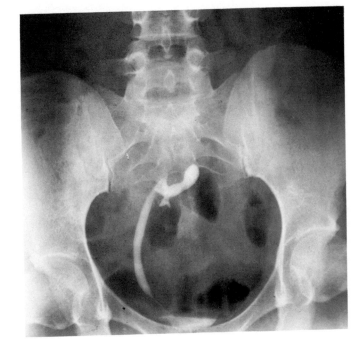

Figure 19–86. Retrograde pyelogram demonstrating a solitary pelvic kidney.

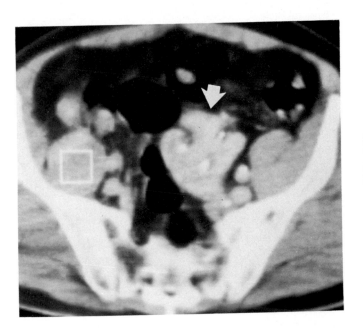

Figure 19–87. CT scan with contrast material at the level of the pelvis demonstrates a pelvic left kidney *(arrow)*. (Courtesy Morton Bosniak, M.D., New York University Medical Center, New York.)

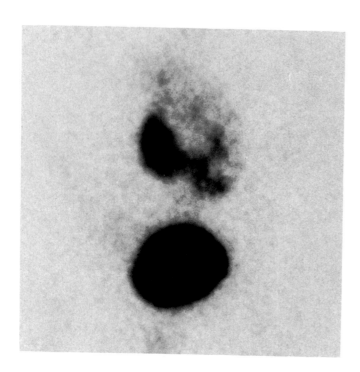

Figure 19–88. Tc-99m-DTPA scan demonstrates a solitary pelvic kidney. (Courtesy Massoud Majd, M.D.)

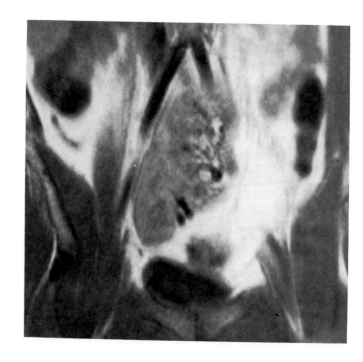

Figure 19–89. Coronal MRI scan demonstrates a pelvic kidney (spin-echo, T1-weighted image). (Courtesy Zoran L. Barbaric, M.D., Department of Radiological Science, The Center for Health Sciences, Los Angeles, California.)

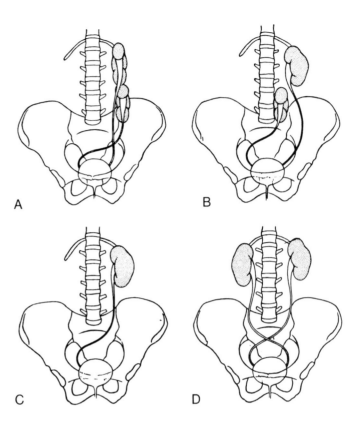

Figure 19–90. Four varieties of crossed ectopia: *A,* with fusion, *B,* without fusion, *C,* solitary, *D,* bilateral. (Redrawn from Mc-Donald JH, McClellan DS: Crossed renal ectopia. Am J Surg 93:995–1002, 1957; as reproduced by Abeshouse BS, Bhisitkul I: Crossed renal ectopia with and without fusion. Urol Int [Basel] 9:63–91, 1959. By permission of S Karger AG, Basel.)

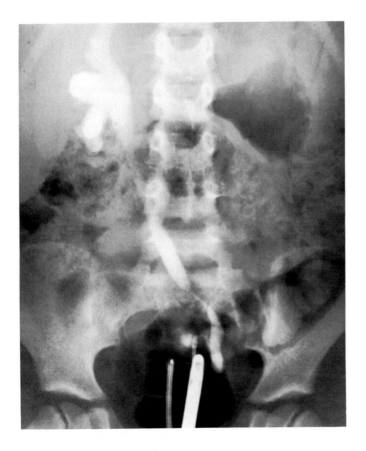

Figure 19–91. Retrograde pyelogram showing solitary crossed ectopia. This is considered to represent agenesis of the right kidney with crossed ectopia of the left kidney to the right—an exceedingly rare anomaly.

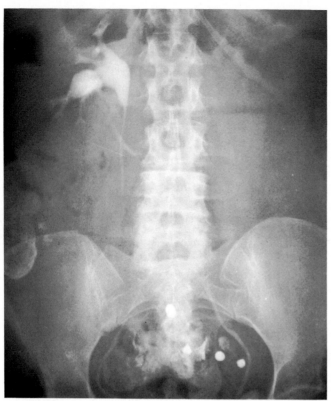

Figure 19—92. Intravenous urogram showing what appears to be a left crossed ectopia without fusion. In fact, the patient had a large left-sided retroperitoneal liposarcoma.

and angiography are helpful in showing whether the kidney is truly solitary; here again, the angiogram proves useful if surgery is considered.

Bilateral crossed ectopia occurs when both the left and the right kidneys are on the wrong side, whereas their attendant ureters arise normally.

Retroperitoneal masses can force a kidney to the opposite side of the body. The resultant appearance can simulate crossed unfused ectopia on an intravenous urogram (Fig. 19—92); however, CT can readily demonstrate the retroperitoneal mass (Fig. 19—93).

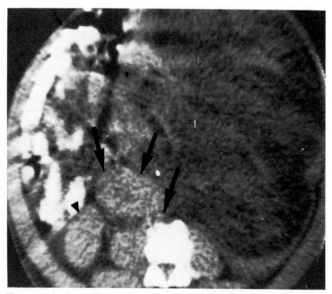

Figure 19—93. CT scan showing a large retroperitoneal liposarcoma forcing the left kidney (arrows) over to the right. Arrowhead identifies the right kidney itself.

Anomalies in Form: Renal Fusion

Renal fusion can take many forms: horseshoe, unilateral, and pelvic. These basic types have many variations.

Horseshoe Kidney

The horseshoe kidney is common, occurring in about 1 in 400 people.[157] Horseshoe kidneys have been reported in identical twins.[172] Because they have also been reported in only one of a set of identical twins,[173] no clear evidence of a hereditary trait exists. The largest number of horseshoe kidneys have been found in stillbirths, while a smaller number have been found in live infants, with the incidence decreasing through childhood and adult life.[174] This gradual decrease occurs because the associated anomalies are usually the reason that the horseshoe kidney is discovered in the first place.[174]

Most of the parenchyma of each kidney lies on the opposite side of the body, and the two kidneys are connected by an isthmus, usually at the lower poles.[175, 176] This isthmus is composed of normal kidney tissue (Fig. 19—94) or connective tissue (Fig. 19—95), and contributes to the characteristic horseshoe shape.

The horseshoe kidney is always ectopic in that it lies lower than the normal kidney. The inferior mesenteric artery always crosses the isthmus. The blood supply usually involves multiple arteries, arising from the aorta, the common iliac, the internal iliac, the external iliac, or the inferior mesenteric arteries (Fig. 19—96).[221]

The isthmus is usually anterior to the aorta and the vena cava (Fig. 19—97), although on rare occasions it may be posterior to both. Alternatively, it may lie between the vena cava and the aorta, where the vena cava is anterior to the isthmus and the aorta is posterior to it. Bifid or double ureters commonly drain horseshoe kidneys (Fig. 19—97).

A rare variant is the upside-down horseshoe, in which the fusion occurs superiorly (Fig. 19—98).

EMBRYOLOGY

At Stage 15, the two metanephrogenic blastemas have grown very close together, and their outer zones virtually touch (Fig. 19—99). This would be the easiest time for fusion to occur. At this point, the kidneys have not yet ascended between the two umbilical arteries. This is important because one currently popular theory regarding the embryological basis of the horseshoe kidney suggests that the umbilical arteries press the lower poles of the kidneys together as the kidneys ascend between them.

This theory was first put forward by Kelly and Burnam[132] in their classic text (Fig. 19—70). They based their theory on an examination of embryos destined to become part of the Carnegie Collection. However, the earliest embryo available to them was from Stage 16. They thus missed all the earlier processes, which we now know contain evidence that the two kidneys can fuse before ascending between the umbilical arteries.

Figure 19—100, for example, illustrates an embryo in which the kidneys fused below the umbilical arteries, before they ascended.[177] For all these reasons it important to keep an open mind regarding the ultimate embryological basis of horseshoe kidney.

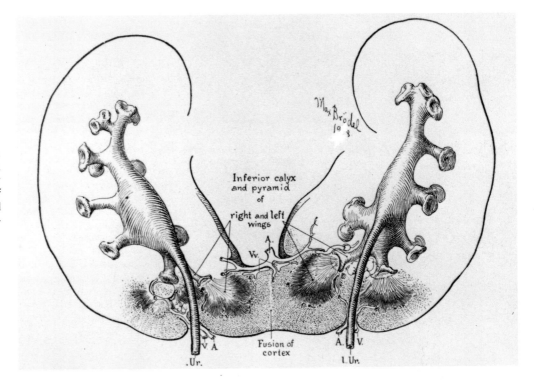

Figure 19–94. Drawing of a coronal section through a horseshoe kidney. (From Kelly HA, Burnam CF: Diseases of the Kidneys, Ureters and Bladder, Vol 2. New York, Appleton Co, 1914, p 313.)

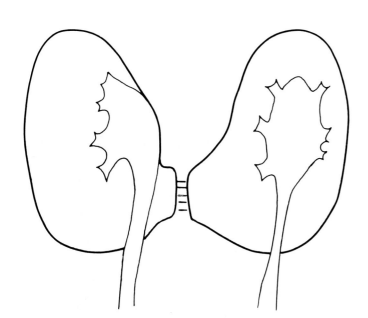

Figure 19–95. Diagram illustrates a horseshoe kidney in which the isthmus is composed of connective tissue.

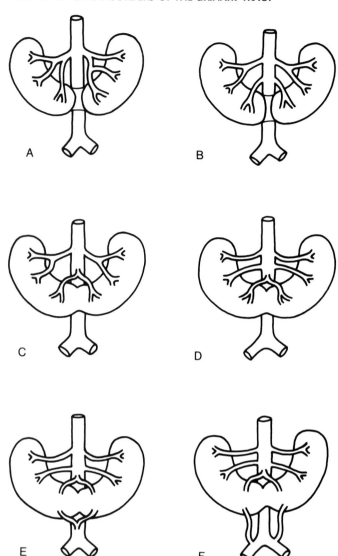

Figure 19–96. Variations in the arterial blood supply to the horseshoe kidney. *A*, A pair of kidneys approximate the midline but are not actually fused in it. Each kidney is supplied by a single artery whose segmental vessels divide early in the pedicle. *B*, The arteries to all segments except the lower segment on both sides are as in a normal kidney. The arteries to the lower segments arise directly from the aorta. They divide into branches, which correspond to the anterior and posterior branches of the normal kidney. *C*, The arterial arrangement is the same as in *B*, except that the two lower segment arteries, instead of arising on either side of the aorta, have fused to form a common trunk and have arisen from its anterior surface. *D*, The middle segment artery as well as the lower segment vessel arises directly from the aorta. *E*, The lower poles of both kidneys receive twin vessels from the aorta both above and below the isthmus. *F* is similar to *E*, except that the posterior branch of the lower segment artery arises from the bifurcation of the aorta or the common iliac arteries. (Modified from Graves FT: The Arterial Anatomy of the Kidney. The Basis of Surgical Technique. © 1971, the Williams & Wilkins Co, Baltimore, pp 39–44.)

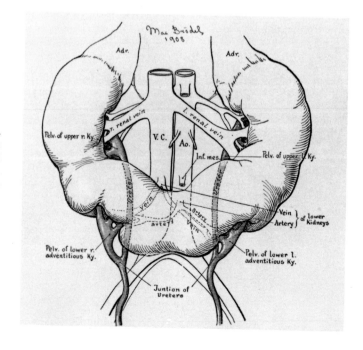

Figure 19–97. Horseshoe kidney and bilateral bifid ureters, with aberrant arterial supply to, and venous drainage of, each of the fused kidneys. The isthmus is anterior to the aorta and vena cava. (From Kelly HA, Burnam CF: Diseases of the Kidneys, Ureters, and Bladder, Vol 2. New York, Appleton Co, 1914, p 316.)

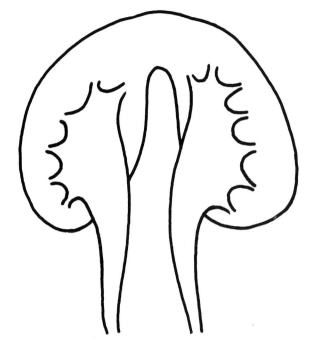

Figure 19–98. Diagram shows upside-down horseshoe kidney, in which the upper poles have fused.

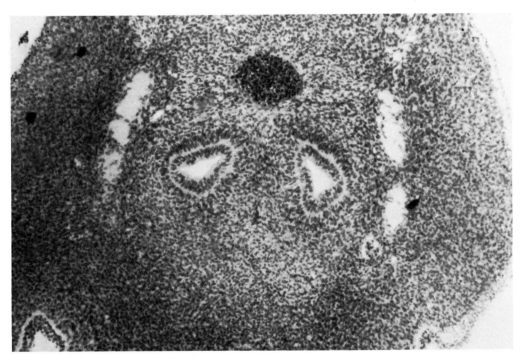

Figure 19–99. Coronal section through Stage-15 embryo showing coapted lower poles of the right and left developing kidneys. They lie below the umbilical arteries. (From the Carnegie Collection.)

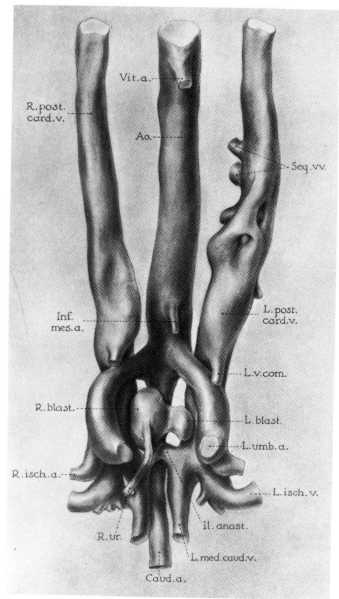

Figure 19–100. Illustration of a wax plate reconstruction of a 10-mm human embryo. The right and left metanephrogenic blastemas are fused below the umbilical vascular girdle. (From Boyden EA: Congenital absence of the kidney, an interpretation based on a 10-mm human embryo exhibiting unilateral renal agenesis. Anat Rec 52:325–349, 1932.)

POSSIBLE POINTS OF FUSION

Horseshoe kidneys can fuse directly in the midline, or they may fuse laterally, in which case some calyces from one side cross the midline and drain some of the renal parenchyma on the opposite side.[178]

POSITION OF THE RENAL PELVIS

The position of the renal pelvis depends on whether the kidney is fused laterally or in the midline. If fusion is in the midline, the position of the renal pelvis depends on whether the isthmus is wide or narrow.[178]

If the width of the isthmus is less than one-third the length of the kidney, the renal pelvis lies somewhere between the normal 30-degree anteromedial angle and the 90-degree direct anterior angle (Fig. 19–101A). However, if the width of the isthmus is one-third the length of the kidney or greater, then the pelvis lies somewhere between the direct anterior and the lateral position (Fig. 19–101B). A rare variation in kidneys fused at the midline occurs when calyces from opposing sides communicate with each other through a common renal pelvis (Fig. 19–102).

In laterally fused kidneys, the part crossing the midline lies approximately in a transverse position. The remaining part is vertical, and the kidney somewhat L-shaped (Fig. 19–103).[178] The pelvis of the part of the kidney that crosses the midline is anterior or lateral; the pelvis of the vertical part is anterior or medial.

The renal pelvis is often large and flabby, and the ureter inserts abnormally high in the pelvis, although small duplicated pelves can occur.

COMPLICATIONS OF HORSESHOE KIDNEYS

The following complications can result from this anomaly:

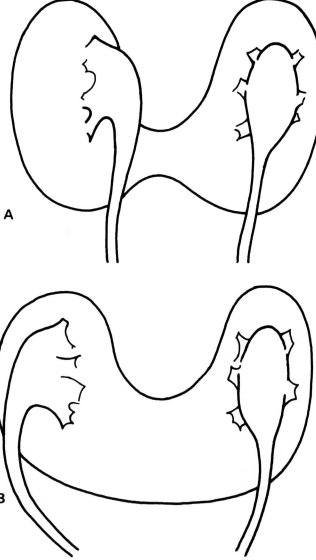

Figure 19–101. Position of the renal pelvis in horseshoe kidney. *A,* Narrow isthmus with pelvis anterior or medial. *B,* Wide isthmus with pelvis anterior or lateral.

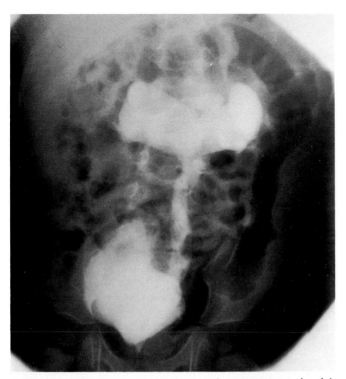

Figure 19–102. Horseshoe kidney with common renal pelvis in a 21-month-old male with anal atresia of the supralevator type. Excretory urogram reveals a horseshoe kidney with both renal pelves joined to form a common pelvis with one ureter. The right ureter was absent. A cutaneous vesicostomy has been performed. (Courtesy Jeffrey Woodside, M.D.)

1. Horseshoe kidneys are prone to injury. The isthmus lies in a very anterior position and is not protected by the ribs. It is easily split by a hard blow to the abdomen. Such kidneys must be protected, especially in patients performing contact sports.

2. Because of the high insertion of the ureter into the renal pelvis, varying degrees of ureteropelvic junction obstruction may accompany the horseshoe kidney.

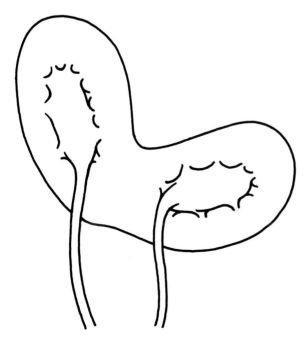

Figure 19–103. Diagram illustrates an L-shaped kidney.

Table 19–19. Congenital Disorders in Which the Incidence of Horseshoe Kidneys is Increased

Chromosomal abnormalities
Turner's syndrome[181, 182]
Trisomy 18[183]
Hematological abnormalities
Fanconi's anemia[148]
Dyskeratosis congenita with pancytopenia[184]
Laurence-Biedl-Moon syndrome
Thalidomide embryopathy[185]

3. Stones are common in horseshoe kidneys. In 75% of patients they are metabolic stones, and in 25% they are struvite stones, resulting from infection with urea-splitting organisms.[179]

4. Wilms' tumors in children are 1.76 to 7.93 times more common in horseshoe kidneys than in the general population.[180]

ASSOCIATED ANOMALIES AND CONGENITAL DISORDERS

Horseshoe kidneys are seen in a great number of heterogeneous congenital disorders (see Table 19–19). Associated anomalies are listed in Table 19–20.

DIAGNOSTIC IMAGING

Plain Abdominal Radiograph. On the plain abdominal radiograph, the following four kinds of abnormalities of the kidney outline(s) may be visible: (1) lower than normal, (2) too close to the spine, (3) vertical long axis, and (4) visible isthmus.

Intravenous Urogram. On the intravenous urogram, the nephrogram is U shaped or L shaped, depending on whether midline or lateral fusion has occurred (Fig. 19–104). Tomograms of horseshoe kidneys can be deceiving. The nephrogram can look normal, because the kidneys are located posteriorly, whereas the isthmus lies anteriorly, outside the area where the tomographic sections are usually made.

The renal pelvis is often large and extrarenal. Its exact orientation depends on whether midline or lateral fusion has occurred (Figs. 19–105 to 19–107). Some degree of ureteropelvic junction obstruction, including delayed

Table 19–20. Anomalies Associated with Horseshoe Kidneys

Organ	Anomaly (in Descending Order of Frequency)[145]
Urinary tract	Ureteropelvic junction obstruction
	Vesicoureteral reflux
	Unilateral or bilateral duplication
	Megaureter
	Ectopic ureter
	Unilateral triplication[188]
	Renal dysplasia[189]
	Retrocaval ureter[190]
	Supernumerary kidney
Gastrointestinal tract[145, 186, 187]	Anorectal malformations[191]
	Esophageal atresia
	Rectovaginal fistula
	Omphalocele
Other	Cardiovascular, vertebral, neurological, peripheral skeletal, facial

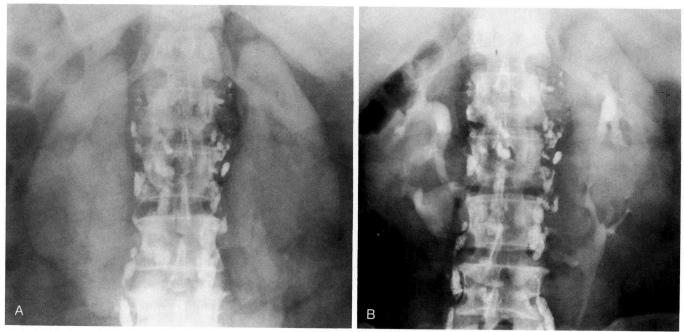

Figure 19–104. Intravenous urogram performed on a patient with a horseshoe kidney. *A,* The nephrogram reveals that the kidney is lower than normal and too close to the spine. The long axis is vertical and the isthmus is visible, with contrast material in lymph nodes from lymphogram. *B,* Later, contrast material outlines bilateral duplex systems.

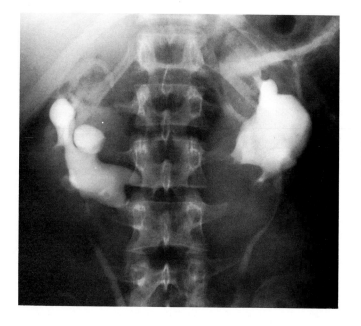

Figure 19–105. Intravenous urogram demonstrates a horseshoe kidney with midline fusion and a narrow isthmus. Both pelves are anterior.

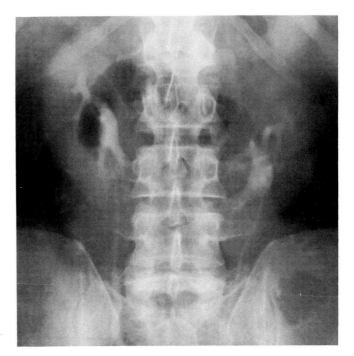

Figure 19–106. Intravenous urogram demonstrates a horseshoe kidney with a wide isthmus. The right pelvis is anterior and the left pelvis is lateral.

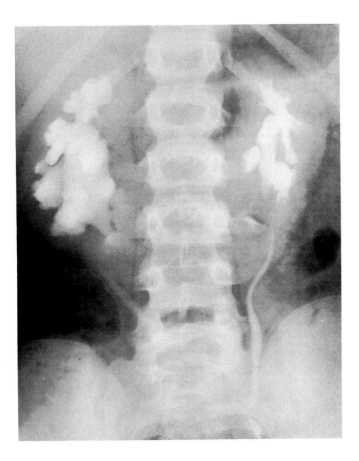

Figure 19–107. Intravenous urogram demonstrates a horseshoe kidney with a wide isthmus. The right renal pelvis is lateral, and the left renal pelvis is anterior. The right renal pelvis is large. As each ureter crosses the isthmus, it curves laterally then medially as it assumes a more normal course after crossing the isthmus (the so-called flower-vase appearance).

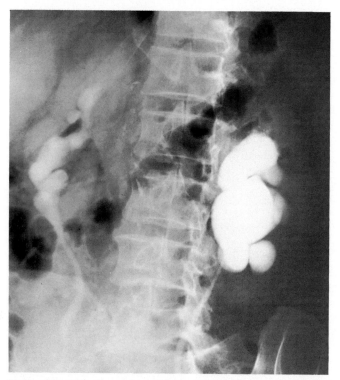

Figure 19–108. Horseshoe kidney with left ureteropelvic junction obstruction. Intravenous urogram, RPO view, shows a markedly distended left pyelocalyceal system.

emptying, is seen in many patients (Figs. 19–108 and 19–109).

In midline fusion, the lower calyces descend toward the midline near the isthmus, resulting in the appearance of the so-called hand-holding calyces. Where lateral fusion has occurred, the lower calyces on one side tend to cross the midline.

The lower calyces are often medial to the ureter on the same side. When this is found, a horseshoe kidney should immediately be suspected, although a similar appearance may be seen in renal malrotation without fusion.

As each ureter crosses the isthmus, it curves laterally. It continues medially and assumes a more normal course after crossing the isthmus. Because of the unusual configuration formed by the ureters, this is called the "flower-vase" appearance (Fig. 19–107). Ascertaining the position of the ureters, which can vary widely, is not required for diagnosis. Gutierrez has pointed out that two lines connecting the lowermost calyces of a horseshoe kidney with a horizontal line drawn through the iliac crest invariably intersect at an acute angle.[222]

A normal kidney on one side and an ectopic, incompletely rotated kidney on the other side can mimic the appearance of a horseshoe kidney.

Some urologists separate horseshoe kidneys, often to treat abdominal pain. The remaining kidneys may look peculiar. A thoracolumbar gibbus deformity can displace the axes of the kidneys in such a way as to cause them to resemble a horseshoe kidney.[193] Scintigraphy, however, can distinguish kidneys with a normal shape from a genuine horseshoe kidney.[193] The false impression of a horseshoe kidney can be gained when both kidneys are huge and their lower poles are forced together, as, for example, in autosomal recessive polycystic kidney disease.

A horseshoe kidney can develop any lesion that can be found in a normal kidney (Figs. 19–109 and 19–110).

Angiography. Angiography may be necessary to provide information about renal arterial supply before surgery or, if hypertension is present, to check for stenosis. It may be needed during the investigation of trauma or for other reasons. When it is performed, however, the normal anatomical variations, some of which may not seem normal, should be remembered.

Scintigraphy, Ultrasonography, Computed Tomography, and Magnetic Resonance Imaging. Scintigraphy (Fig. 19–111) (either Tc-99m-DMSA or glucoheptonate scan), ultrasonography, CT (Fig. 19–112), or MRI can show whether the kidney has a horseshoe shape. In addition, they can show whether the kidney has a wide or narrow isthmus or some other unusual (e.g., L-shaped) configuration.

Special caution is necessary with regard to ultrasonography of the horseshoe kidney, as it will show the isthmus of the kidney anterior to the aorta (Fig. 19–113).[196] This is easily mistaken for a neoplastic abdominal mass, especially in patients with known neoplasms, in whom metastases are suspected.

Scintigraphy is much better than ultrasonography or excretory urography for diagnosing an asymmetrical horseshoe kidney (Fig. 19–114).[197] It may even detect a horseshoe kidney on a bone scan, apart from conventional scintigraphic techniques aimed at the kidney itself.

Voiding Cystourethrography. Vesicoureteral reflux is common in patients with horseshoe kidneys (Fig. 19–115).

Surgical Considerations. It is often desirable to know, prior to surgery, whether the isthmus is composed of functioning renal parenchyma or consists merely of fibrous tissue. Scintigraphy (Tc-99m-DMSA scans) can readily provide this information, as can CT[223] and MRI. Because the unexpected finding of a horseshoe kidney during surgery for an abdominal aortic aneurysm can significantly affect surgical management, such patients should have their kidneys evaluated routinely when they undergo other preoperative abdominal imaging studies for aortic aneurysms. Patients with calculi complicating the horseshoe kidney also present special problems. Percutaneous stone removal requires variations from standard approaches. Even extracorporeal shock wave lithotripsy (ESWL) may be difficult because of the anterior location of these kidneys.

Disc (Cake, Lump) Kidney

A rare variation of midline renal fusion occurs when the kidney is a single disc. This is usually called the disc, cake, or lump kidney. It usually lies lower than a horseshoe kidney, often in the pelvis. A fused pelvic kidney can be drained by a single ureter.[199] Figure 19–100 illustrates how this anomaly can develop embryologically.[177]

In a patient with cancer of the bladder for whom cystectomy is contemplated, a fused pelvic kidney makes access to the bladder more difficult. The urologist will need to exercise great care not to injure the aberrant renal vessels in the process of a lymph node dissection.[200]

On intravenous urography, CT, scintigraphy (Fig. 19–116), or MRI, a single confluent mass of renal tissue is visible, with the two collecting systems lying side by side

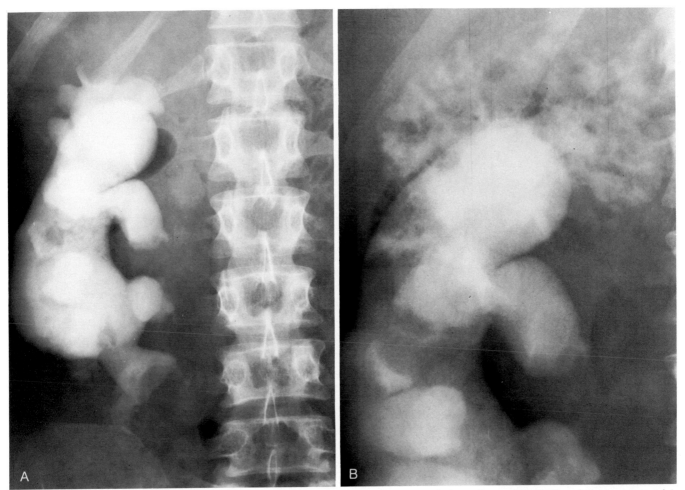

Figure 19–109. Horseshoe kidney in a patient with autosomal dominant polycystic kidney disease (ADPKD) and right ureteropelvic junction obstruction. *A,* Intravenous urogram, with the film coned to the right half of the horseshoe kidney, shows a lateral right renal pelvis and right ureteropelvic obstruction. *B,* Angiogram, performed through a separate artery supplying the right upper pole of this kidney, shows a typical Swiss-cheese nephrogram, characteristic of ADPKD.

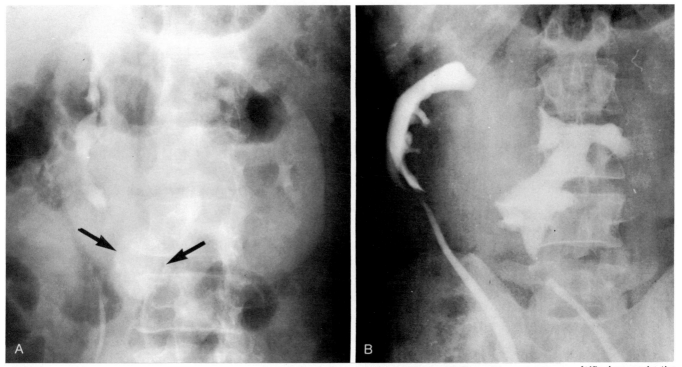

Figure 19–110. Neoplasms occurring in horseshoe kidney. *A,* Excretory urogram, RPO position, shows a calcified mass in the isthmus of a horseshoe kidney *(arrows),* which proved to be a renal cell carcinoma. *B,* Retrograde pyelogram in a second patient reveals a huge renal cell carcinoma originating in isthmus of horseshoe kidney.

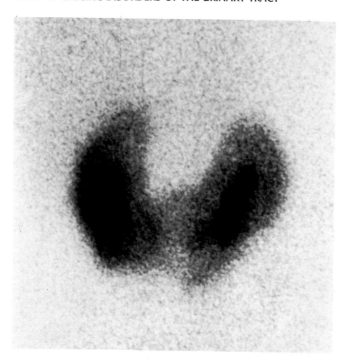

Figure 19–111. Tc-99m glucoheptonate (GHA) scan shows a symmetrical horseshoe kidney with a functioning isthmus. (Courtesy Massoud Majd, M.D.)

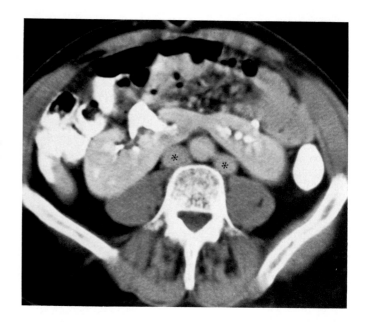

Figure 19–112. CT scan through the isthmus of a horseshoe kidney, in which there is parenchymal fusion. Note the presence of a double inferior vena cava *(asterisks).*

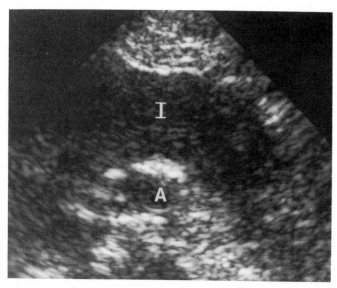

Figure 19–113. Sonogram taken in the transverse direction showing the isthmus (I) of a horseshoe kidney anterior to the aorta (A). This can be very easily mistaken for a neoplasm.

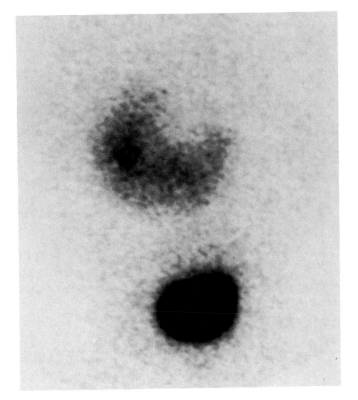

Figure 19–114. Tc-99m-GHA scan shows an asymmetrical horseshoe kidney with uptake in the isthmus. Scintigraphy is much better than ultrasonography or excretory urography for diagnosing an asymmetrical horseshoe kidney. (Courtesy Massoud Majd, M.D.)

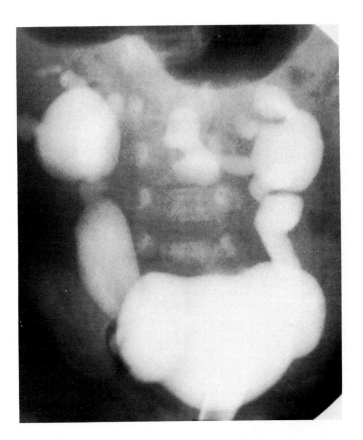

Figure 19–115. Voiding cystourethrogram performed in an infant with a horseshoe kidney shows bilateral vesicoureteral reflux.

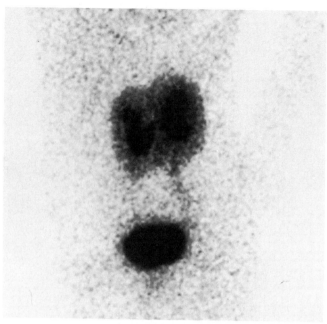

Figure 19–116. Tc-99m-GHA scintigram demonstrates a fused pelvic kidney. (Courtesy Massoud Majd, M.D.)

or with one collecting system anterior to the other. If ultrasonography is used, the disorder is best seen on a transverse scan. A single large confluent mass of renal tissue will be visible, and the two echo complexes will lie side by side, or one will lie anterior to the other (Fig. 19–117).

Unilateral Fused Kidney or Crossed Fused Renal Ectopia

This congenital anomaly occurs when the kidney completely or almost completely crosses the midline to the opposite side of the body and fuses with the kidney on that side. Various series have reported its incidence to be in the range of 1 in 1300 to 1 in 7600.[145] It occurs in males significantly more often than in females and is found on the right side two to three times more often than on the left.[145]

The anomaly has a vast number of classifications, and even more types; however, the following classification is the simplest and most useful.[130] The six varieties are listed in their order of illustration, not in order of frequency (Fig. 19–118).

Superior Ectopia. The kidney crosses over the midline and lies superior to the resident kidney. The pelves of both kidneys are rotated anteriorly.

The Sigmoid or S-Shaped Kidney. The crossed kidney lies inferiorly; the pelvis of the resident kidney is directed medially; the pelvis of the crossed kidney is directed laterally.

The Unilateral Lump Kidney. The two kidneys are completely fused to form a large irregular lump. Both pelves are directed anteriorly. This should not be confused with the midline lump kidney.

The Unilateral L-Shaped Kidney. The kidney that has crossed the midline lies inferiorly and transversely; the resident is oriented normally. This type should not be confused with the L-shaped horseshoe kidney.

The Unilateral Disc Kidney. Each kidney is fused to the other along the medial concave border. The renal pelvis of the resident kidney is located anteromedially, whereas the pelvis of the other is anterolateral. This should not be confused with the midline disc type.

Inferior Ectopia. The kidney that has crossed the midline lies inferior to the resident kidney, and its upper pole has fused with the lower pole of the resident. Both renal pelves are directed anteriorly.

The descending order of frequency for these anomalies is the inferior kidney, the S-shaped kidney, and the lump and disc kidneys. Superior ectopia and L-shaped anoma-

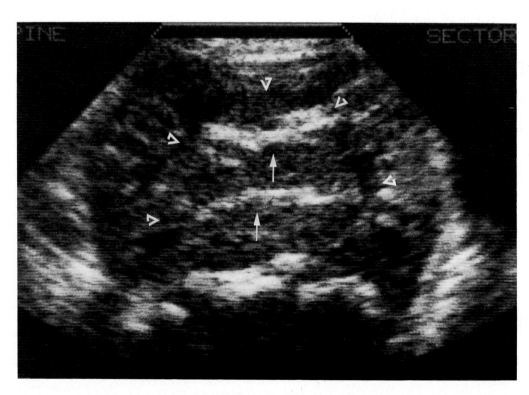

Figure 19–117. Cake kidney. A transverse midabdominal sonogram shows a large confluent mass of renal tissue (arrowheads), with one collecting system echo complex (arrow) anterior to the other (arrow). A few distorted sonolucent medullary rays are discernible. (Courtesy Barry Potter, M.D., and Bruce Markle, M.D.)

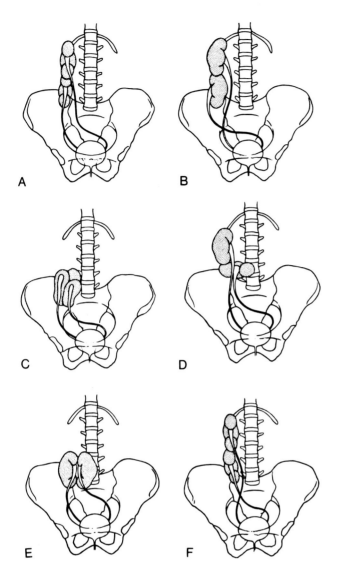

Figure 19–118. Diagram illustrates the types of crossed renal ectopia with fusion: *A,* superior ectopia; *B,* the sigmoid or S-shaped kidney; *C,* the lump kidney; *D,* the unilateral L-shaped kidney; *E,* the unilateral disc kidney; *F,* inferior ectopia. (Modified from McDonald JH, McClellan DS: Crossed renal ectopia. Am J Surg 93:995–1002, 1957; as reproduced by Abeshouse BS, Bhisitkul I: Crossed renal ectopia with and without fusion. Urol Int [Basel] 9:63–91, 1959. By permission of S Karger AG, Basel.)

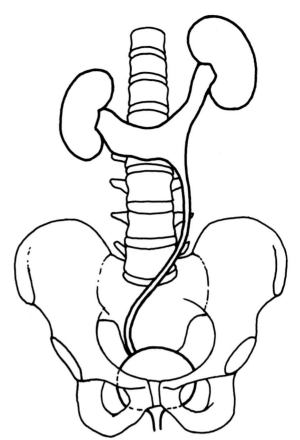

Figure 19–119. Diagram illustrates two separate kidneys on the opposite sides of the spine, which share a single, T-shaped renal pelvis, drained by a single ureter.

lies are rare. The classification can seem arbitrary in practice, because individual cases may not precisely fit any of the categories. For example, an interesting but rare form of crossed fused ectopia can occur when two fused kidneys share a single renal pelvis, which is drained by a single ureter crossing the midline.[201] A similar anomaly can occur when two separate kidneys, on opposite sides of the spine, share a single, T-shaped renal pelvis ("common renal pelvis"), which is also drained by a single ureter (Fig. 19–119).[206, 207]

The crossed fused ectopic kidney has an anomalous blood supply arising from the vessels in the vicinity (Fig. 19–120).

Complications include high insertion of the ureter into the renal pelvis, leading to an increased incidence of ureteropelvic junction obstruction. Stones may occur.

Associated anomalies[204, 205] include nearly all those associated with horseshoe kidneys.

DIAGNOSTIC IMAGING

The intravenous urogram outlines the nephrogram in one of the shapes described, together with an appropriate collecting system (Figs. 19–121 to 19–123). It will be evident that one of the ureters crosses the midline to the opposite side.

Scintigraphy can outline the various kidney shapes described above, as can ultrasonography. A Tc-99m DMSA or glucoheptonate scan clearly reveals the shape of the fused kidney (Figs. 19–124 and 19–125). A Tc-99m-DTPA scan, at about 2 minutes into the series, shows a single irregular mass of functioning kidney tissue on one side of the abdomen. Later, at about 10 minutes, two separate pyelocalyceal systems become visible. At that point, the ureters are also visible, one of which is crossing to the other side of the abdomen.

Sonographically, it is possible to see one or two anterior or posterior notches in the renal parenchyma.[204, 205] These are entirely separate from the sinus, although a similar notch may normally occur in the renal sinus. The two renal sinuses of the fused kidneys lie in different planes and run in different directions, and the echoes reflect these differences (Fig. 19–126).[204, 205] This is in contrast to double collecting systems, in which case the echoes are in the same plane and same direction. If the echoes are in different planes and directions, the opposite renal fossa should be searched, elsewhere in the abdomen and in the pelvis, for another kidney. If none is found, the diagnosis of crossed fused ectopia is strengthened.[204, 205]

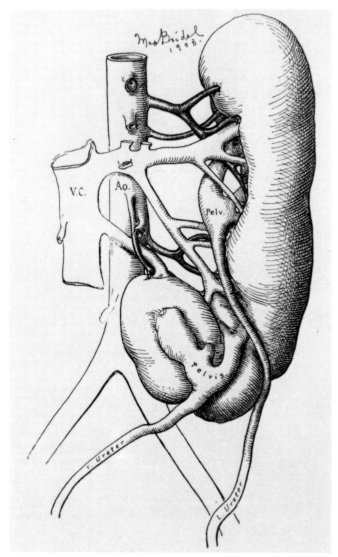

Figure 19–120. Anatomical drawing of crossed fused ectopia with anomalous blood supply. (From Kelly HA, Burnam CF: Diseases of the Kidneys, Ureters and Bladder, Vol 2. New York, Appleton Co, 1914, p 318.)

MRI can also demonstrate the fused kidney and the absence of a kidney on the contralateral side (Fig. 19–127). Arteriography is only routinely performed to show the vascular supply before surgery.

Anomalies in Structure

Congenitally Large Septa of Bertin (Cloisons, Lobar Dysmorphism)

The septa of Bertin consist of cortical tissue, extending from the cortex to the renal sinus, that separates the medulla into segments. They were first described by Bertin as "cloisons," meaning septa, although Bertin's word was mistranslated for many years as "columns." Thanks to Hodson, Bertin's original meaning has been restored.[210, 211]

A congenitally large septum of Bertin consists of normally functioning nephrons. These form a renal mass ranging from 2 to 6 cm in diameter, with an average diameter of 3.5 cm. It lies deep in the kidney, and ex-

tends to the renal sinus. The collecting tubules from this can drain into unusual-looking calyces, which emerge from the mass in strange and unusual directions and shapes.[210, 212–214]

It is crucial to recognize congenitally large septa of Bertin, since patients have had nephrectomies because this innocuous normal variant was misdiagnosed as a neoplasm.[215]

EMBRYOLOGY OF LARGE SEPTA OF BERTIN

The lobes of the kidney can first be identified by the 10th week; by the 14th week, each lobe consists of a medulla and a surrounding cortex. When the cortices of immediately adjacent lobes fuse, they form a septum, ultimately the septum of Bertin. The most prominent septa occur in the midzone of the kidney, especially at the junction of the upper pole and the midzone; these septa enlarge toward and intrude on the renal sinus. Figures 19–128 and 19–129 illustrate the cranial primary septum of Bertin, which is the most prominent of the septa and occurs at the junction of the upper pole and the midzone. The first and most prominent lobar groove is found at this point (Figs. 19–128 and 19–129). Here also, excessive infolding of cortical tissue is most likely to occur.[212] It is thus the most frequent site of a congenitally large septum of Bertin, and of partial division of a

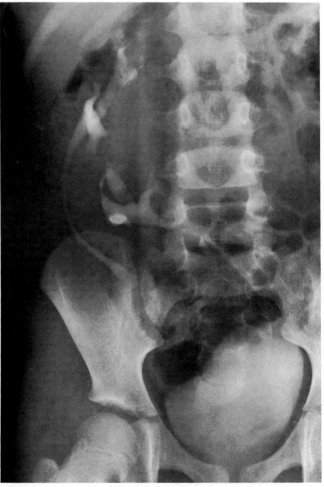

Figure 19–121. Intravenous urogram showing unilateral L-shaped kidney, in which the uncrossed kidney has undergone reverse rotation.

calyces emerge like small teats, deep within the kidney near the renal pelvis. This occurs because the papillae are small and the calyces have short infundibula (Fig. 19–130).

The Aberrant Papilla. This is a tiny papilla draining directly into either the middle of a long infundibulum or the renal pelvis (Fig. 19–130).

An aberrant papilla can look exactly like a small transitional cell carcinoma. If the diagnosis is doubtful, multiple oblique views and tomograms with good ureteral compression should be obtained. If calyceal fornices surround the papilla, the diagnosis can be made with confidence (see page 656).

The Factory Siren Sign. Two or more calyces curve around a congenitally large septum of Bertin and face one another. Each drains into a T-shaped infundibulum. The papillae are sometimes complex. This sign can occur without a large septum of Bertin and by itself is not diagnostic.

Although the mass caused by the large septum may displace the infundibula of the calyces, it never stretches or deforms calyces. In addition, infundibula not immedi-

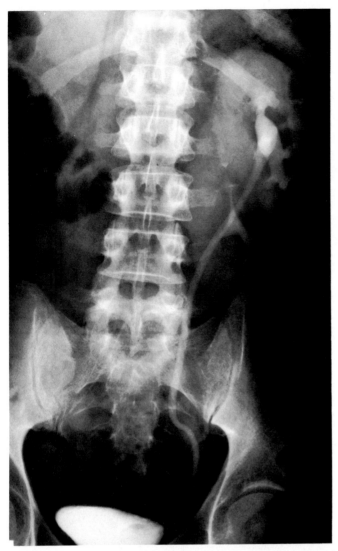

Figure 19–122. Excretory urogram shows inferior crossed ectopia and obstruction of the distal ureter of the uncrossed kidney by a ureteral calculus. (Courtesy of George Harell, M.D., East Jefferson General Hospital, Metairie, Louisiana.)

duplex kidney. Indeed, partial duplication of the kidney is common in kidneys with a congenitally large septum of Bertin.[212]

DIAGNOSTIC IMAGING

Intravenous Urography. The intravenous urogram shows that the mass has exactly the same nephrographic appearance as the rest of the kidney, because it is composed of normal cortical tissue. If nephrotomograms are obtained, a lobulated mass projecting into the renal sinus fat is visible.

Congenitally large septa of Bertin characteristically occur between the upper and middle infundibula in 93% of patients. The anomaly is bilateral in 60% of patients, a significant finding since it is unusual to find bilaterally symmetrical neoplasms deforming the kidneys in the same way on opposite sides.[210] Also characteristic are Hodson's three signs, which are as follows:[210]

The Teat and Udder Sign. The congenitally large septum has an udder shape, from which the papillae and

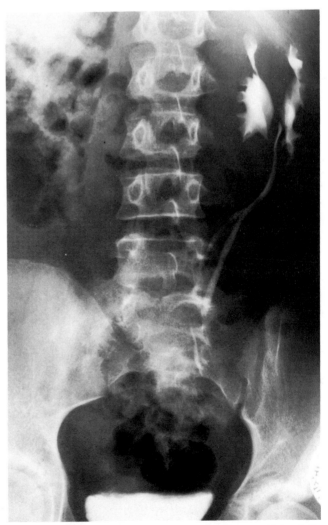

Figure 19–123. Intravenous urogram showing a unilateral disc kidney. The crossed kidney is medial. (Courtesy Richard Silberstein, M.D., Santa Clara Valley Medical Center, San Jose, California.)

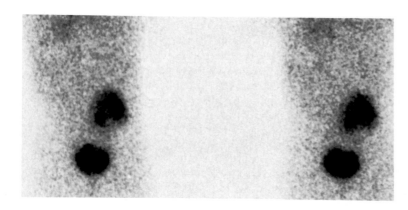

Figure 19–124. Two frames from a Tc-99m-GHA scan showing crossed fused ectopia. (Courtesy Massoud Majd, M.D.)

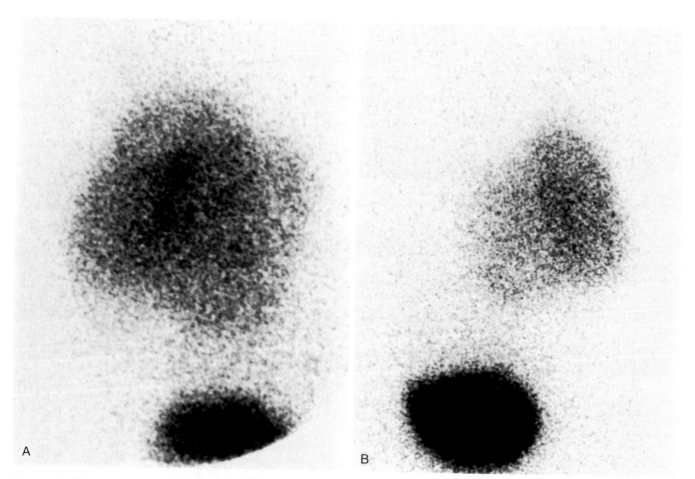

Figure 19–125. Tc-99m-GHA scan shows a unilateral lump kidney: *A*, anterior view; *B*, posterior view. (Courtesy Massoud Majd, M.D.)

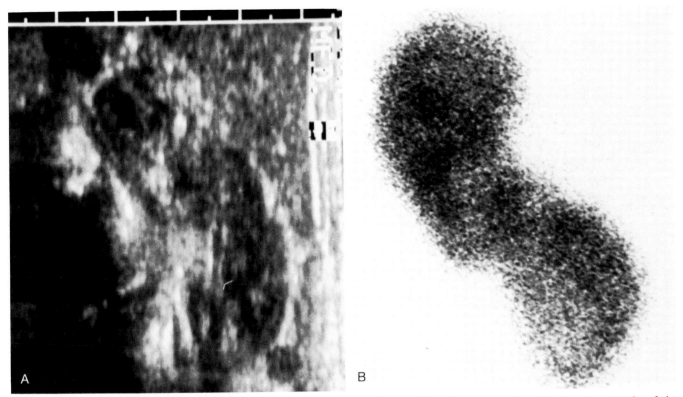

Figure 19–126. Sonographic findings in the most common form of crossed fused ecotopia, in which the lower pole of the uncrossed kidney is fused with the crossed kidney. It is important to perform scans in multiple different planes. It is only on oblique views *(A)* that fusion of the lower pole to another kidney is evident. A radionuclide renal cortical scan *(B)* shows the lower pole of the right uncrossed kidney fused to the upper pole of the left crossed kidney. (Courtesy Barry Potter, M.D., and Bruce Markle, M.D.)

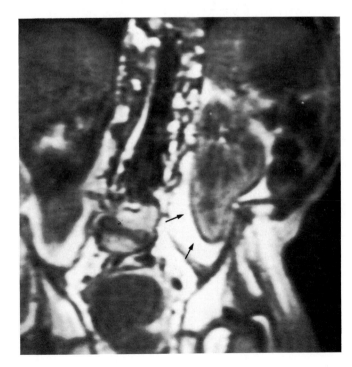

Figure 19–127. Coronal MRI scan showing crossed fused ectopia. The crossed right kidney *(arrows)* is fused to the lower pole of the left kidney. (Spin-echo, T1-weighted image at 1.5 T.)

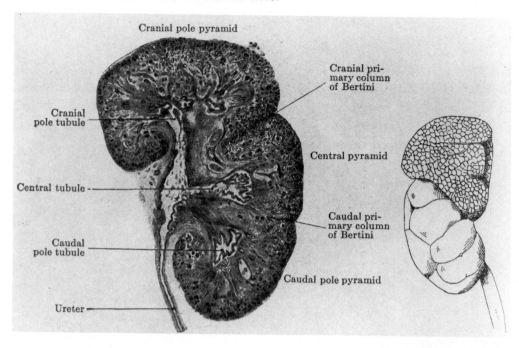

Figure 19–128. *Left,* a frontal section of the kidney of a 160-mm human fetus, 3.75-month-old is illustrated. *Right,* illustration shows the right kidney of a 5-month-old human fetus seen from the ventral surface. The figure on the left illustrates the cranial primary septum of Bertin, which at this stage of development is the most prominent of the septa, and which occurs at the junction of the upper pole and the midzone. The first and most prominent lobar groove occurs at this point. The figure on the right shows that the surface of this kidney is distinctly lobed. (From Keibel F, Mall FP (eds): Manual of Human Embryology, Vol II. Philadelphia, JB Lippincott, 1912, p 844.)

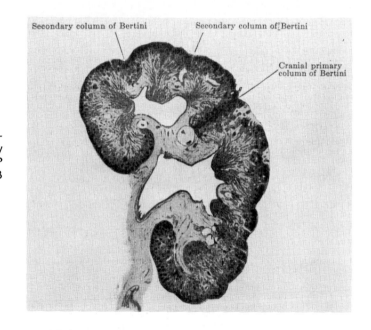

Figure 19–129. Frontal section through the kidney of a 19-week-old human fetus, 175 mm long. The cranial primary septum of Bertin remains prominent. (From Keibel F, Mall FP (eds): Manual of Human Embryology, Vol II. Philadelphia, JB Lippincott, 1912, p 845.)

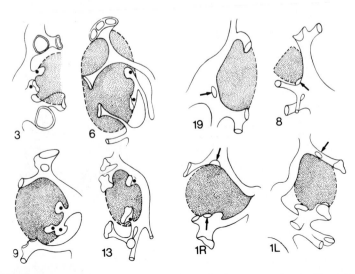

Figure 19–130. Congenitally large septa of Bertin. Cases 3, 6, 9, and 13 show the small midzone short-stemmed calyces that make up the teat-and-udder sign. Cases 19, 8, 1R, and 1L are examples of aberrant papillae *(arrows).* (From Hodson CJ, Mariani B: Large cloisons. AJR 139(2):327–332, © by Williams & Wilkins, 1982.)

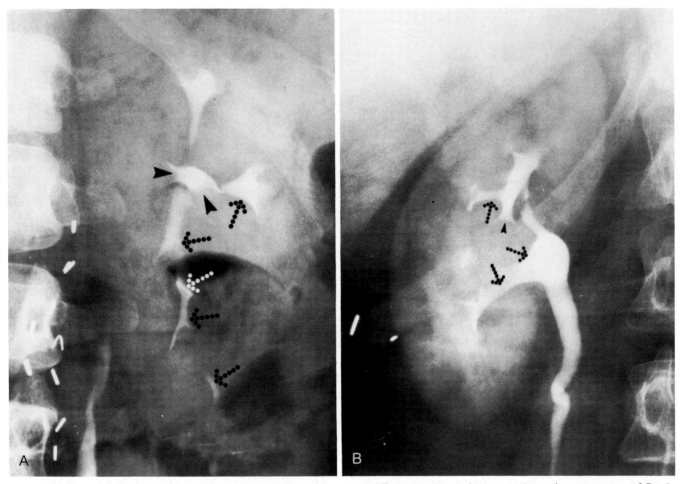

Figure 19–131. *A* and *B,* Intravenous urograms performed on two different patients demonstrating a large septum of Bertin *(stippled arrows).* The arrowheads point to the draining calyces. (From Friedland GW, Filly R, Goris ML, et al: Uroradiology: An Integrated Approach. New York, Churchill Livingstone, pp 1658, 1659, 1983. By permission.)

ately adjacent to the mass are often unusually long (Figs. 19–131 and 19–132).

Congenitally large septa are more common in duplicated kidneys, but, since nonduplicated kidneys are more common, the average practitioner sees more large septa in nonduplicated kidneys.

Arteriography. The artery supplying the cloison usually divides into a wide fork and is larger than normal, supplying the cloison from the medial side. The branches all appear normal and are accompanied by a similar vein (Fig. 19–132). There is no evidence of tumor vessels.

Computed Tomography, Ultrasonography, and Scintigraphy. Contrast-enhanced CT and ultrasonography will show normal renal parenchyma with no mass. The septum can be seen projecting into the sinus fat (Fig. 19–133). Scintigraphy with Tc-99m-DMSA or glucoheptonate will show normal uptake and no photopenic area in the region of the suspected renal mass. Thus, if there is any doubt, scintigraphy is the most helpful examination.

Fetal Lobation

The degree of surface lobation varies among individuals, but by 10 weeks the deep grooves that overlie the septa of Bertin appear, at about 40-mm crown–rump length. These grooves become more marked in fetuses at 24 weeks (200+ mm). They start to fuse as birth ap-

proaches (Fig. 19–134) and continue to do so up to the age of 4 years. Fetal lobation occurs when this fusion is incomplete, and indentations remain on the renal outline (Fig. 19–135).

Diagnostic Imaging

Intravenous Urography, Angiography, and Computed Tomography. Characteristically, these indentations are sharp. They do not overlie the calyces but occur between them. Sometimes, a sharp indentation between the upper and lower pole is seen in a duplex kidney.

Ultrasonography. It is simple to detect fetal lobation on a sonogram of the newborn, although the defect can be seen at any age. The characteristic finding is sharp clefts on the surface of the kidney overlying the septa of Bertin (Fig. 19–136).

Scintigraphy. Fetal lobation can sometimes create a pseudotumor. Scintigraphy can prove that no tumor exists (Fig. 19–137).

Congenital Polar Enlargement

One of the poles is diffusely enlarged. This is almost always the upper pole of the left kidney. There is no associated deformity of the calyces and the infundibula.

Text continued on page 648

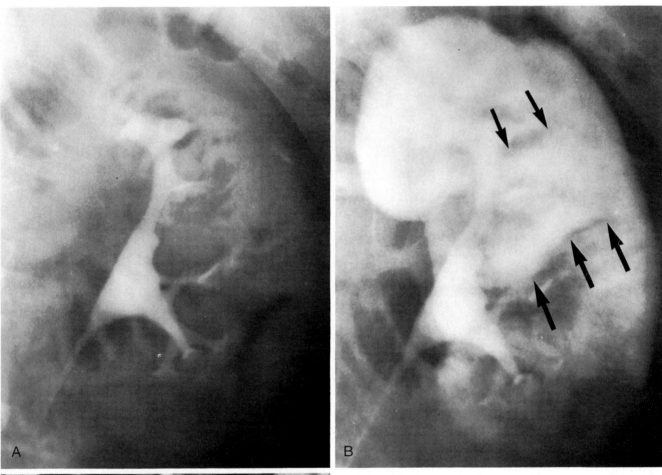

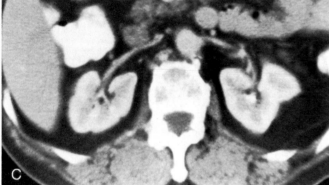

Figure 19–132. Congenitally large septum of Bertin. *A,* Intravenous urogram shows what appears to be a midzone mass. *B,* Nephrogram phase of an arteriogram shows the large septum of Bertin *(arrows).* A prominent fetal lobation is seen in the upper pole. *C,* Dynamic CT scan shows normal renal parenchyma and very prominent fetal lobation.

Figure 19–133. Septum of Bertin. Sonogram of the left kidney performed in the coronal plane demonstrates a septum of Bertin (B) intruding into the left renal sinus *(arrowheads)*. The echogenicity of septa of Bertin is identical to that of normal adjacent renal parenchyma and the edges of the septum ("cloison") tend to join the renal parenchyma at obtuse, rather than acute, angles. Nonetheless, it may be very difficult, and in some cases impossible, to differentiate these benign cortical formations from small intrarenal parenchymal neoplasms by ultrasonography alone.

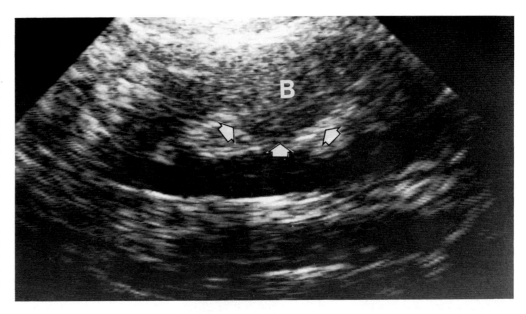

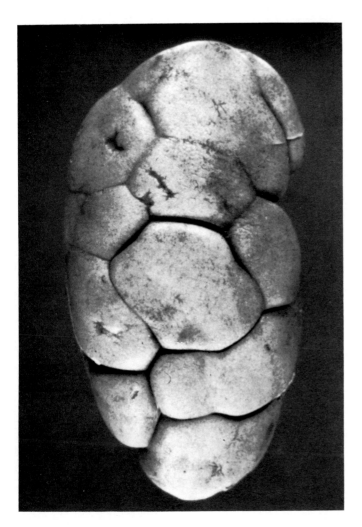

Figure 19–134. The outside of a fetal kidney, illustrating fetal lobation, as denoted by the deep grooves on the surface of the kidney. (From Hodson CJ: The lobar structure of the kidney. Br J Urol 44:246, 1972, Churchill Livingstone, publishers.)

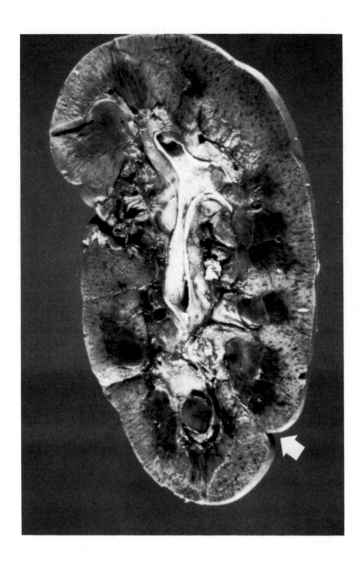

Figure 19–135. Longitudinal section of an adult kidney. The white arrow points to a persistent fetal lobation. The grooves always directly overlie a septum of Bertin. (From Friedland GW, Filly R, Goris ML, et al: Uroradiology: An Integrated Approach. New York, Churchill Livingstone, 1983, p 13. By permission. Courtesy of John Hodson, M.D., Yale University School of Medicine.)

Figure 19–136. Sonogram from a newborn, showing fetal lobation. The lobes, consisting of hypoechoic triangular medullary pyramids surrounded by cortex of medium echogenicity, are separated by clefts *(arrows)* on the surface of the kidney. The echogenicity of the renal cortex is the same as that of the liver, which is normal in a newborn. In addition, the central hilar echoes are relatively small, which is also normal in a newborn.

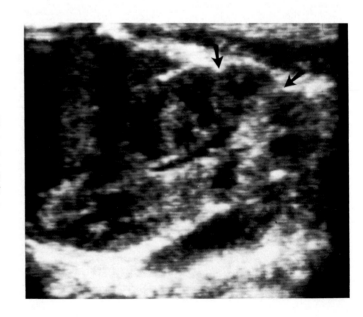

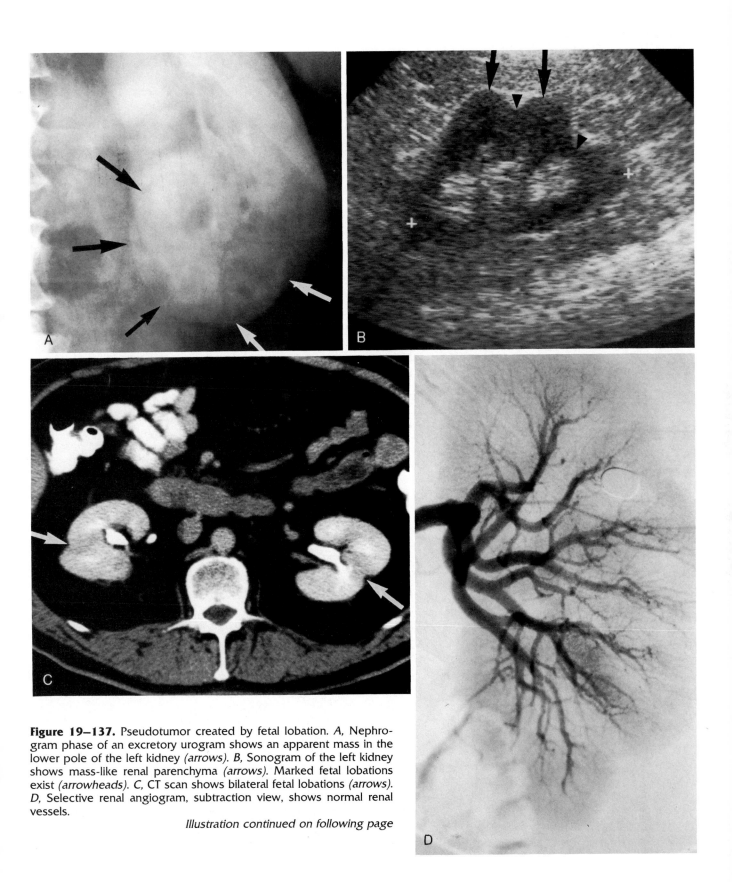

Figure 19–137. Pseudotumor created by fetal lobation. *A,* Nephrogram phase of an excretory urogram shows an apparent mass in the lower pole of the left kidney *(arrows)*. *B,* Sonogram of the left kidney shows mass-like renal parenchyma *(arrows)*. Marked fetal lobations exist *(arrowheads)*. *C,* CT scan shows bilateral fetal lobations *(arrows)*. *D,* Selective renal angiogram, subtraction view, shows normal renal vessels.

Illustration continued on following page

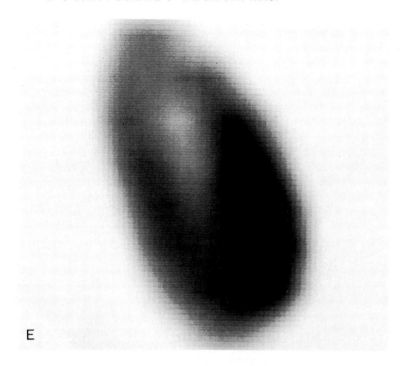

Figure 19–137 *Continued E,* Tc-99m-DMSA scan with tomography, anterior view, shows normal renal parenchyma.

It was once claimed that this congenital anomaly occurred because of congenital absence of the spleen, but in most cases the spleen is present.

Angiography shows that the renal vessels and the nephrogram are normal. Ultrasonography shows a normal kidney with a bulbous renal pole (see Fig. 19–139A). Scintigraphy with Tc-99m-DMSA or Tc-99m-GHA shows completely normal uptake, demonstrating that the bulbous pole is normal renal parenchyma (see Fig. 19–139B).

Other Congenital Renal Masses Composed of Normal Renal Parenchyma

In addition to the upper pole of the kidney, congenital abnormalities of renal contour can occur in other areas, simulating renal masses. This occurs especially in the lower pole of either kidney, where a rounded prominent renal parenchyma can mimic a mass on an intravenous urogram (Fig. 19–137). Sometimes, however, an extra

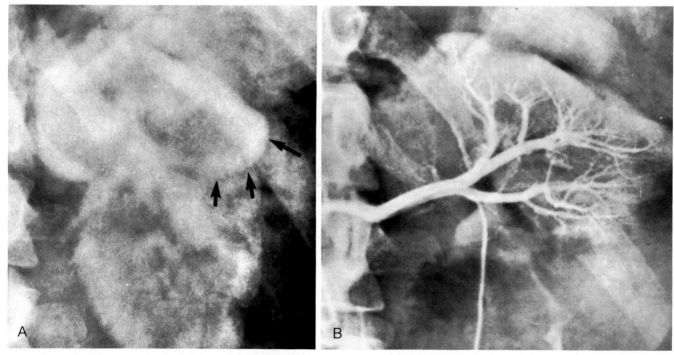

Figure 19–138. Pseudotumor supplied by aberrant renal artery. *A,* Nephrogram phase of an excretory urogram showing an extra bump on the outline of the left kidney *(arrows). B,* Selective angiogram performed on an aberrant renal artery shows that the mass is composed of normal tissue. (From Friedland GW, Goris ML, Gross D, et al: Uroradiology: An Integrated Approach, New York, Churchill Livingstone, 1983, p 1665. By permission.)

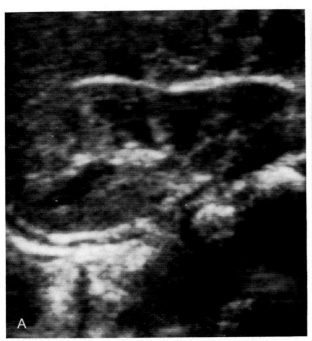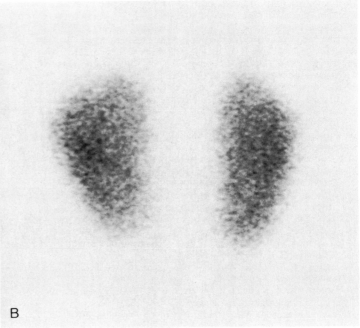

Figure 19–139. Congenital polar enlargement. *A,* Sonogram shows enlargement of the upper pole of the right kidney, but the renal parenchyma is otherwise normal. *B,* Tc-99m-DTPA scintigraphy, anterior view, shows normal uptake in the right kidney, but enlargement of the upper pole of this kidney.

bump or lump anywhere on the renal outline may do the same (Fig. 19–138).

As indicated in Chapter 6, variations in renal parenchymal architecture that are severe enough to cause concern about the possibility of a pseudotumor should be investigated by either radionuclide scintigraphy or dynamic CT scanning. Angiography may reveal that the mass is supplied by a separate renal artery. The common normal variant of the left kidney, the dromedary hump, usually has a single renal artery.

Congenital Indentation of the Left Kidney

The midzone of the left kidney may have a deep indentation laterally resembling a scar, often associated with splaying of the calyces. Such kidneys are often also supplied by two renal arteries, one for each pole.

Cystic Diseases

Congenital cystic diseases of the kidney are considered in the section on cystic disease (Chapters 34 to 42). Likewise, anomalies in the renal blood supply are discussed in the section on vascular disease (Chapters 65 to 69).

References

1. Burns RK: Urogenital system. *In* Willier BH, Weiss PA, Hamburger V (eds): Analysis of Development. Philadelphia, WB Saunders Company, 1955.
2. Streeter GL: Development of the mesoblast and notochord in pig embryos. Carnegie Inst Publ 380, Contrib Embryol 19:73–92, 1927.
3. Fraser EA: The development of the vertebrate excretory system. Biol Rev 25:159–187, 1950.
4. Torrey TW: The early development of the human nephron. Carnegie Inst Wast Publ 603, Contrib Embryol 1954; 35:175–197.
5. Felix W: The development of the urogenital organs. *In* Keibel F, Mall FP (eds): Manual of Human Embryology, Vol 2. Philadelphia, JB Lippincott, 1912, pp 752–976.
6. deVries, PA: Personal observation.
7. Boyden EA: Experimental obstruction of the mesonephric ducts. Proc Soc Exp Biol Med 24:572–576, 1927.
8. Gruenwald P: Zur Entwicklungsmechanik des Urogenitalsystems Geim Huhn. Roux Arch Entwmech Org 136:786–813, 1937.
9. Grobstein C: Inductive interaction in the development of the mouse metanephros. J Exper Zool 130:319–339, 1955.
10. Saxen L: Failure to demonstrate tubule induction in heterologous mesenchyme. Dev Biol 23:511, 1970.
11. Schreiner KE: Uber die Entwicklung der Amniotenniere. Z Wissen Zool 71:1–188, 1902.
12. Friedland GW, deVries PA: Renal ectopia and fusion. Embryological basis. Urology 5:698–706, 1975.
13. Huber CC: On the development and shape of uriniferous tubules of certain of the higher mammals. Am J Anat 4:1–98, 1905.
14. Osathanondh V, Potter EL: Development of human kidney as shown by microdissection. Arch Pathol 76:271–302, 1963.
15. Carlson HE: Supernumerary kidney: A summary of fifty-one reported cases. J Urol 64:221–229, 1950.
16. N'Guessan G, Stephens FD: Supernumerary kidney. J Urol 130:649–653, 1983.
17. McPherson RI: Supernumerary kidney: Typical and atypical features. J Can Assoc Radiol 38:116–119, 1987.
18. Conrad GA, Loes DL: Ectopic supernumerary kidney. Functional assessment using radionuclide imaging. Clin Nucl Med 12:253–257, 1987.
19. Pohlman AG: Abnormalities in the form of the kidney and ureter dependent on the development of the renal bud. Bull Johns Hopkins Hosp 16:51–60, 1905.
20. Geisinger JF: Supernumerary kidney. J Urol 38:331–356, 1937.
21. Cope JR, Trickey SE: Congenital absence of the kidney: Problems in diagnosis and management. J Urol 227:10–12, 1982.
22. Stojanov D, Lovasi'c I, Dujmovi'c M, Bobinac D: Unilateral renal agenesis in the angiographic material and renovascular hypertension. Rontgenblatter 40:179–181, 1987.
23. Fernbach SK, Holland EA, Benuck I, Young S: Hypertension induced by occult renal tissue. J Urol 138:842–844, 1987.
24. Loendersloot EW, Verjaal M, Leschot NJ: Bilateral renal agenesis (Potter's syndrome) in two consecutive infants. Eur J Obstet Gynecol Reprod Biol 8:137–142, 1978.
25. Sangal PR, Feinstein SJ, Chandra PC, Spence MR: Recurrent bilateral renal agenesis. Am J Obstet Gynecol 155:1078–1079, 1986.

26. Wilson RD, Hayden MR: Bilateral renal agenesis in twins. Am J Med Genet 21:147–152, 167–169, 1985.

27. Moore D, Tudehope D, Lewis B, Masel J: Familial renal abnormalities associated with the oligohydramnios tetrad secondary to renal agenesis and dysgenesis. Aust Paediatr J 23:137–141, 1987.

28. McPherson E, Carey J, Kramer A, et al: Dominantly inherited renal adysplasia. Am J Med Genet 26:863–872, 1987.

29. Dicker D, Samuel N, Feldberg D, Goldman JA: The antenatal diagnosis of Potter syndrome (Potter sequence). A lethal and not-so-rare malformation. Eur J Obstet Gynecol Reprod Biol 18:17–24, 1984.

30. Keibel F: Zur Entwick des Mensch Urogenitolapparates. Arch Anat Phys 55:55, 1896.

31. Boyden EA: Experimental obstruction of the mesonephric ducts. Proc Exp Biol Med 24:572–576, 1927.

32. Brown AL: An analysis of the developing metanephros in mouse embryos with abnormal kidneys. Am J Anat 47:117–171, 1931.

33. Boyden EA: Congenital absence of the kidney. An interpretation based on a 10-mm human embryo exhibiting unilateral agenesis. Anat Rec 52:325–349, 1932.

34. O'Connor RJ: Experiments on the development of the amphibian mesonephros. J Anat 74:34–44, 1939.

35. Gruenwald P: Development of the excretory system. Ann NY Acad Sci 55:142–146, 1952.

36. Gruenwald P: Stimulation of nephrogenic tissue by normal and abnormal inductors. Anat Rec 86:321–339, 1943.

37. Wolf EL, Berdon WE, Baker DH, et al: Diagnosis of oligohydramnios–related pulmonary hypoplasia (Potter Syndrome): Value of portable voiding cystourethrography in newborns with respiratory distress. Radiology 125:769–773, 1977.

38. Swischuk LE, Richardson CJ, Nichols MM, Ingman MJ: Bilateral pulmonary hypoplasia in the neonate. AJR 133:1057–1063, 1979.

39. Yokoyama M, Bekku T, Ochi K: Spontaneous rupture of solitary functioning kidney. Br J Urol 53:480, 1981.

40. Muller F, O'Rahilly R: Somitic-vertebral correlations and vertebral levels in the human embryo. Am J Anat 177:3–19, 1986.

41. Longo VJ, Thompson GJ: Congenital solitary kidney. J Urol 68:63–68, 1952.

42. Ashley DJB, Mostofi FK: Renal agenesis and dysgenesis. J Urol 83:211–230, 1960.

43. Kenney PJ, Spirt BA, Leeson MD: Genitourinary anomalies: Radiologic-anatomic correlations. Radiographics 4:233–260, 1984.

44. Matsuoka LY, Wortsman J, McConnachie P: Renal and testicular agenesis in a patient with Darier's disease. Am J Med 78:873–877, 1985.

45. Karamchetti A, Berg G: Seminal vesical cyst associated with ipsilateral renal agenesis. Urology 12:572–574, 1978.

46. Lantz EJ, Berquist TH, Hattery RR, et al: Seminal vesicle cyst associated with ipsilateral renal agenesis: A case report. Urol Radiol 2:265–266, 1981.

47. Fisher JE, Jewett TC Jr, Nelson SJ, Jockin H: Ectasia of the rete testis with ipsilateral renal agenesis. J Urol 128:1040–1043, 1982.

48. Elder JS, Jeffs RD: Suprainguinal ectopic scrotum and associated anomalies. J Urol 127:336–338, 1982.

49. Uthmann U, Terhorst B: Dermoid cyst of the prostate with contralateral renal agenesis. Br J Urol 53:479, 1981.

50. Ataya KM, Mroueh AM: Urologic anomalies associated with an absent uterus. J Urol 127:1125–1127, 1982.

50a. D'Alberton A, Reschini E, Ferrari N, Candiani P: Prevalence of urinary tract abnormalities in a large series of patients with uterovaginal atresia. J Urol 126:623–624, 1981.

51. Vinstein AL, Franken EA Jr: Unilateral hematocolpos associated with agenesis of the kidney. Radiology 102:625–627, 1972.

52. Griffin JE, Edwards C, Madden JD, et al: Congenital absence of the vagina. The Mayer-Rokitansky-Küster-Hauser syndrome. Ann Intern Med 85:224–236, 1976.

53. Tarry WF, Duckett JW, Stephens FD: The Mayer-Rokitansky syndrome: Pathogenesis classification and management. J Urol 136:648–652, 1986.

54. Acci'en P, Armi-nana E, Garcia-Ontiveros E: Unilateral renal agenesis associated with ipsilateral blind vagina. Arch Gynecol 240:1–8, 1987.

55. Wright JE: Failure of mullerian duct development. The Mayer-Rokitansky-Küster-Hauser syndrome. Aust Paediatr J 20:325–327, 1984.

56. Sayer T, O'Reilly PH: Bicornuate and unicornuate uterus associated with unilateral renal aplasia and abnormal solitary kidneys: Report of three cases. J Urol 135:110–111, 1986.

57. Miyazaki Y, Ebisuno S, Uekado Y, et al: Uterus didelphys with unilateral imperforate vagina and ipsilateral renal agenesis. J Urol 135:107–109, 1986.

58. Hamlin DJ, Pettersson H, Ramey SL, Moazam F: Magnetic resonance imaging of bicornuate uterus with unilateral hematometrosalpinx and ipsilateral renal agenesis. Urol Radiol 8:52–55, 1986.

59. Yoder IC, Pfister RC: Unilateral hematocolpos and ipsilateral renal agenesis: Report of two cases and review of the literature. AJR 127:303–308, 1976.

60. Swane LC, Rubenstein JB, Mitchell B: The Mayer-Rokitansky-Küster-Hauser syndrome: Sonographic aid to diagnosis. J Ultrasound Med 5:287–289, 1986.

61. Stephens FD: The Mayer-Rokitansky syndrome. J Urol 135:106, 1986.

62. Gadbois WF, Duckett JW Jr: Gartner's duct cyst and ipsilateral renal agenesis. Urology 4:720–721, 1974.

63. Currarino G: Single vaginal ectopic ureter and Gartner's duct cyst with ipsilateral renal hypoplasia and dysplasia (or agenesis). J Urol 128:988–993, 1982.

64. Johnson J, Hillman BJ: Uterine duplication, unilateral imperforate vagina and normal kidneys. AJR 147:1197–1198, 1986.

65. Morgan WC: Inherited congenital kidney absence in an inbred strain of rats. Anat Rec 115:635–639, 1953.

66. Silverman PM, Carroll BA, Moskowitz PS: Adrenal sonography in renal agenesis and dysplasia. AJR 134:600–602, 1980.

67. Kenney PJ, Robbins GL, Ellis DA, Spirt BA: Adrenal glands in patients with congenital renal anomalies: CT appearance. Radiology 155:181–182, 1985.

68. Benjamin JA, Tobin CE: Abnormalities of the kidneys, ureters and perinephric fascia: Anatomic and clinical study. J Urol 65:715–733, 1951.

69. Braedel HU, Schindler E, Moeller JF, Polsky MS: Renal phlebography: An aid in the diagnosis of the absent or nonfunctioning kidney. J Urol 116:703–707, 1976.

70. Whiting JC, Stanisic TH, Drach GW: Congenital ureteral valves: Report of two patients, including one with a solitary kidney and associated hypertension. J Urol 129:1222–1224, 1983.

71. Limkakeng AD, Retik AB: Unilateral renal agenesis with hypoplastic ureter. Observations on the contralateral urinary tract and report of four cases. J Urol 108:149–152, 1972.

72. Gupta NP, Gill IB: Skeletal anomalies associated with unilateral renal agenesis. Br J Urol 59:15–16, 1987.

73. Strubbe EH, Thign CJ, Willemsen WN, Lappohn R: Evaluation of radiographic abnormalities of the hand in patients with the Mayer-Rokitansky-Küster-Hauser syndrome. Skeletal Radiol 16:227–231, 1987.

74. Currarino G: Association of congenitally small pelvic outlet with hypoplasia of bladder and urethra, and absent kidneys. AJR 109:399–402, 1970.

75. Rabinowitz JG, Pelzman H, Robinson T: Small pelvic outlet associated with underdevelopment of the urinary tract and other anomalies. Radiology 101:629–630, 1971.

76. Fellows RA, Berdon WE, Baker DH: Size of pelvic bony outlet in renal agenesis. AJR 121:159–165, 1974.

77. Sinnassamy P, Yazbeck S, Brochu P, O'Regan S: Renal anomalies and agenesis associated with total intestinal aganglinosis. Int J Pediatr Nephrol 7:1–2, 1986.

78. Valdivieso EM, Scholtz CL: Diffuse meningocerebral angiodysplasia and renal agenesis: A case report. Pediatr Pathol 6:119–126, 1986.

79. Dubbins PA, Kurtz AB, Wapner J, Goldberg BB: Renal agenesis: Spectrum of in utero findings. J Clin Ultrasound 9:189–193, 1981.

80. McGahan JP, Myracle MR: Adrenal hypertrophy: Possible pitfall in the sonographic diagnosis of renal agenesis. J Ultrasound Med 5:265–268, 1986.

81. Majd M: Nuclear medicine NM. In Kelalis PP, King LR, Belman AB (eds): Clinical Pediatric Urology. Philadelphia, WB Saunders Company, 1985, pp 145–150.

82. Howard WH III, Bunker SR, Karl RD, et al: Unilateral renal agenesis and other causes of the solitary photopenic renal fossa. Clin Nucl Med 10:270–273, 1985.

83. Mascatello V, Lebowitz RL: Malposition of the colon in left renal agenesis and ectopia. Radiology 120:371–376, 1976.

84. Meyers MA, Whalen JP, Evans JA, et al: Malposition and displacement of the bowel in renal agenesis and ectopia: New observations. AJR 117:323–333, 1973.

85. Curtis JA, Sadhu V, Steiner RM: Malposition of the colon in right renal agenesis, ectopia, and anterior nephrectomy. AJR 129:845–850, 1977.

86. Hadar H, Gadoth N, Gillon G: Computed tomography of renal agenesis and ectopy. CT 8:137–143, 1984.
87. Kenney PJ, Robbins GL, Ellis DA, Spirt BA: Adrenal glands in patients with congenital renal anomalies: CT appearance. Radiology 155:181–182, 1985.
88. Cussen LG, Stephens FD: Renal dysgenesis: A "urologic" classification. In: Stephens FD (ed): Congenital Malformations of the Urinary Tract. New York, Praeger, 1983, pp 463–482.
89. Schwarz RD, Stephens FD, Cussen LJ: The pathogenesis of renal dysplasia. I. Quantification of hypoplasia and dysplasia. Invest Urol 19:94–96, 1981.
90. Gilboa N, Bartoletti A, Urizar RE: Severe hypertension in a newborn associated with increased renin production by a hypoplastic kidney. J Urol 128:570–571, 1982.
91. Tokunaka S, Osanai H, Hashimoto H, Takamura T, Yachiku S, Mori Y: Severe hypertension in infant with unilateral hypoplastic kidney. Urology 29:618–620, 1987.
92. Sommer JT, Stephens FD: Morphogenesis of nephropathy with partial ureteral obstruction and vesicoureteral reflux. J Urol 125:67–72, 1981.
93. Royer P, Habib R, Mathieu H, Courtecuisse V: L'hypoplasie renale bilaterale congenitale avec reduction du nombre et hypertrophie des nephrons chez l'enfant. Ann Pediatr (Paris) 9:133–146, 1962.
94. Scheinman JI, Abelson HT: Bilateral renal hypoplasia with oligonephronia. J Pediatr 76:369–376, 1970.
95. Carter JE, Lirenman DS: Bilateral renal hypoplasia with oligomeganephronia: Oligomeganephroic renal hypoplasia. Am J Dis Child 120:537–542, 1970.
96. Kusuyama Y, Tsukino R, Oomori H, et al: Familial occurrence of oligomeganephronia. Acta Pathol Jpn 35:449–457, 1985.
97. Smith PK, Hodson J: Lesions in the pig kidney with chronic reflux nephropathy. In Hodson J, Smith PK (eds): Reflux Nephropathy. New York, Masson, 1979, pp 197–212.
98. Zezulka AV, Arkell DG, Beevers DG: The association of hypertension, the Ask-Upmark kidney and other congenital abnormalities. J Urol 135:1000–1001, 1986.
99. Bailey RR, Janus E, McLoughlin K, et al: Familial and genetic data in reflux nephropathy. Contrib Nephrol 39:40–51, 1984.
100. Royer P, Habbi R, Broyer M, et al: Segmental hypoplasia of the kidney in children. Adv Nephrol 1:145–159, 1971.
101. Ljungqvist A, Lagergren C: The Ask-Upmark kidney: A congenital renal anomaly studied by micro-angiography and histology. Acta Pathol Microbiol Scand 56:277–283, 1962.
102. Arant BS Jr, Sotelo-Avila C, Bernstein J: Segmental "hypoplasia" of the kidney (Ask-Upmark). J Pediatr 95:931–939, 1979.
103. Shindo S, Bernstein J, Arant BS Jr: Evolution of renal segmental atrophy (Ask-Upmark kidney) in children with vesicoureteric reflux: Radiographic and morphologic studies. J Pediatr 102:847–854, 1983.
104. Johnston JH, Mix LW: The Ask-Upmark kidney. A form of ascending pyelonephritis? Br J Urol 48:393–398, 1976.
105. Bailey RR, Lynn KL, McRae CU: Unilateral reflux nephropathy and hypertension. Contrib Nephrol 39:116–125, 1984.
106. Gotoh T, Koyanagi T, Tokunaka S: Pathology of ureterorenal units in various ureteral anomalies with particular reference to the genesis of renal dysplasia. Int Urol Nephrol 19:231–243, 1987.
107. Avni EF, Thoua Y, Van Gansbeke D, et al: Development of the hypodysplastic kidney: Contribution of antenatal US diagnosis. Radiology 164:123–125, 1987.
108. Schwarz RD, Stephens FD, Cussen LJ: The pathogenesis of renal dysplasia. II. The significance of lateral and medial ectopy of the ureteric orifice. Invest Urol 19:97–100, 1981.
109. Schwarz RD, Stephens FD, Cussen LJ: The pathogenesis of renal dysplasia. III. Complete and incomplete urinary obstruction. Invest Urol 19:101–103, 1986.
110. Henneberry MO, Stephens FD: Renal hypoplasia and dysplasia in infants with posterior urethral valves. J Urol 123:912–915, 1980.
111. Hoover DL, Duckett JW Jr: Posterior urethral valves, unilateral reflux and renal dysplasia: A syndrome. J Urol 128:994–997, 1982.
112. Greenfield SP, Hensle TW, Berdon WE, Wigger HJ: Unilateral vesicoureteral reflux and unilateral nonfunctioning kidney associated with posterior urethral valves—a syndrome? J Urol 130:733–738, 1983.
113. Hodson CJ, Craven JD: The radiology of obstructive atrophy of the kidney. Clin Radiol 17:305–320, 1966.
114. Winberg J, Claesson L, Jacobsson B, et al: Renal growth after acute pyelonephritis in childhood: An epidemiological approach. In Hodson J, Smith PK (eds): Reflux Nephropathy. New York, Masson, 1979, pp 309–322.
115. Lebowitz RL, Colodny AH: Urinary tract infection in children. Crit Rev Clin Radiol Nucl Med 4:457–475, 1973.
116. Greene A, Cromie WJ, Goldman M: Computerized body tomography in neonatal renal vein thrombosis. Urology 20:213–215, 1982.
117. Friedland GW, Filly R, Brown BW: Distance of upper pole calyx to spine and lower pole calyx to ureter as indicators of parenchymal loss in children. Pediatr Radiol 2:29–38, 1974.
118. Pickney LE, Currarino G, Weinberg WG: Parenchymal reflux in renal dysplasia. Radiology 141:681–686, 1981.
119. Templeton AW, Thompson IM: Aortographic differentiation of congenital and acquired small kidneys. Arch Surg 97:114–117, 1968.
120. Cha EM, Kandzari S, Khoury GH: Congenital renal hypoplasia: Angiographic study. AJR 114:710–714, 1972.
121. Effman EL, Ablow RC, Siegel NJ: Renal growth. Radiol Clin North Am 15:3–17, 1977.
122. Silber SJ: Renal transplantation between adults and children: Differences in renal growth. JAMA 228:1143–1145, 1974.
123. Hodson CJ: Radiology of the kidney. In Black D (ed): Renal Disease. Oxford, Blackwell, 1972, pp 213–249.
124. Orecklin JR, Craven JD, Lecky JW: Compensatory renal hypertrophy: A morphologic study in transplant donors. J Urol 109:952–954, 1973.
125. Dossetor RS: Renal compensatory hypertrophy in the adult. Br J Radiol 48:993–995, 1975.
126. Tapson JS, Owen JP, Robson RA, et al: Compensatory renal hypertrophy after donor nephrectomy. Clin Radiol 36:307–310, 1985.
127. Heideman HD, Rosenbaum HD: A study of renal size after contralateral nephrectomy. Radiology 94:599–601, 1970.
128. Laufer I, Griscom NT: Compensatory renal hypertrophy. AJR 113:464–467, 1971.
129. Kaye KW, Reinke DB: Detailed caliceal anatomy for endourology. J Urol 132:1085–1088, 1984.
130. Witten DM, Meyers GH, Utz DC: Emmett's Clinical Urography, 4th Ed. Philadelphia, WB Saunders Company, 1977, pp 565–801.
131. Gray SW, Skandalakis JE: The kidney and ureter. In Gray SW, Skandalakis JE (eds): Embryology for Surgeons: The Embryological Basis for the Treatment of Congenital Defects. Philadelphia, WB Saunders Company, 1972.
132. Kelly HA, Burnam CF: Diseases of the kidneys, ureters, and bladder. New York, D Appleton and Company, 1914, p 92.
133. Pohlman AG: Abnormalities in the form of the kidney and ureter dependent on the development of the renal bud. Bull Johns Hopkins Hosp 16:51–60, 1905.
134. Priman J: A consideration of normal and abnormal positions of the hilum of the kidney. Anat Rec 42:355–363, 1929.
135. Braasch WF: Anomalous renal rotation and associated anomalies. J Urol 25:9–21, 1931.
136. Brockman AW: Form- und Lageentwicklung der Niere. Morphol Jahrb 77:605–665, 1936.
137. Vereb J, Tischler V, Pavkovcekova O: Differential x-ray diagnosis of renal dystopias and ectopias in children. Pediatr Radiol 7:205–210, 1978.
138. Thompson GJ, Pace JM: Ectopic kidney: A review of 97 cases. Surg Gynecol Obstet 64:935–943, 1937.
139. Anderson GW, Rice GG, Harris BA Jr: Pregnancy and labor complicated by pelvic ectopic kidney. J Urol 65:760–776, 1951.
140. Dretler SP, Olsson C, Pfister RC: The anatomic, radiologic, and clinical characteristics of the pelvic kidney. An analysis of 86 cases. J Urol 105:623–627, 1971.
141. Bergquist A: Ectopic kidney as a complication of pregnancy and labour. Acta Obstet Gynecol Scand 44:289–303, 1965.
142. Lantos I, Bajor G, Fornet B, N'anay A: Screening the familial accumulation of kidney malposition and malrotation. Int Urol Nephrol 19:41–48, 1987.
143. Fanizza-Orphanos A, Bendion RW: Simple ectopia of the kidney in monozygotic twins. J Urol 137:706, 1987.
144. Malek RS, Kelalis PP, Burke EC: Ectopic kidney in children and frequency of association with other malformations. Mayo Clin Proc 46:461, 1971.
145. Kelalis PP, Malek RS, Segura JW: Observations on renal ectopia and fusion in children. J Urol 110:588–592, 1973.
146. Wiener ES, Kiesewetter WB: Urologic abnormalities associated with imperforate anus. J Pediatr Surg 8:151–157, 1973.

147. Meyers MA: The reno-alimentary relationships. Anatomic-roentgen study of their clinical significance. AJR 123:386–400, 1975.
148. Nilsson LR: Chronic pancytopenia with multiple congenital abnormalities (Fanconi's anemia). Acta Paediatr 49:518–529, 1960.
149. Paul ATS, Uragoda CG, Jaywardene FLW: Thoracic kidney. Br J Surg 47:395–397, 1959.
150. N'Guessen G, Stephens FD, Pick J: Congenital superior ectopic (thoracic) kidney. J Urol 24:219–228, 1984.
151. Aliotta PJ, Seidel FG, Karp M, Greenfield SP: Renal malposition in patients with omphalocele. J Urol 137:942–944, 1987.
152. Gruenwald P: The normal changes in the position of the embryonic kidney. Anat Rec 85:163–176, 1943.
153. Lewis FT, Papez JW: Variations in the early development of the kidney in pig embryos with special reference to the production of anomalies. Anat Rec 9:105–106, 1915.
154. Carter TC: Embryology of the Little and Bagg x-rayed mouse stock. J Genet 56:401–435, 1959.
155. Bretler SP, Pfister R, Hendren WH: Extra renal calyces in the ectopic kidney. J Urol 103:406–410, 1970.
156. Fischelovitch J, Jancu J: Bilateral pelvic ectopic kidneys. Br J Urol 50:51, 1978.
157. Kelalis PP: Anomalies of the urinary tract: The kidney. In Kelalis PP, King LR (eds): Clinical Pediatric Urology. Philadelphia, WB Saunders Company, 1976, pp 475–503.
158. Ataya KM, Mroueh AM: Urologic anomalies associated with an absent uterus. J Urol 127:1125–1127, 1982.
159. Nalle BC Jr, Crowell JA, Lynch KM Jr: Solitary pelvic kidney with vaginal aplasia: Report of a case. J Urol 61:862–865, 1949.
160. Hendren WH, Donahoe PK, Pfister RC: Crossed renal ectopia in children. Urology 7:135–144, 1976.
161. Hertz M, Rubenstein ZJ, Shahin N, Melzer M: Crossed renal ectopia: Clinical and radiological findings in 22 cases. Clin Radiol 28:339–344, 1977.
162. Marshall FF, Freedman MT: Crossed renal ectopia. J Urol 119:188–191, 1978.
163. Gruber GB: Missbildungen der Hamorgane. In Schwalbe E, Gruber GB (eds): Die Morphologie der Messbildungen des Menschen und der Tiere. Jena, Fischer, 1927. (Cited by Gruenwald P, Anat Rec 75:237–247, 1939.)
164. Lendon RG, Mehroo F: Deformities of the renal tract associated with spina bifida in trypan blue treated rats. J Anat 110:383–391, 1971.
165. Rubenstein ZJ, Hertz M, Shahin N, Deutsch V: Crossed renal ectopia: Angiographic findings in six cases. AJR 126:1035–1038, 1976.
166. Alexander JC, King KB, Fromm CS: Congenital solitary kidney with crossed ureter. J Urol 64:230–234, 1950.
167. Cranidis A, Terhorst B: Crossed renal ectopia with solitary kidney. Urol Radiol 4:45–46, 1982.
168. Lane V: Congenital patent urachus associated with complete (hypospadiac) duplication of the urethra and solitary crossed renal ectopia. J Urol 127:990–991, 1982.
169. Maatman TJ, DeOreo GA Jr, Kay R: Solitary pseudo-crossed renal ectopia. J Urol 129:128–129, 1983.
170. Marshall VF, Keuhnelian JG: Crossed ureteral ectopia with solitary kidney. J Urol 110:176–177, 1973.
171. Miles BJ, Moon MR, Bellville WD, Kiesling VJ: Solitary crossed renal ectopia. J Urol 133:1022–1023, 1985.
172. Bridge RAC: Horseshoe kidneys in identical twins. Br J Urol 32:32–33, 1960.
173. Kalra D, Broomhall J, Williams J: Horseshoe kidney in one of identical twin girls. J Urol 134:113, 1985.
174. Zondek LH, Zondek T: Horseshoe kidney and associated congenital malformations. Urol Int 18:347–356, 1964.
175. Segura JW, Kelalis PP, Burke EC: Horseshoe kidney in children. J Urol 108:333–336, 1972.
176. Grainger R, Murphy DM, Lane V: Horseshoe kidney: A review of presentation, associated congenital anomalies and complications in 73 patients. Ir Med J 76:315, 1983.
177. Boyden EA: Congenital absence of the kidney. An interpretation based on a 10-mm human embryo exhibiting unilateral renal agenesis. Anat Rec 52:325–349, 1932.
178. Cook WA, Stephens FD: Fused kidneys: Morphologic study and theory of embryogenesis. Birth defects 12:327–340, 1977.
179. Evans WP, Resnick MI: Horseshoe kidney and urolithiasis. J Urol 125:620–621, 1981.
180. Mesrobian H-G Jr, Kelalis PP, Hrabovsky E, et al: Wilms tumor in horseshoe kidneys: A report from the National Wilms Tumor Study. J Urol 133:1002–1003, 1985.
181. Reveno JS, Palubinskas AJ: Congenital renal abnormalities in gonadal dysgenesis. Radiology 86:49–51, 1966.
182. Matthias F, Macdiasmid WD, Rallesom M, Taylor FH: Renal anomalies in Turner's syndrome. Types and suggested embryogenesis. Clin Pediatr 10:561, 1971.
183. Warkany J: Congenital Malformations. Chicago, Year Book Medical Publishers, 1971, pp 1050–1053.
184. Ross SR, Keeling RP, Gingold MP, Pinkerton JV: Dyskeratosis congenita with pancytopenia and horseshoe kidney. South Med J 77:527–528, 1984.
185. Smithells RW: Thalidomide and malformations in Liverpool. Lancet 2:1270, 1962..
186. Boatman DL, Kolln CP, Flocks RH: Congenital anomalies associated with horseshoe kidney. J Urol 107:205–207, 1972.
187. Segura JW, Kalalis PP, Burke EC: Horseshoe kidney in children. J Urol 108:333–336, 1972.
188. Pode D, Shapiro A, Lebensart P: Unilateral triplication of the collecting system in a horseshoe kidney. J Urol 130:533–534, 1983.
189. Feldman SL, Lome LG: Renal dysplasia in horseshoe kidney. Urology 20:74–75, 1982.
190. Kumeda K, Takamatsu M, Sone M, et al: Horseshoe kidney with retrocaval ureter: A case report. J Urol 128:361–362, 1982.
191. Wiener ES, Kiesewetter WB: Urologic abnormalities associated with imperforate anus. J Pediatr Surg 8:151–157, 1973.
192. Whitehouse GH: Some urographic aspects of the horseshoe kidney anomaly—a review of 59 cases. Clin Radiol 25:107–114, 1975.
193. Fernback SK, Davis TM: The abnormal renal axis in children with spinabifida and gibbus deformity—the pseudohorseshoe kidney. J Urol 136:1258–1260, 1986.
194. Boatman DL, Cornell SH, Kolln CP: The arterial supply of horseshoe kidneys. AJR 113:447–451, 1971.
195. Graves FT: The Arterial Anatomy of the Kidney. The Basis of Surgical Technique. Baltimore, Williams & Wilkins Company, 1971, pp 39–44.
196. Mendelson DS, Mitty HA, Janus C, Cohen BA: Horseshoe kidney mimicking adenopathy. Urol Radiol 5:121–122, 1983.
197. Gradone CH, Haller JO, Berdon WE, Friedman AP: Asymmetric horseshoe kidney in the infant: Value of renal nuclear scanning. Radiology 154:366, 1985.
198. Gray WH: Horseshoe kidney simulation by para-aortic metastases from a testicular tumor. Clin Nucl Med 12:75–76, 1987.
199. Goren E, Eidelman A: Pelvic cake kidney drained by a single ureter. Urology 30:492–493, 1987.
200. Vaughn W, Hickey D, Milam WH, Soloway M: Radical cystectomy in the presence of a fused "cake" kidney. Urology 29:552–554, 1987.
201. Aragona F, Serretta V, Fiorentini L, et al: Combined renal and pyelic fusion with crossed ectopia of single ureter. Urology 28:339–341, 1986.
202. McDonald JH, McClellan DS: Crossed renal ectopia. Am J Surg 93:995–1002, 1957.
203. Abeshouse BS, Bhisitkul I: Crossed renal ectopia with and without fusion. Urol Int 9:63–91, 1959.
204. Fishman M, Borden S: Crossed fused renal ectopia with single crossed ectopic ureterocele. J Urol 127:117–118, 1982.
205. Rosenberg HK, Snyder HM III, Duckett J: Abdominal mass in a newborn: Multicystic dysplasia of crossed fused renal ectopia—ultrasonic demonstration. J Urol 131:1160–1161, 1984.
206. Rose G, Vaughn ED Jr: Common renal pelvis. A case report. J Urol 113:234, 1975.
207. Cass AS, Vitko RJ: Unusual variety of crossed renal ectopy with only one ureter. J Urol 107:1056, 1972.
208. McCarthy S, Rosenfield AT: Ultrasonography in crossed renal ectopia. J Ultrasound Med 3:107–112, 1984.
209. Goodman JD, Norton KI, Carr L, Yeh HC: Crossed fused renal ectopia: Sonographic diagnosis. Urol Radiol 8:13–16, 1986.
210. Hodson CJ, Mariani S: Large cloisons. AJR 139:327–332, 1982.
211. Hodson CJ: The lobar structure of the kidney. Br J Urol 44:246, 1972.
212. King MC, Friedenberg RM, Tena LB: Normal renal parenchyma simulating tumor. Radiology 91:217–222, 1968.
213. Popky GL, Bogash M, Pollack H, Longacre AM: Focal cortical hyperplasia. J Urol 102:657–660, 1969.
214. Prando A, Pereira RM, Marins JLC: Sonographic evaluation of hypertrophy of septum of Bertin. Urol 24:505–510, 1984.

215. Charghi A, Dessureault P, Drouin G, et al: Malposition of a renal lobe (lobar dysmorphism): A condition simulating renal tumor. J Urol 105:326–329, 1971.

216. Begg RC: Sextuplicitas renum: A case of six functioning kidneys and ureters in an adult female. J Urol 70:686, 1953.

217. Dietrich RB, Kangarloo H: Pelvic abnormalities in children—assessment with MR imaging. Radiology 163:367, 1987.

218. Kneeland JB, Auh YH, McCarron JP, et al: Computed tomography, sonography vesiculography and MR imaging of a seminal vesical cyst. J Comput Assist Tomogr 9:964, 1985.

219. Heaney JA, Pfister RC, Meares EM Jr: Giant cyst of the seminal vesicle with renal agenesis. AJR 149:139, 1987.

220. Roehrborn CG, Schneider HJ, Rugendorff EW, Hamann W: Embryological and diagnostic aspects of seminal vesicle cysts associated with upper urinary tract malformation. J Urol 135:1029, 1986.

221. Graves FT: The Arterial Anatomy of the Kidney. Baltimore, Williams & Wilkins Company, 1971.

222. Gutierrez R: The Clinical Management of Horseshoe Kidney. New York, Paul Hoeber, 1934.

223. Simpson EL, Mintz MC, Pollack HM, et al: Computed tomography in the diagnosis of renal pseudotumors. CT 10:341, 1986.

224. Sanders RC, Nussbaum AR, Solez K: Renal dysplasia: Sonographic findings. Radiology 167:623–626, 1988.

225. Greenberg CR, Trevenen CL, Evans JA: The BOR syndrome and renal agenesis—prenatal diagnosis and further clinical delineation. Prenat Diagn 8:103–108, 1988.

226. Kaneti J, Lissmer L, Smailowitz Z, Sober I: Agenesis of the kidney associated with malformations of the seminal vesicle. Various clinical presentations. Int Urol Nephrol 20: 29–33, 1988.

227. Liddell RM, Rosenbaum DM, Blumhagen JD: Delayed radiologic appearance of bilateral thoracic kidneys. AJR 152:120, 1989.

CONGENITAL ANOMALIES OF THE PAPILLAE, CALYCES, RENAL PELVIS, URETER, AND URETERAL ORIFICE

CLASSIFICATION OF CONGENITAL ANOMALIES OF THE PAPILLAE, CALYCES, RENAL PELVIS, URETER, AND URETERAL ORIFICE

Table 19–21 shows the classification of the major congenital anomalies of the papillae, calyces, renal pelvis, ureter, and ureteral orifice. Lesions that are primarily obstructive are covered elsewhere (Chapters 55 and 56). The table lists those lesions with appropriate chapter numbers, if further information is sought.

Table 19–21. Classification of the Major Congenital Anomalies of the Papillae, Calyces, Renal Pelvis, Ureter, and Ureteral Orifice

I. Papillae and calyces
  A. Anomalies in number
    1. Unipapillary kidney
    2. Polycalicosis
  B. Anomalies in size
    1. Microcalyx
    2. Megacalyx and hydrocalycosis (see Chapter 56)
  C. Anomalies in position and form
    1. Aberrant or ectopic papilla
    2. Pyelocalyceal diverticulum
    3. Extrarenal calyces (see Chapter 6)
II. Renal pelvis and ureter
  A. Anomalies in number
    1. Bifid, trifid, and multifid renal pelves
    2. Bifid, trifid, and multifid ureters
  B. Anomalies in position and form
    1. Blind-ending ureters
    2. Ureteral diverticula
    3. Retrocaval ureters
    4. Congenital ureteral strictures
    5. Ureteral valves
    6. Ureteral diverticula
  C. Anomalies of the ureteropelvic junction (Chapter 56)
III. Ureteral orifice
  A. Ectopic ureteral orifices
  B. Ureteroceles
  C. Ureterovesical junction obstruction (see Chapter 56)
  D. Reflux (see Chapter 21)

EMBRYOLOGY OF THE PAPILLAE, CALYCES, AND RENAL PELVIS

The ureteral bud has an ampullary end, which divides dichotomously to form tubules. Each tubule also has an ampullary end, and it too divides dichotomously.

At the end of the first period of dichotomous division, four to five generations of tubules are at the poles, and three generations are at the interpolar regions. Afterwards, a second period of dichotomous division occurs, resulting in an additional three to five generations of tubules (Fig. 19–140).

After the second period of dichotomous division, the tubules generated in the first period expand and become confluent to form the renal pelvis and the major calyces (Fig. 19–141). During the second period, very short tubules form rapidly and expand, flatten out and coalesce to form the minor calyces (Fig. 19–140).

Pressure of urine from the functioning nephrons expands the tubules, including the terminal ends of the papillary ducts. The openings of these ducts form the cribriform plate on the papillae.

As each pyramid grows, the pressure becomes higher in the center of the pyramid than in the periphery, so that the central portion intrudes into the minor calyx to form a papilla. Because the pressure in the periphery of the pyramid is lower, that part of the pyramid does not intrude into the minor calyx. The papilla indents only the center of the minor calyx, so the perimeter of the minor calyx remains as the fornix.

PAPILLAE AND CALYCES

Anomalies in Number

Unipapillary Kidney

A unipapillary kidney has only one papilla without a calyx.[1–3] There is a single renal lobe, and the ducts of

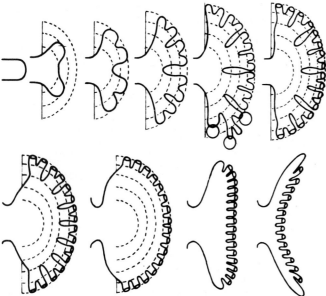

Figure 19–140. Development of the minor calyx and papilla. The proximal portions of the multiple short branches gradually expand and become confluent forming a single cavity. Circles indicate attachments of collecting tubules at the level of the third-, fourth-, or fifth-generation branches distal to the generation initiating calyceal formation. (From Osathanodh V, Potter EL: Development of human kidney as shown by microdissection. Arch Pathol 76:271–302, 1963, p 285. Copyright 1963, American Medical Association.)

Bellini drain directly into the renal pelvis. Unipapillary kidney occurs equally often in males and females. It is important to recognize that a unipapillary kidney in humans is not analogous to the normal solitary calyx found in the kidneys of many animals. Numerous other anomalies can occur in association with unipapillary kidney (Table 19–22).

EMBRYOLOGY

The current hypothesis regarding the genesis of a unipapillary kidney is that if only one of all the tubules formed after the first period of dichotomous division undergoes a second period of dichotomous division, a single papilla will result. One or more of the remaining tubules frequently becomes a "blind ureter," a "blind-ending medial expansion," or a "diverticulum" from the renal pelvis or ureter. A single calyx or diverticulum can develop at either pole or in the interpolar region. All of these changes will have occurred before the 11th week.

Table 19–22. Abnormalities Associated with Unipapillary Kidney

Organ System	Abnormality
Urinary tract	General reduced renal function, hypertension, proteinuria
	Ipsilateral kidney: hypoplasia, blind-ending medial expansion or diverticulum of pelvis
	Contralateral kidney: agenesis, hypoplasia, ectopia
	Oligomeganephronia, if anomaly is bilateral
	Ureter: stricture, multiple diverticula, additional blind-ending ureter
	Urethra: posterior valves
Genital	Unicorn uterus, absent fallopian tube, hypospadias
External ear	Deafness
Branchial arch	Branchial arch anomalies
Vertebrae	Hemivertebrae, scoliosis
General	Goldenhar's syndrome

DIAGNOSTIC IMAGING

Intravenous urography will reveal a small kidney with a single papilla (Fig. 19–142); it will sometimes show a poor nephrogram without excretion, and sometimes an additional blind-ending ureter. The opposite kidney may be absent, hypoplastic, or ectopic. Retrograde urography is necessary, only if the renal function is poor, to demonstrate the involved anatomy. A renal arteriogram shows small, sparse arteries leading to the involved kidney.

Polycalycosis

In this congenital anomaly an inordinate number of calyces (40 or more) are present. The phenomenon occurs normally in certain mammals, such as cows and seals, but is rare in humans (see Fig. 6–61). It occurs in the Rubinstein-Taybi syndrome, and may be associated with megacalyces. Aside from these associations, it is relatively free from complication.

Anomalies in Size

Microcalyx

A microcalyx is a calyx that looks normal in every respect but is tiny. On an intravenous urogram, it is

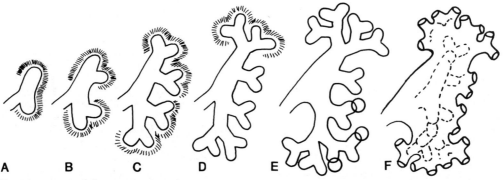

Figure 19–141. Development of the renal pelvis. Diagram shows generations of dichotomous branching: *(A)*, first; *B*, second; *C*, third; *D*, fourth; *E*, fifth. The circles *(E)* indicate the possible location of minor calyces at the level of the third-, fourth-, or fifth-generation branches. *F* indicates the ureteral bud branches that may dilate to form the renal pelvis. (Modified from Osathanodh V, Potter EL: Development of human kidney as shown by microdissection. Arch Pathol 76:271–302, 1963. Copyright 1963, American Medical Association.)

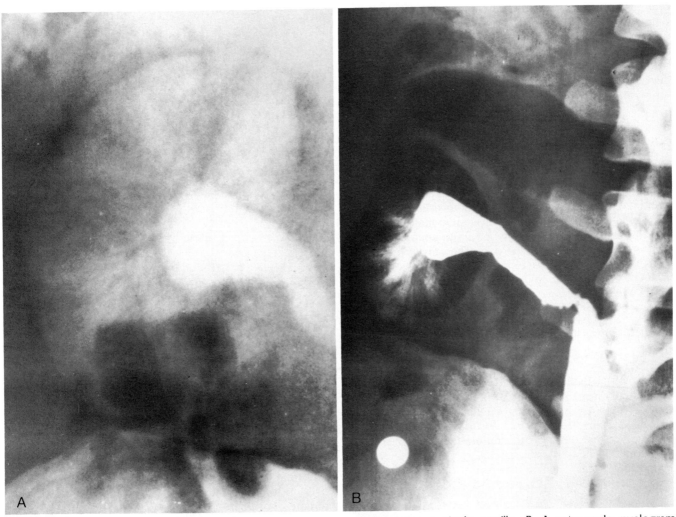

Figure 19–142. Unipapillary kidney. *A,* Intravenous urogram demonstrates a single papilla. *B,* A retrograde pyelogram demonstrates the single papilla and pyelotubular backflow. (From Demos TC, Malone A, Schuster GA: Unicaliceal kidney associated with posterior urethra valves. J Urol 129:1034–1035, © 1983, The Williams & Wilkins Co., Baltimore.)

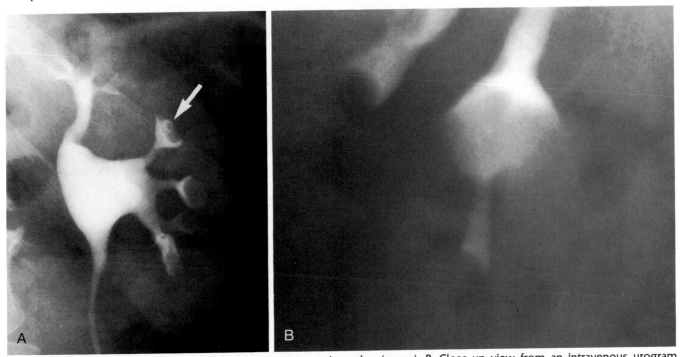

Figure 19–143. *A,* Intravenous urogram demonstrates a microcalyx *(arrow). B,* Close-up view from an intravenous urogram (another patient) reveals a normal right lower-pole calyx from which a tiny microcalyx originates. The smaller calyx appears to extend into the near center of a medullary pyramid. It contains its own papilla, which differentiates it from similar-appearing structures such as cavities, diverticula, and cystically dilated collecting ducts.

present as a tiny projection of contrast material, representing an infundibulum easily mistaken for disease. If ureteral compression is good, it is possible to see a tiny cup at the end of the projection, marking it as a microcalyx (Fig. 19–143A,B). Diverticula, dilated collecting ducts, and cavities do not have a tiny papilla at their termination.

Anomalies in Position and Form

Aberrant or Ectopic Papilla

These papillae occur in one of two typical locations: opening directly into the renal pelvis[6] or draining directly into a long infundibulum.[7] Such papillae may be normal sized or small. They may have no infundibulum of their own or perhaps a very short one. They may be difficult to identify and differentiate from significant lesions, such as small transitional cell carcinomas.

Whenever an ectopic or aberrant papilla exists, a calyx is always associated (Fig. 19–144). This means that when there is a smooth rounded filling defect in the infundibulum or in the renal pelvis (Fig. 19–144), it is important to achieve good ureteral compression to fill any calyx that may be present, and to obtain multiple oblique views and tomograms. These papillae are often associated with a congenitally large septum of Bertin, which may be a clue that an ectopic or aberrant papilla is present.[7] When viewed en face, the calyceal fornix presents as a thin opaque rim of contrast surrounding the papilla, the so-called halo sign.

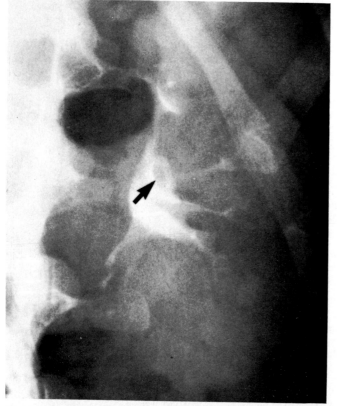

Figure 19–144. Intravenous urogram demonstrates an ectopic papilla opening directly into the renal pelvis *(arrow)*. (From Friedland GW, Goris ML, Gross D, et al: Uroradiology: An Integrated Approach. New York, Churchill Livingstone, 1983, p 72. By permission.)

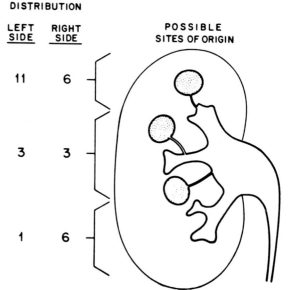

Figure 19–145. Origin and distribution of 30 cases of pyelocalyceal diverticula. Half of diverticula are located in the upper third of the kidneys. (From Middleton AW Jr, Pfister RC: Stone-containing pyelocaliceal diverticulum: Embryogenic, anatomic, radiologic and clinical characteristics. J Urol 111:2–6, © Williams & Wilkins, 1974.)

Pyelocalyceal Diverticulum (Pyelogenic Cyst)

A pyelocalyceal diverticulum is an intraparenchymal cavity filled with urine and lined by transitional epithelium. It communicates with the fornix or infundibulum of a normal calyx or the renal pelvis by means of a narrow neck (Fig. 19–145).[8] It may be single or multiple, or unilateral or bilateral, with a single lobe or multiple lobes and up to four partial septa. The diverticulum varies in size from 0.5 to 5 cm and usually involves the upper pole of the kidney. The prevalence is 3.3 per 1000 pediatric intravenous urograms.[9] Males and females are equally affected. An older term for pyelocalyceal diverticulum that is no longer used is "pyelogenic cyst."

EMBRYOLOGY

One of the last generation of tubules in the first period of dichotomous division fails to expand as it normally would to form the infundibulum of a minor calyx, and remains as a diverticulum. Most congenital calyceal diverticula occur in the upper pole, apparently because that is where the largest number of these generations of tubules form before they dilate and develop into the infundibulum of a minor calyx.

ASSOCIATED ANOMALIES

Calyceal diverticula are usually incidental findings, although they may be associated with the Beckwith-Wiedemann syndrome (Fig. 19–146),[10] vesicoureteral reflux in children,[8, 11] and butterfly vertebrae.[12]

COMPLICATIONS

Complications of pyelocalyceal diverticula include persistent infections,[13] stone formation (especially milk of calcium) (Fig. 19–147),[14–17] and rarely malignancy, organ-

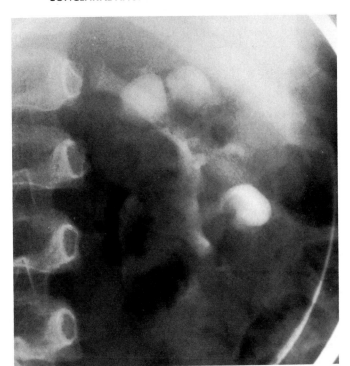

Figure 19–146. Intravenous urogram demonstrates multiple left-sided calyceal diverticula in a child with Beckwith-Wiedemann syndrome. Similar changes were present in the right kidney. (From Taylor WN: Urological implications of the Beckwith-Wiedemann syndrome. J Urol 125:439–441, © 1981, The Williams & Wilkins Co., Baltimore.)

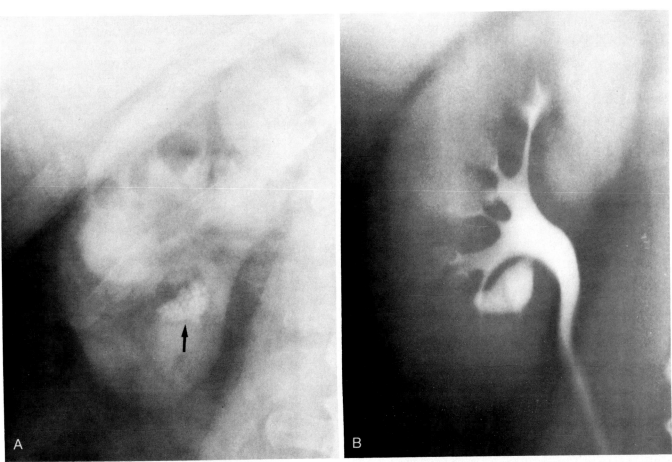

Figure 19–147. Multiple calculi in a calyceal diverticulum. *A*, Preliminary radiograph shows multiple seedlike calculi in the lower pole of the right kidney *(arrow)*. *B*, Intravenous urogram demonstrates the calyceal diverticulum.

ized fibrin clot formation,[18] rupture during an intravenous urogram,[19] xanthogranulomatous pyelonephritis,[8] or renal abscess, if the neck becomes occluded.[8]

DIAGNOSTIC IMAGING

On intravenous urography, the diverticulum usually fills with contrast material via the channel between it and the fornix or infundibulum of the calyx or the renal pelvis. The diverticulum appears round or oval, and smooth walled (Figs. 19–148 and 19–149). It may have two or more lobes and one or more partial septa. If it does not fill, it will present as a fluid-filled intrarenal mass.

Complications of calyceal diverticula may be demonstrated, including stones (Fig. 19–147) that may be single or multiple, are usually mobile, and may occur in 10% to 50% of diverticula, or fluid-calcium level due to milk of calcium. If more detail about the nature of intralesional abnormalities is necessary, retrograde pyelography often provides it, presuming the neck is patent (Fig. 19–149). Calyceal diverticula are also demonstrable by ultrasonography and computed tomography (CT).

Voiding cystourethrography may show reflux in children.[8–11]

DIFFERENTIAL DIAGNOSIS

Rupture of a cyst or abscess into a calyx can resemble a calyceal diverticulum;[8] such ruptures do not usually communicate with the fornix. If tissue is available, microscopic examination shows the cyst lined by flat cuboidal epithelium, rather than the transitional epithelium that lines calyceal diverticula. Microcalyces may be confused with diverticula, but are usually recognized by a small papilla at their tip.[8]

Stenosis of a calyceal infundibulum due to prior infection or stone (hydrocalyx) may also resemble a diverticulum. This is usually central, not derived from the fornix, and the resulting cavity is not deep in the parenchyma.

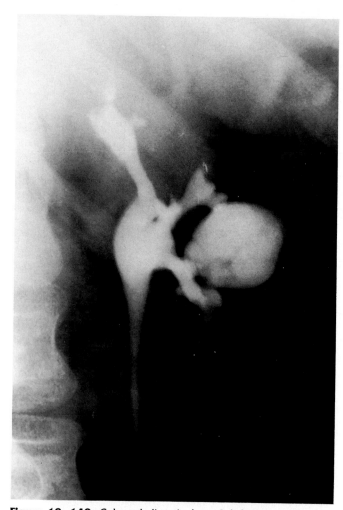

Figure 19–149. Calyceal diverticulum. A left retrograde pyelogram demonstrates filling of a large smooth-walled multilobed diverticulum, which communicates with one of the lower-pole calyces. Filling defects within the diverticulum represent septa.

Papillary necrosis may also be confused with calyceal diverticula, and a history may be helpful in the differential diagnosis. In papillary necrosis, the calyx is flame shaped or clubbed.

Finally, calyceal diverticula can resemble the ruptured calyceal fornices seen in hydronephrosis, which are nevertheless much more irregular than calyceal diverticula.

Extrarenal Calyces

In extrarenal calyces, the major calyces and the renal pelvis are external to the kidney, which is itself disc shaped. The vessels are anomalous, and enter the kidney around the circumference of a flat, wide hilus.

As extrarenal calyces are usually asymptomatic they are discussed in greater detail in the chapter on normal anatomy of the kidney (see Chapter 6).

RENAL PELVIS AND URETER

Anomalies in Number: Duplex Systems, Ectopic Ureters, and Ureteroceles

Current Terminology

This section uses the terminology recommended by the Committee on Terminology, Nomenclature, and Classi-

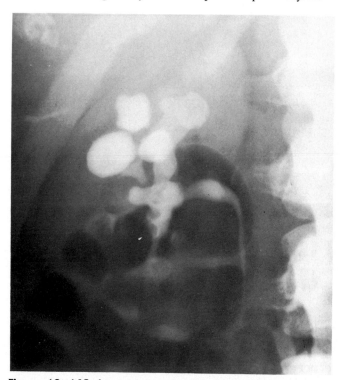

Figure 19–148. Intravenous urogram demonstrates multiple calyceal diverticula in the upper pole of the right kidney.

fication, Section on Urology of the American Academy of Pediatrics.[20]

A duplex kidney is a kidney drained by two pyelocalyceal systems. The term double kidney should not be used, because the two segments are rarely identical. An ectopic ureter opens on the proximal lip of the bladder neck or beyond. Under such circumstances it is ectopic, regardless of whether it is associated with a single ureter or multiple ureters. A ureterocele is a ballooning of the distal end of the ureter. Two types of ureterocele can exist: intravesical and ectopic. The term intravesical ureterocele replaces the designation simple ureterocele. An intravesical ureterocele can develop on a single ureter or on one of two ureters. A ureterocele is ectopic if some part of it lies in the bladder neck or urethra.

The Committee on Terminology developed the following glossary relevant to duplex systems, ectopic ureters, and ureteroceles:

Duplex kidney—a kidney in which two pyelocalyceal systems are present.

Upper (lower) pole—one of the components of a duplex kidney.

Duplex (duplicated) system—a renal unit in which the kidney has two pyelocalyceal systems and is associated with a single ureter or bifid ureters (partial or incomplete duplication), or two ureters (double ureters) that empty separately into the bladder (complete duplication).

Bifid system—a form of duplication in which two pyelocalyceal systems join at the ureteropelvic junction (bifid pelvis) or where two ureters join before emptying into the bladder (bifid ureters).

Double ureters—the two ureters associated with complete duplication. Each independent ureter drains a separate pyelocalyceal system and opens separately into the urinary or genital tract.

Upper (lower) pole ureter—the ureter draining the upper (lower) pole of a duplex kidney.

Upper (lower) pole orifice—the orifice associated with the ureter draining the upper (lower) pole of a duplex kidney; the orifice of an upper (lower) pole ureter.

Caudal or medial ectopia (of ureteral orifice)—an orifice situated at or beyond the proximal lip of the bladder neck.

Ectopic ureter—a ureter draining to an abnormal site. However, because the term has been used so widely to mean a ureter in which the orifice is ectopic caudally, the latter definition is still acceptable.

Intravesical ureterocele—a type of ureterocele located entirely within the bladder. An intravesical ureterocele may be associated with a single system; it may be associated with the upper-pole ureter of a completely duplicated system; rarely is it associated with a lower-pole ureter.

Ectopic ureterocele—a type of ureterocele in which some portion of the ureterocele is situated permanently at the bladder neck or in the urethra. The orifice may be situated in the bladder, at the bladder neck, or in the urethra.

Ureteroceles can be characterized as stenotic, sphincteric, or sphincterostenotic; cecoureteroceles, blind and nonobstructive.

Duplex Kidneys

A duplex kidney has a single renal parenchyma drained by two pyelocalyceal systems.[21] It occurs in 12% of the population and may be unilateral or bilateral. A duplex kidney may be drained by a single ureter or by two ureters that unite to form a single ureter (duplex ureters). Alternatively, the kidney may be drained by two ureters that remain separate to their point of insertion in the bladder or beyond (double ureters).[21] The kidney has an upper pole and a lower pole, each with its separate collecting system; the ureter draining the upper pole is the upper-pole ureter, and the one draining the lower pole is the lower-pole ureter.[20]

Usually the lower-pole system is dominant, draining most of the kidney. However, the upper-pole system may be dominant, or the two collecting systems may share dominance in a variety of ways (Fig. 19–150). In a dominant lower-pole collecting system, for example, a large renal pelvis drains the lower pole via multiple calyces, whereas the upper-pole pyelocalyceal system might have only a single calyx with a single infundibulum and practically no renal pelvis, simply draining directly into the ureter. With a dominant upper-pole collecting system, this situation may be reversed. Between these two extremes, however, any number of combinations is possible.

A duplex kidney is usually larger than normal, although it may be normal in size. The renal parenchyma is usually thinner than normal.

A duplex kidney is often associated with a congenitally

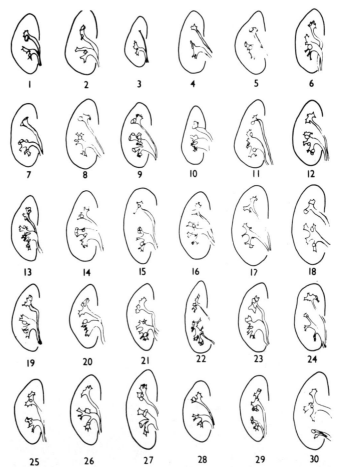

Figure 19–150. Tracings of intravenous urograms of patients with duplex kidneys. The illustration demonstrates the variety of ways in which two collecting systems may share dominance. It is numbered from 1 to 30 in decreasing order of frequency. (From Hartman G, Hodson CJ: Duplex kidney and related anomalies. Clin Radiol 20:387–400, 1969.)

large septum of Bertin between the upper and lower poles. Such large septa may be mistaken for renal masses, leading to unnecessary studies. The duplex kidney may have pronounced fetal lobations between the upper and lower poles, giving the appearance of a deep cleft on an intravenous urogram, which can easily be mistaken for scarring or another disorder.

Ureteropelvic junction obstruction is more common when a duplex kidney exists.[22–24] A duplex kidney with congenital ureteropelvic junction obstruction is inherited by an autosomal dominant gene of variable penetrance.[22] Obstruction usually occurs with the lower-pole renal pelvis, commonly the larger one, and is usually extrarenal. Rarely, it can occur in the upper-pole renal pelvis, when the upper-pole pelvis is larger. Ureteropelvic junction obstruction in a nonexcreting pole of a duplex kidney can be mistaken for a renal mass. Given the availability of ultrasonography, however, this error should no longer occur.

In patients with complete ureteral duplication, hydronephrosis and dysplasia may occur in the upper pole, or dysplasia or chronic pyelonephritis may be found in the lower pole.

Solitary kidneys, hypoplastic kidneys, and fused kidneys of every variety may be duplex. Either or both poles of a duplex kidney may be malrotated.

Duplex kidney is associated with uterus didelphys. This association has been reported in identical twins.[25]

EMBRYOLOGY

If a single ureteral bud bifurcates before the usual time that the ampulla bifurcates, a duplex kidney with a bifid pelvis or bifid ureter results. If two ureteral buds arise from the wolffian duct, a duplex kidney with complete ureteral duplication results.

DIAGNOSTIC IMAGING

Intravenous Urography. A duplex kidney differs from a nonduplex kidney in a number of ways (Fig. 19–151).[21]

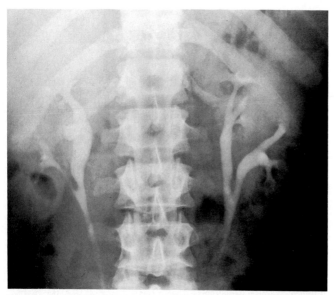

Figure 19–151. Intravenous urogram demonstrating bilateral duplex kidneys. There is a congenitally large septum of Bertin between the upper and the lower poles on both sides.

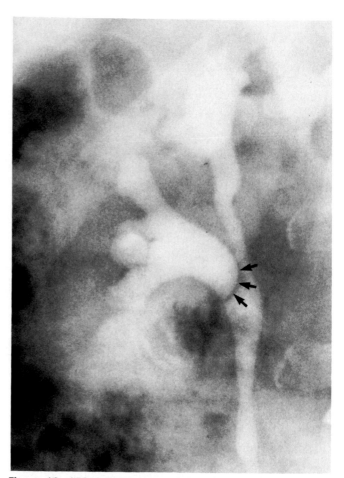

Figure 19–152. Intravenous urogram demonstrating a duplex right kidney. There is a septum within the renal pelvis, partially separating the upper- and lower-pole collecting systems (arrows).

In nonduplex kidneys, the calyces are symmetrical on the two sides in 85% of normal people, and the parenchymal thickness on both sides is usually equal. The four poles are usually thicker than the midzone, but all four poles are normally of equal thickness. The left kidney may be up to 2 cm longer than the right in 80% of normal adults. The right kidney may be up to 1.5 cm longer than the left in 20% of normal adults.

A duplex kidney is nearly always longer than the opposite normal kidney, by as much as 3 cm. One pole of a duplex kidney may have a parenchymal thickness of up to 1 cm less than the other pole; and, if the parenchymal thicknesses of the poles of a duplex kidney are summated, the result is much less than the summated thickness of the poles of a nonduplex kidney. The calyces of a duplex kidney are asymmetrical, compared with the calyces of the nonduplex kidney on the opposite side. A duplex kidney displays any of the varieties of collecting system illustrated in Figure 19–150.

An unusual finding on intravenous urography is the presence of a septum within the renal pelvis, partially separating the upper-pole and lower-pole collecting systems (Fig. 19–152). If this septum is prominent, it can obstruct the lower-pole collecting system (Fig. 19–153).

Intravenous urography can also demonstrate ureteropelvic junction obstruction involving the lower or the upper pole (Fig. 19–154).

Angiography. Almost invariably, a separate artery sup-

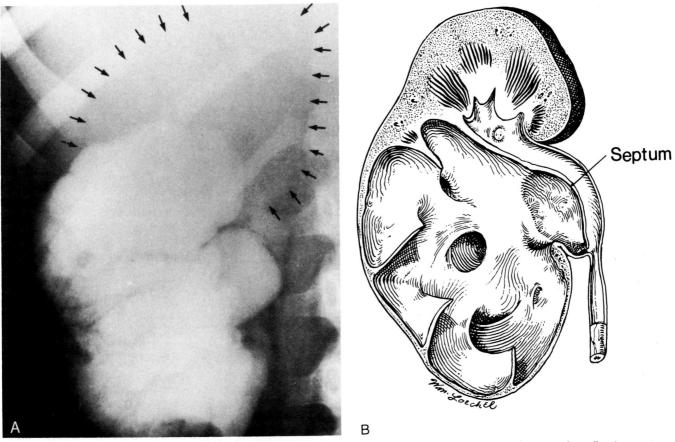

Figure 19–153. Prominent septum within the renal pelvis of a duplex kidney has obstructed the lower-pole collecting system. *A*, Delayed film shows marked hydronephrosis of the lower-pole collecting system. The upper pole is outlined by arrows. *B*, Diagram shows the findings at surgery. (From Broecker BH, Perlmutter AD: Segmental hydronephrosis with a bifid intrarenal pelvis. J Urol 127(4):754–755, © by Williams & Wilkins, 1982.)

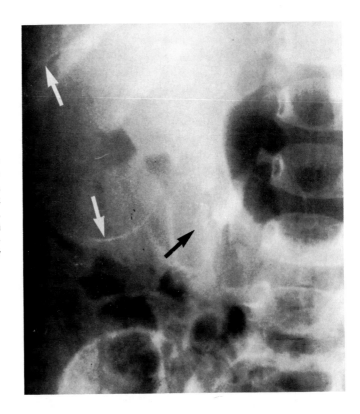

Figure 19–154. Ureteropelvic junction obstruction of the upper pole of a duplex kidney. Intravenous urogram demonstrates Dunbar crescents in the upper pole of the right kidney, indicating hydronephrosis *(white arrows)*. The hydronephrotic upper pole has displaced the lower pole inferiorly and medially. Black arrow points to the lower-pole collecting system. (From Friedland GW, Filly R, Goris ML, et al: Uroradiology: An Integrated Approach. New York, Churchill Livingstone, 1983. By permission.)

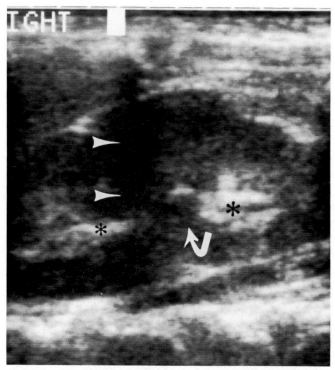

Figure 19–155. Duplex kidney. A coronal sonogram shows two separate central echo complexes *(asterisks)*, with intervening renal parenchyma *(curved arrow)*. A sonographic acoustical shadowing artifact *(arrowheads)* from an overlying rib should not be mistaken for true separation of the central echo complex. These findings do not differentiate a bifid renal pelvis from a bifid ureter or two complete ureters. (Courtesy Barry Potter, M.D., and Bruce Markle, M.D.)

plies each of the poles. In most cases, the vessels arise independently from the aorta.

Ultrasonography. The most important finding on sonograms is two central echo complexes with intervening renal parenchyma (Figs. 19–155 and 19–156; see also Fig. 19–168A).[26] These separate central echo complexes rep-

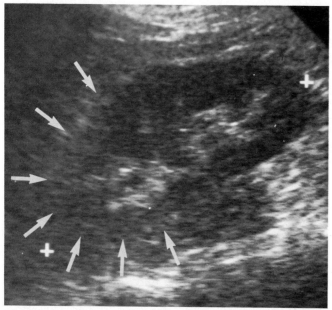

Figure 19–156. Duplex kidney. The sonogram shows two central echo complexes. (Same kidney as shown in Fig. 19–152.) Arrows outline upper pole of kidney.

resent two separate systems, which constitute evidence of a duplex kidney, although they do not necessarily differentiate a bifid renal pelvis from a bifid ureter or two complete ureters. Although this sonographic finding is very specific, it is unfortunately also very insensitive; it occurs in only about 17% of duplex kidneys.[27] It is sometimes possible to see a sharp notch in the outline of the kidney between the two central complexes.

Hydronephrosis of one pole only is suggestive of a duplex kidney and may occur in either pole, although the upper pole is more commonly involved (Fig. 19–157). Upper-pole hydronephrosis is commonly caused by an ectopic, obstructed upper-pole ureter. When the lower pole is hydronephrotic, the most common causes are reflux and ureteropelvic junction obstruction (Fig. 19–158). These findings can be especially suggestive with fetal ultrasound.[28]

If the upper-pole collecting system is very hydronephrotic because of an ectopic ureterocele, a large sonolucent upper-pole mass will displace the lower-pole collecting system, inferiorly and, usually, laterally.

It is sometimes possible to see two distinct collecting systems and two ureters on the same side. This finding is diagnostic.

An ectopic ureterocele in the bladder is also suggestive of a duplex kidney, although it is possible to have an ectopic ureterocele with a single collecting system on that side.

Scintigraphy. Scintigraphy can perform two functions in regard to a duplex kidney:[29] (1), it can confirm the diagnosis suspected on an intravenous urogram or ultrasonogram, or (2), if scintigraphy is the first examination, it can lead to the initial diagnosis. The finding will be two clearly recognizable collecting systems on the same side (Fig. 19–159).

If either a single pole of a duplex kidney, or the entire duplex kidney itself, is dysplastic and therefore nonfunctioning, scintigraphy may show reflux up one or both ureters, thereby demonstrating the presence of a nonfunctioning pole or kidney.[29, 30]

Computed Tomography. When transverse cuts are made through a duplex kidney, the area between the two collecting systems will eventually be reached. This area lacks major vessels and collecting system elements, so that only renal parenchyma is visible. This appearance, which has been called the "faceless kidney," is diagnostic of a partial or complete duplication of the renal collecting system (see Fig. 19–182).[31] It should not be considered to indicate a mass.

CT is excellent for detecting obstruction in either pole of a duplex kidney (Fig. 19–160)[24] for several reasons. First, the findings do not depend on renal function. It is possible to determine whether the system is obstructed or not, and the examination can help to assess how much renal tissue remains in the obstructed part of the kidney. It can also help to determine whether the orifice of an obstructed upper-pole ureter is intravesical or extravesical, and it can be used to examine the retroperitoneum, to determine whether there is some other cause of obstruction of the ureter.[24]

NUBBIN SIGN

The nubbin sign refers to the urographic appearance of a tiny nonfunctioning or poorly functioning lower pole of

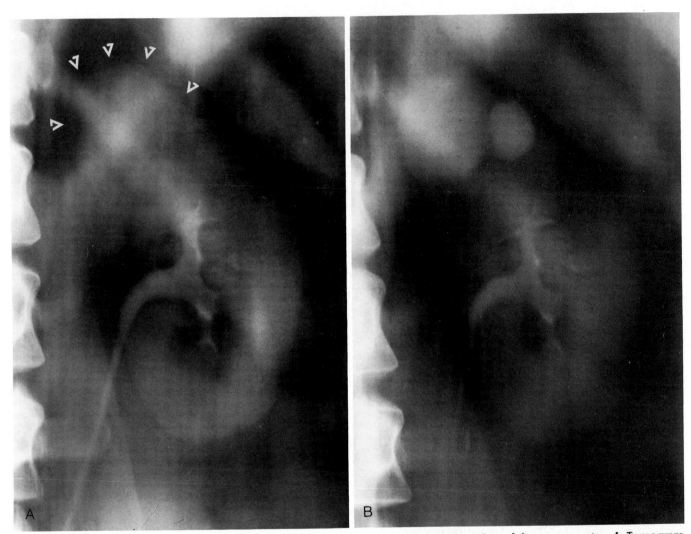

Figure 19–157. Duplex kidney with hydronephrosis of the upper half and ectopic insertion of the upper ureter. *A,* Tomogram from an intravenous urogram demonstrates a mass *(arrowheads)* in the upper pole of the left kidney. The extracalyceal soft-tissue distance at the upper pole of the kidney is abnormally thick, suggesting the presence of a mass in this area. Sonography (not shown) demonstrated that the mass was cystic. *B,* A tomogram of a delayed film from the same study now demonstrates accumulation of contrast medium in the hydronephrotic upper pole. The mass was aspirated under sonographic guidance, and an antegrade pyelogram was performed. The ureter was found to empty into the prostatic urethra.

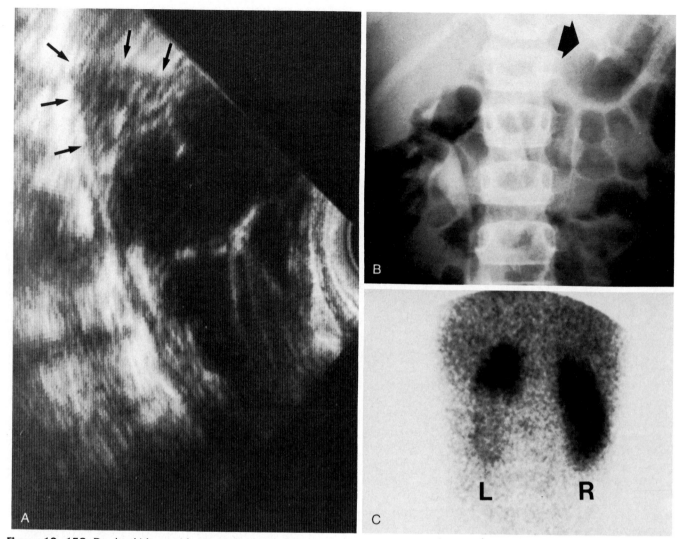

Figure 19–158. Duplex kidney with congenital obstruction of the lower-pole ureteropelvic junction. *A,* Coronal sonogram shows a hydronephrotic lower pole and a small, normal upper pole *(arrows).* Hydronephrosis of one pole only, as in this case, is suggestive of a duplex kidney. *B,* Excretory urogram, shows that only the upper-pole calyces on the left *(arrow)* excrete contrast material. *C,* Renal scan (posterior view) shows that there is no excretion by the lower pole of the left kidney. A left heminephrectomy was performed, which revealed a ureteropelvic junction obstruction involving the lower pole. (Courtesy Massoud Majd, M.D., Barry Potter, M.D., and Bruce Markle, M.D.)

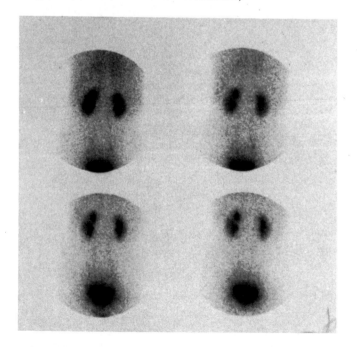

Figure 19–159. Four frames from a Tc-99m-DTPA scan showing a left duplex kidney. Posterior view. (Courtesy Massoud Majd, M.D.)

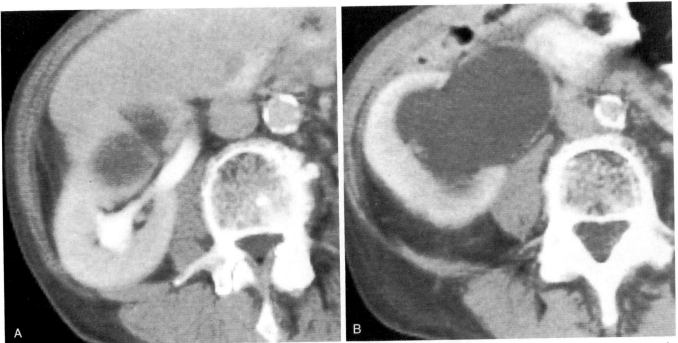

Figure 19–160. Duplex right kidney with ureteropelvic junction obstruction in lower moiety. *A,* CT scan shows the upper-pole collecting system on the right and what appears to be a renal cyst anteriorly. *B,* A lower cut shows that the apparent cyst was a dilated calyx in a patient with ureteropelvic junction obstruction. (Courtesy Roy Bean, M.D., Oakland, California.)

a duplex kidney.[32] This small aggregate of renal tissue may be confused with other disorders. For example, a duplex kidney with a lower-pole nubbin may resemble a nonduplicated kidney with a mass in its lower pole. To differentiate a lower-pole nubbin from a renal mass, it is

important to look for a tiny collecting system, although this may not be possible if the nubbin is nonsecreting (Fig. 19–161). An additional clue is the lack of a full complement of calyces in the rest of the kidney, although this feature may not always be present. In this entity, the

Figure 19–161. Intravenous urogram demonstrating the nubbin sign. The lower-pole collecting system is diminutive and almost no discernible parenchyma surrounds it. (Courtesy Arthur Rosenfield, M.D., Yale University School of Medicine.)

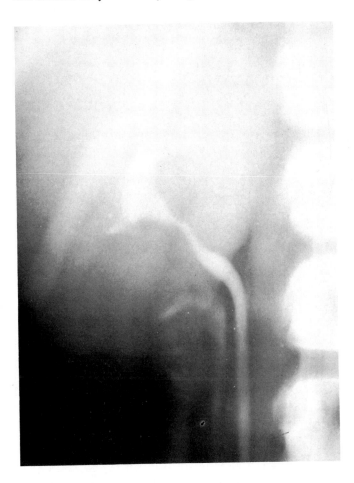

inferior border of the kidney is straight, rather than convex, the nubbin being visible as a bump on this straight lower surface. This appearance is pathognomonic and is unlike the picture that would be expected if a mass were present in the lower pole of a nonduplicated kidney. In that case, the lower pole would appear bulbous—not straight.

This abnormality can resemble a segmental renal infarction that is rarely as severe and in which the kidney retains the normal number of calyces. Arteriography reveals the lack of occlusion of large or medium-sized arteries in a kidney with a nubbin.

Possible causes of the nubbin include parenchymal atrophy secondary to vesicoureteral reflux, infection, or dysplasia secondary to aberrant ureteral bud induction during development. Ninety per cent of duplicated kidneys with a nubbin show reflux into the lower-pole ureter.[33] Cystoscopy to evaluate the presence of a second ureteral orifice and voiding cystourethrography to rule out reflux are helpful procedures when a nubbin is suspected. However, failure to demonstrate reflux, especially in the adult, does not rule out the possibility of reflux nephropathy, since the reflux may long since have ceased. Arguably, the nubbin may also, in some cases, be congenital.

Scintigraphy may show two clearly recognizable collecting systems on the same side. Scintigraphy may also show reflux up the lower-pole ureter, thereby demonstrating its presence.[29]

It is difficult to make the diagnosis with ultrasonography (Fig. 19–162A).[34] CT, however, can be very useful in showing the tiny lower pole of the kidney and two normal-sized ureters (Fig. 19–162B,C).[34] It may also be able to show the faceless kidney between the two collecting systems of the kidney; finally, if the ureter to the lower pole is refluxing, the lower end of the ureter may be distended, and it may be possible to see this on a CT scan.[34]

Bifid, Trifid, and Multifid Renal Pelves

Here the kidney is drained by two, three, or more renal pelves, which unite distal to the normal expected position of the ureteropelvic junction. A common anomaly, it occurs in 10% of the population. At least one infundibulum usually drains into each pelvis. The lower pole is usually larger than the other pelvis or pelves, and drains a larger number of calyces. Many variations of this basic configuration are possible. One pelvis may be obstructed[35] or blind-ending,[36] with no calyces.

Peristaltic dysfunction, similar to the one that occurs with bifid ureters, may occur when these multiple pelves exist, including pyelopelvic reflux.[37]

Bifid Ureters

Bifid ureters draining a duplex kidney join to form a single ureter, usually emptying into the bladder, although they can be ectopic.[38] The ureters may join outside the bladder (i.e., extravesical junction—the most common) or inside the bladder wall (i.e., intravesical junction). If the junction is extravesical, the ureters most often join at the lower third of the distance from the bladder to the kidney. Distally, both ureters travel within a common (Waldeyer's) sheath, share a common blood supply, and may be adherent to each other.

EMBRYOLOGY

A single ureteral bud bifurcates early into two ureters, before the usual time that the ampulla bifurcates. Thus, there is no fundamental embryological difference between duplicated kidneys and supernumerary kidneys; the time that the duplication of the bud occurs affects how buds subsequently induce the metanephrogenic blastema.

Y AND V JUNCTIONS

If the junction is extravesical, it is called a Y junction, sometimes just "Y" or "fork." If the junction is intravesical, it is V shaped.[38]

There are three types of Y junctions (Fig. 19–163).[38] Both bifid ureters and their common chamber may be of normal size. The bifid ureters may be of normal size and the common chamber large. The bifid ureters may be dilated, but the common chamber is bigger than either. These relative calibers have functional significance.

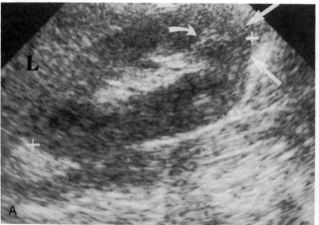
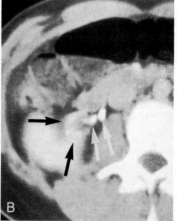
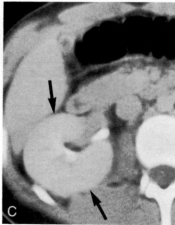

Figure 19–162. Lower-pole nubbin. *A,* Ultrasonography demonstrates small, eccentric aggregate of parenchymal tissue *(arrows)* that constitutes atrophic lower-pole moiety of duplex right kidney ("nubbin"). (L = liver.) *B,* CT scan through the right lower pole nicely demonstrates the nubbin *(black arrows)* with its renal pelvis *(white arrow)* and ureter *(medial white arrow). C,* The upper pole *(arrows)* is hypertrophic and appears healthy. The hypertrophy is related to hypoplasia of the left kidney (not shown). (From Blair D, Rigsby C, Rosenfield AT: The nubbin sign on computed tomography and sonography. Urol Radiol 9:149, 1987.)

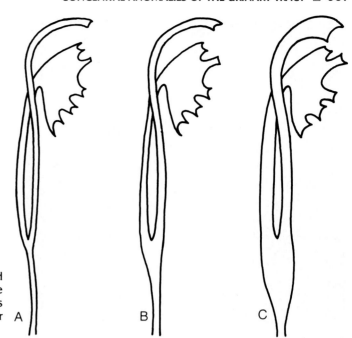

Figure 19–163. The three types of Y junction. *A,* Both bifid ureters and their common chamber are of normal size. *B,* The bifid ureters are of normal size, and the common chamber is large. *C,* The bifid ureters are dilated, but the common chamber is larger than either.

Ureteroureteral Reflux (Yo-Yo Phenomenon)

This phenomenon occurs with an extravesical junction, and involves peristalsis down one limb of a bifid ureter, forcing urine via reflux up the other (Fig. 19–164).[38-40]

It is usually a functional abnormality, although a true distal obstruction may also exist, owing to stenosis or ureterocele. The resting pressure in the common chamber is always higher than in either of the two ureters above it, even if the common chamber is larger than either of the two ureters. Peristalsis down the two ureters is almost always asymmetrical, so that urine, flowing to the site of lowest pressure, may easily progress up the other ureter. The wider the common chamber, the easier it is for urine to flow into the other ureter, because of pressure gradients. Peristalsis down one ureter may cross the common chamber and proceed up the other ureter. At irregular intervals, this peristalsis proceeds down the common ureter; otherwise, the kidney would never empty at all.

As these ureters can serve as a site of persistent infection,[50] surgery has sometimes been performed to alleviate the abnormal situation, which usually involves anastomosing the upper-pole ureter to the lower-pole renal pelvis.[41]

Associated Anomalies

Almost 50% of extravesical junctions have some associated anomaly. Those involving the lower common ureter include vesicoureteral reflux in one-third of cases, ureterocele at the distal end of the ureter, stenosis, and atresia (resulting in multicystic dysplasia of the duplex kidney). Anomalies associated with the bifid ureters include ureteropelvic junction obstruction, usually of the lower-pole pelvis, and stenosis of one of the two ureters.

Intravesical Junctions

Intravesical junctions have none of these associated problems. Ureteroureteral reflux is absent because pressure in the common stem is low, owing to the muscle surrounding the intramural ureter.

Figure 19–164. Diagram illustrates ureteroureteral reflux (the "yo-yo" phenomenon).

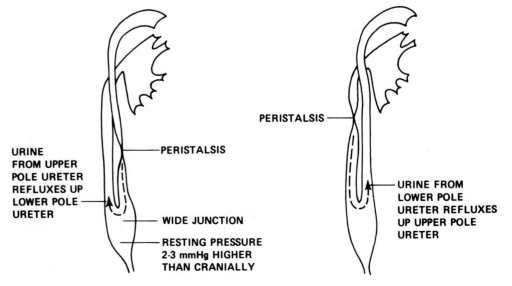

URINE FROM UPPER POLE URETER REFLUXES UP LOWER POLE URETER

PERISTALSIS

WIDE JUNCTION

RESTING PRESSURE 2-3 mmHg HIGHER THAN CRANIALLY

PERISTALSIS

URINE FROM LOWER POLE URETER REFLUXES UP UPPER POLE URETER

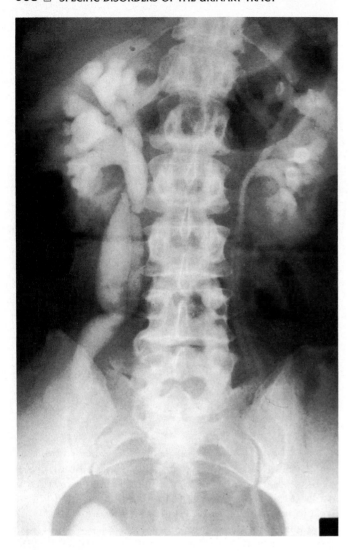

Figure 19–165. Intravenous urogram showing Type A bifid (but otherwise normal) ureters on the left and Type C bifid (dilated) ureters on the right.

Figure 19–166. Ureteroureteral reflux. *A,* Intravenous urogram showing Type C bifid ureters on the left. *B,* The upper-pole ureter has emptied via peristalsis, and reflux of urine is occurring into the distal end of the lower-pole ureter. (From Friedland GW: Hydronephrosis in infants and children. Part I. Curr Prob Diagn Radiol 7:48, 1978.)

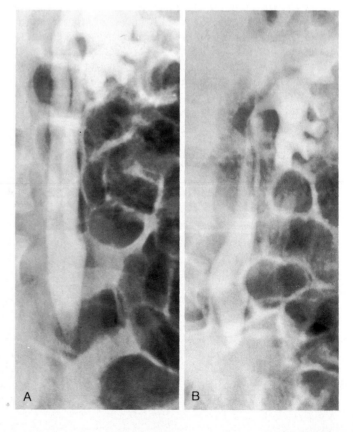

A   B

DIAGNOSTIC IMAGING

Intravenous urography shows all the anatomical findings previously described (Fig. 19–165). Fluoroscopy with videotape recording demonstrates and records ureteroureteral reflux (Fig. 19–166).

Scintigraphy demonstrates two collecting systems on the same side, as well as the presence of ureteroureteral reflux.

Duplex ureters reflux more frequently than do single ureters. This can be demonstrated by a radiological (Fig. 19–167) or scintigraphic voiding cystourethrogram.

Renal ultrasonography occasionally shows two central echo complexes, with intervening renal parenchyma, and sometimes also reveals two distinct collecting systems and two ureters on the same side (Fig. 19–168).

Duplicated Segment within a Single Ureter

This is a rare congenital anomaly. The proximal and distal ends of the ureter form a single tube, but the segment between them is duplicated, forming two tubes.[42]

Inverted Y Ureter

About 30 well-documented cases describe a single proximal ureter that splits distally to form an inverted Y.[43–45] There are usually two ureteral orifices in the bladder on the same side, but it is possible for one ureter to be ectopic[46] and to have an associated ectopic ureterocele (Fig. 19–169).[44, 45]

Double Ureters

Double ureters, by definition, are those that remain completely separate to the point where they insert in the bladder or beyond. In virtually every case, both ureters pass through the bladder wall through a common tunnel,

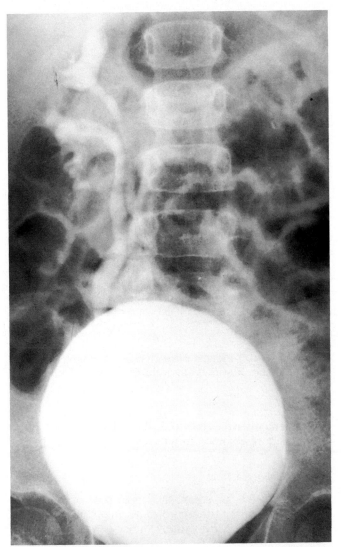

Figure 19–167. Cystogram shows reflux into bifid right ureter.

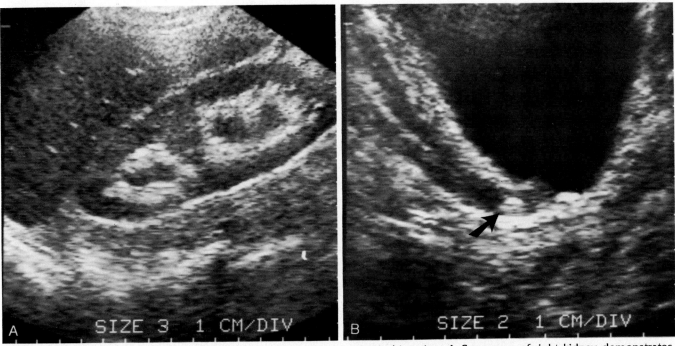

Figure 19–168. Bifid ureter with V junction and calculus at ureterovesical junction. *A*, Sonogram of right kidney demonstrates two central echo complexes separated by normal renal parenchyma. There is hydronephrosis of both calyceal systems. *B*, Sonogram of distal right ureter and bladder demonstrates the V junction, and the calculus (*arrow*) immediately beyond the junction. (Courtesy Professor Dr. A. L. Baert, Universitare Ziekenhuizen, Katholieke Universiteit Leuven, Belgium.)

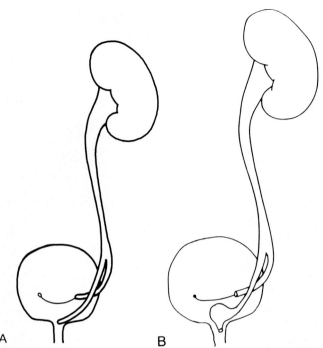

Figure 19–169. Diagrams illustrate inverted Y ureter: *A,* without ureterocele, *B,* with ureterocele, on ectopic ureter.

even when one ureter is ectopic. Double ureters are about 10 times more common in females.

WEIGERT-R MEYER RULE

In about 85% of cases, the upper-pole ureter opens below and medial to the lower-pole ureter; this is known as the Weigert-R Meyer rule.[47]

ECTOPIC PATHWAY

In about 15% of cases, the upper-pole ureter can open anywhere along the so-called ectopic pathway,[46] which is in the shape of a shepherd's crook, circling the superior and medial aspect of the lateral angle of the trigone, then extending across the trigone and down the urethra (Fig. 19–170).

When one ureter is ectopic and opens in the urethra, it always travels in the submucosa of the bladder and the urethra. In the female, it can open anywhere in the posterior wall of the urethra, or in the urethrovaginal septum. In the male, it can open only in the upper third of the prostatic urethra.

In the female, the upper-pole ureter can be extravesical and ectopic and open into the vagina via Gartner's duct or into the hymen. Rarely, it opens into the uterus or fallopian tubes. Rare cases of termination into the rectum have been recorded. In the male, it can be extravesical and ectopic and may open into the seminal vesicle or vas deferens.

ASSOCIATED RENAL DYSPLASIA

The more extreme the location of the orifice, in a cranial or a caudal direction, the more likely it is that the associated pole of the kidney is dysplastic.[48]

INTERVENING URETER

The upper-pole ureter always lies in front of the lower-pole ureter and usually crosses it twice, just below the lower-pole pelvis and just above the bladder. Sometimes, however, this crossing may not occur.

The contralateral ureter is duplicated in 20% of cases, but even if there is a single contralateral ureter, reflux is common. Sometimes the contralateral ureter is dilated, regardless of the presence of reflux.

Urinary tract infections are common, including acute pyelonephritis, which nearly always occurs in females.[21] Usually, the lower pole of the kidney is affected, because it is usually the lower-pole ureter that refluxes,[21] although the upper-pole ureter or both ureters may reflux. If the bladder is infected, the infection is easily carried via this reflux to the kidney.

Persistent urinary tract infections may occur, again most frequently in the female.[50] The upper-pole ureter and the upper pole of the kidney are most commonly affected, because if the upper-pole ureter is ectopic and the upper pole of the kidney is dysplastic, the kidney excretes very little urine. Thus, urine can flow into the ureter only during reflux from the urethra during voiding. If the ectopic segment is infected, antimicrobial agents borne by the urine can be inadequate because of poor or no renal function. Another cause of persistent urinary infection (in this case proteus infection) in patients with double ureters is struvite stone formation.

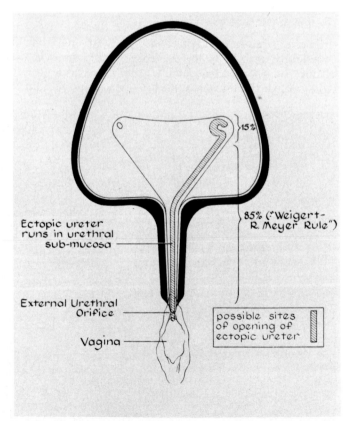

Figure 19–170. Diagram illustrates the Weigert-R Meyer rule and Stephens' ectopic pathway. (From Friedland GW, Cunningham J: The elusive ectopic ureteroceles. AJR 116:792–811, © Williams & Wilkins, 1972.)

Recurrent epididymo-orchitis is the most common presentation of ectopic ureters in the male.[51, 52] The condition arises because of insertion the ureter into the common duct. Because the seminal vesicle and the ejaculatory duct are congenitally abnormal in such patients, Williams calls them the common duct, as there is a common duct for urine and ejaculate.[51] Most ectopic ureters inserting into the common duct are single, not double.

Incontinence occurs only in the female, because in the male the ectopic ureter always opens above the striated external sphincter muscle, insuring continence.[53] Incontinence, when present, is always due to ectopic insertion of the upper-pole, rather than the lower-pole, ureter, especially where that insertion is very ectopic, in the distal half of the urethra or in the vagina itself. Incontinence occurs because neither region is under sphincteric control. The lower-pole ureter is never involved, because it opens into the bladder, where urine is subject to sphincteric control. In girls, incontinence in the presence of normal voiding is highly suggestive of ectopic insertion of an upper-pole ureter.

If the ectopic ureter opens a little higher in the urethra, incontinence is nocturnal (if present). Such patients can maintain control during the day, but not during sleep. Incontinence can occur for the first time later in life, or if childbirth has injured the external sphincter.

Ureteropelvic junction obstruction is more prevalent in patients with double ureters than in the general population and almost always involves the lower-pole pelvis.

Patients with solitary kidneys, hypoplastic kidneys, all varieties of fused kidneys, or posterior urethral valves may have double ureters.

It is currently believed that double ureters are caused by an autosomal dominant trait with low penetrance,[54] but it should be pointed out that double ureters are more prevalent in certain geographic areas as compared with the rest of the country suggesting that environmental factors may also play a role.[55]

Double ureters can occur in patients with multiple congenital anomalies occurring in other systems, as part of the complex of anomalies given the acronyms VATER and VACTERL (see page 560).

EMBRYOLOGY

Instead of only a single ureteral bud arising from the wolffian duct, two are found in the case of double ureters, or three in the case of triple ureters.

If two ureteral buds arise from the primary nephric duct, the bud associated with the future lower pole separates first from the primary nephric duct by a process described in the section on the embryology of the ureteral orifice (page 687). The orifice of the lower-pole ureter then progresses superiorly and laterally, as a result of the growth of the urogenital sinus. The common excretory duct, with the remaining ureter still attached, is meanwhile taken up into the urogenital sinus. When this finally occurs, the orifice of the ureter draining the upper pole opens, medial and inferior to the orifice draining the lower pole. This is the explanation for the Weigert-R Meyer rule.

DIAGNOSTIC IMAGING

The following three general points regarding the imaging of double ureters are important:

1. The ureters usually obey the Weigert-R Meyer rule: the upper-pole ureter opens medial to and caudal to the lower-pole ureter.[47]

2. Both kidneys and ureters may be normal, except for being double.[47, 53]

3. The most common problem found in patients with double ureters is that the upper-pole ureter is ectopic and obstructed and lower-pole ureter refluxes. Reflux occurs three times more often into lower-pole ureters than into upper-pole ureters.

Intravenous Urography. The results of this examination are often normal, apart from the duplex kidney and double ureters (Fig. 19–171). Occasionally, it is possible to see two separate jets of contrast, if both ureters happen to be effluxing in synchrony.

Excretion from the upper pole of a duplex kidney with double ureters can be poor or nonexistent. The causes can be acute if, for example, an acute abscess is in the upper pole or if the upper-pole ureter is obstructed by a stone, or a chronic disorder (Figs. 19–172 to 19–174).

Two problems are associated with poor excretion from the upper pole. The first is the recognition that the lower-pole collecting system, usually clearly visualized, is one of two such systems (Figs. 19–172 to 19–174); the second is the recognition that the upper pole is abnormally large, which can occur whether the obstruction is acute or chronic. If the obstruction is acute, the apparent upper-

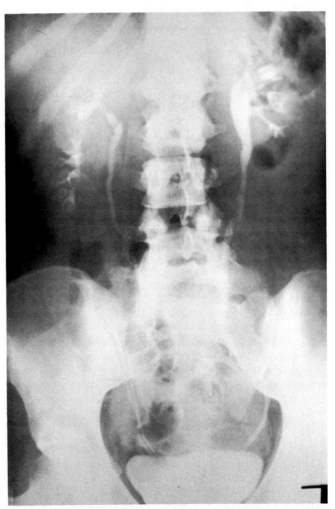

Figure 19–171. Intravenous urogram demonstrating complete ureteral duplication on the right. The appearances are otherwise within normal limits.

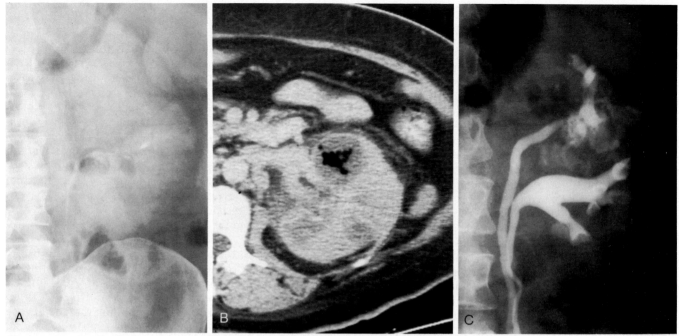

Figure 19–172. Complete ureteral duplication on the left with gas-forming infection in the upper pole of the left kidney. *A*, Intravenous urography shows a decreased nephrogram in the upper pole of the left kidney. The upper pole appears large. The lower-pole calyces appear to be displaced downwardly and laterally. *B*, CT scan through the upper pole of the left kidney shows a large gas-containing mass in the renal parenchyma and diffuse swelling of the upper pole. Some thickening of the tissues in the perinephric space can be seen. *C*, Retrograde pyelograms performed by injecting contrast material into both distal ureters outline the double collecting system. Contrast material is extravasating into the irregular cavities within the parenchyma of the upper pole. The abscess was drained percutaneously, and the patient made an uneventful recovery. (Courtesy Jeffrey Reese, M.D., Division of Urology, Stanford University.)

pole mass is really a nonexcreting upper pole. If the obstruction is chronic, the mass is caused by hydronephrosis and/or cystic dysplasia.

The characteristic features of an upper pole mass due to hydronephrosis and cystic dysplasia are as follows: (1) If the upper pole excretes contrast material, the "crescent" or "rim" sign during the early phase of the intravenous urogram is evidence that hydronephrosis is present, even before the collection system has opacified.[56] (See Chapter 55 for further discussion of crescents and rims.) (2) The ratio of the renal length to the distance between the superior margin of the upper pole and the uppermost calyx is normally approximately 3.3:1. If this ratio falls to less than 2.6:1, a mass becomes a possibility. This finding is best demonstrated on tomography. (3) The so-called drooping lily sign occurs when the lower-pole collecting system resembles a wilting flower (Fig. 19–175). To demonstrate quantitatively that this sign exists, measure the ratio between the uppermost calyx and the nearest pedicle on one side to the distance between the uppermost calyx and nearest pedicle on the opposite side. Normally, these ratios are about equal, but in no case should they be greater than 1.5:1. If the ratio exceeds 1.5:1, a duplication with upper-pole hydronephrosis should be suspected.[57] Ureteral displacement from the midline also occurs on the affected side.

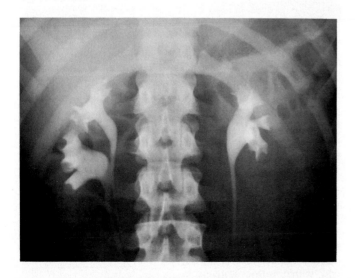

Figure 19–173. Intravenous urogram shows a double collecting system on the right, but only a single collecting system on the left. Note, however, the too few calyces on the left and the short infundibulum of the upper-pole calyx. The patient was found to have a second, ectopic ureter on the left, arising from the upper pole of the left kidney, which did not excrete contrast material during this study.

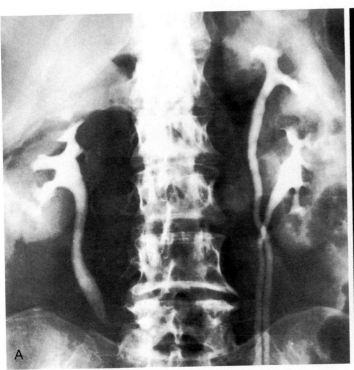

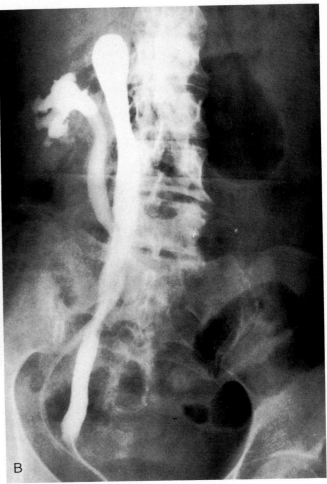

Figure 19–174. Nonvisualizing upper-pole duplication on the right. *A,* Intravenous urogram shows a double collecting system on the left, but only a single ureter on the right. This single ureter is displaced laterally. The renal pelvis on the right appears vertical, and the infundibulum draining the apparent upper pole is short. These features indicate a second, nonfunctioning collecting system draining the upper pole. *B,* Retrograde urogram performed by injecting contrast material into both ureters outlines the hydronephrotic collecting system draining the upper pole of the right kidney. (From Friedland GW, Stamey TA: Recurrent urinary tract infection with persistent Wolffian duct masquerading as duplicated urethra. Urology 4:315–318, 1974.)

When the upper pole is hydronephrotic, the lower-pole renal pelvis is usually more vertical than normal; the upper convex surface may appear flattened. A hydroureter from the upper pole may force the lower-pole ureter laterally into an abnormal, oblique course.[51] The dilated upper-pole ureter may scallop the lower-pole ureter (Fig. 19–175).[51] Finally, the visualized calyces may appear to lack a well-defined upper-pole equivalent.

Two features should cause the examiner to suspect the presence of a lower-pole collecting system, even though it is nonexcreting. First, too few calyces and infundibula are present, although this may not always be obvious. Second, the upper-pole infundibulum is normally the longest. If the apparent upper-pole infundibulum looks short, especially in comparison to that on the opposite side, then a lower-pole collecting system should be suspected (Figs. 19–172 to 19–175).[51]

It may be possible to see that the lower pole is dysplastic, in which case diffuse calyceal clubbing is visible, and thin overlying parenchyma is found. The lower pole is usually somewhat smaller. If it is tiny, the nubbin sign (page 662) may appear. In chronic reflux nephropathy with infection, the calyceal clubbing and overlying paren-chymal scarring are usually patchy and sometimes involve only a single calyx (Fig. 19–176). (See Chapter 21.)

If a struvite stone is present, it usually occurs in the lower pole and is of the staghorn variety (Fig. 19–177).

If a 14 × 17 inch abdominal radiograph is obtained so that the lower edge of the film is below the symphysis pubis and if the upper pole is excreting, it may be possible to see where an ectopic upper-pole ureter inserts.[58] (See later section, Ectopic Ureteral Orifices.) It may be helpful to have a voiding or an immediate postvoiding film, since reflux may occur into, and thus demonstrate, a nonvisualizing nephroureteral unit.[21]

Voiding Cystourethrogram. A voiding cystourethrogram usually fills an ectopic ureter by reflux if the ureter opens into the urethra. It may even demonstrate an ectopic ureterocele by the same method.

Sometimes, especially after nephroureterectomy, in which less than the entire ureter has been removed, only a small segment of ureter fills with contrast material, giving the false impression of a diverticulum (Fig. 19–178A). In a female, any apparent urethral diverticulum should be investigated to be certain it is not an ectopic ureter (Fig. 19–178B).

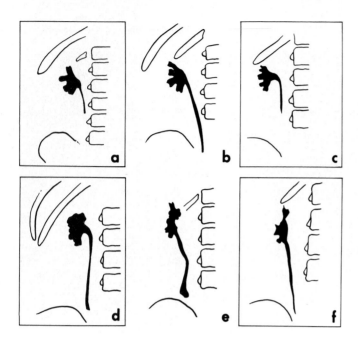

Figure 19–175. Diagram illustrates the ways in which a dilated upper-pole collecting system can displace the lower-pole renal pelvis and ureter. (From Williams DI: Urology in childhood: Encyclopedia of Urology, Vol 15. Berlin, Springer-Verlag 1985.)

Figure 19–176. Intravenous urogram in a patient with complete right ureteral duplication demonstrates calyceal clubbing with overlying parenchymal scarring in the lower pole of the right kidney, which is due to chronic pyelonephritis (reflux nephropathy).

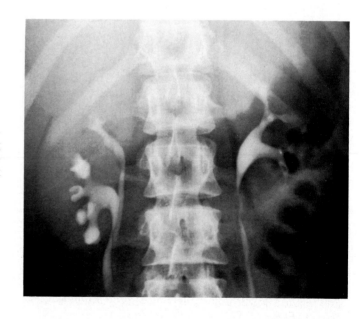

Figure 19–177. Staghorn calculus in lower pole of duplex kidney with complete ureteral duplication. *A,* Preliminary radiograph shows a staghorn calculus with a short upper-pole infundibulum and a wilting-flower appearance. *B,* Outline of the double collecting system is shown, following a retrograde pyelogram with injection of contrast material into both ureters. (From Friedland GW, Filly R, Goris ML, et al: Uroradiology: An Integrated Approach. New York, Churchill Livingstone, 1983, p 512. By permission.)

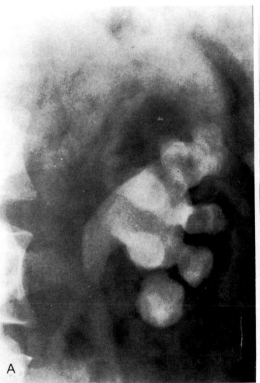
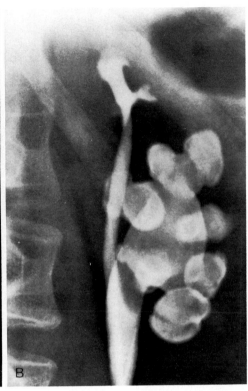

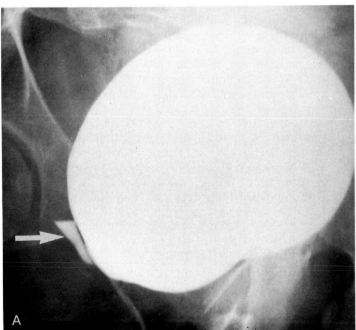
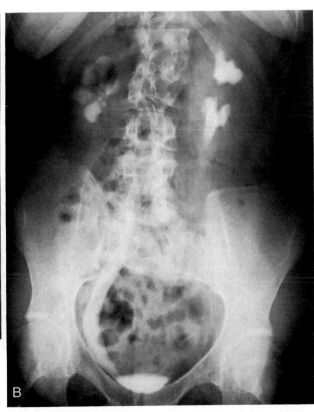

Figure 19–178. Ectopic ureter inserting into the bladder neck. *A,* Cystogram, shows reflux into the distal right ureter *(arrow).* *B,* Intravenous urogram shows right hydroureteronephrosis and a hypoplastic right kidney. The left kidney has not rotated.

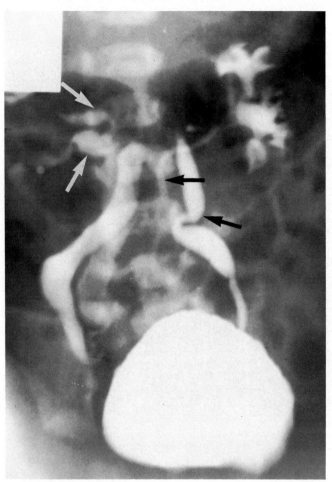

Figure 19–179. Cystogram in an infant with bilateral ureteral duplication shows reflux into all four ureters *(arrows)*.

Reflux may occur if a lower-pole ureter opens in the craniozone of the ectopic pathway (see Fig. 19–207). If a lower-pole ureter happens to open into a diverticulum, the diverticulum is demonstrated. However, reflux may occur into the upper-pole ureter only, both ureters on the same side, or all four ureters, if the duplication is bilateral (Fig. 19–179).

If an ectopic ureter opens into a common duct (a congenitally deformed seminal vesicle or ejaculatory duct) in a male, that duct usually has a wide patulous opening into the urethra, enabling reflux to occur into it as well as the ureter, thereby demonstrating all three structures.

Antegrade Pyelography. Antegrade pyelography is commonly employed in patients with a hydronephrotic upper pole, both for demonstrating the existence of a second ureter and for determining where that ureter terminates. The hydronephrotic sac in the upper pole is first located by means of ultrasonography. Then, under fluoroscopy, a percutaneous needle puncture is performed and contrast material is instilled into the collecting system. Fluoroscopic spot films demonstrate the existence of the ureter and show where it opens. If the involved renal segment excretes contrast medium, direct puncture with fluoroscopy can be done, without the need for ultrasonography.

Retrograde Urogram. The retrograde urogram can be used to opacify one or both duplicated collecting systems, if the ureteral orifices can be adequately visualized endoscopically. An intravenous injection of indigo carmine is useful for this purpose. Presuming that a modicum of renal function exists, a visual inspection is made to see where the colored urine emerges. Once that site is located, a catheter is inserted and contrast material is injected. This is a useful method of demonstrating the junction of the two ureters, if the issue remains in doubt after excretory urography, and of amplifying other findings still indeterminate after that examination. The orifices of many ectopic ureters, however, will prove to be inaccessible to endoscopic catheterization.

Seminal Vesiculogram. Since most ectopic ureteral insertions reflux, this examination should rarely be necessary.

Ultrasonography. The most important finding on renal ultrasonography is two central echo complexes, with intervening renal parenchyma (see Figs. 19–155, 19–156, and 19–168).[26] Although this sonographic finding is very specific, it is unfortunately also very insensitive, as has been previously described on page 662.[27]

Hydronephrosis of one pole only is suggestive of ureteral duplication and may occur in either pole, although more commonly the upper pole is involved (Fig. 19–180).[28] If the upper-pole collecting system is very hydronephrotic, a large sonolucent upper-pole mass will displace the lower-pole collecting system laterally and inferiorly.

It is sometimes possible to see two distinct collecting systems and two ureters on the same side. This finding is diagnostic.

The ureter draining the upper pole may be ectopic. The sonographic appearances of ectopic ureters with ectopic ureteroceles are discussed elsewhere. Ectopic ureters without ectopic ureteroceles are almost always dilated, and transverse sections will show a dilated ureter extending posterior to the bladder base, but usually remaining completely separate from the bladder itself (Fig. 19–180).

Scintigraphy. Scintigraphy can confirm the presence of ureteral duplication suspected on an intravenous urogram or sonogram, or, if scintigraphy is the first examination, it can make the initial diagnosis. The finding will be two clearly recognizable collecting systems on the same side (see Fig. 19–159).

If either a single pole of the associated duplex kidney or the entire duplex kidney itself is dysplastic and therefore nonfunctioning, scintigraphy may show reflux up one or both ureters, thereby demonstrating the presence of a nonfunctioning pole or kidney (Fig. 19–181).

Computed Tomography. CT may show the "faceless kidney" between the two collecting systems of the kidney (Fig. 19–182).[31] It is also excellent for detecting obstruction in either pole of a duplex kidney, for reasons previously described (see page 662).

Triplicate Ureters

In this disorder, three ureters, partial or complete, are present.[53, 59–64] One drains the upper pole, one the lower pole, and one the portion in between (the midzone).

There are three types of triplicate ureters (Fig. 19–183):

Type I. This involves three separate ureters with three separate orifices. There are two subvarieties, each occurring in about half the cases. In the first subvariety, the orifices obey the Weigert-R Meyer rule. The lower-pole

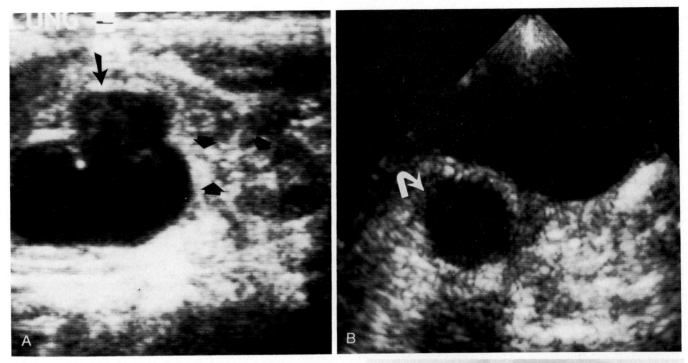

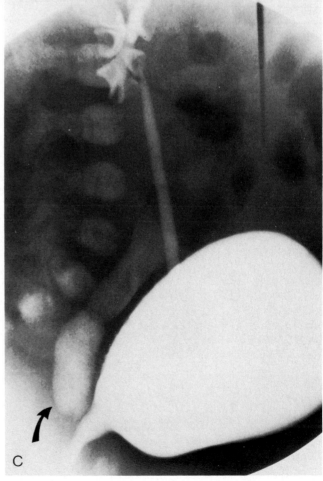

Figure 19–180. Double collecting system with ureteral ectopia. *A,* Longitudinal sonogram of the right kidney shows a dilated upper *(long arrow)* and normal lower-pole *(short broad arrows)* collecting system. *B,* Transverse scan through the bladder base shows the dilated upper-pole ureter posteriorly *(curved arrow),* but no intravesical ureterocele. *C,* On a voiding cystourethrogram the dilated ureter *(curved arrow)* fills from the urethra during voiding. There is reflux into the left ureter and upper collecting system. (Courtesy Barry Potter, M.D., and Bruce Markle, M.D.)

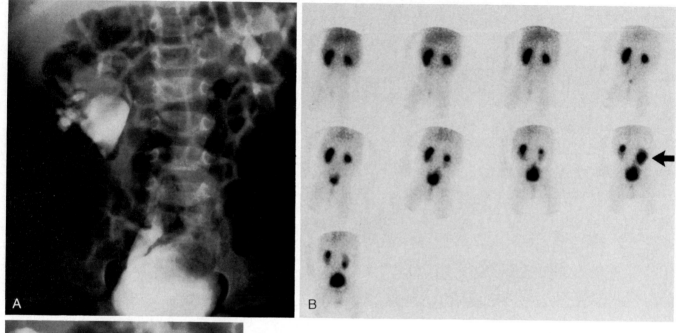

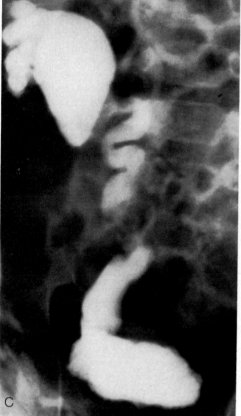

Figure 19–181. An example of the superiority of scintigraphy over intravenous urography in detecting reflux. *A,* An intravenous urogram shows complete ureteral duplication on the right and a single system on the left. The lower-pole renal pelvis is capacious. *B,* A Tc-99m-DTPA scan, posterior view, shows that the lower pole of the right kidney does not function and that it fills by reflux *(arrow).* Thus, scintigraphy can distinguish reflux from function, which was not possible on the intravenous urogram. *C,* A voiding cystourethrogram shows high-grade reflux into the right lower-pole collecting system. (Courtesy Massoud Majd, M.D.)

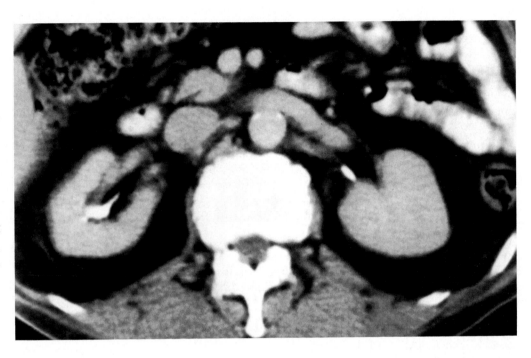

Figure 19–182. "Faceless" kidney. CT scan through the junction of the upper- and lower-pole moieties of a duplex left kidney reveals the faceless appearance produced by a lack of a renal sinus or collecting system structures at this level. Compare with normal right kidney. (From Hulnick DH, Bosniak MA: "Faceless" kidney: CT sign of renal duplicity. J Comput Assist Tomogr 10:771, 1986.)

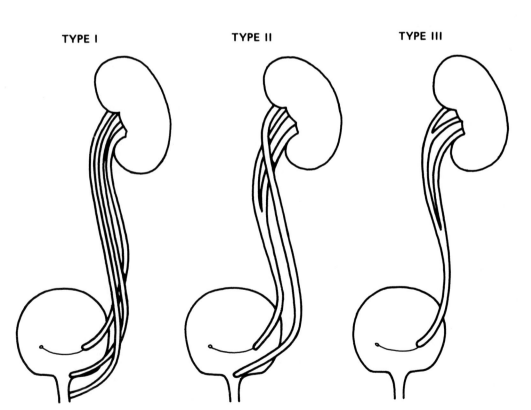

TYPE I   TYPE II   TYPE III

Figure 19–183. Diagram illustrating the three types of ureteral triplication.

ureter opens into the lateral angle of the trigone; the upper-pole ureteral orifice lies medial and caudal to the lower-pole ureteral orifice and is usually ectopic, opening into the urethra or the vagina. If the ureter opens into the urethra, the orifice is stenotic with a ureterocele, or it is incompetent. If the upper-pole ureter is ectopic (usually the case), the function of the upper pole is poor. If it opens in the trigone, the function is usually good.

The second subvariety does not obey the Weigert-R Meyer rule. The lower-pole ureter opens in the lateral angle of the trigone, and the lower pole of the kidney functions well. The upper-pole ureter opens on the trigone medial and caudal to the lower-pole ureter, and the upper pole of the kidney functions well. The midzone ureter, however, opens caudal to both and is usually ectopic, draining a poorly functioning midzone and opening into the urethra or the vagina. Thus, if the upper pole has poor function, then the ureters obey the Weigert-R Meyer rule; if the midzone of the kidney has poor function, the ureters do not obey the Weigert-R Meyer rule.

Type II. This type of ureteral triplication involves a double ureter with one bifid ureter and occurs in about one-third of cases. Usually the bifid ureter drains the midzone and the lower pole, whereas a single separate ureter drains the upper pole. This system usually obeys the Weigert-R Meyer rule.

Type III. These ureteral triplications involve trifid ureters with a single orifice, usually occurring in about one-third of cases. Usually the dominant ureter drains the lower pole, and branches either high or low. There are two varieties. One occurs when a ureter branches off the lower pole ureter, which then divides, in order to drain the upper pole and midzone. Alternatively, two ureters may branch off the lower-pole ureter. When this occurs, the following three possibilities exist:

1. The lowermost branch drains the upper pole; second or highest branch drains the midzone.
2. The lowest branch drains the midzone; the highest drains the upper pole.
3. The lowest branch ends blindly; the highest drains the midzone.

Ureteral triplication can also occur in crossed fused ectopia, in which the uncrossed kidney has three ureters and the crossed kidney has one or two ureters (Fig. 19–184).

DIAGNOSTIC IMAGING

In Type I ureteral triplication, the upper pole or the midzone may appear hydronephrotic or nonexcreting on an intravenous urogram, although occasionally both may appear to be normal. In any type of ureteral triplication, it is possible for the upper pole, the midzone, and the lower pole to excrete normally. This makes possible visualization of three separate ureters (Type I triplication), or the branching of a duplex ureter (Type II triplication), or a single distal ureter (Type III triplication). In the last case, the kidney sometimes appears hydronephrotic.

Other Types of Multiple Ureters

Four,[65] five, six, and even seven ureters have been reported, but instances of these anomalies are rare.

Anomalies in Position and Form

Blind-ending Ureteral Bud (Blind-ending Ureteral Duplication)

A blind-ending ureteral bud is a blind-ending hollow structure the wall of which has all the layers of the normal ureter.[66–79, 141] Always more than twice as long as its greatest diameter, it joins the ureter at an acute angle.[66] The term "ureteral diverticulum," which has been applied to this entity, is incorrect and should be reserved for structures more appropriately conforming to diverticula elsewhere in the body.

A blind-ending ureteral bud can arise from a single ureter (Fig. 19–185) or from one branch of a double or triple ureter. Two blind-ending ureters can arise from a single ureter (Fig. 19–186). The disorder can occur in association with a horseshoe, ectopic, or crossed fused ectopic kidney. Such a bud may arise independently from the urinary bladder (Figs. 19–185 and 19–187). Almost invariably, ureteral buds are oriented so that their blind ends are directed cranially. Rare examples of inverted buds are known, however, as are other curious and sometimes unclassifiable anomalies of the blind-ending ureter (Fig. 19–188).

Blind-ending ureteral buds may first be detected at any age, usually as an incidental finding on an intravenous urogram.[68] The ureters associated with long blind-ending ureteral buds have a higher-than-normal incidence of vesicoureteral reflux.[69] If there is infection and reflux, a blind-ending ureteral bud can become acutely inflamed, although it is not commonly a source of persistent infection, because it is bathed by the urine and by antimicrobial agents when they are present in the urine.[50] It is twice as common in females. A familial occurrence of blind-ending buds has been reported.[79]

Blind-ending ureteral buds can arise with equal frequency from all parts of the ureter. A fibrous cord may extend from the blind end of the bud to the kidney.[70] A common sheath surrounds the ureter and its associated blind-ending bud.[69] Sometimes this sheath binds the ureter and its associated bud together tightly, but sometimes they are widely separated.[69] The anomalous ureteral bud and the normal ureter share a common blood supply.[70]

EMBRYOLOGY

Blind-ending ureters can arise either from the bladder or from the ureter. Those that arise in the bladder do so because a second ureteral bud grows out from the wolffian duct, in the same way that double ureters grow out. However, this second bud probably arises from the wolffian duct much later than do buds that may form a double ureter. Because this occurs later, the growing bud fails to induce the metanephrogenic blastema, and there is no subsequent connection with kidney tissue. The result is a blind-ending ureter arising from the bladder.

A blind-ending ureter can also arise from a ureter, owing to the fact that when the ampullary end of the ureter bifurcates, one branch either fails to induce the metanephrogenic blastema or fails to become associated with it.

DIAGNOSTIC IMAGING

Intravenous Urography. The intravenous urogram reveals a blind-ending hollow structure, often with a bul-

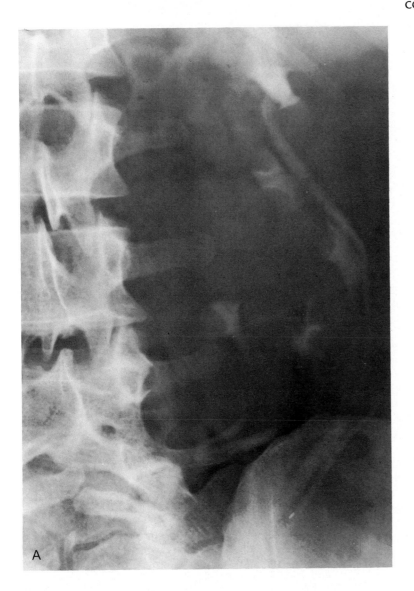

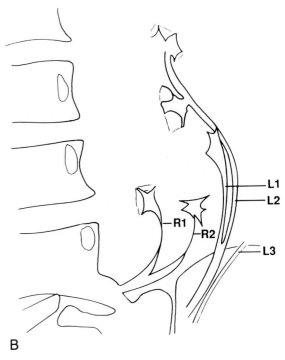

Figure 19–184. *A,* Intravenous urogram demonstrates a crossed fused ectopia. Three ureters drain the uncrossed left kidney, and two ureters drain the crossed right kidney. *B,* Diagram of *A.* (From Friedland GW, Filly R, Goris ML, et al: Uroradiology: An Integrated Approach. New York, Churchill Livingstone, 1983, p 1642. By permission.)

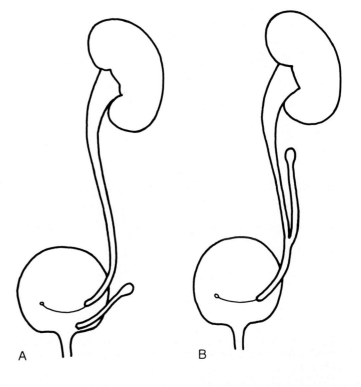

Figure 19–185. *A,* Blind-ending ureteral bud arises from the bladder. *B,* Blind-ending ureteral bud arises from the ureter.

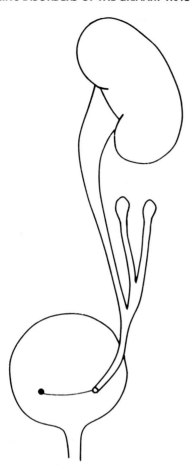

Figure 19–186. Diagram illustrates two blind-ending ureteral buds arising from a ureter.

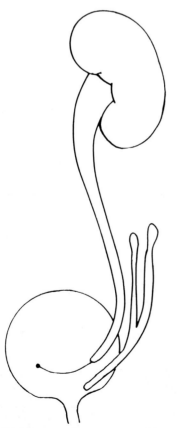

Figure 19–187. Diagram illustrates two blind-ending ureteral buds arising from a single ureter, which in turn arises from the bladder.

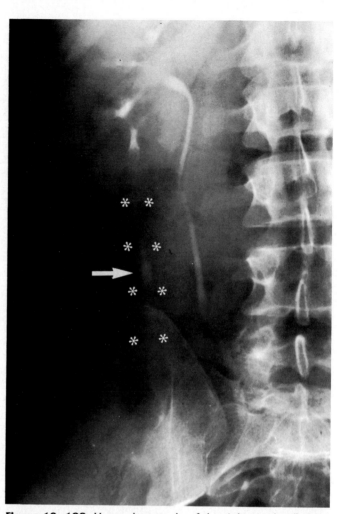

Figure 19–188. Unusual anomaly of the right renal collecting system and ureter. The intravenous urogram demonstrates a long tubular structure filling with contrast medium *(asterisks)*, originating from the lower-pole calyx and extending caudally to end blindly over the iliac bone. This ureter-like structure filled from the lower-pole calyx and contained a calculus *(arrow)*.

bous blind end, the length of which is more than twice the diameter. The structure arises from the bladder (Fig. 19–189) or joins the ureter at an acute angle (Fig. 19–190).[68–72] The blind-ending ureteral bud fills by ureterouretereal reflux, in a manner similar to that of a bifid ureter. Because it is only intermittently opacified, it may be easily overlooked, especially if it is only a few centimeters in length. An extremely long ureteral bud may extend cranially to the base of the renal pelvis or higher.

Retrograde Urography. An intravenous urogram usually adequately demonstrates a blind-ending ureteral bud, rendering retrograde ureterography unnecessary in most cases. Retrograde studies are valuable to confirm a suspected diagnosis or to definitively rule out possible intraureteral abnormalities.

Computed Tomography. A blind-ending bud can create a very confusing picture on CT scans. The cuts through the kidney will show an unduplicated system, and, as cuts are made further down, one ureter becomes visible. Suddenly, as if from nowhere, a second ureter appears.[75]

With this appearance, it is possible to take advantage of the fact that the patient has already been given contrast material and obtain an abdominal radiograph to demonstrate the blind-ending ureteral bud.

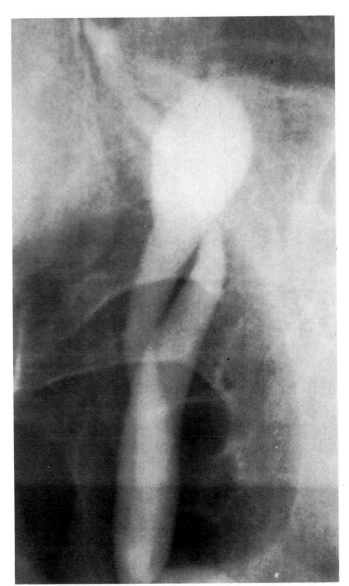

Figure 19–189. Intravenous urogram demonstrates a blind-ending ureteral bud arising from the bladder. (From Friedland GW, Filly R, Goris ML, et al: Uroradiology: An Integrated Approach. New York, Churchill Livingstone, 1983, p 1450. By permission.)

Congenital Ureteral Strictures

The normal ureter has three narrow segments: at the ureteropelvic junction, at the point where the ureters cross the common iliac arteries, and at the ureterovesical junction. Between these narrow segments, the ureter is more dilated. The normal narrow areas occur because the ureters grow more slowly at these points, whereas the more dilated areas occur because the ureters grow faster in the area in between the narrowings.

Kelly and Burnam found a circular muscular coat in the upper collecting system of the embryo that can become thickened in eight different areas (Fig. 19–191).[80] They called these "little ring" muscles. Brown later found narrowings at identical sites in the embryos of a genetic strain of mice that could develop strictures at any of these points.[81] She further found that the upper collecting system was growing more slowly at these points. If one or more of these narrow areas stop growing, and if the ureter above and below that point continues to grow, the

result is a stricture that, in this genetic strain of mice, could cause hydronephrosis. Strictures in humans can develop at these identical sites and result from failure of these areas to grow, coupled with normal growth in surrounding areas of the ureter above and below the point of nongrowth.[82–85] In addition, the arteries supplying the ureter may fail to develop, which may also cause the ureter to remain narrow.

Ureteral Valves

Ureteral valves are true valves because they obstruct the antegrade flow of fluid, causing proximal hydronephrosis, although they allow free retrograde flow.[86–89] They are composed of mucosa and muscle, but not adventitia.[86]

About 35% of ureteral valves occur at the ureteropelvic junction; 60% occur near the ureterovesical junction, and 5% occur in the upper ureter.[86] Valves are three times more common in males. They are usually unilateral, although they may be bilateral, and, if so, usually lead to renal failure. Seventy-five per cent of valves occur on the left side, 25% on the right. Some are associated with intrinsic ureteral stenosis at the site of the valve.

Two anatomical types are identified: single pleat and double pleat (Fig. 19–192).[86]

Single-pleat valves can occur at the uteropelvic junction

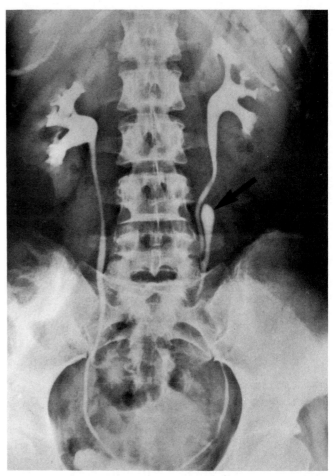

Figure 19–190. Intravenous urogram shows a blind-ending ureteral bud arising from the left ureter *(arrow).* (From Friedland GW, Filly R, Goris ML, et al: Uroradiology: An Integrated Approach. New York, Churchill Livingstone, 1983, p 1449. By permission.)

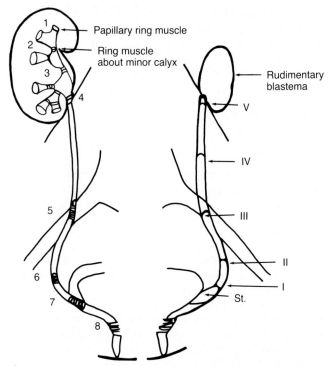

Figure 19–191. Diagram illustrates the position of Kelly's little ring muscles compared with retardation points found in ureters of mouse embryos in Brown's study of abnormal kidneys. Arabic numbers show the position of Kelly's ring muscles. Roman numerals I through V show strictures of the ureteral wall from growth retardation in Brown's genetically abnormal mice. (From Brown AL: An analysis of the developing metanephros in mouse embryos with abnormal kidneys. Am J Anat 47:117–171, 1931, p 127.)

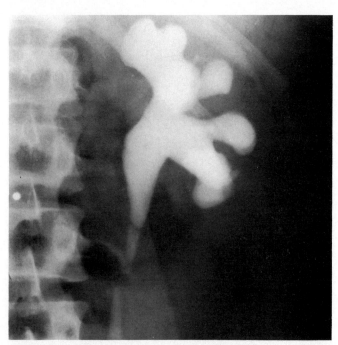

Figure 19–193. Intravenous urogram demonstrates a valve of the left ureter at the level of the transverse process of L3.

or lower, usually near the ureterovesical junction (Fig. 19–193).

A valve of the ureteropelvic junction consists of a crescentic or circular spur or pleat composed of mucosa and muscle, with an extra flap of mucosa at the top. It projects into the lumen. Under pressure from above, it acts as a flap-valve, flapping closed and occluding the ureteral orifice at the ureteropelvic junction. The ureter inserts high into the renal pelvis, and the most proximal undilated part of the ureter distal to the ureteropelvic junction lies close alongside the renal pelvis. The dilated renal pelvis presses on the proximal ureter, closing it and increasing the effectiveness of the valve.

The situation is very similar in the distal ureter, near the ureterovesical junction. There, the situation is complicated by the fact that this entire structure is surrounded by adventitia, so it is not visible at surgery and can be missed.

A *double-pleat ureteral valve* occurs in two parts (Fig. 19–194). The first part has the same anatomy described previously. In addition, the undilated ureter kinks acutely just distal to the first pleat, which acts as a second valve. The entire structure is thereby even more effective against antegrade flow. Because, as with single pleat valves, the structure is completely surrounded by adventitia, the valves themselves are invisible externally, emphasizing the crucial diagnostic role of imaging.

EMBRYOLOGY

About 20% of newborns have prominent transverse mucosal folds in their ureters.[90] These folds arise because of kinking in the underlying muscular coat of the ureter.[90–92]

At about the fourth and fifth month, in some fetuses, the muscle coat at certain locations on one side of the ureter grows more rapidly than the adventitia. The result is a kink in the ureter itself, but since the adventitia bridges the kink, the wall of the ureter appears smooth from the outside.[90–92] The mucosal folds that form as a result of this process are called Wolfler-Englisch-Östling folds, because of the work of the investigators who first described the phenomenon.[90–92]

The most common site for this kinking is just below the ureteropelvic junction, although it can occur anywhere in the ureter.

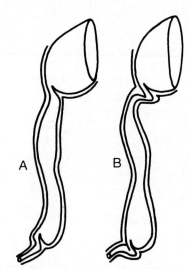

Figure 19–192. Diagrams illustrate single-pleat (A) and double-pleat (B) ureteral valves.

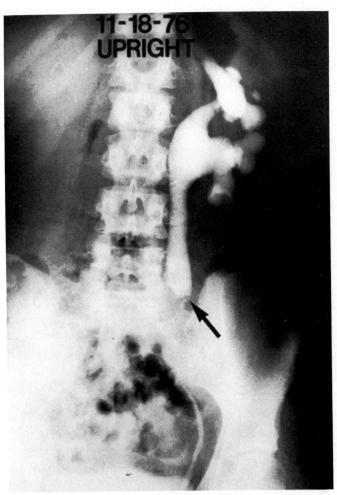

Figure 19–194. Intravenous urogram, upright film, demonstrates a valve in the left ureter at the upper margin of the sacrum *(arrow).* (From Whiting JC, Stanisic TH, Drach GW: Congenital ureteral valves: Report of two patients, including one with a solitary kidney and associated hypertension. J Urol 129:1222–1224, © 1981, The Williams & Wilkins Co., Baltimore.)

Normally, the adventitia grows very much faster again in the postnatal period, and any kinks that may be present straighten out. If the adventitia does not grow in the postnatal period, or if it grows even more slowly than the underlying muscle, these kinks may persist, become prominent, and form valves. If valves develop, they have the same histological appearance as the normal folds in the ureter.

DIAGNOSTIC IMAGING

On an intravenous urogram, hydronephrosis or hydroureteronephrosis appears above the point of obstruction (Figs. 19–193 and 19–194). The actual filling defect attributable to the valve itself is only occasionally seen at urography. Retrograde urography is almost always required.

On a retrograde urogram, it is possible to visualize the valve with appropriate oblique views. In the case of a single pleat valve, there is a sharp ledgelike filling defect at the inferior margin of the ureteropelvic or ureteroureteral orifice (Fig. 19–195). A double pleat valve displays an acute kink in the ureter just distal to the pleat representing the first valve.

The differential diagnosis includes normal mucosal folds. In infants and children, it is common to see transverse filling defects—the results of normal mucosal folds—but such cases involve no obstruction, and the folds disappear in time. Rarely, persistent fetal folds are encountered (Fig. 19–196). Kinks in a tortuous dilated ureter are a diagnostic possibility, but in this case the ureter is dilated below and above the kink, so the kink cannot be a valve. Simple ureteral stenosis must be taken into consideration.

Ureteral Diverticula

Ureteral diverticula may be true or false.

TRUE DIVERTICULA

True diverticula are usually large, containing from 5 to 3500 ml.[66, 93] They are saccular, round or oval, and usually solitary. The wall of the diverticulum contains all the

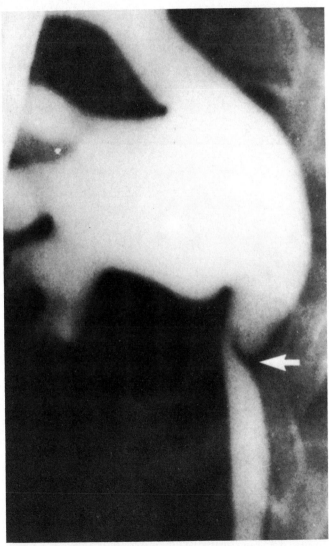

Figure 19–195. Single-pleat valve in the upper right ureter. Right retrograde pyelogram, right anterior oblique position, shows a single filling defect due to a valve in the lumen of the ureter *(white arrow).* (From Maizels M, Stephens FD: Valves of the ureter as a cause of primary obstruction of the ureter: Anatomic, embryologic, and clinical aspects. J Urol 123:742, © 1983, The Williams & Wilkins Co., Baltimore.)

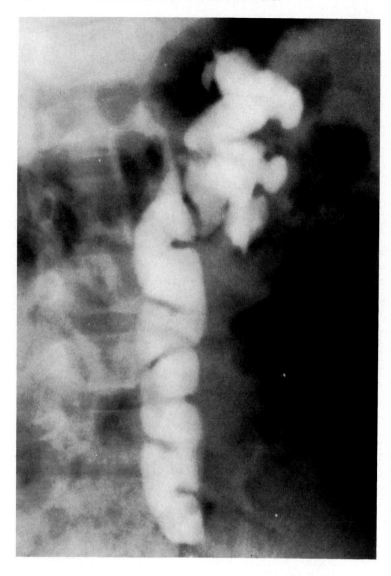

Figure 19–196. Persistent fetal folds in the ureter. During a voiding cystourethrogram, there was massive reflux into the left ureter and kidney of this 3-year-old boy. The ureter has a corkscrew appearance typical of so-called fetal Wolfler-Englisch-Östling folds. These are normal in the fetus but generally disappear before or shortly after birth.

layers of the ureteral wall, and the diverticulum communicates with the ureteral lumen through a stoma.[66, 94] If the communication is obliterated, they present as a paraureteral "cyst," rather than as a diverticulum.[95]

Diagnostic Imaging. On an intravenous urogram, the diverticulum fills slowly from the lumen. It is large and round or oval. It is easily confused with a bladder diverticulum, large ureterocele, or marked hydroureter.

A retrograde urogram is usually necessary to delineate adequately a true diverticulum.

FALSE DIVERTICULA (PSEUDODIVERTICULA)

False diverticula are small. They compress but do not penetrate the full thickness of the muscular wall of the ureter, and they are lined by hyperplastic benign epithelium.[96] They occur predominantly in older men at a mean age of 72 years.[96] The most common presenting symptom is hematuria.

The cause of false diverticula remains unknown. It is not known whether they are congenital or acquired.

False diverticula are multiple in 90% of cases ("ureteral diverticulosis").[96] They are bilateral in 75% of cases, and in 85% of cases they are located in the upper and middle third of the ureter.[96] They are discussed further in Chapter 23.

Controversy still exists as to whether false diverticula are premalignant.[96, 97] Because stasis of urine occurs in these diverticula, and an increased incidence of malignancy could result because of prolonged contact with carcinogens, the best current advice is to follow the patient carefully, clinically and using intravenous urograms.

Diagnostic Imaging. The intravenous urogram shows only about 60% of false diverticula, even with good ureteral compression.[96] Occasionally, they are best seen following release of compression, because, although the ureter has emptied, the diverticula have not. The findings usually include multiple small outpouchings of the lumen in the upper and middle third of the ureter, usually bilaterally.[96]

The retrograde urogram is the best method of proving the existence and the total number of false diverticula (Fig. 19–197). The examination reveals an additional 40% not seen on an intravenous urogram, since these diverticula usually only show up with marked distension of the ureter.[96]

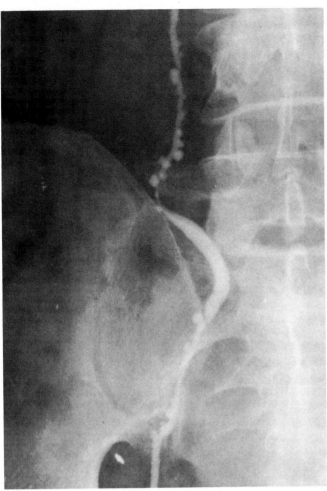

Figure 19–197. Ureteral pseudodiverticulosis. Retrograde pyelogram shows the spectrum of changes seen in ureteral pseudodiverticulosis. (From Wasserman NF, La Pointe S, Posalaky I: Ureteral pseudodiverticulosis. Radiology 155:561–566, 1985.)

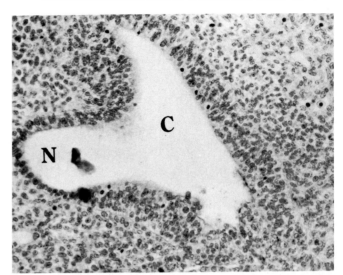

Figure 19–198. Section through an early Stage-14 embryo shows the dilated primary nephric duct (N) orifice opening into the cloaca (C). The thick epithelium is the cloacal wall, and the bottom of the photograph shows the cloacal membrane; the single-layered epithelium is part of the primary nephric duct. (From the Carnegie Collection.)

URETERAL ORIFICE

Embryology

We can arbitrarily divide the development of the distal ureter into two parts. The division is arbitrary because the process is continuous, but for clarity we can describe that process as follows.

In the first part of the development of the distal ureter, four events occur. First, the distal end of the primary nephric duct (also called the wolffian duct or the mesonephric duct) contacts the cloaca (Figs. 19–198 and 19–199) where there are two outpouchings known as the cloacal horns (Fig. 19–200). This contact is not end-to-end, but rather side-to-side, which is why the primary nephric duct extends caudally for some distance relative to the cloaca (Fig. 19–201). Subsequently, the wall between the primary nephric duct and the cloaca breaks down, and the two lumina communicate.

Second, the ureteral bud comes off the primary nephric duct; that portion of the nephric duct between the ureteral bud and the cloaca is now called the common excretory duct. The epithelium of the cloaca and the epithelium of the common excretory duct can be easily distinguished, since the latter is lined by a single layer of cylindrical epithelium, whereas the cloaca is lined with multiple layers of endodermal epithelium. Initially, the ureteral bud branches off dorsally and medially from the wolffian duct.

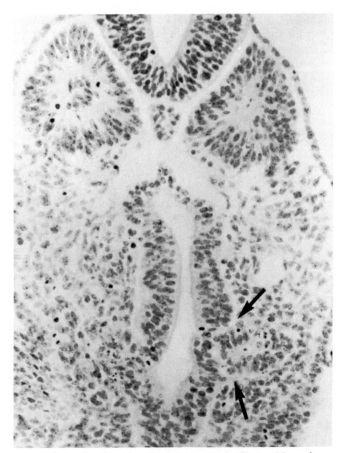

Figure 19–199. Section through an early Stage-13 embryo shows the contact of the primary nephric duct *(arrows)* with the cloacal wall prior to communication of their lumina. (From the Carnegie Collection.)

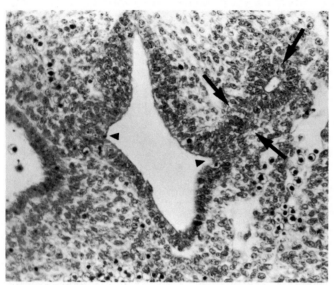

Figure 19–200. Cross section just below the junction of the hindgut with the cloaca shows the "cloacal horns" *(arrowheads)* and the adjoining primary nephric duct on the left *(arrows)*. (From the Carnegie Collection.)

Third, as the ureter grows, it rotates laterally, relative to the wolffian duct, and comes to lie dorsolateral, rather than dorsomedial, to it. This is important because (1) this rotation is simultaneous with the rotation of the kidneys, and if the ureters fail to rotate, the kidneys fail to rotate; and (2) it explains why the orifice of the ureter in the bladder is ultimately lateral to the orifice of the wolffian duct in the bladder, after the common excretory duct has disappeared.

Fourth, the common excretory duct dilates, and the epithelium of the cloaca (the epithelium of the future bladder) begins to replace the epithelium of the common excretory duct. The epithelium of the cloaca grows underneath the epithelium of the common excretory duct, as a result of which the epithelium of the common excretory duct dies and sloughs off (see Fig. 19–204).

The distal end of the common excretory duct is then taken into the cloaca by a process, regarding which two theories are offered. Figure 19–202*B* illustrates one such theory,[98] which states that where the common excretory duct enters the cloaca, the cloaca grows out and surrounds the common excretory duct. The alternate theory is illustrated in Fig. 19–202, in which the distal end of the common excretory duct slides into the cloaca. Figure 19–202*C* shows the result of either process. A nipple projects into the cloacal lumen. The nipple has a common wall that is composed of the walls of the cloaca and the common excretory duct. Subsequently, that wall sloughs off. The net result, illustrated in Figure 19–202*D*, is that the orifice of the ureter and the wolffian duct open next to one another in the cloaca. The orifice of the ureter, however, the ureter already having rotated, is lateral to the orifice of the wolffian duct.

All the sloughed epithelium associated with the processes described above (Figs. 19–203 to 19–205) can temporarily obstruct the distal end of the orifice of the ureter in the cloaca. Chwalle called this sloughed epithelium a membrane,[99] subsequently known as Chwalle's membrane.

At this point a problem arises, however. The development we have been describing occurs in Stages 12 to 14. But three earlier investigators, who also described this process, including Chwalle himself, studied either one embryo,[100] two embryos,[98] or, in Chwalle's case,[99] four embryos from this early stage. The earliest that any investigator had was late Stage 13 or early Stage 14. The processes we have described begin at late Stage 12, so that each earlier investigator, including Chwalle, was not able to accurately determine the cause of the obstruction at the ureteral orifice. It is apparent, however, that Chwalle's membrane does not exist and consists only of sloughed epithelium that temporarily obstructs the ureteral orifice.

At the beginning of the second phase of development, illustrated in Figure 19–206*A*, the orifices of the wolffian duct and the ureter separate. When the tubes of the wolffian duct and the ureter first open into the cloaca,

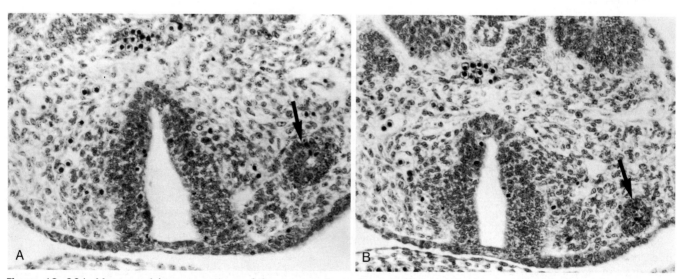

Figure 19–201. More caudal cross sections of the same embryo shown in Figure 19–199. In *A* the left primary nephric duct, after joining the cloaca, continues caudally as a lumened structure *(arrow)*. In *B*, further caudally, the terminal solid primary nephric duct *(arrow)* lies just above the ectoderm.

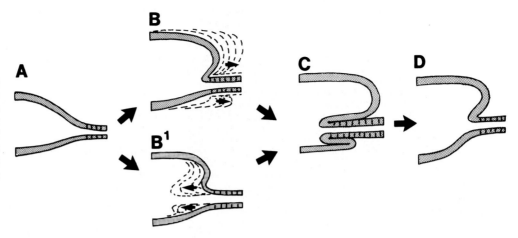

Figure 19–202. Contrasting views regarding the manner in which the primary nephric duct is incorporated into the primitive urogenital sinus. In *B*, the primary nephric duct is taken up into the advancing cavity of the bladder. B₁ is an alternative view of the primary nephric duct intussuscepting into the primitive urogenital sinus.

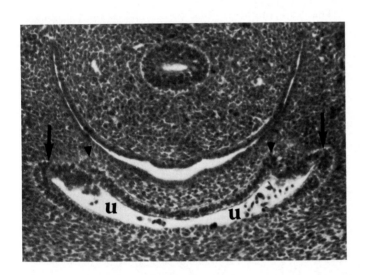

Figure 19–203. Cross section of a Stage-18 embryo, showing the more medial orifices of the primary nephric (wolffian) ducts into the urogenital sinus *(arrowheads)* and those more lateral to the ureters *(arrows)*. The epithelial cells in the lumen of the urogenital sinus (U) were sloughed from the common duct. (From the Carnegie Collection.)

Figure 19–204. Cross section of this Stage-18 embryo shows the epithelium of the urogenital sinus *(arrowhead)* growing beneath the epithelium of the primary nephric (wolffian) duct *(arrow)*, leading to the incorporation of this terminal portion into the urogenital sinus (U). (From the Carnegie Collection.)

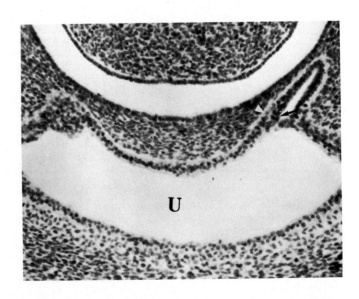

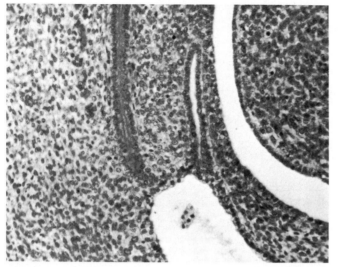

Figure 19–205. Cross section of a late Stage-18 embryo. The primary nephric duct is medial on the right. Lateral to the duct, the ureter is apparently obstructed at its junction with the urogenital sinus. Sloughed "common-duct" epithelium can be seen in the urogenital sinus. (From the Carnegie Collection.)

they are separated by mesoblast, and each tube is covered with a single layer of epithelium (Fig. 19–206A). As this mesoblast grows, however, the growth is much faster distally than proximally, so that the distal end expands caudally. This expansion causes the distal end of the wolffian duct to elongate, grow, and loop caudally as the growing mesoblast pushes it in that direction (Fig. 19–206B).

Thus, a common wall separates the looped distal end of the wolffian duct from the urogenital sinus. This wall is composed of the epithelium lining the wolffian duct,

the epithelium lining the urogenital sinus, and the mesoblast in between (Fig. 19–206B). Subsequently, the common wall breaks down (Fig. 19–206C), and the orifice of the wolffian duct, which was medial to the ureteral orifice, is now also caudal to it.

An ectopic ureter is created if the ureter is dragged caudally by a persisting association with the müllerian duct.[53]

Ectopic Ureteral Orifices

An ectopic ureteral orifice is located on the proximal lip of the bladder neck or beyond. It is ectopic, regardless of whether associated with a single ureter or with duplex, double, or triple ureters. Most of these anomalies obey the Weigert-R Meyer rule.

POSSIBLE LOCATIONS OF ECTOPIC ORIFICES

Working primarily with double ureters, Mackie and Stephens mapped out the places where ureteral orifices can insert (Figs. 19–207 and 19–208).[101]

The map comprises three zones. The first is the normal zone, in the trigone. The second is cranial and lateral to the normal zone. The last is caudal and medial to the normal zone. In 55% of renal poles the ureter opens in the normal zone; in 30% it opens in the craniozone, and in 15% it opens in the caudal zone (Fig. 19–207).

These three zones are divided into eight specific situations. The normal zone contains situations A, E, and F; situation A is in the lateral angle of the trigone, situation E is medial and inferior to A, and situation F is still more medial and inferior. The cranial zone has situations B, C, and D; B and C are cranial and lateral to the outer angle of the trigone, and D is more lateral still, outside the bladder in a diverticulum. Situations G and H are in

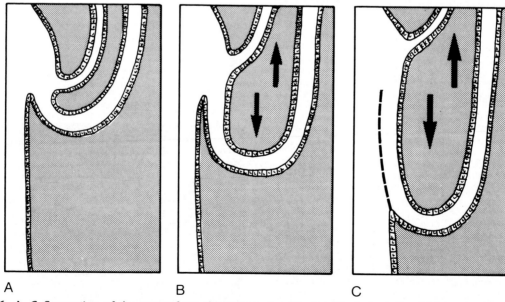

A   B   C

Figure 19–206. A–C, Separation of the ureter from the primary nephric (wolffian) duct. Cranial lateral migration of the ureter relative to the caudomedial migration of the duct is shown. Regardless of whether the ureters grow craniolaterally away from the ducts, or the ducts grow caudomedially away from the ureters, interstitial growth of the intervening mesoblast and of the duct to form a caudal loop undoubtedly has a role in this change. C, The breakdown of the threshold (*dotted line*) represents a sloughing of the epithelium during the second stage similar to that in the first-stage incorporation of the "common" nephric duct into the primitive urogenital sinus.

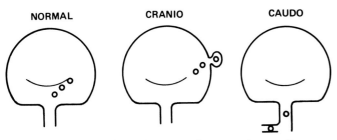

Figure 19–207. Diagram illustrates the normal zone, the craniozone, and the caudozone.

the caudal zone. In the male, G is in the upper third of the prostatic urethra and H is in the vas. In the female, G is anywhere on the posterior aspect of the urethra, or on the urethrovaginal septum. H is at Gartner's duct in the wall of the vagina, or in the hymen.

Patients with double ureters fall into two groups, those in whom both orifices lie in the normal zone (45% of cases), and those in whom one or both orifices open in one of the other zones (55% of cases). In about 25% of the latter group, the orifices open into the normal and caudal zones, respectively; 25% open in the normal and cranial zone, respectively. In 25% both orifices open in the cranial zone, and in 25% one opens in the cranial zone, the other in the caudal zone.

ASSOCIATED RENAL DYSPLASIA

The degree of renal dysplasia usually correlates with the zone where a double ureter opens. The following classification of this renal dysplasia is basically radiological:[102]

1. Alpha (α)—completely normal.
2. Beta (β)—thin parenchyma, clubbed calyces, impaired excretion, smooth or irregular outline.
3. Gamma (γ)—minimal, absent, or cystic parenchyma, irregular or invisible renal outline, poor or no excretion of contrast material on intravenous urography.

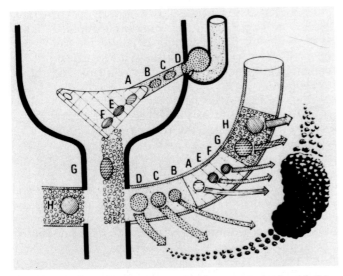

Figure 19–208. Relationships of orifice zones in the bladder and the urethra to points of origin in the ureteral bud from the wolffian duct. Bud positions relative to the nephrogenic blastema are also shown. (From Mackie GG, Stephens FD: Duplex kidneys: A correlation of renal dysplasia with position of the ureteral orifice. J Urol 114(2):274–280, © by Williams & Wilkins, 1975.)

On a voiding cystogram or retrograde urogram, the calyces appear large and clubbed and merge into one another or into the renal pelvis.

Renal poles associated with ureters opening into the normal zone are α poles in 95% of cases, and β poles in 5% of cases. All β poles have orifices in the F position bordering on the caudal zone. About 30% of ureters in this group reflux, and, where a grading system employing three grades (I, II, and III) is used, Grade I reflux is found in 25%, and Grade II reflux in 75%.

Renal poles associated with ureters opening into the cranial zone are 40% α, 55% β, and 5% γ. The ureteral orifices are usually abnormally wide, and the ureteral tunnel is short. Eighty per cent of the ureters reflux, and, where a grading system employing three grades (I, II and III) is used, Grade I is found in 70% of cases and Grade III in 30% of cases.

When renal poles are drained by ureters opening in the caudal zone, 75% of the attendant ureters have ectopic ureteroceles. Forty per cent of these poles are β poles; 60% are γ poles. No α poles have been reported. Reflux occurs in 25% of the attendant ureters.

ECTOPIC URETERAL ORIFICES ASSOCIATED WITH UNDUPLICATED URETERS

Unduplicated ectopic ureters are more common than previously recognized,[103–107] and many may have been missed.[108, 109] Kidneys associated with unduplicated ectopic ureters are usually dysplastic; the more ectopic the position of the ureteral orifice, the more dysplastic the kidney.[105] Unduplicated ectopic ureters may be associated with ureteroceles,[110, 111] posterior urethral valves,[111] and multiple congenital anomalies in other systems.[112, 113]

Unduplicated ectopic ureters most commonly present with persistent urinary infections and incontinence in females, and recurrent epididymo-orchitis in males. In either sex, they may present with an abdominal or pelvic mass due to hydronephrosis or hydroureter.[108, 114]

Because the situations are so different, unduplicated ectopic ureters in males and females are discussed separately.

Unduplicated Ectopic Ureter in the Female. An unduplicated ectopic ureter may occur on one or both sides.

Unilateral. On the side where the ureter is ectopic, the bladder neck and trigone do not develop normally. This is unlike double ureters, in which case one ureter inserts into the trigone, and the bladder neck and trigone are normally developed.[51]

A unilateral unduplicated ectopic ureter can drain one of two kidneys, a solitary kidney, or a fused kidney of any type or with any type of renal ectopia, including crossed fused ectopia. It may have an ectopic ureterocele or ureteral stenosis. These ureters most commonly open into the lower third of the urethra or into the vagina; rarely, they may open into the uterus or fallopian tubes.[143]

INTRAVENOUS UROGRAPHY. Kidneys associated with unduplicated ectopic ureters may be so dysplastic that they do not excrete contrast material at all. Those that do excrete often show marked hydronephrosis, possibly because in its ectopic pathway, the ureter is subjected to compression by the muscles and other tissues through which it passes. In the presence of poor excretion, it can be difficult or impossible to find the ureteral orifice.

VOIDING CYSTOURETHROGRAPHY. On a voiding cystourethrogram it may be possible to demonstrate an ectopic ureter rather easily, because, if it opens into the urethra, it usually refluxes.[51] The risk of mistaking it for a urethral diverticulum has been described (see Fig. 19–178). Interestingly enough, at times the urethral catheter fortuitously finds its way directly into the ectopic ureteral orifice.

RETROGRADE UROGRAPHY. Pyeloureterography by the antegrade approach is usually more expedient than retrograde studies, given the difficulty in endoscopically identifying the ectopic orifice and the fact that a dilated collecting system makes sonographically guided puncture rather straightforward.

ULTRASONOGRAPHY. An ectopic ureter is almost always dilated, and transverse sections show a dilated ureter extending posterior to the bladder base, while remaining completely separate from the bladder itself (see Fig. 19–180). Sometimes an ectopic ureter is very tortuous, so much so that on a sonogram it can look like a cystic abdominal mass with multiple septa.[137] Interestingly, the proximal parts of even severely dilated ectopic ureters are often surprisingly small.

Ectopic ureters may sometimes press on the lower wall of the bladder, simulating a ureterocele, even though none is present.

The kidney associated with an ectopic ureter can be very difficult or impossible to find, either because it is very dysplastic, or because it has been destroyed by chronic pyelonephritis. The parenchyma of these kidneys, once located, is very echogenic. There is no corticomedullary differentiation, and the kidney may have cysts, which can occasionally be huge.[137]

COMPUTED TOMOGRAPHY. The value of CT in patients with unduplicated ectopic ureters is that it can show whether or not a dysplastic kidney is present, even if the kidney is nonfunctioning; moreover, it can show the urine-filled ureter draining a nonfunctioning kidney, and may often show exactly where the ureter drains.[115, 116]

Bilateral. This congenital anomaly is much more common in females. Neither ureter opens into the bladder, and the bladder neck and trigone are poorly developed. Most commonly, the ureters open just inside the external urethral meatus; in this case, the urethra is short. A large number of variations are possible. The ureters can open higher in the urethra or at the bladder neck itself, in which case the patient has some urethra. Alternatively, they can open directly into the vagina, in which case the bladder is very ill-formed, and for all practical purposes the urethra is nonexistent. Under such circumstances, simple implantation of the ureters into the bladder may not constitute adequate treatment, because incontinence is a very real possibility, even if the urethra is present.

INTRAVENOUS UROGRAPHY. The intravenous urogram often shows poor or no excretion with bilateral hydronephrosis. Because the trigone and bladder neck are missing, the bladder base becomes funnel-shaped and the bladder neck becomes patulous. Contrast material outlines this inverted pear-shaped structure, part of which lies across the top of the symphysis pubis. Because the bladder is not used to store urine, it is small. With distal ureteral insertions it may not fill at all. When renal excretion permits, it is often possible to trace the ureters further caudally than is possible

with orthotopically inserting ureters (Fig. 19–209). When attempting to do so, the caudal projection of the normal ureter, which occurs in the prone position, must be kept in mind.

VOIDING CYSTOURETHROGRAPHY. A cystogram shows a small-capacity bladder, with a shape as described above. Reflux frequently occurs.

ULTRASONOGRAPHY. A sonogram shows a small bladder. Both ectopic ureters are dilated, and transverse sections show two dilated ureters extending posterior to the bladder.

Unduplicated Ectopic Ureters in the Male. These disorders may be either unilateral or bilateral.

Unilateral. Unduplicated ectopic ureters in the male can open into the urethra or the genital tract. When they open into the urethra, they almost always do so in its upper third, near the verumontanum.[51]

Most ectopic ureters opening into the genital tract in the male are part of an unduplicated system.[51] Rarely is an ectopic ureter opening in the genital tract in the male part of a double system.[142]

The terminal ureter dilates in a saccular fashion, most often when it opens in the urethra, although it can occur when the ureter opens into the genital tract. This is not an ectopic ureterocele because the saccular dilatation lies outside the bladder muscles. Ectopic ureteroceles, by definition, lie in the submucosa, internal to the bladder muscles.[51]

The terminal ureter can open into the common duct. It is frequently stated that the ureter can open into the seminal vesicle or the vas; the involved structure is not really either, however, but is instead a common duct for urine and ejaculate. It may be short and straight or may consist of a mass of tortuous tubules and cysts. It is often dilated with a wide orifice (which is why it is frequently mistaken for the end of a dilated ureter) opening into the urethra. When the orifice of this common chamber is stenotic, it becomes cystically dilated, producing the so-called seminal vesicle cyst. The associated kidney is usually dysplastic and ectopic.

INTRAVENOUS UROGRAPHY. Intravenous urography usually shows a single functioning hypertrophied kidney. If the patient is old enough to cooperate and can void on demand, it may be possible to achieve reflux into the common duct, demonstrating that structure and the ectopic ureter.

VOIDING CYSTOURETHROGRAPHY. Because the orifice of an ectopic ureter or the orifice of a common duct is usually wide, both usually reflux freely,[111] outlining the ectopic ureter or the duct and the ureter (Fig. 19–210).

RETROGRADE UROGRAPHY AND SEMINAL VESICULOGRAPHY. These studies are sometimes used to show the anatomy, if the other examinations are unsuccessful. When a seminal vesicle cyst is present and bulges into the bladder, it is often possible to inject contrast material into it endoscopically (or suprapubically), further defining the abnormality.

ULTRASONOGRAPHY. An ectopic ureter is almost always dilated, and will be revealed by ultrasonography to extend posterior to the bladder base, but separate from it. A seminal vesicle cyst may be identified.

COMPUTED TOMOGRAPHY. The unique attributes of CT in examining for the presence of a dysplastic kidney and a dilated ureter are described above.[115, 116] The dilated

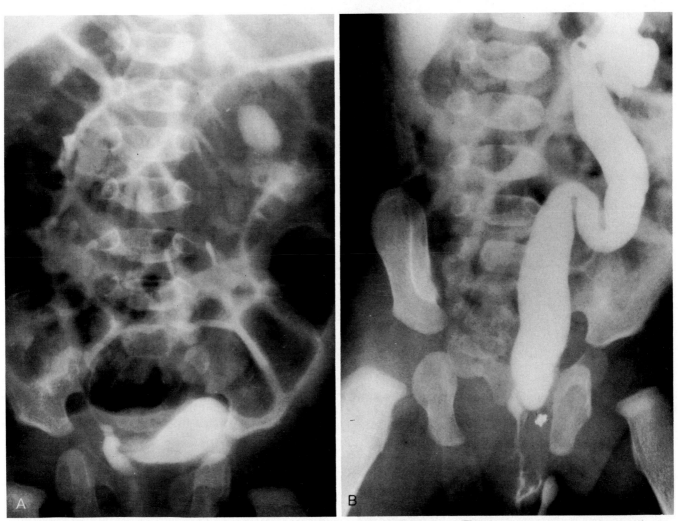

Figure 19–209. Bilateral nonduplicated ectopic ureters. *A,* Excretory urography demonstrates excretion from both kidneys. The left kidney is hydronephrotic. Contrast material fills the distal right ureter, which appears to terminate distal to the opacified urinary bladder. *B,* A left retrograde pyeloureterogram reveals that the urinary bladder does not fill as the ureter empties. This ureter emptied into the urethra.

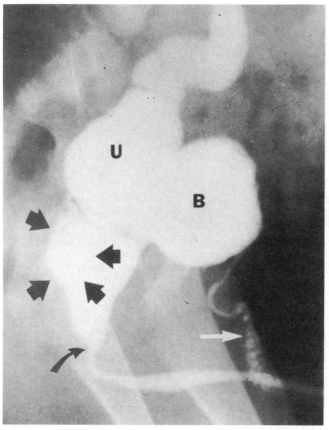

Figure 19–210. Ectopic left ureter draining into the left common excretory duct (seminal vesicle). Voiding cystourethrogram shows ectopic ureter *(black arrows)* and dilated ureter (U) above it, the bladder (B), a posterior urethral valve *(curved arrow)*, and reflux into the right vas deferens *(white arrow)*. (From Cremin BJ, Friedland GW, Kottra JJ: Ectopic ureterocele in single non-duplicated collecting system. Urology 5:154–157, 1975.)

coiled ureter can sometimes reach huge proportions in both solitary and duplicated ectopic ureters (Fig. 19–211). It can also detect an ectopic ureter draining into a seminal vesicle cyst (Fig. 19–212).

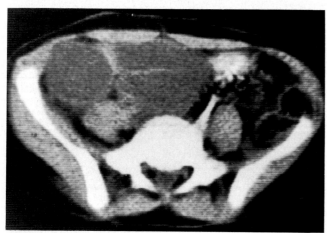

Figure 19–211. CT demonstration of a giant cystically dilated tortuous ureter. CT scan through the pelvis of a 12-year-old boy demonstrates an enormously dilated tortuous ureter occupying the right side of the pelvis. This ureter drained the upper moiety of a right duplex kidney and terminated in an ectopic location within the prostatic urethra.

Bilateral. Bilateral ectopic ureters usually open just above the verumontanum,[118] and only rarely into the genital tract. The renal dysplasia and hydronephrosis that occur are the same as in the female, as are the bladder deformities due to the absent trigone and bladder neck.[51] Male patients with bilateral and unduplicated ectopic ureters are usually not incontinent, since insertion is above the external striated sphincter, which remains unaffected.[51]

DIAGNOSTIC IMAGING. The results of an intravenous urogram, voiding cystourethrogram, and sonogram are the same as in the female.[51]

Ureteroceles

A ureterocele is a ballooning of the distal end of the ureter. Ureteroceles may occur with single or duplex ureters and may be of two types: (1) intravesical, in which the orifice of the ureter and the ureterocele itself are intravesical, and (2) ectopic, in which the ureterocele lies in the submucosa of the bladder, and some part of the ureterocele extends into the bladder neck or urethra.

EMBRYOLOGY

Most theories regarding the embryology of ureteroceles assume that the primary abnormality causing the development of the ureterocele is an abnormality of the mucosa.[130] Indeed, according to the most popular theory, ureteroceles arise because of persistence of the so-called Chwalle's membrane,[99] which temporarily obstructs the ureteral orifice. However, as discussed on page 688, it is clear that Chwalle's membrane does not exist.

Ureteroceles, especially ectopic ones, involve a defect of the muscular coat of the ureter and often a defect in the bladder wall itself. This lack of muscle in the bladder wall is called *poor detrusor backing.*

The muscle coats in the ureter and bladder wall develop from mesoblast. When the ureter and the bladder are finally formed, the muscle wall of the ureter actually forms the inner wall of the bladder at the ureteral orifice and extends downward to form the inner layer of the trigone of the bladder. Thus, the development of the ureter and the bladder are interrelated.

The mesoblast itself induces epithelium.[139] It is likely that ureteroceles result from a local defect in the development of mesoblast, which in turn leads to a defective development of muscle. Because mesoblast also induces epithelium,[139] this defect may also lead to impaired development of the mucosa at the ureteral orifice, resulting in stenosis of the orifice.

Ureteroceles are commonly associated with ectopic ureters. The reason is unknown, but ectopic ureters are possibly more likely to have defects in their mesoblast, and hence in their muscle coats, than normal ureters.

Stephens[46] has attempted to explain the embryology of an intravesical ureterocele with a wide ureteral orifice by speculating that an abnormally wide ureteral bud has led to the wide orifice. As yet, no evidence supports this assertion.

URETEROCELES ON SINGLE URETERS

These too may be intravesical or ectopic (Fig. 19–213). The term intravesical ureterocele replaces the older term,

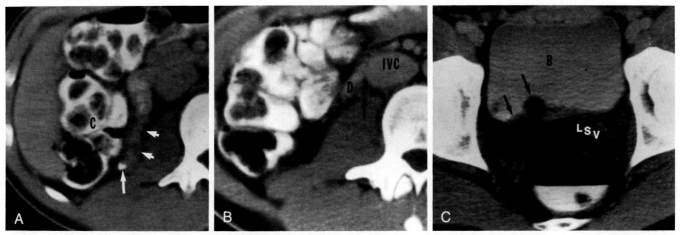

Figure 19–212. Ectopic ureter with seminal vesicle cyst. *A,* Enhanced CT scan of right renal fossa shows a small soft-tissue mass (*short arrows*) containing calcification (*long arrow*). There is no excretion of contrast material. The left kidney was hypertrophied but otherwise normal. (C = colon.) *B,* Urine-filled right ureter (*arrow*) is shown extending inferiorly from dysplastic right kidney. (D = duodenum, IVC = inferior vena cava.) *C,* Right ureter extends into right seminal vesicle, which shows mild cystic dilatations (*arrows*). (B = bladder, LSV = left seminal vesicle.) (From Schwartz ML, Kenney PJ, Bueschen AJ: Computed tomographic diagnosis of ectopic ureter with seminal vesicle cyst. Urology 31:55–56, 1988.)

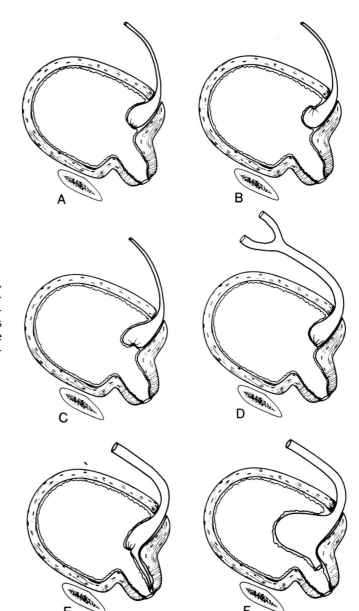

Figure 19–213. Ureteroceles on a single ureter are shown: *A,* intravesical ureterocele with stenotic orifice at its tip; *B,* intravesical ureterocele with stenotic orifice on its superior surface; *C,* intravesical ureterocele with stenotic orifice on its inferior surface; *D,* Intravesical ureterocele with stenotic orifice at its tip—bifid ureter, superiorly; *E,* cecoureterocele; *F,* sphincteric ectopic ureterocele.

simple ureterocele. The anatomy of the ectopic ureterocele itself is similar to the anatomy of that anomaly on a double ureter (see page 669). It may be associated with renal ectopia and fusion.[140] We concentrate here on the intravesical ureterocele on the end of a single ureter.

Intravesical Ureteroceles. The orifice of an intravesical ureterocele opens in the normal zone (see page 690), but is stenotic. There is usually only a slight dilatation of the lower end of the ureter above the ureterocele. The ureterocele may be unilateral or bilateral, and it occurs more often in females.

In distinction to most ureteroceles seen in children, those on single ureters are usually discovered in adults (although numerous examples have been recorded in children) and insert orthotopically, rather than ectopically. Indeed, these ureteroceles are sometimes called "adult type" ureteroceles. This is not an accurate designation, however, since ectopic ureteroceles in duplicated systems may first present late in life. In truth, any type of ureterocele can present at any age. Because one of the causes is a narrowed ureteral orifice, it is reasonable to conclude that not all ureteroceles on single ureters need be congenital. Inflammation or trauma leading to fibrosis can lead to the development of such a ureterocele. Differences between ureteroceles of single and double ureters are summarized in Table 19–23.

Complications. Most examples of intravesical ureterocele are incidental findings, but when the ureterocele is large, it may obstruct the bladder neck, or, if highly obstructive, it may cause hydronephrosis. The incidence of stones,[119] milk of calcium, and persistent infections is increased.

Diagnostic Imaging. Because kidney function is usually normal with an intravesical ureterocele, it is usually distended with urine and protrudes into the bladder lumen; on intravenous urography, the lumen of the ureterocele is usually filled with contrast material. Because the bladder is also filled with contrast material, the wall of the ureterocele is visible as a thin lucent line or halo outlining its lumen, which has the shape of a cobra head or spring onion (Figs. 19–214 to 19–216). Only very obstructive ureteroceles causing poor kidney function are not so outlined. Instead, they are visible as a lucent filling defect, although the ureterocele usually fills with contrast material on delayed films.

Stones, impacted or unimpacted, may be visible inside the ureterocele (Fig. 19–217).

An apparent thick (rather than thin) halo around the ureterocele raises the suspicion of the so-called pseu-

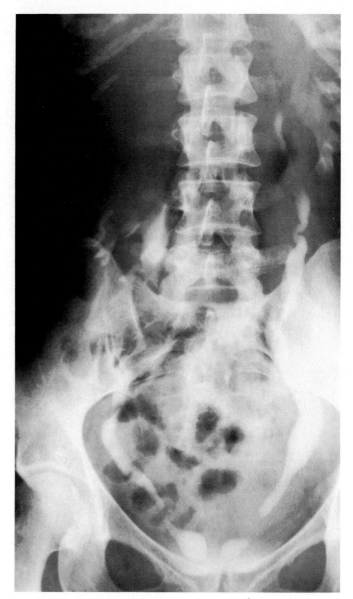

Figure 19–214. Intravenous urogram shows bilateral intravesical ureteroceles in a near-empty bladder. Note the absence of hydronephrosis.

doureterocele, a term referring to dilatation of the intramural ureter in response to contiguous disease. The possibility of nonopaque ureteral calculi, bullous edema, or even infiltrating carcinoma should be excluded when an atypical halo surrounding what appears to be a ureterocele is seen.[120–122]

On a voiding cystourethrogram, the ureterocele forms a lucent filling defect in the bladder, if it is tense. During voiding, it may intussuscept up the ureter, projecting outside the lumen of the bladder and resembling a diverticulum.

Ultrasonography may demonstrate the wall of the ureterocele projecting into the lumen of the bladder (Fig. 19–218).

URETEROCELES ON DUPLEX URETERS

Ureteroceles on duplex systems may occur in the following locations, in descending order of frequency: (1) on the ureter draining the upper pole of the kidney, (2)

Table 19–23. Differences Between Ureteroceles Occurring with Single and Double Ureters

	Single Ureter	Double Ureter
Age first detected	Adult (usually)	Childhood (usually)
Etiology	Congenital or acquired	Congenital
Ureteral insertion	Orthotopic (usually)	Ectopic (usually)
Excretion of contrast	Good	Poor to absent (upper pole usually dysplastic)
Hydronephrosis	Absent to mild (usually)	Severe
Urographic appearance (bladder)	"Halo" ("cobra-head," "spring-onion")	Lucent filling defect

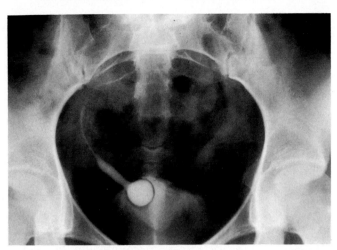

Figure 19–215. Intravesical ureterocele. Coned view of the bladder from an intravenous urogram demonstrates the typical appearance of an intravesical ureterocele on a single ureter in an adult. The dilated ureterocele protrudes into the urinary bladder but is separated from it by a thin radiolucent halo ("cobra-head" or "spring-onion" sign).

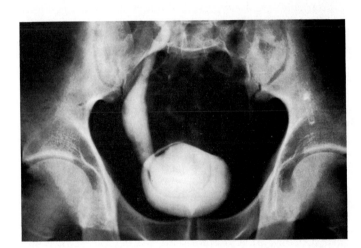

Figure 19–216. Intravenous urogram showing a large intravesical ureterocele. There is an obvious cobra-head sign. The right ureter is mildly dilated.

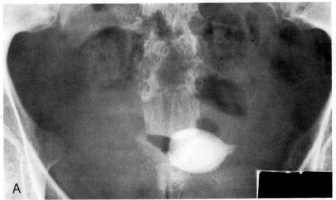

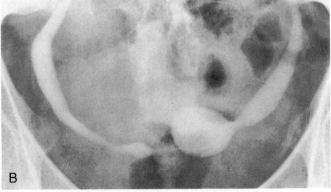

Figure 19–217. Calculus in an intravesical ureterocele. *A,* Preliminary radiograph shows a calculus in the pelvis. It has an oval shape and a spike on the left. The stone did not move with the patient in the right lateral decubitus position, indicating that it was not in the bladder, but more likely in the distal left ureter. *B,* Intravenous urogram proves that the calculus lies in a left intravesical ureterocele. There is probably a small intravesical ureterocele on the right, as well.

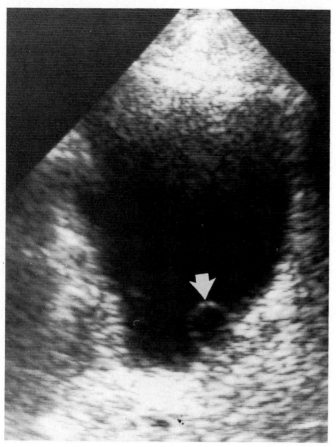

Figure 19–218. Transverse sonogram of the bladder shows an intravesical ureterocele (arrow).

at the lower end of the common stem of a bifid ureter, or (3) on a ureter draining the lower pole of the kidney.[123]

In adults, ureteroceles on duplex ureters are often incidental discoveries on an intravenous urogram or sonogram. Alternatively, an investigation of persistent infections in an adult may reveal the anomaly.[50]

In infants and children ureteroceles are more dangerous, because they are bigger and can cause more problems than those that manage to linger into adulthood.[123–127] They are the most common cause of acute bladder outlet obstruction in infant girls.[125] Over a longer time period, they may be responsible for chronic ureteral obstruction, renal back-pressure atrophy, or persistent urinary infections.[50, 126]

Females develop ureteroceles on duplex ureters seven times more frequently than do males.[126] Ninety per cent are unilateral, and 10% are bilateral.

Ureteroceles on duplex ureters are sometimes difficult to diagnose by any imaging technique currently available, since various physical mechanisms allow them to change size, shape, and position (see Fig. 19–224).[125, 127, 128–130]

Classification. Ureteroceles on duplex ureters can be stenotic, sphincteric, sphincterostenotic, blind, or nonobstructive.[123] To these categories should be added cecoureterocele[123] and pseudoectopic ureterocele.[130] The latter can mimic a true ureterocele. Stenotic and nonobstructive ureteroceles are intravesical (Fig. 19–219).[123]

Intravesical Ureteroceles (Fig. 19–220)

Stenotic ureteroceles: These account for about 40% of ureteroceles on double ureters and involve a congenitally small ureteral orifice, which obstructs the ureter. Stenotic ureteroceles on the upper-pole ureter are the most common; ureteroceles on the lower-pole ureter or on a bifid ureter are rare.

Nonobstructed ureteroceles: Nonobstructed ureteroceles on the upper-pole ureter account for about 5% of the ureteroceles on double ureters and, for reasons discussed in the section on embryology, the characteristic ballooning of the distal ureter occurs without any ureteral obstruction. The ureteral orifice is large and opens into the bladder.[123]

Ectopic Ureteroceles (Fig. 19–221)

Ectopic ureteroceles always arise on the upper-pole ureter.

Sphincteric ureteroceles account for about 40% of ureteroceles on double ureters. They are ectopic because the

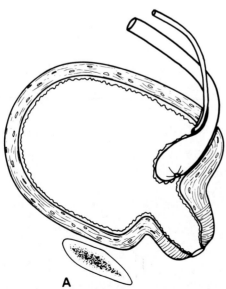
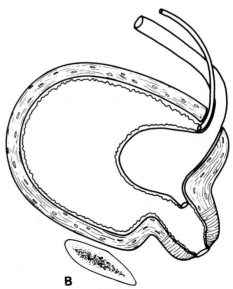

Figure 19–219. Diagram illustrating the two main types of ureteroceles on double ureters. *A,* Intravesical ureterocele on the upper-pole ureter. *B,* Ectopic ureterocele on the upper-pole ureter.

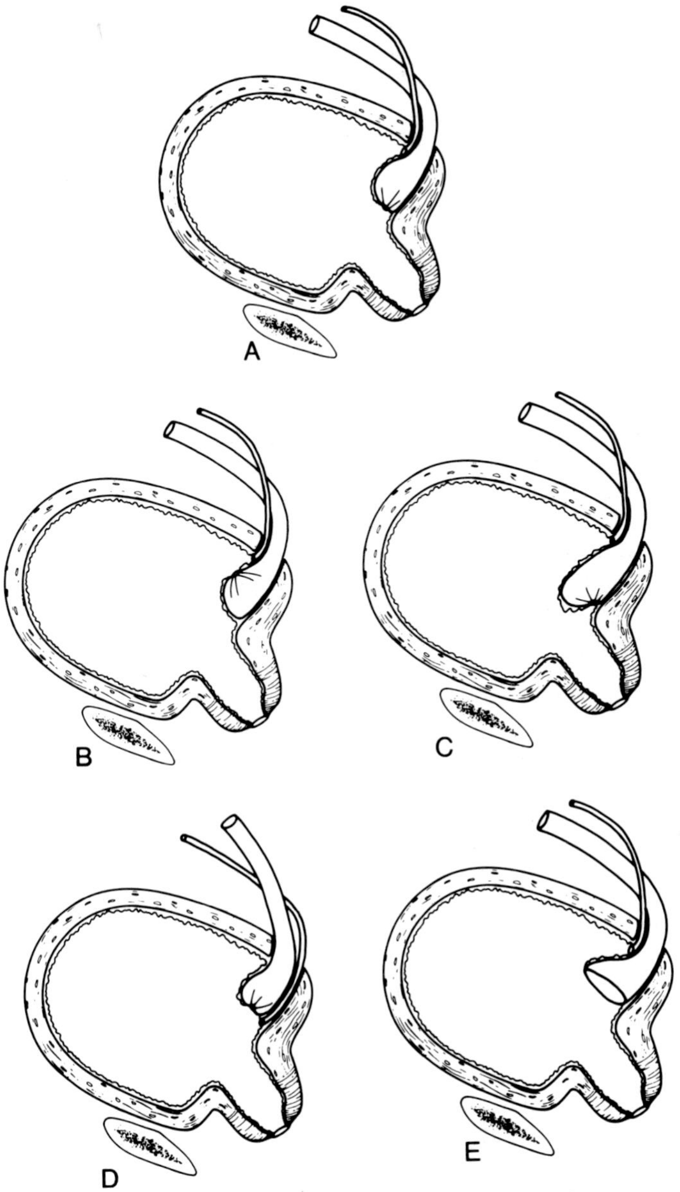

ilar to the sphincteric type, except that the ureteral orifice is stenotic.[123]

Cecoureteroceles account for about 5% of ureteroceles on double ureters. There is a large orifice opening into the bladder, but the ureterocele extends into the submucosa of the urethra as a blind pouch or cecum. When the cecum distends with urine, it may obstruct the urethra.[123, 131]

Blind ectopic ureteroceles account for about 5% of ureteroceles on double ureters and are similar to the sphincteric type, except that there is no ureteral orifice.[123]

Pseudoectopic ureteroceles are rare. They are formed by a coiled, uniformly dilated distal ureter, forming a submucosal mass at the bladder base. Because the ureter is uniformly dilated, a ureterocele "proper" cannot be said to exist, although on an intravenous urogram it can at times be indistinguishable from a true ureterocele; hence its name.[130]

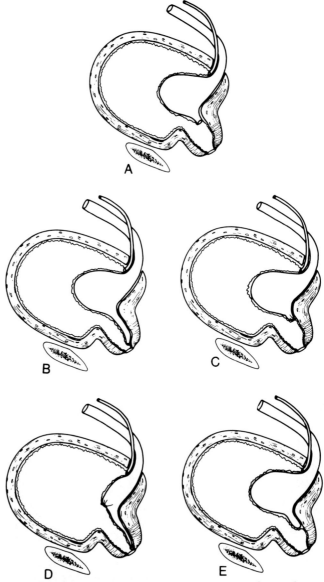

Figure 19–220. Diagram illustrates the main types of intravesical ureteroceles on double ureters: *A,* intravesical ureterocele with stenotic orifice at tip; *B,* intravesical ureterocele with stenotic orifice on superior surface; *C,* intravesical ureterocele with stenotic orifice on inferior surface—in *A, B,* and *C,* the ureterocele is on the upper-pole ureter; *D,* intravesical ureterocele with stenotic orifice on the lower-pole ureter; *E,* wide-mouthed intravesical ureterocele on upper-pole ureter.

orifice opens outside the bladder, and they extend into the bladder neck and urethra. The size of the ureteral orifice is normal or large, and in either sex it may open into the urethra proximal to the external sphincter. In females, but never in males, the ureter may also open distal to the external sphincter.

When voiding is not occurring, the bladder neck, and the external sphincter (if the ureteral opening is in the distal urethra) contract on the ureter and the ureteral orifice and obstruct them. The obstruction is caused by the normal operation of sphincters and not by ureteral meatal stenosis; hence the name.[123]

Sphincterostenotic ureteroceles account for about 5% of ureteroceles on double ureters and are anatomically sim-

Figure 19–221. Diagram illustrates the types of ectopic ureteroceles on a double ureter: *A,* sphincteric ectopic ureterocele, with orifice at bladder neck; *B,* sphincteric ectopic ureterocele, with orifice in distal urethra, in the female—the orifice never extends distal to the openings of the ejaculatory ducts in the male; *C,* sphincterostenotic ureterocele; *D,* cecoureterocele; *E,* blind-ending ectopic ureterocele.

Table 19–24. Pathophysiological Effects of an Ectopic Ureterocele

Affected Structure	Pathophysiological Effect
Upper-pole ureter bearing the ureterocele	Obstruction
	Upper-pole dysplasia
	Reflux
	Prolapse into urethra
	Persistent infection
	Calculi and milk of calcium
Ipsilateral lower-pole ureter	Obstruction
	Reflux
Contralateral ureter(s)	Obstruction
	Reflux
Bladder neck	Obstruction

FUNCTIONAL ABNORMALITIES RESULTING FROM A URETEROCELE

The pathophysiological effects of a ureterocele are listed in Table 19–24, and applies to ureteroceles in duplex systems, although similar effects can sometimes occur with other types of ureterocele.

Approximately 80% of sphincteric ureteroceles have muscle in the ureter and in the ureterocele, which may contract and empty them when the bladder neck opens. Mild cases of stenotic ureterocele may empty at any time, because they have a very hypertrophied muscular wall that can contract.

Intravenous Urogram. Three features are diagnostic of an ureterocele on a duplex ureter (Fig. 19–222). First, a mass is visible in the upper pole of the affected kidney. Second, a radiolucent filling defect is seen in the bladder.

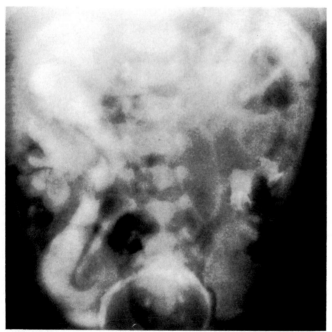

Figure 19–222. Large ectopic ureterocele arising from the upper pole on the left. Intravenous urogram shows a large round filling defect in the bladder. The lower-pole collecting system on the left has a wilting-flower appearance, and a huge mass is seen in the upper pole of the left kidney. Complete ureteral duplication is visible on the right, and the ureterocele has obstructed both right ureters, but not the lower-pole ureter on the left. (From Friedland GW, Cunningham J: The elusive ectopic ureteroceles. AJR 116:792–811, 1972, © by Am Roentgen Ray Soc.)

Third, there are changes in the rest of the urinary tract.[132, 133] Because the ureterocele constantly changes in size, shape, and position, these features are characteristic when detected, even though they may be perplexing at first.[129, 130]

The Mass in the Upper Pole of the Kidney. This mass is usually due to a hydronephrotic upper-pole collecting system surrounded by dysplastic, cystic, parenchyma. Only 10% of these systems excrete contrast material.

The Radiolucent Filling Defect in the Bladder. Little or no excretion of contrast material occurs from the hydronephrotic upper pole early in the examination. Accordingly, the ureterocele contains urine with little or no contrast material. The bladder, however, is contrast-filled, enabling the ureterocele to be visualized as a radiolucent filling defect in the bladder (Fig. 19–223).

If the ureterocele is large, the defect is spherical. If the ureterocele is smaller, however, the defect lies eccentrically in the bladder, on the same side of the bladder as the upper-pole mass, and it is oval-shaped. Because it is oriented along the axis of the upper-pole ureter, the longer axis of this oval points directly to the affected kidney.

Finally, the filling defect may appear bilobed. This can occur when there are bilateral ureteroceles or if a unilateral ureterocele has blown out in two different places.

The Remainder of the Urinary Tract. Bilateral hydronephrosis may occur, owing to bladder outlet obstruction, or to obstruction and/or reflux, which may affect the lower-pole ureter on the same side and the ureter or ureters on the opposite side (see Fig. 19–222).

Dynamic Effects (Fig. 19–224). Infants may void at any time during an intravenous urogram, and if so, the ureterocele may reflux. This causes it to assume the same radiopacity as the bladder itself, making the ureterocele difficult or impossible to visualize. If the ureterocele prolapses, it will lie in the urethra, rather than the bladder. It may become invisible. As the bladder fills during an intravenous urogram, it may compress and empty the ureterocele, rendering it invisible (Fig. 19–225), or, if the urine is opacified, it may become very radiopaque and obscure the ureterocele.

Unusual Presentations. Hydronephrosis may be absent on the lower pole on the same side, but gross hydronephrosis may exist on the opposite side (Fig. 19–222). This may occur, particularly, if the degree and extent of the ballooning is away from, rather than toward, the affected side. The ureterocele may spontaneously rupture, in which case the upper pole may atrophy. The upper pole may undergo back-pressure atrophy. Rarely hydronephrosis and hydroureter may be lacking in the upper pole ("ureterocele disproportion").[144]

Voiding Cystourethrogram. The ureterocele is best seen as a filling defect on the filling phase of the voiding cystourethrogram, with only a small amount of contrast material present in the bladder, as it is seen on an intravenous urogram. Once more contrast material is present in the bladder, the ureterocele may become obscured. When voiding begins, reflux may occur into the ureterocele itself (Fig. 19–226), the lower-pole ureter on the same side, and even the ureter or ureters on the opposite side. During this time, the ureterocele may change in size, shape, and even position (Fig. 19–226). It can contract, empty, and seem to disappear (Fig. 19–227). More confusingly, a ureterocele can invert, project

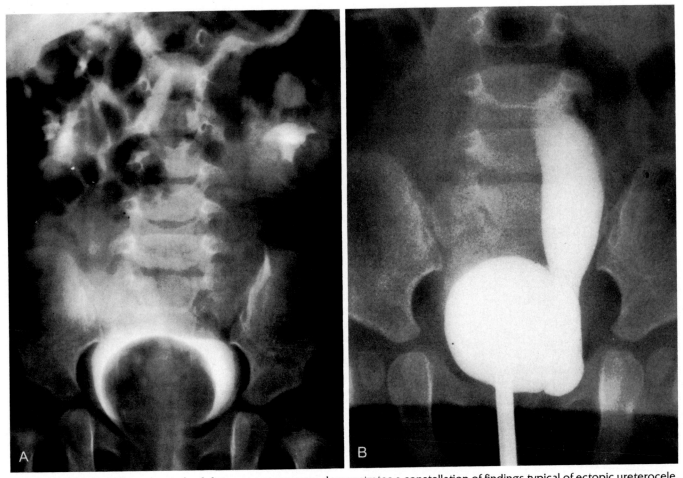

Figure 19–223. Ectopic ureterocele. *A,* Intravenous urogram demonstrates a constellation of findings typical of ectopic ureterocele. Bilateral duplex kidneys are present, but the left upper collecting system does not fill. The lower-pole system demonstrates a wilting-flower appearance. The opacified left ureter draining the lower-pole segment is displaced laterally by a dilated nonopacified ureter draining the upper pole. Both segments of the right renal collecting system appear normal. A large radiolucent filling defect within the urinary bladder represents the ureterocele draining the left upper-pole ureter. *B,* The ureterocele has been injected with contrast medium through a cystoscopic needle puncture. The large ureterocele is opacified, and contrast refluxes into the distal portion of the huge upper-pole ureter leading into it.

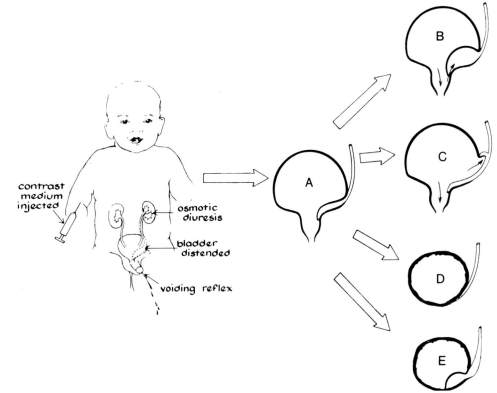

Figure 19–224. Diagram illustrates the changes in size and shape of a ureterocele that can occur during voiding: *A,* Both the ureterocele and the bladder empty; *B,* the ureterocele refluxes; *C,* the ureterocele protrudes outside the bladder, resembling a diverticulum; *D,* the ureterocele is collapsed; *E,* the ureterocele fills from above. (From Friedland GW, Cunningham J: The elusive ectopic ureteroceles. AJR 116:792–811, 1972, © by Am Roentgen Ray Soc.)

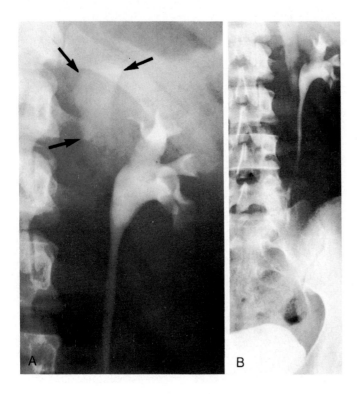

Figure 19–225. Left ectopic ureterocele, with no filling defect in the bladder. *A,* Intravenous urogram shows the lower-pole collecting system; the upper-pole collecting system is faintly visualized *(arrows). B,* A coned film taken later shows the bladder, but no filling defect within the bladder.

Figure 19–226. Voiding cystourethrogram shows reflux of contrast material into an ectopic ureterocele *(arrows).*

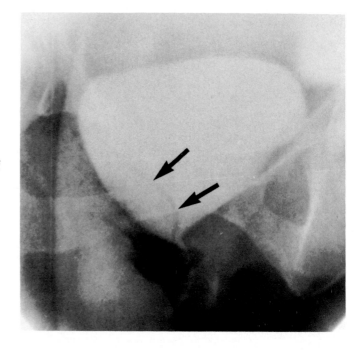

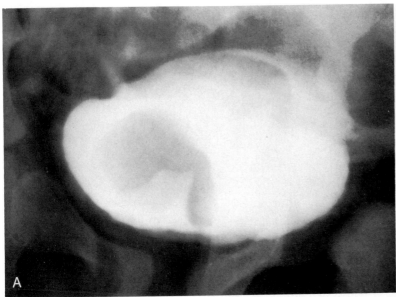

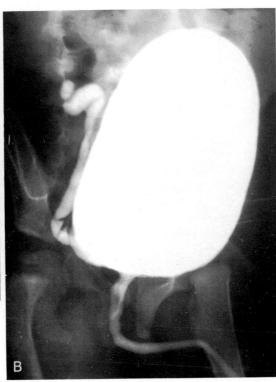

Figure 19–227. Dynamic changes in a ureterocele during voiding. *A,* Cystogram shows ectopic ureterocele on the right. *B,* During voiding, the ureterocele is invisible and reflux is occurring into the upper-pole ureter.

outside the bladder, and resemble a diverticulum (Fig. 19–228).[125, 128–130] This can occur because of a congenital defect in the muscle of the bladder behind the ureterocele, a situation commonly referred to as *poor detrusor backing.* Because the pressure in the bladder is higher during voiding than at other times, once voiding begins, increased pressure forces the ureterocele through the defect, causing it to appear outside the lumen of the bladder.

The ureterocele may intussuscept into the ureter, causing a bizarre and often confusing picture.[128]

If prolapse into the urethra occurs, the bladder neck is wide and a lucent filling defect is seen in the urethra. Alternatively, it may simply obstruct the urethra completely (Figs. 19–229 and 19–230).[133, 134]

Percutaneous Puncture. To demonstrate an ectopic ureterocele it is possible to puncture it cystoscopically or

Figure 19–228. Voiding cystourethrogram in a patient with bilateral ectopic ureteroceles. Reflux into both lower-pole collecting systems has occurred; these have a wilting-flower appearance. The ureterocele (E) protrudes outside the bladder lumen and simulates a diverticulum. (From Friedland GW, Cunningham J: The elusive ectopic ureteroceles. AJR 116:792–811, 1972, © by Am Roentgen Ray Soc.)

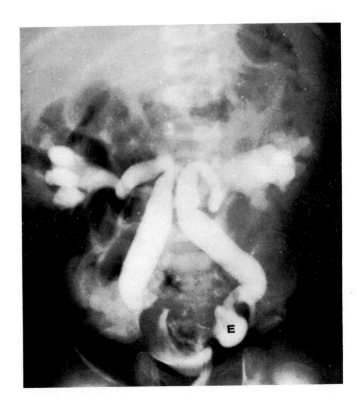

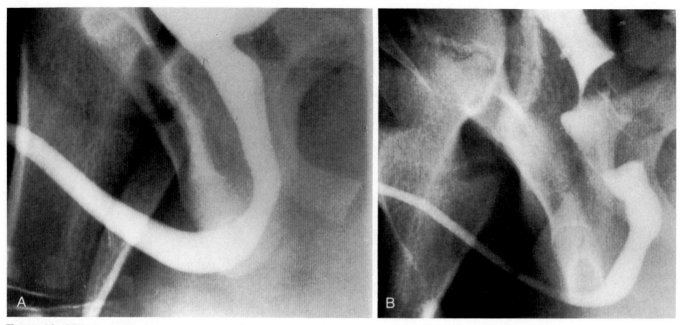

Figure 19–229. Prolapsing ectopic ureterocele. *A,* In this voiding cystourethrogram, the urethra appears normal. *B,* A prolapsing ectopic ureterocele caused sudden cessation of flow during voiding. (From Fenelon MJ, Alton DJ: Prolapsing ectopic ureteroceles in boys. Radiology 140:373–376, 1981.)

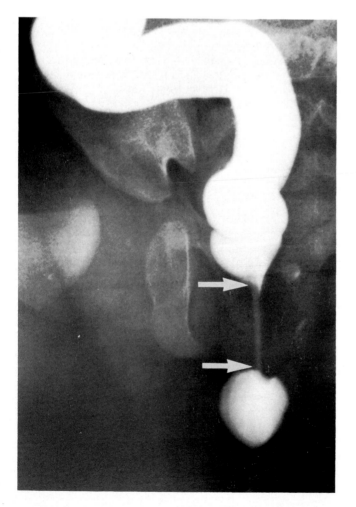

Figure 19–230. Prolapsed ectopic ureterocele presenting as an interlabial mass in a girl. The ureterocele protrudes through the urethral meatus. The ureterocele was inadvertently catheterized during a voiding cystourethrogram, and contrast material was instilled into the ureterocele and the upper-pole ureter. During voiding, the ureterocele prolapsed through the urethra. The ureterocele is very narrow within the confines of the urethra *(between arrows)* but expands as soon as it is through the urethral meatus *(below lower arrow).* (From Nussbaum AR, Lebowitz RL: Interlabial masses in little girls: Review and imaging recommendations. AJR 141(1):65–71, 1983, © by Am Roentgen Ray Soc.)

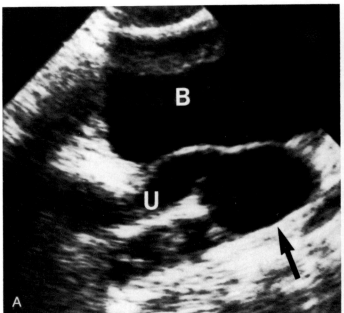
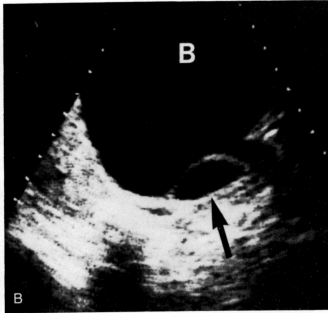

Figure 19–231. Extravesical protrusion of a ureterocele with a dysplastic kidney. *A,* Longitudinal sonogram in the pelvis shows a dilated right ureter (U) that enters a ureterocele *(arrow),* much of which lies outside the bladder (B). *B,* Repeat longitudinal sonogram with the bladder (B) less distended shows the ureterocele in its typical intravesical position *(arrow).* (From Nussbaum AR, Dorst JP, Jeffs RD, et al: Ectopic ureter and ureterocele: Their varied radiographic manifestations. Radiology 159:227–235, 1986.)

percutaneously, and then to image the ureterocele by injecting contrast material (see Fig. 19–223).[136]

Ultrasonography. There are three characteristic findings on ultrasonography of an ectopic ureterocele (Fig. 19–231):[137] (1) The presence of a fluid-filled mass in the upper pole of the kidney. (2) The dilatation of the ureter draining the upper pole on the same side. (3) A fluid-filled mass in the bladder on the same side as the fluid-filled mass in the upper pole of the kidney.

Other findings are that the patient may or may not have obstruction and hydronephrosis of the lower pole on the same side; hydronephrosis can also occur in the opposite kidney.

The same dynamic factors seen on an intravenous urogram or voiding cystourethrogram may affect the appearance of an ectopic ureterocele on ultrasonography.[137] As explained earlier, an ectopic ureterocele may be dynamic, changing significantly in size and shape (Fig. 19–231).

It can be very difficult to find the lower pole of a duplex kidney in which an ectopic ureterocele is at the end of the upper-pole ureter (Fig. 19–232). This is because the dilated ureter and dilated renal pelvis may displace the lower pole inferiorly and laterally, causing difficulty in finding the lower pole.

Many difficulties may also be encountered in the examination of the ectopic ureter bearing the ureterocele.[137] Sometimes this ureter is so tortuous that on a sonogram it may look like a cystic abdominal mass with multiple septa.[137] A similar finding may occur with an ectopic ureter without a ureterocele (Fig. 19–232B).

The sonographic differential diagnosis of ectopic ureterocele includes perivesical cyst.[137] Because an ectopic

ureterocele is usually submucosal and projects into the lumen of the bladder, the angle between the wall of the ureterocele and the wall of the bladder is generally acute. In some cases, however, a cyst may have this appearance, so the rule is not infallible. A dilated ectopic ureter must also be distinguished from a ureterocele.[137] Because a dilated ectopic ureter may indent the posterior wall of the bladder, it may resemble a ureterocele (Fig. 19–233). However, the echoes between the lumen of the bladder and the lumen of the dilated ectopic ureter are thick and irregular, whereas the echoes from an ectopic ureterocele are thin-rimmed.[137] It is also difficult, at times, to distinguish the bladder from a very dilated distal ureter. Given all these considerations, it is clear that ultrasonography alone cannot always establish the diagnosis. Additional studies are often needed.

Scintigraphy. Scintigraphic findings include delayed and decreased function of the upper pole. As the collecting system begins to fill with the radiopharmaceutical, it is shown to be hydronephrotic. The hydronephrotic upper-pole mass tilts the lower-pole collecting system inferiorly and laterally. In addition, in the earlier phases of the examination, the typical oval filling defect characteristic of an ectopic ureterocele in the bladder may be visible (Fig. 19–234).

If the lower pole of the affected kidney happens to be dysplastic and nonfunctioning, it may fill via ureteral reflux during the examination, and thereby become visible.

Computed Tomography. CT demonstrates the hydronephrotic upper pole of the kidney, and the hydronephrotic upper-pole ureter and fluid-filled mass in the bladder on the same side (Fig. 19–235).[138]

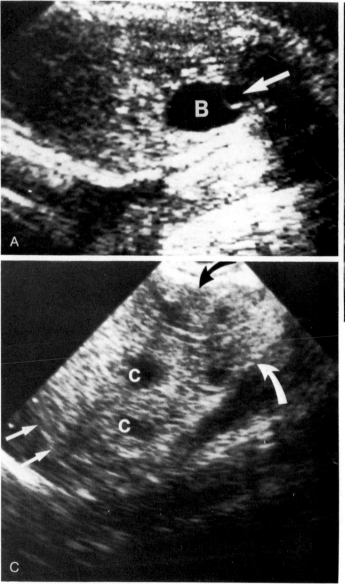

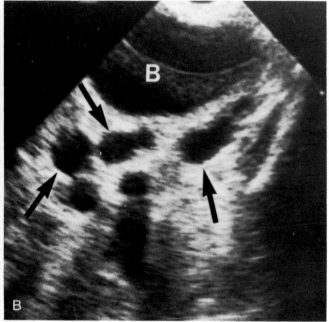

Figure 19–232. A dysplastic kidney and ureterocele detected in utero. *A,* This longitudinal sonogram was obtained at 23 weeks of gestation. A ureterocele *(arrow)* can be seen in the fetal bladder (B). *B,* Longitudinal sonogram obtained after birth. A dilated tortuous ureter *(arrows)* is present behind the bladder (B). *C,* This longitudinal sonogram was obtained after birth. The left kidney is 8 cm long, and the renal parenchyma in the lower pole is normal *(curved arrows)*. The upper-pole renal parenchyma *(straight arrows)* is highly echogenic with no corticomedullary differentiation, and it contains two small cysts (c). (From Nussbaum AR, Dorst JP, Jeffs RD, et al: Ectopic ureter and ureterocele: Their varied radiographic manifestations. Radiology 159:227–235, 1986.)

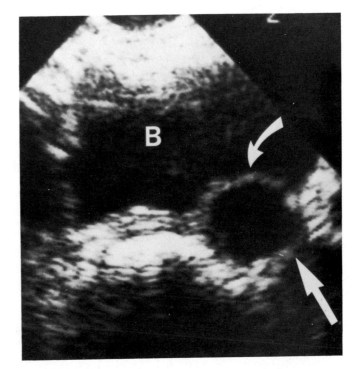

Figure 19–233. Dilated ectopic ureter that simulates a ureterocele. Transverse sonogram in the pelvis. The dilated extravesical ectopic ureter *(straight arrow)* indents the posterior wall of the bladder (B) such that it simulates a ureterocele. The interface *(curved arrow)* is thicker and more irregular than in an ectopic ureterocele. (From Nussbaum AR, Dorst JP, Jeffs RD, et al: Ectopic ureter and ureterocele: Their varied radiographic manifestations. Radiology 159:227–235, 1986.)

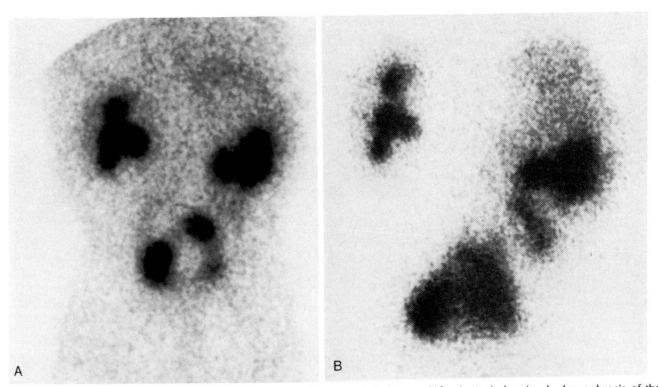

Figure 19–234. Ectopic ureterocele shown by a Tc-99m-DTPA scan. *A,* Early scan (10 minutes) showing hydronephrosis of the right upper pole. There is an oval filling defect in the bladder, delayed appearance of radioactivity in the upper pole of the right kidney, and inferior displacement of the lower pole. This combination is characteristic of ectopic ureterocele. *B,* Delayed scan (30 minutes) shows a duplicated right collecting system. (Courtesy Massoud Majd, M.D.)

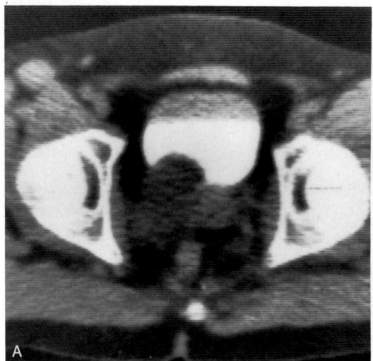

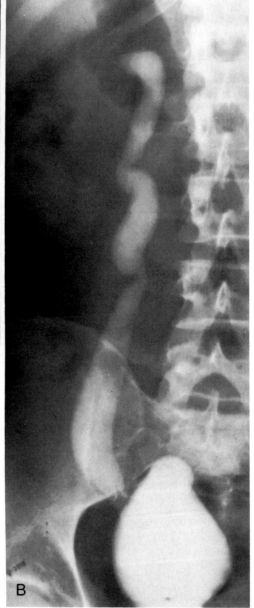

Figure 19–235. *A,* CT scan features of an ectopic ureterocele. *B,* A voiding cystourethrogram shows reflux into the right upper-pole ureter. (Courtesy Alan Davidson, M.D., Department of Radiologic Pathology, Armed Forces Institute of Pathology, Washington, D.C.)

References

1. Smith SJ, Cass AS, Aliabadi H, et al: Unipapillary kidney: A case report and literature review. Urol Radiol 6:43–47, 1984.
2. Demos TC, Malone A, Schuster GA: Unicaliceal kidney associated with posterior urethral valves. J Urol 129:1034–1035, 1983.
3. Peterson JE, Pinckney LE, Rutledge JC, Currarino G: The solitary renal calyx and papilla in human kidneys. Radiology 144:525–527, 1982.
4. Beraud C, David M, Cruaud D, Savoix C: Rein multicaliciel et syndrome de Rubinstein-Taybi. J Radiol Electrol 51:187, 1970.
5. Hanaghan J, Munro T: Megacalyces with polycalyces. J Can Assoc Radiol 32:131–132, 1981.
6. Kumar D, Cigtay OS, Klein LH: Aberrant renal papilla. Br J Radiol 50:141–142, 1977.
7. Hodson CJ, Mariani S: Large cloisons. AJR 139:327–332, 1982.
8. Siegel MJ, McAlister WH: Calyceal diverticula in children: Unusual features and complications. Radiology 131:79–82, 1979.
9. Timmons JW Jr, Malek RS, Hattery RR, et al: Caliceal diverticulum. J Urol 114:6–9, 1975.
10. Taylor WN: Urological implications of the Beckwith-Wiedemann syndrome. J Urol 125:439–441, 1981.
11. Amar AD: The clinical significance of renal caliceal diverticulum in children: Relation to vesicoureteral reflux. J Urol 113:255–257, 1975.
12. Johnson DE: Calyceal diverticulum: Report of 31 cases with reference to associated anomalies. South Med J 62:220, 1969.
13. Stamey TA: Pathogenesis and Treatment of Urinary Tract Infections. Baltimore, Williams & Wilkins, 1980, pp 524–531.
14. Middleton AW Jr, Pfister RC: Stone-containing pyelocaliceal diverticulum: Embryogenic, anatomic, radiologic, and clinical characteristics. J Urol 111:2–6, 1974.
15. Berg RA: Milk of calcium renal disease. Report of cases and review of the literature. AJR 101:708–713, 1967.
16. Rosenberg MA: Milk of calcium in a renal caliceal diverticulum: Case report and review of literature. AJR 101:714–718, 1967.
17. Nicholas JL: An unusual complication of calyceal diverticulum. Br J Urol 47:370, 1975.
18. Conrad M, Newton J, Harkins J: Growing caliceal diverticular defect. Urol Radiol 9:194–196, 1987.
19. Ulreich S, Lund DA, Jacobson JJ: Spontaneous rupture of a calyceal diverticulum during urography. AJR 131:337–338, 1978.
20. Glassberg KI, Braren V, Duckett JW, et al: Suggested terminology for duplex systems, ectopic ureters and ureteroceles. J Urol 132:1153–1154, 1984.
21. Hartman GW, Hodson CJ: Duplex kidney and related anomalies. Clin Radiol 20:387–400, 1969.
22. Atwell JD: Familial pelviureteric junction hydronephrosis and its association with a duplex pelvicaliceal system and vesicoureteral reflux. A family study. Br J Urol 57:365–369, 1985.
23. Aaronson IA: Upper moiety pelviureteric obstruction in infant with Turner syndrome. Urology 27:158–159, 1986.
24. Cronin JJ, Amis ES, Dorfman GS: Obstruction of the upper-pole moiety in renal duplication in adults: CT evaluation. Radiology 161:17–21, 1986.
25. Daw E, Toon P: Identical twins with uterus didelphys and duplex kidneys. Postgrad Med J 61:269–270, 1985.
26. Schaffer RM, Shih GH, Becker JA: Sonographic identification of collecting system duplications. J Clin Ultrasound 11:309–312, 1983.
27. Horgan JG, Rosenfield NS, Weiss RM, Rosenfield AT: Is renal ultrasound a reliable indicator of a nonobstructed duplication anomaly? Pediatr Radiol 14:388–391, 1984.
28. Jeffrey B, Laing FC, Wing VW, Hoddick W: Sonography of the fetal duplex kidney. Radiology 153:123–124, 1984.
29. Majd M: Nuclear medicine. In Kelalis PP, King LR, Belman AB (eds): Clinical Pediatric Urology. Philadelphia, WB Saunders Company, 1985, pp 145–148.
30. Wu F, Snow B, Taylor A Jr: Potential pitfall of DMSA scintigraphy in patients with ureteral duplication. J Nucl Med 27:1154–1156, 1986.
31. Hulnick DH, Bosniak MA: Faceless kidney: CT sign of renal duplicity. J Comput Assist Tomgr 10:771–772, 1986.
32. Curtis JA, Pollack HM: Renal duplication with a diminutive lower pole: The Nubbin sign. Radiology 131:327–331, 1979.
33. Privett JTJ, Jeans WD, Roylance J: The incidence and importance of renal duplication. Clin Radiol 27:521–530, 1976.
34. Blair D, Rigsby C, Rosenfield AT: The nubbin sign on computed tomography and sonography. Urol Radiol 9:149–151, 1987.
35. Broeker BH, Perlmutter AD: Segmental hydronephrosis with a bifid intrarenal pelvis. J Urol 127:754–755, 1982.
36. Takahashi K, Miura M, Horiuchi S: Bifid pelvis with a blind ending: A case report. J Urol 118:97–98, 1977.
37. Carris CK, Duikhuizen RF: Yo-yo renal pelvis: An unusual cause of flank pain. J Urol 117:153–155, 1977.
38. Lenaghan D: Bifid ureters in children: An anatomical, physiological, and clinical study. J Urol 87:808–817, 1962.
39. Kaplan N, Elkin M: Bifid renal pelves and ureters: Radiographic and cinefluorographic observations. Br J Urol 40:235–244, 1968.
40. Inamoto K, Tanaka S, Takemura K, Ikoma F: Duplication of the renal pelvis and ureter: Associated anomalies and pathologic conditions. Radiat Med 1:55–64, 1983.
41. Sole GM, Randall J, Arkell DG: Ureteropyelostomy: A simple and effective treatment for symptomatic ureteroureteric reflux. Br J Urol 60:325–328, 1987.
42. Bingham BJ: Duplicate segment within a single ureter. J Urol 135:1234, 1986.
43. Klauber GT, Reid EC: Inverted Y reduplication of the ureter. J Urol 107:362, 1972.
44. Mosli HA, Schillinger JF, Futter N: Inverted Y duplication of the ureter. J Urol 135:126–127, 1986.
45. Beasley SW, Kelly JH: The inverted Y duplication of the ureter in association with ureterocele and bladder diverticulum. J Urol 136:899–900, 1986.
46. Stephens FD: Caecoureterocele and concepts on embryology and etiology of ureteroceles. Aust NZ J Surg 40:239–248, 1971.
47. Meyer R: Normal and abnormal development of ureter in human embryo: Mechanistic considerations. Anat Rec 96:355–371, 1946.
48. Mackie GG, Stephens FD: Duplex kidneys: A correlation of renal dysplasia with position of the ureteric orifice. Birth Defects 13:313–321, 1977.
49. Ahmed S, Pope R: Uncrossed complete ureteral duplication with upper system reflux. J Urol 135:128–129, 1986.
50. Stamey TA: Urinary tract infections: Radiologic aspects of patients at serious risk. In Friedland GW, Filly R, Goris ML, et al (eds): Uroradiology: An Integrated Approach. New York, Churchill Livingstone, 1983, pp 461–464.
51. Williams DI: Urology in Childhood. New York, Springer, 1974, pp 139–145, 195–212.
52. Siegel A, Snyder H, Duckett JW: Epididymitis in infants and boys: Underlying urogenital anomalies and efficacy of imaging modalities. J Urol 138:1100–1103, 1987.
53. Stephens FD: Congenital malformations of the urinary tract. New York, Praeger, 1983, pp 294–295, 350–368.
54. Atwell JD, Cook PL, Howell CJ, et al: Familial incidence of bifid and double ureters. Arch Dis Child 49:390–393, 1974.
55. Phillips DIW, Divall JM, Maskell RM, Barker DJP: A geographic focus of duplex ureter. Br J Urol 60:329–331, 1987.
56. Dunbar JS, Nogrady MB: Calyceal crescent: Roentgenographic sign of obstructive hydronephrosis. AJR 110:520–528, 1970.
57. Lundin E, Riggs W: Upper urinary tract duplication associated with ectopic ureterocele in childhood and infancy. Acta Radiol (Diagn) 7:13–24, 1968.
58. Friedland GW, Filly R: Demonstration of vestibular implantation of ectopic ureter on an excretory urogram. Pediatr Radiol 2:137–138, 1974.
59. Patel NP, Lavengood RW Jr: Triplicate ureter. Urology 5:242–243, 1975.
60. Patel NP, Lavengood RW Jr: Triplicate duplicate ureters. Br J Urol 54:436, 1982.
61. Logo CM, Casselas JG, Gonzales FC, et al: Ureteral triplication and duplicated opposite kidney with refluxing ureterocele. J Ped Surg 18:614–616, 1983.
62. Perkins PJ, Kroovand RL, Evans AT: Triplication of ureter: A case report. Radiology 108:533, 1973.
63. Bloom RA, Crooks KK, Wise HA II: Complete ureteral triplication with ectopia. Urology 25:176–178, 1985.
64. Smith I: Triplicate ureter. Br J Surg 34:182, 1946.
65. Sonderdah DW, Shiraki IW, Schamber DT: Bilateral ureteral quadruplication. J Urol 116:255–256, 1976.
66. Culp OS: Ureteral diverticulum: Classification of the literature and report of an authentic case. J Urol 58:309–326, 1947.
67. Dolan LM, Alford BA, Bray ST, et al: Crossed fused ectopia with a blind left ureter in a young woman with Turner's syndrome: Sonographic and radiological demonstration of a previously undescribed variant. J Urol 132:1175–1176, 1984.
68. Finder CA, Love L, Rich JI: Blind ending ureters—clinical significance? Urol Radiol 4:235–238, 1984.

69. Marshall FF, McLoughlin MG: Long blind-ending ureteral duplications. J Urol 120:626–628, 1978.
70. Peterson LJ, Grimes JH, Weinerth JL, Glenn JF: Blind-ending branches of bifid ureter. Urology 5:191–195, 1975.
71. de Filippi G, dal Fosno S, Bianchi M: Blind ureteric buds. Pediatr Radiol 5:160–163, 1977.
72. Nishimura T, Akimoto M, Kawai H: Long blind-ending bifid ureter. Br J Urol 55:578–579, 1983.
73. Muraro GB, Pecori M, Biusti G, Masini CG: Blind-ending branch of bifid ureter: Report of seven cases. Urol Radiol 7:12–15, 1985.
74. Muller SC, Riedmiller H, Walz PH, Hohenfellner R: Blind-ending bifid ureter with an intravesical ectopic orifice. Eur Urol 10:416–419, 1984.
75. Rubenstein DJ, Brenner RJ: Misleading features of blind-ending bifid ureter on computerized tomography examination. J Urol 134:342–343, 1985.
76. Coughlan JD: Blind-ending branch of a trifid ureter. Urol Radiol 7:172–173, 1985.
77. Hawas N, Noah M, Pattel PJ: Blind-ending bifid ureter—clinical significance? An analysis of 13 cases with review of literature. Eur Urol 13:39–43, 1987.
78. Keane TE, Fitzgerald RJ: Blind-ending duplex ureter. Br J Urol 60:275, 1987.
79. Aragona F, Glazel GP, Zacchello G, Andreetta B: Familial occurrence of blind-ending bifid and duplicated ureters. Inst Urol Nephrol 19:137–139, 1987.
80. Kelly HA, Burnam CF: Diseases of the kidneys, ureters, and bladder, Vol 1. New York, Appleton and Company, 1914.
81. Brown AL: An analysis of the developing metanephros in mouse embryos with abnormal kidneys. Am J Anat 47:117–171, 1931.
82. Bazy P: Contribution a la pathogenie de l'hydronephrose intermittente; bassinets et ureterls des nouveauz-ns. Rev de chir 27:1–27, 1903.
83. Kermauner F: Fehlbildungen der weiblichen Geschlechtsergane, des Harn-apparates und der Kloake. In Halban J, Seitz L (eds): Biologie und pathologie des weibes, Vol III, Berlin, Urban and Schwarzenberg, 1924, pp 282–620.
84. Hellstrom J: Zur Kenntnis der isolierten dilatation des pelvinen oder juxtavesikalen harnleitenabschnittes. Acta Radiol 18:141–156, 1937.
85. Ayyat F, Adams G: Congenital midureteral strictures. Urology 26:170–172, 1985.
86. Maizels M, Stephens FD: Valves of the ureter as a cause of primary obstruction of the ureter: Anatomic, embryologic and clinical aspects. J Urol 123:742, 1980.
87. Sant GR, Barbalias GA, Klauber GT: Congenital ureteral valves—an abnormality of ureteral embryogenesis? J Urol 133:427–431, 1985.
88. Reinberg Y, Aliabadi H, Johnson P, Gonzalez R: Congenital ureteral valves in children: Case report and review of the literature. J Pediatr Surg 22:379–381, 1987.
89. Whiting JC, Stanisic TH, Drach GW: Congenital ureteral valves: Report of two patients, including one with a solitary kidney and associated hypertension. J Urol 129:1222–1224, 1983.
90. Wolfler A: Neue Beitrage zur chirurgischen. Pathologie der Nieren. Arch Klin Chir 21:694–723, 1877.
91. Englisch J: Uber primare hydronephrose. Deutsche Zeischr Chir 11:252, 1879.
92. Ostling K: The genesis of hydronephrosis particularly with regard to the changes at the ureteropelvic junction. Acta Chir Scand 86 (Suppl) 72:1–122, 1942.
93. Richardson EH: Diverticulum of the ureter: A collective review with a report of a unique example. J Urol 47:535–570, 1942.
94. Gettel RR, Lee F, Ratliff RK: Ureteral diverticula. J Urol 108:392–395, 1972.
95. Orr PS, McGregor CGA: Congenital ureteric cyst—rare anomaly. Urology 12:699–700, 1978.
96. Wasserman NF, La Pointe S, Posalaky LP: Ureteral pseudodiverticulosis. Radiology 155:561–566, 1985.
97. Kenny PJ, Wasserman NF: Ureteral pseudodiverticulosis associated with carcinoma of renal pelvis. Urol Radiol 9:161–163, 1987.
98. Frazer JE: The terminal part of the wolffian duct. J Anat 69:455–468, 1935.
99. Chwalle R: Uber die Entwicklkung der Harnblase und der primaren Harnrohre des Menschen mit besonderer Berviksichtigung der Art und Weiss, in der sich die Uniteren von den Urnierengangen trenen, nebst Bemerkungen uber die Entwicklung der Mullerschen Gange und des Mastdarms. Zeitschr Anat Entwickl Gesch 83:615–733, 1927.
100. Gyllensten L: Contributions to the embryology of the urinary bladder. Acta Anat 7:305–344, 1949.
101. Mackie GG, Stephens FD: Duplex kidneys: A correlation of renal dysplasia with position of ureteral orifice. J Urol 114:274, 1975.
102. Mackie GG, Awang H, Stephens FD: The ureteric orifice: The embryologic key to radiologic status of duplex kidneys. J Pediatr Surg 10:473, 1975.
103. Gotoh T, Marita H, Tokunaka S, et al: Single ectopic ureter. J Urol 129:271–274, 1983.
104. Kesavan P, Ramakrishnan MS, Fowler R: Ectopia in unduplicated ureters in children. Br J Urol 49:481–493, 1977.
105. Scott JES: The single ectopic ureter and the dysplastic kidney. Br J Urol 53:300–305, 1981.
106. Sorenson CW Jr, Middleton AW Jr: The single ectopic ureter: Three case reports. J Urol 129:132–134, 1983.
107. Weiss JP, Duckett JW, Snyder HM: Single unilateral vaginal ectopic ureter: Is it really a rarity? J Urol 132:1177–1179, 1984.
108. Prewitt LH Jr, Lebowitz RL: The single ectopic ureter. AJR 127:941–948, 1976.
109. Persky L, Noseworthy J: Adult ureteral ectopia. J Urol 116:156–160, 1976.
110. Blacklock ARE, Shaw RE, Geddes JR: Late presentation of ectopic ureter. Br J Urol 54:106–110, 1982.
111. Cremin BJ, Friedland GW, Kottra JJ: Ectopic ureterocele in a single nonduplicated collecting system: Diagnosis by radiography. Urology 5:154–157, 1975.
112. Sotolongo JR Jr, Rose J, Strauss L, Gribetz M: Single vaginal ectopic ureter and the VATER syndrome. J Urol 127:1181–1182, 1982.
113. Cobb LM, Panagiotou E, Bowen A, Price SE: Ectopic ureter with seminal vesicle insertion in an infant with tracheoesophageal fistula and possible adult polycystic kidney disease. J Urol 129:1038–1039, 1983.
114. Finan BF, Mollitt DL, Golladay ES, Redman JF: Giant ectopic ureter presenting as abdominal mass in infant. Urology 30:246–247, 1987.
115. Utsunomiya M, Itoh H, Yoshioka T, et al: Renal dysplasia with a single vaginal ectopic ureter: The role of the computerized tomography. J Urol 132:98–100, 1984.
116. Korogi Y, Takahashi M, Fujimura N, et al: Computed tomography demonstration of renal dysplasia with a vaginal ectopic ureter. J Comput Assist Tomogr 10:273–275, 1986.
117. Schwartz ML, Kenney PJ, Bueschen AJ: Computed tomographic diagnosis of ectopic ureter with seminal vesicle cyst. Urology 31:55–56, 1988.
118. Glasser J, Lefleur R, Subramanyam B, Al-Askari S: Ectopic duplicated ureter opening into ipsilateral vas deferens. Urology 23:309–312, 1984.
119. Golomb J, Korazak D, Lindner A: Giant obstructing calculus in the distal ureter secondary to obstruction by a ureterocele. Urol Radiol 9:168–170, 1987.
120. Thornbury JR, Silver TM, Vinson RK: Ureteroceles versus pseudoureteroceles in adults. Radiology 122:81–84, 1977.
121. Mitty HA, Schapira HE: Ureterocele and pseudoureterocele: Cobra versus cancer. J Urol 117:557–561, 1977.
122. Gordon NSI: The cobra raises its head—transitional cell tumor progressing as acquired ureterocele. Br J Urol 60:271–278, 1987.
123. Stephens FD: Caecoureterocele and concepts on embryology and aetiology of ureteroceles. Austr NZ J Surg 40:239–248, 1971.
124. Ericsson NO: Ectopic ureterocele in infants and children: Clinical study. Acta Chir Scand (Suppl) 197:5–92, 1954.
125. Williams DI, Fay R, Lillie JG: The functional radiology of ectopic ureterocele. Br J Urol 44:417–433, 1972.
126. Williams DI: Urology in childhood. New York, Springer Verlag, 1974, pp 146–161.
127. Thornbury JR: Roentgen diagnosis of ureterocele in children. AJR 90:15–25, 1963.
128. Cremin BJ, Funston MR, Aaronson LA: The intraureteric diverticulum. A manifestation of ureterocele intussusception. Pediatr Radiol 6:92, 1977.
129. Koyanagi T, Hisajimas, Goto T, et al: Everting ureteroceles: Radiographic and endoscopic observation and surgical management. J Urol 123:538, 1980.
130. Friedland GW, Cunningham J: The elusive ectopic ureteroceles. AJR 116:792–811, 1972.
131. Shappley NP, Keeton JE: Unusual presentation of cecoureterocele. Urology 6:605, 1975.
132. Berdon WE, Baker DH, Becker JA, Uson AC: Ectopic ureterocele. Radiol Clin North Am 6:205–214, 1968.

133. Churchill BM, Abara EO, McLorie GA: Ureteral duplication, ectopy and ureteroceles. Pediatr Clin North Am 34:1273–1289, 1987.
134. Nussbaum AA, Lebowitz RL: Interlabial masses in little girls: Review and imaging recommendations. AJR 141:65–71, 1983.
135. Fenelon MJ, Alton DJ: Prolapsing ectopic ureteroceles in boys. Radiology 140:373–376, 1981.
136. Diament MJ, Stanley P: Two unusual duplication anomalies of the upper urinary tract: Use of percutaneous urography. Urol Radiol 9:185–187, 1987.
137. Nussbaum AR, Dort JP, Jeffs RD, et al: Ectopic ureter and ureterocele: Their varied radiographic manifestations. Radiology 159:227–235, 1986.
138. Hinman CG, Older RA, Cleeve DM, et al: Computerized tomographic diagnosis of massive hydronephrosis of duplicated system in an adult. Urology 12:92, 1978.

139. Cunha GR: Epithelial–stromal interactions in the development of the urogenital tract. Int Rev Cytol 47:137–194, 1976.
140. Pak K, Konishi T, Tomoyoshi T: Noncrossed renal ectopia with fusion associated with single ectopic ureterocele. Urology 32:246–249, 1988.
141. Tilley EA, Dow CJ: Cranial blind-ending branch of a bifid ureter. Report of 3 cases. Br J Urol 62:127–130, 1988.
142. Brown DM, Peterson NR, Schultz RE: Ureteral duplication with lower pole ectopia to the epididymis. J Urol 140:139–142, 1988.
143. Fisk NB, Bayliss A: Hysterosalpingographic diagnosis of a single cervical ectopic ureter. Obstet Gynecol 71:1041–1043, 1988.
144. Share JC, Lebowitz RL: Ectopic ureterocele without ureteral and calyceal dilatation (ureterocele disproportion): Findings on urography and sonography. AJR 152:567–571, 1989.

CONGENITAL ANOMALIES OF THE URACHUS AND BLADDER

CLASSIFICATION OF CONGENITAL ANOMALIES OF THE URACHUS AND BLADDER

Table 19–25 shows the classification of the major congenital anomalies of the urachus and bladder.

URACHUS

Embryology

In Stage 13, a diverticulum grows out of the cloaca in a cranioventral direction (Fig. 19–236). This structure is called the urachus.[1-5] The cranioventral end of the urachus opens into the allantois at the level of the umbilicus;[6-8] thus, initially, the bladder extends all the way to the umbilicus.

In late embryonic, fetal, and early postnatal life, the urachal portion, which is still microscopic, fails to grow; therefore, its lumen remains narrow. It may even be visible in adults as a microscopic structure. However, functionally it can be considered closed by the last one-half of fetal life.

Initially, both the cloaca and the urachus are lined by cuboidal epithelium. Later, cloacal epithelium is replaced

Table 19–25. Classification of Congenital Anomalies of the Urachus and Bladder

I. Urachal anomalies
A. Patent urachus
B. Urachal cyst
C. Urachal sinus
D. Urachal diverticulum
II. Bladder anomalies
A. Anomalies in number
1. Agenesis
2. Duplication
B. Anomalies in size
1. Hypoplasia
2. Megacystis
C. Anomalies in form
1. Exstrophy-epispadias complex
2. Congenital bladder diverticula

by transitional epithelium in 70% of individuals, while in the remainder, the cloacal epithelium is replaced by columnar epithelium.[9]

Normal Urachus

At birth, three structures are visible on the posterior aspect of the anterior abdominal wall, running from the pelvis to the umbilicus: (1) the two umbilical arteries, one on each side, which become obliterated soon after birth, and are sometimes termed the lateral umbilical ligaments, and (2) the urachus itself, which is located on the midline and originates from the anterior surface—sometimes from the apex of the bladder—and lies between the two umbilical arteries (Fig. 19–237).[1, 5] The obliterated urachus is also known as the median umbilical ligament.

The urachus has three parts: intramucosal, intramuscular, and supravesical.[9] It communicates with the lumen of the bladder microscopically in one-third of adults.[9] This communication is of three types:[9] (1) serpiginous tubes with parallel walls, (2) serpiginous tubes with dilated and narrow areas, and (3) serpiginous tubes with dilated and narrow areas and with side branches (Fig. 19–238). These tubes are lined with transitional epithelium in 70% of cases, and columnar epithelium in 30%.[9]

In its path from the bladder to the umbilicus, the urachus lies between the transversalis fascia and the peritoneum in the space of Retzius.

Congenital Anomalies

There are four types of congenital urachal anomalies.[1, 10-16] They are twice as common in males as in females.

1. Patent urachus (about 50% of cases) (Fig. 19–238A)
2. Urachal cyst (about 30% of cases) (Fig. 19–238B)
3. Urachal sinus (about 15% of cases) (Fig. 19–238C)
4. Urachal diverticulum (about 5% of cases) (Fig. 19–238D)

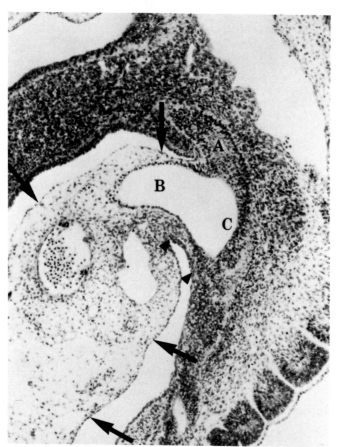

Figure 19–236. Stage-13 embryo showing *A*, the confluence of the hindgut, and *B*, the expanded allantois with *C*, the cloaca. The cloacal membrane *(arrowheads)* can be seen between the upper portion of the lumen of the cloaca and its terminal portion below its junction with the tailgut. Arrows point to the body stalk (the future umbilical cord). (From the Carnegie Collection.)

Patent Urachus

Here the urachus is patent between the bladder and the umbilicus. In 15% to 30% of patients, the patent urachus is associated with urethral atresia or very obstructive posterior urethral valves. The bladder empties through the patent urachus, rather than through the urethra. Because urine still enters the amniotic fluid, there is no oligohydramnios. The evolving lungs are protected from the direct pressure of the uterus. Consequently, no pulmonary hypoplasia or pneumothoraces are present, as they are in other cases of urethral atresia or very obstructive posterior urethral valves. In these patients, the patent urachus serves as a protective mechanism.

If the patent urachus is large, the umbilical cord is large and tense at birth. If the patent urachus is smaller, urine pours out of it at the umbilicus when the cord becomes detached.

Patent urachus may be associated with multiple congenital anomalies.

Diagnostic Imaging

A fistulogram (Fig. 19–239*A*) or voiding cystourethrogram (Fig. 19–239*B*) in the lateral view, or a sonogram (Fig. 19–239*C*) shows the patent urachus.[85] The voiding cystourethrogram will reveal whether the urethra is obstructed.

Urachal Cyst

A urachal cyst develops if the urachus closes both at the umbilicus and the bladder, but remains patent between these two areas. The cyst is usually found in the lower third of the urachus, and much less frequently in the upper third.[11] Rarely, it may be intramural.[11] The lining is usually transitional epithelium but may be glandular epithelium; the epithelium may calcify.

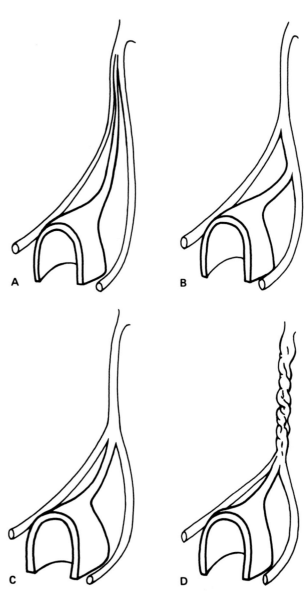

Figure 19–237. The urachus and umbilical arteries as viewed from inside the peritoneal cavity. *A,* The urachus extends independently to the umbilicus. *B,* The urachus joins one umbilical artery, continuing with it toward the umbilicus. *C,* The urachus and both umbilical arteries join and course to the umbilicus as a single ligament. *D,* The urachus is very short, and the common structure forms a fibrous plexus. (From Duckett JW, Caldamone AA: Bladder and urachus. *In* Kelalis PP, King LR, Belman AB (eds): Clinical Pediatric Urology. Philadelphia, WB Saunders, 1985, p 744).

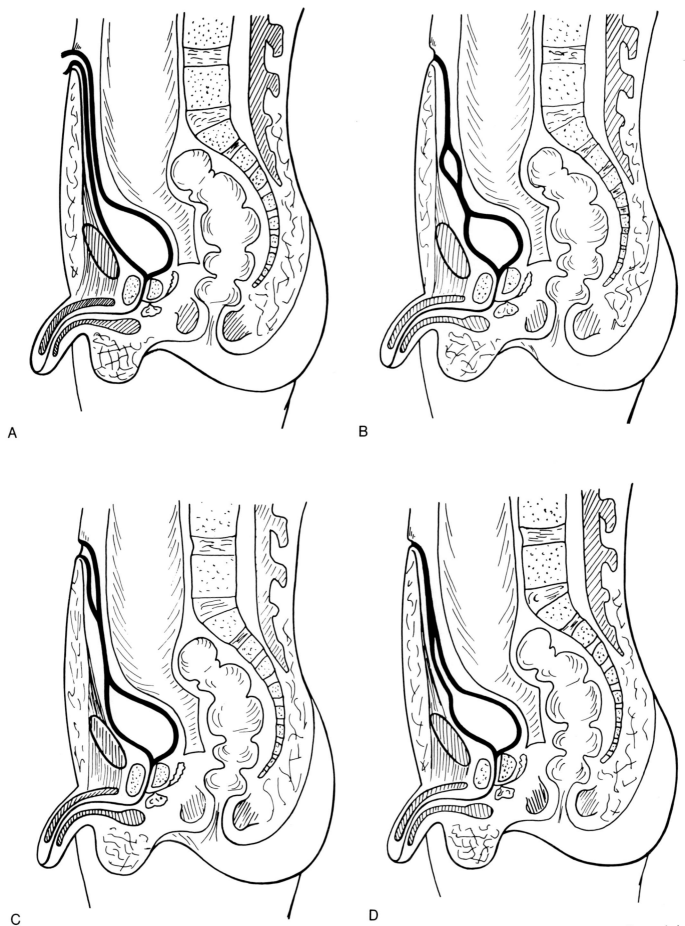

A

B

C

D

Figure 19–238. Congenital urachal anomalies are shown: *A,* patent urachus, *B,* urachal cyst, *C,* urachal sinus, *D,* urachal diverticulum. (From Schnyder PA, Candardjis G: Vesicourachal diverticulum. CT diagnosis in two adults. AJR 137(5):1063–1065, 1981, © by Am Roentgen Ray Soc.)

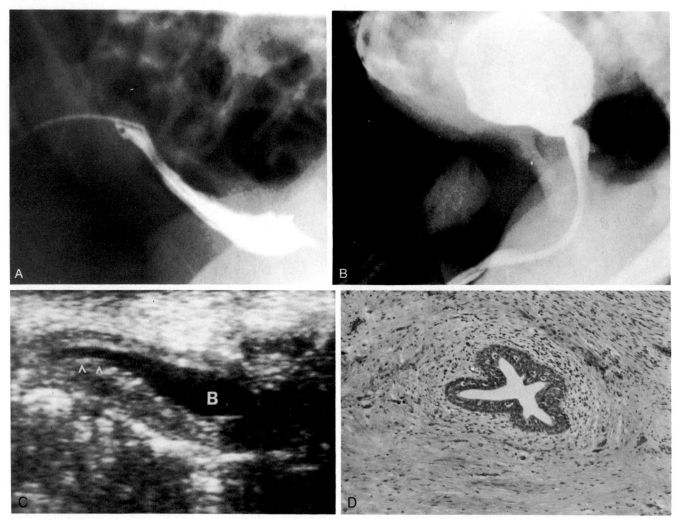

Figure 19–239. Patent urachus demonstrated by *A*, fistulogram, *B*, voiding cystourethrogram, and *C*, sonogram (*arrowheads*; B = bladder), in the same child. *D*, A histological cross section of the resected urachus is shown. (Courtesy Jeffrey Reese, M.D., Division of Urology, Stanford University.)

The contents of the cyst are usually mucinous or serous fluid, although it may be packed with cells shorn off the lining. The cyst is usually small, but varies considerably in size; it may create a large abdominal mass.

Complications

The complications of urachal cyst are as follows:

1. The most common complication is a staphylococcal infection. This occurs usually in adults, only occasionally in childhood. (An infected urachal cyst is demonstrated in Chapter 24.) When the cyst is infected, it may rupture into the bladder, out at the umbilicus, or into the peritoneal cavity.

2. A large cyst may lead to urinary retention and azotemia.[17]

3. There is an increased incidence of carcinoma, particularly adenocarcinoma (see Fig. 19–244; see also Chapter 46).

4. The cyst can bleed after relatively minor trauma.

Diagnostic Imaging

The intravenous urogram and voiding cystourethrogram are not a good means of visualizing a urachal cyst, because typically only an extrinsic impression on the fundus of the bladder is seen. Rarely, eggshell calcification is visible.[18]

The preferred methods of diagnostic imaging are ultrasonography and/or computed tomography (CT),[11, 12] followed by percutaneous puncture under sonographic guidance. Abscesses and cysts can be drained in this way; unfortunately, cysts tend to recur.

Urachal Sinus

If a small urachal cyst becomes infected, it may drain via a sinus at the umbilicus or into the bladder. One particularly interesting variety is the alternating urachal sinus, in which the drainage shifts alternately between the umbilicus and the bladder (Fig. 19–240).[19]

If the drainage is at the umbilicus, a fistulogram in the lateral view is preferable; if the bladder is suspect, a cystogram in the lateral view will better reveal the disease (Fig. 19–240).

Urachal Diverticulum

A urachal diverticulum, common in prune-belly syndrome, forms when the urachus closes at the umbilicus but not at the bladder. It is usually asymptomatic, and may be discovered incidentally during a CT examination of the pelvis.

Diverticula are often found at the fundus of the bladder in patients with chronic bladder-outlet obstruction. It is conceivable that they are remnants of a microscopically patent urachus forced open as a result of the obstruction.

Complications

Complications include (1) an increased incidence of carcinoma, usually after puberty, (2) a tendency toward

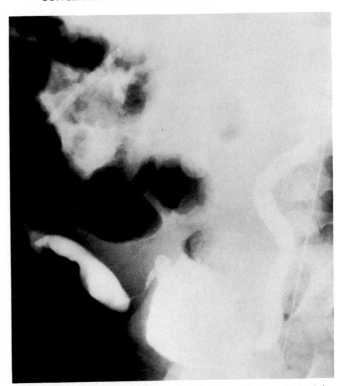

Figure 19–240. Alternating urachal sinus, demonstrated by voiding cystourethrography. Vesicoureteral reflux is present. (Courtesy Jeffrey Reese, M.D., Division of Urology, Stanford University.)

stone formation, and (3), in patients with Crohn's disease of the small bowel or colon or with diverticulitis of the sigmoid colon, formation of a fistula between these segments of the bowel and the urachal diverticulum.

Diagnostic Imaging

It may be possible to see the calcification of an adenocarcinoma or calcification due to stones on a plain abdominal radiograph.

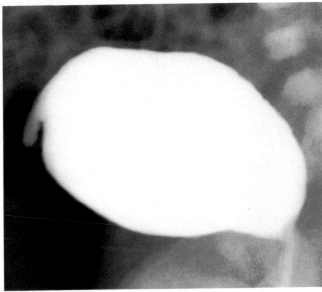

Figure 19–241. Lateral cystogram demonstrates a small urachal diverticulum.

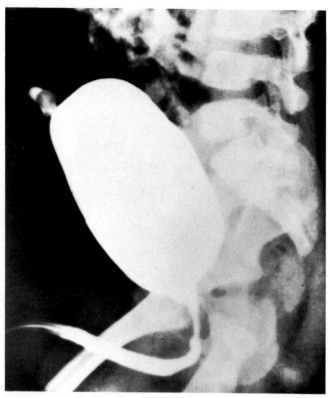

Figure 19–242. Voiding cystourethrogram demonstrating a urachal diverticulum. The sacrum is hypoplastic. The Foley balloon appears to be within the diverticulum. (From Cacciarelli AA, Lucas B, McAlister WH: Multichambered bladder anomalies. AJR 126:642–646, © 1976, by Am Roentgen Ray Soc.)

On an *intravenous urogram* or *voiding cystourethrogram*, a urachal diverticulum has the typical appearance of a diverticulum, but arises from the fundus of the bladder (Figs. 19–241 and 19–242).

A barium enema or small-bowel series may show the etiology of *fistulas*, such as Crohn's disease or diverticulitis, and may outline the fistulas themselves. After a barium enema or small-bowel series, urine can always be radiographed for barium, which indicates the presence of a fistula (Bourne test).

CT identification requires[10] (1) the use of large amounts of oral contrast material, (2) multiple sections before and after the administration of intravenous contrast material. A lateral digital radiograph is extremely valuable (Fig. 19–243). Calcification due to an adenocarcinoma (Fig. 19–244) or stones may be visible.

Magnetic resonance imaging (MRI) may be useful in demonstrating urachal diverticula, and any carcinoma that may be present.

BLADDER

Embryology

The development of the bladder takes place in two stages. The first is between Stages 13 and 17, and the second is between Stages 18 and 23.

At the beginning of the first stage of development, a structure called a cloaca exists. *Cloaca* is the Latin word for "drain," appropriate in this case because the structure drains both the gastrointestinal and urinary tracts. The cloaca is separated into two structures, the rectum and the primitive urogenital sinus, although the mechanism of separation is still controversial.

The modern concept[6, 20, 27] is that the hindgut starts above the cloaca and the rectum is formed largely from the hindgut, which is brought to the perineal region by differential growth. Mesoblast between the evolving bladder and the evolving rectum proliferates in all directions; the result is the formation of the so-called urorectal septum (for want of a better term), which actually represents the elongating dorsal wall of the urogenital sinus, and the elongating ventral wall of the hindgut.[6, 20–27]

The urorectal septum forms at the same time that the ventral body wall develops below the body stalk (Fig. 19–245).[6] The separation of the cloaca into the urogenital sinus and the rectum starts cranially and proceeds caudally (Figs. 19–245 and 19–246).[6] This separation is unequal, so that most of the cloaca eventually forms the urogenital sinus and, eventually, the bladder; it thus contributes little to the formation of the rectum, which develops mainly from the hindgut.

Also in this first stage, the common excretory duct dilates. The cloacal epithelium grows into the common excretory duct, and the epithelium of the common duct sloughs off (preceding section of this chapter). The common excretory duct thus becomes part of the bladder,[28] and it is later absorbed into the bladder as described on page 688.

During the second stage of bladder development, the primitive urogenital sinus becomes differentiated into a bladder portion, a trigonal portion, and a urethral portion. At the same time, the ureteral orifices and the wolffian duct orifices separate, as described previously (page 688).

The bladder portion of the primitive urogenital sinus develops mainly from the cloaca, although the allantoic orifice may contribute to the development of the dome.[6, 7] The trigonal portion is a composite structure, formed partially by the cloaca and partially by the common excretory duct. The latter gives rise to the muscle layers that extend from the distal end of the ureter caudally to form the superficial muscle layer of the trigone. Because the cloacal epithelium replaces that within the common excretory duct, this new trigonal epithelium is derived from the cloaca—not the common excretory duct.

The ventral portion of the urogenital sinus grows distally, forming the entire urethra in the female and all but the distal end of the urethra in the male. Initially, the ureterovesical junction is arbitrarily defined at the point where the wolffian ducts open. Just before the end of the embryonic period (Stage 23), however, the müllerian tubercle becomes visible. This forms the arbitrary point at which the bladder becomes urethra.

Anomalies in Number

Agenesis

Here there is no bladder and no urethra.[29, 30] Infants with agenesis of the bladder are usually stillborn, but virtually all surviving infants are female.[29, 83, 86]

The ureters open ectopically in an area where the external urethral meatus might be expected, opening on

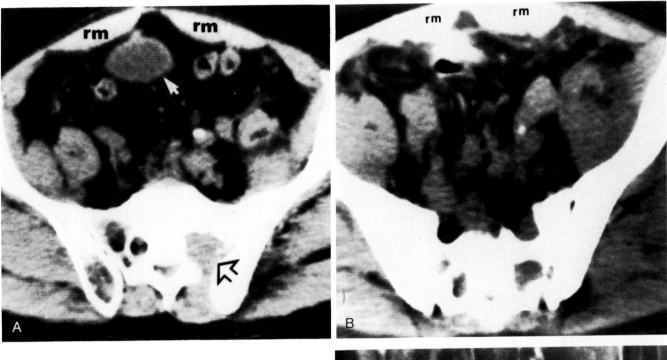

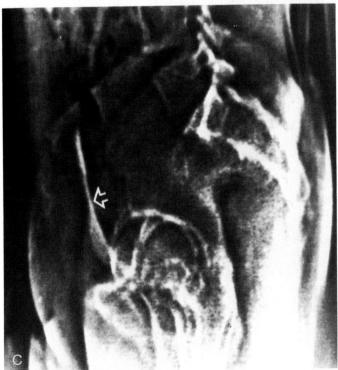

Figure 19–243. Urachal diverticulum in an adult demonstrated by CT. *A* to *C* show a patient with Hodgkin's lymphoma. *A,* Before the administration of intravenous contrast, urachal diverticulum is visible as a gasless tubular structure *(white arrow)* posterior to the rectus muscles (rm) at the level of the umbilicus and extending downward into the pelvis. Partial destruction of the left half of the sacrum *(open arrow)* is seen. *B,* Lower CT scan and *C,* lateral digital radiograph, 1 hour after intravenous contrast is given, demonstrate the diverticulum filled with contrast material *(open arrow).* (*A–C* From Schnyder P, Candardjis G: Vesicourachal diverticulum: CT diagnosis in two adults. AJR 137(5):1063–1065, 1981, © by Am Roentgen Ray Soc.)

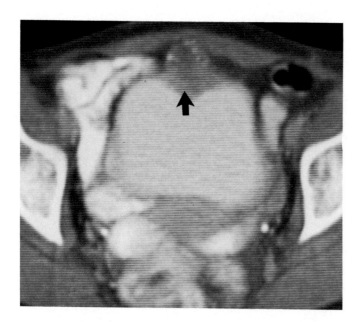

Figure 19–244. CT scan showing a calcified urachal adenocarcinoma *(arrow)*. (Courtesy Robert Mindelzun, M.D., Santa Clara Valley Medical Center, San Jose, California.)

Figure 19–245. Sagittal sections through embryos, Stage 14 through Stage 18, showing the evolution of the urogenital sinus and rectum during the apparent division of the cloaca by the *perineal fold,* commonly called the *urorectal septum.* (From Friedland GW, deVries PA: Renal ectopia and fusion, embryologic basis. Urology 5:698–706, 1975.)

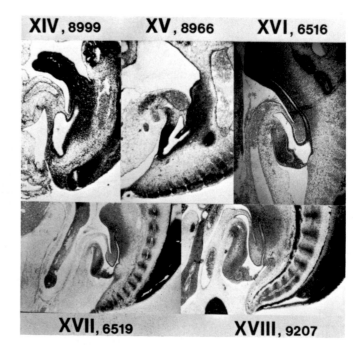

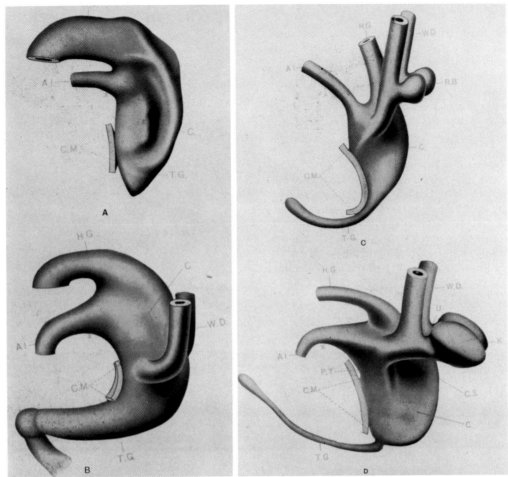

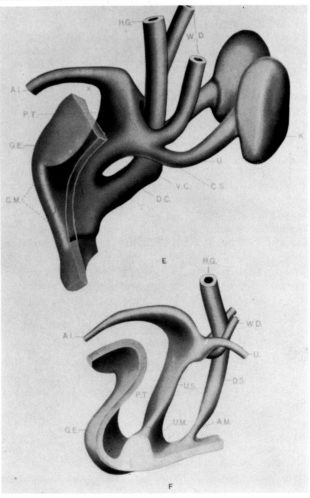

Figure 19–246. Illustrations of wax-plate reconstructions of the hindgut, lower primary nephric (wolffian) duct, and their derivatives. *A,* Stage-11 embryo with the hindgut positioned cranially, and allantois ventrally leading into the precloaca. *B,* Stage-13 embryo with the primary nephric ducts now fused to the cloaca, and the tailgut extending caudally. *C,* Stage-14 embryo with the ureteral buds extending dorsally from the primary nephric ducts. *D,* Stage-15 embryo showing the beginning of sequestration of the primitive urogenital sinus from the dorsal gut primordium. The tailgut is atrophying. *E,* Stage-16 embryo showing the separation of the lumen of the evolving rectum from the urogenital sinus. *F,* Complete separation of the urogenital sinus from the anorectum and the early separation of the ureters from the primary nephric ducts. (From Pohlman AG: The development of the cloaca in human embryos. Am J Anat 12:1–26, 1911, pp 24–26.)

each side. Alternatively, the ureters may unite and open through a single orifice. The presenting complaint is usually persistent incontinence. The major complications are infection, which can result in chronic pyelonephritis and hydronephrosis.

Associated anomalies include agenesis of the kidney,[83] ureteral duplication,[83] and the VATER association.[84]

DIAGNOSTIC IMAGING

A sonogram and an intravenous urogram show no bladder. If it is possible to find the openings of the ureters, they may be catheterized, contrast material may injected, and the diagnosis may be made by retrograde urography. A retrograde urethrogram may also fill the ureters and serves as well to differentiate vesical agenesis from bilateral ureteral ectopia, in which case a small bladder should be present.

Duplication

The three main types of duplicated bladders are as follows:[31-41]

Type I. The duplication involves the mucosa and the muscle wall. A peritoneal fold of varying depth separates the two bladders. Subtypes are (1) complete duplication (Fig. 19–247A) and (2) incomplete duplication (Fig. 19–247B).

Type II. An internal septum, of mucosa only or of mucosa and muscle, divides the bladder. A shallow groove may or may not be visible on the outside of the bladder, marking the location of the internal septum. Subtypes are (1) sagittal septum: complete (Fig. 19–247C) and incomplete (Fig. 19–247D), (2) frontal septum: complete (Fig. 19–247E) and incomplete (Fig. 19–247F), (3) multiple septa (Fig. 19–247H).

Type III. There is a transverse band of thick muscle dividing the bladder into two unequal cavities, giving it a characteristic hourglass shape (Fig. 19–247G).

EMBRYOLOGY

All suggestions to explain the embryology of duplicated bladders are speculative at this point. Chwalle[42] theorized that completely duplicated bladders may form, if one ureter remained obstructed at the ureterovesical junction, owing to the membrane named after him. This would lead to cystic dilatation at the lower end of the ureter. Muscle and fibrous tissue would develop around the structure, which would then be forced over to the median line, resulting in a bipartite bladder. The hourglass bladder has been theorized to be a result of a dysplastic junction between the urachus and the bladder.

The Danforth strain of mice is unfortunately now extinct, but had developed duplication of the body as well as of the gonads and bladder, and other internal organs.[43] These duplications are no longer available for study, and we have no idea how congenital bladder septations develop.

COMPLETE DUPLICATION

Complete duplication involves two completely separate bladders, each with its own wall of muscle and mucosa,

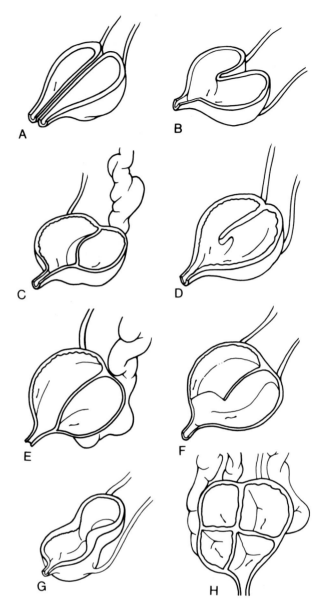

Figure 19–247. Duplicated bladders are shown: *A,* complete duplication, *B,* incomplete duplication, *C,* complete sagittal septum, *D,* incomplete sagittal septum, *E,* complete frontal septum, *F,* incomplete frontal septum, *G,* hourglass bladder, and *H,* multiseptate bladder.

separated by a peritoneal fold of varying depth. The right and left kidneys drain into the right and left bladders, respectively, via single ureters. There are two urethras, one for each bladder.

In the male, there are often two penises, or a partially duplicated penis, or one penis with two urethras. Commonly, the scrotum is bifid.

In the female, there are usually two urethras, two vaginas, and two uteri, each commonly having one horn and fallopian tube. A rare variation involves the development of one introitus, a septated vagina, and a uterus with two horns.

Abnormalities associated with completely duplicated bladders are listed in Table 19–26.

Rarely, the accessory bladder lies in front of the normal bladder, with an accessory urethra extending from it dorsally to a penile epispadiac meatus.[39] Neither ureter drains into the accessory bladder (Fig. 19–248).

Table 19–26. Anomalies Associated with Complete Duplication of the Bladder

Renal ectopia (50%)
Duplicated colon with an anorectal malformation of the lateral colon and rectourethral fistula (50%)
Duplicated anus
Duplicated appendix
Duplicated ileum from Meckel's diverticulum to ileocecal valve
Duplicated sacrum and coccyx
Wide separation of pubic rami

Intravenous Urography. An intravenous urogram shows two kidneys with two bladders. The left ureter drains into the left bladder, and the right ureter drains into the right bladder.

Voiding Cystourethrography. It is usually possible to catheterize both urethras and fill both bladders (Figs. 19–248 to 19–250). When the patient voids, both bladders usually contract simultaneously, so the urethras are outlined with contrast material simultaneously. However, percutaneous puncture is sometimes necessary to outline one of the two bladders.[44]

Barium Enema. A barium enema sometimes shows the two colons.

INCOMPLETE DUPLICATION

Incomplete duplication involves two separate fundi, composed of mucosa and muscle with overlying peritoneum. Only a single base and only one urethra are present. There are no associated anomalies.

Diagnostic Imaging. An intravenous urogram, static cystogram, or voiding cystourethrogram shows a valentine-shaped bladder.

COMPLETE SAGITTAL SEPTUM

A septum composed of mucosa only or of mucosa and muscle, located on either side of the midline, divides the bladder completely into two unequal portions. One portion is drained by the urethra, but the other is not. Two kidneys are present; the left drains into the left portion, and the right into the opposite side. The kidney draining into the obstructed portion, which is not drained by the urethra, is hydronephrotic and dysplastic.

Diagnostic Imaging. An intravenous urogram shows only one functioning kidney draining into a hemibladder. A cystogram or voiding cystourethrogram shows half of a bladder on either the left side or the right.

INCOMPLETE SAGITTAL SEPTUM

This is similar to a complete sagittal septum, except that the septum is incomplete inferiorly, where it has a crescentic lower edge. The size of the resultant opening between the two bladder halves varies significantly. There are no associated anomalies.

Diagnostic Imaging. An intravenous urogram, cystogram, or voiding cystourethrogram shows the incomplete septum.

COMPLETE FRONTAL SEPTUM

An oblique septum runs from the posterior wall of the fundus to the base of the bladder. It is united with the base in front of or behind the bladder neck, dividing the bladder into an anterosuperior segment and a posteroinferior segment. One or the other segment is completely obstructed, depending on whether the septum opens in front of or behind the bladder neck.

Each kidney drains via a single ureter into one or the other bladder segment, respectively. The ureters open into the bladder at different levels, because the bladder segments lie at different levels. The kidney draining into the obstructed segment is hydronephrotic and dysplastic. Occasionally, an obstructed bladder segment becomes so distended that it bulges into the opposite segment, sometimes obstructing the opposite ureter and causing acute renal failure.

Diagnostic Imaging. An intravenous urogram shows one functioning kidney, with contrast material in one or the other bladder segment. The results of a voiding cystogram are similar in bladder appearance.

INCOMPLETE FRONTAL SEPTUM

The anatomy of incomplete frontal septum is similar to that of a complete frontal septum, except that the septum is incomplete inferiorly and has a crescentic lower edge. One ureter from each kidney opens into each segment, but at different levels. Duplication of the kidney is commonly associated with an incomplete frontal septum.

An incomplete frontal septum can be pushed into the urethra during voiding, obstructing the urethra.

Diagnostic Imaging. An intravenous urogram, cystogram, or voiding cystourethrogram shows an incomplete frontal septum as a filling defect in the bladder.

MULTIPLE SEPTA (Multiseptate Bladder)

Here fibromuscular septa divide the bladder into four unequal segments. There is always complete bilateral ureteral duplication, so one ureter drains into each segment; however, only one segment actually opens into the urethra. The other three bladder segments are obstructed, and only one pole of one duplex kidney is unobstructed. The remaining part of that kidney and the entire opposite kidney are hydronephrotic and dysplastic.

Diagnostic Imaging. An intravenous urogram demonstrates one pole of one kidney draining into a tiny, deformed chamber. The appearance is similar to that of the near-empty bladder on a voiding cystourethrogram.

HOURGLASS BLADDER

A thick transverse band of muscle incompletely divides the bladder into two unequal segments in this anomaly. The ureters usually open into the lower portion, but may open into the upper portion. As there are no associated anomalies, hourglass bladders are often not detected until adult life.

Diagnostic Imaging. An intravenous urogram, cystogram or voiding cystourethrogram shows a characteristic hourglass-shaped bladder.

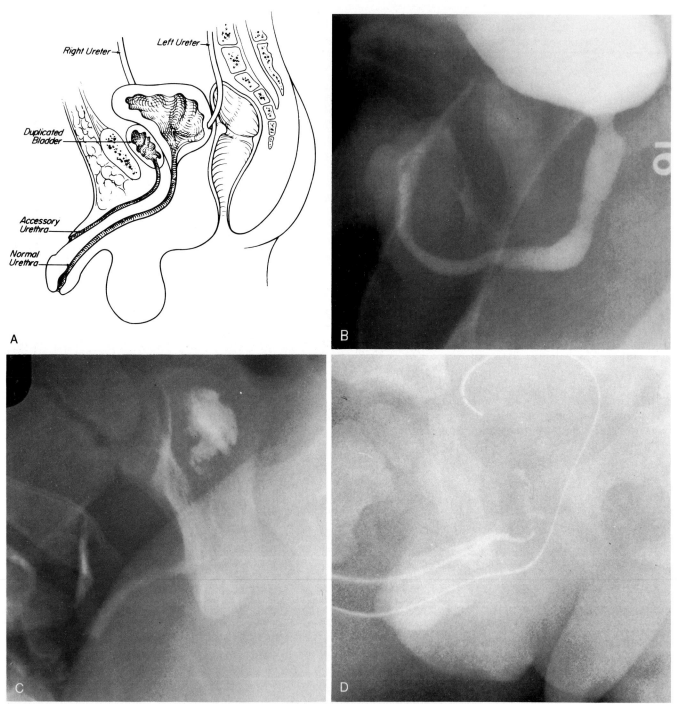

Figure 19–248. Accessory bladder with accessory urethra in front of normal bladder. *A,* Diagram of anomaly shows that neither ureter drains into the accessory bladder. *B,* Voiding cystourethrogram through normal urethra is shown. *C,* Retrograde urethrogram was taken through accessory urethra. *D,* Radiopaque wires are seen in both bladders and both urethras. (From Dunetz GN, Bauer SB: Complete duplication of bladder and urethra. Urology 25:179–182, 1985.)

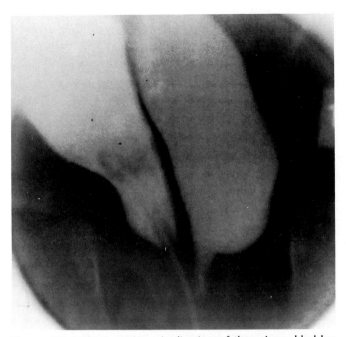

Figure 19–249. Complete duplication of the urinary bladder. Simultaneous cystograms are performed on each half of a completely duplicated urinary bladder. Two bladder necks are seen; both urethras are separate and nonfused.

Anomalies in Size

Hypoplasia

This is a small or tiny bladder, usually seen in infants with sacral agenesis who are often children of diabetic mothers (Fig. 19–251). Hypoplasia of the bladder also occurs in some patients with hypospadias and bilateral renal agenesis, and, for reasons previously described, in children with bilateral ectopia of nonduplicated ureters.

Megacystis

Megacystis means simply "large bladder." It can occur in infants and young children for many reasons. The most common cause is congenital bladder outlet obstruction (e.g., posterior urethral valves), although it may be due to areflexia secondary to spinal dysraphism or may accompany prune-belly syndrome. The disorder may be seen in infants who produce very large volumes of urine, such as those with diabetes insipidus, because of vasopressin deficiency or nephrogenic diabetes insipidus, or infants with Bartter's syndrome.

In addition to these entities that all lead to a distended bladder, there are certain congenital anomalies in which infants also have a large bladder. These include congenital

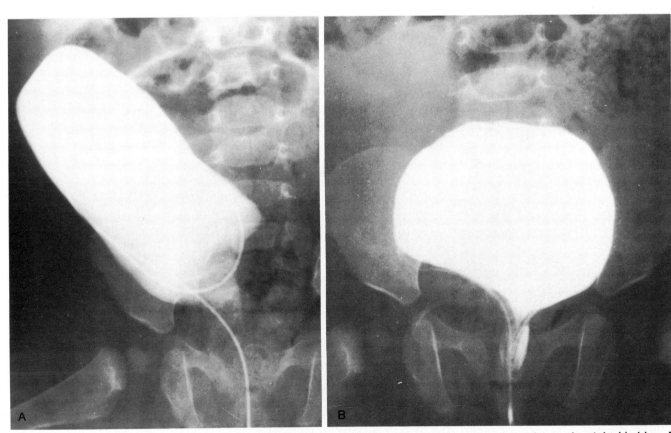

Figure 19–250. Duplicated bladder in a patient with left renal agenesis. The single ureter drained into the right bladder. A, Cystogram demonstrates right-sided bladder. B, Cystogram demonstrates left bladder. (From Cacciarelli AA, Lucas B, McAlister WH: Multichambered bladder anomalies. AJR 126:642, © 1976, by Am Roentgen Ray Soc.)

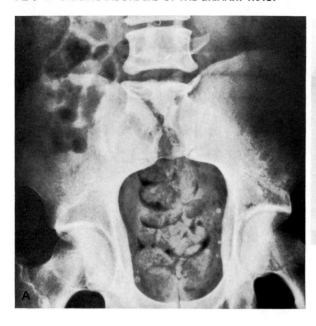

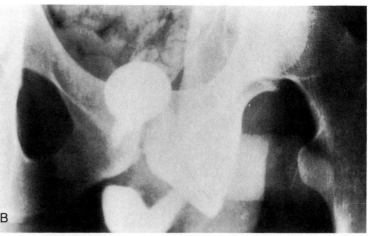

Figure 19–251. Hypoplastic bladder in a child with sacral agenesis born of a diabetic mother. *A,* Abdominal radiograph demonstrates sacral agenesis. *B,* Cystogram demonstrates a tiny bladder and left reflux. (From Friedland GW, Filly R, Goris ML, et al: Uroradiology: An Integrated Approach. New York, Churchill Livingstone, p 1494, 1983. By permission.)

megacystis, the megaureter-megacystis syndrome, and the microcolon-hypoperistalsis-megacystis syndrome.

CONGENITAL MEGACYSTIS (Vesical Gigantism)

Congenital megacystis describes a congenitally huge unobstructed bladder.[45, 46] A normal trigone, normal ureteral orifice, no reflux, and a normal upper urinary tract differentiate the disorder from megaureter-megacystis. In congenital megacystis, large residual volumes follow voiding, although they can usually be significantly reduced or eliminated by reduction cystoplasty.

MEGAURETER-MEGACYSTIS SYNDROME

This entity was first described by Williams,[45, 47] who defined it as a large smooth bladder with a wide trigone, dilated ureteral orifices, and grossly dilated ureters. When the infant voids, the bladder empties completely. During voiding, large volumes of urine reflux up the dilated ureters. When voiding ceases and the ureters contract, urine rapidly refills the bladder.

Histologically, there are a normal number of normal-appearing ganglia in the bladder.[48]

Etiology. The cause of megaureter-megacystis is un-

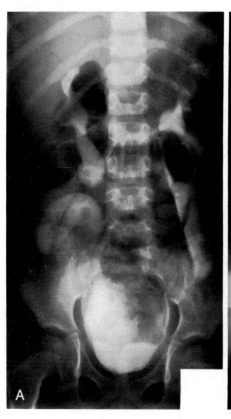

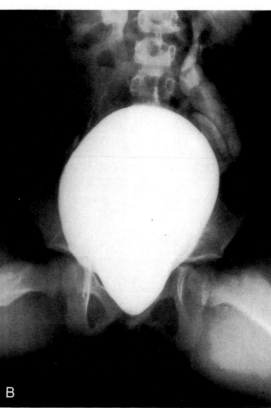

Figure 19–252. Megacystis megaureter syndrome. *A,* Intravenous urogram demonstrates calyceal clubbing and bilateral ureterectasis. *B,* Cystogram shows bilateral reflux, of differing degrees, and megacystis. (From Koefoot RB Jr, Webster GD, Anderson EE, Glenn JF: The primary megacystis syndrome. J Urol 125:232–234, © 1981, The Williams & Wilkins Co., Baltimore.)

known, although Williams[45] postulated a congenital anomaly.

There are two other theories, however; one that the real problem is the massive reflux, so that when infants with megaureter-megacystis void, they reflux at least as much urine as they void, meaning the urine is continually recycled. The bladder is always overfull and distended, eventually becoming decompensated, dilated, and thin-walled.[49] A less prevalent opinion holds that the capacity of the upper urinary tract is too low to lead to bladder decompensation, and suggests some variety of psychogenic voiding dysfunction.[50]

Diagnostic Imaging. On an intravenous urogram there is bilateral hydroureter and hydronephrosis with a huge bladder (Fig. 19–252). A voiding cystourethrogram also shows a huge bladder with massive bilateral reflux (Fig. 19–253).

MEGACYSTIS-MICROCOLON-HYPOPERISTALSIS SYNDROME

As the name suggests, these patients have a huge bladder, often with reflux, and a dilated upper urinary tract. A small colon and a dilated small bowel exist, and hypoperistalsis is seen throughout the gastrointestinal tract.[51] There is incomplete rotation of bowel and lax abdominal musculature. This syndrome is more common in females and is usually detected in the neonate.[52] It is usually fatal during the first year of life.[52] The cause is unknown, although some studies suggest it is due to a degenerative smooth muscle disease.[52]

Diagnostic Imaging. A voiding cystourethrogram shows a huge bladder and often reflux. A barium enema shows a small colon, with the cecum often in the left upper quadrant, because the bowel is incompletely rotated.

Anomalies in Form

Exstrophy-Epispadias Complex

Exstrophy of the bladder and epispadias represent opposite ends of a spectrum of anterior abdominal wall defects, rather than separate entities. For this reason, it is customary to consider the entire group of disorders as a unit.

This group of anomalies is associated with related genitourinary anomalies that share one other characteristic feature: In each, the pubic bones are separated more than 1 cm at the symphysis pubis.[53]

CLASSIFICATION

The most common anomaly in this complex is *exstrophy of the bladder,* occurring in 1 in 30,000 live births; the next is *epispadias,* occurring in 1 in 100,000 live births.

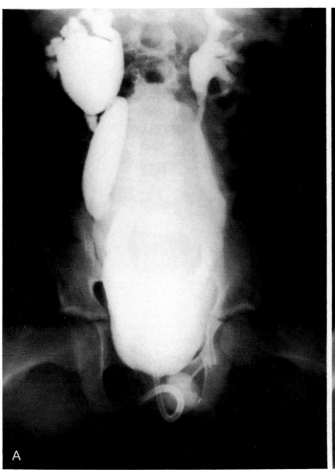
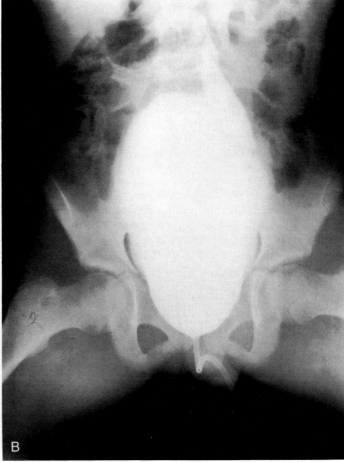

Figure 19–253. *A, B,* Cystograms in different patients show megacystis with reflux. (From Koefoot RB Jr, Webster GD, Anderson EE, Glenn JF: The primary megacystis syndrome. J Urol 125:232–234, © 1981, The Williams & Wilkins Co., Baltimore.)

Table 19–27. Rare Forms of the Exstrophy-Epispadias Complex

Pubic umbilicus
Covered exstrophy
Covered exstrophy and visceral sequestration
Superior vesical fistula
Superior vesical fissure
Duplicate exstrophy
Exstrophy of the cloaca, including covered exstrophy of the cloaca

The other rare anomalies are listed in Table 19–27, in increasing order of severity.[54, 55]

EMBRYOLOGY OF EPISPADIAS AND EXSTROPHY

The embryology of bladder exstrophy is not known. The current theory, however, is that the cloacal membrane either persists or is abnormally large.[56]

Immediately beneath the body stalk in a Stage-14 embryo is mesoblast that forms the anterior abdominal wall, the anterior wall of the bladder, and the genital tubercle (see Fig. 19–245). If the cloacal membrane is large or rigid, the mesoblast, instead of growing directly caudad, is deviated to each side of the cloacal membrane. In this case, two genital tubercles, rather than one, are present. After having passed beyond the abnormal cloacal membrane, they fuse caudad to it. In such circumstances, the corpora of the penis or the clitoris are abnormal, and have a tendency to be separate. As a result of this deviation, the developing rectus muscles separate, although they are otherwise normal.

Because the persistent cloacal membrane also separates the developing symphysis pubis, the pelvis is abnormally wide, as a result of which the two mullerian ducts are separated more than usual. The result can be either two completely separate vaginas and uteri, or a bicornuate uterus. In the event of cloacal exstrophy, double inferior vena cavas may result as well.

This persistent cloacal membrane eventually breaks down. When this occurs, all the structures immediately posterior to it turn inside out and protrude through the opening in the anterior abdominal wall.

Several factors may play a crucial role in determining the nature of the exstrophy: (1) which part of the membrane is abnormal—the entire membrane, the caudad portion only, or the cephalad portion only, and (2) the moment at which the membrane, or some part of it, breaks down. If the entire membrane is abnormal and the membrane breaks down after the urogenital sinus and the rectum have separated, the result is exstrophy of the bladder. If the entire membrane is abnormal and the membrane breaks down earlier, the result is exstrophy of the cloaca, in which the cloaca turns inside out and projects through the defect in the anterior walls of the abdomen. Should this occur, the undeveloped hindgut separates the two halves of the bladder. If, on the other hand, only the caudal part of the cloacal membrane persists, epispadias results; if only the cephalad part persists, the result is a superior vesical fissure.

EXSTROPHY OF THE BLADDER

Here the lower abdominal wall is absent, as is the anterior wall of the bladder. The remainder of the bladder

is visible through the resultant opening (Fig. 19–254). In such circumstances, the bladder often turns inside out and protrudes through the opening in the anterior abdominal wall—hence the term *exstrophy,* which originally meant "turned inside out."

The protruding mass of hyperemic mucosa is an unpleasant sight for parents. Despite its terrifying appearance, untreated exstrophy of the bladder is not necessarily incompatible with long life. Indeed, many elderly people live comfortably with the untreated disorder.[57]

Exstrophy of the bladder, after the related genital defects have been treated surgically, is not incompatible with normal fertility. Men can father and women can bear children.[57]

If one parent has exstrophy, the chance of having a child with exstrophy is 1 in 70, significantly higher than the usual frequency.[58]

The obvious bladder problem may be just one of several anomalies requiring surgery. Other areas of concern include the musculoskeletal, gastrointestinal, and genital tracts.

Congenital Musculoskeletal Anomalies. The pubic bones at the symphysis pubis are widely separated. Only in this instance and in some cases of complete bladder duplication are the pubic bones truly congenitally separated. Although the bones can appear to be separated in infants with cleidopubocranial dysostosis and in some who are premature, they have merely failed to ossify. That is, they are not visible radiologically but are not anatomically separated.[53] The pubic bones may be widely separated because of acquired causes—injury, surgery, or childbirth.

Two associated pelvic bone anomalies are always present in cases of exstrophy of the bladder:[59]

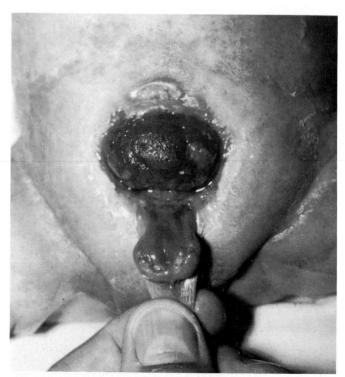

Figure 19–254. Neonate with exstrophy of the bladder and epispadias. (Courtesy Duncan Govan, M.D., Division of Urology, Stanford University.)

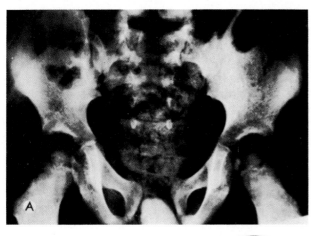

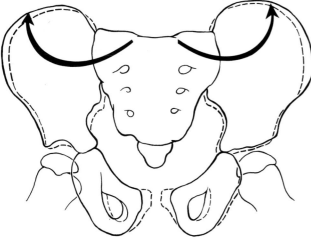

B

Figure 19–255. *A, B,* Pelvic anomalies in epispadias. The innominate bones are rotated outward along the sacroiliac joints, relative to the sagittal plane of the body, and the symphysis pubis is widened. (From Muecke MC, Currarino G: Congenital widening of the pubic symphysis. Associated clinical disorders and roentgen anatomy of affected bony pelves. AJR 103:179–185, 1968, © by Am Roentgen Ray Soc.)

1. The innominate bones are rotated outward along the sacroiliac joints relative to the sagittal plane of the body (Fig. 19–255).

2. Each pubic bone is rotated outward at its junction with the ilium and ischium (Fig. 19–256).

A third pelvic anomaly may be present in severe cases. The inferior parts of the innominate bones separate laterally, and the fulcrum for the separation is at the sacroiliac joints (Fig. 19–257).[59]

Muscular abnormalities accompany exstrophy of the bladder. The lower part of the rectus abdominis muscle is widely separated, and the umbilicus is often low with an accompanying umbilical hernia. Even omphalocele may be associated.[60]

Despite these musculoskeletal anomalies, the gait is usually normal.

Congenital Anorectal Anomalies. The perineum is usually short, and the anus is more anterior than normal. Occasional congenital anal stenosis or rectal prolapse may be mild and easily reduced, or severe, owing to a major congenital defect in the pelvic floor.

Congenital Genital Anomalies. Exstrophy of the bladder is twice as common in males, compared with females. The testes may appear undescended because of the abnormal position of the pubic bones, but in most cases they have descended. The vas and seminal vesicles are normal, as is ejaculation after puberty. A short penis, epispadias, and chordee are present. Prior to penile reconstruction, it is vital to investigate the corpora thoroughly by cavernosography, CT, or MRI to obtain the best possible surgical correction.[61–64]

In the female, the uterus, tubes, and ovaries are usually normal, but the vagina is short, which may lead to uterine prolapse after puberty or childbirth. Occasionally, there is vaginal stenosis or double vagina and uterus (Fig. 19–258).[65] The urethra is short, the labia widely separated, and the clitoris bifid. Unlike men, women can usually maintain a satisfactory reproductive life without surgery, although minor surgery is occasionally required to correct vaginal stenosis or uterine prolapse.

Congenital Urinary Tract Anomalies. The remnant bladder is often small, although the size varies widely.

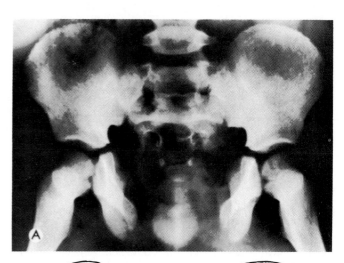

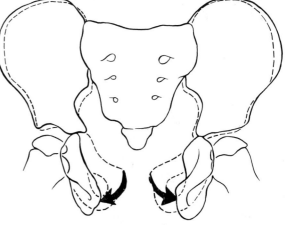

B

1 + 2

Figure 19–256. *A, B,* Pelvic anomalies in exstrophy of the bladder. In addition to the abnormalities noted in Figure 19–255, each pubic bone is rotated outward at its junction with the ilium and ischium. (From Muecke MC, Currarino G: Congenital widening of the pubic symphysis. Associated clinical disorders and roentgen anatomy of affected bony pelves. AJR 103:179–185, 1968, © by Am Roentgen Ray Soc.)

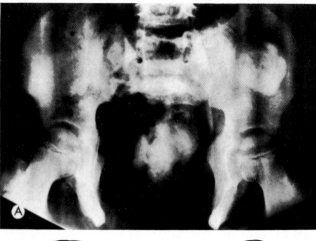

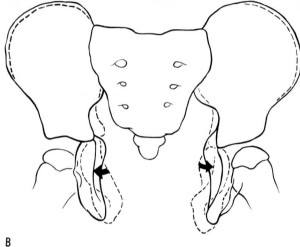

1 + 2 + 3

Figure 19–257. *A, B,* Pelvic anomalies in exstrophy of the cloaca. In addition to the findings described in Figure 19–256, the inferior parts of the innominate bones separate laterally. (From Muecke MC, Currarino G: Congenital widening of the pubic symphysis. Associated clinical disorders and roentgen anatomy of affected bony pelves. AJR 103:179–185, 1968, © by Am Roentgen Ray Soc.)

The capacity after reconstruction may be from zero to almost normal.[55, 63, 67]

The bladder mucosa may range from completely smooth and healthy to ulcerated. It may have undergone squamous metaplasia at the apex or glandular metaplasia at the base of the bladder (cystitis glandularis), possibly resulting in polyps.[54]

The muscles, including the detrusor, the bladder neck, and the external sphincter, may be congenitally abnormal.

The lower ends of the ureters curve widely laterally, and then turn medially and slightly upward. They pass through the bladder wall perpendicularly, not obliquely as is normal. The last short segment of the ureter is always dilated, causing the so-called hurley-stick appearance on urograms, named after the stick used in the Irish game of hurley (Fig. 19–259).[53]

Carcinoma of the bladder is 200 times more common in untreated patients than in the general population. Ninety per cent are adenocarcinomas; however, most are of low grade.

DIAGNOSTIC IMAGING

Sixty-five per cent of upper tracts appear normal on intravenous urograms, except for those with the typical hurley-stick appearance (Figs. 19–259 and 19–260).[53] The rest show hydronephrosis, one possible cause being that the ureters are caught between the everted bladder and the anterior abdominal wall and are obstructed. A gloved hand pushing back the bladder may free the ureter and cause the hydronephrosis to disappear. In other cases, the hydronephrosis may be due to fibrosis or other abnormalities of the bladder wall, in which case the hydronephrosis is permanent.

An intravenous urogram before surgery shows no bladder. After bladder reconstruction, a voiding cystourethrogram usually shows that the ureters reflux permanently. In the past, most children were treated by ileal loop diversion, but this procedure is performed less frequently today. One of the reasons is that postoperative compli-

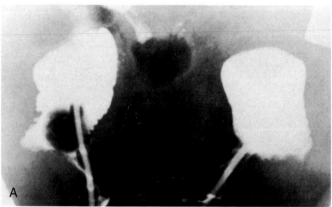

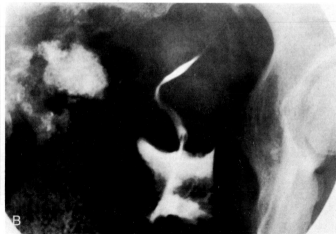

Figure 19–258. Exstrophy of the bladder with duplicated vaginas and uteri. *A,* Contrast material introduced via Foley catheters into both vaginas. *B,* Left hysterosalpingogram demonstrates a hypoplastic left uterus. (Courtesy Helen Redman, M.D., University of Texas, Southwestern Medical Center.)

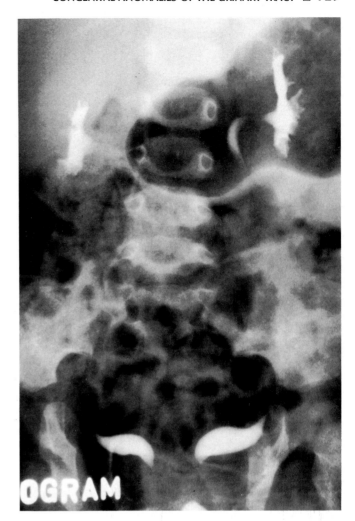

Figure 19–259. "Hurley-stick" appearance in exstrophy of the urinary bladder. An intravenous urogram in this 15-month-old boy with bladder exstrophy demonstrates relatively normal-appearing upper urinary tracts. The distal ureters terminate in a characteristic appearance, resembling the sticks used in the Irish game of Hurley (hurley-stick ureters).

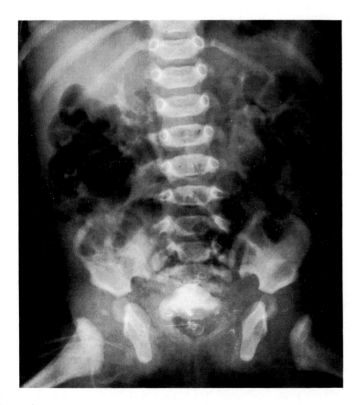

Figure 19–260. Intravenous urogram performed on an infant after repair of exstrophy of the bladder. Note the normal upper urinary tracts and the anomalies of the bony pelvis.

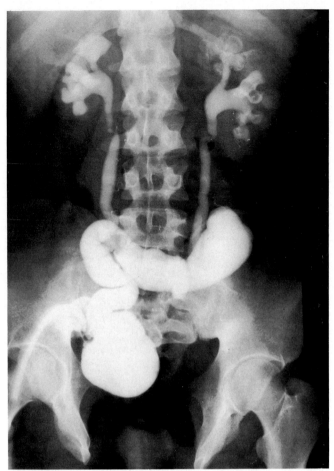

Figure 19–261. Complications of an ileal loop in a patient with exstrophy of the bladder. Loopogram outlines the loop and both upper collecting systems. Note the multiple filling defects in the left kidney, attributable to calculi, and the typical appearance of the pelvic bones.

cations, including calculi (Fig. 19–261) and deterioration of renal function, are common.

Coronal MR images can show separation of the pubic bones.[68] Sagittal MR images after surgery can show absence of the rectus abdominis muscles in the midline and help to determine the capacity of the bladder (Fig. 19–262).[68] These lesions are best seen on T1-weighted sequences because they result in better anatomical resolution.[68]

A corpus cavernosogram (Fig. 19–263),[61] CT (Fig. 19–264),[61] and MRI (Fig. 19–265)[69] are useful for demonstrating corporeal length preoperatively.

EPISPADIAS

An epispadias is a congenital fissure in the upper wall of the female urethra or a congenital defect of the male urethra where it opens on the dorsum of the penis.

In females with epispadias, the clitoris is divided, the bladder is small and thin-walled, and the bladder neck is congenitally absent. The urethra is short and wide, the greatest diameter running transversely (Fig. 19–266). The patient is incontinent,[70–72] although appropriate surgery establishes urinary control in about 85% of patients.[71]

An intravenous urogram usually shows typical widening of the symphysis pubis and a funnel-shaped bladder base extending to just below the top of the symphysis pubis.

The separation of the pubes tends to be less severe than that occurring in classical exstrophy (see Chapter 5). The upper urinary tract is usually normal.

In the male, the roof of the distal urethra is absent, and the proximal urethra may open anywhere from the base of the penis to the glans. The external sphincter is intact in one-third of patients. In the two-thirds who are incontinent, the success rate of surgery for urinary control is only about 33%; 70% of these patients become continent at puberty, because the prostate enlarges.[71]

The results of intravenous urography are the same as in females.

PUBIC UMBILICUS

This umbilicus is extremely low and the symphysis pubis is widely separated. These patients are usually continent and their intravenous urogram is normal, apart from the widely separated pubic bones.

COVERED EXSTROPHY

This is the mildest form of anterior abdominal wall defect. A thin-walled bladder and wide symphysis pubis are present. The lower part of the rectus abdominis muscles are widely separated, through which the bladder herniates.[54]

Males have a micropenis and females a normal clitoris. Both males and females are incontinent, and apart from the wide symphysis pubis, both have a normal-appearing intravenous urogram.

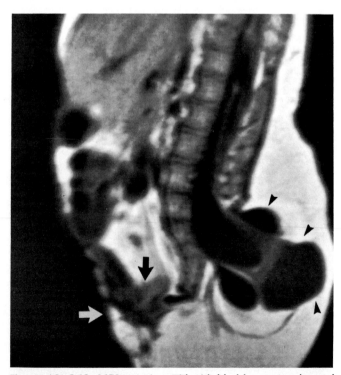

Figure 19–262. MRI scan in a girl with bladder exstrophy and meningocele. Sagittal image (SE 500/28) shows the absence of the rectus abdominis muscles and the symphysis pubis anteriorly, and the small reconstructed bladder *(arrows)*. The arrowheads point to the meningocele. (From Dietrich RB, Kangarloo H: Pelvic abnormalities in children: Assessment with MR imaging. Radiology 163:367–372, 1987.)

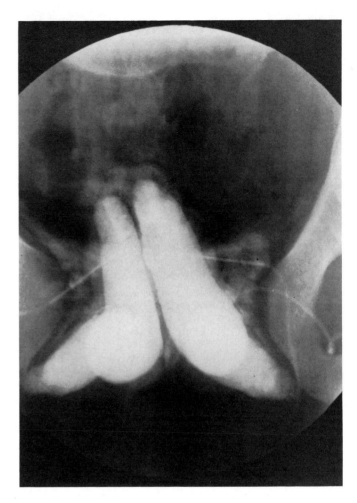

Figure 19–263. Cavernosograms for comparison of corporeal length. In AP view of exstrophy patient, note the markedly decreased corporeal lengths. (From Woodhouse CRJ, Kellet MJ: Anatomy of the penis and its deformity in exstrophy and epispadias. J Urol 132:1122–1124, © 1984, The Williams & Wilkins Co., Baltimore.)

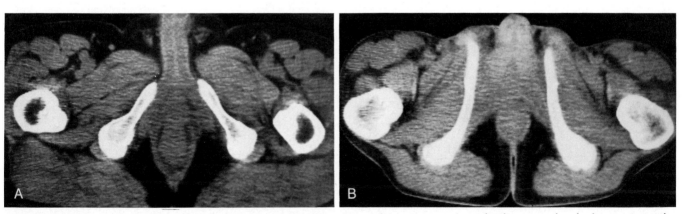

Figure 19–264. CT scans of *A,* normal pelvis, and *B,* epispadiac pelvis, at approximately the same level, demonstrate the shortness of the deep part of the corpora in *B.* (From Woodhouse CRJ, Kellet MJ: Anatomy of the penis and its deformity in exstrophy and epispadias. J Urol 132:1122–1124, © 1984, The Williams & Wilkins Co., Baltimore.)

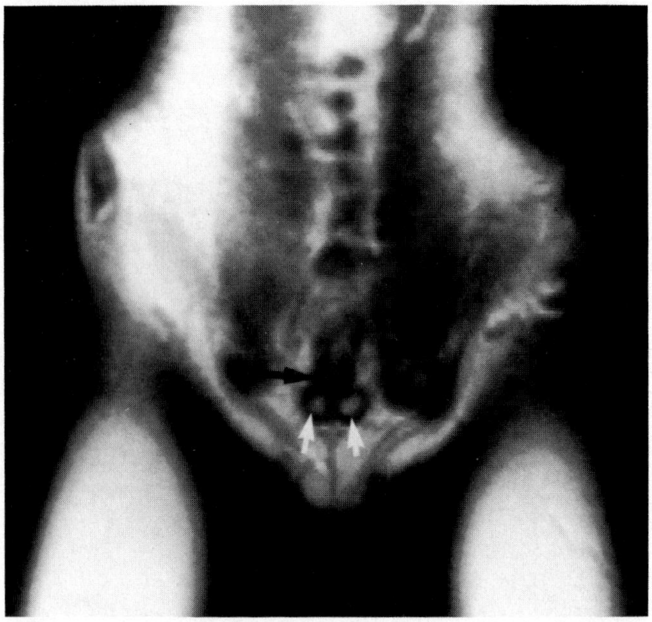

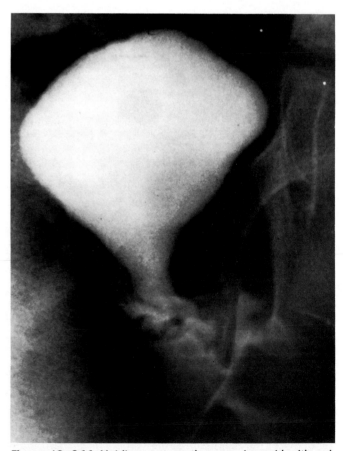

Figure 19–265. Coronal MR image of the pelvis with the penis in transverse section, showing corpus spongiosum *(black arrow)* above the corpora cavernosa *(white arrows)* in a patient with epispadias (0.35 T; SE 500/30 msec). (Hricak H, Marotti M, Gilbert TJ, et al: Normal penile anatomy and abnormal penile conditions. Radiology 169:683–690, 1988.)

COVERED EXSTROPHY AND VISCERAL SEQUESTRATION

In this disorder, an isolated segment of bowel lies on the surface of the abdominal wall of a patient with covered exstrophy.[54, 73] There is a wide symphysis pubis with or without epispadias. The bladder neck is usually poorly formed, so the patient may be incontinent. The intravenous urogram closely resembles that of epispadias. Simple excision of the ectopic bowel is usually curative.

SUPERIOR VESICAL FISTULA

This is a tiny fistulous tract running from the top of the bladder to a small area of transitional epithelium on the anterior wall of the abdomen. There is a wide symphysis pubis. Patients are usually continent.

The fistula is best shown on a fistulogram. An intravenous urogram shows, in addition to the wide symphysis pubis, a normal upper urinary tract.

SUPERIOR VESICAL FISSURE

Here there are only two abnormal findings—a wide symphysis pubis and a large opening between the upper part of the bladder and the anterior abdominal wall.

DUPLICATE EXSTROPHY

In this defect two bladders exist, one normal and the other exstrophied.[54] The size of the exstrophied bladder varies from tiny to almost normal. When the exstrophied bladder is very tiny, it may appear only as a patch of transitional epithelium on the skin, although the wide symphysis pubis is characteristic. In tiny exstrophied bladders, both ureters usually empty into the normal bladder. When the exstrophied bladder is larger, however, one ureter connects to the normal bladder and one to the exstrophied bladder. A related anomaly is bladder duplication with one exstrophy and one cloaca.[74]

In duplicate exstrophy, an intravenous urogram shows a ureter entering a normal-appearing bladder on one side of the midline while the ureter draining the kidney on the opposite side ends abruptly with a hurley-stick lower end, the characteristic feature of bladder exstrophy.

EXSTROPHY OF THE CLOACA

This is the most severe of the congenital ventral wall defects. The terminal portion of the gut as well as the bladder is exposed. It occurs in 1 in 200,000 live births. Two exstrophied hemibladders are found on either side with an exstrophied cecum between them. As one looks down on the patient, two posterior hemibladder walls are seen, with the posterior wall of the cecum and the terminal ileum visible between them.[53, 75] One ureter enters each hemibladder.[54]

The terminal ileum often prolapses; on an abdominal radiograph it may be mistaken by inexperienced observers for a penis. Radiographically, the terminal ileum often contains bubbles of gas (Fig. 19–267).

The exstrophied cecum continues into the colon, which is short and ends blindly. Often there are two colons, two appendices, and sometimes two abdominal vena cavas.

Figure 19–266. Voiding cystourethrogram in a girl with epispadias, showing the short wide urethra, absence of the bladder neck, and small bladder capacity. (From Hendren WH: Congenital female epispadias with incontinence. J Urol 125:558–564, © 1981, The Williams & Wilkins Co., Baltimore.)

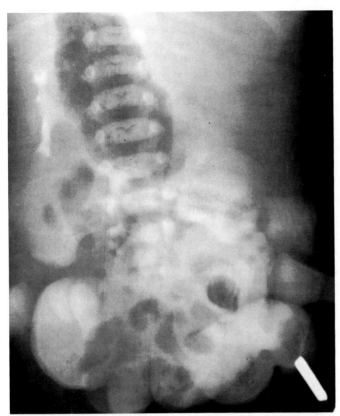

Figure 19–267. Exstrophy of the cloaca. The intravenous urogram demonstrates the ectopic left kidney, common in cloacal exstrophy, and the prolapsed gas-containing terminal ileum (opaque marker).

In 80% of cases, one or both kidneys are ectopic.[76] Several other congenital anomalies are usually found.

One patient managed to live comfortably for 18 years with untreated cloacal exstrophy.[77]

In covered cloacal exstrophy all visceral changes described previously are present, but the abdominal wall remains intact, although thin.

Congenital Bladder Diverticula

Diverticula and saccules are anatomically identical, except that diverticula are larger.[78] Diverticula measure more than 2 cm in diameter on a postvoid film of an intravenous urogram or voiding cystourethrogram, whereas saccules have diameters of 2 cm or less. Both are hernias of the bladder mucosa through the detrusor muscle of the bladder. Diverticula have only small amounts of detrusor muscle and adventitia in their walls.

The majority (98%) of congenital bladder diverticula occur in males.[78] They are most common in the region of the bladder base, most frequently in the region of the ureteral hiatus, in which case they are known as Hutch's diverticula (Figs. 19–268 and 19–269).[79] They can give rise to obstruction or reflux.

Congenital diverticula may occur, however, at a point more posterior and lateral to the ureteral hiatus. Here they may obstruct the urethra in boys.[78, 80, 81] Because the diverticulum has a wide mouth, more urine may enter the diverticulum during voiding than passes through the urethra. As a result, the diverticulum may enlarge and press on the posterior wall of the urethra, thereby obstructing it (Fig. 19–270).

Diverticula may also occur, although with less frequency, in the fundus of the bladder. Diverticula in this location are sometimes bilateral and symmetrical, giving rise to the "Mickey-Mouse" appearance. Another form of congenital diverticulum of the fundus, the urachal diverticulum, is discussed in the section on congenital anomalies of the urachus (see page 715). Congenital diverticula of the bladder have been reported in Menke's syndrome ("kinky-hair" syndrome), a disease of copper metabolism.[82] It is not clear whether this is due to a primary bladder wall disturbance or secondary to neuropathic bladder.

All these diverticula are best shown on a voiding cystourethrogram, although they may be visible by ultrasonography, CT, or MRI.

DIFFERENTIAL DIAGNOSIS[78]

Congenital bladder diverticula must be differentiated from bladder ears, which are transitory bladder pouches projecting anteriorly into the inguinal rings in males under 6 months of age. Bladder ears differ from congenital bladder diverticula because of their anterior position and because there is no obvious neck connecting the pouching sac to the bladder.

These bladder diverticula must also be distinguished from an outpouching from the bladder in girls posterolateral to the ureteral orifices. In girls this is an area of anatomically thin muscle cover, so that the bladder bulges during voiding. Most investigators regard this as a normal anatomical variation, although some suggest that it is a true diverticulum.

Third, bladder diverticula are to be distinguished from wide-mouthed lateral pouches in the bladder with a normal thickness of muscle, which contract when the bladder contracts (Fig. 19–271). This is unlike a true diverticulum, which tends to enlarge as the bladder contracts, and is considered a normal anatomical variation.

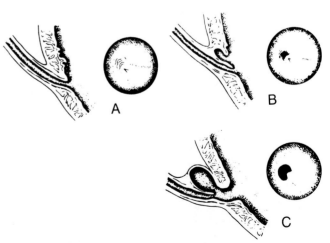

Figure 19–268. Diagrams illustrating A, B, the development of saccules and diverticula at the ureteral hiatus in the bladder, and C, their enlargement during voiding. (From Williams DI: Paediatric Urology. New York, Appleton-Century-Crofts, 1968, p 221.)

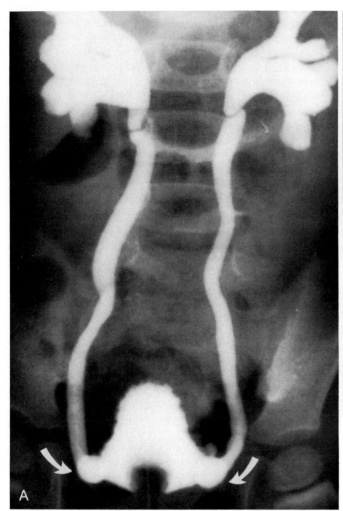

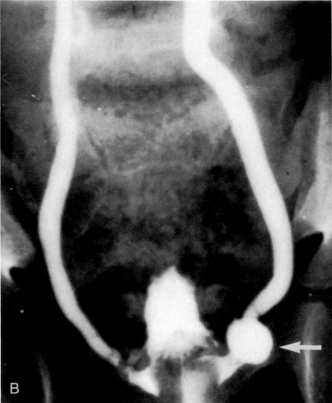

Figure 19–269. Hutch's diverticula. *A,* Cystogram in 3.5-year-old female with recurrent urinary tract infections showing bilateral Hutch's diverticula *(curved arrows).* Associated Grade-3 reflux is present bilaterally. *B,* Cystogram in a 5-year-old female with recurrent urinary tract infections. A large Hutch's diverticulum is present on the left *(arrow).* A right-sided diverticulum has just emptied.

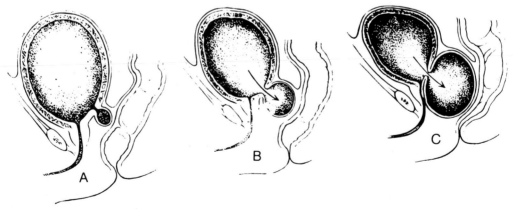

Figure 19–270. Diagram shows the mechanism of acute retention due to a bladder diverticulum in a male infant. (From Williams DI: Paediatric Urology, New York, Appleton-Century-Crofts, 1968, p 225.)

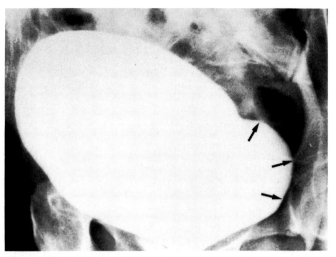

Figure 19–271. Cystogram shows a normal wide-mouthed lateral bladder pouch *(arrows)*. (From Friedland GW, Filly R, Goris ML, et al: Uroradiology: An Integrated Approach. New York, Churchill Livingstone, 1983, p 125. By permission.)

Finally, bladder diverticula should be distinguished from a disorder in which, after surgery or injury, urine has extravasated and then become walled off. A cavity lined with granulation tissue remains and communicates with the bladder. The patient's previous history is necessary in order to make the diagnosis.

References

1. Cullen TS: Embryology, anatomy and diseases of the umbilicus together with diseases of the urachus. Philadelphia, WB Saunders Company, 1946.
2. Keibel F: Zur Entwickelungsgeschichte der Harnblase. Anat Anz 6:186, 1891.
3. Reichel P: Die Entwickelung der Harnblase und Haröhre. Phys-Med Gesellch zu Würzb pp 147–189, 1893.
4. Pohlman AG: The development of the cloaca in human embryos. Am J Anat 12:1–26, 1911.
5. Begg RC: The urachus: Its anatomy, histology and development. J Anat 64:170–183, 1930.
6. deVries PA, Friedland GW: The staged sequential development of the anus and rectum in human embryos and fetuses. J Pediatr Surg 9:755–796, 1974.
7. Born G: Die Entwicklung der Ableitungswege des Urogenital—apparates und des Dammers bei den Saugetierern. Anat Hefte 3:490–516, 1893.
8. Florian J: The formation of the connecting stalk and the extension of the amniotic cavity towards the tissue of the connecting stalk in young human embryos. J Anat 64:454–476, 1930.
9. Schubert GE, Pavkovic MB, Bethke-Bedurftig BA: Tubular urachal remnants in adult bladders. J Urol 127:40–42, 1983.
10. Schnyder PA, Candarjia G: Vesicourachal diverticulum. CT diagnosis in two adults. AJR 137:1063–1065, 1981.
11. Spataro RF, Davis RS, McLachlan MSF, et al: Urachal abnormalities in the adult. Radiology 149:659–663, 1983.
12. William BD, Fisk JD: Sonographic diagnosis of giant urachal cyst in the adult. AJR 136:417–418, 1981.
13. Blichert-Toft M, Koch F, Nielsen DV: Anatomic variants of the urachus related to clinical appearance and surgical treatment of urachal lesions. Surg Gynecol Obstet 137:51–54, 1973.
14. Bauer SB, Retick AB: Urachal anomalies and related umbilical disorders. Urol Clin North Am 5:195, 1978.
15. Berman SM, Tolia BM, Laor E, et al: Urachal remnants in adults. Urology 31:17–21, 1988.
16. Lane V: Congenital patent urachus associated with complete (hypospadiac) duplication of the urethra and solitary crossed renal ectopia. J Urol 127:990–991, 1982.
17. Standfield NJ, Shearer RJ: Prostatism, obstructive uropathy and uraemia associated with a urachal cyst. Br J Urol 53:482, 1981.
18. Leyson JFJ: Calcified urachal cyst. Br J Urol 56:438, 1984.
19. Hinman F Jr: Surgical disorders of the bladder and umbilicus of urachal origin. Surg Gynecol Obstet 113:604–614, 1961.
20. Henneberg B: Beitrag Zur Entwicklung der ausseren Genitalorgane beim Sauger. Anat Hefte 55:227–415, 1917.
21. Krasna FC: Die Entwicklungsgeschichte des Urogenital-systems beim Maulwurf. Anat Hefte 55:443–509, 1918.
22. Politzer G: Uber die Entwicklung des Dammes beim Menschen. A Ges Anat 95:734–768, 1931.
23. Wijnen HP: Hypothesen oven enkele congenitale vitia van het menselijk lichaam aan een morphologische embryologish onderzoek getoetst. Thesis, Universiteit Van Amsterdam, 1964.
24. Van der Putte SCJ, Neetson FA: The normal development of the anorectum in the pig. Acta Morphol Neerl-Scand 21:107–132, 1983.
25. Fleischmann A: Morphogenetische Studien uber Kloake und Phallus der Amnisten. Morph Jarb 32:21–103, 1904.
26. Dimpfl H: Die Teilung der Kloake bei Cavia cobaya. Morph Jarb 35:17–65, 1906.
27. Forsberg J: On the development of the cloaca and the perineum and the formation of the urethral plate in female rat embryos. J Anat 95:423–435, 1961.
28. Gyllensten L: Contributions to the embryology of the urinary bladder. Acta Anat 7:305–344, 1949.
29. Tortosa FL Jr, Lucey DT, Fried FA, Mandell J: Absence of the bladder. J Urol 1235–1237, 1983.
30. Metoki R, Orikassa S, Kanetoh H: A case of bladder agenesis. J Urol 136:662–664, 1986.
31. Abrahamson J: Double bladder and related anomalies: Clinical and embryological aspects and a case report. Br J Urol 33:195–214, 1961.
32. Satter EJ, Mossman HW: A case report of a double bladder and double urethra in a female child. J Urol 79:274–278, 1958.
33. Woodhouse CRJ, Williams DL: Duplications of the lower urinary tract in children. Br J Urol 51:481–487, 1979.
34. Cacciarelli AA, Lucas B, McAlister WH: Multichambered bladder anomalies. AJR 126:642–646, 1976.
35. Veeraraghaven KA, Gonazales ET Jr, Gibbons D, et al: Cloacal duplication: Genitourinary and lower intestinal implications. J Urol 129:389–391, 1983.
36. Scholtmeijer RJ, Molenaar JC: Three cases of bladder duplication. Z Kinderchir 40:108–113, 1985.
37. Millikarjunaiah GS, Solomon B, Reddy DG: Double bladder (report of two unusual cases). Aust Radiol 30:51–53, 1986.
38. Kapoor R, Saha MM: Complete duplication of the bladder, urethra and external genitalia in a neonate—a case report. J Urol 6:1243–1244, 1987.
39. Dunetz GN, Bauer SB: Complete duplication of bladder and urethra. Urology 25:179–182, 1985.
40. Retick AB, Bauer SB: Bladder and urachus. *In* Kelalis PP, King LR (eds): Clinical Pediatric Urology. Philadelphia, WB Saunders Company, 1976, pp 557–564.
41. Richman TS, Taylor KJW: Sonographic demonstration of bladder duplication. AJR 139:604, 1982.
42. Chwalle R: Process of formation of cystic dilatations of vesical end of ureter and of diverticula at ureteral ostium. Urol Cut Rev 31:499–504, 1927.
43. Danforth CH: Development anomalies in a special strain of mice. Am J Anat 45:275–288, 1930.
44. Diament MJ, Stanley P: Two unusual duplication anomalies of the upper urinary tract: Use of percutaneous urography. Urol Radiol 9:185–187, 1987.
45. Williams DI: Megacystis and megaureter in children. Bull NY Acad Med 35:317, 1959.
46. Inamdar S, Mallouh C, Ganguly R: Vesical gigantism or congenital megacystis. Urology 24:601–603, 1984.
47. Williams DI: Urology in childhood. New York, Springer-Verlag, 1974, pp 132–133.
48. Leibowitz S, Bodian M: A study of the vesical ganglia in children and the relationship to the mega-ureter megacystis syndrome and Hirschsprung's disease. J Clin Pathol 16:342, 1963.
49. Burbige KA, Lebowitz RL, Colodny AH, et al: The megacystis-megaureter syndrome. J Urol 131:1133–1136, 1984.
50. Koefoot RB Jr, Webster GD, Anderson EE, Glenn JF: The primary megacystis syndrome. J Urol 125:232–234, 1981.
51. Berdon WE, Baker DH, Blanc WA, et al: Megacystis microcolon—intestinal hypoperistalsis syndrome: A new cause of intestinal obstruction in the newborn. Report of radiologic findings in five newborn girls. AJR 126:957–964, 1976.
52. Redman JF, Jimenez JF, Golladay ES, Seibert JJ: Megacystis-

microcolon-intestinal hypoperistalsis syndrome: Case report and review of the literature. J Urol 131:981–983, 1984.
53. White P, Lebowitz RL: Exstrophy of the bladder. Radiol Clin North Am 15:93–107, 1977.
54. Williams DI: Urology in childhood. New York, Springer-Verlag, 1974, pp 266–279.
55. Jeffs RD: Exstrophy, epispadias and cloacal and urogenital sinus abnormalities. Pediatr Clin North Am 34:1233–1257, 1987.
56. Muecke EC: The role of the cloacal membrane in exstrophy: The first successful experimental study. J Urol 92:659, 1964.
57. Woodhouse CRJ, Ransley PG, Williams DI: The patient with exstrophy in adult life. Br J Urol 55:632–635, 1983.
58. Shapiro E, Lepor H, Jeffs RD: The inheritance of the exstrophy-epispadias complex. J Urol 132:308–310, 1984.
59. Muecke MC, Currarino G: Congenital widening of the symphysis pubis. Associated clinical disorders and roentgen anatomy of affected bony pelves. AJR 103:179–185, 1968.
60. Zivkovic SM: Variations in the bladder exstrophy complex associated with large omphalocele. J Urol 118:440–442, 1977.
61. Woodhouse CRJ, Kellet MJ: Anatomy of the penis and its deformity in exstrophy and epispadias. J Urol 132:1122–1124, 1984.
62. King LR: Exstrophy and epispadias. J Urol 132:1159–1160, 1984.
63. Lepor H, Shapiro E, Jeffs RD: Urethral reconstruction in boys with classical bladder exstrophy. J Urol 131:512–515, 1984.
64. Schillinger JF, Wiley MJ: Bladder exstrophy: Penile lengthening procedure. Urology 24:434–438, 1984.
65. Gilsanz V, Cleveland RH: Duplications of the Mullerian ducts and genitourinary malformations. Part I: The value of excretory urography. Radiology 146:793–796, 1982.
66. Jeffs RD, Guice SL, Oesch L: The factors in successful exstrophy closure. J Urol 127:974–976, 1982.
67. Lepor H, Jeffs RD: Primary bladder closure and bladder neck reconstruction in classical bladder exstrophy. J Urol 130:1142–1144, 1983.
68. Dietrich RB, Kangarloo H: Pelvic abnormalities in children: Assessment with MR imaging. Radiology 163:367–372, 1987.
69. Hricak H, Marotti M, Gilbert TJ, et al: Normal penile anatomy and abnormal penile conditions. Radiology 169:683–690, 1988.
70. Hendren WH: Congenital female epispadias with incontinence. J Urol 125:558–564, 1981.
71. Kramer SA, Kelalis PP: Assessment of urinary continence in epispadias: Review of 94 patients. J Urol 128:290–293, 1982.
72. Saltzman B, Mininberg DT, Muecke EC: Epispadias: Contending with continence. Urology 26:256–264, 1985.
73. Narasimharao KL, Chana RS, Mitra SK, Pathak IC: Covered exstrophy variant. J Urol 133:274–275, 1985.
74. Feins NR, Cranley W: Bladder duplication with one exstrophy and one cloaca. J Pediatr Surg 21:570–572, 1986.
75. Mee S, Hricak H, Kogan BA, Molnar JJ: An 18-year-old woman born with cloacal exstrophy. J Urol 762–764, 1986.
76. Herman TE, Cleveland RH, Kushner DC: Pelvic kidney in cloacal exstrophy. Pediatr Radiol 16:306–308, 1986.
77. Remigailo RV, Woodard JR, Andrews HG, Patterson JH: Cloacal exstrophy: 18 year survival of untreated case. J Urol 116:811–813, 1976.
78. Williams DI, Eckstein HB: Bladder disorders: Diverticula. In Williams DI (ed): Paediatric Urology. New York, Appleton-Century-Crofts, 1968, pp 220–227.
79. Stephens FD: The vesicoureteral hiatus and paraureteral diverticula. J Urol 121:786, 1979.
80. Lebowitz RL, Colodny AH, Crissey M: Neonatal hydronephrosis caused by vesical diverticula. Urology 13:335, 1979.
81. Taylor WN, Alton D, Toguri A, et al: Bladder diverticula causing posterior urethral obstruction in children. J Urol 122:415, 1979.
82. Harcke HT Jr, Capitanio MA, Grover WD, Valdes-Dapena M: Bladder diverticula and Menkes' syndrome. Radiology 124:459, 1977.
83. Akdas A, Iseri C, Ozgur S, Kirkali Z: Bladder agenesis. Int Urol Nephrol 20:261–263, 1988.
84. Dusmet M, Fiete F, Crusi A, Cox JN: VATER association: Report of a case with three unreported malformations. J Med Genet 25:57–60, 1988.
85. Avni EF, Matos C, Diard F, Schulman CC: Midline omphalovesical anomalies in children: contribution of ultrasound imaging. Urol Radiol 10:189, 1988.
86. Aragona F, Glazel GP, Zaramella P, et al: Urol Radiol 10:207, 1988.

CONGENITAL ANOMALIES OF THE URETHRA

CLASSIFICATION OF CONGENITAL ANOMALIES OF THE URETHRA

Table 19–28 shows the classification of the major congenital anomalies of the urethra. This chapter does not include congenital anomalies that are primarily obstructive. They are discussed elsewhere. (See Chapter 55.)

Table 19–28. Classification of Congenital Anomalies of the Urethra

A. Anomalies in number
  1. Duplication
  2. Trifurcation
  3. Quadruplication
B. Anomalies in form
  1. Posterior urethral valves (see Chapter 56)
  2. Congenital urethral stricture (see Chapter 56)
  3. Congenital polyp
  4. Congenital diverticulum
  5. Epispadias
  6. Hypospadias
C. Anomalies of the urethral glands of Cowper
  1. Cowper's syringocele
  2. Duct enters back of bulbous urethra
  3. Orifice of duct stenosed or occluded

Nevertheless, the table lists those lesions with appropriate chapter numbers if further information about them is desired.

URETHRA

Embryology

The point at which the wolffian ducts open into the urethrovesical canal is arbitrarily designated the urethrovesical junction. The urethra distal to this point is divided into two portions: a narrow pelvic portion, and a wider phallic portion, which is widest in the dorsoventral direction.

In the male, the pelvic portion forms the urethra from the verumontanum to the bulbous urethra, while the phallic portion forms the bulbous urethra. In the female, the pelvic part forms the entire urethra, and the phallic part forms the vaginal vestibule.

The lower end of the ventral abdominal wall forms a prominence called the genital tubercle, which in turn forms a phallus. The epithelium of the urogenital sinus grows into the tubercle (Fig. 19–272), where it forms the

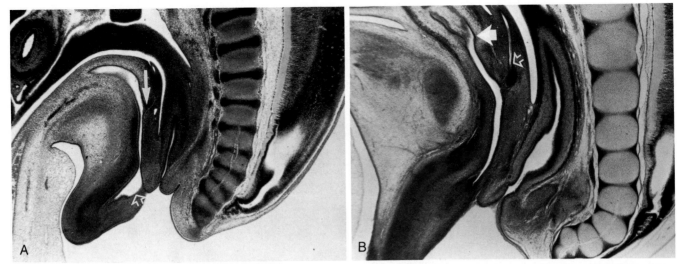

Figure 19–272. Sagittal sections, *A*, Stage-20 embryo, and *B*, Stage-23 embryo, at the same magnification. In *A* the primary nephric duct is apparent *(arrow)*. The dilated vesicourethral primordium is above, and the pelvic urogenital sinus below, the duct. Further caudally, the dorsoventrally expanded phallic portion of the urogenital sinus *(open arrow)* can be seen. In *B* the primary nephric duct *(open arrow)* can be seen extending into the müllerian tubercle. The solid arrow points to the level of the ureteral orifices.

urethral plate (so named because it is fused sagittally) extending to the tip of the phallus.[1] Because the cloacal epithelium is of endodermal origin, most of the epithelium of the urethral plate is also endodermal, although it is covered on the surface by ectoderm. Therefore, it really is an extension of the cloacal membrane, which is also composed of endoderm covered by ectoderm.

Beginning at Stage 18, low folds arise on either side of the urethral plate and form the primary urethral groove between them, lined entirely by ectoderm. By Stage 22, the cloacal membrane begins to break down, while the buds of Cowper's glands develop at the junction of the pelvic and phallic portions of the urethra.

The embryonic period ends at Stage 23, at which point the fetal period begins. Two modern theories explain what happens next.

The first theory[1, 2] is that the ectodermally lined floor of the primary urethral groove—which is also the ventral portion of the urethral plate—breaks down, probably a continuation of the breakdown of the cloacal membrane. As a result, a secondary urethral groove forms; it is deeply lined by endoderm, since it had been the original urethral plate, and is superficially lined by ectoderm.

In the male, the two remaining superficial folds fuse at the 40- to 50-mm stage, beginning proximally and proceeding distally. After this fusion has occurred, mesoblast grows in and separates the tubular urethra from the surface. By the 65-mm stage, the orifice of the tubular urethra has moved to the undersurface of the glans.

In the 70-mm stage, the urethral plate extends near the tip of the glans. As it nears the tip of the glans, the ectoderm from the tip of the glans grows inward, and the two contact.

The male distal urethra is a composite structure formed of ectodermal and endodermal epithelia. The ingrowth of ectodermal epithelium may extend proximally, dorsal to the urethral plate. In the distal glans, the urethral plate atrophies, and the ectodermal invagination excavates to form a ventral groove lined by ectoderm.

This groove closes at about the 150-mm stage and produces the frenulum and the ectodermally lined terminal urethra. At the 115- to 135-mm stage, the dorsal portion of the ectoderm excavates, and the lumen becomes the lacuna magna, or sinus of Guerin. There is a normal breakdown of tissue between this dorsal sinus and the ventral urethra. If the breakdown is incomplete, it can lead to the formation of a valve or a dorsal diverticulum extending proximally.

In the female, the same process occurs, but the urethral folds do not fuse. Rather, they remain separate, forming the labia.

The second modern theory is that the penile urethra is not formed by the fusion of the urogenital folds covering the urethral groove. Rather, the penile orifice is forced forward by the rapidly growing perineum.[3, 4]

Both theories are correct. The urethral plate does grow ventrally, and the genital folds do fuse, but that fusion is not the primary factor leading to the closure of the urethra. Instead, the ventral growth of the perineum is the primary factor in forcing the urethra outward.

Figure 19–273 shows the appearance of the urethra in a 52-mm fetus and a 131-mm female fetus, respectively.

Anomalies in Number

Urethral Duplications in the Male

This congenital anomaly has two urethras, either partial or complete. One urethra is usually normal, and the other is an accessory urethra.

Urethral duplications are completely different in males and females. Males may have the following three main types of urethral duplication:[5] *Type I*—blind-ending accessory urethra (Fig. 19–274); *Type II*—patent accessory urethra (Figs. 19–275, 19–276, and 19–277)—Types I and II are not associated with duplicated or septated bladders; *Type III*—accessory urethras arising from duplicated or septated bladders.

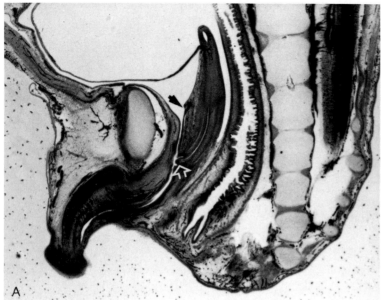

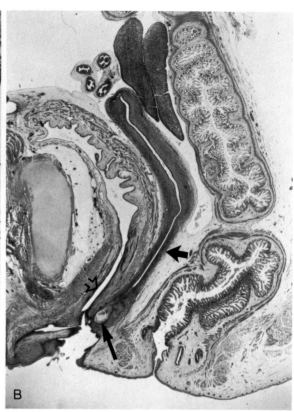

Figure 19–273. *A,* Sagittal section of a 52-mm fetus, where the müllerian duct and tubercle *(open arrow)* can be seen widely separated from the ureteral orifice *(black arrow). B,* Sagittal section of a 131-mm female fetus, showing the elongated uterovaginal canal *(broad arrow)* caudally obstructed by a "plug" or large "epithelial pearl" *(long arrow)* at its hymenal junction. The derivatives of the phallic portion of the urogenital sinus are above the vestibule. The urethra *(open arrow)* is elongated, keeping pace with the elongating vagina.

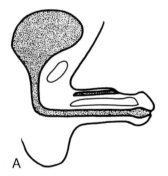

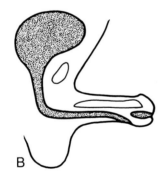

Figure 19–274. Blind-ending accessory urethra. *A,* Epispadiac accessory blind-ending urethra is shown. *B,* Blind-ending urethra opening is in normal position. Hypospadiac urethra is patent.

Figure 19–275. Patent accessory urethra. The main channel opens in the hypospadiac position. *A* shows the distal opening. *B* shows the proximal opening.

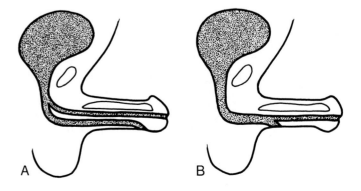

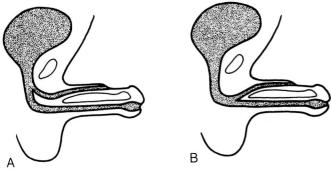

Figure 19–276. Patent epispadiac accessory urethra is shown: A, complete, B, incomplete.

Table 19–29. Classification of Congenital Urethral Duplication in the Male

Type I: blind incomplete urethral duplication (accessory urethra)
  A. Distal—opening on the dorsal or ventral surface of the penis but not communicating with the urethra or bladder (most common type)
  B. Proximal—opening from urethral channel but ending blindly in the periurethral tissue; may be difficult to differentiate from urethral diverticula or Cowper's ducts (rare)

Type II: completely patent urethral duplication
  A. Two meati—(1) two noncommunicating urethras arising independently from the bladder; (2) second channel arising from the first and coursing independently into a second meatus
  B. One meatus—two urethras arising from the bladder or posterior urethra and uniting into a common channel distally

Type III: Urethral duplication as a component of partial or complete caudal duplication

Accessory urethras may be found dorsal to, ventral to, or side by side with the normal urethra.[6-10] When the accessory urethra is in the dorsal position, the normal urethra is located ventrally. The glans and penis usually appear normal, although an accessory meatus is found near the tip of the glans, just dorsal to the normal meatus. Proximal to the two meati, the accessory urethra runs parallel to the normal urethra. As it courses proximally, one of three possibilities may occur: the accessory urethra may end blindly; the accessory urethra may unite with the normal urethra; or the accessory urethra may remain independent all the way to the bladder, where a separate urethral orifice is found at the bladder neck. Very rarely, the accessory urethra may communicate with the prostatic ducts[62] or the seminal vesicle (Fig. 19–278).[63]

When the accessory urethra is in the dorsal position, it is possible that its external meatus can be epispadic, opening anywhere from the coronal sulcus of the glans to the base of the penis. Should this occur, the distal penis is usually broad and recurved. The accessory urethra may course all the way to the bladder, where it opens independently, or it may unite with the normal proximal urethra. In any epispadiac type, the symphysis pubis is abnormally wide.

A dorsal accessory urethra may rarely drain a completely separate small bladder anterior to the normal bladder. No ureters drain into this extra bladder.[11]

A dermoid sinus may sometimes be confused with a dorsal accessory urethra. However, the dermoid sinus is a small hollow tube arising from the base of the penis, where it runs behind the symphysis pubis, in front of the prostatic urethra and bladder, and then up to the umbilicus with a blind or open ending.

When the accessory urethra is in the ventral position, the normal urethra lies dorsally. The accessory urethra is usually hypospadiac, and the external urethra can open anywhere from the glans to the penoscrotal junction. As the accessory urethra extends proximally, it too may develop in one of three ways: it may end blindly; it may unite with the normal urethra; or it may travel independently to the bladder. In some patients the accessory urethra opens in the anal canal or at the anorectal junction,[5, 12] but this congenital anomaly is better called an H-type fistula, rather than an accessory urethra.[13, 14] Rarely, the accessory ventral urethra forms a cyst, without cutaneous or rectal communication.[15]

The two urethras may lie side by side. This is usually associated with a duplicated bladder or a multiseptate bladder. The two urethras are usually the same size.

All these factors involving urethral duplication are classified as shown in Table 19–29.[5]

Associated anomalies include bladder exstrophy,[16] posterior urethral valves,[17] and congenital anterior urethral polyps.[18]

Embryology

A number of theories are offered about the cause of complete duplication of the urethra with separate orifices into the bladder. Currently the most widely accepted theory is that of Patten and Barry,[19] which is supported by, among others, Gray and Skandalakis.[20]

The theory holds that there is an abnormal relationship between the lateral anlagen of the genital tubercle and the ventral end of the cloacal membrane. Normally, these anlagen fuse in front of the genital part of the cloacal membrane, thereby preventing the membrane from extending further ventrally. If the tubercles lie more posteriorly or the membrane extends more ventrally than usual, a part of the membrane remains in front of the tubercle and interferes with its subsequent growth, causing the lesion.

This hypothesis is similar to that explaining the embryological basis of epispadias and exstrophy of the bladder. The similarity was noted by Patten and Barry themselves. Indeed, they argue that abnormalities involving the cloacal membrane result in epispadias, exstrophy of the bladder, and duplicated urethras (the mildest of the three).

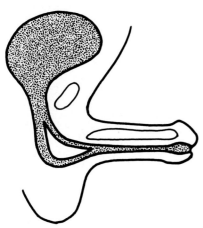

Figure 19–277. Patent accessory urethra with one external meatus is demonstrated.

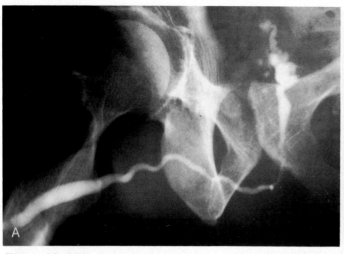 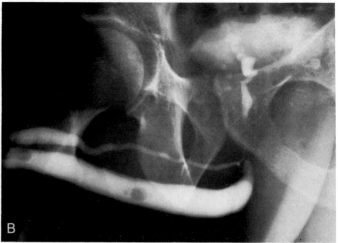

Figure 19–278. Duplicated urethra with accessory urethra opening into the seminal vesicle. *A,* Retrograde urethrogram demonstrates the accessory dorsal channel opening into the seminal vesicle. *B,* Retrograde urethrogram performed after *A* shows the accessory and the normal channels. (*A, B,* from Linsenmeyer TA, Friedland GW: Duplicated urethra communicating with the seminal vesicle. Urol Radiol 10:210–212, 1988.)

Clinical Features

Most patients have no symptoms, except for perhaps a double stream and rarely incontinence.

Diagnostic Imaging

A voiding cystourethrogram and a retrograde urethrogram, both performed in the lateral projection, are necessary for demonstrating the size, shape, and position of the two channels (Figs. 19–278 and 19–279).[5] Regardless of the relative positions of the normal and accessory urethras, it has been found in practice that catheterization of the ventral channel is always easier.[5] Films made in the frontal projection may also be advantageous, especially when the urethras are laterally paired.

An intravenous urogram shows a wide symphysis pubis, if the accessory urethra is epispadiac. There may be unilateral renal agenesis or ureteral duplication, and, in some varieties, a duplicated or septated bladder.

The differential diagnosis includes the lacuna magna, which is a problem especially in patients with hypospadias (see page 743), where the lacuna lies distal to the meatus. Other possibilities include urethral diverticula, dilated Cowper's duct, or acquired fistulas. MRI can demonstrate the two channels (Fig. 19–280).

Urethral Duplications in the Female

Six types of urethral duplication are found in the female (Table 19–30, Figs. 19–281 and 19–282).[6, 21]

The patients have no evidence of virilization. Other genital anomalies may be present, however, including abnormal-appearing labia, introital stenosis, absent vaginal vestibule, absent hymen, and vaginal introitus more

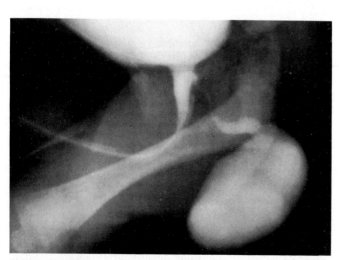

Figure 19–279. Voiding cystourethrogram shows an accessory ventral urethra that forms a cyst, without cutaneous or rectal communication. (From Lawrence D, Howard ER, Harris RF: A case of congenital urethral duplication cyst and its embryological significance. Br J Surg 70:565–566, 1983.)

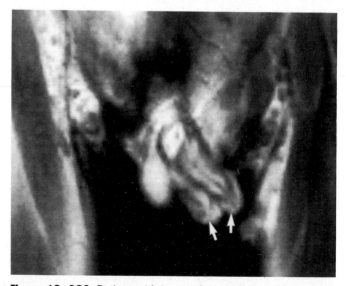

Figure 19–280. Patient with incomplete diphallus. Coronal MR image (0.35 T; 500/30 msec) shows two penile shafts *(arrows),* with urethras visible. (From Hricak H, Marotti M, Gilbert TJ, et al: Normal penile anatomy and abnormal penile conditions. Radiology 169:683–690, 1988.)

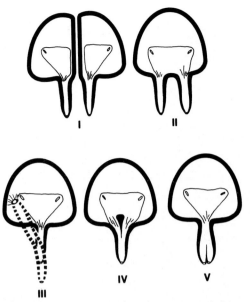

Table 19–30. Classification of Urethral Duplications in the Female

Double urethra and double bladder. Often patients have a double genital tract, a double lower vertebral column, and other anomalies.

Double urethra, single bladder. There is a bifid clitoris and widely separated pubic bones.

The accessory urethra opens in the bladder on one side of the normal urethra. As it travels distally, the accessory urethra goes behind the normal urethra and the external meatus is posterior to the meatus of the normal urethra.

A septum divides the proximal urethra into two channels, although the septum does not extend distally. The septum has a valvelike action, and can partially obstruct the urethra during voiding.

A single proximal urethra and a duplicated distal urethra.

An accessory phallic urethra (Figure 19–283). This has the appearance of a male urethra and opens on the clitoris. The clitoris is prominent, and there is no ventral curve.[22] The other urethra may open into the vagina.[23] The dorsal urethra may be obstructed and dilated.[24]

Figure 19–281. Urethral duplications in the female. *(I)* Double urethra and double bladder. *(II)* Double urethra, single bladder. *(III)* Accessory urethra posterior to normal channel. *(IV)* Double proximal urethra and single distal urethra. *(V)* Single proximal urethra and duplicated distal urethra. (From Friedland GW, Stamey TA: Recurrent urinary tract infection with persistent wolffian duct masquerading as duplicated urethra. Urology 1974; 4:315–318.)

posterior than normal.[22] The perineal body may be deficient. Accessory female phallic urethra may be associated with a persistent cloaca (Fig. 19–283).[25]

Trifurcation of the Urethra

Urethral trifurcation, which is limited to males, exists in the following three types:[26–28] (1) three penile urethras; (2) two penile urethras, and a third ending in a perineal hypospadias (Fig. 19–284); (3) two penile urethras and a third opening at the anorectal junction. This is probably best described as an H-type fistula.

Urethral trifurcation may be associated with congenital unilateral absence of the kidney and of the testis.[27]

Quadruplication of the Urethra

In this anomaly, four urethras lie one behind another.[6] Quadruplicate urethras may occur in males with complete duplication of the bladder.

Anomalies in Form

Congenital Urethral Polyp (Congenital Polyp of the Verumontanum)

Nearly all cases of congenital urethral polyp occur in males.[28–36] Although they may occur any time after birth, they are most often discovered between the ages of 3 and 6 years.

Pathologically, congenital urethral polyps are covered by transitional epithelium. The underlying stroma is composed of vascular fibrous tissue and smooth muscle, although it may contain some small cysts and neural tissue. The mean diameter is about 1 cm, and the mean length of the stalk is about 1.5 cm. Although there is usually only one stalk, the periphery of a polyp can be multilobated, and contain many finger-like projections, rather than being smooth.

The base of the stalk is usually attached to the verumontanum and there may be a slightly enlarged utriculus masculinus. On rare occasions, the polyp may be attached to the floor of the anterior urethra.[37] Occasionally in females, the base of the stalk is attached to the posterior wall of the distal urethra.

Complications include obstructive uropathy and bladder calculi.[31]

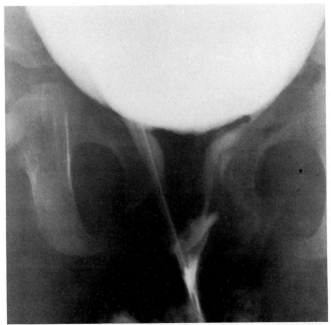

Figure 19–282. Duplication of female urethra. This 11-month-girl had complete urethral duplication, with two separate external urethral orifices. The bladder was normal. A catheter in the right-sided urethra was used to fill the bladder. Both urethras filled during micturition, as seen here.

EMBRYOLOGY

The mesonephric ducts fuse and open into the urethra at Müller's tubercle, which is also the point at which the

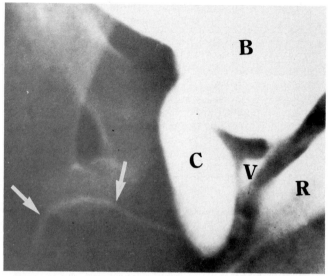

Figure 19–283. Accessory female phallic urethra in a patient with a persistent cloaca. Voiding cloacagram demonstrates accessory phallic urethra *(arrows)*. The bladder (B), vagina (V), and rectum (R) drained into the cloaca (C). (From Sotolongo JR Jr, Gribetz ME, Saphir RL, Begun GR: Female phallic urethra and persistent cloaca. J Urol 130:1186–1187, © 1983, The Williams & Wilkins Co., Baltimore.)

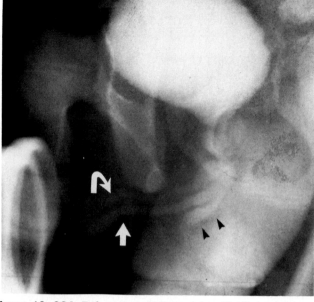

Figure 19–284. Trifurcation of the urethra. Voiding cystoure-throgram on a 12-year-old boy with urethral triplication. The functioning dorsal urethra *(curved arrow)*, ventral urethra *(straight arrow)*, and perineal hypospadiac urethra *(arrowheads)* all opacify and emit urine during micturition.

müllerian ducts fuse and open into the urethra at the end of the embryonic period. At the same time, the epithelial cells and the subepithelial tissue undergo hyperplasia, forming Müller's tubercle. If the tubercle persists and remains large, the urinary stream elongates it, thus forming a congenital urethral polyp.

CLINICAL FEATURES

Congenital urethral polyps are rare. In males, symptoms include intermittent obstruction of the stream during voiding, and more rarely hematuria. In females, the polyp is so distal that it protrudes during voiding and is visible.

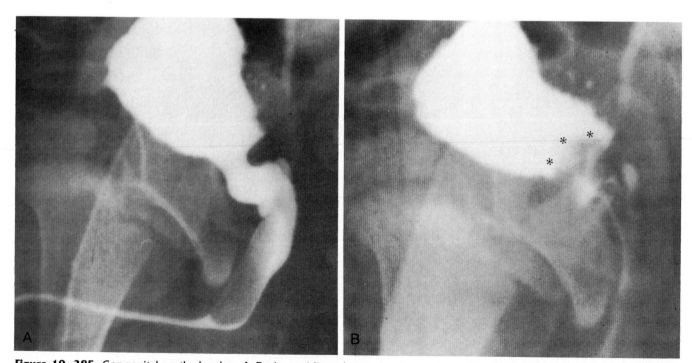

Figure 19–285. Congenital urethral polyp. *A,* During voiding, the stream forces the polyp distally. The polyp is seen as a filling defect, occupying the entire dilated posterior urethra. *B,* After voiding, the polyp retracts *(asterisks)*, and its tip occupies the bladder neck.

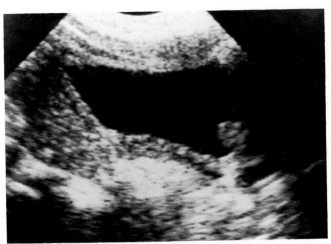

Figure 19–286. Urethral polyp demonstrated sonographically. Suprapubic ultrasonography in the sagittal midline demonstrates a urethral polyp that has prolapsed into the urinary bladder of this 3-week-old male. The polyp now rests on the trigone.

DIAGNOSTIC IMAGING

On a voiding cystourethrogram in males, a polypoidal filling defect is visible in the urethra. The stalk is attached to the verumontanum.

Sometimes the utriculus masculinus is visible, in which case the stalk is attached just below the utriculus.

During voiding, the stream forces the polyp distally, where it can partially obstruct the flow of urine. After voiding or on a retrograde study, the polyp retracts and its tip occupies the region of the bladder neck or even the trigone. This "flip-flop" appearance is pathognomonic for posterior urethral polyp (Fig. 19–285). Congenital urethral polyps occasionally calcify, and, if the tip of the polyp lies in the bladder, it may simulate a bladder calculus. Urethral polyps have been detected sonographically (Fig. 19–286).[61]

Congenital Anterior Urethral Diverticula

Five types of these diverticula have been identified: (1) diverticulum in the roof of the anterior urethra (the lacuna magna), which is common; (2) the narrow-mouthed saccular diverticulum, (3) the wide-mouthed saccular diverticulum; (4) the scaphoid megalourethra, which occurs in the floor of the anterior urethra, and is rare; and (5) fusiform megalourethra, which involves the entire circumference of the anterior urethra and is also rare.

DIVERTICULA IN THE ROOF OF THE ANTERIOR URETHRA (LACUNA MAGNA; SINUS OF GUERIN; VALVE OF GUÉRIN)

This common finding occurs in 30% of all males[38] and consists of a diverticulum 4 to 6 mm long in the roof of the fossa navicularis (Fig. 19–287).[38–40] It is the only congenital diverticulum in the roof of the urethra.

The diverticulum extends proximally parallel to the urethra and is lined by squamous epithelium, although a few mucous glands may be present. A leaflet at the orifice of the diverticulum may prevent filling. The diverticulum is usually asymptomatic, although rare complaints include hematuria, bloody spotting, and pain.

Embryology. The male distal urethra is a composite structure formed of ectodermal and endodermal epithelia. The ingrowth of ectodermal epithelium may extend proximally dorsal to the urethral plate. In the distal glans, the urethral plate atrophies, and the ectodermal invagination excavates to form a ventral groove, lined by ectoderm.

This groove closes at about the 150-mm stage, and produces the frenulum and the ectodermally lined terminal urethra. At the 115- to 135-mm stage the dorsal portion of the ectoderm excavates, and the lumen becomes the lacuna magna, or sinus of Guérin. There is a normal breakdown of tissue between this dorsal sinus and the ventral urethra. If this breakdown is incomplete, it can lead to the formation of a valve or a dorsal diverticulum extending proximally.

Diagnostic Imaging. A voiding cystourethrogram shows a smooth spherical diverticulum (Fig. 19–288) or tubular structure projecting from the roof of the fossa navicularis. The leaflet at the orifice of the diverticulum may prevent filling, as can the use of a Zipser clamp, which is why it is rarely visualized on a voiding cystourethrogram. An incorrect diagnosis may occur if radiopaque droplets of urine are on the skin (Fig. 19–289), if the film is not made at a distance sufficient to include the fossa navicularis, if the film is overpenetrated, or if the observer does not illuminate the end of the urethra with a bright light.

Figure 19–287. Common configurations of the lacuna magna. (From Duszlak EJ Jr, Bellinger MF, Boal DK, Stanford A: Dorsal diverticulum of the distal male urethra. AJR 138(5):931–933, 1982, © by Am Roentgen Ray Soc.)

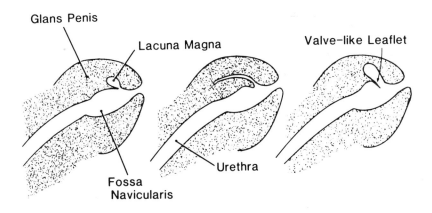

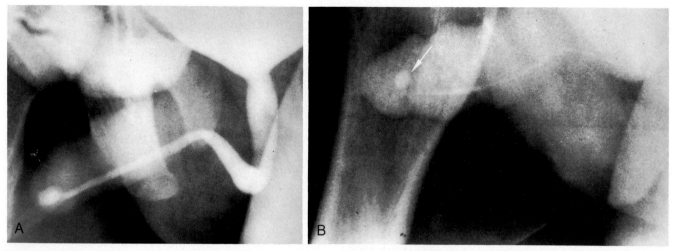

Figure 19–288. A, B, Spectrum of findings in patients with a spherical lacuna magna *(arrow)*. (A, B, From Duszlak EJ Jr, Bellinger MF, Boal DK, Stanford A: Dorsal diverticulum of the distal male urethra. AJR 138(5):931–933, 1982, © by Am Roentgen Ray Soc.)

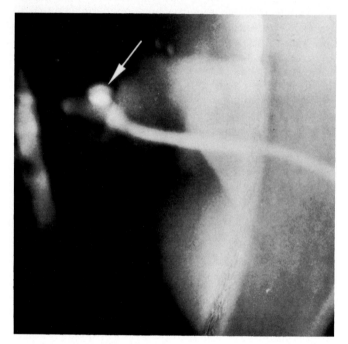

Figure 19–289. Radiopaque droplets of urine on the penile skin *(arrow)*, simulating a lacuna magna. (From Duszlak EJ Jr, Bellinger MF, Boal DK, Stanford A: Dorsal diverticulum of the distal male urethra. AJR 138(5):931–933, 1982, © by Am Roentgen Ray Soc.)

Figure 19–290. Congenital saccular diverticulum is demonstrated. (Modified from Dorairajan: Defects of spongy tissue and congenital diverticula of the penile urethra. Aust NZ J Surg 32:209–214, 1963.)

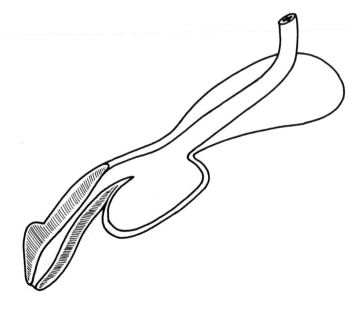

It can be missed on a retrograde study because the catheter has been inserted past the diverticulum.

DIVERTICULA OF THE FLOOR OF THE ANTERIOR URETHRA

Three types of this disorder exist: (1) narrow-mouthed saccular diverticulum, (2) wide-mouthed saccular diverticulum, and (3) scaphoid megalourethra. These three types are due to small, larger, and very large defects, respectively, in the corpus spongiosum. Scaphoid megalourethra is due to a defect in the corpora cavernosa as well.

The varieties of saccular diverticula are narrow-mouthed and round, and wide-mouthed, round, or elongated (in a cephalocaudal direction) (Fig. 19–290).[41–48] The latter is also referred to—perhaps erroneously—as an anterior urethral valve (Fig. 19–291). These varieties are due to small and somewhat larger (respectively), defects in the corpus spongiosum. Both varieties can distend with urine during voiding, partially occluding the urethral lumen. Although anterior urethral valves are said to occur,[59] the vast majority (if not all) of the obstructive ones probably represent the anterior lip of saccular diverticula.

The wide-mouthed variety of saccular diverticulum is the most common congenital lesion obstructing the anterior urethra during voiding. Urine lifts up the distal lip of the diverticulum during voiding, forcing it against the roof of the urethra, where it acts as a valve, partially obstructing the urethra (Fig. 19–291).

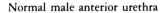

Normal male anterior urethra

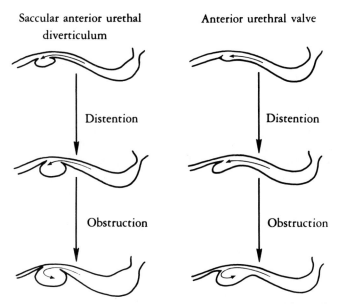

Saccular anterior urethal diverticulum | Anterior urethral valve

Distention | Distention

Obstruction | Obstruction

Figure 19–291. Diagram illustrates how urine can lift up the distal lip of a saccular diverticulum during voiding, forcing it against the roof of the urethra; there, it simulates a valve, partially obstructing the urethra. (From Kirks DR, Grossman H: Congenital saccular anterior urethral diverticulum. Radiology 140:367–372, 1981.)

Clinically, these patients have a poor stream, and, if the diverticulum is large, a palpable or even visible swelling may be found on the ventral surface of the penis or the perineum during voiding.

On a voiding cystourethrogram the urethra is usually dilated proximal to the diverticulum, which is seen as either a narrow or a wide-mouthed protrusion from the round or elongated urethral lumen (Fig. 19–292). The urethra distal to a wide-mouthed diverticulum may be narrow or invisible; if it is invisible, the distal lip of the diverticulum may be interpreted as the external urethral meatus and the diagnosis may be missed. Ultrasonography has been described as a method of visualizing acquired diverticula of the anterior urethra.[60] If a high-frequency small-parts scanner is used, it is reasonable to assume that the technique may also be of some use in evaluating selected cases of anterior urethral diverticula.

The third type of diverticulum in the floor of the anterior urethra is the scaphoid megalourethra (Fig. 19–293). The term megalourethra indicates that during voiding, the urethra is not only wide but also elongated. It has recently been recognized that scaphoid and fusiform megalourethra are at opposite ends of a single continuum, representing two versions of the same congenital anomaly.[49] Moreover, there can be intermediate lesions not precisely like either version. For descriptive purposes, each is discussed separately, although this fundamental kinship should always be borne in mind.

Scaphoid megalourethra describes a large defect in the corpus spongiosum. This produces a congenitally long penis with a completely flaccid ventral surface because there is no corpus spongiosum along that surface. When the patient voids, the anterior urethra swells through the defect in the ventral surface of the penis, and the penis elongates (Fig. 19–294).

Because both the corpora cavernosa are present, the roof of the anterior urethra is supported and does not bulge, causing the diverticulum to be scaphoid. The proximal and distal ends are funnel-shaped, with gently sloping walls, so there is no valvular obstruction.

Clinically, the anterior urethra in patients with scaphoid megalourethra can present in a wide spectrum of sizes, from almost normal to huge. Associated anomalies are listed in Table 19–31.

These patients should not be catheterized for a voiding cystourethrogram, since it is easy to introduce an infection not readily eradicated. Rather, the urethra can be outlined by asking the patient to void after an intravenous urogram, if the patient is old enough. In young patients, a suprapubic puncture can be performed and an antegrade voiding cystourethrogram can be obtained.

Table 19–31. Anomalies Associated with Scaphoid Megalourethra[41, 50–53]

Prune-belly syndrome (50%)[50–52]
Hypospadias[53]
Urethroperineal fistula
Dilated prostatic urethra
Bladder diverticula
Congenital reflux
Megaureters
Hypoplastic or dysplastic kidneys
Ventricular septal defects
Supernumerary digits[41, 50]

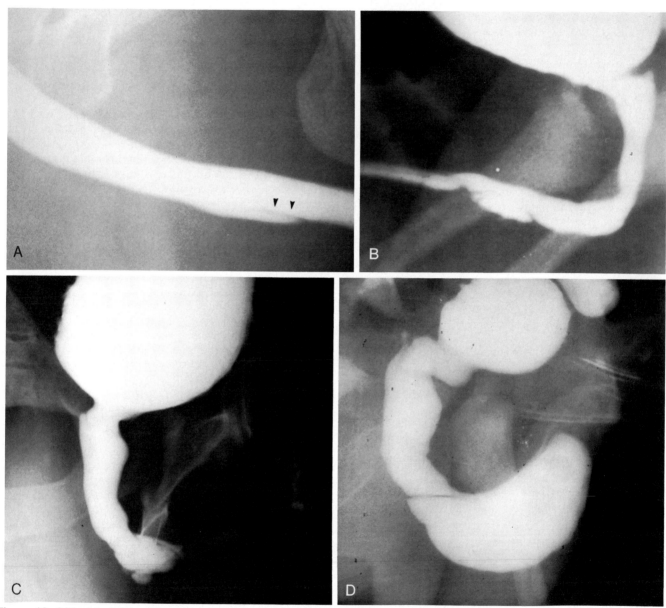

Figure 19–292. *A* to *F,* Five different patients, showing the range of appearances and sizes of saccular anterior urethral diverticula *(arrowheads* in *A, white arrow* in *F).* Note how in *D* the proximal flaplike edge of the diverticulum simulates a valve. *E* is a sonogram of patient in *D,* demonstrating an enormously thickened bladder and a dilated posterior urethra. In *F,* there is right-sided vesicoureteral reflux, and contrast material has extravasated from a ruptured fornix of a calyx *(open arrow)* into the perinephric space *(solid black arrow).* (*A, C,* courtesy Robert Mindelzun, M.D., Santa Clara Valley Medical Center, San Jose, California; *B, F,* from Kirks DR, Grossman H: Congenital saccular anterior urethral diverticulum. Radiology 140:367–372, 1981.)

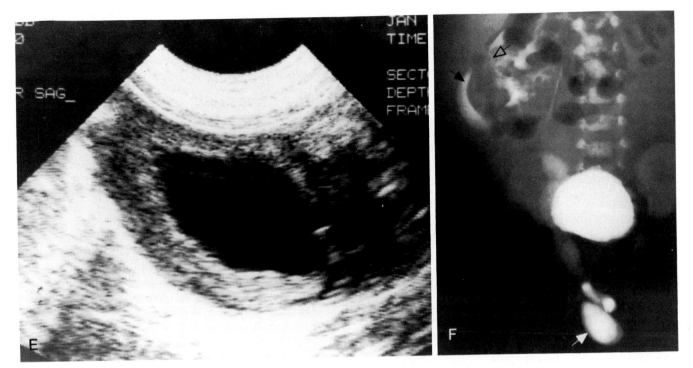

Figure 19–292 *Continued*

The mortality rate is about 20%, most often due to renal failure.

DIVERTICULA INVOLVING THE ENTIRE CIRCUMFERENCE OF THE ANTERIOR URETHRA: FUSIFORM MEGALOURETHRA

Fusiform megalourethra is a congenital anomaly involving the entire circumference of the anterior urethra. Large defects are present in the corpus spongiosum and in both corpora cavernosa (see Fig. 19–293).

Clinical Features. The entire penis is flabby, flaccid, and long. When the patient voids, the entire penis elongates and swells in a fusiform manner.

Associated Anomalies. Fusiform megalourethra is associated with covered exstrophy of the bladder and congenital rectovesical fistula, with usually fatal results.

Diagnostic Imaging. On a voiding cystourethrogram, the entire anterior urethra dilates in a fusiform manner. There is no valve or obstruction.

URETHRAL DIVERTICULA IN THE FEMALE

Urethral diverticula in the female are acquired and are discussed in Chapter 25.

Congenital Anomalies of the Periurethral Glands of Cowper

The paired Cowper's glands are imbedded in the urogenital diaphragm and drain into the proximal bend of the bulbous urethra through ducts that run distally immediately below and lateral to the bulbous urethra. On rare occasions, the normal duct and gland are visible on a voiding cystourethrogram (Fig. 19–295).

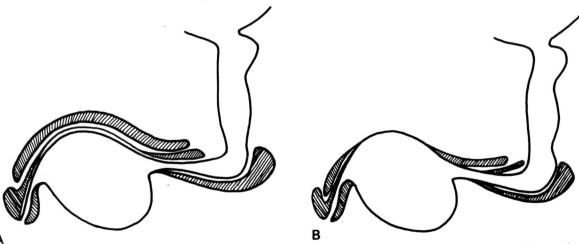

Figure 19–293. *A,* Scaphoid, and *B,* fusiform, types of megalourethra. In *A,* the corpus spongiosum is deficient, whereas in *B* both the corpus spongiosum and the corpora cavernosa are deficient. (Modified from Stephens FD: Congenital Malformations of the Urinary Tract. [Copyright © 1983 by Praeger Publishers, New York, a division of Greenwood Press, Inc. p 139].)

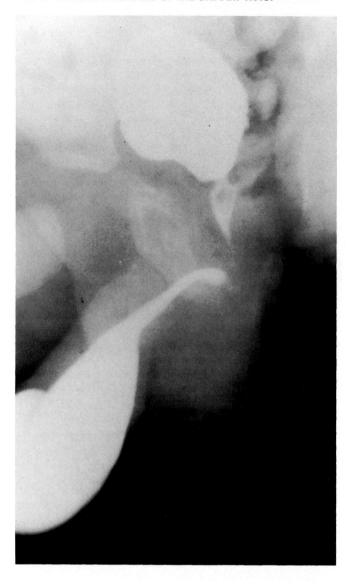

Figure 19–294. Megalourethra. A voiding cystourethrogram in a newborn male with a scaphoid megalourethra demonstrates enormous dilatation of the entire ventral surface of the distal (penile) urethra. The verumontanum is seen as a prominent filling defect in the prostatic urethra, but is probably within normal limits.

Three major kinds of congenital anomalies occur in Cowper's glands.[56] The first consists of an abnormally wide orifice of the gland, while the duct is abnormally dilated (Fig. 19–296). In the latter instance, the dilatation may be smooth or may have multiple lobulations and is called Cowper's syringocele. If the ducts are abnormally dilated, they may impinge upon the urethral lumen and partially obstruct the urethra. Second, there may be an abnormal entry of the duct into the back of the bulbous urethra (Fig. 19–296). Finally the orifice of the duct may be congenitally stenosed or occluded. If so, the duct dilates and presses on the lumen of the urethra.

A voiding cystourethrogram or retrograde urethrogram demonstrates a Cowper's syringocele (Figs. 19–297 and 19–298) or abnormal entry of the duct.[56, 57] If the orifice of the duct is stenosed or occluded, the radiological finding is a filling defect due to a mural lesion (the dilated duct) (Fig. 19–299).[58]

Congenital Urethral Atresia and Stenosis

Congenital atresia of the entire urethra is usually found in cases of the prune-belly syndrome.[54] Congenital atresia of the proximal urethra with a patent distal urethra may occur with bilateral renal agenesis[55] and with vesical

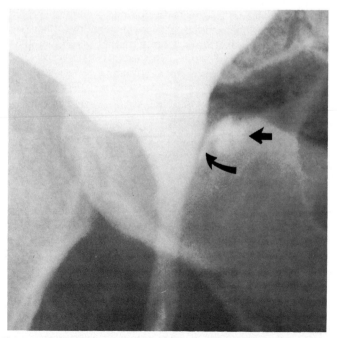

Figure 19–295. Normal Cowper's gland *(straight arrow)* and duct *(curved arrow)* are opacified during voiding cystourethrogram.

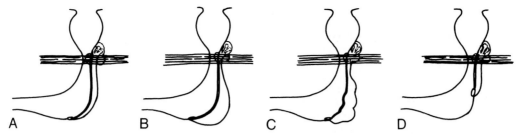

Figure 19–296. Cowper's gland and duct. *A* is normal. *B, C* show Cowper's syringocele. *D* shows abnormal entry site of the duct into the ventral aspect of the bulbous urethra. (Modified from Stephens FD: Congenital Malformations of the Urinary Tract. [Copyright © 1983 by Praeger Publishers, New York, a division of Greenwood Press, Inc. p 142].)

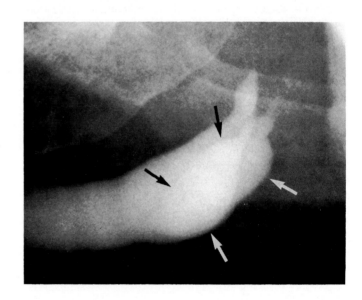

Figure 19–297. Retrograde urethrogram shows Cowper's syringocele *(arrows).*

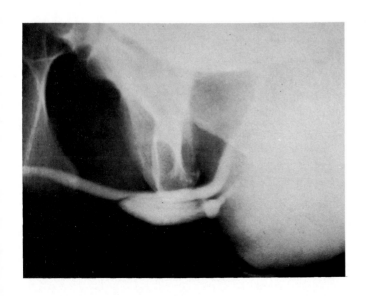

Figure 19–298. Voiding cystourethrogram demonstrates a Cowper's syringocele. (From Kirks DR, Grossman H: Congenital saccular anterior urethral diverticulum. Radiology 140:367–372, 1981.)

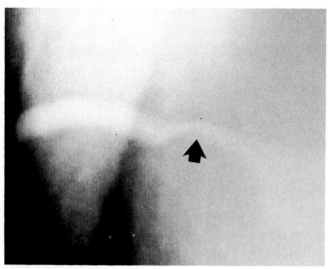

Figure 19–299. Filling defect in the urethra *(arrow)* due to a dilated, obstructed Cowper's duct. (From Redman JF, Rountree GA: Pronounced dilatation of Cowper's gland duct manifest as a perineal mass: A recommendation for management. J Urol 139:87–88, © Williams & Wilkins, 1988.)

agenesis. The patent distal portion of the urethra probably represents that part of the urethra derived from ectoderm.[55]

Congenital stenosis is found in the prune-belly syndrome[54] and some cases of congenital H-type anourethral fistula.[14] These congenital stenoses, however, are found at a very specific site: the junction of the anterior and posterior urethra. Strictures found elsewhere in the urethra are not congenital. Urethral meatal stenosis is rarely, if ever, congenital. It is seen almost exclusively in circumcised males, as a result of recurrent animoniacal meatitis.

References

1. Glenister TW: The origin of the urethral plate in man. J Anat (London) 88:413–425, 1954.
2. Glenister TW: Development of the penile urethra in the pig. J Anat (London) 90:461–477, 1956.
3. Van der Putte SCJ, Neetson FA: The normal development of the anorectum in the pig. Acta Morphol Neerl-Scand 21:107–132, 1983.
4. Van der Putte SCJ: Normal and abnormal development of the anorectum. J Pediatr Surg 21:434–440, 1986.
5. Effman EL, Lebowitz RL, Colodny AH: Duplication of the urethra. Radiology 119:179–185, 1976.
6. Woodhouse CRJ, Williams DL: Duplications of the lower urinary tract in children. Br J Urol 51:481–487, 1979.
7. Das S, Brosman SA: Duplication of the male urethra. J Urol 117:452–454, 1977.
8. Stephens FD: Congenital malformations of the urinary tract. New York, Praeger, 1983, pp 22–24.
9. Veeraraghaven KA, Gonzales ET Jr, Gibbons D, et al: Cloacal duplication: Genitourinary and lower intestinal implications. J Urol 129:389–391, 1983.
10. Psihramis KE, Colodny AH, Lebowitz RL, et al: Complete patent duplication of the urethra. J Urol 136:63–67, 1986.
11. Dunetz GN, Bauer SB: Complete duplication of bladder and urethra. Urology 25:179–182, 1985.
12. Williams DI, Bloomberg S: Bifid urethra with preanal accessory tract (Y duplication). Br J Urol 47:877–882, 1976.
13. Stephens FD, Donnellan WL: "H-type" urethro-anal fistula. J Pediatr Surg 12:95–102, 1977.
14. deVries PA, Friedland GW: Congenital "H-type" anourethral fistula. Radiology 113:397, 1974.
15. Lawrence D, Howard ER, Harris RF: A case of congenital urethral duplication cyst and its embryological significance. Br J Surg 70:565–566, 1983.
16. Schulze KA, Pfister RR, Ramsley PG: Urethral duplication and complete bladder exstrophy. J Urol 133:276–278, 1985.
17. Fernbach SK, Maizels M: Posterior urethral valves causing urinary retention in an infant with duplication of the urethra. J Urol 132:353–355, 1984.
18. Redman JF, Robinson CM: Anterior urethral polyp in a child. J Pediatr Surg 12:735–737, 1977.
19. Patten BM, Barry A: The genesis of exstrophy of the bladder and epispadias. Am J Anat 90:35–57, 1952.
20. Gray SW, Skandalakis JE: Embryology for surgeons. Philadelphia, WB Saunders Company, 1972, p. 548.
21. Friedland GW, Stamey TA: Recurrent urinary tract infection with persistent wolffian duct masquerading as duplicated urethra. Urology 4:315–318, 1974.
22. Bellinger MF, Duckett JW: Accessory phallic urethra in the female patient. J Urol 127:1159–1164, 1982.
23. Hurwitz RS, Fitzpatrick TY: Vaginal urethra, clitoral hypertrophy, and accessory phallic urethra: A rare syndrome of female pseudohermaphroditism. J Urol 127:1165–1168, 1982.
24. Feins NR, Cranley WR: Urethral duplication with the dorsal urethra presenting as a perineal mass. J Pediatr Surg 17:743–744, 1982.
25. Sotolongo JR Jr, Gribetz ME, Saphir RL, Begun GR: Female phallic urethra and persistent cloaca. J Urol 130:1186–1187, 1983.
26. Zattoni F, Gennari T, Rovasio A: Y-type urethral triplication. Br J Urol 54:195, 1982.
27. Schmeller NT, Schirmer HKA: Trifurcation of the urethra: A case report. J Urol 127:545–546, 1982.
28. Downs RA: Congenital polyps of the prostatic urethra. Br J Urol 42:76–85, 1970.
29. De Wolf WC, Fraley EE: Congenital urethral polyp in the infant: Case report and review of the literature. J Urol 109:515–516, 1973.
30. Kimche D, Lask D: Congenital polyp of the prostatic urethra. J Urol 127:134, 1982.
31. Dalena B, Vanneuville G, Vincent L, Fabre JL: Congenital polyp of the posterior urethra and vesical calculus in a boy. J Urol 128:1034–1035, 1982.
32. Eakins M, Crooks KK: Congenital polyp of the verumontanum. Urol Radiol 4:49–50, 1982.
33. Zulian RAS, Brito RR, Borges HJ: Transurethral resection of pedunculated congenital polyps of the posterior urethra. Br J Urol 54:45–48, 1982.
34. Vereecken RL, Dewaele HM, Marshall GJ, Baert AC: Pedunculated polyp of posterior urethra in a child. Br J Urol 55:575–576, 1983.
35. Hutchinson I, McGeorge A, Garland L, Abel BJ: Congenital urethral polyp in an adult. Br J Urol 55:576–577, 1983.
36. Stephens FD: Congenital malformations of the urinary tract. New York, Praeger, pp 105–106, 1983.
37. Redman JF, Robinson CM: Anterior urethral polyp in a child. J Pediatr Surg 12:735–737, 1977.
38. Sommer JT, Stephens FD: Dorsal urethral diverticulum of the fossa navicularis; symptoms, diagnosis, and treatment. J Urol 124:94–97, 1980.
39. Duszlak EJ Jr, Bellinger MF, Boal DK, Stanford A: Dorsal diverticulum of the distal male urethra. AJR 138:931–933, 1982.
40. Bellinger MF, Purohit GS, Duckett JW, Cromie WJ: Lacuna magna: A hidden cause of dysuria and bloody spotting in boys. J Pediatr Surg 18:163–166, 1983.
41. Stephens FD: Congenital malformations of the urinary tract. New York, Praeger, 1983, pp 22–24.
42. Netto NR, Lemos GC, Claro JF de A, Hering FLO: Congenital diverticulum of male urethra. Urology 24:239–242, 1984.
43. Lima SVC, Pereira CS: Giant diverticulum of the anterior urethra. Br J Urol 56:335–336, 1984.
44. Kirks DR, Grossman H: Congenital saccular anterior urethral diverticulum. Radiology 140:367–372, 1981.
45. Kirks DR: Practical pediatric imaging: Diagnostic radiology of infants and children. Boston, Little, Brown & Company, 1986, pp 728–730.
46. Baker AR, Neoptolemas JP, Wood KF: Congenital anterior urethral diverticulum: A rare cause of lower urinary tract obstruction in childhood. J Urol 134:751–752, 1985.
47. Smith SEW: Unexpected anterior urethral diverticula. Clin Radiol 37:55–58, 1986.
48. Tank ES: Anterior urethral valves resulting from congenital urethral diverticula. Urology 30:467–469, 1987.

49. Appel RA, Kaplan GW, Brock WA, Streit D: Megalourethra. J Urol 135:747–751, 1986.
50. Shrom SH, Cromie WJ, Duckett JW Jr: Megalourethra. Urology 17:152–156, 1981.
51. Sellers BB Jr, McNeal R, Smith RV, et al: Congenital megalourethra associated with prune-belly syndrome. Urology 116:814–815, 1976.
52. Kroovand RL, Al-Ansari RM, Perlmutter AD: Urethral and genital malformations in prune-belly syndrome. J Urol 127:94–96, 1982.
53. Wilson JA, Walker RD III: Megalourethra and hypospadias. J Urol 129:556–557, 1983.
54. Berdon WE, Baker DH, Wigger HJ, Blank WA: The radiologic and pathologic spectrum of the prune-belly syndrome. The importance of urethral obstruction in prognosis. Radiol Clin North Am 15:83–92, 1977.
55. Katz SM, Chatten J: The urethra in bilateral renal agenesis. Arch Pathol 97:269–270, 1974.
56. Maizels M, Stephens FD, King LR, Firlit CF: Cowper's syringocele: A classification of dilatations of Cowper's duct based upon clinical characteristics of eight boys. J Urol 129:111, 1983.
57. Sant GR, Kaleli A: Cowper's syringocele causing incontinence in an adult. J Urol 133:279–280, 1985.
58. Redman JF, Rountree GA: Pronounced dilatation of Cowper's gland duct manifest as a perineal mass: A recommendation for management. J Urol 139:87–88, 1988.
59. King LR: Editorial comment. J Urol 128:378, 1982.
60. Kauzlaric D, Barmeir E, Peyer P, Tschuor S: Sonographic appearance of urethral diverticulum in the male. J Ultrasound Med 7:107, 1988.
61. Caro P, Rosenberg H, Snyder HM: Congenital Urethral Polyp. AJR 147:1041, 1986.
62. Schmidt JD: Congenital urethral duplication. J Urol 105:397–399, 1971.
63. Linsenmeyer TA, Friedland GW: Duplicated urethra communicating with the seminal vesicle. Urol Radiol 10:210–212, 1988.

CONGENITAL ANOMALIES OF THE MALE GENITALIA

CLASSIFICATION OF CONGENITAL ANOMALIES OF THE MALE GENITALIA

Table 19–32 shows the classification of the major congenital anomalies of the male genitalia.

CONGENITAL ANOMALIES OF THE PROSTATE GLAND

Embryology

In an adult, the prostate is divided into a glandular portion and the anterior fibromuscular portion.[1] The glandular portion is further divided into the peripheral zone, the central zone, and the transitional zone.[1] In the early embryos of humans and experimental animals, when the ducts of the various lobes are traced to the urethral openings, it is apparent the prostate develops from five lobes that later fuse into the three adult zones.[2, 3] This typically occurs in fetuses between 50 and 55 mm[2, 3] and is largely caused by the mesenchyme of the urogenital sinus, which plays a dominant role in the interaction necessary to the development of the prostate.[4–6] The mesenchymal cells induce the urethral epithelium to form various ducts.[4–6] They are largely responsible for the way cells differentiate in order to form the prostate.[4–6]

The five lobes in the embryonic prostate[3, 7, 8] are as follows: (1) those arising from the rectal surface of the urethra above the orifices of the wolffian ducts (the middle lobe); (2) those arising from the rectal surface below the wolffian ducts (the posterior lobe); (3 and 4) those arising from the right and left lateral walls of the urethra (the right and left lateral lobes); and (5) those arising from the ventral walls of the urethra (the anterior lobe). These lobes and their associated branching tubules are most pronounced at the 16-week stage or when they are about 125 mm, at which time an average of 63 tubules open into the urethra. The medial, lateral, and posterior lobes

fuse, and give rise to the various adult zones. The anterior lobe atrophies in the fetus after the 16th week and forms the anterior fibromuscular zone of the prostate.

Table 19–32. Classification of Congenital Anomalies of the Male Genitalia

I. Congenital anomalies of the prostate
A. Hypoplasia
B. Utriculus (vagina) masculinus
C. Müllerian duct cyst
D. Congenital prostatic cysts
II. Congenital anomalies of the ejaculatory ducts
A. Congenital diverticulum
B. Congenital cyst
III. Congenital anomalies of the seminal vesicles
A. Anomalies in number
1. Agenesis
2. Duplication
B. Anomalies of position
1. Ectopia
2. Crossed ectopia
C. Anomalies of form or structure
1. Ectopic ureter entering seminal vesicle
2. Congenital diverticulum
3. Congenital cyst
IV. Congenital anomalies of the vas deferens
A. Anomalies in number
1. Congenital absence
2. Double or bifid vas
B. Anomalies of position
1. Congenital vasoureteral communication
2. Other types of ectopic vas
V. Congenital anomalies of the testis
A. Anomalies in size
1. Rudimentary testis
2. Congenitally large testis
B. Anomalies in number
1. Monorchia
2. Polyorchia
C. Anomalies of position
1. Undescended testis
D. Anomalies of form
1. Splenogonadal fusion

Congenital Hypoplasia

Congenital prostatic hypoplasia is most often seen in prune-belly syndrome.[9-13, 123] It is more fully discussed in that section (see page 771). Briefly, recent studies show that some prostatic tissue always remains in prune-belly syndrome, although earlier studies alleged the possibility of complete agenesis. In the posterior glandular part of the prostate, prostatic tubules are present in about 15% of cases; anteriorly, where smooth muscle should have developed, connective tissue predominates. The verumontanum is small or completely absent, and instead of projecting into the lumen it may project outward as a small dimple. The prostatic utricle is sometimes enlarged.

Embryology

Congenital hypoplasia of the prostate is most often due to a defect of the mesenchyme surrounding the urethra. It may also arise from urethral obstruction distal to the developing prostate.

Diagnostic Imaging

The prostatic urethra is usually dilated and elongated on a voiding cystourethrogram. A diverticulum-like projection may arise from the posterior wall of the prostatic urethra.

Congenitally Large Prostatic Utricle (Utriculus Masculinus)

All males have a tiny prostatic utricle, which is generally not visible on a voiding cystourethrogram or on genitography. It can become visibly enlarged in cases of hypospadias, ambiguous genitalia, undescended testis, or congenital urethral polyp. It is called a prostatic utricle or utriculus masculinus if no cervix or uterus is attached; if a uterus or cervix is attached, this structure is a vagina masculina.

Embryology

It is likely that the prostatic utricle develops from the müllerian ducts, the wolffian ducts, and the epithelium of the urogenital sinus. The cranial portion develops from the müllerian ducts, and the caudal portion from the wolffian ducts and the urogenital sinus.

At the end of the embryonic period, at approximately 60 days, the two terminal ends of the müllerian ducts fuse. They unite, via a solid cord of cells called the vaginal plate, with the urogenital sinus at the müllerian tubercle, between the orifices of the wolffian ducts.

In male fetuses, at about the 45-mm stage, the Sertoli cells of the developing testicles secrete antimüllerian factor (AMF), as a result of which the cranial portion of the müllerian ducts involute.[14, 15] The lowest duct remnant persists as a shorter, well-defined tube, which unites with the posterior wall of the urogenital sinus via the solid cord of cells described above. This cord is now called the utricular plate in the male.

The wolffian duct epithelium grows over the urogenital sinus epithelium of the müllerian tubercle. In embryos of about 65 mm, two sinoutricular bulbs develop from the surface epithelium of the müllerian tubercle. These bulbs grow toward the utricular plate, fusing at the midline at about the 90-mm stage to form the sinoutricular cord.

The urethrovaginal segment of the fused müllerian ducts develops a lumen, which lies entirely within the prostate. At about 150 mm, the solid cord develops a lumen, which communicates with the prostatic urethra. This cord is believed to arise from the wolffian ducts, the urogenital sinus, and the müllerian ducts.

By 175 mm, the utricle is huge and extends to the prostatic capsule. Glandular buds extend out from the caudal portion near its opening into the urethra; these buds eventually form the central zone of the prostate.

The development of the prostate and the tubularized penis depends on the presence of a hormone called 5-α reductase, which converts testosterone to dihydrotestosterone.[8, 16, 17] This hormone develops from the urogenital sinus mesoblast. A variable deficiency in this enzyme may account for a spectrum of cases, ranging from hypospadias associated with an enlarged prostatic utricle to severe hypospadias associated with severe enlargement of the utricle.

Grades

Three grades of congenitally large prostatic utricle are identified, varying with position and size (Fig. 19–300).[18] Grades 0, I, and II open in the center of the verumontanum; Grade III opens in the bulbous urethra. Grade 0 does not extend above the verumontanum. Grade I is above the verumontanum but short of the bladder neck, and grade II extends above the bladder neck.

In patients with hypospadias, the prostatic utricle is more likely to be congenitally large and the grade of enlargement higher, as the severity of the hypospadias increases. About 15% of patients with glandular hypospadias, 20% with penile hypospadias, 30% with penoscrotal hypospadias, and 40% with perineal and scrotal hypospadias have an enlarged prostatic utricle. Those with glandular and penile hypospadias usually have utricles of Grades 0 to I; those with penoscrotal hypospadias usually have Grades 0 to II; those with scrotal hypospadias have Grades 0 to II and occasionally III; those with perineal hypospadias usually have Grade III congenitally enlarged prostatic utricle.

Differential Diagnosis

Enlarged prostatic utricle is often confused with müllerian duct cyst. Although both are congenital, the utricle is usually discovered before the age of 20 years, since the patient has abnormal genitalia. Patients with müllerian duct cysts have normal external genitalia, and do not usually present clinically until above the age of 20 years. If it is necessary to excise the utricle, moreover, it is generally less difficult to do so than to excise a müllerian duct cyst.

Complications

Complications are rare, because the utricle is usually incidental; however, persistent infections or stones may develop.

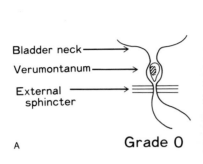

Bladder neck
Verumontanum
External sphincter

Grade 0

A

Figure 19–300. *A–H,* Classification of congenitally large prostatic utricle by urethrography. (From Ikoma F, Shima H, Yabumoto H: Classification of enlarged prostatic utricle in patients with hypospadias. Br J Urol 57:334–337, 1985.)

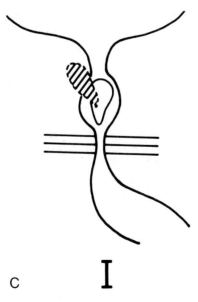

C

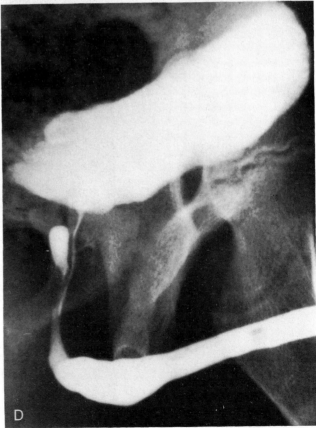

B

D

Illustration continued on following page

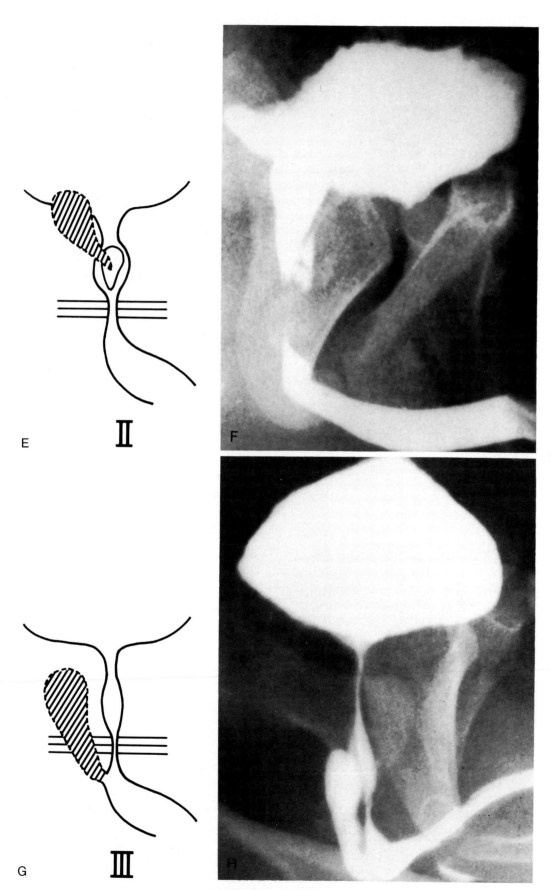

E   II

F

G   III

H

Figure 19–300 *Continued*

Diagnostic Imaging

It is often easy to outline a utricle on a voiding cystourethrogram, but some cases may require a flushing technique on genitography. Direct catheterization of a prominent utricle through the cystoscope is feasible in selected cases.

The structure appears as a tubular projection extending cephalad from the middle of the verumontanum, except in rare Grade III cases where the utricle extends from the bulbous urethra. Whatever the grade, there is always a typical dome-shaped fundus; if the fundus has a cervical indentation, the structure is a vagina masculina. This is discussed in the section on ambiguous genitalia (see page 779).

Müllerian Duct Cyst (Cyst of the Prostatic Utricle)

Müllerian duct cyst is a single midline cyst arising behind the verumontanum and extending above the base of the prostate.[19-24] It occasionally communicates with the urethra at the verumontanum, where a typical beaklike projection appears at the inferior edge of the cyst.

Müllerian duct cysts are shaped like an inverted pear or a simple oval (Fig. 19–301). They may vary significantly in volume, from only a few milliliters to several liters; the fluid may be serous, mucoid or purulent, and the colors are brown, yellow, or green. Unlike seminal vesical cysts with which they are sometimes confused, they contain neither spermatozoa nor fructose.

Embryology

The most likely explanation for the development of a müllerian duct cyst is that prostatic secretions from the

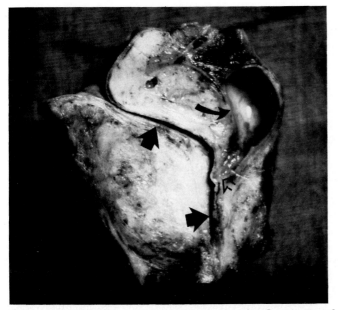

Figure 19–301. Cyst of the prostatic utricle. Specimen of prostate opened sagittally shows a müllerian duct cyst, which is shaped like an inverted pear *(curved arrow)* and ends with a typical beaklike projection at the verumontanum *(open arrow)*. The urethra *(broad arrows)* angulates anteriorly at its midpoint at an angle of about 45 degrees. (Courtesy John McNeal, M.D., Division of Urology, Stanford University.)

middle-lobe ducts and acini that arise from the sinoutricular plate become blocked because the plate was not canalized.[25] This leads to cystic dilatation of the utricle but is a different process than that causing enlarged prostatic utricle.[25] Its difference explains why patients with cysts of the prostatic utricle do not have associated anomalies of the external genitalia and why cysts of the prostatic utricle develop after the onset of puberty.[25]

Clinical Features

Patients present over the age of 20 years with symptoms mimicking those of benign prostatic hyperplasia. The patient complains of frequency and a decrease in the size and force of the stream. A very large cyst may push the bladder base and urethra upward and forward, causing acute retention.

A rectal examination shows a cystic mass at the midline above the base of the prostate. The characteristic feature is a midline mass, unlike seminal vesicle cyst, which would be located on either side, or a prostatic cyst, which lies within the prostate. This is the only cyst in the area that can be at the midline, except an ejaculatory duct cyst, which is rare, or an atypical prostatic cyst.

There are usually no associated anomalies.

Complications

Complications include stones, characteristically located behind the bladder and urethra. Müllerian duct cyst is the only condition in which stones occur in this position. The exception is the remnant of a rectourethral fistula, left behind after surgery.

An increased incidence of carcinoma, either adenocarcinoma or squamous cell carcinoma, may be associated with müllerian duct cyst.

The structure is not easily removed surgically, because it is near the pelvic nerves. If damaged, they may affect bladder function and erections.

Diagnostic Imaging

An intravenous urogram reveals normal upper urinary tracts. However, if the cyst is large enough, a rectovesical midline mass is apparent, causing anterior and sometimes cranial displacement of the bladder.

An excellent method of imaging a müllerian duct cyst is by means of transrectal ultrasonography, using a radial or linear array transducer. The latter generally provides more information, since it can produce images in the sagittal plane (Fig. 19–302).

A central pear-shaped cystic mass extends cephalad from the verumontanum. It may be possible to see a small stalklike projection pointing in the direction of the verumontanum.

A müllerian duct cyst is also visible on CT or MRI. With its extreme contrast sensitivity in the detection of fluid collections, MRI promises to become an important method of imaging these lesions (Fig. 19–303).

Congenital Prostatic Cysts

Congenital prostatic cysts are usually small, are sometimes seen incidentally on transrectal prostatic ultraso-

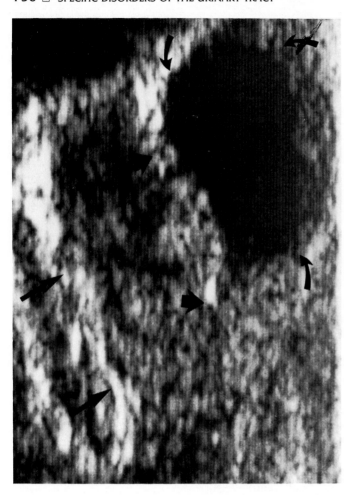

Figure 19–302. Transrectal sonogram, performed with a linear array transducer, showing a hypoechoic müllerian duct cyst *(curved arrows)*, which has a typical beaklike projection at the inferior edge of the cyst, near the verumontanum. Short arrows point to the urethra. Long arrows point to the prostatic capsule.

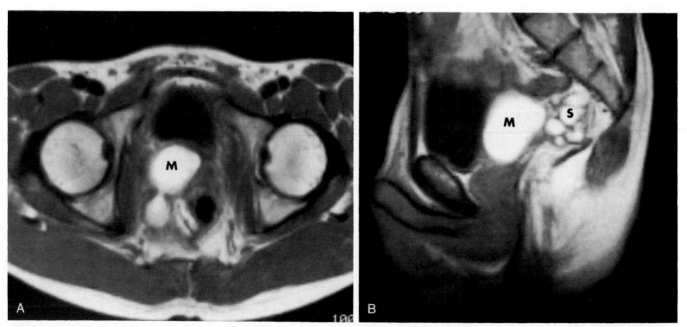

Figure 19–303. Hemorrhagic müllerian duct cyst with hemorrhage into the right seminal vesicle. MRI at 0.35 T. *A,* Axial T1-weighted image (TR = 500 msec, TE = 30 msec) shows a large cystic mass (M) anterior and superior to the right seminal vesicle (S). The lesion and the right seminal vesicle show high-signal intensity on the T1-weighted image, consistent with subacute blood. *B,* Sagittal view is shown. (From Higgins CB, Hricak H: Magnetic Resonance Imaging of the Body. New York, Raven Press, 1988.)

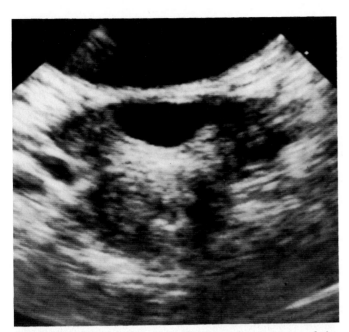

Figure 19–304. Prostatic cyst. Transrectal sonogram of the prostate gland in the axial plane demonstrates the typical sonographic appearance of fluid within a cyst of the prostate located posteriorly in the midline. The differential diagnosis would include a cyst of the utricle. Müllerian duct cysts are usually situated cranial to the prostate.

nography, and result from focal dilatation of prostatic ducts. Large cysts are rare. Prostatic cysts may be acquired.

They usually occur on either side of the midline, although they commonly cannot be palpated unless they are large; paradoxically, they may feel hard on palpation and may mimic prostatic carcinoma.

Transrectal sonography is the best method for demonstrating prostatic cysts (Fig. 19–304). If present, they are well defined, exhibit no internal echoes, and transmit sound well.[26] They are usually small; if large, they can sometimes be aspirated under sonographic control. Characteristically, there are no spermatozoa in the fluid.

Large prostatic cysts may be visible on CT or MRI. An intravenous urogram or voiding cystourethrogram is usually negative, except when large cysts displace the bladder upward, forward, and to the opposite side. They may displace the urethra toward the opposite side and forward.

Seminal vesiculography was formerly the diagnostic method of choice for examining large cysts, but transrectal ultrasonography has supplanted it.

CONGENITAL ANOMALIES OF THE EJACULATORY DUCT

The only important anomaly is a diverticulum or cyst (the urogenital sinus cyst).[27, 28] The three types are as follows: (1) both ejaculatory ducts enter a single midline cyst; (2) bilateral cysts or diverticula arise from both ejaculatory ducts; and (3) unilateral diverticulum or cyst arises from one of the ejaculatory ducts.

Symptoms are those of acute prostatitis, but may include hemospermia or painful ejaculation. A cystic mass is palpable just above the base of the prostate on a rectal examination.

Diagnostic Imaging

In most reported cases, seminal vesiculograms have been obtained, but the cyst is also demonstrated on transrectal ultrasonography or CT. If transrectal ultrasonography is available, the cyst can be punctured under sonographic control, aspirated, filled with contrast material, and adequately outlined on a subsequent radiograph.

CONGENITAL ANOMALIES OF THE SEMINAL VESICLES

Embryology

The seminal vesicles first appear in fetuses of about 80 mm in length (at 13 weeks) as small lateral outpouchings of the lower end of the wolffian ducts, just above the base of the prostate. During the following week they grow significantly, and by the 19th week (170 mm) the lower end of the wolffian ducts dilates to form the ampullae of the vas deferens. At this stage, each seminal vesicle has 3 to 8 sacculations, but by 25 weeks (220 mm), the vas deferens is well developed, and the seminal vesicles and ampullas approach their adult appearance.

The virilization of the wolffian ducts to form the vas deferens and seminal vesicles is largely caused by testosterone. Thus the seminal vesicles are normal in testicular feminization and in the Reifenstein syndrome.

An absent kidney and absent seminal vesicle on the same side may occur for one of two reasons: (1) The nephric duct fails to grow down to the level at which the ureteral bud would arise, in which case the kidney, the seminal vesicle, and the trigone would not develop on that side. (2) The wolffian duct grows to the cloaca, but produces neither a ureteral bud nor a seminal vesicle.

If the ureteral bud arises from the wolffian duct but the seminal vesicle does not, an absent seminal vesicle and a normal kidney may be on the same side.

Anomalies in Number

Agenesis and Duplication

The seminal vesicles can be congenitally absent on one or both sides (see Fig. 19–47).[29–33] Patients with bilateral agenesis characteristically have a volume of ejaculate less than 1.5 ml. Unilateral agenesis is often an incidental finding on CT or transrectal ultrasonography performed for some other purpose. However, it may occur in patients with renal agenesis, congenital absence of the vas, or congenital vasoureteral communications.

The seminal vesicles may be duplicated and are often discovered in the same way.

The diagnosis of both types of anomaly can be made by means of CT,[29] MRI,[32] or transrectal ultrasonography.[33] Seminal vesiculography is not required.

Anomalies in Position: Ectopia

Anomalies of position include ectopia, and, in particular, crossed ectopia. This may be associated with renal

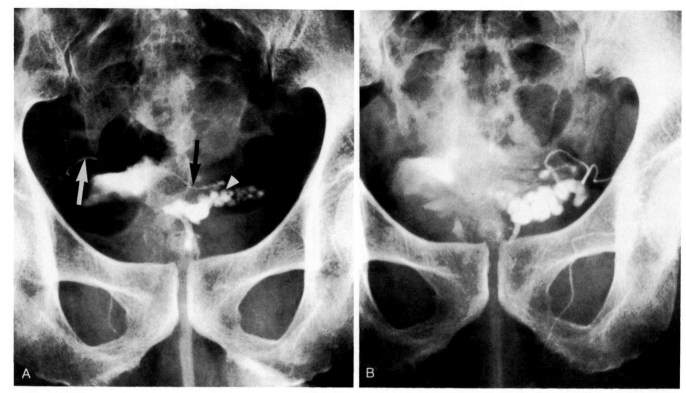

Figure 19–305. Crossed ectopia of the right seminal vesicle. *A,* Right vasovesiculogram shows that the right vas deferens crosses over to the left side *(arrows)* and empties into a seminal vesicle on the left *(arrowhead). B,* Left vasovesiculogram shows a normal-appearing left vas deferens and seminal vesicle. (From Wakatsuki A, Oda T, Ochi K: Case profile: Crossed ectopia of seminal vesicles and blind-ending ureter. Urology 24:291–292, 1984.)

agenesis on the same side, or with an ectopic ureter entering a common duct for the ureter and the seminal vesicles.[34]

Ectopia is usually demonstrated by ultrasonography or CT, but a seminal vesiculogram may sometimes be necessary for confirmation (Fig. 19–305).

Anomalies of Form or Structure

An ectopic ureter can enter a common duct with the seminal vesicle (Fig. 19–306) (described in the section on

single ectopic ureters in the male, page 692), or diverticula can occur in the seminal vesicle, usually discovered incidentally on a seminal vesiculogram.

Congenital Seminal Vesicle Cyst

Congenital seminal vesicle cysts are usually unilocular, but may, rarely, be multilocular.[31, 35–40] They involve one or more convolutions of the seminal vesicle, or the entire organ. Usually, they are unilateral, although they may be bilateral. They may be small or large with huge cysts that fill the entire pelvis.[40]

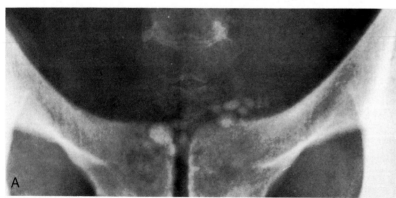

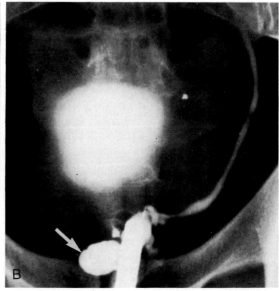

Figure 19–306. Ectopic left ureter terminating in a left common duct with the seminal vesicle. *A,* Preliminary radiograph of the pelvis shows calculi in the left common duct and the left seminal vesicle, which extends over to the right. *B,* Transurethral injection of contrast material into the left common duct outlines the left seminal vesicle, which extends over to the right *(arrow),* as well as the distal end of the left ectopic ureter.

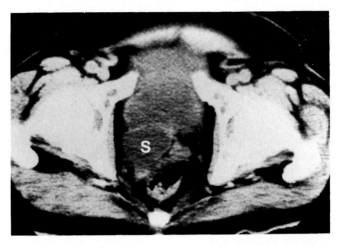

Figure 19–307. Seminal vesicle cyst in a patient with renal agenesis. CT section through the pelvis in a 15-year-old boy with right renal agenesis demonstrates a cystic malformation, incorporating the right seminal vesicle (S). The cystic mass actually represents a dysplasia of the common excretory duct, involving the anlagen of both the right seminal vesicle and the abortive ureteral bud. There was no kidney on this side.

The cysts may be lined by stratified or low cuboidal epithelium. Macroscopically, they are filled with red cells, nonmobile spermatozoa, white cells, and epithelial cells.

CLINICAL FEATURES

Patients have been ages 15 through 60 years at the time of diagnosis, with the peak incidence occurring between the ages of 20 and 30 years.

If the cyst is small, symptoms are usually absent. If the cyst is large, it may irritate the bladder, causing frequency and urgency. It may also obstruct the bladder, causing difficulty in voiding, or it may obstruct the vas, causing pain on ejaculation.

On rectal examination, a cystic mass can be palpated above the prostate on one side of the midline.

ASSOCIATED ANOMALIES

Anomalies associated with seminal vesicle cysts are always ipsilateral and include renal agenesis, absent ureter and trigone, and a fibrous band or dilated blind-ending ureter instead of a normal ureter. This close association between seminal vesical cysts and renal agenesis or dysgenesis has been emphasized in many published reports.[125] Not as well appreciated, however, is the fact that such cysts may occur in the presence of healthy kidneys and ureters.

DIAGNOSTIC IMAGING

Ultrasonography, transabdominal or transrectal, depending on available equipment, is the method of choice for diagnostic imaging.[36–38]

If the cyst is large enough, it is possible to puncture it under sonographic control using the suprapubic, transperineal, or even endoscopic approach. Vasovesiculography is an alternate route of opacification. The cyst may be aspirated and injected with contrast material, at which point it is clearly outlined—usually as a small, single, smooth, and round cyst. On rare occasions, it can be multilocular, as shown on ultrasonography, and several injections and punctures may be needed to visualize it. Contrast material may outline a typical-appearing seminal vesicle, or a structure only remotely resembling one. A vas deferens may or may not be identifiable. Seminal vesicle cysts are rarely bilateral; if they are, bilateral punctures may be required.

During sonographic examination for seminal vesicle cysts, possible renal agenesis on the affected side can be assessed.

CT (Fig. 19–307; see also Fig. 19–48)[31, 37–40] or MRI demonstrates renal agenesis and the presence of the cyst or cysts, but is more expensive, elaborate, and not necessarily more sensitive than ultrasonography.

The intravenous urogram is the least sensitive examination. Since the cyst is typically small, the intravenous urogram is usually normal or shows one absent kidney on the affected side. On rare occasions when the seminal vesicle cyst is large enough, it may displace the bladder upward, forward, and to the opposite side; these effects may be visible on an intravenous urogram.

CONGENITAL ANOMALIES OF THE VAS DEFERENS

Anomalies of Number

Congenital Absence of the Vas

This congenital anomaly is bilateral in 80% of cases; the bilateral form accounts for 1% to 2% of all cases of sterility in men.[41–44] A common cause of bilateral congenital absence of the vas is cystic fibrosis.[41]

This congenital anomaly is unilateral in 20% of cases, affecting, for some unknown reason, the left side four times more often than the right.[44]

When the vas is absent, the ejaculatory duct is absent. The seminal vesicle itself is not necessarily absent,[126] and it may be cystic or rudimentary. The tail and body of the epididymis is absent, but not the head.[45]

ASSOCIATED ANOMALIES

Bilateral congenital absence is associated with cystic fibrosis (as noted previously),[41] single-system ectopic ureteroceles, and bilateral intra-abdominal testes.[46] If the vas is unilaterally absent, 50% of cases are associated with congenital anomalies of the kidney or ureter on the same side or both sides. These may include renal agenesis, renal ectopia (simple, crossed, or fused), horseshoe kidney, polycystic kidneys, or single ectopic ureter.[43]

If a patient undergoing vasectomy has a renal abnormality on one side, and if no vas is palpable on that side, the vasectomy need only be unilateral; incisions on the opposite side are unnecessary.

DIAGNOSTIC IMAGING

Diagnostic imaging is usually not necessary, because the clinician can palpate the absence of the vas. If necessary, the absence can be confirmed if CT is performed with 4-mm sections, or with MRI. If infertility is present, however, further evaluation by vasovesiculography may be indicated if a portion of the vas can be located.

An intravenous urogram, CT, or ultrasonography shows the associated anomalies described previously. Unless there are compelling reasons to do otherwise, excretory urography should be performed in all men for whom one or both vasa cannot be palpated.

Double or Bifid Vas

This is a rare congenital anomaly, associated with an absence of the kidney and with multiple testes on the same side.

Anomalies of Position

Congenital Vasoureteral Communication (Persisting Mesonephric Duct; High Junction of Vas and Ureter)

This is a rare congenital anomaly in which the vas joins the ureter.[46–48] The resulting structure is also called a persisting mesonephric duct,[49] which can open anywhere from the normal position of the ureteral orifice in the lateral angle of the trigone to the verumontanum. The anomaly may be unilateral or bilateral.

Histologically, the persisting mesonephric duct is exactly the same as the ureter above the point of junction of the vas. The seminal vesicle on the same side is always absent.

In most cases the vas joins the ureter just above the base of the bladder (Figs. 19–308 and 19–309). However, it may join at the ureteropelvic junction or lower down, just above the common iliac artery.

EMBRYOLOGY

The most likely reason for the development of congenital vasoureteral communications is that the wolffian duct, which gives rise to the epididymis, the ureteral bud, and the seminal vesicles, develops aberrant structures in one place or another.

A number of theories have been developed to explain why these aberrant structures form, but the facts remain scarce.

ASSOCIATED ANOMALIES

Associated anomalies include anorectal malformations, blind-ending distal ureter, ureteral valve above the junction, ureteropelvic junction obstruction or atresia, bifid urethra, vesicoureteral reflux, and renal ectopia.

The kidney on the same side is always hypoplastic or dysplastic. If that kidney is completely obstructed, the

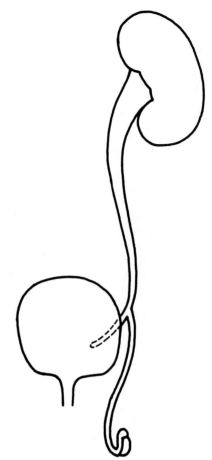

Figure 19–308. Illustration of a left vasoureteral communication. (Modified from Aaronson IA, Cremin BJ: Clinical paediatric uroradiology. Edinburgh, Churchill Livingstone, p 161, 1984.)

result is either multicystic renal dysplasia or a completely nondescript small solid piece of tissue.

DIAGNOSTIC IMAGING

Findings on an intravenous urogram include a small kidney on the same side and a collecting system that varies from well visualized to nonvisualized. The connection to the vas is not usually seen.

The best way to demonstrate a persisting mesonephric duct is usually a voiding cystourethrogram, because nearly all such ducts reflux, at which point the duct itself and the reflux into the vas and ureter can be demonstrated.

Other Types of Vasoureteral Communication and Ectopic Vas

Other types of vasoureteral communications (Fig. 19–310) or of ectopic vas are rare.[50, 51] The latter occurs when the vas opens on the trigone, below and medial to the ureteral orifices (Fig. 19–311). Sometimes peristalsis is visible between the scrotum and the inguinal canal. Associated anomalies include anorectal malformations and cleft palate.

A voiding cystourethrogram is the best method for demonstrating an ectopic vas opening on the trigone, because free reflux occurs between the bladder and the vas.

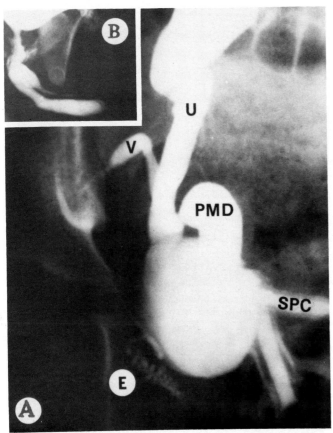

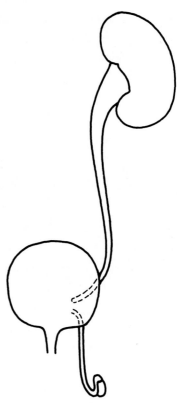

Figure 19–309. Congenital vasoureteral communication. *A,* Postvoid film of a voiding cystourethrogram showing reflux into a right vasoureteral communication, a dilated tortuous ureter, the vas deferens and the epididymis. (PMD = vasoureteral communication, U = ureter, V = vas deferens, E = epididymis.) *B,* View of the urethra shows a bifid urethra. (From Schwarz R, Stephens FD: The persisting mesonephric duct: High junction of the vas deferens and ureter. J Urol 120:592–596, © 1978, The Williams & Wilkins Co., Baltimore.)

Figure 19–311. Anomalous termination of the vas deferens into the bladder. (Modified from Aaronson IA, Cremin BJ: Clinical paediatric uroradiology. Edinburgh, Churchill Livingstone, p 161, 1984.)

Ultrasonography is the method of choice to show the difference in testicular volume. One or both testes may be congenitally large, an anomaly that can be discovered at any time but most often at puberty,[54, 55] and ultrasonography is useful in showing the presence of one or two such testes.

CONGENITAL ANOMALIES OF THE TESTES

Anomalies of Size

A testis can be congenitally small (rudimentary testis). This is usually detected either at birth or at puberty. The anomaly is nearly always unilateral. The bilateral form sometimes occurs in several members of the same family[52] and may be associated with micropenis.[53]

Anomalies of Number

One or both testes may be congenitally absent, one of the causes of nonpalpable testes.[56, 57] About 3% to 5% of patients with an apparent undescended testis have a congenital absence of the testis (monorchia).[57] The diagnostic imaging of congenitally absent testes is discussed in the section on undescended testes.

Congenital duplication of a testis can also occur (polyorchia),[58–65] most commonly involving a bifid or duplicated testis and a single epididymis or vas deferens. A uniform tunica albuginea surrounds the duplicated or bifid testis.

Complete duplication of the testis, together with duplication of the epididymis and vas deferens, may occur, but is less common.

Congenitally duplicated testes are usually discovered when an apparent mass is palpated in the testis. Ultrasonography is the method of choice for diagnostic imaging.[57, 61, 63, 118] In view of the high radiofrequency signal returned by the testis, especially on T2 weighted images, MRI is rapidly becoming an accepted mode of imaging a variegated group of testicular disorders (Fig. 19–312).[66, 124]

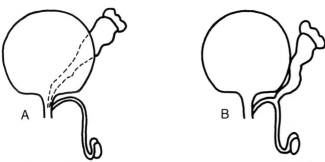

Figure 19–310. *A,* Distal, and *B,* proximal, insertion of an ectopic ureter into the vas deferens. (Modified from Aaronson IA, Cremin BJ: Clinical paediatric uroradiology. Edinburgh, Churchill Livingstone, p 161, 1984.)

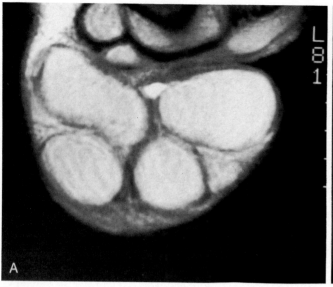
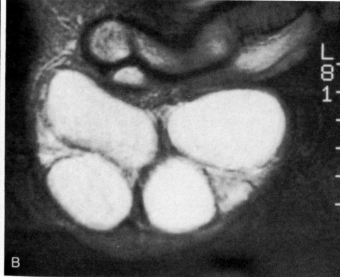

Figure 19–312. Bilateral testicular duplication. Coronal MRI scans show four testes: *A*, T1-weighted image (TR 2000 msec; TE 25 msec). *B*, T2-weighted image (TR 2000 msec, TE 70 msec). (From Baker LL, Hajek PC, Burkhard TK, Mattrey RF: Polyorchidism: Evaluation by MR. AJR 148:305–306, 1987, © by Am Roentgen Ray Soc.)

Anomalies of Position

Undescended Testes

Undescended testes is one of the most common genitourinary anomalies occurring in male infants.[67, 68] Its exact occurrence rate depends on the maturity and weight of the infant; for example, the incidence at birth in otherwise normal boys is 3.5%,[67] but in premature infants weighing under 2 pounds, the incidence is virtually 100%. From birth to the age of 1 year, many undescended testes spontaneously descend, so at the age of 1 year the prevalence falls to 0.8%. Beyond the age of 1 year, however, spontaneous descent is unlikely to occur and the prevalence, if the defect is left untreated, remains at 0.8%.[67] About 10% of undescended testes are bilateral.

Cryptorchism is clinically important for a number of reasons. (1) An increased incidence of malignant testicular neoplasms occurs in these testes. (2) There is a high rate of infertility in cryptorchism. (3) Patients are more likely to undergo testicular torsion than those with normal testes. (3) There is a greater risk of trauma to an undescended testis. (4) An associated inguinal hernia with its potential complications is present in all cases. Gender can be erroneously assigned. (5) Obviously important cosmetic and psychological factors affect the boy and his family.

EMBRYOLOGY OF TESTICULAR DESCENT

The early development of the testis is described in the section on ambiguous genitalia (see page 779). This section focuses on descent of the testis.

In Stage 18 (44 to 48 days), a ridge of mesoblast exists, which eventually extends from the genital ridge through an opening in the ventral abdominal wall (the future inguinal canal) to the genital swelling (the future scrotum). This ridge is the future gubernaculum.[69]

By Stage 17 (42 to 44 days) in the male the indifferent

gonad begins to become a testis. The exact process by which this occurs is unknown; it is perhaps due to the secretion of H-Y antigen by the X-Y primordial germ cells, but views on this are conflicting.

By the end of the embryonic period (Stage 23, 57 to 60 days), the testis begins to secrete two hormones—testosterone and the müllerian inhibiting factor.[15–17, 69] Testosterone is secreted by the Leydig cells, and induces the wolffian duct on the same side to become the vas deferens and the epididymis. The Sertoli cells secrete the müllerian inhibiting factor, which causes the müllerian ducts to regress, until only the appendix testis remains.

At this point the peritoneum pouches out ventral to the gubernaculum, forming the processus vaginalis. Androgens cause the genital swelling to begin its transformation into the scrotum, and the gubernaculum runs from the tail of the epididymis through the inguinal canal into the genital swelling cum scrotum.

From the 12th week to the seventh month the processus vaginalis gradually grows downward into the scrotum. At the seventh month, just before the descent of the testis, the vas deferens and the testicular vessels enlarge, the gubernaculum swells, and the processus vaginalis starts growing even more rapidly.

The gubernaculum separates from the wall of the scrotum. It distends the scrotum and the inguinal canal, the process allowing first the epididymis and then the testis to pass through the inguinal canal into the scrotum. Next, the upper part of the processus vaginalis becomes obliterated, and the remainder within the scrotum becomes the tunica vaginalis. Finally, the gubernaculum atrophies.

Two kinds of theories are offered regarding the causes of testicular descent. One type includes various mechanical theories, and the other suggests that an endocrine factor (especially dihydrotestosterone) is responsible.[72] Of the mechanical theories, the most popular, and probably the most important, is that intra-abdominal pressure rises immediately prior to testicular descent, forcing the testis into the scrotum.[69, 72] The second theory is that the gubernaculum pulls the testis into the scrotum. In experiments on animals, however, the transected gubernaculum does not prevent the testis from descending. Furthermore, the gubernaculum is so weakly attached to the scrotum that its ability to pull the testis downward seems unlikely. According to the third theory, the gubernaculum pulls the testis into the scrotum as the rest of the abdomen grows away from it. This theory is contradicted by the fact that, at the time of testicular descent, the gubernaculum is growing faster than the abdomen as a whole. Finally, it has been suggested that the maturation of the epididymis pulls the testis[70] into the scrotum, but little support for this hypothesis is currently available.

CLASSIFICATION

The two main groups of undescended testes are the retractile testis, accounting for 70% of cases, and the truly maldescended testis (cryptorchism), accounting for 30%.[74, 75] A retractile testis lies in the scrotum intermittently or can be manipulated into the scrotum. Its high position is thought to be due to contraction of the cremaster muscle, although in some cases a patent processus vaginalis is present.[76]

Of the truly maldescended testes, some 20% are obstructed in their caudal descent, 80% are functionally dystopic, and less than 1% are ectopic.[77] A testis is called obstructed when it lies in the superficial inguinal pouch of Browne[119], which lies anterior to the aponeurosis of the external oblique muscle. In patients with an obstructed testis, the cord is of normal length and the testis is grossly normal.

A testis is functionally dystopic if it has never reached its final destination in the scrotum, but nevertheless lies in the natural pathway of descent.[77] It is located less than 4 cm below the pubic tubercle. Fifty per cent of maldescended testes are in the high scrotal positions; 20% are in the canalicular position, somewhere between the external and internal ring; and 10% are in the abdominal position, lying somewhere in the abdomen inside the internal inguinal ring.[77] The highest point in the abdomen at which a testis can be located is the level of the lower pole of the ipsilateral kidney, a fact of some significance for surgeons and radiologists. Even if a testis cannot be palpated, the chance is high (96%) that it is present.[120, 121]

Ectopic testes are testes that lie in the groin, perineum, root of the penis, the femoral triangle, or the opposite side (crossed ectopia).

PATHOLOGY

Progressive testicular abnormalities develop from 1 year onward, which is one reason that surgeons currently recommend surgery at 9 to 12 months in order to forestall later fertility problems.[78]

Pathological abnormalities occur in all undescended testes, regardless of position.[78–80] In individuals with this disorder, the following are found:

1. A progressive decrease in the number of germ cells, so that by the age of 13 years, most undescended testes have no discernible germ cells remaining.

2. A decrease in the size of the seminiferous tubules, and thickening of the basement membrane of the seminiferous tubules. By the age of 13 years, most of the seminiferous tubules are sclerotic.

3. The number of Leydig's cells increases or decreases, sometimes increasing so much that they form nodules.

4. The number of Sertoli's cells usually increases, and they may form nodules. Less frequently, they disappear entirely.

Unfortunately, similar findings of varying degrees of severity are found in the opposite testis in two-thirds of patients with an undescended testis.[81] The reason is unknown, although there are several unproven hypotheses.[81, 82] The first is that an associated congenital anomaly is in the opposite testis, and the second is that some hormonal anomaly is at fault, although the hormonal profiles in all these patients have been normal.[82] The third is an autoimmune phenomenon, arising since the undescended testis, because of its higher position, has a higher temperature, disrupting the Sertoli cells, and causing a reaction in the opposite testis because of the escape of antigens.[82] Supporting this hypothesis is the fact that similar findings are reported in spinal cord injury patients whose testes are also exposed to a higher than normal temperature.

Because there are frequently bilateral histological problems, even when only one testis is undescended, only 60% of males with surgically repaired unilateral undescended testes are fertile as adults. One reason surgery is performed much earlier now than formerly is to try to prevent damage to the opposite testis.

COMPLICATIONS

Infertility. The leading complication of an undescended testis is infertility.

In untreated bilateral undescended testes, the infertility rate is 100%. If both testes are successfully brought down, about 40% become fertile.

If the disorder is unilateral, the mean fertility rate is 60% when the undescended testis is successfully brought down surgically. However, about one-third of undescended testes also have anomalies of the epididymis, vas, seminal vesicle, and ejaculatory duct, which can independently cause infertility.[83] Even in fertile males with surgically treated undescended testes, the mean sperm density is only one-third of normal.[78, 81] This is much worse than one would expect from an apparently unilateral anomaly, but this arises because the pathological abnormalities are bilateral in two-thirds of patients, although they may be less severe on the contralateral side.

Recently, men who had unilateral undescended testis successfully treated surgically were studied.[86] Each had fathered children and had sought a vasectomy, which was performed on the normal side only. After the surgery, a large percentage had no sperm. The conclusion was that a unilaterally undescended testis usually does not produce sperm, even after it has been brought down. This is perhaps because the operation was performed when the patient was too old; another 20 years may be necessary to determine if earlier surgery can help prevent the loss of sperm.

Malignant Testicular Neoplasms. Malignant testicular neoplasms also occur with greater frequency in these patients. The prevalence for patients with untreated undescended testis is 30 to 50 times higher than usual. As the usual prevalence is 2 to 3 per 100,000 men per year, this prevalence indicates a figure of 50 to 150 per 100,000 men. The prevalence most commonly agreed upon is about 100 per 100,000 men. This means that a patient with an untreated undescended testis faces odds of about 1 in 1000 that he will develop a malignant testicular neoplasm.

The earliest detectable lesion is carcinoma in situ.[85] In one series, testicular biopsies were done in subfertile men, one-third with an undescended testis treated surgically. Carcinoma in situ developed in some, characterized by large cells, more vacuolated cytoplasm, irregular nuclei, an increase in the diameter of the nuclei, and an increase in the number of nucleoli. Fifty per cent with carcinoma in situ later developed invasive carcinoma.[87]

Once malignant neoplasms develop, in most series the most frequent histological type is seminoma. In others, there seems to be an equal chance of seminoma, embryonal cell carcinoma, and teratocarcinoma.

There is an increased risk of developing a malignant neoplasm only if the undescended testis is untreated after the age of 5 years, so current policy is to bring down the undescended testis if the patient is not yet 5 years old, and to remove it if the patient is 5 years or over.[88]

Torsion of the Testis. There is an increased risk of torsion of the testis, especially if a testicular neoplasm has developed. If torsion is untreated for more than 24 hours, spermatogenic capability is usually lost. For this reason, even in patients without an undescended testis, it is customary to remove a testis that has undergone torsion for more than 24 hours.

ASSOCIATED ANOMALIES

Without Somatic Abnormalities. Diagnostic imaging studies show that the incidence of other congenital anomalies in the urinary tract in patients with undescended testes is about 3%, the same for age-matched and otherwise healthy cohorts.[89] Although contrary opinions have been expressed,[128] there would seem to be no scientifically valid indication for routine diagnostic imaging of the rest of the urinary tract in a patient with undescended testis.[129] About one-third of undescended testes have anomalies of the mesonephric duct.[83] These include agenesis of all mesonephric duct derivatives, anomalies of the epididymis (agenesis, nonunion between head and testis, agenesis of midepididymis, agenesis of the tail, [elongated or looped, cyst]), anomalies of the vas deferens (agenesis or ureter entering vas), anomalies of the seminal vesicle (agenesis, cyst, or ureter entering seminal vesicle), and agenesis of the ejaculatory duct.

Chromosomal Abnormalities. Undescended testis is associated with abnormal sex chromosomes: XXY, XXYY, XXXY, XYY, XO/XY, XX male.[90]

Undescended testis is associated with abnormal autosomes: 13, 18, 21, 9, 14, 4p−, rq+, 5p−, 21q−.

Nonchromosomal Abnormalities and Syndromes. Practically all patients with prune-belly syndrome have bilateral cryptorchism.[123] The theory is that abdominal pressure is necessary to force descent into the scrotum and that with prune-belly syndrome the abdominal musculature is not sufficient to force the testes into the scrotum.

Undescended testis is also associated with large omphaloceles, possibly for the same reason. The incidence of undescended testes in a hospitalized population with mental deficiency is 33%.[91]

Undescended testis is associated with a large number of syndromes, including the following:[90] Prader-Willi syndrome, Aarskog's syndrome, Beckwith-Wiedemann syndrome, Noonan's syndrome, Silver-Russel syndrome, Laurence-Moon-Biedl syndrome, and Kallman's syndrome. Undescended testis can be associated with other syndromes, although most are too rare to list here.

Ambiguous Genitalia, Including Hypospadias. Undescended testes are associated with ambiguous genitalia, including abnormalities in gonadal differentiation (mixed gonadal dysgenesis and true hermaphroditism), and with female and male pseudohermaphroditism.[90] These anomalies are discussed later (page 779).

DIAGNOSTIC IMAGING

Physical examination is the most important guide. About 20% to 30% of undescended testes are nonpalpable.

The use of diagnostic imaging for nonpalpable undescended testes is very controversial.[122] Many surgeons prefer to explore the patient without diagnostic imaging and regard surgery as the most efficient and cost-effective way to proceed.[92] Others use laparoscopy,[93–95] claiming it is more helpful than diagnostic imaging. If the testis is not found, they do not explore the patient further; if it is found, they evaluate the anatomy and plan the surgical approach.

The goal of diagnostic imaging is to aid the therapy, hormonal or surgical. There are two types of hormonal therapy:[73, 96–98] human chorionic gonadotropin, (hCG) given by intramuscular injection or an intranasal spray of gonadotropin-releasing hormone; the latter is not FDA approved. Both work excellently with retractile testes, but not with truly undescended testes, for which reason hormonal treatment may help to select retractile from maldescended testis. The problem with either variety of hormonal therapy is that it can interfere with growth and later testicular function. Moreover, the long-term effects are unknown. Diagnostic imaging shows whether the testis is high or low; if it is low, it could be retractable, and the hormonal therapy may work.

Surgery for truly undescended testis is normally easy and can usually be done on an outpatient basis.[99] It is currently performed at between 9 and 12 months. This avoids operating too early, since many undescended testes spontaneously descend up to the age of 12 months, and also avoids operating too late, in order to prevent later infertility problems.

Between the ages of 12 months and puberty, the normal procedure is orchiopexy. After the onset of puberty, because of the risk of neoplasm, an orchiectomy is normally performed.

Gonadal Phlebography. Weiss and Glickman[100] advocate gonadal phlebography as a method of searching for the undescended testis. Gonadal vein catheterization is usually successful in 90% of cases. The left side is easier to catheterize than the right. The authors classified their findings in 43 cases of impalpable testis into three basic groups:[100]

Group I. The internal spermatic vein terminates in a mesh of vessels Weiss and Glickman call the pampiniform-like plexus. Although in their series a testis was always present at this site, other authors report a different experience (Fig. 19–313).[101]

Group II. There are two subgroups: *Group IIA*—the internal pelvic spermatic vein ends blindly without a valve. The testis is absent in 90% of cases (Fig. 19–314), but *it may still be present,*[101] *Group IIB*—there is a blind-ending spermatic vein, and a valve prevents contrast material from filling the terminal part of the vein. The testis is present in 75% of cases, absent in 25%.

Group III. There is no gonadal vein. The testis is absent in 70% of cases, present in 30%.

The results of phlebography are undependable;[101] the examination is invasive, uses radiation, requires a general anesthetic in an infant or small child, and is technically difficult in a child under the age of 1 year.[101] It does not prevent exploration, except perhaps in Group IIA; the examination might possibly be indicated in post pubertal males with asymptomatic nonpalpable testis or in a patient with a prior negative exploration in whom another exploration is contemplated, but even in these patients other less invasive techniques are probably more appropriate for the initial evaluation.

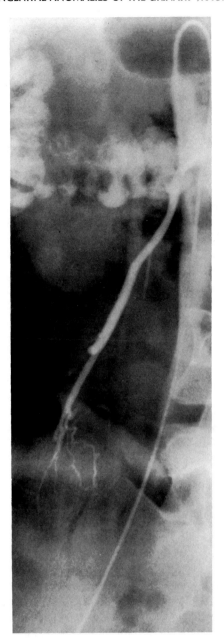

Figure 19–314. Absent pampiniform plexus in testicular agenesis. A right testicular phlebogram demonstrates a high termination of the gonadal vein. Although there are a few small filamentous venous tributaries, a well developed pampiniform plexus is absent. At surgery no right testis was found.

Ultrasonography. This method (Fig. 19–315) is very sensitive if the testis is in the inguinal canal.[102, 127] It is less adequate if the testis is in the pelvis or abdomen.[102] In either case, it is important to find the mediastinum testis.[102] Finding it can confirm that the structure is the testis; otherwise the structure may be, for example, an enlarged lymph node.

Computed Tomography. Computed tomography (CT)[103, 104] is sometimes useful, although there is a size limitation—no testis smaller than 1 cm in diameter can be detected. If it is important to find a high testis, this limitation may be significant, because high testes are occasionally smaller than 1 cm in diameter and can be difficult to detect. The higher and smaller the testis, the more difficult to differentiate it from bowel loops, lymph

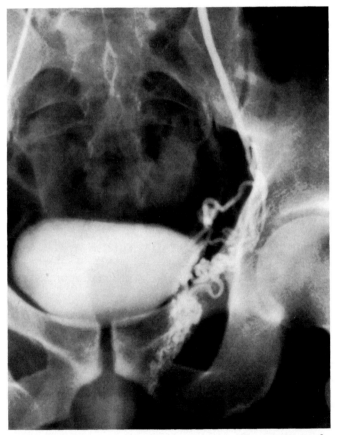

Figure 19–313. Left testicular agenesis in the presence of a normal pampiniform plexus. A left testicular phlebogram demonstrates a relatively normal appearing pampiniform plexus although the location of the plexus is somewhat more coronal than usual and is primarily within the inguinal canal, suggesting the presence of an undescended testis. In spite of the well developed pampiniform plexus however, no testis was found either in the inguinal canal or in the abdomen at the time of surgery.

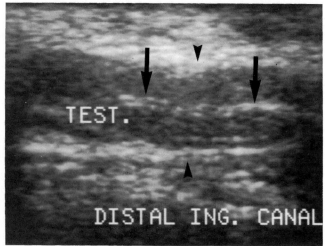

Figure 19–315. Sonogram of undescended testis. The testis *(arrowheads)* is smaller than normal, but the mediastinum testis *(arrows)* is clearly depicted. (From Friedland GW, Chang P: The role of imaging in the management of the impalpable undescended testis. AJR 151:1107–1111, 1988, © by Am Roentgen Ray Soc.)

nodes, and vessels. Computed tomography involves radiation, which is a consideration in this generally young age group. It has proved to be most successful in the postpubertal male and when the testes lie close to the internal inguinal ring. Obviously, CT will be of great value if neoplastic degeneration in an undescended testis is suspected (Fig. 19–316).

CT findings show a mass on the side on which the testis is not palpable (Fig. 19–317). Its density is the same as soft tissue, it is oval in shape, and it lies in a place where an undescended testis might be expected (e.g., inguinal canal). If it is large, malignancy or infection (Fig. 19–318) should be suspected. The absence of a normal spermatic cord in the inguinal canal should also raise the suspicion of cryptorchism.

Cuts should be made at 0.5-cm intervals, with a 0.5-cm thickness, beginning at the upper scrotum. The examination should stop as soon as the testis is identified. There is no need to continue higher than the lower pole of the

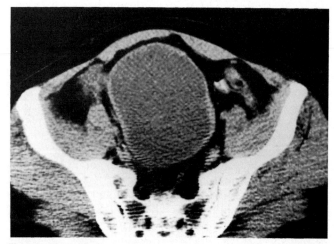

Figure 19–316. Tumor in an undescended testis. An axial CT section through the pelvis in this 54-year-old man demonstrates a huge, cystic, necrotic mass, which originated in the retroperitoneum and extended caudally to terminate above the urinary bladder. The mass was determined to be seminoma.

kidney, since an undescended testis does not occur any higher. Finally, it is important to have the bowel well-filled with contrast material to differentiate it from testis.

Magnetic Resonance Imaging. MRI (Fig. 19–319) clearly shows an undescended testis in both transaxial and coronal planes.[115] If a 1.5-T unit is used, the testis is best seen with long TR/TE sequences, whereas if a 0.35-T unit is used, short TR/TE sequences are most useful. As with ultrasonography, it is important diagnostically to find the mediastinum testis.

Some problems are associated with MRI for the purpose of detecting undescended testes. It is much more expensive than either ultrasonography or CT. Moreover, for CT it is possible to administer oral contrast, which can help to distinguish parts of the gastrointestinal tract from an undescended testis. This is not possible with MRI, in which it can sometimes be difficult to distinguish testis from bowel. Under these circumstances, CT is clearly the preferable imaging modality. Finally, children do not usually tolerate the long scanning times that MRI requires.

Problems Caused by the Pars Infravaginalis Gubernaculi and Associated Structures. In patients who have undescended testis, the remaining gubernaculum sometimes ends in a bulbous swelling.[106] The swelling may be located some distance from an undescended testis on the same side, and it may even be present if the same-side testis is congenitally absent. Compounding the problem is the fact that the pars infravaginalis gubernaculi (PIG) often has the same size and shape as the testis and may appear exactly like a testis on a sonogram, CT scan or MRI scan. The importance of this fact is that by mistaking the PIG for a testis, one might localize the testis inappropriately. Moreover, the pampiniform plexus and the PIG can both be in the inguinal canal, whereas the testis is located higher up, so that if phlebography is performed, the testis may be incorrectly localized.

Once again, the testis can be firmly localized by ultrasonography or MRI once a mediastinum testis is detected (see Fig. 19–315). This is the only known way to ascertain clearly whether the structure is a testis.

SPLENIC-GONADAL FUSION

The two basic types of this congenital anomaly are continuous and discontinuous.[107–109]

In the continuous form, a band of tissue unites the normally located spleen with the gonad. In the male, this band unites the spleen with the testis and epididymis, and in the female, with the ovary and mesovarium. The band is either splenic or fibrous tissue, or both. In the male cryptorchism is usually associated.

In the discontinuous form, there is no connection between the abnormally located splenic tissue and the spleen.

Embryology

Embryologically, the spleen forms in the left dorsal mesogastrium in the 6th week, very close to the mesonephros and the developing left gonad, until the 8th week when the left gonad descends.

Some fusion between the gonad and the spleen may

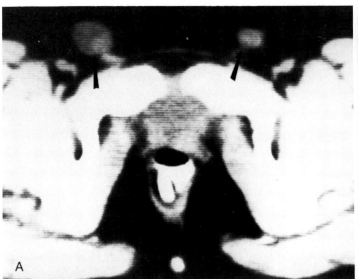

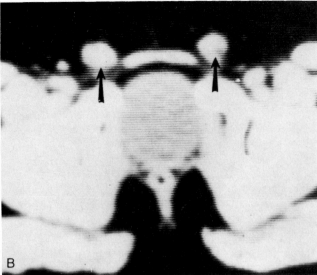

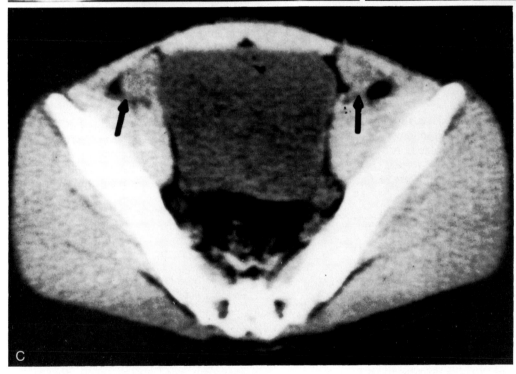

Figure 19–317. The use of CT to localize the impalpable testes. CT scans performed on different patients show *A,* bilateral undescended testes *(arrows)* at the external inguinal ring, *B,* bilateral retractile testes *(arrows)* in superficial inguinal pouch and *C,* bilateral undescended testes *(arrows)* at internal inguinal ring. (From Rajfer J, Tauber A, Zinner M, et al: The use of computerized tomography scanning to localize the impalpable testis. J Urol 129: 972–974, © 1983, The Williams & Wilkins Co., Baltimore.)

Figure 19–318. Acute and chronic epididymitis associated with an undescended right testicle. CT scan at the level of the inguinal canal near the external ring shows a 4-cm soft-tissue mass in the right inguinal canal. A focal area of low density is consistent with inflammation. (From Katz ME, Glazer HS, Menon M: Groin pain and swelling in a unilaterally cryptorchid adult. Urol Radiol 5:275–278, 1983.)

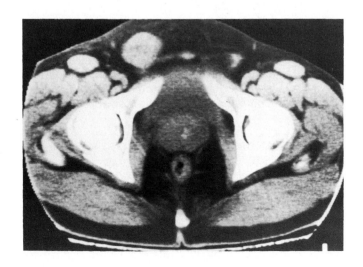

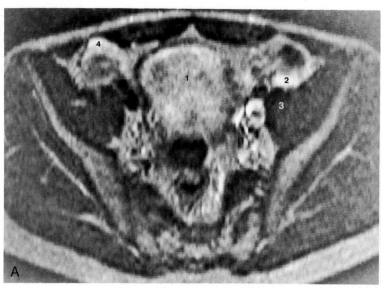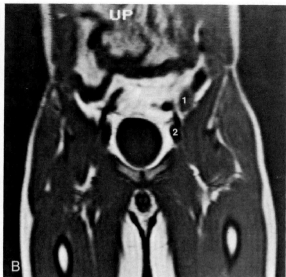

Figure 19–319. Bilateral intra-abdominal testes. *A*, Transverse MR image (SE 1500/90 msec) through the pelvis near the top of the bladder (1). The undescended testis on the left (2) is located immediately anterior to the psoas muscle (3) and lateral to the iliac vessels. The high signal of the testis is similar to the high signal noted in the fluid filled bowel (4) on the right. The similarity in signal intensity at this TR/TE indicates the importance of triangulating structures on the multiple planes. *B*, Coronal MR image (SE 700/28 msec). The left intra-abdominal testis is intermediate in signal (1) and immediately lateral to the iliac vessels (2). The intra-abdominal testis on the right is not visible because it is at a different plane. (From Fritzsche PJ: MRI of the scrotum. Urol Radiol 10:52–57, 1988.)

occur between the 6th and the 8th week. As the gonad descends, it may pull out a long cord from the spleen that remains, linking the gonad and the spleen. Alternatively, it pulls some tissue away from the spleen, and carries it through the descent, although it no longer has any structural connection with the spleen.

with urinary tract, gastrointestinal, and skeletal anomalies.[111, 117] Of cases of suprainguinal ectopic scrotum, 70% have had significant urinary tract anomalies on the same side.[115] When these scrotal anomalies are encountered, it is advisable to examine the patient carefully for other anomalies.

Clinical Features

Most commonly, the discovery of this condition is an incidental finding when the surgeon is operating for inguinal hernia or cryptorchism. It can cause a swelling that may become painful if the patient had been involved with vigorous exercise or has had a splenic infection. The condition is usually discovered in adults, although it may be found in children. It is nine times more common in males than in females, and is, for obvious reasons, always found on the left side. The incidence of other anomalies, including ectromelia and micrognathia, is higher as well.

Diagnostic Imaging

The diagnosis can be made using a radionuclide liver-spleen study (Fig. 19–320). Using this method, it may be possible to visualize the tail between the spleen and the testis, or an abnormal uptake in the testis itself.

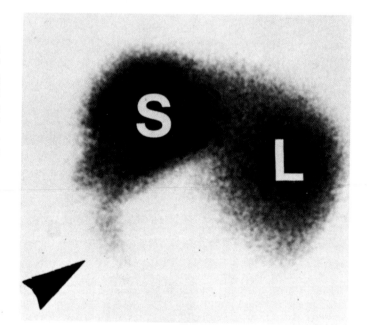

Figure 19–320. Splenic-gonadal fusion. Tc-99m-sulfur colloid liver-spleen scan obtained in the posterior view shows that the lower pole of the spleen extends inferomedially *(arrowhead)* for about 3 cm. This "tail" of activity outlines the proximal portion of the anomalous splenogonadal fusion. The liver (L) and upper portion of the spleen (S) are normal. (From McLean GH, Alavi A, Ziegler MM, et al: Splenic-gonadal fusion: Identification by radionuclide scanning. J Pediatr Surg 16:649–651, 1981.)

ANOMALIES OF THE SCROTUM

The scrotum can be bifid, particularly in the case of intersex problems.[110] It may be transposed, along with the penis,[111, 112] or may be ectopic in one of the following ways: (1) infrainguinal (on one or both sides),[113, 114] (2) suprainguinal,[115] (3) perineal.[116]

Anomalies of the scrotum are commonly associated

References

1. McNeal JE: The zonal anatomy of the prostate. Prostate 2:35–49, 1981.
2. Johnson FP: The later development of the urethra in the male. J Urol 4:447–501, 1920.
3. Lowsley OS: The development of the human prostate gland with reference to the development of other structures at the neck of the urinary bladder. Am J Anat 13:299–349, 1912.
4. Cunha GR: Epithelial-stromal interactions in development of the urogenital tract. Int Rev Cytol 47:137–194, 1976.
5. Cunha GR, Lung B: The possible influence of temporal factors in androgenic responsiveness of urogenital tissues recombinants from wild type and androgen insensitive (Tfm) mice. J Exp Zool 205:181–194, 1978.
6. Chung LWR, Cunha GR: Stromal-epithelial interacts: Regulations of prostatic growth by embryonic urogenital sinus mesenchyme. Prostate 4:503–511, 1983.
7. Glenister TW: The development of the utricle and the so-called "middle" or "median" lobe of the human prostate. J Anat (London) 96:443–455, 1962.
8. Price D: Comparative aspects of development and structure of the prostate. Natl Cancer Inst Monogr 12:1–27, 1963.
9. Nunn IN, Stephens FD: The triad syndrome: A composite anomaly of the abdominal wall, urinary system, and testes. J Urol 86:782, 1961.
10. Woodward JR: The prune-belly syndrome. Urol Clin North Am 5:75–93, 1978.
11. Berdon WE, Baker DH, Wigger HJ, Blanc WA: The radiologic and pathologic spectrum of the prune-belly syndrome. The importance of urethral obstruction in prognosis. Radiol Clin North Am 15:83–92, 1977.
12. Kroovand RL, Al-Ansari RM, Perlmutter AD: Urethral and genital malformations in prune-belly syndrome. J Urol 127:94–96, 1982.
13. Cremin BJ: The urinary tract anomalies associated with agenesis of the abdominal walls. Br J Radiol 44:767, 1971.
14. Wilson JD, Griffon JE, George FW, Leshin M: The role of gonadal steroids in sexual differentiation. Rec Prog Horm Res 37:1–39, 1981.
15. Donahoe PK, Budzik GP, Tretslad R, et al: Müllerian-inhibitory substance: An update. Recent Prog Hormone Res 38:279–330, 1982.
16. Wilson JD, Lasnitzki I: Dihydrotestosterone formation in fetal tissues of the rabbit and rat. Endocrinology 89:659, 1971.
17. Lasnitski I, Mezuno T: Role of mesenchyma in the induction of the rat prostate by androgens in organ culture. J Endocrinol 82:171–178, 1979.
18. Ikoma F, Shima H, Yabumoto H: Classification of enlarged prostatic utricle in patients with hypospadias. Br J Urol 57:334–337, 1985.
19. Culbertson LR: Müllerian duct cyst. J Urol 58:134–136, 1947.
20. Deming CL, Bernecke RR: Müllerian duct cysts. J Urol 51:563–568, 1944.
21. Landes RR, Ransom CL: Müllerian duct cysts. J Urol 61:1089–1093, 1949.
22. Lloyd FA, Bennet D: Müllerian duct cysts. J Urol 64:777–782, 1950.
23. Ruschec, Butler OW: Müllerian duct cysts. J Urol 59:962–965, 1948.
24. Spence HM, Chenoweth VC: Cysts of the prostatic utricle (mullerian duct cysts): Report of two cases in children, each containing calculi, cured by retropubic operation. J Urol 79:308–314, 1958.
25. deVries PA: Personal observation.
26. Rifkin MD: Diagnostic imaging of the lower genitourinary tract. New York, Raven Press, 1958, pp 162–166.
27. Elder JS, Mostwin JL: Cyst of the ejaculatory duct/urogenital anus. J Urol 132:768–771, 1984.
28. Yamashita T, Watanabe K, Ogawa A: Retroprostatic midline cyst involving both ejaculatory ducts. Urol Radiol 7:178–179, 1985.
29. Kenny PJ, Spirt BA, Leeson MD: Genitourinary anomalies: Radiologic-anatomic correlations. Radiographics 4:233–266, 1984.
30. Okuyama A, Sonoda T, Miyagawa M: Absence of both seminal vesicles associated with hypospermatogenesis. Br J Urol 53:188, 1981.
31. Kenny PJ, Leeson MA: Congenital anomalies of the seminal vesicles: Spectrum of computed tomographic findings. Radiology 149:247–251, 1983.
32. McClure RD, Hricak H: Magnetic resonance imaging: Its application to male infertility. Urology 27:91–98, 1986.
33. Patel MR, Dulabon D, Roth R: Absent seminal vesicle diagnosed by transrectal ultrasound. Urology 29:332, 1987.
34. Wakatsuki A, Oda T, Ochi K: Case profile: Crossed ectopia of seminal vesicles and blind-ending ureter. Urology 24:291–292, 1984.
35. Lantz EJ, Berquist TH, Hattery RR, et al: Seminal vesicle cyst associated with ipsilateral renal agenesis: A case report. Urol Radiol 2:265–266, 1981.
36. Rifkin MD, Needleman L, Kurtz AB, et al: Ultrasound of non-gynecological cystic masses of the pelvis. AJR 142:1169–1174, 1984.
37. Rifkin MD: Diagnostic imaging of the lower urinary tract. New York, Raven, 1985, pp 95, 201–203.
38. Roehrborn CG, Schneider HJ, Rugenderf EW, Hamann W: Embryological and diagnostic aspects of seminal vesicle cysts associated with upper urinary tract malformations. J Urol 135:1029–1032, 1986.
39. Steers WJ, Corriere JN: Seminal vesicle cyst. Urology 27:177–178, 1986.
40. Heaney JA, Pfister RC, Meares EM: Giant cyst of the seminal vesicle with renal agenesis. AJR 149:139–140, 1987.
41. Jequier AM, Ansell ID, Bullimore NJ: Congenital absence of the vasa deferentia presenting with infertility. J Androl 6:16–19, 1985.
42. Malatinsky E, Labady F, Lepies P, et al: Congenital anomalies of the seminal ducts. Int Urol Nephrol 19:189–194, 1987.
43. Emery CB, Goldstein AMB, Morrow JW: Congenital absence of the vas deferens with ipsilateral urinary anomalies. Urology 4:201–203, 1974.
44. Deane AM, May RE: Absent vas deferens in association with renal abnormalities. Br J Urol 54:298–299, 1982.
45. Van Wingerden JJ, Franz L: The presence of a caput epididymidis in congenital absence of the vas deferens. J Urol 131:764–766, 1984.
46. Johnson DK, Perlmutter AD: Single system ectopic ureteroceles with anomalies of the heart, testis, and vas deferens. J Urol 123:81–83, 1980.
47. Schwarz R, Stephens FD: The persisting mesonephric duct: High junction of the vas deferens and ureter. J Urol 120:592–596, 1978.
48. Redman JF, Sulieman JS: Bilateral vasoureteral communications. J Urol 116:808–809, 1976.
49. Vodermark JS: The persisting mesonephric duct syndrome: The description of a new syndrome. J Urol 130:958–961, 1983.
50. Gibbons MD, Cromie WJ, Duckett JW Jr: Ectopic vas deferens. J Urol 120:597, 1978.
51. Aaronson IA, Cremin BJ: Clinical paediatric uroradiology. Edinburgh, Churchill Livingstone, 1984, pp 160, 161.
52. Najjar SS, Takla RJ, Nassar VH: The syndrome of rudimentary testes: Occurrence in five siblings. J Pediatr 84:119, 1974.
53. Glass AR: Identical twins discordant for the "rudimentary testes" syndrome. J Urol 127:140–141, 1982.
54. Lee PA, Marshall FF, Greco JM, Jeffs RD: Unilateral testicular hypertrophy: An apparently benign occurrence without cryptorchidism. J Urol 127:329–331, 1982.
55. Breen DH, Braunstein DG, Neufeld N, Kudish H: Benign macroorchidism in a pubescent boy. J Urol 125:589–591, 1981.
56. Connors MH, Styne DM: Functional familial anorchism: A review of etiology and management. J Urol 133:1049–1051, 1985.
57. Goldberg LM, Skaist LB, Morrow JW: Congenital absence of the testes: Anorchism and monorchism. J Urol 111:840, 1974.
58. Rifkin MD, Kurtz AB, Pasto ME, Goldberg BB: Polyorchidism diagnosed preoperatively by ultrasound. J Ultrasound Med 2:93–94, 1983.
59. Butz RE, Croushore JH: Polyorchidism. J Urol 119:289–291, 1978.
60. Pelander WM, Luna G, Lilly JR: Polyorchidism. Case report and literature review. J Urol 119:705–706, 1978.
61. Finkelstein MS, Rosenberg HK, Snyder H M III, Duckett WJ: Ultrasound evaluation of scrotum in pediatrics. Urology 27:1–9, 1986.
62. Hancock RA, Hodgins TE: Polyorchidism. Urology 24:303–307, 1984.
63. Giyanani VL, McCarthy J, Venable DD, Terkeurst J, Fowler M: Ultrasound of polyorchidism: Case report and literature review. J Urol 138:863–864, 1987.
64. McAlister WH, Manley CB: Bilobed testicle. Pediatr Radiol 17:82, 1987.
65. Rogus BJ: Polyorchidism and testicular torsion. Urology 31:137, 1988.

66. Baker LL, Hajek PC, Burkhard TK, Mattrey RF: Polyorchidism: Evaluation by MR. AJR 148:305–306, 1987.
67. Rajfer J, Walsh PC: Testicular descent: Normal and abnormal. Urol Clin North Am 5:223–235, 1978.
68. Elder JS: Cryptorchidism: Isolated and associated with other genitourinary defects. Pediatr Clin North Am 34:1033–1053, 1987.
69. Frey HL, Rajfer J: Role of the gubernaculum and intra-abdominal pressure in the process of testicular descent. J Urol 131:574–579, 1984.
70. Mininberg DT, Scholosaberg S: The role of the epididymis in testicular descent. J Urol 129:1207–1208, 1983.
71. Rajfer J, Walsh PC: Testicular descent. Birth Defects 13:107–122, 1977.
72. Frey HL, Peng S, Rajfer J: Synergy of abdominal pressure and androgens in testicular descent. Biol Reprod 29:1233–1239, 1983.
73. Hadziselimovic F: Pathogenesis and treatment of undescended testes. Eur J Pediatr 139:255–265, 1982.
74. Schoorl M: Classification and diagnosis of undescended testes. Eur J Pediatr 139:253–254, 1982.
75. Weiss RM, Glickman MG: Localization and management of nonpalpable undescended testes. Surg Clin North Am 60:1253–1263, 1980.
76. Robertson JFR, Azmy AF, Cochran W: Assent to ascent of the testis. Br J Urol 61:146–147, 1988.
77. Lipshultz LI: Crytorchidism in the subfertile male. Fertil Steril 27:609–620, 1976.
78. Hadziselimovic F: Histology. Dial Pediatr Urol 4:3–4, 1981.
79. Muller J, Shakkebaek NE: Abnormal germ cells in maldescended testes: A study of cell density, nuclear size, and deoxyribonucleic acid content in testicular biopsies from 50 boys. J Urol 131:730–731, 1984.
80. Hedinger CE: Histopathology of undescended testes. Eur J Pediatr 139:266–271, 1982.
81. Kogan SJ: Cryporchidism and infertility: An overview. Dial Pediatr Urol 4:2–3, 1981.
82. Lipshultz LL: Cryptorchidism and infertility: Theoretical observations on endocrine and immunological aspect. Dial Pediatr Urol 4:7–8, 1981.
83. Kroovand RL: Cryptorchidism and infertility: Mesonephric system anomalies. Dial Pediatr Urol 4:5–6, 1981.
84. Rajfer J: Endocrine aspects of cryptorchidism. Dial Pediatr Urol 5:5–8, 1982.
85. Whitaker RH: Cryptorchidism and malignancy: Carcinoma in situ and tumor formation. Dial Pediatr Urol 4:4–5, 1981.
86. Alpert PF, Klein RS: Spermatogenesis in the unilateral cryptorchid testis after orchiopexy. J Urol 129:301–302, 1983.
87. Martin DC: Cryptorchidism and malignancy. Tumors after orchiopexy. Dial Pediatr Urol 10:8, 1981.
88. Batata MA, Whitmore WFJ, Hilaris, et al: Cryptorchidism and testicular cancer. J Urol 124:382, 1980.
89. Fallon B, Welton M, Hawtrey C: Congenital anomalies associated with cryptorchidism. J Urol 127:91–93, 1982.
90. Visser HKA: Associated anomalies in undescended testes. Eur J Pediatr 139:272–274, 1982.
91. Cortada X, Kouseff BG: Cryptorchidism in mental retardation. J Urol 131:674–676, 1984.
92. Martin DC: Testis (editorial). J Urol 124:388, 1980.
93. Lowe DH, Brock WA, Kaplan GW: Laparoscopy for localization of nonpalpable testes. J Urol 131:728–729, 1984.
94. Hamidinia A, Nold S, Amankwah KS: Localization and treatment of nonpalpable testes. Surg Gynecol Obstet 159:439–441, 1984.
95. Manson AL, Terhune D, Jordan G, et al: Preoperative laproscopic localization of the nonpalpable testis. J Urol 134:919–920, 1985.
96. King LR: Optimal treatment of children with undescended testes. J Urol 131:734–735, 1984.
97. Bierich JR: Undescended testes: Treatment with gonadotropin. Eur J Pediatr 139:275–279, 1982.
98. Hagberg S, Westphal O: Treatment of undescended testes with intranasal application of synthetic LH-RH. Eur J Pediatr 139:285–288, 1982.
99. Caldamone AA, Rabinowitz R: Outpatient orchiopexy. J Urol 127:286–289, 1982.

100. Weiss RM, Glickman MG: Venography of the undescended testis. Urol Clin North Am 9:387–395, 1982.
101. Greenberg SH, Ring EJ, Pollack HM, Wein AJ: The falsely positive gonadal venogram: Presence of a pampiniform plexus without a gonad. J Urol 125:887–888, 1981.
102. Weiss RM, Carter AR, Rosenfield AT: High resolution real-time ultrasonography in the localization of the undescended testis. J Urol 135:936–938, 1986.
103. Rajfer J, Tauber A, Zinner M, et al: The use of computerized tomography scanning to localize this impalpable testis. J Urol 129:972–974, 1983.
104. Lee JKT, Glazer HS: Computed tomography in the localization of the nonpalpable testis. Urol Clin North Am 9:397–404, 1982.
105. Fritzsche PJ, Hricak H, Kogan BA, et al: Undescended testis: Value of MR imaging. Radiology 164:169–173, 1987.
106. Rosenfield AT, Blair DN, McCarthy S, et al: The pars infravaginalis gubernaculi and associated structures: An imaging pitfall in the identification of the undescended testis (Abstr) Society of Uroradiology, Member's Scientific Program, Uroradiology 1988.
107. McLean GH, Alavi A, Ziegler MM, Pollack HM, Duckett JW: Splenic-gonadal fusion: Identification by radionuclide scanning. J Pediatr Surg 16:649–651, 1981.
108. Heloury Y, Valayer J, Leborgne J, et al: Splenogonadal fusion: Anatomic and angiographic study of a case. Surg Radiol Anat 8:147–151, 1986.
109. Tank ES, Forsyth M: Splenic gonadal fusion. J Urol 139:798–799, 1988.
110. Walsh PC: The differential diagnosis of ambiguous genitalia in the newborn. Urol Clin North Am 5:213–221, 1978.
111. Glenn JF, Anderson EE: Surgical correction of incomplete penoscrotal transposition. J Urol 110:603, 1973.
112. Cohen-Addad N, Zarafu IW, Hanna MK: Complete penoscrotal transposition. Urology 26:149–152, 1985.
113. Bajaj PS, Bailey BN: Ectopic scrotum—a case report. Br J Plast Surg 22:87, 1969.
114. Mininberg DT, Richman A: Bilateral scrotal testicular ectopia. J Urol 108:652, 1972.
115. Elder JS, Jeffs RD: Suprainguinal ectopic scrotum and associated anomalies. J Urol 127:336–338, 1982.
116. Takayasu H, Ueno A, Tsukada O: Accessory scrotum: A case report. J Urol 112:826–827, 1974.
117. Lamm DL, Kaplan GW: Accessory and ectopic scrota. Urology 9:149, 1977.
118. Goldberg RM, Chilcote W, Kay R, Bodie BH: Sonographic findings in polyorchidism. J Clin Ultrasound 15:412, 1987.
119. Browne D: The diagnosis of the undescended testicle. Br Med J 2:168–171, 1938.
120. Kogan SJ, Gill B, Bennett B, et al: Human monorchism: A clinicopathological study of unilateral absent testes in 65 boys. J Urol 135:758–761, 1986.
121. Levitt SB, Kogan SJ, Schneider KM, et al: Endocrine tests in phenotypic children with bilateral impalpable testes can reliably predict "congenital" anorchism. Urology 11:11–17, 1978.
122. Friedland GW, Chang P: The role of imaging in the management of the impalpable undescended testis. AJR 151:1107–1111, 1988.
123. Greskovich FJ III, Nyberg LM Jr: The prune-belly syndrome: A review of its etiology, defects, treatment and prognosis. J Urol 140:707–712, 1988.
124. Fritzche PJ: MRI of the scrotum. Urol Radiol 10:52–57, 1988.
125. Oyen R, Gielen J, van Poppel H, Baert L: Seminal vesical cyst and ipsilateral renal agenesis. Eur J Radiol 8:122–124, 1988.
126. Golstein M, Schlossberg S: Men with congenital absence of the vas deferens often have seminal vesicles. J Urol 140:85–86, 1988.
127. Johansen TE, Larmo A: Ultrasonography in undescended testes. Acta Radiol 29:159–163, 1988.
128. Pappis CH, Argianas SA, Bousgas D, Athanasiades E: Unsuspected urological anomalies in asymptomatic cryptorchid boys. Pediatr Radiol 18:51–53, 1988.
129. Lebowitz RL, Ben-Ami T: Trends in pediatric uroradiology. Urol Radiol 5:135–147, 1983.

MISCELLANEOUS CONGENITAL ANOMALIES OF THE GENITOURINARY TRACT

Table 19–33 lists the miscellaneous congenital anomalies of the genitourinary tract that are discussed in this chapter.

PRUNE-BELLY SYNDROME (EAGLE-BARRETT-SYNDROME; TRIAD SYNDROME)

Prune-belly syndrome is usually diagnosed in the newborn and consists of a congenital deficiency or hypoplasia of the abdominal muscles, undescended testes, a generalized dilatation of the urinary tract, and associated renal anomalies.[1–7] It is also known as Eagle-Barrett syndrome and abdominal musculature deficiency syndrome (AMDS),[3] and it is called triad syndrome, because it involves three separate regions—the abdominal muscles, the testes, and the urinary tract.

The prevalence varies between 1 in 350,000 and 1 in 500,000 live births.[4] Nearly all cases are in boys, although a few cases of prune-belly syndrome in girls have been reported.[9, 10]

The prognosis is poor in the more severe forms. Twenty per cent of affected infants die in the neonatal period, and 30% die within the first 2 years, usually of renal failure.[6, 7] In the milder forms, however, survival into adulthood is quite possible.

Prune-belly syndrome takes its name from the fact that the newborn's thin-walled abdomen is very wrinkled and creased.[11] If the child gets older, the skin gradually becomes smooth, and in time the belly looks like a potbelly.

The degree of absence of the abdominal muscles varies considerably, from almost 0% through 100%. The degree of absence can vary between the two sides. The most commonly involved part is the lower rectus.

The absence of abdominal muscle has affects on the rest of the body, notably the thorax and the spine.[4] As a result of the absence of abdominal muscles pulling downward, the lower rib cage flares out. The patient may develop a pectus deformity and difficulty breathing and coughing. Deficiency of lower abdominal muscles anteriorly, to counterbalance the paraspinal muscles, may result in kyphosis.

Pathology in the Urinary Tract

Kidneys

Hydronephrosis is common in patients with prune-belly syndrome, as is renal dysplasia, some degree of which occurs in 50% of cases. The dysplastic kidneys are small.

Table 19–33. Miscellaneous Congenital Anomalies of the Genitourinary Tract

I	Prune-belly syndrome
II	Intersex problems
III	Gartner's duct cyst
IV	Fused labia

The degree of dysplasia and the location of the orifice of the attendant ureter are related; the more laterally displaced the orifice, the more dysplastic the kidney,[12] although the kidneys in some of these patients may be normal.

The calyces are often clubbed, given the hydronephrosis, but the clubbing may be patchy, leaving some intervening normal calyces. Other calyces may be tiny. Some infundibula are long and narrow. The renal pelvis may vary from dilated to very tiny. There is often a disproportion between the size of the ureters (see below) and the relatively less voluminous renal pelves.

Ureters

The ureters may show areas of extreme dilatation as well as areas of marked narrowing, either or both of which may be combined with an extraordinary tortuosity. They sometimes wander all over the abdomen, which is a characteristic feature. The walls are usually thick but are often patchily deficient in muscle, which has been replaced by collagen tissue. The ureteral orifices are often laterally displaced.

Bladder

The bladder is usually large and the wall can vary from thick to thin. Some patients may show a mixture of thick, normal, and thin walls. The muscle tends to be replaced by collagen, and there is almost never any trabeculation. In most cases, the bladder is very elongated and attached to the umbilicus, where a urachal diverticulum, cyst, or patent urachus may be found.

Urethra

The prostatic urethra is longer and wider than normal, quite possibly as a result of the hypoplastic prostate gland accompanying the condition. The verumontanum is small or completely absent or is in the form of a dimple. An enlarged protruding prostatic utricle may be present.

Some prostatic tissue always remains in prune-belly syndrome. In the posterior glandular part of the prostate, prostatic tubules are present in about 15% of cases. Anteriorly, where smooth muscle should have developed, connective tissue predominates.[13]

The anterior urethra is abnormal in about 70% of cases, often in the form of a scaphoid megalourethra.[13–15]

Testes

The testes rarely descend in patients with prune-belly syndrome.

Associated Anomalies

A number of nonurological anomalies are associated with prune-belly syndrome (Table 19–34).[3, 21, 59]

Table 19–34. Anomalies Associated with the Prune-Belly Syndrome

Site	Anomaly
Musculoskeletal	Common: metatarsus varus, congenital lip dislocation Uncommon: polydactylism, webbing, arthrogryposis, scoliosis, lumbar lordosis, clover-leaf skull
Gastrointestinal	Common: intestinal malrotation, universal mesentery Uncommon: anorectal malformations, gastric duplication, wandering spleen
Thoracic	Flaring rib cage, pectus excavatum, pectus carinatum
Cardiac	Common: patent ductus arteriosis, intraventricular septal defect Uncommon: patent foramen secundum, tetralogy of Fallot

Embryological Basis of Prune-Belly Syndrome

The embryological basis of the prune-belly syndrome is completely unknown, although a number of theories are offered.[54]

The most popular current theory is that a transient, very severe abdominal distention prevents the development of the abdominal muscles. This transient condition might be caused in the following way.[16-18] Every patient with the prune-belly syndrome has prostatic hypoplasia and dilatation of the prostatic urethra. The smooth muscle of the prostate is absent, so that the weak prostate wall bulges, especially dorsally and caudally. The membranous urethra, in turn, faces in a more frontal direction. As a result, the membranous urethra twists at its junction with the prostatic urethra, creating a flap valve that obstructs the flow of urine. This obstruction causes the bladder to become distended; the upper urinary tract becomes hydronephrotic and ruptures, causing transient urine ascites. In support of this hypothesis is the fact that the histologic findings of the abdominal muscle wall show atrophy, not primitive muscle. This theory would explain why the prune-belly syndrome occurs almost exclusively in males.

The second major theory is that a primary defect is in the mesoblast.[19] The abdominal wall develops from the mesoblast, as do the kidneys, the muscular walls of the ureters, bladder, and urethra, and part of the prostate. Thus, a primary defect in the mesoblast would cause all these areas to show developmental defects.

The third theory is that prune-belly syndrome is caused by complex chromosomal mutations.[20]

A number of theories also attempt to explain the undescended testes, which are almost universally associated with the prune-belly syndrome. The most popular current theory is that, since one factor thought to cause normal descent of the testes is intra-abdominal pressure, the absence of abdominal muscles would lessen the intra-abdominal pressure. The likelihood of undescended testes would thereby be increased.

Finally, if the bladder is very distended because of a urethral obstruction, it may itself prevent the testes from descending.

Diagnostic Imaging

Radiological presentation of prune-belly syndrome has been arbitrarily divided into three groups.[5]

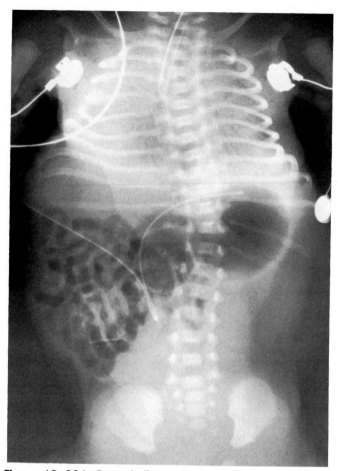

Figure 19–321. Prune-belly syndrome, Group I. Abdominal and chest radiograph of neonate with urethral atresia, prune-belly (bulging flanks) and pulmonary hypoplasia.

Group I: Potter's Syndrome (Oligohydramnios)

This is the most severe form. Infants are usually stillborn or die shortly after birth. The cause of death is pulmonary dysplasia and a resultant failure to oxygenate the blood (Fig. 19–321). When resuscitation is attempted, the patient develops interstitial pulmonary emphysema, pneumomediastinum, and pneumothorax.

The apparent basic reason for the severe lung hypoplasia is oligohydramnios during pregnancy. In these infants, the kidneys may be severely dysplastic or there may be complete urethral obstruction, so that little or no urine is produced. Because the basis of the amniotic fluid is fetal urine, oligohydramnios is the result of this dysplasia or obstruction.

It is thought that the lung changes in the fetus may result from the dry uterus pressing against the chest of the developing fetus.

Most of these patients demonstrate talipes equinovarus, also postulated to be due to the direct pressure of the uterus on the fetus.

Scintigraphy can demonstrate that the ureters are tortuous, and that portions of the ureters are hugely dilated. Delayed films demonstrate the large bladder, which often lies to one side.

Group II: Severe Neonatal and Infantile Urinary Tract Involvement

Patients in Group II include those born with severe urinary tract involvement. However, the lungs ventilate

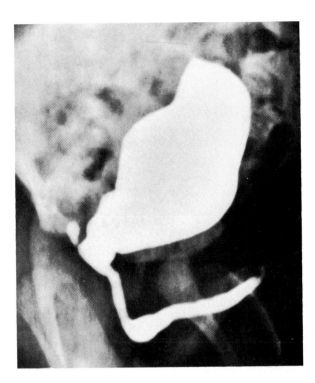

Figure 19–322. Voiding cystourethrogram in a boy with the prune-belly syndrome, showing a huge smooth bladder, dilated prostatic urethra, and enlarged prostatic utricle. (From Berdon WE, Baker DH, Wigger HJ, Blanc WA: The radiologic and pathologic spectrum of the prune-belly syndrome. The importance of urethral obstruction in prognosis. Radiol Clin North Am 15:83–92, 1977.)

reasonably well, and the kidneys are not so involved that the infant dies immediately.

Nevertheless, these patients show dramatic changes in the chest wall. The lower sternum is pulled in, the upper sternum bulges out, and the lower rib cage flares. There are rapid respiration and acidosis; however, the condition improves as the child gets older.

A chest radiograph shows both domes of the diaphragm as low and flat. It also possibly shows the flaring rib cage, the drawn-in lower sternum, and the bulging upper sternum (Fig. 19–321).

Because the deficient abdominal muscles do not support the flanks, both flanks bulge markedly, readily detectable on an abdominal radiograph (Fig. 19–321; see also Fig. 19–328).

The voiding cystourethrogram usually shows a huge bladder with a very unusual shape, although the bladder may be hypoplastic (Fig. 19–322). At the dome of the bladder, a urachal cyst (which may calcify) or a patent urachus may be present. The bladder dome may occasionally calcify (Fig. 19–323).[22] Often the bladder neck is wide, and a long and wide prostatic urethra may be found. An enlarged prostatic utricle may project posteriorly (Fig. 19–322). Unlike the sausage-shaped prostatic urethra seen in children with posterior urethral valves, the dilated urethra in prune-belly patients tends to be

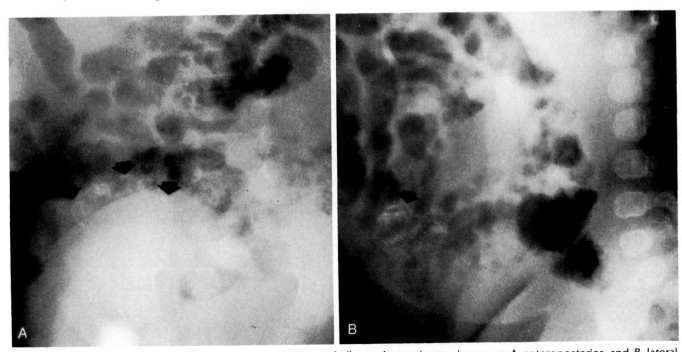

Figure 19–323. Calcified bladder in an infant with the prune-belly syndrome (arrows) seen on A, anteroposterior, and B, lateral, radiographs of the abdomen. (From Kirschner SG, Kirschner FK Jr, Jolles H, et al: Bladder calcification in the prune-belly syndrome. Radiology 138:597–600, 1981.)

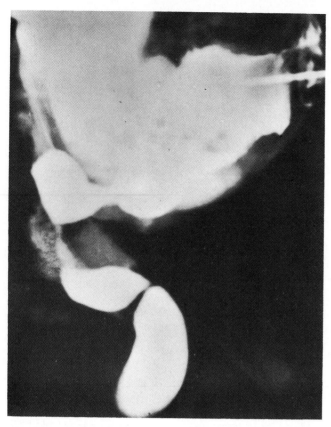

Figure 19–324. Voiding cystourethrogram in an infant with the prune-belly syndrome, showing a fusiform megalourethra. (From Berdon WE, Baker DH, Wigger HJ, Blanc WA: The radiologic and pathologic spectrum of the prune-belly syndrome. The importance of urethral obstruction in prognosis. Radiol Clin North Am 15:83–92, 1977.)

triangular. There may be a fusiform megalourethra (Fig. 19–324).

Sometimes reflux into the vas and the seminal vesicles occurs. Vesicoureteral reflux is common, during which it may be possible to observe the strange ureters, hugely dilated in some areas and greatly narrowed in others (Figs. 19–325 and 19–326).

A combination of posterior urethral valves and prune-belly syndrome has been noted in some patients.[23]

On the intravenous urogram the entire collecting system generally seems to fill, so that a reasonable examination is possible. The findings, described in the previous section on pathology, include dramatic changes throughout the urinary tract, particularly of the ureters, which

may be more dilated than the colon in some areas of some patients and which may wander throughout the abdomen. A markedly lateral course at the level of the pelvic inlet is quite suggestive of prune-belly. Usually, contrast material will enter the ureters, opacifying them.

The kidneys frequently have an unusual appearance, although they may be normal. Their size may be normal or small (Fig. 19–327), in which case one kidney is often smaller than the other. They can have a lobulated outline, and may be hydronephrotic (Fig. 19–328). Sometimes, however, only some of the calyces are clubbed, while some are tiny, and others normal. The infundibula may be long and spidery or normal, and the renal pelvis varies from tiny to normal to hydronephrotic. These changes

Figure 19–325. Voiding cystourethrogram in a newborn with the prune-belly syndrome, shows bulging flanks and reflux into a hugely dilated right ureter. (From Friedland GW: Hydronephrosis in infants and children, Parts I and II. *In* Moseley RD Jr (ed): Current problems in diagostic radiology. Chicago, Year Book Medical Publishers, 1978.)

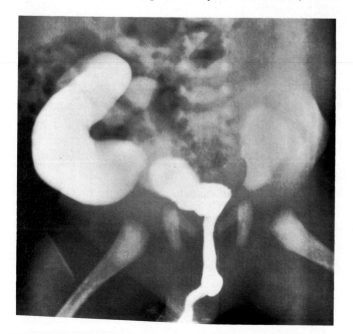

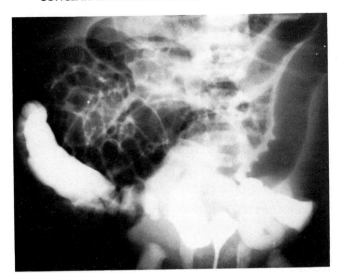

Figure 19–326. Voiding cystourethrogram in a newborn with the prune-belly syndrome, showing bulging flanks and bilateral reflux into hugely dilated, tortuous ureters, so characteristic of the syndrome.

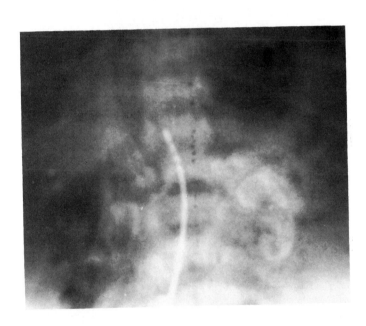

Figure 19–327. Bilateral renal hypoplasia in the prune-belly syndrome. Nephrogram obtained by injecting contrast material through an umbilical artery catheter reveals two tiny kidneys. (From Friedland GW: Hydronephrosis in infants and children, Parts I and II. *In* Moseley RD Jr (ed): Current problems in diagnostic radiology. Chicago, Year Book Medical Publishers, 1978.)

Figure 19–328. Intravenous urogram on an infant with the prune-belly syndrome shows bulging flanks and poor excretion with bilateral hydronephrosis.

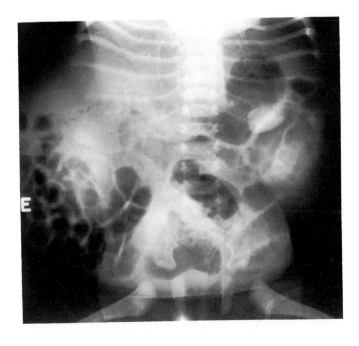

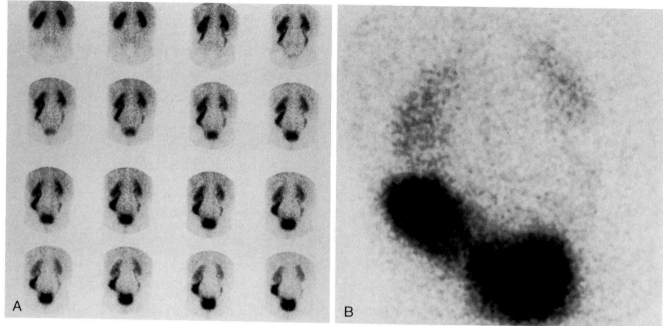

Figure 19–329. Tc-99m-DTPA scan in a neonate with the prune-belly syndrome. *A,* Both ureters are dilated and tortuous. *B, A* delayed image shows a huge bladder lying to one side. (Courtesy Massoud Majd, M.D.)

are usually asymmetrical and randomly distributed throughout the urinary tract.

Scintigraphy shows the ureteral dilatation and tortuosity, as well as the large bladder (Fig. 19–329).

Both computed tomography (CT) and magnetic resonance imaging (MRI) demonstrate the abdominal musculature deficiency and the undescended testes.

Group III: Mild Involvement

The abdominal wall in Group III patients can at times be nearly normal. Indeed, these patients may initially be seen simply for undescended testes, if the clinical features are sufficiently mild.

An examination may show mild wrinkling of the abdominal wall or mild separation of the rectus muscle, which may require abdominal straining to demonstrate. An intravenous urogram, however, may show the characteristic unusual kidneys and bizarre ureters, although the examination can vary from normal to milder versions of the features noted previously in Group-II prune-belly syndrome. One typical combination may involve a small kidney on one side and a large unusual kidney on the opposite side, although kidney function and blood pressure may be normal. Individuals with this form of prune-belly may easily live into adulthood (Fig. 19–330).

DISORDERS OF SEXUAL DIFFERENTIATION

Intersex problems are common, occurring once in every 1000 live births. The exception is hypospadias, which occurs once in every 650 births. From the radiologist's and urologist's point of view, it is easiest to separate disorders of sexual differentiation into those with and those without ambiguous genitalia. Because the results of chromosomal and hormonal studies are not likely to be available to the radiologist at the time of the imaging examination, given that these studies usually take place when the patient is first admitted to a hospital, the

following discussion emphasizes what the radiologist is likely to observe.

At this point it may be useful to recall and summarize earlier discussions of the relevant embryology.

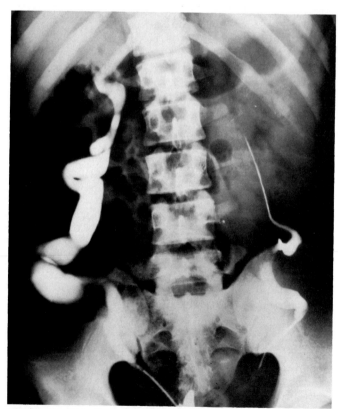

Figure 19–330. Prune-belly syndrome in a 28-year-old man. Bilateral retrograde pyeloureterograms demonstrate a tortuous dilated right ureter that has the course and appearance usually associated with the ureter in patients with prune-belly syndrome. The right kidney functioned well, in spite of the abnormal appearance of the ureter. The left ureter is atretic in its proximal portion, and the left kidney was dysplastic and essentially nonfunctioning.

Embryology of the Genital Tract

Urogenital Fold

The mesonephros develops on the posterior wall of the coelomic cavity. Only in the earliest stages is there sufficient space for this structure in the retroperitoneum.[24] As it expands, it projects as a fold into the coelomic cavity. Later this fold contains the müllerian duct and the reproductive glands as well as the mesonephros;[24] hence its name—the urogenital fold. It is an area within which a number of important processes take place.[24]

Development of the Indifferent Gonad

The anlagen of the gonads appear in the urogenital folds lateral to the mesonephros in Stage 16 (37 to 42 days).[24] When the indifferent gonads develop to their maximum length, they extend from the T6 to the S2 segments.[24]

When the gonads first develop, they contain no germ cells. However, germ cells do exist. After forming in the 4.5-day-old blastocyst,[56, 57] they can be found in the endoderm of the yolk sac by the 13th day,[55] and the endoderm of the allantois by the 17th day.[55] From the allantois, the germ cells migrate to the gonads.[25, 26] During this migration, these cells divide and increase in number. By late Stage 16 (42 days), the germ cells reach the gonads.

At this point, the gonads of the male and female are identical, and consist of three types of cells. In addition to the germ cells, supporting cells are present, originally from the coelomic epithelium of the genital ridge. These later become Sertoli's cells in the male and the granulosa cells of the ovary in the female. The third component of these indifferent gonads are stromal or interstitial cells, originating from the mesoblast of the urogenital fold.

Development of the Testis and Ovary

At Stage 17 (42 to 44 days) in the male and Stage 18 (44 to 48 days) in the female, differentiation of the indifferent gonad into the testis or the ovary, respectively, becomes evident.

The testis grows very rapidly. The rete (seminiferous) tubules develop, and by the end of the embryonic period (Stage 23, 56 to 60 days) the testis begins to have an endocrine function.

During the same period the ovaries also grow, but undergo fewer changes. Only at 75 to 80 days do the germ cells in the ovaries begin to cluster and undergo division by meiosis. Follicular cells then surround the germ cells, and by about 15 weeks a definite ovary with follicles and stroma is visible. Interestingly, this final gonadal differentiation occurs 8 weeks later in the female than in the male.[27, 28]

Development of the Müllerian Duct System

The müllerian ducts form symmetrically in both sexes on both sides of the body, although they develop completely in the female only, and they degenerate in the male fetus.

Each müllerian duct is divided into a short cranial portion, known as the ostium abdominale, and a longer caudal portion, which is the tube proper.[24]

The ostium abdominale is formed as coelomic epithelium invaginates into the summit of the urogenital fold, and the tube proper develops as an independent outgrowth of the blind end of this invagination. At this point the müllerian duct lies lateral to the primary nephric duct.[24] The first anlagen of the ostium abdominale is seen in Stage 16 (37 to 42 days).

In both sexes the right and left müllerian ducts unite. The resultant canal is called the uterovaginal canal,[24] and it may be seen in embryos of Stages 20 to 23. This union first takes place in the second quarter segment, as measured from above, of what becomes the uterovaginal canal.[24] From that point the union advances cranially and caudally and is frequently discontinuous, especially in the caudal portion. The caudal end of the uterovaginal canal fuses with the wolffian duct so completely that the epithelial cells of either structure lie immediately adjacent, with no intervening basement membrane.

Just before the ovary and testis can be differentiated, both sexes have two wolffian ducts and two müllerian ducts.

Almost immediately after the union of the müllerian ducts in the male, at the end of the embryonic period, they and the uterovaginal canal begin to degenerate, because Sertoli's cells of the developing testes secrete antimüllerian factor (AMF).

In the female, the uterovaginal canal becomes the uterus and cephalic portion of the vagina, while the rest of the müllerian ducts become the fallopian tubes. The distal portion of the vagina first appears at 9 weeks and consists of a solid mass of cells between the caudal end of the uterovaginal canal and the dorsal wall of the urogenital sinus. This mass of cells grows, and by 11 weeks a lumen forms. By 20 weeks the lumen is completely formed, and the hymen separates the vagina from the urogenital sinus.

Urogenital Union

The ducts of the mesonephros and the tubules of the testis unite in a process called urogenital union.[24]

It is recalled that there are two periods during which the mesonephros degenerates. Urogenital union occurs in the second period, so that part of the mesonephros has already disappeared. The remnant is divided into the upper-genital and lower-gland portions by this urogenital union; the upper-genital portion is called the epigenitalis, and the lower-gland portion is known as the paragenitalis.

Each glomerulus of the mesonephros has a secretory tubule, draining into a collecting ductule. All such collecting ductules drain independently into the wolffian duct. During the total time the mesonephros is present, a grand total of 83 glomeruli, secretory tubules, and collecting ductules will have developed. However, as the mesonephros is serially degenerating, not all these glomeruli and ductules will be present at the same time (Fig. 19–331).[24]

When the glomeruli and the secretory ducts degenerate, the ends of the collecting ductules seal off and become blind-ending diverticula off the wolffian ducts. Some then unite with the rete tubules, which are ducts that had previously developed in the gonads (Fig. 19–331). As soon as the collecting ductules have broken through as a result of this union, they are called the efferent ducts of the testis.[24] In the 4th fetal month, the wolffian duct just caudal to the efferent ducts lengthens, coils, and forms

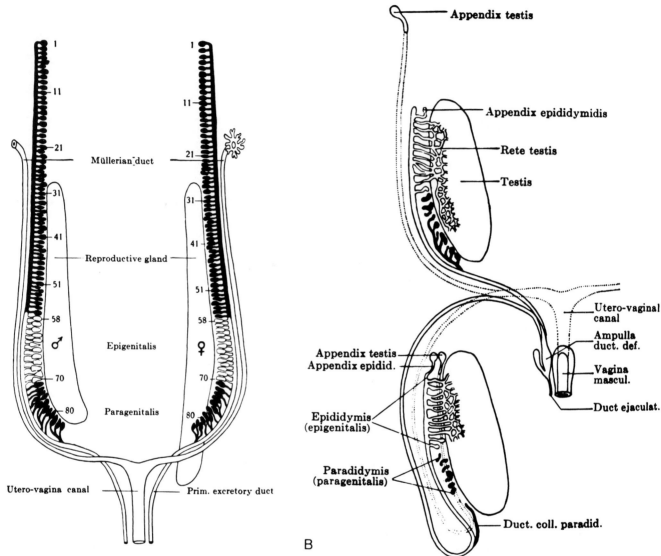

Figure 19–331. Diagram of the entire renal organ, gonad, and efferent ducts. The numbers are the serial numbers of the ductules. Solid lines represent area that persists, and dotted lines represent area that degenerates. White represents changes in position, and black represents whatever has reached its final position. *A*, structures are shown before descent of the gonads. The male gonad is on the left, and the female gonad is on the right. *B* shows development of the accessory organs of reproduction in the male after testicular descent. The müllerian duct degenerates throughout the greater part of its extent, and the closed ostium abdominale persists as the appendix testis (hydatid of Morgagni), and the lowest portion of the uterovaginal canal persists as the vagina masculina (utricle). All the tubules of the epididymis are not employed in the urogenital union: the first tubule remains free and becomes the appendix epididymis; the other unemployed tubules persist as appendices retis. The paradidymis is separated into its individual parts—some, for the collecting ductules, persist as the organs of Giraldes; the terminal portions of the ductules, united to form a canal, persist as the collecting duct of the paradidymis (the hallerian duct).

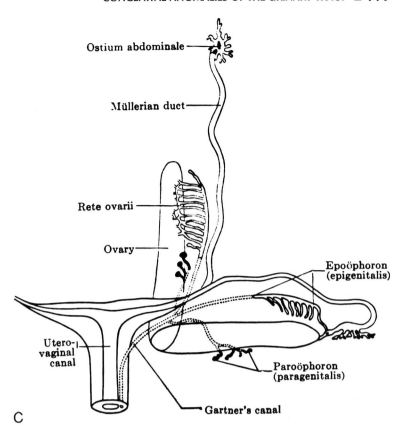

Figure 19–331 *Continued C* shows the development of the accessory organs of reproduction in the female, after descent of the ovary. The ovary remains in the body cavity, but rotates through 90 degrees in such a way that its cranial pole, through which the axis of rotation passes, remains where it was and becomes the medial pole. The urogenital fold is rotated at the same time around the müllerian duct, and, as a result, the tube comes to lie cranial to the ovary. The mesonephros and primary excretory duct degenerates; of the mesonephros, the epigenitalis persists as the epo-ophoron and parts of the paro-ophoron. Of the wolffian duct, only the portion that receives the tubules of the epo-ophoron is retained, although portions of the rest may persist at Gartner's canal. (From Felix W: The development of the urogenital organs. *In* Keibel F, Mall FP (eds): Manual of Human Embryology, Vol II. Philadelphia, JB Lippincott Company, 1912.)

C

the epididymis.[24] The wolffian duct adjacent to the testis remains straight. The embryology of the vas, seminal vesicles, and ejaculatory duct are discussed on page 757.

Development of the Accessory Organs of Reproduction After Gonadal Descent

Both the testis and ovary descend.[24] Testicular descent is described on page 762. After the testis descends, the closed ostium abdominale of the müllerian duct persists as the appendix testis, and the uterovaginal canal persists as the utriculus masculinus (vagina masculina) (Fig. 19–331).[24]

All the tubules of the epididymis are not used during the process of urogenital union. The first tubule remains free and becomes the appendix epididymis.[24] Other such tubules persist as the appendices retis. Some of the collecting ductules of the paradidymis persist as the organ of Giraldes; the terminal portions of the ductules unite to form a canal that persists as the collecting ductules of the paradidymis (the duct of Haller) (Fig. 19–331).[24]

In the female, the ovary rotates through 180 degrees. As a result, the müllerian duct lies cranially, and the ovary caudally.[24] After the mesonephros degenerates, the epigenitalis persists as the epo-ophoron; the paragenitalis persists as the paro-ophoron. Portions of the wolffian duct may persist as Gartner's canal.[24]

Seven Components of Sex

There are seven major components of sex (Table 19–35).[29] The role of the radiologist is usually limited to defining the internal genital anatomy by ultrasonography, CT, radiography, or whatever imaging studies are appro-

priate. Regardless of the modality employed, the goal is accurate definition of the internal genital anatomy to allow for the proper classification of the disorder and the proper sex assignment.

It should be emphasized that achieving the latter goal requires close cooperation with medical and surgical specialists. Since the patient's family faces an unexpected and certainly unwanted crisis, patience, tact, and delicacy are required to enable them to face this enormously difficult time.

Ambiguous Genitalia

Ambiguous genitalia are usually discovered in the neonate. Although congenital adrenal hypospadia constitutes a genuine medical emergency, most forms of ambiguous genitalia are not actually medical emergencies. However,

Table 19–35. Seven Components of Sex

Component	Variables	Comment
Chromosomal sex	Chromatin positive (XX) Chromatin negative (XY)	
Gonadal sex	Testes: neither or both Ovaries: neither or both	Morphological intersex
Internal genital anatomy	Müllerian (female) Wolffian (male)	
External genital anatomy		
Hormonal sex	Androgenic Estrogenic	Effect at puberty
Rearing sex	Sex assignment	Governed by genital anatomy
Gender	Sex orientation	Governed by rearing sex

Modified from Shopfner C: Genitography in intersexual states. Radiology 82:664–674, 1964.

they are considered psychological emergencies, and the prompt diagnosis can help the family, and later the child, to adjust.

Disorders involving ambiguous genitalia are classified into the following four categories:

Female Pseudohermaphrodite. The patient has ovaries, a 46 XY karyotype, and androgen excess.

Male Pseudohermaphrodite. The patient has testes and a 46 XX karyotype. There is decreased synthesis of, or sensitivity to, androgen.

Mixed Gonadal Dysgenesis. The patient has chromosomal abnormalities and abnormal testes.

True Hermaphrodite. The patient possesses testicular as well as ovarian tissue.

Female Pseudohermaphroditism

Female pseudohermaphrodites are genetic females, with a normal 46 XX karyotype and normal female internal genitalia.

These patients present with a variable degree of virilization, ranging from minimal clitoral hypertrophy to a fairly well-developed penis with some degree of hypospadius and a scrotal sac, into which the ovaries have not descended. The task of the radiologist is to examine the anatomy of the vagina and urogenital sinus (if present). The examination of choice is genitography, as discussed below.

The underlying cause of female pseudohermaphroditism is prenatal exposure to excess androgen in the first few months of gestation. The following kinds of exposure can occur.

Congenital Adrenal Hyperplasia. The most common cause of female pseudohermaphroditism is congenital adrenal hyperplasia, an inherited deficiency of an enzyme involved in corticosteroid synthesis.[30] This is discussed more fully in Chapters 84 and 85. Low levels of cortisol induce increased adrenocorticotropic hormone (ACTH) production through a feedback mechanism, which causes an excess of intermediate metabolites and androgens. Virilization results.

Of this group, there are two main subtypes. Of patients with congenital adrenal hyperplasia, 90% to 95% have 21 hydroxylase deficiency, which in 50% of cases is associated with severe salt wasting. A neonate with ambiguous genitalia who is dehydrated and perhaps is vomiting should be immediately evaluated for salt-losing congenital adrenal hyperplasia and treated on an emergency basis. The less common form, 11 hydroxylase deficiency, occurs in 5% to 10% of cases and is associated with hypertension.

Several other enzyme deficiencies can cause congenital adrenal hyperplasia. In all cases of enzyme deficiency, however, the diagnosis is made by measuring levels of steroid metabolites in the blood and urine.

Maternal Ingestion of Androgens. The second most common cause of ambiguous genitalia is the maternal ingestion of androgens, which will usually be progestational agents, with some androgenic activity.

Maternal Virilizing Tumor of the Ovary or Adrenal. A rare cause of female pseudohermaphroditism is a maternal virilizing tumor of the ovary or adrenal.[31, 32]

Male Pseudohermaphroditism

Male pseudohermaphrodites are genetic males with a 46 XY karyotype. Generally also, such patients have ambiguous genitalia, and normal or mildly defective testes. All of which the four major types of the disorder are caused by enzyme deficiencies, or organ resistance to androgen, or both.

The four major types are described below.

Decreased Testosterone Biosynthesis. This rare type may be due to several different enzyme deficiencies leading to a wide range of clinical manifestations.

The Testicular Feminization Syndrome. In this type, the target organs are insensitive to androgens.[33–35] Testicular feminization may be complete or incomplete. In *complete testicular feminization*, the patient is phenotypically female, and reared as such. Subsequent abnormal puberty leads to the discovery that the karyotype is 46 XY, the uterus is absent, and the undescended gonads are testes. These testes are removed after puberty by some clinicians for two reasons: They are at significant risk of developing malignant neoplasms, and their removal makes it more likely that breasts will develop in these phenotypically female patients. Others have advocated earlier removal with hormonal replacement. In *incomplete testicular feminization syndrome* (the Reinfenstein syndrome), a wide spectrum of intersex abnormalities can occur. Genitography and ultrasound will define the internal anatomy and demonstrate that the uterus is absent.

The determination of sex in these patients depends on several factors. Most can be reared as males; those with minimal or no virilization are usually reared as females.

Familial Pseudovaginal Penoscrotal Hypospadias. This disorder, common in the Dominican Republic but not elsewhere, is caused by a deficiency of 5-reductase, the enzyme that converts testosterone to dihydrotestosterone, which is required in order to induce masculinization of the phallus and urogenital sinus. It is also involved in the development of the prostate gland.

The internal genitalia in such patients are normal, because the production of testosterone and of müllerian inhibitor factor is unaffected. The testes may be cryptorchid and lie either in the abdomen or the inguinal canals.

Prior to puberty, the phallus is small to intermediate in size, and may resemble a large clitoris; a perineal hypospadias and a vagina of variable size opening into the urogenital sinus also exist. The prostate gland is undeveloped.

At puberty, however, the patient begins to appear more masculine, sperm production begins, the phallus enlarges, and, frequently, the testes descend into the scrotum. The breasts do not enlarge. This change may be so startling that in the Dominican Republic, for example, affected patients who are initially reared as females change to male identities after puberty.

Male Hypospadias. Male hypospadias is a mild form of male pseudohermaphroditism, as discussed in the preceding section of this chapter on page 567.

Mixed Gonadal Dysgenesis

Patients with mixed gonadal dysgenesis have rudimentary or dysgenetic gonads, or both, and also have associated chromosomal abnormalities.[36] The most common karyotype is XO/XY, although multiple mosaic forms also occur.

A range of clinical virilization may occur, depending on the amount of testicular tissue present and on androgen production. Many patients have phenotypic signs of Turner's syndrome. Some virilization, however, should suggest mixed gonadal dysgenesis.

Most patients have ambiguous genitalia, ranging from almost normal female anatomy to male hypospadias.

This condition is called mixed gonadal dysgenesis because there is a streak gonad (or the gonad is absent) on one side and a testis on the other side. The side with the streak gonad or an absent gonad usually has a fallopian tube; the side with the testicular tissue has a vas deferens. Often a rudimentary uterus is present.

Patients with mixed gonadal dysgenesis who also have a Y chromosome component are at high risk of developing malignant germ cell carcinoma; therefore, when a patient with mixed gonadal dysgenesis and a Y chromosome is identified, the gonads should be removed (Fig. 19–332). Such patients are also at risk of developing Wilms' tumor,[37] which occurs in association with nephritis (the Drash syndrome),[38] so that the kidneys should be followed throughout childhood by ultrasound examination.

True Hermaphroditism

True hermaphrodites have both ovarian and testicular tissue, either in an ovotestis, or in a separate testis and ovary.[39, 40] The most common variation is an ovotestis on one side with either an ovary, testis, or another ovotestis on the opposite side.

The external genitalia are usually ambiguous, although the patient may look more male than female, owing to the presence of androgens.

The internal genitalia are variable and depend primarily on the amount of androgen and müllerian inhibiting factor produced by the ipsilateral testicular tissue.

True hermaphroditism occurs much less frequently than the other conditions described above.

Disorders of Sex Differentiation without Ambiguous Genitalia

Turner's Syndrome

Turner's syndrome[41] patients are phenotypic females with a 45 XO karyotype.[42] The external genitalia are female; the uterus is small, and the gonads range from streaks to dysplastic or hypoplastic ovaries. In the newborn period these patients present with a webbed neck and lymphedema of the hands and feet. The incidence of cystic hygromas is higher, and these can be diagnosed by prenatal ultrasonography. Affected individuals show a distinctive facies, a short broad neck, and a shieldlike chest. They are often short.

Radiographic features include normal or near-normal bone age, short metacarpals, abnormal distal tufts, abnormal carpal bones, cubitus valgus, coarctation of the aorta, and horseshoe kidney.

Maturation at puberty is poor, and hormonal treatment is required for improved breast development and other secondary sex characteristics.

Mosaic Forms of Turner's Syndrome. Mosaic forms of Turner's syndrome are distinguished from classic Turner's syndrome by the facts that (1) the karyotype is XO/XX, and (2) clinical manifestations are less severe.

Pure Gonadal Dysgenesis

Pure gonadal dysgenesis is distinguished from Turner's syndrome by the fact that (1) the karyotype is XX/XY or mosaic, and (2) some clitoral enlargement may occur.[43] The patients are otherwise clinically similar to those with Turner's syndrome, and, like many such patients, they also have bilateral streak gonads. As in mixed gonadal dysgenesis, moreover, the presence of a Y chromosome component increases the risk of gonadal malignancy.

Klinefelter's Syndrome

Patients with Klinefelter's syndrome[44] are phenotypic males with an XXY karyotype.[45] They are usually tall with relatively small genitalia, especially the testes. Gynecomastia is common. The genitalia and pubic hair do not mature normally at puberty. Most patients are sterile and about 25% are mentally retarded.

XX Male (Sex Reversal Syndrome)

These patients are phenotypic males, and their karyotype is XX.[46] They have normal male internal genitalia and normal or small male external genitalia. Hypogonadism, hypospadias, and gynecomastia may be associated with this rare disorder.

Persistent Müllerian Ducts Syndrome (Hernia Uteri Inguinalis)

This rare disorder is caused by a deficiency of müllerian inhibiting factor. In addition to male internal and external genitalia, affected patients have a small uterus and fallopian tubes and a vagina that connects to the posterior urethra. Cryptorchidism and inguinal hernias may be present. The uterus may enter such a hernia. Patients with intra-abdominal testes may develop testicular tumors.[47, 48] Transverse testicular ectopia may be present.[49] A urethrogram can be normal, but, if contrast material is directed into the vagina (utriculus), the uterus and fallopian tubes may be visualized.

Complete Testicular (Feminization) Syndrome

These patients are phenotypic females but have an XY karyotype.[50] The disorder is caused by an X-linked androgen receptor binding defect that does not allow virilization, even though androgens are present. The incidence is about 1 in 20,000 to 60,000 females but rises to about 1% to 2% of females with inguinal hernias. These patients have no uterus or fallopian tubes. The vagina is short and blind-ending. Half the patients have no inguinal hernias; all have intra-abdominal gonads and testes. For the remaining 50% of patients, the testis may often be in the inguinal hernia—not the abdomen. After puberty, the likelihood of testicular tumors increases. Because of the androgen receptor binding defect, feminization occurs at puberty (although obviously menstruation is absent) and

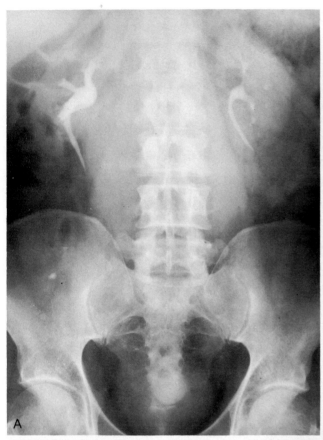

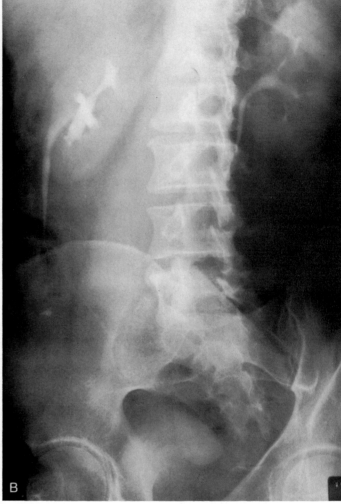

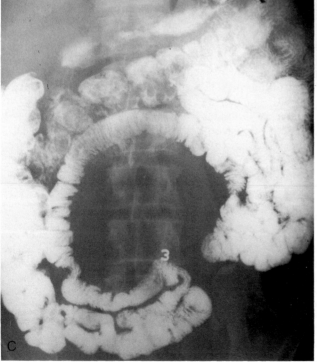

Figure 19–332. A 19-year-old male with mixed gonadal dysgenesis, who developed a malignant germ cell carcinoma on the right. The patient presented clinically with volvulus of the tumor-bearing gonad. An intravenous urogram, with AP *(A)* and oblique *(B)* views shows anterolateral ureteral displacement due to enlarged para-aortic nodes. A small-bowel series *(C)* shows displacement of small-bowel loops by an abdominal mass. The patient was found to have huge para-aortic nodes and developed large pulmonary metastases, but he responded to therapy and is alive and well, 21 years later.

is actually enhanced by the presence of testes; indeed, this is why the testes in such patients are not removed until sufficient feminization has occurred. After the testes are removed, the patients should receive exogenous female hormones.

Incomplete forms (see previous discussion) may present with ambiguous genitalia.

IMAGING EVALUATION

A basic understanding of the internal disorders enables the radiologist to plan an appropriate imaging evaluation. Any plan, however, should be coordinated with several pediatric and surgical specialists. A thorough history, physical examination, and laboratory tests, together with the imaging evaluation, usually provide the information required for a correct diagnosis. An accurate imaging evaluation of the anatomy of the lower genitourinary tract is essential, moreover, to help the surgeon plan reconstructive surgery.

A wide variety of imaging modalities are available. Contrast examinations such as genitography and voiding cystourethrography are still mainstays, but MRI and ultrasonography have become increasingly useful. CT is useful in selected cases.

Genitography

The term *genitography* refers to the identification and the injection with contrast material of all external orifices, including an ectopic anus and fistulous tracts.[29] A catheter is often appropriate for this purpose (see the first section of this chapter). If that fails to yield useful results, the "flush" technique should be used, which involves inserting the nozzle of a syringe into an available orifice and flushing the contrast material into the internal structure. For either technique, the most useful projection is the lateral one. Barium paste or some other marker on the perineum is a useful way to mark the outside of the body in relation to the internal structure.

The radiologist should fill the bladder, urethra, vagina (or utriculus masculinus), or any fistulous tract or anal anomaly with contrast material. Findings are variable, but frequently the urethra and vagina join internally to form a urogenital sinus; if the rectum or the anus also joins the urethra, a cloaca is visualized.

A filling defect at the top of the vagina suggests a cervix, which in turn suggests the presence of a uterus, as does the filling of the uterine cavity. Similarly, a small defect on the floor of the proximal urethra usually represents a verumontanum, suggesting the patient is a genetic male.

The appearance on genitography varies from that of a normal female to a near-normal male with hypospadias. The radiographic appearance may determine the degree of virilization and consequently the decision regarding sex assignment (Figs. 19–333 and 19–334).

Ultrasonography

This method is used to establish the presence of a uterus, to define congenital abnormalities of the genitourinary tract, and to evaluate the kidneys. Because of maternal hormonal stimulation in utero, the uterus can usually be seen within the first few weeks of life, provided the bladder contains enough urine to serve as a sonic window. The length of the uterus in a newborn is approximately 3.5 cm. If it is difficult to visualize, a catheter may be placed in the bladder to assist the sonographic imaging. This is also useful because later in infancy, the uterus is more difficult to identify, particularly since it decreases to about 2.5 cm in length. Ovaries are variably seen and may occasionally contain cysts. Because renal anomalies are frequently associated with lower genitourinary anomalies, screening renal ultrasonography is useful, together with whatever other examinations are necessary.

Figure 19–333. Diagram illustrating the appearances on genitography in patients with disorders of sexual differentiation. They vary from near-normal female (A) to near-normal male with hypospadias (F). (Modified from Shopfner CE: Genitography in intersexual states. Radiology 82:664–674, 1964.)

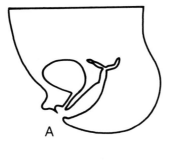
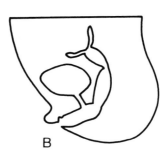
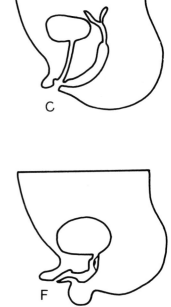
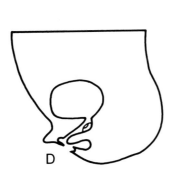
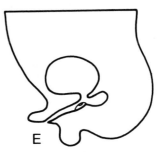

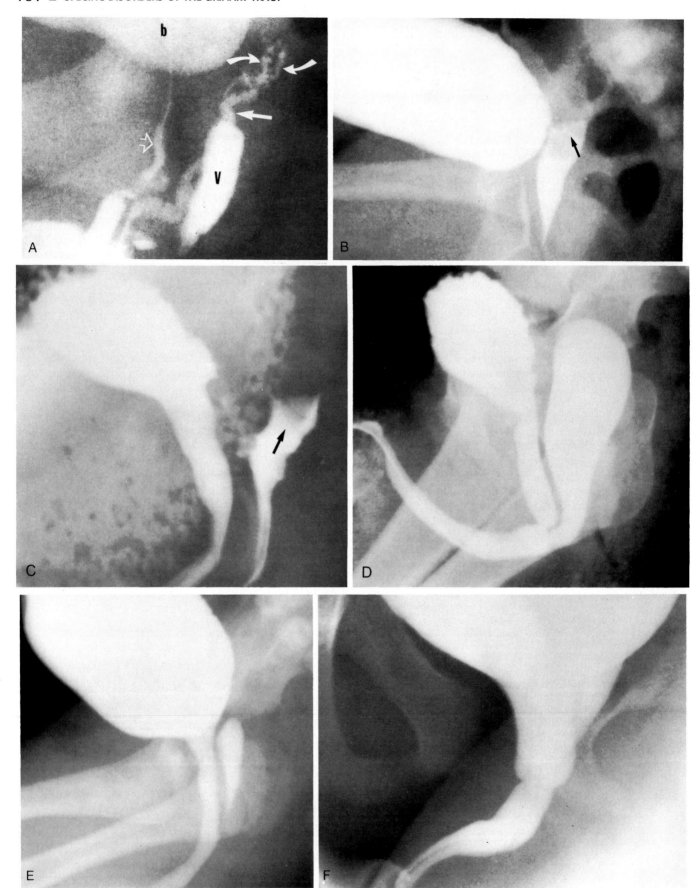

Figure 19–334. The appearances on genitography in patients with disorders of sexual function. They vary from *A*, near normal female, to *F*, near normal male with hypospadias. Note filling of uterus *(straight white arrow)*, fallopian tubes *(curved arrows)* and urethra *(open arrow)* in *A*, the cervical indentation *(arrow)* in *B* and *C*, and the lack of a cervical indentation in *D* and *E* (b = bladder, v = vagina.)

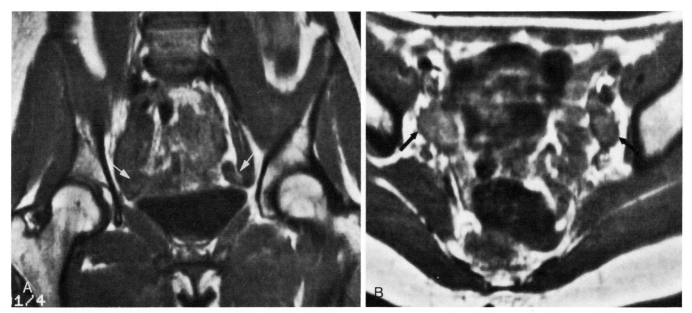

Figure 19–335. Testicular feminization in a 19-year-old woman. *A,* Coronal image (SE 500/28) shows absence of the uterus with primitive gonads *(arrows)* where normal ovaries should be located. *B,* Axial image (SS 500/28) shows primitive gonads *(arrows)* adjacent to internal obturator muscle. (From Dietrich RB, Kangarloo H: Pelvic abnormalities in children: Assessment with MR imaging. Radiology 163:367–372, 1987.)

Computed Tomography and Magnetic Resonance Imaging

MRI is clearly superior to ultrasonography in the evaluation of intersex disorders[51] and penile anatomy[60] and should be used whenever the information provided by ultrasound and contrast examinations is ambiguous (Figs. 19–335 and 19–336). CT is also helpful,[40] especially for evaluating the adrenal glands.

Other Examinations

Other examinations, such as hysterosalpingograms, pneumopyelography, and arteriography are rarely indicated.[52] The location of an undescended gonad may be identified by methods described in the preceding section of this chapter on page 764.

GARTNER'S DUCT CYSTS

Gartner's ducts are the remainders of the wolffian ducts left in the cervix,[58] the wall of the vagina,[53] or the leaves of the broad ligament.

An ectopic ureter may open into Gartner's duct, or the duct may dilate and form a cyst. Usually the cyst is small and has no effect on the urinary tract, although it may be large and displace the ureter upward. It may be well demonstrated by ultrasonography.[53] Gartner's duct cysts

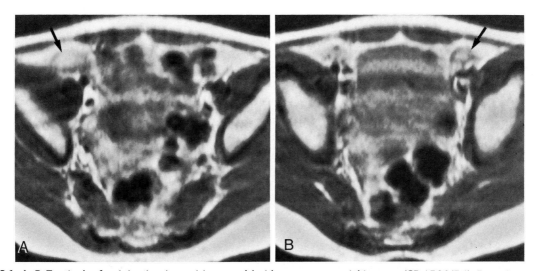

Figure 19–336. *A, B,* Testicular feminization in an 11-year-old girl, as seen on axial images (SE 1500/56). Ectopic gonads *(arrows),* seen in inguinal canals bilaterally, show central high signal intensity with surrounding mantle of low signal intensity. (From Dietrich RB, Kangarloo H: Pelvic abnormalities in children: Assessment with MR imaging. Radiology 163:367–372, 1987.)

occurring in the broad ligament may present in a fashion similar to other cystic pelvic masses. A Gartner's duct cyst may communicate with the cervical canal and fill with contrast during a hysterosalpingogram.[58]

FUSED LABIA

Fused labia may be congenital and familial, or acquired. The major clinical problem is that they are sometimes confused with congenital absence of the vagina. The condition is sometimes not discovered until later in life because of enuresis or dysuria. The radiologist examining for these symptoms may be the first to discover the disorder. Dribbling of urine is another symptom that is sometimes encountered. The adherent labia may form a nearly watertight compartment in contact with the urethra. Retention of urine in this space may lead to post-micturitional incontinence.

Regardless of whether they are partially or completely fused, the labia can usually be pried apart with lateral pressure of the thumbs, after which normal anatomy should be revealed underneath.

References

1. Nunn IN, Stephens FD: The triad syndrome: A composite anomaly of the abdominal wall, urinary system, and testes. J Urol 86:782, 1961.
2. Williams DI, Burkholder GV: The prune belly syndrome. J Urol 98:224–251, 1967.
3. Welch KJ, Kearney GP: Abdominal musculature deficiency syndrome: prunebelly. J Urol 111:693, 1974.
4. Woodward JR: The prune belly syndrome. Urol Clin North Am 5:75–93, 1978.
5. Berdon WE, Baker DH, Wigger HJ, Blanc WA: The radiologic and pathologic spectrum of the prune belly syndrome. The importance of urethral obstruction in prognosis. Radiol Clin North Am 15:83–92, 1977.
6. Barnhouse DH: Prune belly syndrome. Br J Urol 44:356, 1972.
7. Burke EC, Shin MH, Kelalis PP: Prune-belly syndrome. Am J Dis Child 117:668, 1969.
8. Carter TC, Tomskey GC, Ozog LS: Prune-belly syndrome. Urology 3:279–282, 1974.
9. Aaronson ZA, Cremin BJ: Prune belly syndrome in young females. Urol Radiol 1:151, 1980.
10. Rabinowitz R, Schillinger JF: Prune belly syndrome in the female subject. J Urol 118:454, 1977.
11. Jacobson Y: Passing Farms: Enduring Values. Los Altos, William Kaufmann, 1984, pp 89–90, 186, 187.
12. Schwarz RD, Stephens FD, Cussen LJ: The pathogenesis of renal dysplasia. II: The significance of lateral and medial ectopy of the ureteric orifice. Invest Urol 19:97, 1981.
13. Kroovand RL, Al-Ansari RM, Perlmutter AD: Urethral and genital malformations in prune-belly syndrome. J Urol 127:94–96, 1982.
14. Cremin BJ: The urinary tract anomalies associated with agenesis of the abdominal walls. Br J Radiol 44:767, 1971.
15. Sellers BB: Congenital megalourethra associated with prune belly syndrome. J Urol 116:814–815, 1976.
16. Monie IW, Monie BJ: Prune belly syndrome and fetal ascites. Teratology 19:111–118, 1979.
17. Pagon RA, Smith DW, Shepard TH: Urethral obstruction malformation complex: A cause of abdominal muscle deficiency and the "prune belly." J Pediatr 94:900–906, 1979.
18. Moerman P, Fryns JP, Goddeeris P, Lauweryns JM: Pathogenesis of the prune-belly syndrome: A functional urethral obstruction caused by prostatic hypoplasia. Pediatrics 73:470–475, 1984.
19. Williams DI: Paediatric urology. New York, Appleton-Century-Crofts, 1968, pp 282–286.
20. Riccardi VM, Grum CM: The prune-belly anomaly: Heterogeneity and superficial X-linkage mimicry. J Med Genet 14:266, 1977.
21. Teramoto R, Opas LM, Andrassy R: Splenic torsion with prune-belly syndrome. J Pediatr 98:91–92, 1981.
22. Kirschner SG, Kirschner FK Jr, Jolles H, et al: Bladder calcification in the prune belly syndrome. Radiology 138:597–600, 1981.
23. Aaronson IA: Posterior urethral valve masquerading as the prune belly syndrome. Br J Urol 55:508–512, 1983.
24. Felix W: The development of the urogenital organs. II. The development of the reproductive glands and their ducts. In Keibel F, Mall FP (eds); Manual of Human Embryology, Vol III. Philadelphia, JB Lippincott, 1912, pp 881–975.
25. Witschi E: Migration of germ cells of human embryos from the yolk sac to the primitive gonadal folds. Carnegie Contrib Embryol 209 32:69–80, 1948.
26. Peters H: Migration of gonocytes into the mammalian gonad and their differentiation. Philos Trans R Soc Lond (Ser B) 259:91, 1970.
27. Gillman J: The development of the gonads in man, with a consideration of the role of fetal endocrines and the histogenesis of ovarian tumors. Carnegie Contrib Embryol 210 32:83, 1948.
28. Gondos B, Bhinaleus P, Habel CJ: Ultrastructural observations on germ cells in human fetal ovaries. Am J Obstet Gynecol 110:644, 1971.
29. Shopfner CE: Genitography in intersexual states. Radiology 82:664–674, 1964.
30. Quazi QM, Thompson MW: Genital changes in congenital virilizing adrenal hyperplasia. J Pediatr 80:653–654, 1972.
31. Malinak LR, Miller GV: Bilateral multicentric ovarian leutinomas of pregnancy associated with masculinization of a female infant. Am J Obstet Gynecol 91:251–256, 1965.
32. Veincens E, Martinez-Mora J, Potau N, et al: Masculinization of a female fetus by Krukenberg tumor during pregnancy. J Pediatr Surg 15:188–190, 1980.
33. Aiman A, Griffin JE: The frequency of androgen receptor deficiency in infertile men. J Clin Endocrinol Metab 54:725, 1982.
34. Giffin JE, Durant LJ: Qualitative receptor defects in families with androgen resistance: Failure of stabilization of fibroblast cytosol androgen receptor. J Clin Endocrinol Metabl 55:465, 1982.
35. Imperato-McGinley J, Peterson RE, Gautier T, et al: Hormonal evaluation of a large kindred with complete androgen insensitivity. Evidence for secondary 5-alpha reductase deficiency. J Clin Endocrinol Metab 54:931, 1982.
36. Davidoff F, Federman DD: Mixed gonadal dysgenesis. Pediatrics 52:725–742, 1973.
37. Rajfer J: Association between Wilms' tumor and gonadal dysgenesis. J Urol 125:388–390, 1981.
38. Goldman SM, Garfinkel DJ, Oh KS, Dorst JP: The Drash syndrome: Male pseudohermaphroditism, nephritis, and Wilms' tumor. Radiology 141:87–91, 1981.
39. Aaronson IA: True hermaphroditism. A review of 41 cases with observations on testicular histology and function. Br J Urol 57:775–779, 1985.
40. English RE, Tulloch DN, Blaquiere RM: The demonstration of true hermaphroditism by computed tomography. Clin Radiol 37:593–594, 1986.
41. Turner HH: A syndrome of infantilism, congenital webbed neck, and cubitus valgus. Endocrinology 23:566, 1938.
42. Ford CE, Jones KW, Polani PE, et al: A sex-chromosome anomaly in a case of gonadal dysgenesis (Turner's syndrome). Lancet 1:711, 1959.
43. Judd HL, Scully RE, Atkins L, et al: Pure gonadal dysgenesis with progressive hirsutism. Demonstration of testosterone production by gonadal streaks. N Engl J Med 282:881–885, 1970.
44. Klinefelter HF Jr, Reifenstein EC Jr, Albright F: Syndrome characterized by gynecomastia, aspermatogenesis with A-leydigism, and increased secretion of follicle-stimulating hormone. J Clin Endocrinol 2:615, 1942.
45. Jacobs PA, Strong JA: A case of human intersexuality having a possible XXY sex-determining mechanism. Nature 183:302, 1959.
46. Raspa RA, Burige KA, Hensle TW: The sex reversal syndrome (the XX male patient). J Urol 134:152–153, 1985.
47. Kazim E: Intra-abdominal seminomas in persistent müllerian duct syndrome. Urology 26:290–292, 1985.
48. Snow BW, Rowland RC, Seal CM, Williams SD: Testicular tumor in patient with persistent müllerian duct syndrome. Urology 26:495–497, 1985.
49. Mouli K, McCarthy P, Ray P, et al: Persistent müllerian duct syndrome in a man with transverse testicular ectopia. J Urol 139:373–375, 1988.

50. Schwimer SR, Rubinstein L, Lebovic J: Sonographic evaluation of the testicular feminization syndrome. J Ultrasound Med 4:503–504, 1985.
51. Dietrich RB, Kangarloo H: Pelvic abnormalities in children: Assessment with MR imaging. Radiology 163:367–372, 1987.
52. Cremin BJ: Intersex states in young children: The importance of radiology in making the correct diagnosis. Clin Radiol 25:63–73, 1974.
53. Klein FA, Vick CW III, Broecker BH: Neonatal vaginal cysts. Diagnosis and management. J Urol 135:371–372, 1986.
54. Greskovich FJ III, Nyberg LM Jr: The prune-belly syndrome: A review of its etiology, defects, treatment and prognosis. J Urol 140:707–712, 1988.
55. Jirásek JE: Development of the genital system and male pseudo-hermaphroditism. Baltimore, The Johns Hopkins Press, 1971.
56. Hertig AT, Rock J, Adams EC: A description of 34 human ova within the first 17 days of development. Am J Anat 98:435–493, 1956.
57. Hertig AT, Adams EC, McKay DG, et al: A thirteen-day ovum studied histochemically. Am J Obstet Gynecol 76:1025–1040, 1958.
58. Katz Z, Bernstein D, Lancet M: A possible causal relationship between mesonephric remnants and infertility of uterine origin. Int J Fertil 27:125–128, 1982.
59. Bracero LA, Clark D, Pieffer M, Fakhry J: Sonographic findings in a case of cloverleaf skull deformity and prune belly. Am J Perinatol 5:239–241, 1988.
60. Hricak H, Marotti M, Gilbert TJ, et al: Normal penile anatomy and abnormal penile conditions. Radiology 169:683–690, 1988.

Inflammatory Disease

BRUCE L. McCLENNAN
Editor

20 Urinary Tract Inflammation: An Overview

WILLIAM R. FAIR

The recognition and treatment of urinary tract infection (UTI) have changed dramatically in the era of antibiotic therapy and improved diagnostic techniques. Proper radiological consultation, including the appropriate selection and sequence of imaging studies, requires that physicians treating these patients have a thorough knowledge of the changing trends as well as an awareness of the most efficient and cost-effective methods for establishing a timely and correct diagnosis.

Historically, Avicenna (ca. 980–1037) described renal abscess and "hard inflammation" of the kidney, which is thought to be a reference to nephritis, in his *Canon Medicare*.[1] One of the earliest implications that renal damage could be the result of infection was in the thirteenth century by Guglielmo Salicetti (ca. 1201–1277),[2] who suggested that chronic "nephritis" and "sclerosis of the kidneys" could be either due to infection or secondary to a "fever in the kidney."[2]

In Bright's classic description of renal disease, which bore his name for succeeding generations of medical students, the sequelae of renal inflammation are well described.[3] However, it was not until 1870 that Klebs actually identified microorganisms in the renal tubules and recognized their etiological significance in some cases of nephritis.[4]

The credit for distinguishing the clinical and pathological features of pyelonephritis, as distinct from other forms of Bright's disease, belongs primarily to Wagner,[5] who described in detail five cases of contracted kidneys secondary to cystitis and pyelitis and documented the pathological changes characteristic of pyelonephritis.[6] The difficulty in reaching a consensus about the diagnosis and management of UTI in the years that followed was emphasized by Crabtree and Cabot in 1916,[7] who noted "there is no subject in which there is so little uniformity of opinion and so much confusion."

Over the decades that followed, the gradual delineation of the role of infection in the pathogenesis of urinary tract disease became more focused. With the advent of the antibiotic era, the morbidity and mortality long recognized as the natural sequelae of untreated UTI began to yield to modern diagnostic and therapeutic interventions. The recognition that effective prophylaxis was possible in many patients prone to UTI and the changing concepts regarding the amount and duration of antimicrobial therapy needed have radically altered treatment options and outcome. The observation that alterations on the cell surface of both the microbe and the host cell in the urinary tract can dramatically affect the adherence and subsequent infectivity of a given bacterium paved the way for even more effective preventive strategies.

At the same time, however, the efficacy of short-course therapy—as little as a single dose of an appropriate antibiotic in many patients may be effective—raises the intriguing question of whether or not prophylactic antibacterial therapy should even be considered for most adult females prone to recurrent infections.

DEFINITIONS

Urinary Tract Infection

This term implies the presence of bacteria within the urinary tract (bacteriuria). It also suggests that the microorganisms are actually colonizing the urinary tract and are not simply contaminants present as a result of a break (flaw) in the collection or culture technique. Significant bacteriuria is generally defined as a bacterial colony count of greater than 100,000 organisms/ml voided midstream urine.[8] Although this "magic number" is helpful in defining the significance of a particular urine culture result, there are serious limitations in applying this figure to assess the clinical implications of culture results with fewer than 1,000,000 bacteria/ml. This is especially true in patients receiving antibiotics at the time of culture. Obviously *any* bacteria in a direct renal or bladder aspirate indicate a UTI. A UTI may be further classified as an *upper tract* (kidney) or *lower tract* (bladder-urethra) infection and may be *symptomatic* or *asymptomatic*.

Pyuria

The term *pyuria* refers to the presence of an abnormal number of pus cells (polymorphonuclear leukocytes) in the urine. Although urinary tract infections are far and away the most common cause of pyuria, noninfectious causes such as chemical irritation (e.g., cyclophosphamide), stones, interstitial nephritis, and so forth, occur also. Pyuria associated with a failure to grow organisms on routine culture media is known as "sterile" pyuria.

Tuberculosis, fungus infections, and viral cystitis are some causes of sterile pyuria.

Upper Tract Infection

This term is used to indicate an infection above the level of the bladder and usually includes signs or symptoms of fever, chills, and flank pain.

Lower Tract Infection

This term is limited to describing infections that occur at the level of the urinary bladder or below; it is a generalized term including patients with symptoms of cystitis, prostatitis, urethritis, and so forth. The symptoms of lower tract infection reflect the site of the infection and typically consist of urinary frequency, painful or difficult urination (dysuria), and suprapubic pain. Fever does not often accompany lower tract infections, except in male patients with documented bacterial prostatitis. At times, lower urinary symptomatology may be the only indication of upper tract disease (e.g., tuberculosis).

Cystitis

This is more restrictive than the term lower tract infection and indicates an inflammatory condition of the bladder, often accompanied by irritative symptoms. Cystitis may be bacterial or nonbacterial in origin.

Urethritis

Inflammation of the urethra, particularly in the female, causes symptoms of urethritis, which are often indistinguishable from those of cystitis and may be secondary to bacterial or nonbacterial causes.

In patients presenting with symptoms of urethral irritation when no bacterial cause can be elicited, the term *urethral syndrome* is often applied. Urethritis in males is commonly accompanied by a urethral discharge and may be symptomatic or asymptomatic.

Prostatitis

This term is used to indicate a symptom complex usually manifested by irritative symptoms such as suprapubic, perineal, or low back pain, dysuria, frequency, and nocturia. Prostatitis may be further subdivided into conditions with a known bacterial origin and those for which no bacterial cause has been firmly established.

Acute Bacterial Prostatitis. This condition presents as an acute urinary infection. The patient frequently manifests systemic signs or symptoms of chills, fever, back pain, and lower tract complaints. The urine culture is invariably positive.

Chronic Bacterial Prostatitis. As the name implies, this is a bacterial infection localized in the prostate gland. Typically, these patients have a history of recurrent UTI, usually with the same strain of microorganism; when the patient is symptomatic, the urine culture will be positive.

The diagnosis of chronic bacterial prostatitis requires the demonstration of bacteria in the cultured, expressed prostatic secretion (EPS) or the postprostatic massage urine specimen, in between episodes of bladder bacteriuria, when the bladder urine is sterile.

Nonbacterial Prostatitis. This term refers to an inflammatory reaction in the prostate demonstrated by the presence of irritative symptoms and an increase in the number of white blood cells found in the EPS. The EPS and urine cultures are sterile.

Prostatodynia. Also known as the *painful prostate,* prostatodynia is a symptom complex suggestive of prostatitis without confirmatory evidence of prostatic inflammation (no increase in the number of leukocytes in the EPS), sterile urine, and prostatic fluid cultures.

From a radiological standpoint, the intravenous urogram (IVU) will be normal in patients with prostatitis but is often useful in excluding other causes of urinary tract inflammation. Conversely, infected urine in men with a normal urogram usually indicates bacterial prostatitis as a source of the UTI.[9]

Pyelonephritis. This is a term with both clinical and pathological connotations (Fig. 20–1). Clinically, it describes an acute illness characterized by fevers, chills, flank pain, and infected urine. In the histological sense, the term *chronic pyelonephritis* describes the findings of renal scarring thought to be the sequelae of kidney infection. The disease is characterized by patchy areas of involvement with the base of the triangular area of involvement at the cortical margin extending toward the papilla, thereby accounting for the broad scarring characteristics seen at urography (Fig. 20–2). Histologically, the striking colloid-filled tubules (thyroidization), found particularly in the proximal convoluted tubules, are characteristic.[10] The term has limited histological usefulness because a variety of renal diseases, particularly those resulting from obstruction and infarction, can produce virtually identical histological changes in the renal cortex. In its broadest sense, *pyelonephritis* does not imply any specific etiology. The term is used to describe tuberculous, fungal, viral, and other infections of the kidney. Bacterial pyelonephritis implies that the kidney is, or has been, affected specifically by bacteria.

Just as the term pyelonephritis should be used judiciously in describing pathological changes resulting from infection, it should also be carefully considered when describing radiographic findings. During acute bacterial pyelonephritis, the involved kidney may appear swollen or with nonspecific changes in some patients but is normal in most.[11, 12] Focal renal enlargement, termed acute focal bacterial nephritis (AFBN) (sometimes referred to as acute lobar nephronia), may appear as a renal mass.[13, 14]

The radiographic changes resulting from chronic bacterial infection of the kidney are the findings of focal, coarse, broad scars overlying a calyx and invariably associated with calyceal distortion (Fig. 20–2).[15] The intervening areas of normal renal tissue may undergo hypertrophy presenting the appearance of a mass, often described as a *pseudotumor,* which may require additional imaging techniques such as radionuclide and ultrasound scans for proper delineation.

As employed clinically, the term acute pyelonephritis usually implies acute bacterial pyelonephritis. Acute clinical pyelonephritis does not cause scarring in most adults with a normal, unobstructed, urinary tract,[16] but in some

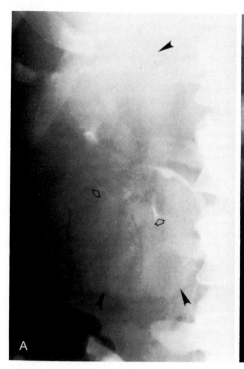
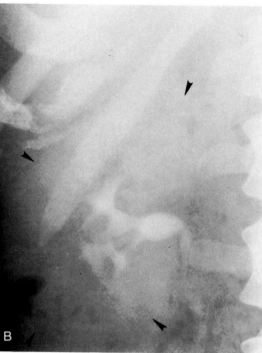

Figure 20–1. Acute pyelonephritis. *A,* Coned view of the right kidney on a 10-minute film from an intravenous urogram. A patchy involvement of the kidney is seen throughout, most marked in the lower pole. Global renal swelling is present (*arrowheads*). The collecting system is poorly filled (attenuated), owing to decreased urine flow and renal edema (*open arrowheads*). *B,* A follow-up IVU 6 weeks after antibiotic treatment for clinically acute pyelonephritis shows a normal right kidney (*arrowheads*), reduced to normal size.

patients a focal or global cortical atrophy with resultant overall renal shrinkage has been documented.[17] When found in association with vesicoureteral reflux, the term "reflux nephropathy" has been used to describe the changes of atrophy and pyelonephritis, although the actual role of reflux alone (in the absence of concomitant obstruction or infection) in the pathogenesis of the renal changes remains controversial. As a result, the term reflux nephropathy is limited and does not always accurately reflect the cause of the upper tract changes. In adult

bacteriuric females, radiographic findings consistent with reflux nephropathy are found in approximately 1% of patients.[18, 19]

Xanthogranulomatous Pyelonephritis

Xanthogranulomatous pyelonephritis represents an unusual reaction to chronic renal infection often associated with stones or obstruction. The typical presentation at

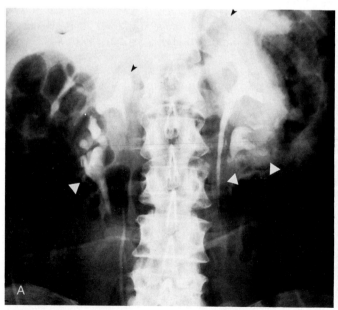
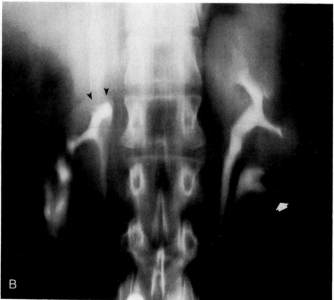

Figure 20–2. Chronic atrophic pyelonephritis (reflux nephropathy). *A,* A 36-year-old female with history of recurrent urinary tract infections since childhood. IVU shows bilateral duplication with calyceal deformity (clubbing) and cortical atrophy, most marked in lower poles (*white arrowheads*). The left upper-pole cortex is normal (*black arrowhead*), but severe cortical scarring is present in the right upper pole (*black arrowhead*) as well as in both lower poles. *B,* Tomogram shows similar findings but shows right upper-pole caliectasis and scarring to better advantage. Reflux is presumed to have occurred in childhood.

excretory urography is of an enlarged, poorly functioning or nonfunctioning renal mass with an associated calculus, although not all three characteristic features are found in every patient (Fig. 20–3). The bacteria most commonly involved are those found to produce urease (typically *Proteus*)[20, 21] with resulting urinary alkalinization and the subsequent formation of struvite (ammoniomagnesium phosphate) calculi. Because of their low calcium content, these stones may be poorly visualized by urography. Xanthogranulomatous pyelonephritis has been termed "the great imitator,"[22] as it may be misdiagnosed as a renal neoplasm, especially if it occurs as a focal process.[23] In addition to intensive antibacterial therapy, extirpative surgery is invariably required to completely eradicate the infection and the accompanying stone and/or obstruction (Table 20–1).

Interstitial Nephritis

Interstitial nephritis is a term describing the results of nonspecific renal interstitial inflammation and scarring that are not of infectious origin. It is often found associated with obstruction, analgesic or antibiotic abuse, diabetes mellitus, hyperuricemia, and other generalized conditions. Forms of interstitial nephritis may also result from adverse reactions to a wide variety of drugs including antibiotics (especially methicillin and rifampin), cimetidine, phenindione, fenoprofen, and many others.

CLASSIFICATION

Many classifications of UTI incorporate terms that are often inappropriate or misleading. Thus, when the term

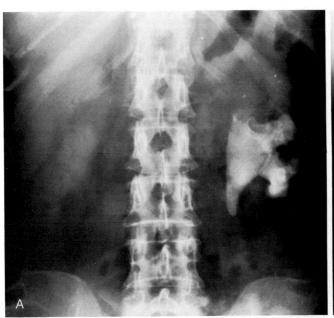

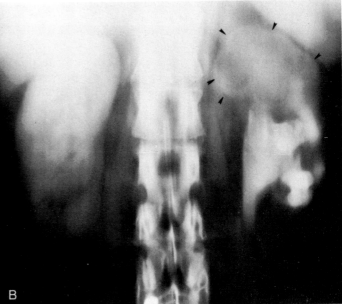

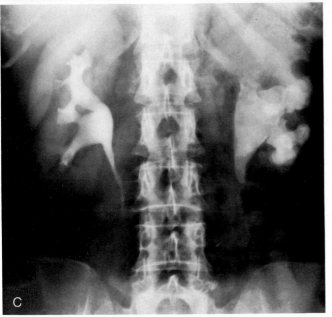

Figure 20–3. Staghorn calculus with focal (tumefactive) xanthogranulomatous pyelonephritis (XGPN). *A,* An IVU from a 69-year-old female with acute (*Escherichia coli*) urinary tract infection revealed a large staghorn calculus in the left kidney on the preliminary film. *B,* Tomography shows a slightly enlarged right kidney and focal hydronephrosis of left upper pole. Enhancement of residual cortex (rims) is noted (*arrowheads*) on left during nephrogram phase. *C,* Ten-minute film shows a normal right kidney. No excretion was seen on the left. Diffuse cortical atrophy, with focal XGPN and large struvite staghorn calculus, was found at surgery (left nephrectomy).

Table 20–1. Indications for Intravenous Urography (IVU) in Patients with Real or Suspected Urinary Tract Infection

Clinical pyelonephritis
Renal colic (history of stones or obstruction)
Urinary infection with a urea-splitting organism
Multiple UTIs caused by the same organism
History of childhood infections
Painless hematuria
Persistent microscopic hematuria after infection is
    adequately treated
Neuropathic bladder
Systemic disease associated with renal damage:
    diabetes mellitus, sickle cell anemia, analgesic
    abuse

chronic is applied to most UTIs it often fails to distinguish between continuous persistence of the same strain of bacteria, such as is the case in men with chronic bacterial prostatitis, and patients with rapid reinfection with a different bacterial species or strain, as is typical of women or children often labeled as suffering from *chronic cystitis*. The Stanford classification[24] divides all urinary tract infections into the following four simple categories:

I. First infection
II. Bacteriuria: unresolved during therapy
III. Recurrent infection
   A. Bacterial persistence: rapid relapse or infection with the *same organism* following antimicrobial treatment; bacteria are found mainly within the urinary tract.
   B. Reinfection: due to *different organisms* each time; the infection is from outside the urinary tract.

First Infection

The significance of the initial infection in nonhospitalized women is minimal; they are usually caused by organisms (predominantly *Escherichia coli*) that are pansensitive to antibacterial drugs. Uncomplicated initial infections may also occur in the male, but with much less frequency. About 25% of these women will have a subsequent infection over the next 18 months.[25]

Bacteriuria: Unresolved During Therapy

This term is applied to infections in patients for whom the initial therapy to sterilize the urine was not successful. Obviously, if the clinician fails to ensure that follow-up urine cultures during or immediately following therapy are sterile, it will be impossible to determine if any subsequent bacteriuria is the result of a new infection or inadequate therapy of the initial infection. The most common cause of unresolved bacteriuria during treatment is the selection of an antibiotic to which the bacteria are resistant. Although antimicrobial sensitivity testing to select the proper agent is theoretically appealing, a comparison of in vitro sensitivity testing and the therapeutic response to treatment has shown little correlation.[26] In fact, by simply identifying the organism responsible for the infection, the knowledgeable clinician can select the proper treatment without the cost and time delay inherent in the performance of antimicrobial sensitivity studies.[27]

Although bacterial resistance to the drug initially selected for treatment is the primary explanation, others, in decreasing order of frequency, are as follows:

1. Drug resistance during therapy due to resistant clones
2. Unsuspected mixed bacterial infection
3. Rapid reinfection with a completely different organism before completion of therapy
4. Azotemia (inadequate urinary antibiotic levels)
5. Papillary necrosis
6. Staghorn calculi
7. Patient noncompliance
8. Inaccessibility of organism to antibiotic (e.g., thick-walled abscesses).

Recurrent Infections

Recurrent infections, as the term implies, are repeated UTIs *after the initial bacteriuria has been adequately treated and resolved*. Recurrent infections may be further subdivided into (1) those due to bacterial persistence within the urinary tract and (2) those that result from entirely different bacteria at each infection, the microorganisms arising outside the urinary tract.

Recurrent infections can result from a chronic focus of infection seeding the urinary tract with infecting organisms, which may be quite sensitive to antibiotic therapy but are not totally eradicated by antimicrobial treatment, thus causing a recurrent infection once the antibiotic is stopped. The most common examples of bacterial persistence are patients with poorly visualized struvite renal calculi and the relatively rare patients with chronic bacterial prostatitis. Stamey[28] has identified the most common urological abnormalities responsible for bacterial persistence and recurrent infection. The following is a modification of his list:

1. Infection stones
2. Chronic bacterial prostatitis
3. Unilateral infected atrophic kidneys
4. Vesicovaginal and vesicoenteric fistulae
5. Ureteral duplication and ectopic ureters
6. Foreign bodies within the urinary tract
7. Urethral diverticula and infected paraurethral glands
8. Unilateral medullary sponge kidney
9. Nonrefluxing, normal-appearing, infected ureteral stumps after nephrectomy
10. Infected urachal cysts
11. Infected communicating calyceal diverticula
12. Papillary necrosis
13. Paravesical abscess with bladder fistula
14. Renal abscess

Reinfections due to a new organism as the cause of each infection are by far the most common cause of UTI and account for 95% of all recurrent infections in females.[29]

INCIDENCE AND EPIDEMIOLOGY

Except for the immediate postnatal period of life, when the frequency of UTI in male babies is 10 times greater than it is in female babies, urinary tract infections are many times more common in females than males. Bergstrom and colleagues[30] considered the hematogenous route to be the primary mode of renal infection in the newborn. Beyond the first few weeks of life, UTIs are uncommon in males. Kunin and coworkers[31, 32] in an epidemiology study of Virginia school children found a prevalence rate of only 0.03% among males, compared with a 1% rate in females. Following puberty, the prevalence rate in females increases sharply, with about 5% to 6% of sexually active women of childbearing age found to have a urinary tract infection at any given time.[33] The rate increases as age increases; in women over 60 years, UTI can be found in 10% to 12% of the female population.[34, 35] In contrast, UTI in males is rare below the age of 50. In Freedman's study,[34] the infection rate among Japanese men was 1.5% in those over the age of 60 and rose to 3.6% in those beyond the age of 70.

ETIOLOGY

Most UTIs are caused by gram-negative enteric bacteria. *Escherichia coli* is the most common pathogen recorded and accounts for most UTIs.[36] Other organisms commonly responsible include *Proteus, Klebsiella, Pseudomonas,* and enterococcus (*Streptococcus faecalis*). Less commonly, gram-positive organisms, notably *Staphylococcus* and *Streptococci,* are etiological agents. Recently, coagulase-negative staphylococci (*Staphylococcus saprophyticus*) have been implicated as an important pathogen in young females with recurrent UTI.[37, 38]

Particular attention should be given to infections caused by organisms capable of producing the enzyme urease. These organisms, usually *Proteus, Klebsiella,* or *Staphylococcus,* are frequently associated with stone formation. The role of anaerobic bacteria in causing UTI has not been totally defined but they appear to be responsible for fewer than 1% of all infections.[39]

PATHOGENESIS

It now appears conclusive that the primary incident in the chain of events leading to bladder bacteriuria in women is a biological alteration in the normal bacterial flora of the urethra and vagina, but the factors that cause vaginal colonization are *not* directly related to vaginal pH, electrolyte composition, glucose content, or the presence or absence of vaginal lactobacilli. These variables do not distinguish women with a susceptibility to recurrent UTI from those apparently resistant to this problem.[16] The finding of decreased cervicovaginal antibody in vaginal fluid of females susceptible to recurrent UTI may imply that a local immune response may be involved in vaginal colonization.[40]

The mechanisms by which bacteria adhere to urothelial cells lining the urethra may provide some answers regarding bacterial colonization, as well as providing a potential avenue for future investigation concerning prophylaxis. Bacteria capable of causing UTI appear to attach to urothelial cells, or to the uromucoid coating the cells through microfibrillar cell surface attachments known as pili or fimbriae. These protein structures are found on most gram-negative bacteria and appear to attach to specific epithelial cell receptors.[36] These receptors may be glycoproteins or glycolipids found on the host cell.

Type I bacteria pili adhere to a mannose-like receptor[41] and bacterial adherence may be prevented by competitive inhibition with mannose[42] or the Tamm-Horsfall protein.[43] P-pili (fimbriae) appear to attach to specific P blood group antigen related glycosphingolipids.[44] Patients with the P_1 blood group antigen may possess increased susceptibility to uncomplicated pyelonephritis.[45] Only 10% to 15% of *E. coli* responsible for UTIs possess fimbriae, yet 75% to 100% of cases of nonobstructive pyelonephritis are caused by P-fimbriated *E. coli*.[46, 47] More recently, Roberts and coworkers demonstrated that immunization with purified P-fimbriae prevented both acute and chronic pyelonephritis in monkeys.[48]

The administration of analogues of glycolipid cell membranes will prevent ascending infections in experimental animals.[49] Thus P-fimbriated *E. coli*, as opposed to organisms possessing only Type I pili, or those without pili, appear to be nephropathogenic.

In males, the antibacterial activity of normal prostatic fluid may be a significant factor in explaining the relative resistance of men to UTI, as compared with women.[50] This antibacterial activity appears to be due to the high zinc content of prostatic fluid.[51] In men with documented chronic bacterial prostatitis, the zinc level of the expressed prostatic secretions is markedly reduced, compared with normal controls or men with benign prostatic hyperplasia.[52]

The sequence of events leading to renal parenchymal damage once the bacteria ascend to the kidney has been studied in great detail by Roberts.[53] An early host response aimed at eliminating the bacteria involves complement activation, which probably occurs by the alternate pathway, leading to subsequent leukocyte demargination.

Phagocytosis, which is the ingestion of bacteria by activated leukocytes and macrophages, leads to lysozyme release and a marked increase in the oxidative metabolism of the phagocytes. During that time, oxygen is converted to the free radicals: superoxide, hydrogen peroxide, and hydroxyl radical (the radical respiratory burst).[54] These free radicals and their metabolites are powerful oxidizing agents that can exert toxic effects not only on the bacteria but on other cells as well.[55] When the free radical scavenger superoxide dismutase is administered to monkeys, it protects the renal tubules from ultrastructural damage caused by experimental pyelonephritis.[56]

These and other studies suggest that events leading to irreversible renal damage are related to the interaction between the infecting bacteria and the host's attempt to counteract or control the infection. If this is so, diagnosis and treatment directed at controlling the effects of bacterial invasion must be initiated early, because the reactions responsible for cell damage occur within 24 to 48 hours after onset of the infection.[57] This hypothesis is consistent with experimental observations that antibacterial treatment of experimental pyelonephritis was effective in preventing renal scarring only if it was started within 1 to 4 days after initiation of the infection.[58, 59]

RISK FACTORS

Sex

As described previously, beyond the neonatal period UTIs occur much more frequently in women than in men.[30, 32, 34, 35] Unlike their female counterparts, no dramatic increase in the prevalence of UTI is seen in postpubertal males; the incidence slowly increases with time, so that at age 60 the prevalence of UTI in the male population is approximately 1%.

Sexual Intercourse

The suggestion that sexual intercourse plays a pathogenic role is supported by several pieces of evidence. As already noted, females show a marked increase in the prevalence of UTI after puberty and the onset of sexual activity. Kunin and McCormack[33] contrasted the frequency of bacteriuria in nuns with age matched control groups of black and white women. At every age group from 15 to 55 years, the incidence of UTI in the control women was significantly higher than in the nuns. In the group between 15 and 34 years of age, the incidence of bacteriuria was more than 22 times higher in the white control group than in white nuns and 25 times higher in black controls than in black nuns.[33]

Of interest is the fact that the overall incidence in the 15- to 34-year-old nuns was the same as that found in prepubertal females, that is, approximately 1%.

Pregnancy

No data support the frequent suggestion that pregnant women are more susceptible to UTI than nonpregnant women. The prevalence of bacteriuria in the pregnant population is approximately 4% to 6%, the same as in nonpregnant women of similar ages.[60] It now appears that most women who have UTI in pregnancy actually acquire their asymptomatic bacteriuria before the pregnancy. Gamans and colleagues[61] documented that symptomatic infection in pregnant women occurs three times more frequently than symptomatic infections in a nonpregnant control group. In addition, the dilatation of the collecting system and the relative ureteral obstruction that may occur as the uterus enlarges appear to raise the incidence of acute clinical pyelonephritis in pregnant females.[62–64]

Obstruction

Little evidence exists to show that obstruction, in the absence of urological instrumentation that may result in iatrogenic infection, leads to a higher incidence of UTI.[28] In this regard, it should be noted that the postvoid film of the intravenous urogram may be adequate for roughly estimating the volume of residual urine in most patients. Of course, this assumes that micturition has been accomplished physiologically, a factor that, unfortunately, is subject to a number of modifying influences. The practice of quantifying the residual urine by urethral catheterization as an indicator of the need for relief of prostatic obstruction in older men is conceptually unsound and potentially dangerous. Infection in the presence of obstruction is a potential cause of septicemia and death. It is one of the few true emergencies in urological practice. In systemically ill patients with infected urine and a distal obstruction, the primary goal of the physician should be to relieve the obstruction or to temporarily divert the urine.

Urinary Tract Calculi

Most urinary tract calculi are composed of calcium oxalate and are unrelated to infection. However, infection stones composed of ammoniomagnesium phosphate (struvite) present a unique risk factor to afflicted patients, since the potential for obstruction and infection may be relatively high. Infection stones are formed as a result of the action of the bacterial enzyme urease. This enzyme, produced by the "urea-splitting bacteria," acts to degrade the abundant amounts of urea in urine to produce ammonium ion and a resulting alkalinization of the urine. At a urinary pH above 5.6, struvite readily precipitates. The organisms most commonly responsible for the formation of infection stones are most *Proteus mirabilis*, *Klebsiella*, and *Staphylococcus aureus*. It should be noted that *E. coli* does not produce urease and hence cannot form infection stones; however, it can secondarily infect calcium oxalate stones and, in the presence of obstruction, can produce symptomatic pyelonephritis. It is not unusual to recover viable bacteria on culture from such calculi.

Azotemia

Decreased renal function, although not a factor predisposing to urinary inflammation, may cause difficulty in definitive treatment, because of a defect in urinary concentrating ability limiting the levels of antimicrobial drug that can be attained in the urine. In addition, adequate urinary output ensures a "wash-out" mechanism in the bladder, which is a very effective means of reducing the likelihood of bacterial growth and colonization.

Foreign Body

The most common foreign body encountered in the urinary tract is the indwelling catheter. Infection almost always occurs in patients requiring long-term catheterization.[65, 66] Despite a variety of measures to maintain sterility, urethral-catheter–associated infections remain those most commonly acquired in the hospital. Most patients with a UTI and a freely draining urethral catheter are asymptomatic and infected with *E. coli* or a similar non–urease-producing organism. Well-intentioned attempts to render the urine sterile, despite the continued use of Foley's catheter, are doomed to failure and often lead to the emergence of an antibiotic-resistant or urea-splitting organism and subsequent stone formation. As discussed below, the therapeutic principle should be to culture the urine of patients with an indwelling catheter frequently and treat (with a short course of therapy) only the infections that are caused by urea-splitting bacteria or that produce symptoms. If a freely draining catheter is used, a non–urease-producing organism in the urine of an asymptomatic patient requires no therapy.

Diabetes Mellitus

It appears that diabetes mellitus may predispose to UTI, especially in women. Such infections may be particularly difficult to eradicate. Forland and colleagues[67] found a greater-than-twofold increase in bacteriuria in women with diabetes, compared with age-matched controls; in men, 2% of the study population had UTI. The reasons for the increased susceptibility to infection are unknown; however, these patients often have glomerulopathy. Diabetes is the systemic disease most commonly associated with papillary necrosis and may therefore render the renal medulla and papillae particularly susceptible to infection.[68] Although any case of acute pyelonephritis is potentially serious and should never be taken lightly, those occurring in diabetic patients are even more threatening. Emphysematous pyelonephritis is a grave complication of acute pyelonephritis occurring in diabetic patients. Clinically, it is characterized by acute pyelonephritis that fails to respond to appropriate therapy; the finding of *intraparenchymal* gas on a plain abdominal film, IVU, sonogram, or CT scan of the kidney is diagnostic. The gas may be produced by any bacteria that ferments lactose, although *E. coli* is the most common etiological agent. Ten per cent of cases are bilateral. Aggressive treatment is required, including surgical or percutaneous drainage or nephrectomy in some cases. This is a particularly serious complication, and the mortality rate may exceed 40%.[69]

Vesicoureteral Reflux

It now appears, on the basis of both clinical and experimental evidence, that the role of infection in the subsequent development of reflux nephropathy is primarily associated with the demonstration of intrarenal reflux in children below 4 years of age; the resulting scars appear to develop in the area where the intrarenal reflux was previously demonstrated.[70, 71] Ransley and Risdon,[72] using the pig kidney, which possesses a renal pyramid system similar to that of humans, demonstrated that intrarenal reflux occurred primarily in areas drained by papillae of a particular configuration. These studies documented that the papillae prone to reflux are those in the upper and, less commonly, the lower renal poles. These papillae are composed of papillary ducts that enter almost directly at right angles into the calyx and consequently were not occluded when the intracalyceal pressure rose. The nonrefluxing papillae, however, are composed of smaller-diameter ducts, thought to enter at a more oblique angle. When intracalyceal pressure rises, these ducts are compressed sufficiently to close and prevent intrarenal reflux.[73] In considering the implications of the excellent studies of Hodson and Ransley, two points must be kept in mind: (1) intrarenal reflux occurred only in the presence of distal obstruction, and (2) renal scarring subsequent to reflux occurred only in piglets with infected urine—in the absence of infection, reflux did not lead to scarring. In children without demonstrated urinary tract infection, sterile reflux does not appear to cause renal deterioration (see page 853).[16, 74] The converse also appears to be true: children with infected urine but no reflux appear to be at little risk of developing upper tract

damage.[75] In children with vesicoureteral reflux, the cure of a UTI is no more difficult, and the rate of reinfection no higher, than in children without reflux.[76] In adult women screened for bacteriuria, radiographic evidence of reflux nephropathy was found in 0.6% to 1%.[18, 19]

SELECTED OBSERVATIONS ON TREATMENTS

General Considerations

A detailed discussion of treatment is beyond the scope of this presentation; nevertheless, a few general observations concerning the principles of treatment are in order. Although it appears obvious, the statement that adequate treatment of a UTI must result in a *sterile* urine is often not appreciated in clinical practice. Thus, in a patient being evaluated for repeated UTI, failure to culture the urine while the patient is on therapy to ensure that the urine is actually sterile and that small numbers of pathogenic bacteria do not persist will make it impossible to document that the therapy chosen was appropriate and effective. A second major observation made in recent years is that more than 90% of UTIs in children and women are due to reinfection (with a different strain of pathogenic organism each time), rather than due to a relapse from a chronic source of infection.[77] This means that the biggest challenge in the control of UTI in women and children lies in the area of prophylaxis—not therapy.

Recent observations have demonstrated that the successful treatment of UTI is nearly always accompanied by sterilization of the urine within 24 hours after the start of treatment.[78] Conversely, prolonged therapy, such as a 28-day course of treatment, is no more effective in eradicating UTI than shorter treatment regimens.[79–84]

Other considerations notwithstanding, the economic savings are considerable with shorter-term therapy. In one study,[81] 3 days and 10 days of treatment were equally effective. Considerable effort has been expended to devise various means of bacteriologically, biochemically, or immunobiologically differentiating upper tract from lower tract infection, on the assumption that upper tract infection may require longer periods of therapy. However, in studies utilizing fluorescence antibody coating to distinguish between upper and lower tract bacteriuria, no difference in cure rate between upper and lower tract infections was demonstrated.[82, 83]

The therapy of asymptomatic bacteriuria (ABU) very much depends on the clinical setting in which it is discovered. In young children with vesicoureteral reflux, treatment of ABU is encouraged as a means of preventing the development of upper tract scarring. In pregnant females, it is now clear that treatment of bacteriuria in early pregnancy markedly reduces the subsequent incidence of acute pyelonephritis.[62, 63, 84, 85]

In adult females, about one-third of patients with ABU will develop symptoms of UTI within 12 months.[86] The likelihood of these infections producing renal damage is quite low. Patients with urethral catheters, suprapubic tubes, or percutaneous nephrostomy tubes present special problems in therapy. In patients with nephrostomy tubes, as well as those with bladder catheters, the physician must accept that after a given period virtually all will have infected urine. However, there is no evidence that freely draining infected urine in the adult kidney leads to deterioration of renal function. What is important is that all steps be taken to prevent stone formation or the emergence of a bacterial species resistant to antimicrobial agents.

Vigorous attempts to keep the urine sterile with a succession of antimicrobial agents will eventually lead to a greater therapeutic challenge—an infection that is resistant to most antibiotics. Such an infection often requires the use of potentially nephrotoxic antimicrobial agents to sterilize the urine, resulting in a loss of renal function secondary to antibiotic therapy that is greater than that due to the original infection. The stones that form in patients with catheters or nephrostomy tubes are almost always struvite stones, which can be prevented by prompt treatment and eradication of urea-splitting bacteria. Since the most common of these organisms is *Proteus mirabilis,* and since the vast majority of *P. mirabilis* strains are exquisitely sensitive to small doses of oral penicillin,[87] treatment of these organisms usually presents no major problems.

IMPLICATIONS FOR RADIOLOGICAL EVALUATION

In general, most adult patients presenting with acute lower urinary tract infections will not require imaging studies. (This in contrast to children, most of whom *will* require such evaluation) (see Chapter 21). However, for patients in whom stones, obstruction, underlying renal disease, or congenital abnormalities are suspected, radiological imaging is warranted (Table 20–1). Intravenous urography is the most commonly performed radiological imaging study of the urinary tract in adult patients with real or suspected urinary tract infection. The most serious and potentially life-threatening conditions that require definitive diagnosis and treatment are infections associated with stones, obstruction, or diabetes mellitus. Infected urine in the presence of obstruction is a urological emergency that must be diagnosed and treated to prevent the subsequent development of generalized sepsis. Opaque stones are generally easily visualized on a plain film of the abdomen. The plain film of the kidney, ureters, and bladder (KUB) may also be useful to detect the presence of unusual gas patterns, such as those found in emphysematous pyelonephritis, or to demonstrate a large kidney displacing the normal gas pattern of the upper abdomen (e.g., tumor, polycystic kidney, abscess).

Plain film tomograms are of value in permitting visualization of poorly calcified or cystine stones not seen on conventional radiographs. These stones, usually struvite calculi, may be easily missed on the routine urogram without plain film tomograms but would be readily documented by renal ultrasound or CT scanning of the kidneys. Uric acid stones, if not detected by urography, will also be readily apparent on the latter studies.

The urogram is of little value in the routine evaluation of women presenting with symptoms of an acute lower UTI. In 164 patients studied with a history of recurrent UTIs, 11 (6.7%) were found to have minor anatomical variations. Nine (5.5%) were considered to have positive findings, but in no patient did a significant finding require surgical intervention or alter the therapeutic approach.

In this small study the total cost to the patients was $17,930. In view of the extremely negative cost-benefit ratio, it was concluded that the routine use of excretory urograms as part of the evaluation of women with a UTI is expensive and unrewarding, and it has little justification.[88]

Other studies have subsequently confirmed these findings and documented the limited usefulness of routine cystograms or voiding cystourethrography in similar adult populations.[89, 90]

The IVU is of primary value in ruling out obstruction, stones, and abscesses in patients presenting with symptoms of acute pyelonephritis. In patients with azotemia, or other conditions that may make the performance of a urogram hazardous to the patient, a conventional radiograph or a plain film tomogram of the abdomen, plus renal ultrasound to eliminate the possibility of obstruction, is usually a rapid, safe, efficient, and relatively inexpensive way of establishing the diagnosis.[12]

Renal ultrasonography is also of value in serial studies of renal growth in children and patients with polycystic kidneys. However, ultrasonography is the most operator dependent of all the renal imaging studies; the proper performance, and later the interpretation, of the examination depends on the skill of the individual. Lesions such as papillary necrosis, tuberculosis, and minimal dilation hydronephrosis may easily be overlooked by ultrasonography, making this at best a limited technique for urinary tract screening.

The use of CT in the evaluation of patients with UTI is hampered by cost considerations, but for delineating renal structure and anatomy it is the gold standard against which the other modalities are measured. It is particularly useful in detecting poorly visualized calculi (*no non-opaque stones are shown by CT*) but must compete with ultrasonography in this regard. The size, location, and density of renal and perinephric masses found on CT allow for accurate delineation of cysts, tumors, and renal and perinephric abscesses in most patients without the need for more invasive imaging tests.[91] In the evaluation of patients with renal infection, CT is usually reserved for those failing to respond therapeutically as expected or for those with particularly virulent clinical courses. It is in this highly select subgroup of patients that complications likely to require surgical or radiological intervention will be seen.

At this writing, experience with MRI imaging in renal inflammation is insufficient to permit specific recommendations regarding its sphere of usefulness. With its extreme sensitivity to changes in renal parenchymal integrity, and with its potential for spectroscopic imaging, it is safe to say that MRI will soon find an important place in the evaluation of patients with UTI.

References

1. Murphy LJT: The History of Urology. Springfield, Illinois, Charles C Thomas, 1972, p 35.
2. Kincaid-Smith P: Pyelonephritis, chronic interstitial nephritis and obstructive uropathy. *In* Hamburger J, Crosnier J, Grumfeld JP (eds): Nephrology. New York, John Wiley & Sons, 1979, pp 553–582.
3. Bright R: Reports of medical cases. London, 1827.

4. Klebs E: Handbuch der Pathologischen Anatomie Berlin. A Hirschwald, 1870.

5. Wagner E: Der Morbus Brightii. *In* Handbuch der Krankheiten des Harnapparates. 1 Halfte. Leipzig, FCW Vogel, 1882.

6. Mobley JE, Schlegel JU: Pyelonephritis. *In* Landes RR, Bush RB, Zorgeniotti AW (eds): Perspectives in Urology, Vol. 1. Nutley, New Jersey, Roche Laboratories, 1976.

7. Crabtree EG, Cabot H: Pyelonephritis: Its nature and possible prevention. Trans Sec Genitourin Dis Am Med Assoc 67:209–217, 1916.

8. Kass EH, Finland M: Asymptomatic infections of the urinary tract. Trans Assoc Am Physicians 69:56, 1956.

9. Meares EM, Jr: Prostatitis—a review. Urol Clin North Am 2:3, 1975.

10. Heptinstall RH: Pathology of the Kidney. Boston, Little, Brown & Company, 1966.

11. Little PJ, McPherson DR, de Wardener HE: The appearance of the intravenous pyelogram during and after acute pyelonephritis. Lancet 1:1186, 1965.

12. Silver TM, Cass EM, Thornbury JR, et al: The radiologic spectrum of acute pyelonephritis in adults and adolescents. Radiology 118:65–71, 1976.

13. Rosenfield A, Glickman M: Acute focal bacterial nephritis (acute lobar nephronia). Radiology 132:553, 1978.

14. Sotonongo JR, Schiff H, Wulfsohn MA: Radiographic findings in acute segmental pyelonephritis. Urology 19:335, 1982.

15. Witten EM, Myers GH, Utz DG: Emmett's Clinical Urography. Philadelphia, WB Saunders Company, 1977.

16. Stamey TA: Pathogenesis and Treatment of Urinary Tract Infections. Baltimore, Williams & Wilkins, 1980.

17. Davidson AJ, Talner LB: Rare sequelae of adult onset of acute bacterial nephritis. Radiology 127:367, 1978.

18. Alwall N: Screening for urinary tract infection in non-pregnant women. Kidney Int 8:107, 1975.

19. Kincaid-Smith P, Becker GJ: Reflux nephropathy in the adult. *In* Hodson J, Kincaid-Smith P (eds): Reflux Nephropathy. New York, Masson Publishing USA, 1979.

20. Anhalt MA, Cawood D, Scott R: Xanthogranulomatous pyelonephritis: A comprehensive review with report of 4 additional cases. J Urol 105:10, 1971.

21. Tolia BM, Newman HR, Fruchtman B, et al: Xanthogranulomatous pyelonephritis: Segmental or generalized disease? J Urol 124:122, 1980.

22. Malek RS, Elder JS: Xanthogranulomatous pyelonephritis: A critical analysis of 26 cases and of the literature. J Urol 119:589, 1978.

23. Gerber WL, Catalona WJ, Fair WR, et al: Xanthogranulomatous pyelonephritis masquerading as occult malignancy. Urology 11:466, 1978.

24. Stamey TA: Editorial: A clinical classification of urinary tract infections based upon origin. South Med J 68:934, 1975.

25. Kraft JK, Stamey TA: The natural history of symptomatic recurrent bacteruria in women. Medicine 56:55, 1977.

26. Eudy WW: Correlations between in vitro sensitivity testing and therapeutic response in urinary tract infections. Urology 2:519, 1973.

27. Fair WR, Fair WR III: Clinical value of sensitivity determination in treating urinary tract infections. Urology 19:565, 1982.

28. Stamey TA: Urinary Tract Infections. Baltimore, Williams & Wilkins, 1980.

29. Shortliffe LMD, Stamey TA: Infections of the urinary tract: Introduction and general principles. *In* Walsh P, Gittes R, Perlmutter A, Stamey TA (eds): Campbell's Urology, 5th Ed. Philadelphia, WB Saunders Company, 1985.

30. Bergstrom T, Larson H, Lincoln K, Windberg J: Studies of urinary tract infections in infancy and childhood. XIII. Eighty (80) consecutive cases with neo-natal infection. J Pediatr 80:858, 1972.

31. Kunin CM, Zacha E, Paquin AJ: Urinary tract infections in school children. I. Prevalence of bacteriuria and associated urologic findings. N Engl J Med 266:1287, 1962.

32. Kunin CM, Southall I, Paquin AJ: Epidemiology of urinary tract infections: A pilot study of 3057 school children. N Engl J Med 263:817, 1960.

33. Kunin CM, McCormack RC: An epidemiologic study of bacteriuria and blood pressure among nuns and working women. N Engl J Med 278:635, 1968.

34. Freedman LR, Phair JP, Seki M, et al: The epidemiology of urinary tract infections in Hiroshima. Yale J Biol Med 37:262, 1965.

35. Miall WE, Kass EH, Ling J, Stuart KL: Factors influencing arterial pressure in the general population in Jamaica. Br Med J 2:497, 1962.

36. Glauser MP: Urinary tract infection and pyelonephritis. *In* Bruade AI, Davis CE, Fierer J (eds): Infectious Diseases and Medical Microbiology. Philadelphia, WB Saunders Company, 1986.

37. Stamm WE, Wagner KF, Amsel R, et al: Causes of the acute urethral syndrome in women. N Engl J Med 303:409, 1980.

38. Maskell R: Importance of coagulase negative staphylococci as pathogens in the urinary tract. Lancet 1:1155, 1974.

39. Segura JW, Kelalis PP, Martin WJ, Smith LH: Anaerobic bacteria in the urinary tract. Mayo Clin Proc 47:30, 1972.

40. Stamey TA, Wehner H, Mihara G, et al: The immunologic basis of recurrent bacteriuria: Role of cervicovaginal antibody in enterobacterial colonization of the introital mucosa. Medicine 57:47, 1978.

41. Ofek I, Mierlman D, Sharon N: Adherence of *Escherichia coli* to human mucosal cells mediated by mannose receptors. Nature 265:623, 1977.

42. Aronson M, Medalia O, Schori L, et al: Prevention of colonization of the urinary tract of mice and *Escherichia coli* by blocking the bacterial adherence with methyl alpha-D-mannopyranoside. J Infect Dis 139:329, 1979.

43. Orskov I, Ferencz A, Orskov F: Tamm-Horsfall protein or uromucoid is the normal urinary slime that traps Type I fimbriated *Escherichia coli*. Lancet 1:887, 1980.

44. Kallenius G, Mollby R, Svenson SB, et al: Occurrence of P-fimbriated *Escherichia coli* in urinary tract infections. Lancet 2:1369, 1981.

45. Lomberg H, Hanson LA, Jacobsson B, et al: Correlation of P blood group, vesicoureteral reflux, and bacterial attachment in patients with recurrent pyelonephritis. N Engl J Med 308:1189, 1983.

46. Vaisanen V, Elo J, Tallgren LG, et al: Mannose resistant haemagglutination and P antigen recognition are characteristic of *Escherichia coli* causing primary pyelonephritis. Lancet 2:1366, 1981.

47. Svanborg-Eden C, Haigberg L, Leffler H, et al: Recent progress in the understanding of the role of bacterial adhesion in the pathogenesis of urinary tract. Infection 10:327, 1982.

48. Roberts JA, Hardaway K, Kaack B, et al: Prevention of pyelonephritis by immunization with P-fimbriae. J Urol 132:602, 1984.

49. Svanborg-Eden C, Freter R, Haigberg L, et al: Inhibition of experimental ascending urinary tract infection by an epithelial cell surface receptor analogue. Nature 298:560, 1982.

50. Fair WR, Stamey TA: Bactericidal properties of prostatic fluid in bacterial infections of the male genital system (workshop). Warrenton, National Research Council, National Academy of Science. October, 1967, pp 199–211.

51. Fair WR, Couch J, Wehner H: Prostatic antibacterial factor: Identity and significance. Urology 7:169–177, 1976.

52. Fair WR, Parrish RF: Antibacterial substances in prostatic fluid in the prostatic cell: Structure and function. New York, Allan R Liss, 1981.

53. Roberts JA: Infections in surgery. 633, November, 1986.

54. Johnston RB, Lehmeyer JE: Neutrophil and monocyte oxidative metabolism in inflammation: Stimulation by surface contact and suppression by antiinflammatory agents. *In* Movement, Metabolism and Bactericidal Mechanisms of Phagocytes. Padua, Piccin Medical Books, 1977, p 243.

55. McCord JM, Wong K: Phagocytes produced free radicals: Roles in cytotoxicity and inflammation. *In* Oxygen Free Radicals and Tissue Damage. Amsterdam, Elsevier, 1979, p 343.

56. Roberts JA, Roth JK Jr, Domingue G, et al: Immunology of pyelonephritis in the primate model. V. Effect of superoxide dismutase. J Urol 128:1394, 1982.

57. Fussell EN, Roberts JA: The ultra-structure of acute pyelonephritis in the monkey. J Urol 133:179, 1984.

58. Slotki IN, Asscher AW: Prevention of scarring in experimental pyelonephritis in the rat by early antibiotic therapy. Nephron 30:262, 1982.

59. Miller T, Phillips S: Pyelonehritis: The relationship between infection, renal scarring and antimicrobial therapy. Kidney Int 19:654, 1981.

60. Shortliff LMD, Stamey TA: Urinary infections in adult women. *In* Walsh P, Giddes R, Perlmutter A, Stamey TA (eds): Campbell's Urology, 5th Ed. Philadelphia, WB Saunders Company, 1985.

61. Gamans R, Haverkorn MJ, Valkenburg HA, et al: A prospective study of urinary tract infections in a Dutch general practice. Lancet 2:674, 1976.

62. Condie AP, Williams JD, Reeves DS, Brumfitt (eds): Urinary Tract Infection. London, Oxford University Press, 1968, p 148.
63. Kincaid-Smith P, Bullen M: Bacteriuria in pregnancy. Lancet 395, 1965.
64. Whalley PJ: Bacteriuria of pregnancy. Am J Obstet Gynecol 97:723, 1967.
65. Turck M, Stamm W: Nosocomial infection of the urinary tract. Am J Med 70:651, 1981.
66. Garibaldi RA, Burke JP, Britt MR, et al: Meatal colonization and catheter associated bacteriuria. N Engl J Med 303:316, 1980.
67. Forland M, Thomas V, Shelokov A: Urinary tract infections in patients with diabetes mellitus. JAMA 238:1924, 1977.
68. Eknoyan G, Qunibi WY, Grissom TR, et al: Renal papillary necrosis: An update. Medicine 61:55, 1982.
69. Freiha FS, Messing EM, Gross DN: Emphysematous pyelonephritis. J Urol 18:9, 1979.
70. Hodson CJ: The effects of the disturbance of flora on the kidney. J Infect Dis 120:54, 1969.
71. Rolleston GL, Maling TMJ, Hodson CJ: Intra-renal reflux and the scarred kidney. Arch Dis Child 49:531, 1974.
72. Ransley PG, Risdon RA: Renal papillae and intra-renal reflux in the pig. Lancet 2:1114, 1974.
73. Ransley PG, Risdon RA: Pathogenesis of reflux nephropathy. Contrib Nephrol 16:90, 1970.
74. Heale WF, Feurguson RS: The pathogenesis of renal scarring in children. In Kass EH, Brumfitt W (eds): Infections of the Urinary Tract. Chicago, University Press, 1978, p 201.
75. Fair WR, Govan DE, Friedland GW, Filly RA: Urinary tract infections in children. Part I. Young girls with non-refluxing ureters. West J Med 121:366, 1974.
76. Fair WR, Govan DE: Influence of vesico-ureteral reflux on the response to treatment of urinary tract infections in female children. Br J Urol 48:111, 1976.
77. McGeachie J: Recurrent infection of the urinary tract: Re-infection or recrudescence? Br Med J 5493:952, 1966.
78. Stamey TA, Govan DE, Palmer JN: The localization and treatment of urinary tract infections: The role of bactericidal urine levels as opposed to serum levels. Medicine 44:1, 1965.
79. Cosgrove MD, Gault C, Fiorentino N, Ivlar D: Twenty-eight day courses of antibiotics for urinary tract infection. Urology 7:156, 1956.
80. Lincoln K, Janson G, Winberg J: Treatment trials in urinary tract infection with special reference to the effects of antibiotic on the fecal flora. In Kincaid-Smith P, Fairley KF (eds): Renal Infection and Renal Scarring. Melbourne, Australia, Mercedes Publishing Company, 1971, p 151.
81. Fair WR, Crane DP, Peterson LJ, et al: Three-day treatment of urinary tract infections. J Urol 123:717, 1980.
82. Buckhold FJ, Ludwig P, Godfrey KN, et al: Therapy for acute cystitis in adult women: Randomized comparison of single dose sulfisoxazole vs trimethoprim-sulfamethoxazole. JAMA 247:1839, 1982.
83. Tolkoff-Rubin NE, Weber D, Fang LST, et al: Single dose therapy with trimethoprim-sulfamethoxazole for urinary tract infection in women. Rev Infect Dis 4:444, 1982.
84. Savage WE, Hajj SN, Kass EH: Demographic and prognostic characteristics of bacteriuria in pregnancy. Medicine 46:385, 1967.
85. Little PJ: The incidence of urinary infection in 5000 pregnant women. Lancet 2:925, 1966.
86. Asscher AW, Sussman W, Waters WE, et al: The clinical significance of asymptomatic bacteriuria in the non-pregnant woman. J Infect Dis 120:17, 1969.
87. Fair WR, Feit RM: The treatment of infection stones with penicillin. J Urol 122:592, 1979.
88. Fair WR, McClennan BL, Jost RG: Are exploratory urograms necessary in evaluating women with urinary tract infections? J Urol 121:313, 1979.
89. Engel G, Schaeffer AJ, Grayhack JT, et al: The role of exploratory urography in cystoscopy in the evaluation and management of women with recurrent urinary tract infection. J Urol 123:190, 1980.
90. Fowler JE, Polaski ET: Exploratory urography, cystography and cystoscopy in the evaluation of women with urinary tract infection. N Engl J Med 304:462, 1981.
91. Benson M, Li Puma JP, Resnick MI: The role of imaging studies in urinary tract infection. Urol Clin North Am 13:605, 1986.

21 Renal Inflammation

RICHARD PALMER GOLD □ BRUCE L. McCLENNAN □ PHILIP J. KENNEY
EAMANN S. BREATNACH □ ROBERT J. STANLEY □ ROBERT L. LEBOWITZ

ACUTE INFECTIONS OF THE RENAL PARENCHYMA
RICHARD PALMER GOLD □ BRUCE L. McCLENNAN

Acute pyelonephritis is a general term and refers to any inflammatory process affecting the renal interstitium. The adjacent collecting system is often involved as well; hence, the prefix *pyelo* is used to further categorize the nephritis. The renal interstitium refers to the connective tissue elements separating the tubules in the cortex and medulla. Inflammation of the interstitium can be due to both infectious (usually bacterial) and noninfectious insults. The latter are usually drug related and are often referred to simply as interstitial nephritis (Table 21–1).

Most cases of acute infectious pyelonephritis affect women from 15 to 40 years of age, originating in the lower urinary tract and then ascending to the kidney. Bacteria that infect the urinary tract, such as *Escherichia coli*, come from the fecal flora. *E. coli* is thought to be a less common pathogen in older patients because of the increased incidence of catheterization and instrumentation in this age group, which results in infections with other bacteria (e.g., *Proteus*).[1] The routes described are either via subepithelial lymphatic channels of the bladder and ureter or by direct ascent through the lumen of the ureter. The demonstration of gross vesicoureteral reflux (VUR) in these individuals is difficult, and in fact reflux is *not* common in adult women with recurrent infections. The incidence of reflux rises slightly in patients with bacteriuria at the time of cystography. Reflux in the patient without bacteriuria probably causes no significant renal damage, although the issue has been debated.[2, 3] The precise causal factors in most uncomplicated cases of acute pyelonephritis are incompletely understood. Predisposing conditions include neuropathic bladder, prolonged catheter drainage, reflux, bladder malignancy, obstruction, calculus disease, altered host resistance, congenital anomalies, analgesic abuse, diabetes mellitus, and pregnancy.[4, 5]

The information regarding the histopathology of acute pyelonephritis has been derived from the severe infections seen at autopsy or renal biopsy. Involved kidneys are usually enlarged by inflammatory edema and contain multiple foci of intense inflammation. The distribution of the infection is very patchy, with extensive areas of parenchyma showing no inflammation. Infected regions may assume discrete wedge shapes corresponding to the medullary rays with no spread of infection outside them (Fig. 21–1). Infiltration with polymorphonuclear leukocytes is typical, as is the presence of microabscess formation, which may range from the size of a pinhead to 5 to 6 mm or larger in diameter. Purulent casts may occur within the collecting tubules. These tubules have been described pathologically as yellowish streaks extending from the cortex to the medullary papilla. The inflammation typically involves the pelvic and calyceal epithelium,[6, 7] spreading from the medullary region out to the cortex.[8] The renal medulla, which has a lower oxygen tension and lower blood flow compared with renal cortex, is where the critical battles between host defenses and bacteria are fought.

In patients with additional complications such as immunosuppression, corticosteroid therapy, or diabetes mellitus, the usually well-controlled infection of pyelonephritis may progress to a more intense inflammatory response called bacterial nephritis, which may be focal or diffuse. This is also occasionally called lobar nephronia, but not without objection.[9] Organisms implicated may include *Klebsiella* or *Proteus* as well as the more usual *E. coli*. Patients are female, febrile, and septic, and the process may be diffuse or very focal[10, 11] throughout the kidney with occasionally bilateral findings. Hematogenous or blood-borne transmission of bacteria to the kidney is much less common than transmission by the ascending or urogenous route, but nonetheless may be an important clinical entity. Because of its proportionately high blood supply, the kidney can be seeded by organisms from the blood stream, producing a focal, bacterial nephritis. Staphylococcal septicemia in particular has a propensity for renal involvement, but any organism, including fungi, may be the offending agent. Unlike ascending pyelonephritis, the infection resulting from hematogenous spread is primarily cortical in distribution. With appropriate treatment, the focal areas of inflammation resolve completely (see Fig. 21–3). However, if treatment is inadequate or the host's resistance is overwhelmed, small cortical abscesses followed by coalescence into one or more larger abscesses can result. Perinephric abscess is a recognized complication of this chain of events (Fig. 21–2).

Table 21–1. Acute Renal Interstitial Inflammation

Nephritis (interstitial)—infectious (bacterial)
  Acute pyelonephritis
  Acute *focal* bacterial nephritis
  Acute *diffuse* bacterial nephritis
Nephritis (interstitial)—noninfectious
  Acute nephritis (e.g., drug induced)

ACUTE FOCAL BACTERIAL NEPHRITIS

A recently described architectural alteration in acutely infected kidneys is the focal edematous mass. It is seen

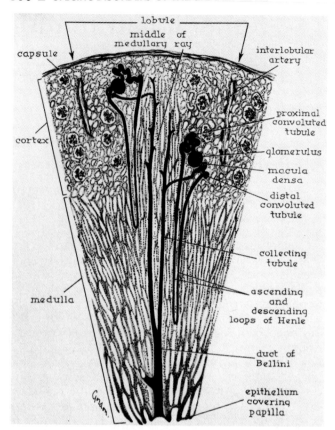

Figure 21–1. The medullary ray with its central collecting tubules forms the core of each renal lobule. The central collecting tubules are shown diagrammatically as they project into the renal cortex. Ascending infection from the calyceal mucosa extends through this tubular system to the overlying cortex. Associated vascular spasm, edema, and infiltrate (inflammatory) can create wedge-shaped (lobular) zones of low attenuation on computed tomographic (CT) scans. (From Ham WA: Histology. Philadelphia, Lippincott, 1979.)

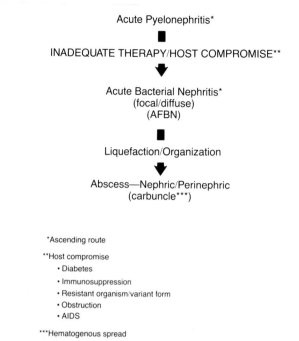

Figure 21–2. Acute renal infection is a spectrum ranging from clinically evident pyelonephritis to a more organized inflammatory response (e.g., renal abscess).

in uncomplicated cases of acute pyelonephritis as well as in the more severe infections of bacterial nephritis; nevertheless, the mass is referred to as acute focal bacterial nephritis (AFBN) or acute lobar nephronia (ALN). Older terms include renal phlegmon or cellulitis. The term ALN is used largely because the masses appear to be in the distribution of discrete renal lobes.[12–14]

No clinical characteristics appear to predict who might develop a focal renal mass as a component of pyelonephritis, but incompletely or inadequately treated urinary tract infections seem to predispose patients to the condition. When such a mass is detected at intravenous urography, the major concern is whether or not it represents an abscess. Most of these inflammatory masses resolve with medical therapy and without renal damage, even if they contain small areas of liquefaction (Fig. 21–4). However, they are often tenacious, and not uncommonly 6 to 8 weeks of antibiotic therapy may be required before involution is complete. Focal scarring, which is common in children, has also been reported in adults, both with and without underlying calyceal abnormality.[13] Some masses may advance to abscess formation and surgical or percutaneous drainage may be necessary (Figs. 21–4 to 21–6).[15, 16]

First infections—and even reinfections—of the upper urinary tract, when uncomplicated by additional urologi-

cal disease, do not result in significant renal damage as judged by intravenous urography. In the absence of lower urinary tract pathology (neuropathic bladder, vesicoureteral reflux, bladder calculi) or upper tract problems (obstruction, calculi, diabetes, papillary necrosis, congenital anomalies), it is unlikely that acute pyelonephritis causes remarkable renal scarring or calyceal deformity in adults, although some minor diminution in renal size occasionally may occur (Fig. 21–7).[17–19] Acute bacterial nephritis, however, may produce permanent structural damage in the form of papillary necrosis or global renal wasting.[20, 21]

RENAL ABSCESS

Although the vast majority of renal infections undergo resolution with proper treatment, complications sometimes occur, especially in those with the important risk factors described (Table 21–2). One of these complications is renal abscess. It is superimposed on a background of acute pyelonephritis or focal bacterial nephritis that most renal abscesses probably form today. The concept of a suppurative pyelonephritis complicated by many small collections of pus coalescing into one large abscess is popular although not widely accepted.[22] Cases of focal bacterial nephritis progressing to liquefactive necrosis and

Text continued on page 806

Table 21–2. Complications of Acute Bacterial Pyelonephritis

Acute focal bacterial nephritis (AFBN)
Renal abscess
Perinephric abscess
Renal atrophy (focal or global)
    Fatty replacement
Emphysematous pyelonephritis
Papillary necrosis
Pyonephrosis

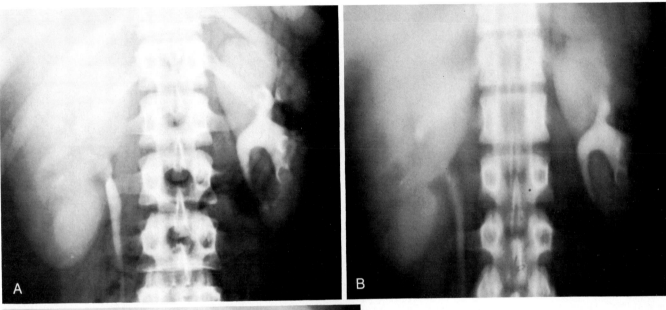

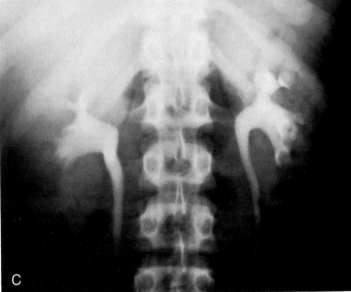

Figure 21–3. Twenty-three-year-old female with clinically acute right-sided pyelonephritis. *A,* A 4-minute film from IVU shows a normal left kidney. The right kidney is slightly enlarged, and the calyces are compressed (poorly filled). *B,* Tomogram at 3 minutes shows a nephrogram but a very poor pyelogram as a result of poor distensibility of the structures. *C,* An 8-minute film shows an optimal pyelogram on the right, but slightly decreased density of the contrast material, compared with the left kidney. Early films during urography may reveal urographic features of pyelonephritis that become less obvious later in the study. Changes resolved completely after treatment.

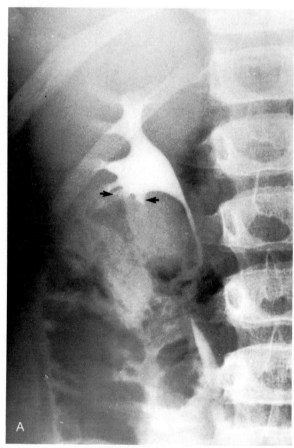

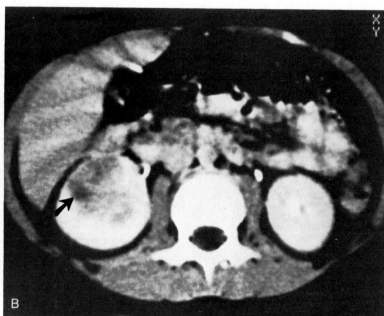

Figure 21–4. Acute focal bacterial nephritis (AFBN). *A,* IVU film shows right lower-pole mass effect with calyceal compression (*arrows*). *B,* CT scan after contrast enhancement shows focal, low-density area with patchy enhancement, corresponding to right lower-pole mass on urogram. Area of liquefaction (*arrow*) or microabscess formation. (From Gold RP, McClennan BL, Rottenberg RR: CT appearance of acute inflammatory disease of the renal interstitium. AJR 141(2):343–349, 1983, © by Am Roentgen Ray Soc.)

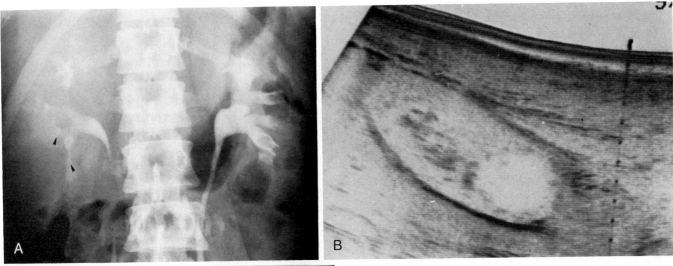

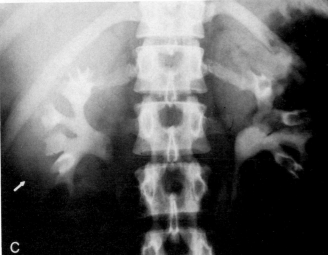

Figure 21–5. AFBN with resolution and cortical scarring. *A,* IVU shows attenuated collecting system on the right with lower-pole mass effect splaying the calyces (*arrowheads*). Nephrogram in lower pole is diminished. *B,* Ultrasound scan shows right lower-pole, hypoechoic mass. Well-defined borders are appreciated, but no real through transmission of sound waves occurs, indicating "solid" nature of mass. *C,* Follow-up IVU 1 month later shows normal excretion on right, but a cortical scar in lower pole (*arrowhead*) is present. No mass effect is seen, and underlying calyces are normal.

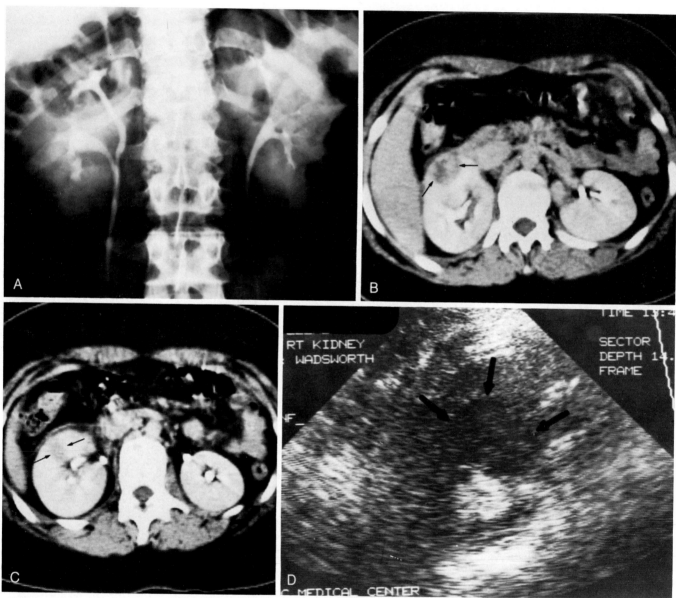

Figure 21–6. AFBN in teenage girl. A 14-year-old female with right-sided pain, fever, and positive urine culture. *A,* On admission, IVU film was normal, except for a duplicated right system. However, symptoms of pyelonephritis persisted. *B,* CT scan revealed 3-cm mass in anterior aspect of right kidney (*arrows*). The mass contains areas of contrast enhancement as well as areas of low density representing necrosis. *C,* CT scan, more caudal than *B,* reveals thickening of anterior paranephric fascia, and the inferior aspect of the mass (*arrows*) is seen. Apparent enlargement of right kidney is due to the duplication. *D,* Ultrasound (transverse) scan through right upper pole shows focal bulge (*arrows*) with a hypoechoic appearance. (Case courtesy Donald E. Wadsworth, M.D., Richland, Washington.)

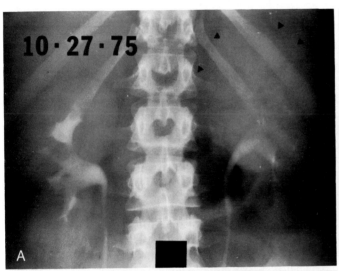

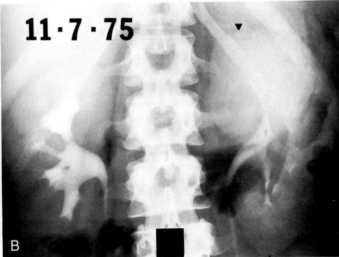

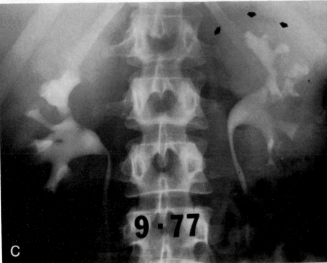

Figure 21–7. AFBN. A 28-year-old female presenting with clinical picture of left-sided pyelonephritis. *A,* IVU shows normal right kidney and bulbous left upper pole (*arrowheads*). Entire left kidney is enlarged, with poor filling of calyces. Little or no filling of left upper-pole calyces is seen. *B,* One month later, 4-minute IVU film shows left kidney to be smaller than before, but with improved excretion. The upper pole is still bulbous (*arrowhead*). Calyceal filling is still less than on the right. Patient had been on antibiotics; urine was sterile and symptoms were gone. *C,* Two asymptomatic years later, kidney has decreased further in overall size. Left upper-pole calyces are blunted with overlying cortical atrophy (*arrowheads*).

collections of drainable pus have been reported.[16] Ascending gram-negative organisms are the current predominant infectious cause, replacing the staphylococcal or streptococcal septicemias of the preantibiotic era, which were thought to be the cause of the so-called renal carbuncle.[23] Intravenous drug abuse and skin infections remain, however, as major sources of vascular contamination and may give rise to hematogenous abscess with *Staphylococcus,* and *Streptococcus*, as well as with *Enterobacteriaceae,* as the offending organisms.[16] Superinfection (secondary infection) of a renal cyst or calyceal diverticulum may simulate the urographic and other imaging features of a renal abscess.

Patients with polycystic disease, or acquired cystic disease of dialysis, may develop renal abscesses if their cysts become infected. The indolent nature of the process and nondescript symptomatology have traditionally hindered early detection. Frequently, renal abscesses cause vague malaise and pain without pyuria, bacteriuria, or bacteremia and may therefore be associated with negative cultures.[24] Abscesses tend to be solitary and may spontaneously drain into the collecting system or perinephric space. As a complication of diagnostic cyst aspiration or alcohol embolization of the kidney,[25] abscesses may result from iatrogenic intervention.[15]

Percutaneous aspiration and drainage, when indicated, provides the optimal nonoperative therapy. Proper diagnosis of a nonlobar, low-attenuation, well-defined intrarenal mass by computed tomography (CT) or a fluid-filled mass by ultrasonography should suggest a renal abscess "ripe" for drainage. After detection, appropriate culture and antibiotic treatment, determination of the proper access route for a needle-catheter system usually requires sonographic and/or CT guidance. Ribs, pleural space, lung, and the peritoneal cavity should be avoided. The general principles of abscess drainage and catheter management obtain in the consideration of percutaneous aspiration and drainage of a renal or perinephric abscess (Figs. 21–8 to 21–10) (see Chapter 125).

IMAGING

Urography

The accepted incidence of urographic abnormalities in acute pyelonephritis is approximately 25%. It is difficult to assess the severity of infections in many studies.[7–11] The usual criteria for inclusion are the clinical signs and symptoms of fever, flank pain and tenderness, and infected urine. Fever and flank pain associated with bacteriuria may often be present with lower urinary tract infection alone and may be absent in elderly females with significant infection.[1] In fact, studies in which patients are defined as having upper urinary tract infection on the basis of symptoms may include a high percentage of those in whom there is no supravesical bacteriuria.[17, 26]

The findings on IVU of acute, infectious pyelonephritis are detectable within the first 24 hours. Smooth renal enlargement, diminished nephrographic density, delayed calyceal appearance time, diminished calyceal contrast density, and attenuated, underfilled pyelocalyceal structures are the most common abnormalities; they may be either focal or diffuse (Table 21–3; see also Figs. 21–3 and 21–11). Additional but less common findings include

Table 21–3. Urographic Findings in Acute Bacterial Pyelonephritis

Urographic Finding	Percentage Patients
Normal	75%
Renal enlargement	20%
Global	
Focal	
Impaired excretion	15%
Delayed appearance time	
Decreased contrast density	
Decreased nephrogram	
Nonhomogeneous nephrogram	5%
Lucent areas	
Streaking and blushing	
Attenuation of collecting system	
Mucosal edema	
Poor definition of renal margins	
Pyeloureteral dilatation	

the following: focal calyceal compression; calyceal, pelvic, or ureteral dilatation (nonobstructive hydronephrosis); focal nephrographic defects, and even ridging or nodular edema of the pelvic and infundibular mucosa; on rare occasion, a striated nephrogram (Fig. 21–12).[27–30] The radiographic picture is relatively specific, renal vein thrombosis being the only entity that can be confused with it. The clinical pictures are quite dissimilar, however, affording ready differentiation in almost all cases.

In the most severe form of acute pyelonephritis (bacterial nephritis) the inflammatory response may be so intense that renal function is significantly impaired. Marked delay or even absence of the nephrogram and calyceal opacification have been reported in kidneys that are, at the same time, enlarged. Both retrograde and antegrade pyelography have been used to exclude obstruction. This condition can now be more efficiently evaluated with ultrasonography or CT (see Fig. 21–7).[31]

Arteriography has been utilized to exclude renal vein thrombosis or replacement of renal tissue with tumor in some rare cases of severe infection with diminished contrast excretion and urographic visualization. Indeed, angiographic findings in cases of renal infection most likely reflect the underlying inflammatory response of renal edema and vascular spasm. Slow flow, attenuation of small and medium-sized arterial branches, and a resultant patchy nephrogram may be seen (Fig. 21–13).[32, 33] A peripheral distribution and a fine neovascularity pattern have been reported to be common angiographic features of focal inflammatory processes (e.g., infected cysts, abscess) (Fig. 21–14).[33, 35]

Ultrasonography

Modern gray-scale ultrasonography has not demonstrated high sensitivity in the detection of the edema and microabscess formation characterizing most cases of uncomplicated acute pyelonephritis, and the sonographic appearance is often normal. With increasing severity of the renal inflammation, diffuse renal enlargement, scattered small- to medium-sized zones of hypoechoic or hyperechoic parenchyma, and the occasional loss of part of the central sinus–renal parenchymal interface may be seen.[36, 37] Zones of diminished reflectivity may represent intense edema or early abscess formation.

Text continued on page 812

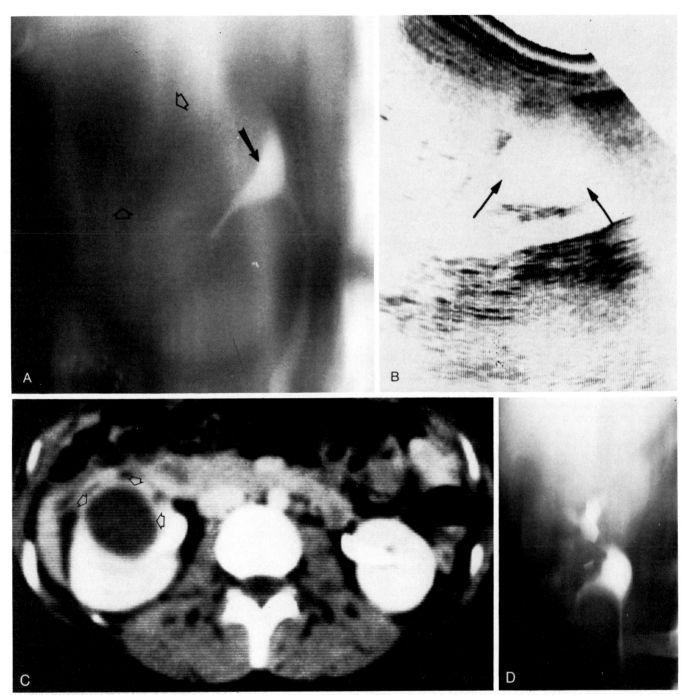

Figure 21–8. Renal abscess. Twenty-eight-year-old nurse with low-grade fever, right flank pain, and positive urine culture. *A,* IVU shows right renal mass, causing effacement (*arrow*) of the renal pelvis, and a lucent mass effect (*arrowheads*) in the nephrogram. *B,* Longitudinal ultrasound scan confirmed anechoic mass (*arrows*) in right kidney. *C,* CT scan obtained 2 weeks later shows persistence of thick-walled, nonenhancing renal mass (*arrows*). Antibiotic treatment was continued, for a total of 6 weeks. *D,* Follow-up IVU after 6 weeks of antibiotics shows right kidney nearly normal and smaller, overall, than in *A. No* residual mass is seen, and renal pelvis appears to be normal.

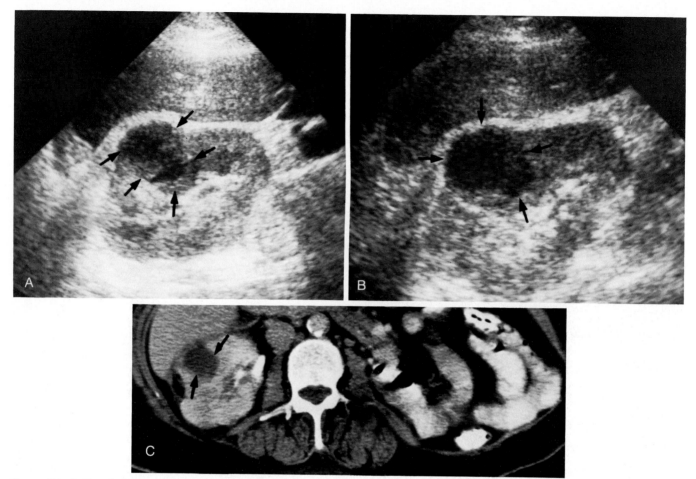

Figure 21–9. Renal abscess. Seventy-two-year-old diabetic female with *E. coli* in blood and urine. *A,* Transverse ultrasound scan through solitary right kidney. Irregular dumbbell-shaped mass deforming (*arrows*) anterior surface of the right kidney has mixed internal echogenicity. *B,* Transverse ultrasound scan 1 week after *A* shows abscess (*arrows*) is more hypoechoic and more round (developed) in appearance. *C,* CT scan at same time as *A* shows nonenhancing mass (*arrows*) with irregular renal border, corresponding to ultrasound findings. CT and ultrasound appearance are consistent with renal abscess.

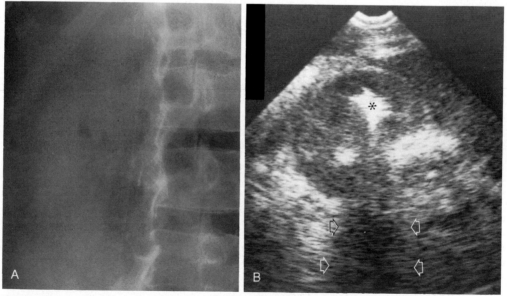

Figure 21–10. Gas-forming renal abscess in 36-year-old diabetic with pyelonephritis that is resistant to treatment. *A,* Plain abdominal film reveals loculated gas collection overlying right kidney. *B,* Ultrasound scan demonstrates extremely echogenic focus (*asterisk*) within kidney, associated with indistinct, acoustical shadow (*arrowheads*) ("dirty" shadowing). The findings indicate a gas-forming renal abscess, producing the "comet" sign.

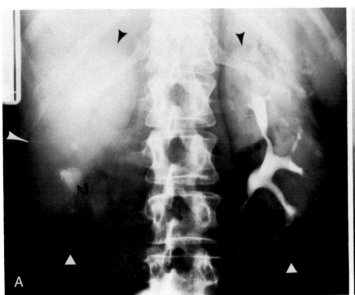

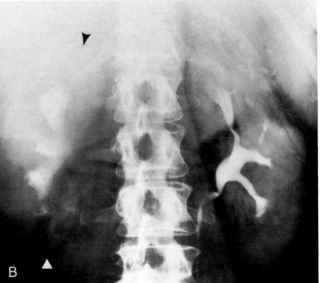

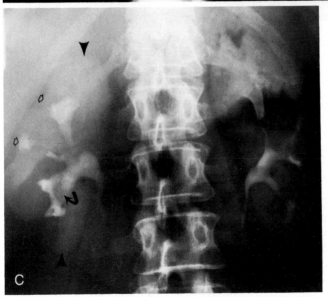

Figure 21–11. Recurrent pyelonephritis (bacterial nephritis). Sixty-nine-year-old female with recent history of recurrent right-sided pyelonephritis. Cultures had been positive for *Proteus.* A right renal calculus was present. *A,* A 4-minute film from an IVU shows a normal but slightly enlarged left kidney (*arrowheads*). The right kidney shows poor excretion but is 15 cm in length (*arrowheads*). A stone (*curved arrow*) is present in the right lower-pole infundibulum. *B,* Eight-minute film from same study shows enlarged kidney on right (*arrowheads*), but poor pyelogram (delayed filling) and decreased density of contrast. *C,* Six months later, the right kidney (*arrowheads*) has decreased in length to 12.3 cm. Clubbed calyces with cortical scars are present (*open arrowheads*). Calculus on right (*curved arrow*) has grown, but patient is asymptomatic.

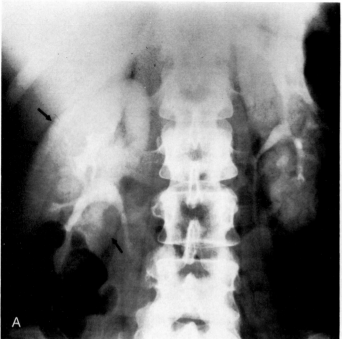

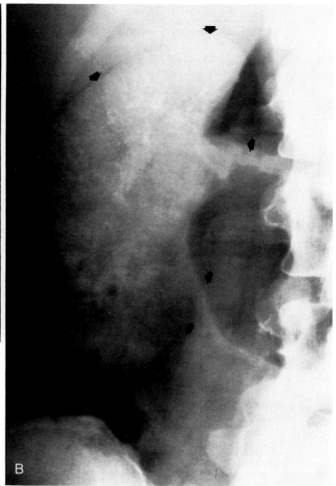

Figure 21–12. Striated nephrogram from acute infection. A 47-year-old female with acute bilateral pyelonephritis. *A,* IVU produces an adequate pyelogram but a striated nephrogram at 10 minutes. These findings are bilateral but are more marked on the right (*arrows*). *B,* A 2.5-hour delayed film results in a striated, persistent nephrogram. A coned view of the right kidney shows the striations to be patchy in distribution. Follow-up IVU 6 weeks later was normal. Renal contour is illustrated with arrows.

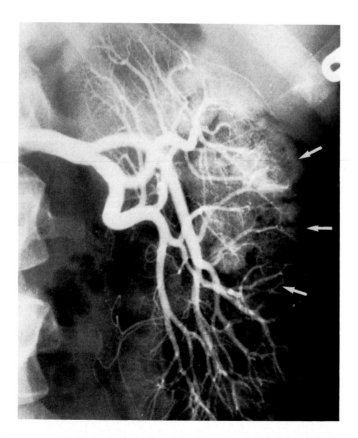

Figure 21–13. Renal angiogram showing changes of acute renal inflammation. Early arterial phase reveals attenuation of distal interlobar and arcuate vessels, most marked in midpolar region (*arrows*). (From Gold RP, McClennan BL, Rottenberg RR: CT appearance of acute inflammatory disease of the renal interstitium. AJR 141(2):343–349, 1983, © by Am Roentgen Ray Soc.)

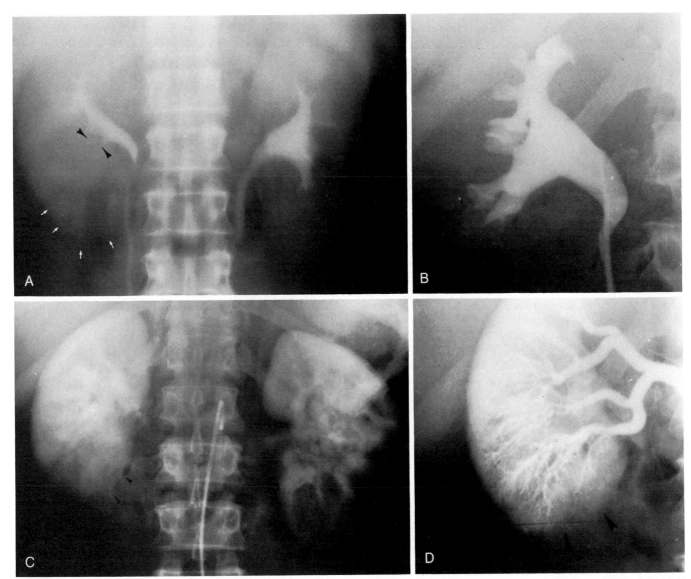

Figure 21–14. AFBN in a fifty-four-year-old diabetic man who presented with acute urinary tract infection. *A*, Film from IVU performed on admission to hospital reveals swollen right lower pole (*arrows*) with poor nephrogram and no filling of lower pole calyces (*arrowheads*). *B*, Retrograde pyelogram shows normal but slightly compressed right lower-pole calyx. *C*, Nephrogram phase from aortography shows poor right lower-pole visualization (*arrowheads*). *D*, Selective right renal angiogram shows a defect in the cortex in the right lower pole (*arrowheads*). Defect in right upper pole was due to accessory vessels. Vascular findings may be subtle in acute renal infection, manifest only as hypovascular masses or cortical defects.

Ultrasonography has proved to be more helpful in the diagnosis and management of focal inflammatory masses and may be more sensitive to their detection than either intravenous urography or radionuclide imaging.[21, 24, 28, 38] Focal bacterial nephritis almost always presents as a hypoechoic mass containing scattered low-level echoes with weak sound transmission (see Figs. 21–5 and 21–6). These masses are poorly marginated and usually disrupt the normal corticomedullary junction. Occasionally they may be multiple and rarely they have been reported as being hyperechoic in children in what may be a hemorrhagic form of acute pyelonephritis.[37, 39] Focal anechoic areas within these masses probably represent early liquefaction, but this development does not mean that continued antibiotic therapy will not result in healing. Occasionally, focal liquefaction has been sonographically demonstrated to progress to abscess formation, in which case either percutaneous or surgical drainage may be required.[16] A renal abscess often has a typical sonographic appearance of a round, thickened, or smooth-walled complex mass. Rarely, such a lesion is anechoic. Low-level echoes that move with change of position may represent internal debris (see Figs. 22–8 and 22–9). Internal septations or loculations may cause the sonographic diagnosis to be more difficult.[39] It is important to remember that these findings are not specific. Hemorrhagic cysts, infected cysts, or necrotic neoplasms may each display sonographic findings similar to those found in a renal abscess. In the absence of enhanced through transmission or refractive artifact, the diagnosis of renal abscess should be made with caution. The thickness and contour of the wall are variable, and internal echo characteristics depend on the amount of debris and/or fluid present. Highly reflective contents within an abscess raise the possibility of gas, especially if associated with "dirty" shadowing.[40]

Computed Tomography

Because CT can register differences in tissue attenuation of as little as 0.5%, it has revealed areas of renal parenchyma involved by acute inflammation that have not been detected by either urography or ultrasonography. The inflammatory edema, microabscess formation, and vasoconstriction of acute pyelonephritis produce sufficient alterations in tissue density to be readily detected, particularly on contrast-assisted CT scans.[41, 42] CT reflects the pathophysiology of renal inflammation in four major ways: (1) alteration in renal contour, (2) alteration of normal parenchymal attenuation, (3) alteration of contrast medium enhancement and excretion, and (4) perinephric abnormalities.[42]

The characteristic CT pattern of acute, uncomplicated pyelonephritis appears to reflect the pathophysiology of the disease. Ascending infection involves the calycine mucosa, and from there the medullary rays, each of which consists of a central collecting tubule and its draining cortical nephrons. The involved cortical tissue is affected as a group of lobules or an entire renal lobe (see Fig. 21–1). Accordingly, the most common CT pattern is that of wedge-shaped zones of diminished attenuation seen only after intravenous contrast administration (Figs. 21–15 and 21–16).[41–43]

These areas have very straight borders, radiate from the collecting system to the renal capsule, demonstrate a modest increase in attenuation after intravenous contrast (although always less than the enhancement of normal parenchyma), and generally are widest at the periphery of the kidney. Delayed scanning, up to 6 hours after intravenous contrast, may reveal dense enhancement in these previously low-density wedge-shaped zones. This phenomenon suggests the eventual filling of tubules that are partially obstructed by surrounding interstitial inflammatory edema—a focal, delayed obstructive nephrogram pattern.[43] Hemorrhage into areas of acute pyelonephritis has been described as echogenic wedge-shaped zones on sonographic images and as foci of high attenuation on noncontrast CT scans.[37] It is important to remember that these zones of acute pyelonephritis do not have rounded contours, do not deform the normal capsular boundary of the kidney, and do not appear as tumefactive masses (see Fig. 21–15).

An additional feature of these low-density, wedge-shaped delayed perfusing zones is the occasional presence of narrow, parallel bands of alternating density within them. The bands probably correspond on a macroscopic level to the microstriations seen at angiography during the capillary nephrogram phase in patients with acute renal inflammation. These striations are most probably a function of slow tubular urine flow secondary to the increased interstitial pressure of diffuse edema and the relatively stagnant capillary blood flow that is partly due to the associated vasospasm (Figs. 21–16 and 21–17).[41] In most cases a mild to moderate perinephric reaction is present, consisting of any or all of the following features: indistinctness of the renal outline, thickening of Gerota's fascia, edematous perinephric fat, and perinephric connective tissue septae (Fig. 21–18).[44]

The inflammatory mass of acute, focal, bacterial nephritis is well demonstrated with CT and frequently accompanies other areas of typical uncomplicated pyelonephritis in the same or contralateral kidney not detected by urography or ultrasonography (see Figs. 21–16 and 21–17). Focal nephritis is always best seen after the administration of intravenous contrast material. Characteristically, the lobar phlegmon is 20 to 40 H less dense than the normal renal parenchyma, and it has irregular boundaries, a rounded contour and, usually, an inhomogeneous appearance. Single or multiple lower-density areas may exist within this mass, consistent with liquefaction. To use the term "abscess" when these small lower-density zones are detected may be misleading, inasmuch as antibiotics alone can lead to total resolution.[13, 41] On precontrast CT scans, abscesses are solitary or multiple, round, well-marginated low-attenuation masses. Their distribution is often random, and bilateral involvement is not rare. The rim or rind sign represents enhancement of the abscess wall, but typically no central enhancement is seen (see Fig. 21–8). Gerota's fascia may be thickened, or perinephric extension of the abscess may be seen. CT is also the best imaging method for determining extrarenal extension of renal inflammatory processes, such as perinephric abscesses. Nevertheless, CT does not always provide the diagnostic specificity one would like in renal inflammation. Other entities that, at times, may provide a somewhat similar CT appearance include: segmental renal infarction, metastases, trauma, lymphoma, and

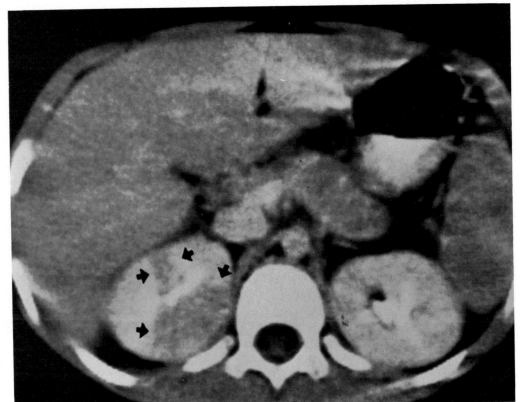

Figure 21–15. Contrast-enhanced CT scan shows large wedge-shaped areas (*arrows*) of poor enhancement, consistent with pyelonephritis. The straight borders suggest renal lobar distribution. (From Gold RP, McClennan BL, Rottenberg RR: CT appearance of acute inflammatory disease of the renal interstitium. AJR 141(2):343–349, 1983.)

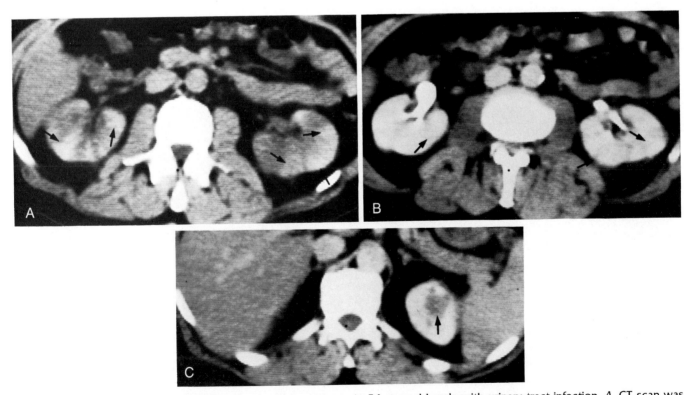

Figure 21–16. Bilateral focal bacterial nephritis—CT appearance in 54-year-old male with urinary tract infection. *A*, CT scan was obtained 24 hours after an IVU that was interpreted as normal. Non–contrast-enhanced scan shows, bilaterally, persistent cortical wedge-shaped areas of high attenuation (*arrows*). These areas correspond to focal "obstructive" nephrograms in areas presumed to be involved by inflammation. The parenchymal opacification is attributable to the contrast given for IVU. *B*, After contrast material was again administered, patchy enhancement (*arrows*) of the high-attenuation areas was noted, although some volume averaging masks their appearance. *C*, CT scan through left upper pole shows rounded area (AFBN) (*arrow*). All CT changes resolved after appropriate antibiotic therapy. (Courtesy Robert Boltuch, M.D., Cleveland, Ohio.)

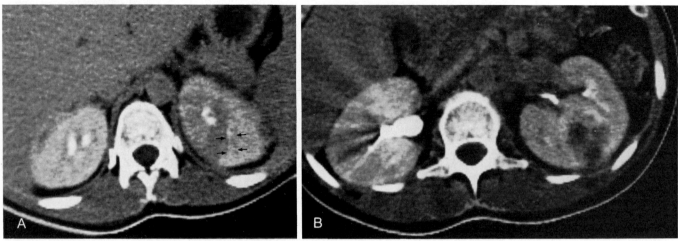

Figure 21–17. Acute bacterial nephritis—multifocal. *A,* Contrast-enhanced CT scan shows low density wedge-shaped area radiating from upper calyx on left. Appearance of striation is suggested (*arrows*). *B,* CT scan, more caudal than *A,* shows rounded, low-attenuation mass deforming midpolar region of left kidney. Central areas of low attenuation and nonenhancement are consistent with some liquefaction or microabscess formation. Streak artifacts through right kidney are present. (From Gold RP, McClennan BL, Rottenberg RR: CT appearance of acute inflammatory disease of the renal interstitium. AJR 141(2):343–349, 1983, © by Am Roentgen Ray Soc.)

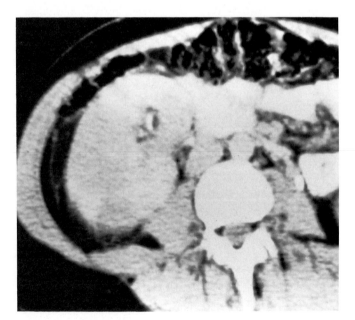

Figure 21–18. CT scan of acute pyelonephritis. Thickening of Gerota's fascia and renal enlargement is seen.

renal vein thrombosis. Appropriate clinicolaboratory correlation with the imaging findings almost always leads to a correct diagnosis.

Magnetic Resonance Imaging

Although some of the characteristic CT and sonographic features have correlates on magnetic resonance imaging (MRI) of the kidney, very few cases of acute renal inflammation have been reported (Fig. 21–19).[45] Because of the intense edema associated with focal infection, the usually low signal intensity of the kidney may be reduced even further. As judged by the behavior of infection in other organs, a markedly increased signal intensity on T2 weighting would be expected. On T1-weighted images, focal enlargement with low signal intensity has been encountered with focal nephritis.[45] For the immediate future, MRI appears to offer few advantages, compared with the modalities discussed above, for evaluating acute inflammation of the renal interstitium.

Radionuclide Imaging

Scintigraphic techniques for the diagnosis of infectious processes of the kidney have become more sensitive and specific over the last decade. Beginning with gallium-67 (Ga-67) citrate studies in the middle 1970s, and more recently with the introduction of indium-111 (In-111)–labeled leukocytes, nuclear medicine methods have become very practical for localizing an infection to the kidney and/or perinephric spaces.[46–48] Combined imaging with a renal cortical labeling agent such as technetium-99m dimercaptosuccinate (DMSA) or glucoheptonate (GHA) permits detection and characterization of underlying renal structural and physiological abnormalities and often leads to a specific diagnosis, such as acute pyelonephritis or abscess, or aids in the choice of further diagnostic or interventional procedures.[45a]

In patients with normal results of excretory urography and renal ultrasonography, Ga-67 imaging often demonstrates accumulation of this tracer in kidneys clinically thought to be involved by an acute inflammatory process (Fig. 21–20).[47, 49] Concomitant cortical imaging in some cases has shown wedge-shaped defects similar to the wedge-shaped zones of poor enhancement noted on contrast-enhanced CT (Fig. 21–20). This is also thought to represent inflammation involving a renal lobe, a typical distribution for acute pyelonephritis.[47] Although generally nonspecific in their patterns of radiopharmaceutical uptake, other inflammatory lesions, such as intrarenal or perinephric abscesses and noninfectious interstitial nephritis, have been detected by scintigraphy.[46, 49, 50] Patients with nonfunctioning kidneys or with fever of unknown origin (FUO) may be shown by radionuclide imaging to have an inflammatory process localized to one or both kidneys.[49]

Problems with renal Ga-67 imaging stem from the fact that this agent is normally excreted by the kidneys during the first 24 hours after injection, and delayed images at 48 or 72 hours are often needed to confirm that renal uptake is abnormal. In addition, gallium imaging is nonspecific, and renal tumors frequently accumulate this agent, as do other inflammatory processes such as acute tubular necrosis and various forms of vasculitis.[47] The scintigraphic differentiation of a renal from a perinephric process is also difficult, as is the localization of an infection to a specific part of the kidney. The latter difficulty can sometimes be handled with the aid of modern scintigraphic instruments (single-photon emission CT), as well as by means of dual-agent or even triple-agent subtraction studies.[47, 48]

In-111–labeled leukocytes are normally not accumulated in the kidneys and appear to be much more specific than gallium for diagnosis of inflammatory processes. Uptake in acute pyelonephritis, acute focal bacterial nephritis, and renal abscesses has been reported, as has the localization of abscesses in patients with polycystic kidney disease or a nonfunctioning kidney.[46, 52, 53] False-negative leukocyte scans do occur, and possible causes include prior antibiotic therapy, walled-off abscesses, and infections with poorly developed inflammatory responses.[54]

The use of radionuclide imaging agents can be a powerful tool for the early detection of renal or perinephric infection.[55–58] The proper use of these scintigraphic techniques and their integration with other diagnostic procedures such as urography, ultrasonography, CT, aspiration biopsy or drainage, and eventually MRI will depend on the local expertise and availability of radiopharmaceuticals and instruments at each institution.

PYELONEPHRITIS IN PREGNANCY

Asymptomatic bacteriuria is found in 2% to 7% of all women during the first trimester of pregnancy.[59] If not properly and promptly treated with antibiotics, a significant percentage (20% to 30%) of women will develop acute pyelonephritis.[59] Clinically significant episodes of acute pyelonephritis are more common in the last trimester,[60] so bacteriuria does place pregnant women at risk for urinary tract infection and its sequelae. Many women (up to 33%) with pyelonephritis of pregnancy have a previous history of urinary infection; many have abnormal radiographic findings.[61] While the kidney increases in size

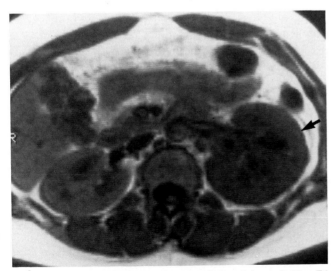

Figure 21–19. MR scan of acute bacterial nephritis, T1-weighted image. The left kidney is enlarged (*arrow*), but the corticomedullary demarcation is preserved.

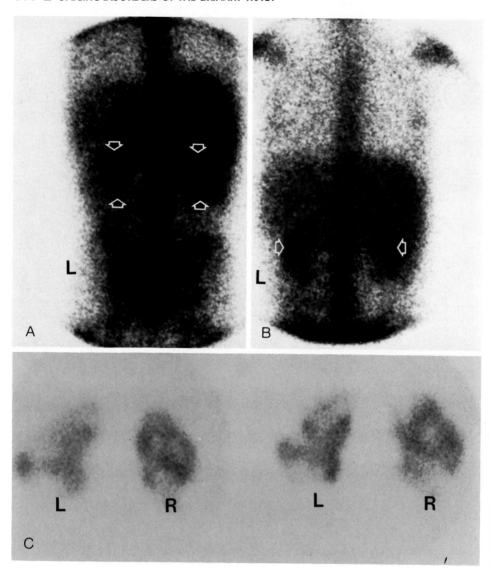

Figure 21–20. Radionuclide imaging in patient with bilateral renal infection. *A,* Fifteen-year-old male with clinical and CT evidence of bilateral acute focal bacterial nephritis (arrowheads indicate kidneys). Gallium-67 citrate scan at 48 hours after a 1.98 mCi dose. *B,* A 72-hour delayed scan shows bilateral persistent retention of radionuclide (arrowheads indicate kidneys). *C,* A technetium-99m glucoheptonate pinhole camera radionuclide image at 72 hours shows diffuse bilateral cortical defects coincident with wedged-shaped areas of lack of enhancement seen on CT scan (not shown). Each view of both kidneys is a 15-degree oblique. Diagnosis is bilateral focal bacterial nephritis.

and develops mild hydronephrosis during pregnancy, ultrasonography has become the preferred primary imaging method for evaluation of the pregnant patient with real or suspected pyelonephritis. Calculi, especially those large enough to be obstructive, complicate the imaging and treatment regimens. Hydronephrosis does not signify urinary tract obstruction, since the gravid uterus and hormonal effects of pregnancy alone can cause dilatation of the collecting system. Dilatation is the rule, and it increases throughout pregnancy, the right side being more dilated than the left. Judicious use of radiographs is recommended, especially early in gestation. If required for diagnosis or therapy, a single delayed film taken 30 minutes to several hours after administration of contrast medium will usually suffice to document urinary tract obstruction and locate a calculus (Fig. 21–21). Percutaneous nephrostomy may be performed primarily under sonographic guidance with minimal fluoroscopic exposure. Ureterorenoscopy with 6- to 9-F flexible, deflectable instruments may obviate the need for complex radiographic evaluation. MRI along with ultrasonography may allow diagnosis and appropriate intervention without the need for ionizing radiation or intravenous contrast material. The follow-up of the symptomatic woman with

pyelonephritis of pregnancy should include ultrasonography and/or voiding cystourethrography at 4 to 6 months postpartum. Urography at that time may reveal typical findings of chronic pyelonephritis, which may or may not be the result of the pyelonephritis during pregnancy.[61] Pregnant patients with ureteral calculi can often be managed by ureteral stenting, with definitive treatment of the stone deferred until the postpartum period.

COMPLICATIONS OF PYELONEPHRITIS

Emphysematous Pyelonephritis

Pyelonephritis encountered in the modern antibiotic era refers to a spectrum of conditions (see Fig. 21–24). Partially or inappropriately treated infections may result in complications such as renal abscess, perinephric abscess, pyonephrosis, xanthogranulomatous pyelonephritis (XGPN), fatty replacement, and emphysematous pyelonephritis (Table 21–3). The latter is a serious complication of upper urinary tract infection, usually limited to patients with ureteral obstruction and/or diabetes mellitus.[62–64] The condition is a very real threat to both patient and renal

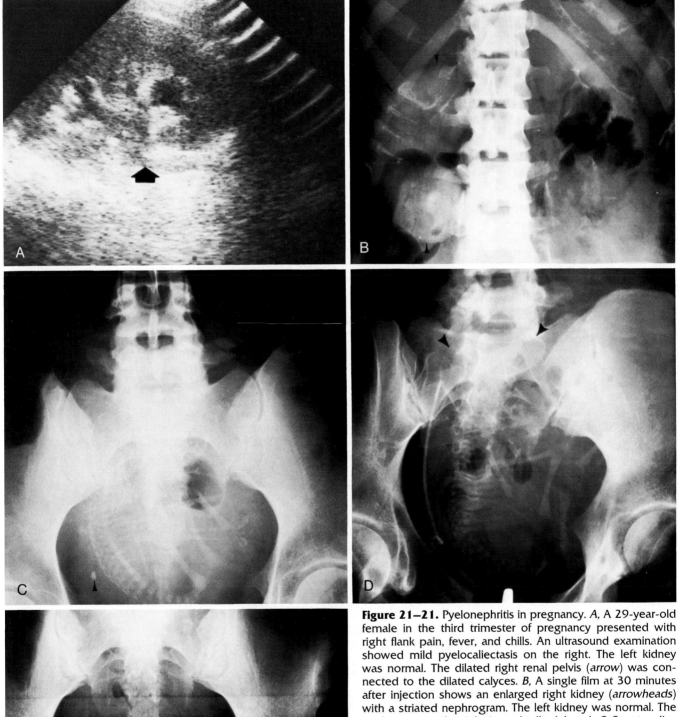

Figure 21–21. Pyelonephritis in pregnancy. *A,* A 29-year-old female in the third trimester of pregnancy presented with right flank pain, fever, and chills. An ultrasound examination showed mild pyelocaliectasis on the right. The left kidney was normal. The dilated right renal pelvis (*arrow*) was connected to the dilated calyces. *B,* A single film at 30 minutes after injection shows an enlarged right kidney (*arrowheads*) with a striated nephrogram. The left kidney was normal. The pyelogram on the right is markedly delayed. *C,* Scout radiograph prior to IVU revealed a right distal ureteral calculus (*arrowhead*) to the right of the fetal spine. *D,* A ureteral catheter was passed beyond the calculus in the right ureter. The fetal head can be seen (*arrowheads*). The patient carried to term with the indwelling catheter, which was cut off and left to drain into the bladder. The stone was passed during the interval. A double-pigtail ureteral stent would have served nicely in this case. *E,* Postpartum radiograph shows stent catheter curled in bladder. No ureteral stone was seen. Stent catheter has calcified.

survival, and it warrants prompt imaging and intervention. Gas within the renal collecting system, parenchyma, and surrounding tissues (perinephric spaces) is considered to be emphysematous pyelonephritis. Although some authors limit the definition to renal parenchymal gas, preferring to classify gas limited to the renal pelvis as emphysematous pyelitis,[64a] gas can appear in the urinary tract consequent to the following: penetrating trauma or interventional procedures, fistulae, infarction, or infection by gas-forming organisms. Patients with emphysematous pyelonephritis are more often female (2:1) and diabetic (Figs. 21–22 and 21–23).[63, 64] The clinical findings most commonly observed at presentation are chills, fever, flank pain, lethargy, and confusion.[61] Abdominal symptoms and shock are less common manifestations. In the review of 55 patients by Michaeli and coworkers,[61] the left kidney was most often involved (53% cases), whereas 35% of cases involved the right kidney and 7% had bilateral involvement. A recent report of 13 cases by Ahlering and colleagues[64] demonstrated right kidney involvement in 53%, left kidney involvement in 38%, and bilateral disease in 7%. Metachronous involvement of the opposite kidney, as well as emphysematous pyelonephritis in a solitary kidney, polycystic kidney, and a transplanted kidney have all been reported (Figs. 21–22 and 21–23).

The association with diabetes mellitus is remarkable (87%),[62] and obstruction is not a necessary prerequisite. However, almost all nondiabetics with emphysematous pyelonephritis do demonstrate obstruction. Infection caused by a known gas-producing organism of the enteric group was present in all cases. Mechanisms postulated to explain the rare formation of gas in these patients include high glucose concentration in tissues of diabetics from which organisms can produce carbon dioxide and hydrogen by fermentation, along with impaired host vascular and tissue response.[67] Gas-forming organisms that cause emphysematous pyelonephritis include *E. coli*, *Klebsiella pneumoniae*, *Aerobacter aerogenes*, and *Proteus mirabilis*. *E. coli* was the causative organism in 71% of cases reviewed by Michaeli and colleagues.[62] *Clostridium*, which characteristically produces gas, has not been reported in this condition. However, emphysematous pyelonephritis secondary to *Candida tropicalis* infection has been observed.[68] On examination, the renal tissue is necrotic and liquefied. Intrarenal vascular bacterial and clot thrombi are present.

Radiological evaluation of the patient is essential to establish the diagnosis of emphysematous pyelonephritis. Important features of identification on plain radiographs include a mottled gas pattern within the region of the renal outline and extension of gas into the perinephric space or through Gerota's fascia into the retroperitoneum. Radial distribution ("streaking") of gas along pyramids and gas extension into the perinephric spaces and Gerota's fascia correspond to an advanced stage of the process equivalent to renal necrosis.[62] Michaeli and coworkers[62] have proposed a staging classification by plain film findings: Stage I—gas in either the renal parenchyma or perinephric tissues; Stage II—gas in both the kidney and its surroundings; Stage III—extension through Gerota's fascia and/or bilateral emphysematous pyelonephritis.

Inability to clearly discern renal parenchymal gas from overlying bowel gas has necessitated intravenous urogra-

phy in some patients. The most common urographic finding is a nonvisualized kidney, although partial function with poor definition of the renal outline can be observed. Retrograde pyelography can be used to establish the presence or absence of ureteral obstruction. Fluoroscopic spot films may also render the diagnosis without the use of intravenous iodinated contrast material in patients with diabetes mellitus and/or renal insufficiency (see Figs. 21–22 and 21–23).

Sonographic examination may be useful when gas is confined to the renal parenchyma. At this stage, dense echoes originating from within the identifiable renal cortex most likely represent gas. If gas has entered the perinephric space and surrounding tissues, the sonographic appearance is more likely to be a "gassed-out" kidney (i.e., the sound beam is almost totally reflected by the highly echogenic gas).

Other imaging modalities have also been employed in the work-up and management of emphysematous pyelonephritis. CT has been proposed as a means of evaluating patients in whom establishing the extent of gas distribution in the soft tissues is difficult. Renal scintigraphy has also been employed to assess renal function, to evaluate the response to antimicrobial therapy, and to evaluate the uninvolved kidney prior to intervention.[17, 69]

Treatments of emphysematous pyelonephritis have varied, including antibiotics only, incision and drainage, and nephrectomy as well as a combination of these modes. Current therapy is aimed at controlling the predisposing factors to emphysematous pyelonephritis. Systemic antibiotics are tried first and combined later with nephrectomy, if necessary. Percutaneous drainage of the infected space and nephrostomy tube placement offers a more conservative method of treatment for the very ill, high-risk patient.[69] It must be emphasized that emphysematous pyelonephritis is a life-threatening situation. Speed in implementing diagnostic and therapeutic measures is critical if lives, let alone kidneys, are not to be lost. Gas-forming infections limited to the renal pelvis can be treated with antibiotics and stent drainage,[64a] but CT examinations must be performed to be certain that the parenchyma is not involved.

SUMMARY: IMAGING APPROACH

Most patients with acute pyelonephritis will not have any diagnostic imaging procedures. Clinical presentation and laboratory investigations are usually the only findings necessary to start appropriate treatment. Urography is usually reserved for symptomatic individuals in whom a urinary tract infection cannot be documented and other pathology is suspected, or for patients in whom an infection is not responding to usual measures or in whom a reinfection with a different organism is documented. When the urogram with tomography is normal in the face of persistent clinical evidence of renal sepsis or when the urogram reveals a mass, further radiographic investigation with either ultrasonography, CT, or radionuclide imaging may be warranted.[24]

The pathophysiology of renal inflammation produces morphological and functional changes in the kidney. These changes are detectable using a variety of imaging studies. Optimally performed, these techniques yield val-

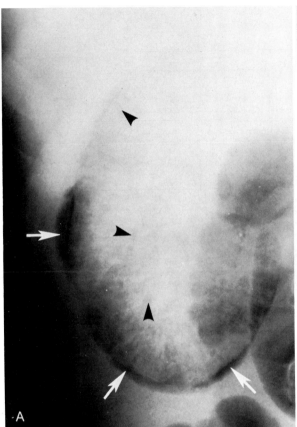

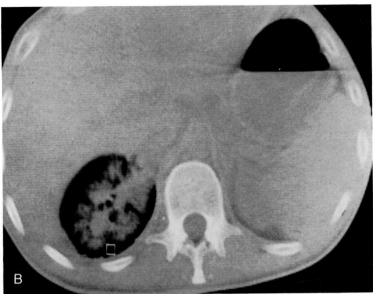

Figure 21–22. Emphysematous pyelonephritis. *A,* Plain radiograph shows gas in renal parenchyma with striated appearance (*arrowheads*). Perinephric and subcapsular gas (*arrows*) is noted as well. *B,* CT scan shows intraparenchymal and perinephric gas on right. (Courtesy Gaston Morillo, M.D., Miami, Florida.)

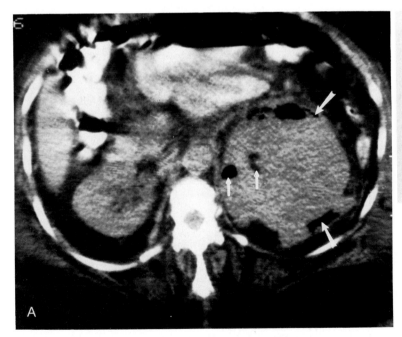

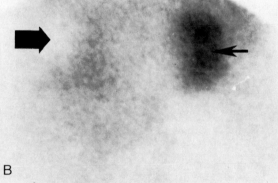

Figure 21–23. Emphysematous pyelonephritis. *A,* CT scan shows marked enlargement of the left kidney with parenchymal (*small arrows*) and perinephric gas collections (*larger arrows*). *B,* Immediate static posterior image from Tc-99m-DTPA renal scan shows radionuclide in the right kidney (*arrow*), with a photopenic area surrounded by background activity in the expected region of the left kidney (*large arrow*).

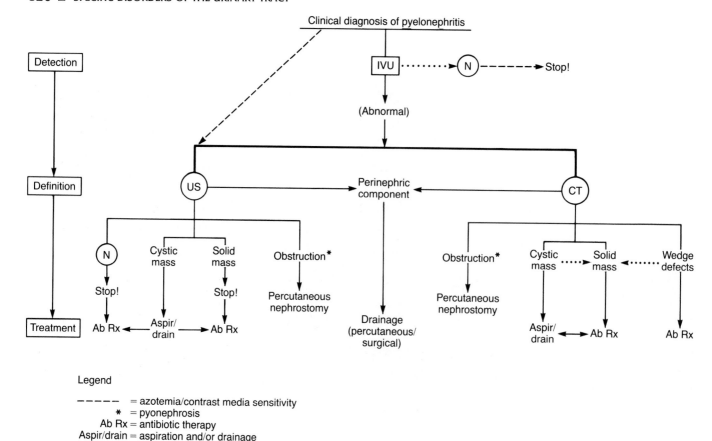

Figure 21–24. Imaging approach to pyelonephritis.

uable information that can be critical to patient management and outcome (Fig. 21–24). Selection of the appropriate test requires knowledge of the clinical and radiological features of pyelonephritis.

References

1. Roberts JA: Pyelonephritis, cortical abscess and perinephric abscess. Urol Clin North Am 13:645, 1986.
2. Stamey TA: Pathogenesis and treatment of urinary tract infections. Baltimore, Williams & Wilkins, 1980.
3. Kunin CM: Detection, Prevention and Management of Urinary Tract Infections. Philadelphia, Lea & Febiger, 1983, p 33.
4. Carrol G: Non-tuberculous infections of the urinary tract. In Campbell MF, Harrison JH, (eds): Urology. Philadelphia, WB Saunders Company, 1970, pp 399–442.
5. Lapides J (ed): Fundamentals of Urology, Philadelphia, WB Saunders Company, 1976.
6. Heptinstal RH: Pathology of the Kidney, Vol 3, 3rd Ed. Boston, Little, Brown & Company, 1983.
7. Dunnill MS (ed): Pathological Basis of Renal Disease. London, WB Saunders Company, 1976.
8. Freedman LR, Beeson PB: Experimental pyelonephritis. IV. Observations on infections resulting from direct inoculation of bacteria in different zones of the kidney. Yale J Biol Med 30:406, 1958.
9. Sarma DP: Re: Acute lobular nephronia (letter). J Urol 137:1007, 1987.
10. Lilienfield RM, Lande A: Acute adult onset bacterial nephritis: Long-term urographic and angiographic follow-up. J Urol 114:14–20, 1975.
11. Davidson AJ, Talner LB: Urographic and angiographic abnormalities in adult onset acute bacterial nephritis. Radiology 106:249–256, 1973.
12. Rosenfield AT, Glickman MG, Taylor KJW, et al: Acute focal bacterial nephritis (acute lobar nephronia). Radiology 132:553–561, 1979.
13. Lee JKT, McClennan BL, Melson GL, Stanley RJ: Acute focal bacterial nephritis: Emphasis on gray scale sonography and computed tomography. AJR 135:87–92, 1980.
14. Sotolongo JR, Schiff H, Wulfsohn MA: Radiographic findings in acute, segmental pyelonephritis. Urology 19:335–337, 1982.
15. Cronan JJ, Amis ES, Dorfman GS: Percutaneous drainage of renal abscesses. AJR 142:351, 1984.
16. McCoy RI, Kurtz AB, Rifkin MD, et al: Ultrasound detection of focal bacterial nephritis (lobar nephronia) and its evolution into a renal abscess. Urol Radiol 7:109–111, 1985.
17. Huland H, Busch R, Riebel TH: Renal scarring after symptomatic and asymptomatic upper urinary tract infection: A prospective study. J Urol 128:682–685, 1982.
18. Little PJ, McPherson DR, deWardener HE: The appearance of the intravenous pyelogram during and after acute pyelonephritis. Lancet 1:1186–1188, 1965.
19. Bailey RR, Little PJ, Rolleston GL: Renal damage after acute pyelonephritis. Br Med J 1:550–551, 1969.
20. Davidson AJ: Radiology of the Kidney. Philadelphia, WB Saunders Company, 1985, pp 255–295.
21. Zayontz MR, Pahira JJ, Wolfman M, et al: Acute focal bacterial nephritis: A systematic approach to diagnosis and treatment. J Urol 133:752–757, 1985.
22. Anderson KA, McAninch JW: Renal abscess: Classification and review of 40 cases. Urology 16:333, 1980.
23. Fernandez JA, Miles BJ, Buck AS, Gibbons RP: Renal carbuncle: Comparison between surgical open drainage and closed percutaneous drainage. Urology 25:142, 1985.
24. Melson GL: Ultrasound and computed tomography in renal infections. In Simeone J (ed): Clinics in Diagnostic Ultrasound, Coordinated Diagnostic Imaging, Vol 14. New York, Churchill Livingstone, 1984.
25. Tupper TB, Cronan JJ, Wald LM, Dorfman GS: Renal abscess: A complication of ethanol embolization. Radiology 161:35, 1986.

26. Hodson J: Radiology in pyelonephritis. Cur Prob Radiol 2:1–32, 1972.
27. Elkin M: Infections of the urinary tract. *In* Radiology of the Urinary System. Boston, Little, Brown & Company, 1980, pp 157–258.
28. Silver TM, Kass EJ, Thornbury JR, et al: The radiological spectrum of acute pyelonephritis in adults and adolescents. Radiology 118:65–71, 1976.
28a. Kuligowska E, Newman B, White SJ, Caldarone A: Interventional ultrasound in detection and treatment of renal inflammatory disease. Radiology 147:521–526, 1983.
29. Teplick JG, Teplick SK, Berinson H, Haskin ME: Unilateral pyelonephritis. Clin Radiol 30:59–66, 1978.
30. Berliner L, Bosniak MA: The striated nephrogram in acute pyelonephritis. Urol Radiol 4:41–44, 1982.
31. Richie JP, Nicholson TC, Hunting D, Brosman SA: Radiographic abnormalities in acute pyelonephritis. J Urol 119:832–835, 1978.
32. Hill GS, Clark RL: A comparative angiographic microangiographic and histologic study of experimental pyelonephritis. Invest Radiol 7:33–47, 1972.
33. Levin DC, Gordon D, Kinkhabwala MN, Becker JA: Reticular neovascularity in malignant and inflammatory renal masses. Radiology 120:61–68, 1976.
34. Jander HP, Vilar JS, Kashlan BM, Witten DM: Selective angiography in renal and perirenal inflammatory lesions: Correlation with histopathology. Br J Radiol 52:536–557, 1979.
35. Caplan LH, Siegelman SS, Bosniak MA: Angiography in inflammatory space occupying lesions of the kidney. AJR 88:14, 1967.
36. Edell SL, Bonavita JA: The sonographic appearance of acute pyelonephritis. Radiology 132:683–685, 1979.
37. Rigsby CM, Rosenfield AT, Glickman MG, Hodson J: Hemorrhagic focal bacterial nephritis: Findings on gray scale sonography and CT. AJR 146:1173–1177, 1986.
38. Kumar B, Bedi DG, Fawcett HD, et al: Indium-111 leukocyte scanning in false negative study in a renal abscess. Clin Nucl Med 11:274, 1986.
39. Siegel MJ, Glaser CM: Acute focal bacterial nephritis in children: Significance of ureteral reflux. AJR 137:257–260, 1981.
39a. Hoddich W, Jeffrey RB, Goldberg HI: CT and sonography of severe renal and perirenal infections. AJR 140:517, 1983.
40. Piccirillo M, Rigsby CM, Rosenfield AT: Sonography of renal inflammatory disease. Urol Radiol 9:66, 1987.
41. Gold RP, McClennan BL, Rottenberg RR: CT appearance of acute inflammatory disease of the renal interstitium. AJR 141:343–349, 1983.
42. Balfe BM, Stanley RJ, McClennan BL: The CT spectrum of renal inflammatory disease. *In* Computed Tomography of the Kidney and Adrenals, Siegelman SS, Gatewood OM, Goldman S (eds): New York, Churchill Livingstone, pp 167–188, 1984.
43. Ishikawa I, Saito Y, Onouchi Z, et al: Delayed contrast enhancement in acute focal bacterial nephritis: CT features. J Comput Assist Tomogr 9:894–897, 1985.
44. Seen E, Zaunbauer W, Bandhauer K, Haertel M: Computed tomography in acute pyelonephritis. Br J Urol 59:118, 1987.
45. Choyke Pl, Kressel HY, Pollock HM, et al: Focal renal masses: Magnetic resonance imaging. Radiology 152:471–477, 1984.
45a. Traisman ES, Conway JJ, Traisman HS, et al: Localization of urinary tract infection with ^{99m}Tc glucoheptonate scintigraphy. Pediatr Radiol 16:403, 1986.
46. Fawcett HD, Goodwin DA, Lantieri RL: In-111 leukocyte scanning in inflammatory renal disease. Clin Nucl Med 6:237–241, 1981.
47. Handmaker H: Nuclear renal imaging in acute pyelonephritis. Semin Nucl Med 12:246–253, 1982.
48. Hampel N, Class RN, Persky L: Value of 67 gallium scintigraphy in the diagnosis of localized renal and perirenal inflammation. J Urol 124:311–314, 1980.
49. Mendez G, Morillo G, Alonso M, Isikoff MB: Gallium-67 radionuclide imaging in acute pyelonephritis. AJR 134:17–22, 1980.
50. Wood BC, Sharma JN, Germann DR, et al: Gallium citrate 67 imaging in noninfectious interstitial nephritis. Arch Intern Med 138:1665–1666, 1978.
51. Myerson PJ, Myerson DA, Spencer PR, Prokop E: 67 GA-citrate identification of inflammation in the perirenal space. Clin Nucl Med 3:434–436, 1978.
52. Fortner A, Taylor A, Alazraki N, Datz FL: Advantage of indium-111 leukocytes over ultrasound in imaging an infected renal cyst. J Nucl Med 27:1147–1149, 1986.
53. Gilbert BR, Cerqueira MD, Eary JF, et al: Indium-111 white blood cell scan for infection complications of polycystic renal disease. J Nucl Med 26:1283–1286, 1985.
54. Kumar R, Bedi DG, Fawcett HD, et al: Indium-111 leukocyte scanning: False-negative study in a renal abscess. Clin Nucl Med 1174–275, 1986.
55. Sty JR, Wells RG, Schroeder BA, Starshak RJ: Diagnostic imaging in pediatric renal inflammatory disease. JAMA 256:895–899, 1986.
56. Conway JJ: Radionuclide imaging of acute bacterial nephritis. Contr Nephrol 39:28–35, 1984.
57. Linton AL, Richmond JM, Clark WF, et al: Gallium-67 scintigraphy in the diagnosis of acute renal disease. Clin Nephrol 24:84–87, 1985.
58. Graham GD, Lundy MM, Moreno AJ: Failure of gallium-67 scintigraphy to identify reliably noninfectious interstitial nephritis: Concise communication. J Nucl Med 24:568–570, 1983.
59. Kass EH: The role of unsuspected infection in the etiology of prematurity. Clin Obstet Gynecol 16:134, 1973.
60. Cunningham FG, Morris GB, Mickal A: Acute pyelonephritis of pregnancy: A clinical review. Obstet Gynecol 42:112, 1973.
61. Shortliffe LD, Stamey TA: Urinary infections in adult women. *In* Walsh P, Gittes R, Perlmutter A, Stamey TA (eds): Campbell's Urology, Vol 1, 5th Ed. Philadelphia, WB Saunders Company, 1986, pp 802–808.
62. Michaeli J, Magle S, Perlberg S, et al: Emphysematous pyelonephritis. J Urol 131:203–208, 1974.
63. Lanston CS, Pfister RC: Renal emphysema. A case report and review of the literature. AJR 110:778, 1970.
64. Ahlering TE, Boyd SD, Hamilton CL, et al: Emphysematous pyelonephritis: A 5-year experience with 13 patients. J Urol 134:1086–1088, 1985.
64a. Evanoff GV, Thompson CS, Foley R, Weinman EJ: Spectrum of gas within the kidney: Emphysematous pyelonephritis and emphysematous pyelitis. Am J Med 8.:149, 1987.
65. Levison ED, Weidner FA: Emphysematous pyelonephritis in a polycystic kidney. J Urol 125:734, 1981.
66. DePauw AP, Ross G: Emphysematous pyelonephritis in a solitary kidney. J Urol 125:734, 1981.
67. Brenbridge AN, Buschi AJ, Cochrane JA, Lees RT: Renal emphysema of the transplanted kidney: Sonographic appearance. AJR 132:656–658, 1979.
68. Godec CJ, Cass AS, Berkseth R: Emphysematous pyelonephritis in a solitary kidney. J Urol 124:119–121, 1980.
69. Chandhuri TK, Venkatesan R, Bobbit JV: The monitoring of renal dysfunction in renal emphysema by dual radiopharmaceutical scintiscanning. J Nucl Med 19:67–68, 1978.
70. Seidenfeld SM, Lemaistre CF, Setiawan H, Munford RS: Emphysematous pyelonephritis caused by *Candida tropicalis*. J Infect Dis 146:569, 1982.
71. Hudson MA, Weyman PJ, van der Vliet AH, et al: Emphysematous pyelonephritis: Successful management by percutaneous drainage. J Urol 136:884, 1986.

CHRONIC INFLAMMATION

PHILIP J. KENNEY □ EAMANN S. BREATNACH □ ROBERT J. STANLEY

CHRONIC URINARY TRACT INFECTION

The pathogenesis of chronic pyelonephritis is uncertain, since the disease may progress without symptoms, obstruction, or bacteriuria. Hodson noted in 1967 that the term chronic pyelonephritis should be reserved for renal inflammation caused by bacterial infections.[1] Histologically chronic pyelonephritis is an interstitial nephritis with inflammatory cellular infiltrates, and the diagnosis is made pathologically without bacteria present. The ability of bacteria to persist in variant forms may contribute to the recurrence and/or progression of infection in cases of chronic pyelonephritis (Fig. 21–25).

The role and significance of vesicoureteral reflux in the pathogenesis of chronic pyelonephritis is covered in the fourth section of Chapter 21. The former term, chronic "atrophic" pyelonephritis, has given way to the more appropriate term *reflux nephropathy,* because most of the morphological changes seen in imaging studies are thought to be due to the combination of reflux and infection. Although little hard evidence exists to show that *acute* urinary tract infection progresses inexorably to *chronic* urinary tract infection, reflux and other predisposing causes (e.g., diabetes, papillary necrosis, obstruction) play major contributory or causal roles (Fig. 21–26).

The onset of chronic pyelonephritis typically occurs in childhood, but it may be unilateral or bilateral and is typically asymmetrical in its renal manifestations. The disease is more predominant in females, and often there is no history of intercurrent symptoms or signs. The involved renal unit typically shows cortical scarring overlying the involved calyx (usually polar), with papillary retraction (clubbing) due to the fibrotic parenchymal response. The urographic appearance is characterized by parenchymal scarring and calyceal distortion, and the hallmark feature is focal change (Fig. 21–27). Global atrophy may occur as a result of growth failure or global scarring, and contralateral hypertrophy is usually present. Acute fulminant bacterial nephritis can also cause the typical urographic changes of reflux nephropathy in adults, although it is rare.

Dilatation of the involved calyces or entire collecting system may be seen in chronic pyelonephritis. In the presence of obstruction, progression to a pyo/hydronephrosis may occur (see third section of this chapter). Calculi may form (e.g., struvite), and the picture of xanthogranulomatous pyelonephritis (XGPN) may supervene (see Fig. 20–3). Sloughed papillae or debris can secondarily calcify, thereby initiating the obstruction, and pre-existing calculi may even become secondarily infected.[2]

Angiographic features of chronic pyelonephritis include decreased vessel caliber, tortuosity, slow flow, poor corticomedullary distinction, loss of arborization, and contour deformities (scars). Because inflammatory involvement is often patchy and polar, areas of normal uninvolved parenchyma may hypertrophy, causing focal mass effects or areas of apparent "hypervascularity."

Chronic inflammation in the adult may take various forms, including fat proliferation, XGPN, malacoplakia, and squamous metaplasia. The differential diagnosis may include papillary necrosis, analgesic abuse, sinus fibrolipomatosis, excessive or persistent fetal lobation, nephrosclerosis, ischemia, radiation change, and hypoplastic kidney.

FAT PROLIFERATION IN THE KIDNEY

One response to chronic inflammation is proliferation of sinus fat. Since the renal sinus fat at the hilus is contiguous with the fat in the perinephric space, fatty

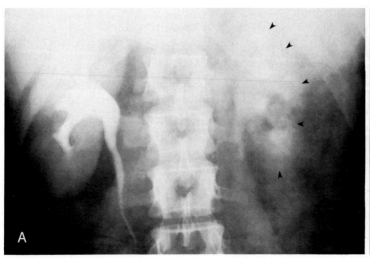
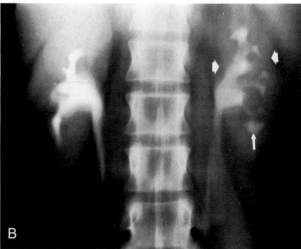

Figure 21–25. Chronic pyelonephritis—unilateral. *A,* A 41-year-old man presented with a clinical picture of acute pyelonephritis. An IVU was performed showing decreased and delayed excretion from a small left kidney at 5 minutes (*arrowheads*). The right kidney appeared normal. *B,* Tomogram shows diffuse calyceal blunting with overlying cortical scarring (*arrowheads*). A left lower-pole calculus was present in a dilated lower-pole calyx (*arrow*). The patient had a long history of urinary tract infections, and VCU had shown no reflux.

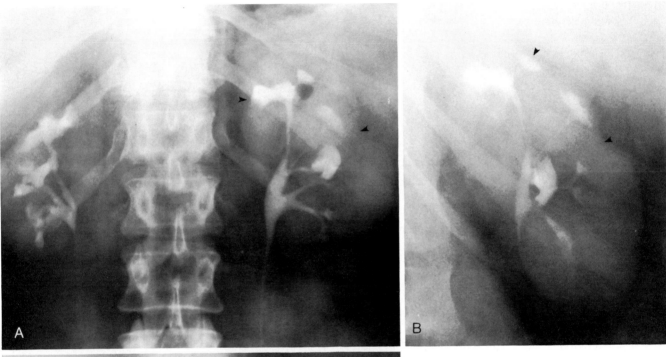

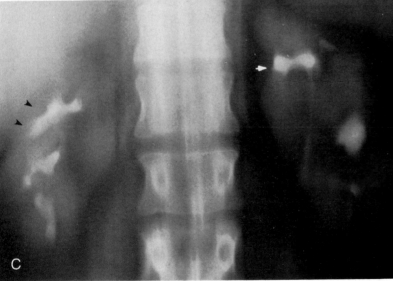

Figure 21–26. Chronic pyelonephritis—bilateral. *A,* The IVU of a 38-year-old diabetic man with a long history of urinary infection shows changes of bilateral (atrophic) pyelonephritis. Focal calyceal blunting with overlying cortical scarring (*arrowheads*) is present. The right kidney appears small. *B,* A left posterior oblique view from the urogram shows left upper-pole calyceal changes and scarring to better advantage. *C,* Tomogram shows bilateral scarring (*arrowheads*) most marked in both upper poles. The right kidney again appears small.

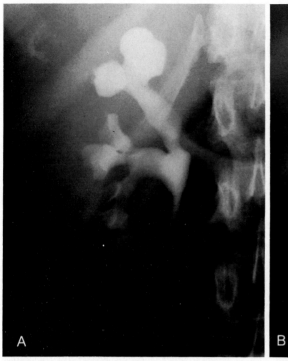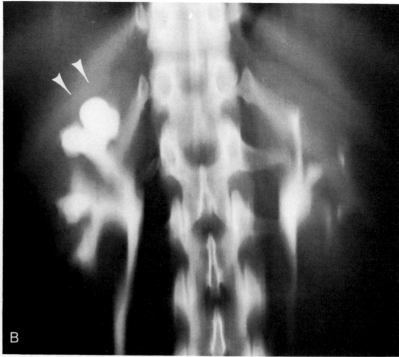

Figure 21–27. Focal atrophic pyelonephritis. *A,* A coned view of right kidney shows urographic features of focal pyelonephritis. Diffuse calyceal clubbing in the upper pole is present, with moderate blunting of the middle calyceal group. The lower-pole calyces are normal. *B,* Tomography shows overlying scarring (*arrowheads*) and calyceal deformity to be most marked in the right upper pole.

proliferation may occur in one or both of these anatomical areas.

In the normal kidney, a variable amount of fibrofatty tissue is always present in the renal sinus, a potential space that separates the renal parenchyma from the collecting system. The renal sinus contains blood vessels and lymphatics and is directly continuous with the renal hilus and perinephric fat. Fat proliferation may occur within the renal sinus, and a number of terms have been used to describe various degrees of this condition. Renal sinus lipomatosis refers to the most common situation, where a moderate increase in fibrofatty tissue is observed, particularly in the aging kidney, with no associated renal abnormality. Renal replacement lipomatosis (or fibrolipomatosis) lies at the other end of the spectrum. In this condition the renal parenchyma is destroyed, most often by infection, and is replaced by massive proliferation of fibrofatty tissue.

Renal Sinus Lipomatosis

A moderate increase in the amount of renal sinus fat is frequently seen in the normal population as a consequence of aging and when obesity is present. Poilly and colleagues[3] in 1969 record an incidence of renal sinus lipomatosis (RSL) in 23 of 3500 consecutive urograms (0.66%). Hadar and Meiraz[4] in 1980 report an incidence of twice that amount (1.25%). The difference between both figures is probably explained by the availability of computed tomography (CT) in the recent series, with its higher sensitivity to fat. The only clinical importance of RSL is that it may simulate a parapelvic mass on imaging, although this is less likely as awareness of its characteristic appearance increases.

Imaging

On the urogram, the condition is commonly associated with an extrarenal pelvis. The calyces appear elongated and stretched, but hydronephrosis is absent, and the kidneys are otherwise normal. Conventional tomography shows that the stretching is the result of a large collection of radiolucent renal sinus fat insinuating between the infundibula and calyces (Fig. 21–28). Angiography is not indicated in such cases; if performed, however, it shows normal vessels coursing through the excess renal sinus fat. It may be impossible to distinguish a parapelvic cyst from RSL on urography. Although the distinction is not of great clinical importance, ultrasonography discriminates these entities. Unusually extensive echogenicity arising from the renal sinus tissues is seen in RSL, whereas parapelvic cysts are sonolucent (Figs. 21–29 and 21–30).

In the vast majority of patients, parapelvic cyst formation can confidently be distinguished from RSL on CT scans (Figs. 21–31 and 21–32). Rarely, sinus lipomatosis mimics a parapelvic cyst or hydronephrosis on a CT scan. This occurs when a large fibrous component raises the attenuation values beyond the negative range, closer to water density. Although scans with intravenous contrast may fail to distinguish between parapelvic cysts and high-density renal sinus fibrolipomatosis, hydronephrosis can be excluded by visualizing an attenuated, nondilated collecting system. In such a rare case, ultrasonography is able to differentiate a parapelvic cyst from a cyst-shaped collection of water-density fibrolipomatous tissue.

Renal Replacement Lipomatosis

This condition represents the other end of the spectrum of fat tissue proliferation in the kidney, and it most often

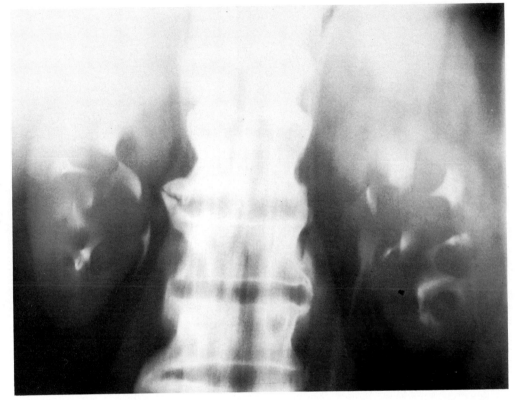

Figure 21–28. Renal sinus lipomatosis. Tomography reveals lucent material filling the renal sinus of both kidneys. (Courtesy George J. Dechet, M.D.)

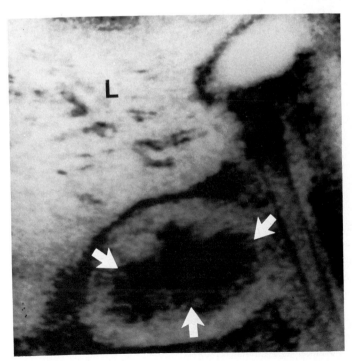

Figure 21–29. Renal sinus lipomatosis. On this sagittal sonogram, excess fat in the right renal sinus is seen as a broad hyperechoic region (*arrows*). The cortex is normal. (L = liver.)

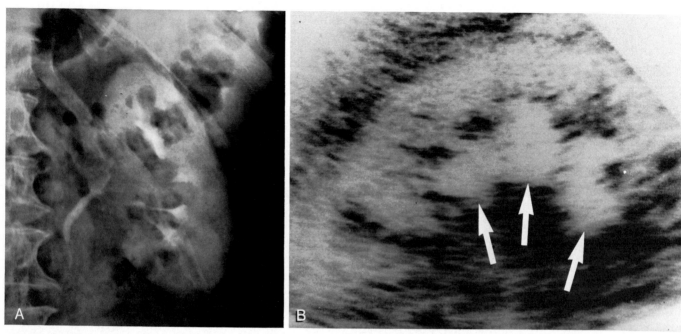

Figure 21–30. Parapelvic cysts mimicking sinus lipomatosis. *A,* Urogram demonstrates stretching and attenuation of calyces. *B,* Sonogram of the left kidney (same patient) reveals multiple sonolucent structures in the renal sinus (*arrows*), representing parapelvic cysts, not renal sinus fat. While this sonogram simulates hydronephrosis, that possibility was excluded by the urogram (*A*).

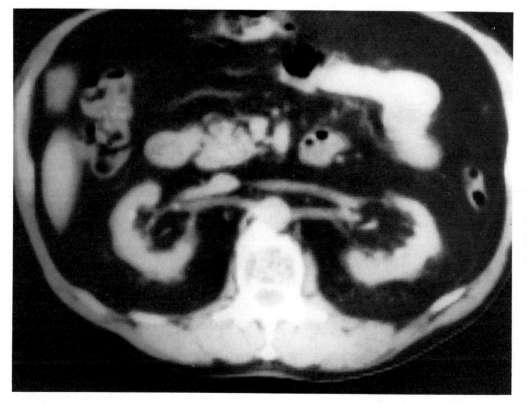

Figure 21–31. Renal sinus lipomatosis. Enhanced CT scan in an elderly male demonstrates slight thinning of the renal parenchyma with large amounts of fat in the renal sinus of both kidneys. Note the normal renal vessels and nondilated calyces.

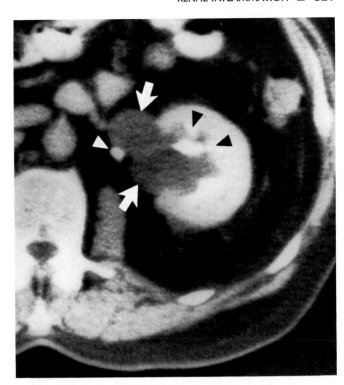

Figure 21–32. Parapelvic cysts. Enhanced CT scan (same patient shown in Figure 21–30) clearly shows fluid-filled structures (*arrows*) in the renal sinus stretching the calyces (*arrowheads*). The opacified, nondilated calyces and ureter are seen as separate from these cysts, thus excluding any possibility of hydronephrosis (compare with Figure 21–31).

results from severe infection, usually being associated with obstruction. Most of the renal parenchyma is destroyed and replaced by fibrofatty tissue. Renal calculi are found in 70% of the cases.[5–7] The degree of fat replacement depends on the stage at which the disease is encountered, and the crossover between renal replacement lipomatosis (RRL) and RSL is not clearcut. Parenchymal loss may occur in the normal aging kidney, where prominent sinus lipomatosis may also be present. RRL is by no means unique to the kidney and has been described in many atrophied organs, including the thymus and senile pancreas.[8] However, in those organs no accompanying inflammation is present. In the kidney, associated long-standing inflammation or stone formation is always present.

Grossly, the kidney appears enlarged but in fact consists primarily of abundant perinephric and renal sinus fat. The renal parenchyma is thin, and hydronephrosis or pyonephrosis with acute and chronic pyelonephritic changes may exist. Microscopically, in addition to the large amount of renal sinus fat, a proliferation of lipid-laden macrophages is found within the sinus. Histological differences between RRL and xanthogranulomatous pyelonephritis (XGPN) include the presence of lipid-laden foam cells actually infiltrating the interstitium of the kidney in XGPN, whereas in RRL the foam cells are contiguous with renal parenchyma but do not directly invade it.

Imaging

On the plain film of the abdomen, renal calculi are frequently demonstrated, and in two series they were reported in 76% and 79% of the patients evaluated.[5, 6] Nephrotomography will show significant renal parenchymal atrophy with a thinned rim of poorly enhancing tissue surrounding the abundant fat. Diminished renal function is manifested by poor or absent excretion of intravenous

contrast material (Fig. 21–33). If the collecting system is visualized by retrograde pyelography, the calyces and infundibula will appear stretched, attenuated, and possibly hydronephrotic. Arteriography is not commonly used to identify the condition, but if performed for other reasons, stretching and attenuation of intrarenal vessels caused by the masses of fat tissue will be seen.[9]

Ultrasonography[9] usually clearly demonstrates the increase in fat, showing hyperechoic areas in a kidney where renal parenchyma is grossly thinned (Fig. 21–33).

CT confirms the presence of abundant fat within the shell of an atrophied kidney and may show stones, even when they are nonopaque on conventional radiography (Fig. 21–33C).[10] Conceivably, a tumor composed primarily of fat could arise centrally and displace various components of the kidney. In that case, however, function would be preserved and a history of chronic inflammatory disease would be lacking.

XANTHOGRANULOMATOUS PYELONEPHRITIS

XGPN is a chronic suppurative form of renal infection characterized by destruction and replacement of renal parenchyma with lipid-containing macrophages (xanthoma cells). The process may be focal or diffuse, and extension of inflammation outside the kidney is not uncommon. Prior to CT and ultrasonography, the preoperative diagnosis was frequently missed, which probably explains the high rate of postoperative complications encountered.[11–13] The condition is of particular interest to radiologists, because, although the focal type mimics renal cell carcinoma, the global form of the disease has characteristic imaging features that are diagnostic.

The condition, which was first described in 1916 by Schlagenhaufer,[14] was at first considered an oddity but has become more frequently reported in the past decade. Malek and colleagues[11] found XGPN in 18 patients during

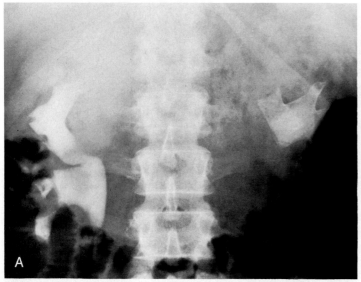

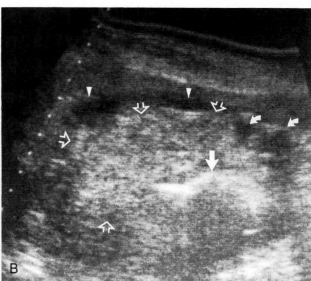

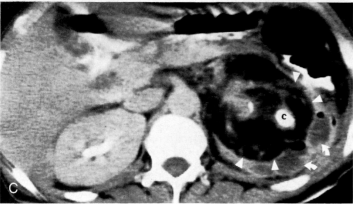

Figure 21–33. Renal replacement lipomatosis. *A,* Staghorn calculus lies within the pelvis of the nonvisualizing left kidney on this urogram. This 43-year-old man presented with fever and left flank pain. *B,* Prone sagittal sonogram of the left kidney also shows the staghorn calculus (*arrow*) and thinning of the cortex (*arrowheads*) with excessive echogenic material extending from the renal sinus (*open arrows*). Perinephric abscess is present (*curved arrows*). *C,* On a CT scan, the replacement of left renal parenchyma by fat proliferation (*arrowheads*) is clearly evident. Perinephric abscesses (*arrows*) with gas (due to fistula to descending colon) is also present. C = calculus. (*A–C* from Subramanyam BR, Bosniak MA, Horii SC, Megibow AJ, Balthazar EJ: Replacement lipomatosis of the kidney: diagnosis by computed tomography and sonography. Radiology 148:791–792, 1983.)

a series of 3000 consecutive nephrectomies and renal biopsies reported in 1972. Gingell and colleagues[15] summarized 100 cases in the world literature in 1973, and in 1981 Tolia and associates[16] reported that more than 400 cases had been described. Since then, Grainger and coworkers[17] have added 80 patients to the world literature. Thus, the condition is by no means a clinical curiosity, being estimated to occur in 1% to 8% of kidneys requiring a nephrectomy for inflammatory conditions.[18]

The disease is more commonly found in women than in men, with a peak incidence in middle life. However, no age group is immune: Gingell and coworkers[15] have reported it in a 10-month infant, and Abbate and Myers in an infant of 48 days;[18] both Goldman[19] and Malek and Elder[20] have described it separately in patients of 82 years.

Most typically, the clinical picture is of a middle-aged woman with a staghorn calculus, a recurrent fever, dysuria, and flank pain that are unresponsive to antibiotics. Surprisingly, urinary symptoms (frequency and dysuria) may be absent, as was true in 55% of those in Gingell's literature survey,[15] and less specific symptoms may predominate. The latter include malaise, nausea, vomiting and weight loss, which may be profound. The reported duration of symptoms prior to presentation is extremely variable, extending from 3 days to over 8 years. Physical findings include tenderness in the renal area and a loin mass. The mass may be nonreniform, a finding that should alert the clinician to possible extrarenal extension of disease. Laboratory investigations show an elevated erythrocyte sedimentation rate (ESR) (frequently above

90 mm/H Westergren), and anemia accompanied by leukocytosis. Proteinuria and pyuria are frequent, with urine cultures yielding, in decreasing order of frequency, *Proteus, Escherichia coli, Klebsiella, Pseudomonas, Enterobacter,* or a variety of other organisms.[21] The urine, however, may be sterile, as in 39% of cases reported by Malek and Elder.[20] The same authors quote from Matz's series, in which up to 30% of patients had sterile urine cultures,[22] which may occur despite positive growth from the infected kidney. Alternatively, different organisms may be isolated from the urine of the removed kidney, underlining the problems of medical management. Reversible hepatic dysfunction, although reported in approximately 15% of patients with renal cell carcinoma, appears to be more closely associated with XGPN. Of 26 patients with XGPN studied by Malek and Elder,[20] all 13 who underwent liver function studies showed evidence of reversible hepatic dysfunction. The abnormality was present in 6 of 29 patients reported by Tolia, although those authors do not state how many of their patients underwent liver function tests (LFT).[16] The syndrome is characterized by a variety of abnormal LFTs and is accompanied in some patients by hepatomegaly. The cause is not known, but LFT results seem to return to normal following treatment.

Pathology

The disease is almost always unilateral, and only one patient with bilateral involvement has been reported.[23] Two major disease forms are recognized: a diffuse variety and a focal, or tumefactive, type. Cases are also described in which small areas of XGPN have been pathologically recognized in kidneys destroyed by pyonephrosis, in association with renal cell or transitional cell carcinoma, or even in a renal cyst wall.[16] Imaging techniques cannot distinguish these microscopic expressions of disease, and without other evidence such XGPN is not radiographically diagnosable.

For both the global and tumefactive types, three stages have described the extent of involvement.[11] In Stage One the lesion is confined to the kidney; in Stage Two it extends to Gerota's space; and in Stage Three it spreads further to involve the paranephric spaces and other retroperitoneal structures.

Macroscopically, in the tumefactive form of the disease, a mass usually develops adjacent to a stone-containing calyx. On section, the "tumor" is a solid or semisolid yellowish-white necrotic conglomerate that is indistinguishable from renal cell carcinoma.

In the diffuse form, the entire kidney is enlarged and the surrounding perinephric fat thickened and indurated. The renal pelvis is usually dilated and frequently contains a staghorn calculus, although it may not be possible to identify any preserved urothelium. Calyces, if preserved, are dilated and clubbed or occasionally are compressed and lined by a yellow zone of tissue. Microscopically, this zone consists of a mixture of large and finely granular foam cells, smaller cells with an eosinophilic granularity, plasma cells, fibroblasts, and polymorphonuclear leukocytes.[21] The renal cortical thickness is reduced, its consistency is softened, and it may contain multiple abscesses surrounded by more xanthoid tissue.

Microscopically, except for the extent of disease, both the global and focal types are similar. Pyelonephritis, both acute and chronic, is seen, again with prominent large foam cells. The foam cells contain lipid consisting of neutral fat and cholesterol ester granules, which stain positively with periodic acid-Schiff (PAS). These staining characteristics differentiate these cells from the clear cells seen in renal cell carcinoma, a diagnosis that, mistakenly, was not infrequently made in the past, especially in focal disease. While similar in name, XGPN should not be confused with renal xanthogranulomatosis, which is a systemic proliferative disorder of histiocytes, which may involve the kidney (sinus histiocytosis).

Imaging

Intravenous Urography

In the typical patient with XGPN, a scout film shows the presence of a staghorn calculus (Fig. 21–34A). Careful inspection may reveal further small calcifications scattered throughout the affected kidney, and a tumefaction may be identified, arising from the renal surface. If perinephric extension has occurred, the renal margins may be ill-defined, and a large soft-tissue mass occupies the renal fossa. Thickened Gerota's fascia is sometimes demonstrable. After intravenous contrast material is administered, findings will vary according to the morphological type of XGPN. If global disease is present, little or no excretion is seen after the administration of intravenous contrast material (Fig. 21–34B). Some opacification of inflammatory tissue may be discernible on nephrotomography, and lucent nonopacified central masses corresponding to xanthomatous collections may be visualized. The renal outline is obscured in areas where the process extends beyond the renal margins. Although arteriography no longer has a major role in establishing the diagnosis of XGPN, features described in global disease have included splayed vessels similar to those seen in hydronephrosis, attenuation of major renal arteries, and lack of arborization of peripheral vessels (Fig. 21–35A, B). Inhomogeneity of the nephrographic phases may also be seen, sometimes mimicking hydronephrosis (Fig. 21–35C).[24, 25] The numbers of reports of patency and thrombosis of renal veins on phlebography appear to be almost equal.[15, 23, 26] Commonly, the intrarenal veins are stretched and compressed by the inflammatory mass or masses (Fig. 21–35D). Thrombosis in the inferior vena cava has not been reported.

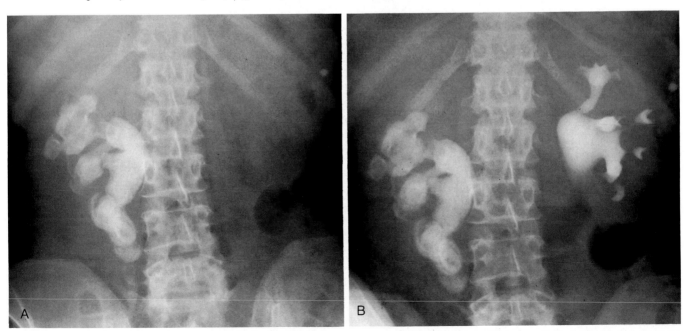

Figure 21–34. Xanthogranulomatous pyelonephritis (XGPN). *A*, Scout radiograph shows staghorn calculus in an enlarged right kidney. *B*, No excretion is evident from the right kidney on urography. (Courtesy Errol Levine, M.D.)

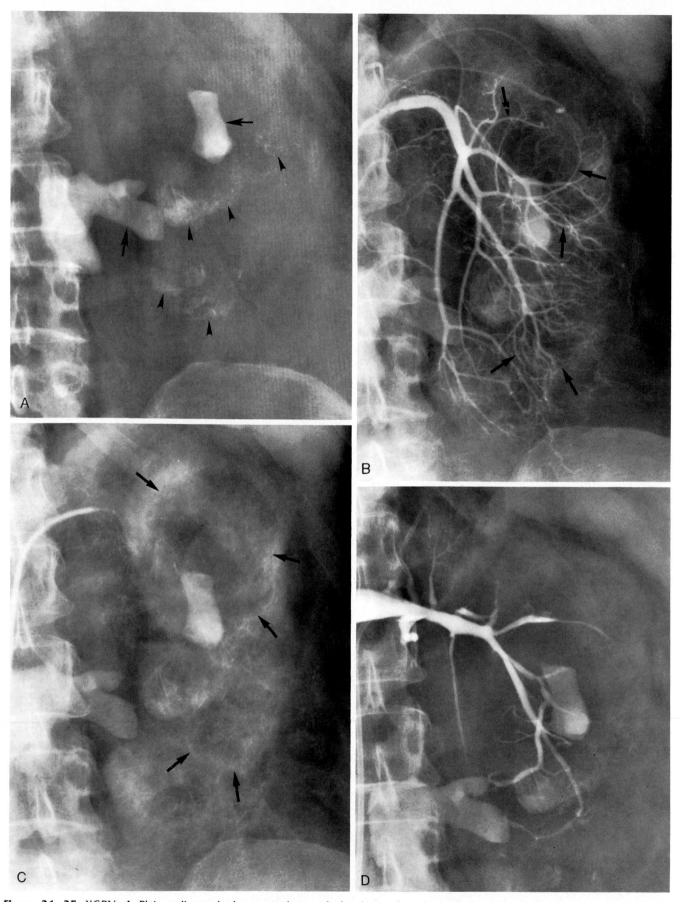

Figure 21–35. XGPN. *A,* Plain radiograph shows staghorn calculus (*arrows*) and stippled calcifications (*arrowheads*) in the left kidney in this 60-year-old female with left upper-quadrant pain. Sonography was interpreted as showing a renal mass. *B,* Selective renal arteriogram demonstrates splaying of intrarenal vessels (*arrows*) with lack of arborization. No neovascularity is evident. *C,* Late phase of this selective arteriogram shows an inhomogeneous nephrogram. Lucent regions are seen with subtle peripheral enhancement (staining) (*arrows*). *D,* Epinephrine phlebogram reveals splaying and compression of intrarenal veins but no thrombosis. Surgical resection confirmed XGPN. (*Courtesy Josef Rosch, M.D., and Frederick S. Keller, M.D.*)

When the disease is focal, findings are similar to those noted earlier, but are confined to a segment of the kidney (Fig. 21–36A, B). The mass is typically hypovascular on arteriography (Fig. 21–36C). Vessels may be stretched by the swelling, but little local alteration in their caliber is identified. Some authors have pointed to the prominent capsular and periureteral vessels that may be seen,[27] but it is not possible to exclude hypovascular neoplasms, such as transitional cell carcinoma or papillary adenocarcinoma, from XGPN on the arteriogram.

Ultrasonography

The reported sonographic findings in patients with XGPN correlate well with the abnormalities seen pathologically.[28–29a] Typically there is enlargement of a kidney, which contains multiple anechoic or hypoechoic areas corresponding to the large cavitary collections seen in the anatomical specimen (Fig. 21–37). Within these areas, central echogenic foci with associated acoustic shadowing may be seen, representing smaller calcifications. Sound

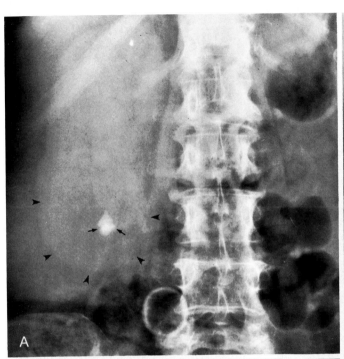

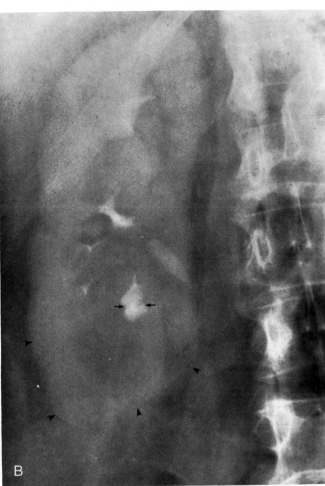

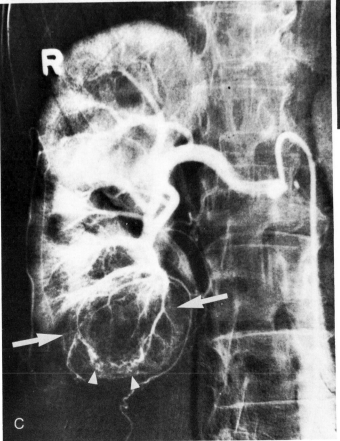

Figure 21–36. Segmental XGPN. *A,* On plain radiograph a calculus (*arrows*) lies within a right lower-pole renal mass (*arrowheads*). *B,* Excretory urography shows the calculus to be at the apex of the mass (*arrowheads*). There is no excretion by the lower pole. Note the calcification conforms to the shape and location of the lower-pole calyx. *C,* The mass (*arrows*) is hypovascular on renal arteriography. Note the peripheral inflammatory neovascularity (*arrowheads*). Surgery confirmed XGPN. (From Hartman DS: Radiologic pathologic correlation of the infectious granulomatous diseases of the kidney. 1985 Monographs in Urology, pp 26–35.)

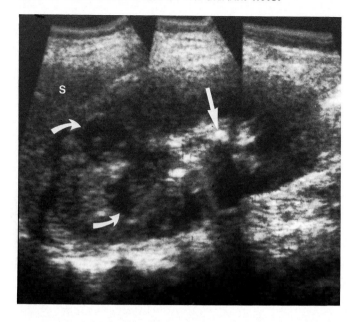

Figure 21–37. XGPN. This 35-year-old woman with fever and left flank pain had calculi in a nonvisualizing left kidney. Longitudinal sonogram reveals an enlarged kidney with a calculus (*arrow*) and several hypoechoic areas in the renal parenchyma (*curved arrows*). There is poor sound transmission through the hypoechoic areas suggesting they are not merely dilated calyces. (S = spleen.) (From Subramanyam RB, Megibow AJ, Raghavendra BN, Bosniak MA: Urol Radiol 4:3–9, 1982.)

transmission is not usually enhanced, because the hypoechoic areas are not simple fluid-filled spaces. The renal parenchyma is markedly thinned and may be interrupted by smaller cystic collections representing intracortical abscesses. Corticomedullary demarcation is usually not discernible. Although this combination of findings in a nonvisualizing kidney with an associated staghorn calculus should alert one to the possibility of XGPN, the findings are by no means specific. The appearance may be mimicked by simple hydronephrosis in association with a renal calculus, nonspecific pyonephrosis, and other inflammatory processes, including tuberculosis, cystic renal cell carcinoma, or even lymphoma. To differentiate between the conditions, it is helpful to remember that the dilated calyces are usually sharply outlined and show enhanced sound transmission in uncomplicated hydronephrosis, while fluid-debris levels are often found in pyonephrosis. Such is usually not the case in XGPN.

Computed Tomography

To date, CT shows the greatest promise in the preoperative identification and assessment of extent of XGPN. CT features characteristic of the disease have been well described.[18, 29, 30] The appearances depend on whether focal or global disease is present. In global disease, a staghorn calculus may be seen in the renal pelvis of an enlarged nonexcreting kidney (Fig. 21–38). Although an overall reniform shape is maintained, the renal architecture is grossly destroyed and replaced by multiple nonenhancing cystic-appearing masses. Attenuation values recorded in these lesions vary from approximately −10 to 30 H (Hounsfield units), depending on the quantity of lipid present. The renal pelvis may or may not be identifiable, and finer calcifications may occur within the xanthomatous masses. Gas pockets are sometimes present (Fig. 21–39).[18] Almost invariably, thickening of Gerota's fascia is found. The perinephric fat may or may not be intact. In very extensive cases, the disease may infiltrate into the psoas muscle, bowel, or flank muscles. After intravenous contrast medium is administered, rim enhancement of these rounded accumulations may occur, reflecting well-vascularized granulation and inflammatory tissue (Fig. 21–40).[31] The xanthomatous material itself

does not enhance, and the accumulations thus become more obvious. Smaller intracortical abscesses may also become more visible with contrast medium. A marginal blush outlining the kidney is frequently prominent, reflecting the enlarged capsular arteries that occur in this condition.

In patients with tumefactive XGPN, a large mass is identified in an otherwise functioning kidney (Fig. 21–41). Such a mass has a low attenuation value and does not change significantly after the injection of contrast medium. However, rim enhancement may again be seen. An associated calculus related to the central portion of the mass is often identified, indicating that a segment of renal parenchyma drained by a single or composite calyx has borne the brunt of the disease. None of the features listed above is diagnostic of XGPN, but they are sufficiently typical of global disease to warrant considering a preoperative diagnosis in the appropriate clinical setting. Tumefactive disease cannot be diagnosed radiologically with confidence, and the presumption of malignancy is paramount until the lesion is histologically proven to be otherwise. The importance of urine cultures in assessing an unexplained renal mass and in excluding inflammation as a cause cannot be overemphasized.

Either pattern of XGPN may demonstrate infiltration into the adjacent perinephric soft tissues, and CT is of particular benefit in making this assessment (Fig. 21–42). Renal fascial thickening is frequently seen on CT scans of any renal infection and should not be interpreted as indicating extrarenal extension. Direct spread will be visible as alteration of the usual fat density in the perinephric space. With extensive perinephric involvement, the overall renal architecture may be destroyed to such an extent that identification of the kidney proper is impossible. In that case, the appearance may simulate other chronic inflammatory conditions, including fungal infection.

Magnetic Resonance Imaging

Only scattered reports of the appearance of XGPN on MRI have appeared.[31a] The findings have been inconsistent, some authors noting greater signal intensity in the involved areas than in normal renal parenchyma, and

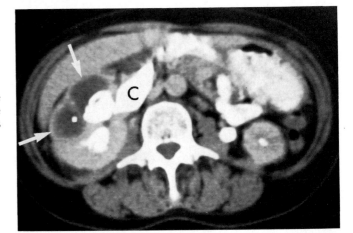

Figure 21–38. XGPN. Staghorn calculus (C) is seen in the large nonexcreting right kidney on contrast-enhanced CT. Note the low-density parenchymal regions (*arrows*) (same patient as Figure 21–34). (Courtesy Errol Levine, M.D.)

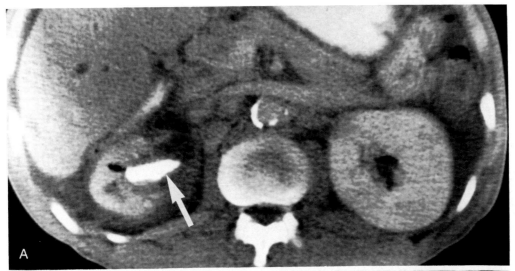

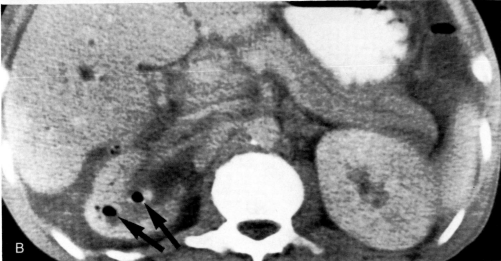

Figure 21–39. XGPN. *A,* Enhanced CT scan in this 52-year-old male with fever, night sweats, and weight loss was done after urogram revealed a nonvisualizing right kidney with a calculus. The calculus (*arrow*) lies in the renal pelvis; the kidney is atrophic. *B,* In the same patient, slightly more superior scan reveals gas in the collecting system (*arrows*). XGPN was confirmed by nephrectomy.

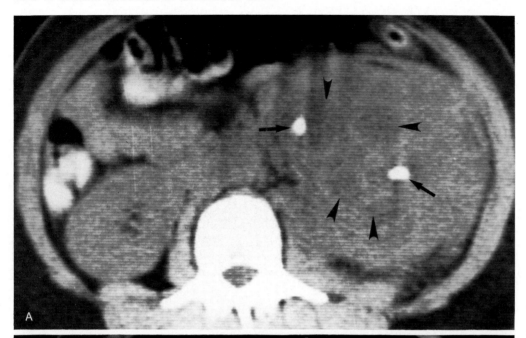

Figure 21–40. XGPN. *A*, This 30-year-old woman with a *Proteus* urinary tract infection had a nonvisualizing left kidney on urography. Nonenhanced CT shows the left kidney is enlarged and contains calculi (*arrows*) and low-density regions (*arrowheads*). *B*, CT after intravenous contrast injection shows no excretion on the left, but enhancement of the rims of the low-density regions has occurred. Note the perinephric extension of the inflammation. At surgery, the kidney was adherent to the psoas, but the muscle itself was not involved.

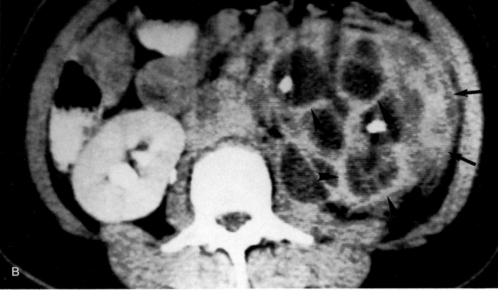

Figure 21–41. Segmental XGPN. On enhanced CT, a solitary low-density mass with an irregular wall lies in the right lower renal pole (*arrows*). Surgery confirmed focal XGPN (same patient as in Fig. 21–36A–C). (Courtesy David S. Hartman, M.D.)

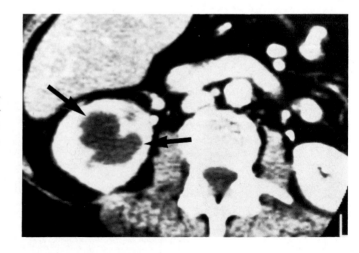

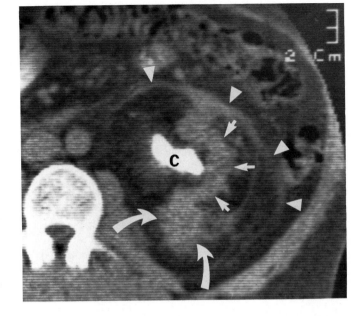

Figure 21–42. XGPN. This 48-year-old female had left flank pain for two months. The left kidney showed no uptake on radionuclide studies. Enhanced CT reveals a calculus (C) in the left renal pelvis. The renal parenchyma (*arrows*) is thin with irregular soft-tissue density material extending into the perinephric space (*curved arrows*). Note the thickening of the renal fascia (*arrowheads*).

others noting less. In general, the results have not been more helpful than those of CT.

Treatment

Surgery is the only therapy proven to be successful in patients with XGPN. Kidney-sparing operations have been suggested if the disease is suitably localized and have been used in Stage I focal disease.[16] Total nephrectomy is required for global disease. Wider excision is necessary for extensive perinephric involvement, and a transabdominal approach—although not desirable—may be advantageous, even in the presence of the renal infection. CT has great value for preoperative planning and its use should reduce complications related to inadequate surgical extirpation.

MALACOPLAKIA

Malacoplakia is a rare granulomatous inflammatory disease found most frequently in the urinary tract, where it is associated with recurrent infections. For more than 50 years after its original description by Michaelis and Gutmann in 1902,[32] it was thought to occur only in the urinary system; however, in 1958 it was described elsewhere[33] and is now known to occur in many extraurinary sites. Of 153 cases reviewed by Stanton and Maxted,[34] the urinary tract was involved in 58%. The disease shows a predilection for involving the bladder; the ureter, renal pelvis, ureteropelvic junction, and urethra also may be affected. The renal parenchyma was involved in 16% of patients. The testes were involved in 12%, and the prostate in 10%. The epididymis was involved in four patients. The gastrointestinal tract and retroperitoneum were affected in 12% of cases, and the skin and vagina in three and two patients, respectively.[50] Other uncommon areas of involvement included the hip joint, buttock, vertebrae, adrenal gland, cerebrum, lungs, pleura, pancreas, endometrium, vulva, broad ligament, tonsils, conjunctiva, and spleen.

Malacoplakia is best known to urologists, to whom it is most commonly manifested as soft, yellowish, plaque-like nodules on the bladder (from the Greek *malakos* [soft] and *plakos* [plaque]). The disease predominates in females in a 4-to-1 ratio, and the peak-incidence age is the 6th decade. However, it has been described in patients from 6 weeks to 85 years.[34]

The pathogenesis is unknown, but an altered host response is probably the cause.[36–39] Its association in some patients with diabetes mellitus, alcoholic liver disease, sarcoidosis, and mycobacterial infection[36] and its occurrence after renal transplantation suggest that an acquired abnormality of the immune system predisposes certain patients to develop malacoplakia as a response to urinary infection. The basic abnormality appears to be a deficiency of cyclic 3′,5′ guanosine monophosphate (GMP) in the intracellular microtubules of monocytes, resulting in decreased lysosomal degradation and enzyme release.[40] Because of this, ingested organisms remain viable and serve as a potential nidus for recurring infections.[41] Bacteria have been demonstrated within the phagocytic vacuoles of involved histiocytes,[42, 43] and abnormal monocyte function with inability to digest phagocytosed *Escherichia coli* has been demonstrated with in vitro studies.[44] Many patients with malacoplakia have infected urine, and a strong correlation with coliform organisms has been noted.

Apart from symptoms and signs relating to urinary tract infection, clinical manifestations of urinary malacoplakia are nonspecific and physical examination is generally unremarkable. Most commonly the bladder is involved, and symptoms of bladder irritability or hematuria may be present.[45] Flank pain, fever, and a palpable mass have been described in renal parenchymal malacoplakia. According to Arnesen and colleagues,[46] if a urinary tract infection resistant to appropriate antibiotics develops in a renal transplant patient, renal parenchymal malacoplakia should be considered. Another entity that is clinically, histopathologically, and radiographically very similar to renal parenchymal malacoplakia is megalocytic interstitial nephritis.[46, 47] The condition is an interstitial nephritis in which the renal cortex is predominantly involved. Radiographic appearances of solid-appearing tumefactions are described: strong internal echoes have been reported on ultrasonography, but convincing neo-vascularity has not been shown on arteriography.[48] Because of the striking similarities between megalocytic interstitial nephritis and renal parenchymal malacoplakia, some believe that the conditions, in fact, represent the same pathological entity.

Pathology

Grossly, lesions of malacoplakia appear as soft nodular or plaquelike yellow tumors that may coalesce to form nodules of substantial size. There may be central ulceration and peripheral hyperemia. Histologically, the characteristic finding is an aggregation of large mononuclear phagocytes called von Hanseman cells, which contain PAS-positive granules. Spherical calcific structures called Michaelis-Gutmann bodies are also characteristic. These range in size from 5 to 10 μm and have a unique ultrastructure. A central core of dense crystals is surrounded by a clear zone of featureless material. Outside this, another layer of crystals is gives the entire structure an "owl's-eye" appearance.[49]

Imaging

The radiological appearance varies according to the site of involvement.[35] With bladder involvement, the IVU shows single or multiple mucosa-based filling defects that are indistinguishable from other sessile tumefactions (see Fig. 24–10). They are usually not more than 5 mm in diameter but may grow to a diameter of 3 cm or larger. Multiple nodules may be seen best on the postvoid film. Serial studies may show disappearance in one area and reappearance at another site. The CT presentation of one such patient has been reported; here again, the appearance was nonspecific.[50]

Ureteral involvement is manifested by nodular filling defects, which may be multiple throughout the entire ureter (Fig. 21–43). Strictures may or may not be present. The lesions are flatter than those of pyeloureteritis cystica and more closely mimic the appearance of transitional cell carcinoma. Little identifiable normal intervening mucosa is found.[51] Tuberculosis also enters the differential diagnosis; however, the characteristic multiple strictures of that disease do not occur in malacoplakia, and the nodular intraluminal defects of malacoplakia are not common in tuberculosis.

Multifocal disease, which is common when the kidney is affected, was found in three of five patients reported by Hartman and colleagues.[52] It was unilateral in all their patients. Urographically, multifocal renal malacoplakia appears as an enlarged kidney containing multiple masses, primarily within the renal cortex (Fig. 21–44). Occasionally, multifocal involvement causes nonvisualization of the affected kidney at urography.[36, 53] Unifocal disease will be evident as a mass, arising from the kidney, that is indistinguishable from any other focal mass (Fig. 21–45). Importantly, radiographic demonstration of calcification is rare.[54] Malacoplakia may involve the renal pelvis and ureteropelvic junction, where severe stricturing may result (Fig. 21–46).

In the few instances where renal angiography has been performed in patients with multifocal disease, stretching

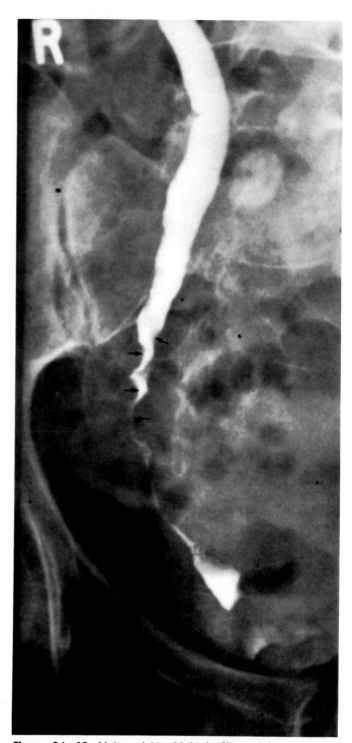

Figure 21–43. Malacoplakia. Multiple filling defects (*arrows*) in the distal right ureter produce a scalloped appearance on this antegrade pyelogram. The distal right ureter is narrowed, producing significant obstruction.

and attenuation of intrarenal arteries was present. The nephrogram was nonuniform and showed numerous irregular filling defects (Fig. 21–44B).[52] Neovascularity has not been reported in multifocal disease, although it has been shown in unifocal disease.[54–56] Arteriography may demonstrate lesions not seen by nephrotomography.[54, 55] Renal vein thrombosis has been reported to complicate renal parenchymal malacoplakia but, as is the case with other causes of renal vein thrombosis, this is infrequently diagnosed based on the urogram.[57]

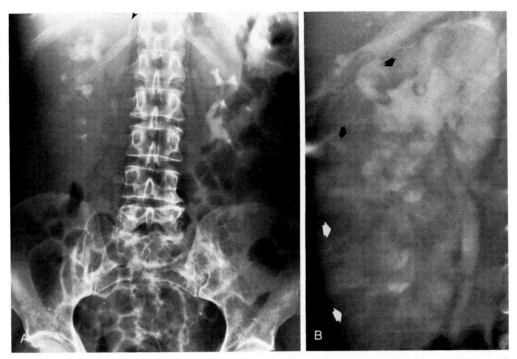

Figure 21–44. Malacoplakia, multifocal. *A,* Urogram in this 68-year-old woman with right flank pain and fever shows an enlarged right kidney (16.5 cm length) (*arrowheads*) with distortion of calyces and pelvis suggesting multiple masses. *B,* Nephrogram phase of angiogram reveals multiple ill-defined cortical defects (*arrowheads*). Nephrectomy specimen documented multiple sites of involvement in cortex and medulla. (From Hartman DS, Davis CJ, Lichtenstein JE, Goldman SM: Renal parenchymal malacoplakia. Radiology 136:33–42, 1980.)

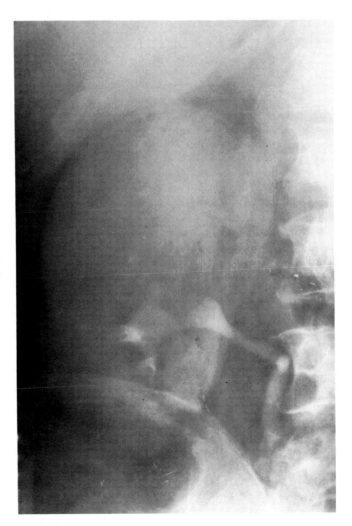

Figure 21–45. Malacoplakia, unifocal in a 58-year-old woman with history of urinary tract infections but no recent infections. Urogram reveals large mass in upper pole of right kidney. The mass is indistinguishable from renal cell carcinoma on this study.

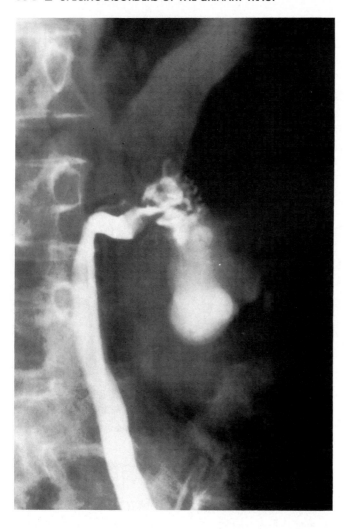

Figure 21—46. Malacoplakia of renal pelvis. Retrograde pyelography reveals strictured renal pelvis with marked irregularity of mucosa. Proximal hydronephrosis is a result of the stenotic renal pelvis.

Sonographic appearances of renal parenchymal malacoplakia have been reported for both the diffuse and the focal type. In diffuse disease, the kidney is enlarged, and the echo pattern of the renal sinus area may be distorted and compressed by many ill-defined tumors.[52] In unifocal disease, the mass is most often echogenic and virtually indistinguishable from other solid tumors,[58, 59] although Lamb and Ayers have described anechoic areas in the renal parenchyma.[60]

Perinephric extension is common in both unifocal and multifocal malacoplakia. This is difficult to identify urographically but can be detected by ultrasonography or CT. Although experience is limited, CT is probably the most accurate means of evaluating the extent of the disease (Fig. 21–47). The CT appearance of malacoplakia is nonspecific, however, showing an inhomogeneous mass or masses arising from the kidney. The spectrum of appearances can overlap with that of renal cell carcinoma.

The prognosis of urinary malacoplakia is related to both the site and extent of disease. When involving the lower urinary tract, long-term antibiotics are used and the outlook appears relatively good.[36, 40, 41] In contrast, renal parenchymal malacoplakia carries a poorer prognosis because of the progressive destruction of functioning renal parenchyma. When the disease is extensive, resection of the affected area with adjuvant antibiotic therapy appears to be the most accepted therapy.[41, 61] Most patients with renal parenchymal malacoplakia involving a transplanted kidney have died within 6 months of diagnosis.[40, 46, 62, 63] Clearly, the disease is not always benign. It should be considered in the differential diagnosis of filling defects seen throughout the urinary tract or of masses in the kidney. This is particularly important in middle-aged women, or in post-transplant patients who have a history of recurrent urinary tract infections resistant to appropriate antibiotics. More recently, cholinergic agonists such as bethanecol have been used in treatment, based on the theory that these agents increase levels of cyclic GMP. The efficacy of this treatment, which is often used in conjunction with ascorbic acid, awaits conclusive proof.

SQUAMOUS METAPLASIA (LEUKOPLAKIA) AND CHOLESTEATOMA

Some confusion exists as to the precise definitions of, and the relationships between, the terms leukoplakia, squamous metaplasia, and cholesteatoma as they apply to the urinary tract. *Squamous metaplasia* is the replacement of normal transitional cell epithelium by squamous epithelium; keratin production may or may not be present. The term *leukoplakia* has no histological significance, but refers to the presence of grossly discernible white patches commonly seen on the mucosal surfaces of areas of squamous metaplasia. The two terms are sometimes used synonymously. A urinary *cholesteatoma* represents a mass of desquamated keratin (i.e., a "keratin ball")

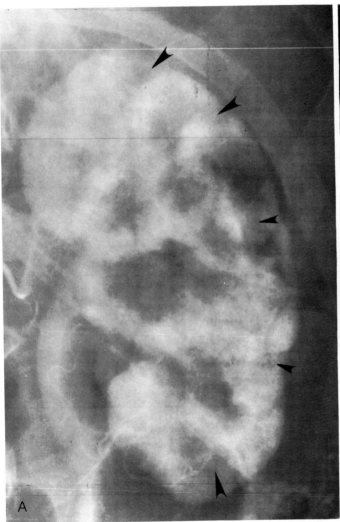

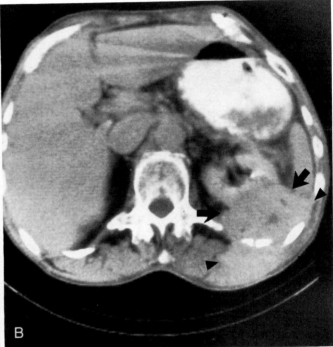

Figure 21–47. Malacoplakia. *A,* Nephrogram phase of arteriogram reveals multiple irregular cortical defects (*arrowheads*). *B,* CT scan of same patient shows the left renal mass (*arrows*) extending through the perinephric space and into the flank (*arrowheads*). (Courtesy David S. Hartman, M.D.)

attached to, or lying free in, the lumen of the renal pelvis, ureter, or bladder. It is not seen in the absence of squamous metaplasia. In an attempt to dispel the confusion surrounding terminology, Hertle and Androulakakis have proposed the unifying term keratinizing desquamative squamous metaplasia (KDSM) of the upper urinary tract to refer to the leukoplakia/cholesteatoma complex.[64]

The etiology of squamous metaplasia is a controversial subject, but the disease appears to be related to chronic infection or irritation. Of less certainty is its relationship, if any, to squamous cell carcinoma of the renal pelvis. Arguments both for and against such an association may be found. Clearly, however, squamous metaplasia of the renal pelvis is not necessarily an ominous condition. The often-associated infections are frequently a greater clinical problem than the threat of malignancy.

Squamous metaplasia is a disease of middle age or older, but cases are reported in young adults as well as in children. The renal pelvis is involved in male and female patients with equal frequency, but vesical leukoplakia is more common in male patients (4:1). Shredlike tissue with a gritty consistency, which represents desquamated keratin and mucosa, is sometimes passed in the urine.

A cholesteatoma of the urinary tract is an intraluminal accumulation of keratin composed of desquamated epithelial cells. It is distinct from the rare primary cholesteatoma of brain, ovary, testicle, or breast and is more akin to the deposition occasionally encountered in the chronically inflamed middle ear or gallbladder.

Urinary cholesteatomata are rare, and fewer than 30 have thus far been reported in the world literature. They have been described in almost equal numbers in men and women and have been found in patients ranging from 12 to 78 years of age, without predilection for any decade.[65]

Cholesteatomata appear to be most common in infections attributable to tuberculosis, schistosomiasis, and syphilis.[66] Urinary obstruction and infection have also been implicated.[67–69] As with other forms of squamous metaplasia, vitamin A deficiency has also been incriminated, although its role is not clearcut.[70–72]

Symptoms are nonspecific, reflecting the wide number of possible causes. Patients may complain of renal colic, hematuria, or other symptoms suggestive of urinary tract infection. Desquamated epithelial cells may be identified in the urine singly or in sheets.

Imaging

Plain film findings are unremarkable in squamous metaplasia, with the exception of renal calculi. Urography may be of limited value if the function of the involved kidney is compromised, but on either excretory urography or especially retrograde pyelography, prominent mucosal thickening is the hallmark of the leukoplakic renal pelvis. This feature is so striking that it has led to the designation "tree-barking" or "corduroy" appearance (Fig. 21–48).

The urographic appearance of cholesteatoma is that of intraluminal, rounded masses. A laminated or onion-skin appearance resulting from contrast material entering the narrow spaces within and around the mass has been described (Fig. 21–49). Irregularity of the remaining urothelium may be present, owing to the underlying squamous metaplasia. Calcification has been reported

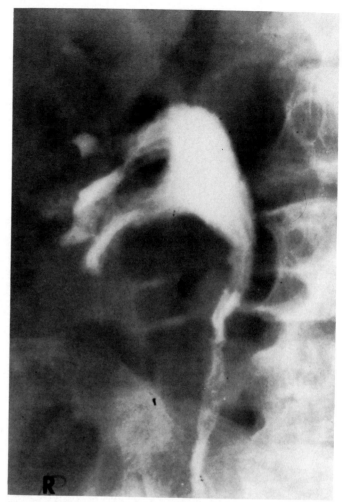

Figure 21–48. Squamous metaplasia of renal pelvis and ureter (leukoplakia): Chronically infected right kidney with no excretion on IVU. Retrograde pyelogram reveals multiple linear radiolucencies in pelvis and ureter, attributable to grossly thickened, hyperkeratotic mucosal folds producing "corduroy" appearance.

within the keratin masses on the scout radiograph,[66, 73] and calculi may be identified elsewhere in the collecting system. Evidence of chronic obstruction may be present.

Wills and colleagues[66] have described the use of CT in the evaluation of two patients with cholesteatomata. In one, they described a relatively high CT number (109 to 120 H) measured over a portion of the lesion. From this, it was inferred that the mass was probably a benign process rather than a collecting-system tumor, for which a lower number (in the range of 30 to 60 H) would be expected. Punctate calcifications were identified in the second lesion, again suggesting a benign lesion (Fig. 21–50). Although ultrasonography was performed, neither acoustic shadowing nor marked echogenicity associated with the masses was identified. The authors surmised that this was because of the very small size of the calcium particles dispersed within the cholesteatoma.

The radiological differential diagnosis of cholesteatoma includes other nonopaque filling defects such as urothelial carcinoma, blood clot, papillomata, sloughed papillae, nonopaque stones, and fungus balls. A high index of suspicion for cholesteatoma should be maintained if such "stringy" or "laminated" intraluminal filling defects are seen and a history of chronic infection is present. High

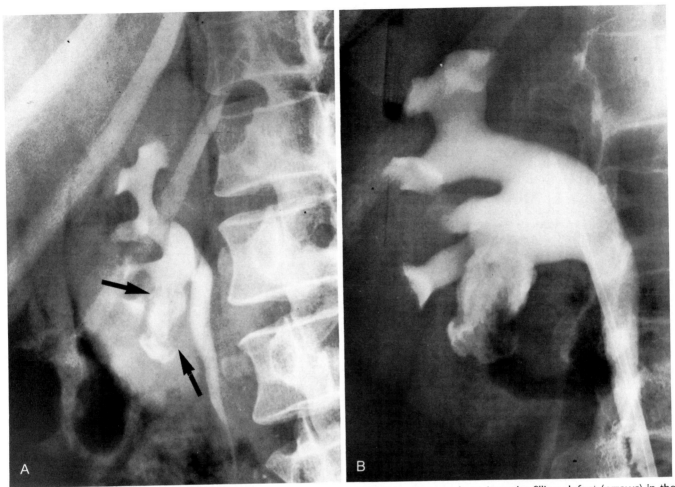

Figure 21–49. Cholesteatoma. *A,* Intravenous urogram in a 49-year-old woman reveals an irregular filling defect (*arrows*) in the right lower-pole infundibulum and calyx. Contrast obscures two small calculi seen on the scout films. *B,* Retrograde pyelogram in the same patient more clearly demonstrates a laminated pattern within the filling defect. Pathologic examination documented squamous metaplasia with hyperkeratosis with masses typical of cholesteatoma. (From Wills JS, Pollack HM, Curtis JA: Cholesteatoma of the upper urinary tract. AJR 136(5):941–944, 1981, © by Am Roentgen Ray Soc.)

Figure 21–50. Cholesteatoma. Nonenhanced CT shows a lightly calcified mass occupying the lower pole collecting system (*arrow*). CT attenuation value = 120 H. Diagnosis was proved by removal via pyelotomy. (From Wills JS, Pollack HM, Curtis JA: Cholesteatoma of the upper urinary tract. AJR 136(5):941–944, 1981, © by Am Roentgen Ray Soc.)

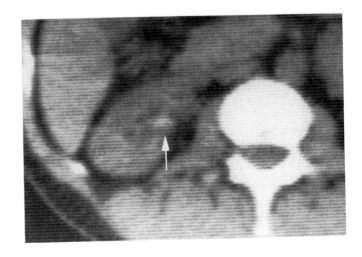

attenuation values found on CT may help differentiate these masses from carcinoma. The distinction is important, as cholesteatomata have not been shown to be premalignant, and when proven they warrant a conservative approach. The differential diagnosis of simple squamous metaplasia encompasses the many causes of mucosal striations, including vesicoureteral reflux, intermittent hydronephrosis, inflammatory edema, submucosal hemorrhage, varices, and epithelial neoplasms.[74]

References

1. Hodson CJ: The radiological contributions toward the diagnosis of chronic pyelonephritis. Radiology 88:857, 1967.
2. Yoder I, Pfister RC: Pyonephrosis: Imaging and intervention. AJR 141:735, 1983.
3. Poilly JN, Dickie J, James WB: Renal sinus lipomatosis: Report of 26 cases. Br J Urol 141:257–266, 1969.
4. Hadar H, Meiraz D: Renal sinus lipomatosis. Differentiation from space-occupying lesion with aid of computed tomography. Urology 15:86–88, 1980.
5. Kutzman A: Replacement lipomatosis of the kidney. Surg Gynecol Obstet 52:690–701, 1931.
6. Roth LJ, Davidson HB: Fibrous and fatty replacement of renal parenchyma. JAMA 111:233–239, 1938.
7. Hamm FC, De Veer JA: Fatty replacement following renal atrophy or destruction: So-called lipomatosis of the kidney. J Urol 41:850–866, 1939.
8. Faegenburg D, Bosniak MA, Evans JA: Renal sinus lipomatosis: Its demonstration by nephrotomography. Radiology 83:987–997, 1964.
9. Ambos MA, Bosniak MA, Gordon R, Madayag MA: Replacement lipomatosis of the kidney. AJR 130:1087–1091, 1978.
10. Subramanyam BR, Bosniak MA, Horii SC, et al: Replacement lipomatosis of the kidney: Diagnosis by computed tomography and sonography. Radiology 148:791–792, 1983.
11. Malek RS, Greene LF, de Weerd JH, Farrow GM: Xanthogranulomatous pyelonephritis. Br J Urol 44:296–308, 1972.
12. McCormack T, Butler M: Xanthogranulomatous pyelonephritis: A comprehensive review with report of additional cases. J Urol 105:10–17, 1971.
13. Bianchi G, Franzolin N: Renojejunal fistula caused by xanthogranulomatous pyelonephritis. Br J Urol 52:66, 1980.
14. Schlagenhaufer F: Uber eigentumlich Staphylomykosen der Neiven und des pararenalen Bindegewebes. Frankfurt Z Pathol 19:139–148, 1916.
15. Gingell JC, Roylance J, Davies ER, Penry JB: Xanthogranulomatous pyelonephritis. Br J Radiol 46:99–109.
16. Tolia BM, Iloretta A, Freed Z, et al: Xanthogranulomatous pyelonephritis: Detailed analysis of 29 cases and a brief discussion of atypical presentations. J Urol 126:437–442, 1981.
17. Grainger RG, Longstaff AJ, Parsons MA: Xanthogranulomatous pyelonephritis: A reappraisal. Lancet 1:1398–1401, 1982.
18. Abbate AD, Meyers J: Xanthogranulomatous pyelonephritis in childhood. J Urol 116:231, 1976.
19. Goldman SM, Hartman DS, Fishman EK, et al: CT of xanthogranulomatous pyelonephritis: Radiologic-pathologic correlation. AJR 141:963–969, 1984.
20. Malek RS, Elder JS: Xanthogranulomatous pyelonephritis: A critical analysis of 26 cases and of the literature. J Urol 119:589–593, 1978.
21. Heptinstall RH: Pathology of the Kidney, 3rd Ed, Vol III. Little, Brown & Company, 1983, p 1381.
22. Matz JA, Elizalde G, Puigvert A: Pielonefritis xantogranulomatosa. Puigvert, An Fund 4:129, 1974.
23. Rossi P, Myers DH, Furey R, Bonfils-Roberts EA: Angiography in bilateral xanthogranulomatous pyelonephritis. Radiology 90:320–321, 1968.
24. Gammill S, Rabinowitz JG, Peace R, et al: New thoughts concerning xanthogranulomatous pyelonephritis (X-P). AJR 125:154–163, 1975.
25. Miller HL, Ney C, Puljic S: Xanthogranulomatous pyelonephritis: With emphasis on angiographic findings. NY State J Med, 76:919–924, 1976.
26. Akintewe RA, Dealier S, Hutcheon AE: Xanthogranulomatous pyelonephritis presenting with unilateral renal vein thrombosis. Postgrad Med J 56:280–281, 1980.
27. Lorentzen M, Overgaard NH: Xanthogranulomatous pyelonephritis. Scand J Urol Nephrol 14:193–200, 1980.
28. Kirk OCV, Go RY, Wedel VJ: Sonographic features of xanthogranulomatous pyelonephritis. AJR 134:1035–1039, 1980.
29. Subramanyam BR, Megibow AJ, Raghavendra BN, Bosniak MA: Diffuse xanthogranulomatous pyelonephritis: Analysis by computed tomography and sonography. Urol Radiol 4:5–9, 1982.
29a. Hartman DS, Davis CJ Jr, Goldman SM, et al: Xanthogranulomatous pyelonephritis: Sonographic-pathologic correlation of 16 cases. J Ultrasound Med 3:481, 1984.
30. McClennan BL, Lee JKT: Kidney. In Lee JKT Sagel SS, Stanley RJ (eds): Computed Body Tomography. New York, Raven Press, 1983, pp 341–378.
31. Claes H, Vereeken R, Oyen R, van Damme BV: Xanthogranulomatous pyelonephritis with emphasis on computerized tomography scan. Urology 29:389, 1987.
31a. Mulopulos GP, Patel SK, Pessis D: MR imaging of xanthogranulomatous pyelonephritis. J Comput Assist Tomogr 10:154, 1986.
32. Michaelis L, Gutmann C: Ueber einschlusse in blasentumoren. Zeitschrift fur dlinische Medizin 47:208–215, 1902.
33. Scott EVZ, Scott WF: A fatal case of malakoplakia of the urinary tract. J Urol 79:52, 1958.
34. Stanton MJ, Maxted W: Malacoplakia: A study of the literature and current concepts of pathogenesis, diagnosis and treatment. J Urol 125:139–146, 1981.
35. Miller OS, Finck FM: Malakoplakia of the kidney: The great impersonator. J Urol 103:712–717, 1970.
36. Maderazo EG, Berlin BB, Morhardt C: Treatment of malakoplakia with trimethoprim-sulfamethoxazole. Urology 13:70–73, 1979.
37. Deridder PA, Koff SA, Gilkas PW, Heidelberger KP: Renal malacoplakia. J Urol 117:428–432, 1977.
38. Lewin KJ, Fair WR, Steigbigel RT, et al: Clinical and laboratory studies into the pathogenesis of malacoplakia. J Clin Pathol 29:354–363, 1976.
39. Lou TY, Teplitz C: Malakoplakia: Pathogenesis and ultrastructural morphogenesis. A problem of altered macrophage (phagolysosomal) response. Human Pathol 5:191–207, 1974.
40. Streem SB: Genitourinary malacoplakia in renal transplant recipients: Pathogenic, prognostic and therapeutic considerations. J Urol 132:10–12, 1984.
41. Qualman SJ, Gupta PK, Mendelsohn G: Intracellular *Escherichia coli* in urinary malakoplakia: A reservoir of infection and its therapeutic implications. Am J Clin Pathol 81:35–42, 1984.
42. McClurg FB, D'Agostino AN, Martin JH, et al: Ultrastructural demonstration of intracellular bacteria in three cases of malakoplakia of the bladder. Am J Clin Pathol 60:780–788, 1973.
43. Lewin KJ, Harell GS, Lee AS, Crowley LG: Malacoplakia. An electron-microscopic study: Demonstration of bacilliform organisms in malacoplakic macrophages. Gastroenterology 66:28–45, 1974.
44. Abdou NI, NaPombejara C, Sagawa A, et al: Malakoplakia: Evidence for monocyte lysosomal abnormality correctable by cholinergic agonist in vitro and in vivo. N Engl J Med 297:1413–1419, 1977.
45. Curran FT: Malacoplakia of the bladder. Br J Urol 59:559, 1987.
46. Arnesen E, Halvorsen S, Skojrten F: Malacoplakia in renal transplant. Report of a case studied by light and electron microscopy. Scand J Urol Nephrol 11:93, 1977.
47. Ravel R: Megalocytic interstitial nephritis: An entity probably related to malakoplakia. Am J Clin Pathol 47:781–789, 1967.
48. Gonzalez AC, Karcioglu Z, Waters BB, et al: Megalocytic interstitial nephritis: Ultrasonic and radiographic changes. Radiology 133:449–450, 1979.
49. Tanaka T, Sakuma H, Takahashi K, et al: Extravesical malacoplakia—possibly originated from a superficial part of the renal cortex. Acta Pathol Jap 31:323–334, 1981.
50. Elliott GB, Moloney PJ, Clement JG: Malacoplakia of the urinary tract. AJR 116:830–837, 1972.
51. Epstein BM, Karf V, Porteous PH: CT appearance of bladder malakoplakia. J Comput Assist Tomogr 7:541–543, 1983.
52. Hartman DS, Davis CR Jr, Lichtenstein JE, Goldman SM: Renal parenchymal malacoplakia. Radiology 136:33–42, 1980.
53. Bowers JM, Cathey WJ: Malacoplakia of the kidney with renal failure. Am J Clin Pathol 55:765–769, 1971.
54. Trillo A, Lorentz WB, Whitley NO: Malakoplakia of kidney simulating renal neoplasm. Urology 10:472–477, 1977.

55. Scullin DR, Hardy R: Malacoplakia of the urinary tract with spread to the abdominal wall. J Urol 107:908–910, 1972.
56. Cavins JA, Goldstein AMB: Renal malacoplakia. Urology 10:155–158, 1977.
57. Clark RA, Wyatt GM, Colley DP: Renal vein thrombosis: An underdiagnosed complication of multiple renal abnormalities. Radiology 132:43–50, 1979.
58. Pamilo M, Kulatunga A: Renal parenchymal malacoplakia. A report of 2 cases. The radiological and ultrasound images. Br J Radiol 57:751–755, 1984.
59. Jander HP, Pujara S, Murad TM: Tumefactive megalocytic interstitial nephritis. Radiology 129:635–636, 1978.
60. Lamb GHR, Ayers AB: Ultrasound findings in a case of renal malacoplakia. Br J Radiol 50:735–754, 1977.
61. Sunshine B: Malacoplakia of the upper urinary tract. J Urol 112:362, 1974.
62. Mullan H, Hesse VE: Malacoplakia of a cadaveric renal allograft: A case report. J Surg Oncol 10:197, 1978.
63. Osborn DE, Castro JE, Ansell ID: Malacoplakia in a cadaver renal allograft: A case study. Human Pathol 8:341, 1977.
64. Hertle L, Androulakakis P: Keratinizing desquamative squamous metaplasia of the upper urinary tract: Leukoplakia–cholesteatoma. J Urol 127:631, 1982.
65. Weitzner S: Cholesteatoma of the calyx. J Urol 108:365–367, 1972.
66. Wills JS, Pollack HM, Curtis JA: Cholesteatoma of the upper urinary tract. AJR 136:941–944, 1981.
67. Gale GL, Kerr WK: Cholesteatoma of the urinary tract. J Urol 104:71–72, 1970.
68. Myrvoid H, Fritjofsson A, Magnosson P: Cholesteatoma of the renal pelvis. Scand J Urol Nephrol 8:69–72, 1974.
69. Carsky EW, Prior JT, Moore R, Hamel J: Cholesteatoma of the kidney: Radiographic findings. Radiology 78:786–798, 1962.
70. Bennington JL, Beckwith JB: Tumors of the kidney, renal pelvis and ureter. In Atlas of Tumor Pathology, 2nd Series. Washington DC, Armed Forces Inst Pathol, 1976, 245–246.
71. Noyes WE, Paulbinskas AJ: Squamous metaplasia of the renal pelvis. Radiology 89:292–295, 1967.
72. Mostofi FK: Potentialities of bladder epithelium. J Urol 71:705–714, 1954.
73. Kutzmann AA: Leukoplakia of the renal pelvis. Arch Surg 19:871–897, 1929.
74. Haugen SG, Wasserman NF: Keratinizing desquamative squamous metaplasia of the upper urinary tract. Urol Radiol 8:211, 1986.
75. Merine D, Fishman EK, Siegelman SS: Renal xanthogranulomatosis: Radiological, clinical and pathological features in two cases. J Comput Assist Tomogr 11:785, 1987.

PYONEPHROSIS

PHILIP J. KENNEY □ EAMANN S. BREATNACH □ ROBERT J. STANLEY

It is well known that an obstructed renal collecting system is predisposed to infection. The term *pyonephrosis* denotes suppurative infection in such an obstructed system.[1] The more restrictive use of the term, limited to hydronephrotic kidneys filled with tenacious gelatinous semisolid pus, seems unnecessarily pedantic. The broader use, here, refers to a hydronephrotic kidney containing infected urine.

Untreated pyonephrosis will eventually lead to destruction of the renal parenchyma as a result of the associated obstruction and pyelonephritis. Typically, a progressive loss of renal function occurs. Because of the poor excretory ability of the pyonephrotic kidney, this diagnosis was difficult to invoke before the development of morphological studies such as ultrasound and computed tomography (CT), and it was not possible to distinguish pyonephrosis from other causes of the nonvisualizing kidney. Percutaneous techniques have led to more rapid diagnosis and accurate microbiological studies, in addition to their use for nonsurgical therapy.

Pyonephrosis can result from virtually any cause of urinary tract obstruction; chronic obstruction is the usual condition. Urinary calculus disease is an especially common cause, and as many as 52% of patients have stones.[2] Malignant disease of the retroperitoneum and pelvis, retroperitoneal fibrosis, postoperative fibrosis, congenital obstruction (e.g., ureteropelvic junction [UPJ] obstruction), and many other causes have been reported.[2, 3]

A patient with pyonephrosis usually presents with some systemic signs and symptoms of infection.[3] The presentation often is acute, with the patient having fever, chills, flank pain, and leukocytosis. Subacute presentation with a low-grade fever, weight loss, anorexia, and dull pain is not uncommon. Patients may also be strikingly asymptomatic; in a recent series of 65 patients, 10 were afebrile and showed no signs of infection except for purulent urine obtained by percutaneous aspiration.[2] Diabetes does not strongly predispose the patient to pyonephrosis. If the obstructive process is bilateral, the patient may be azotemic when first seen. The infecting organism is almost always a common urinary pathogen and is most often a gram-negative bacterium. *Escherichia coli, Proteus mirabilis, Klebsiella pneumoniae,* and *Pseudomonas aeruginosa* accounted for 63% of the cases in Yoder's series, with occasional cases of infection with *Candida, Staphylococcus,* and other *Proteus* species.[2] Gas-forming organisms may also be found.

PATHOLOGY

Pyonephrosis consists of a spectrum of pathologic processes, and its severity depends on their duration. Chronic obstructive changes are almost always present. With acute infection, acute pyelonephritis develops in the renal parenchyma. Because of the obstruction, purulent debris that consists of sloughed urothelium and a mixture of inflammatory cells collects in the calyces and pelvis. The exact constituents of the debris depend on the severity of the inflammatory process.[4] The quality of the exudate changes gradually, depending on the stage and duration of the infection, with viscosity gradually increasing. In longstanding pyonephrosis, the collecting system contents may be too thick to aspirate through even a large-bore needle. In time, the renal changes of chronic pyelonephritis develop, and extensive destruction of the renal parenchyma eventually occurs. Initially, the kidney is enlarged due to hydronephrosis and swelling of the parenchyma. As the parenchyma is destroyed, the kidney may remain large or may decrease in size, sometimes resulting in a small kidney. In some cases, the process extends beyond the kidney itself to produce perinephric abscess. Extension to the flank may occur. No specific pathological changes accompany pyonephrosis, but xanthoma cells are absent, which distinguishes this disease from xanthogranulomatous pyelonephritis.

RADIOLOGY

A variety of findings on plain radiographic studies may suggest the possibility of pyonephrosis. However, these are nonspecific and may be found in patients with other diseases. In nearly one-third of patients, the KUB is normal.[2] Because pyonephrosis can result from a variety of obstructive processes, and since the pathology spans a wide spectrum, urographic findings are also quite variable.

At least 50% of patients will have renal and/or ureteral calculi (Fig. 21–51), including staghorn calculi.[2] Nonopaque calculi may also be present. The renal outline may be enlarged [11%] but often is normal.[2] If there is perinephric extension of inflammation, obscuration of the renal outline and psoas shadow occurs. Gas may be found in the collecting system.[5]

Urographic findings vary, depending on whether residual renal function exists and on whether the infection is acute or chronic. An obstructive nephrogram with delayed opacification of dilated calyces will be seen if the process is relatively acute.[2] Commonly, especially with longstanding disease, urography shows little or no excretion. In such cases, nephrotomography can aid diagnosis, as it may show the lucent hydronephrotic calyces and some enhancement of the residual cortex.[3] Contrast may layer around the thickened debris in the calyces (Fig. 21–51B), producing dense rims. Unless calculi are present, urography rarely is able to show the site and cause of obstruction. Most often, pyonephrosis is unilateral and involves the whole kidney; however, it may be bilateral, or—in the case of an obstructed infundibulum or a portion of a duplicated system—it may be segmental.

It must be emphasized that the plain radiographic and urographic findings are nonspecific. Other causes of a nonvisualizing kidney cannot be distinguished from pyonephrosis. Most of the urographic findings are due to the chronic obstruction. Unless there are previous studies for comparison, lack of excretion may be ascribed purely to the obstructive process. Obscuring of the retroperitoneal planes may, of course, be seen in perinephric abscess without pyonephrosis. Xanthogranulomatous pyelonephritis and pyonephrosis typically show enlargement, nonexcretion of contrast, and calculi.

RETROGRADE PYELOGRAPHY

Retrograde injection of contrast into a pyonephrotic kidney may produce a striking picture, often suggestive of the diagnosis (Fig. 21–52). When the purulent contents of such kidneys are extremely viscous, the poor mixing of contrast with the pelvic pus results in a characteristic picture. A hydronephrotic kidney containing innumerable stringy and particulate filling defects is observed. From a practical standpoint, only an extensive urothelial malignancy and pyonephrosis will produce such a picture. When the intrapelvic urine is only minimally purulent, however, the classical findings are absent. Retrograde pyelography in pyonephrosis is a double-edged sword. On the one hand, it may go a long way toward establishing the correct diagnosis, while perhaps more importantly establishing an avenue of temporary drainage. Conversely, it may be impossible to negotiate a ureteral catheter into the kidney and the possibility of exacerbating symptoms when manipulating or overinjecting into an infected system is a very real one.

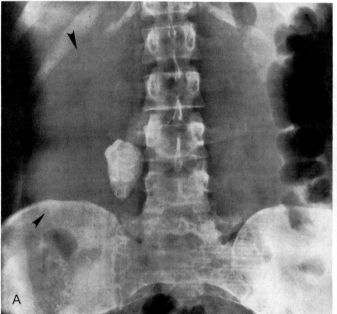 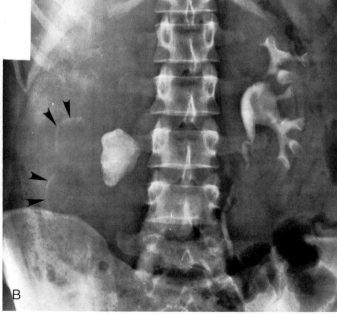

Figure 21–51. Pyonephrosis—urography. *A,* Thirty-nine-year-old diabetic female presented with right flank pain, chills, and weight loss. Scout radiograph reveals calculus in region of right renal pelvis and suggestion of enlargement of the right renal outline (*arrowheads*). *B,* Intravenous urogram shows almost no excretion from the right kidney except for subtle rim enhancement ("crescents") about the calyces (*arrowheads*). Right nephrectomy confirmed pyonephrosis.

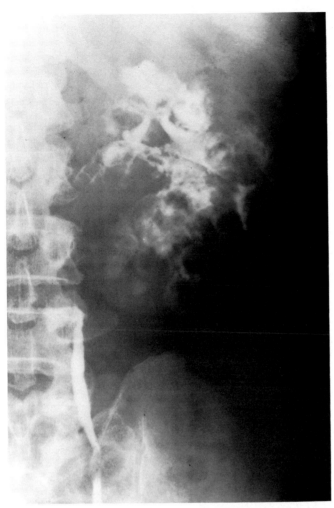

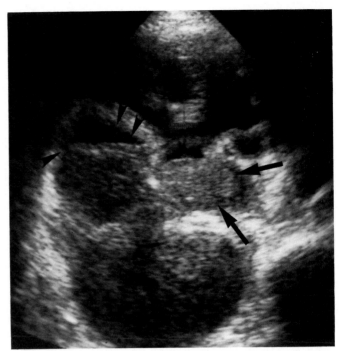

Figure 21–53. Pyonephrosis—sonography. This 22-year-old female had a 3-week history of right upper-quadrant discomfort, 4 days of fever, and right upper-quadrant tenderness. Sonogram shows hydronephrosis with very thin cortex, fluid-debris levels in calyces (*arrowheads*) and echogenic material attributable to debris, and organized pus in the renal pelvis (*arrows*).

diagnosis of pyonephrosis is the character of the material within the collecting system. Unlike simple hydronephrosis, in which the collecting system is anechoic, pyonephrosis is accompanied by echogenic material (Figs. 21–53 and 21–54). Four distinct patterns have been described.[5] Persistent strong or weak echoes seen at the dependent portion of the collecting system (Type I) is the

Figure 21–52. Pyonephrosis—retrograde pyelography. A 48-year-old man with known calculous disease, complained of flank pain, anorexia and weight loss. No excretion on IVU. Retrograde pyelogram reveals pelvis and calyces to be filled with nonopaque material presumed to be thick and viscous, since contrast does not diffuse easily or mix freely with pelvic contents. At surgery, this was found to be due to inspissated, organized pus. Urothelial malignancy could present the same picture. Nephrectomy revealed congenital ureteropelvic junction obstruction with pyonephrosis.

ULTRASONOGRAPHY

Ultrasonography has greatly aided the diagnosis of pyonephrosis. The presence or absence, size, and appearance of the kidney as well as the sonographic character of the contents of the collecting system can be reliably shown by ultrasonography. This of course does not depend upon any residual renal function. Because ultrasonography is quick, noninvasive, relatively inexpensive, and widely available, it is extremely useful in evaluating a patient presenting with suspected urinary infection and/or sepsis.

With pyonephrosis, ultrasonography usually shows moderate to marked hydronephrosis (90%).[2] Dilatation of the ureter may be detected. Calculi in the collecting system and pelvis can usually be documented by ultrasonography. The presence of a pelvic or retroperitoneal mass may be demonstrable. The most important sonographic finding that must be evaluated to permit the

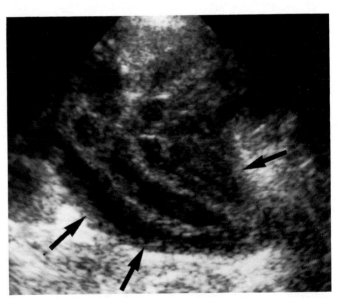

Figure 21–54. Pyonephrosis—sonography. This woman with chronic ureteral obstruction due to unresectable cervical carcinoma became febrile after her nephrostomy tube became dislodged. Laminated echogenic material is seen on sonogram, filling renal pelvis and calyces (*arrows*). Pus was drained upon replacement of nephrostomy tube.

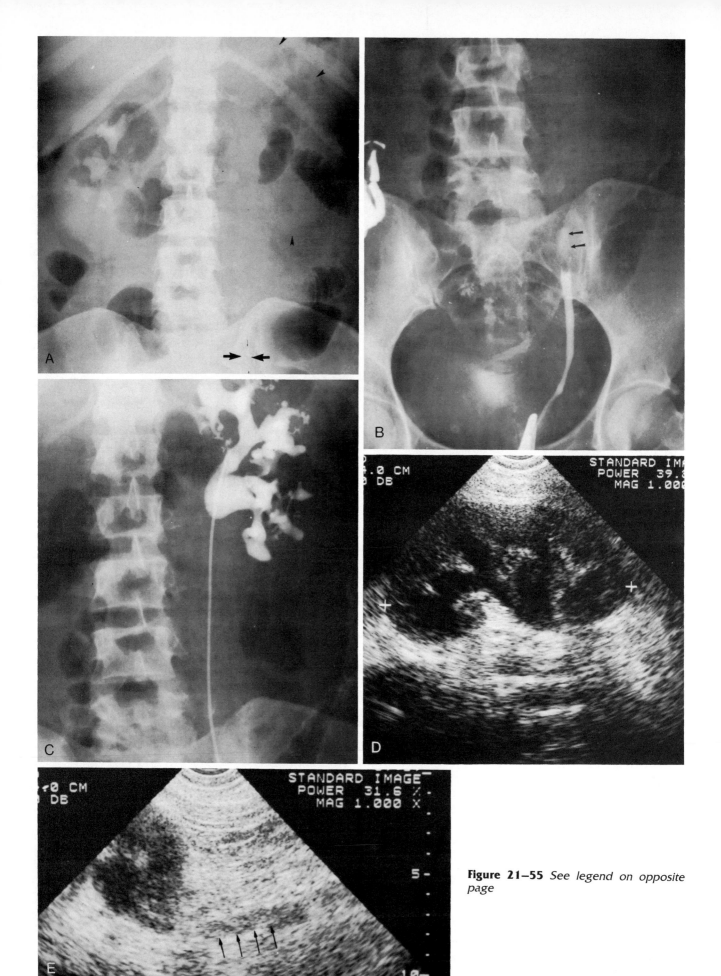

Figure 21–55 *See legend on opposite page*

most frequently encountered. There may be a fluid-debris level (Fig. 21–53) in the collecting system, which shifts when the patient is repositioned (Type II). This (Type II) is uncommon. Type III refers to coarse, strong echoes, with shadowing resulting from gas in the collecting system. Finally, multiple weak echoes throughout the collecting system may be recorded (Type IV). In a patient with clinical signs of infection, such echogenic material in a dilated collecting system is nearly diagnostic of pyonephrosis.[4] However, other considerations are blood clot, matrix material, fungal infection, and urothelial tumor. Renal calculi are another source of difficulty in sonographic diagnosis. Staghorn calculi, in particular, can obscure pus and can make appreciation of hydronephrosis difficult as a result of shadowing.[6] The sonographic findings of pyonephrosis are easily distinguished from the other usual clinical considerations, such as acute pyelonephritis, acute focal bacterial nephritis, and renal abscess. Other causes of a nonvisualizing kidney, such as renal infarction, renal vein thrombosis, renal tumor, and renal agenesis, have sonographic findings that are well described and distinct from those of pyonephrosis.

Some controversy has surrounded the accuracy of sonographic findings of pyonephrosis. In a prospective study of 73 patients, the presence or absence of persistent and reproducible echoes in the collecting system was highly accurate.[4] A sensitivity of 90% for detecting pyonephrosis with a false-positive rate of 3% and a false-negative rate of 10% was described.[4] In a more recent study, a sensitivity of only 62% was found. In this study, Jeffrey and colleagues reported a positive predictive value of 100% when a sonogram detected echogenic material in a hydronephrotic kidney in a patient suspected of pyonephrosis.[7] However, the negative predictive value of an anechoic collecting system in such a patient was only 80%. The discrepancy in these reports is probably due to inclusion of patients with acutely infected hydronephrotic kidneys. In such cases, not enough purulent debris has yet accumulated to produce definitive echoes in the collecting system (Fig. 21–55). Because of this difficulty, diagnostic aspiration of urine from a hydronephrotic kidney may be necessary in a patient with suspected pyonephrosis, even if the sonogram suggests uncomplicated hydronephrosis.

COMPUTED TOMOGRAPHY

CT may be useful in evaluating some cases of pyonephrosis. Usually, it is not needed, because diagnosis and treatment can be effected by plain radiographs and ultrasonography followed by retrograde or percutaneous aspiration and drainage. CT may be performed, however, if pyonephrosis is not the prime clinical consideration. The technique can also be very useful in evaluating the site and cause of obstruction, especially if malignancy is

present. CT is probably more accurate than ultrasonography for detecting or excluding perinephric extension of the infection.[8]

Even without contrast enhancement, CT can detect hydronephrosis quite accurately.[9] If pyonephrosis is present, the density of the contents of the collecting system may be higher than that of uninfected urine (i.e., greater than 20 H) (Fig. 21–56).[10] In many cases, the density of the distended pelvis is the same as that of renal parenchyma or a nonenhanced CT scan. Calculi are easily detectable, even if not calcified, because their density is well above that of soft-tissue range.[11] On enhanced scans, loss of renal function is shown as a decreased enhancement of renal parenchyma, compared with the normal kidney (Fig. 21–57). Little (if any) filling of calyces with contrast material may be seen. If the pus in the collecting system is very dense, the contrast may layer over the debris (Fig. 21–58).[2] This is contrary to the usual situation, in which the contrast layers in the dependent portion of a dilated system. The thickness of renal parenchyma is easily shown by CT. Perinephric extension of infection is indicated by alteration of the perinephric and retroperitoneal fat planes. An increased, streaky density is a result of inflammatory infiltration. Swelling of the psoas muscle and fluid collections in the perinephric space, psoas, or flank indicate development of perinephric abscess.[8]

ANGIOGRAPHY

Although it is not used routinely as a diagnostic procedure for pyonephrosis, angiography may show several typical findings. There may be diminution in caliber of the main renal artery with stretching and attenuation of interlobar vessels due to hydronephrosis and loss of renal parenchyma. In addition, however, clusters of inflammatory hypervascularity ("staining") may be seen in the region of active inflammation rimming the calyces.[12] Although these could be mistaken for the neovascularity of malignancy, the vessels lack the bizarre luminal irregularity and discrepant diameters seen in neoplasms, and arteriovenous shunts are absent.

ROLE OF PERCUTANEOUS TECHNIQUES

The development and widespread availability of percutaneous urinary tract interventional techniques have had a significant impact not only on diagnosis, but also on the treatment of pyonephrosis. Although the diagnosis of pyonephrosis is often made or suggested by noninvasive studies such as ultrasonography or CT, percutaneous aspiration of urine from the collecting system remains a most efficient and accurate means of confirming the diagnosis. Aspiration of purulent urine is diagnostic.

Figure 21–55. Pyonephrosis in a 35-year-old diabetic female with sepsis and left flank pain. *A,* Delayed film (1 hour, 45 minutes) from IVU shows a normal right kidney, but no visualization of left kidney. Left renal outline can be seen (*arrowheads*). A large left ureteral calculus is present (*arrows*). *B,* A retrograde left ureterogram shows obstruction at the level of the large calculus (*arrow*). *C,* After passage of a catheter and injection of contrast, the hydronephrotic, enlarged left kidney is outlined. Numerous abscess cavities communicate with the collecting system. Pus was recovered from the catheter. *D,* Ultrasound scan through long axis of left kidney prior to drainage shows moderate hydronephrosis but no definite debris. *E,* Ultrasound image of left lower pole and proximal left ureter (*arrows*) shows mild dilatation of ureter.

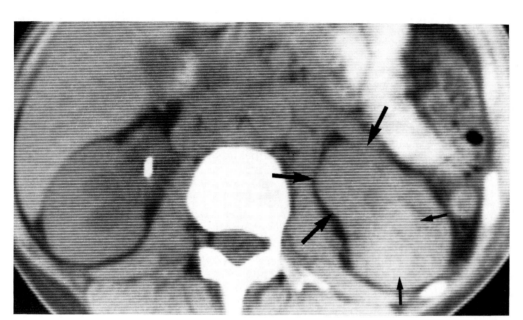

Figure 21–56. Pyonephrosis—CT. This 63-year-old male with colon carcinoma developed oliguria. Sonogram and CT scan showed bilateral hydronephrosis due to recurrent tumor in the pelvis. Noncontrast CT scan shows right hydronephrosis with stent. Stent could not be passed on the left. Note high-density material filling the distended left renal pelvis and calyces (*arrows*). Pyonephrosis was confirmed by percutaneous drainage (metastatic adenopathy is also present in the retroperitoneum).

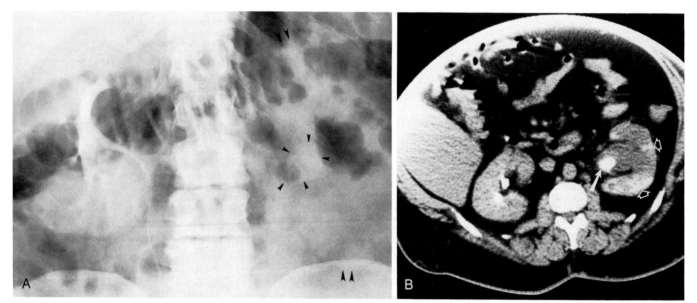

Figure 21–57. Pyonephrosis—acute. Fifty-year-old, 350-pound male with severe left flank pain and sepsis. *A,* Coned view from IVU shows large but normal right kidney. Nonvisualization of the left kidney (*double arrowheads*) at 1 hour and central (pelvic) calculus (*arrowheads*) is noted. *B,* CT scan obtained after IVU shows central obstructing pelvic calculus (*arrow*) and patchy, obstructive nephrogram pattern not discernible on urogram (*arrowheads*). Left percutaneous nephrolithotomy was successfully performed, and the kidney was salvaged.

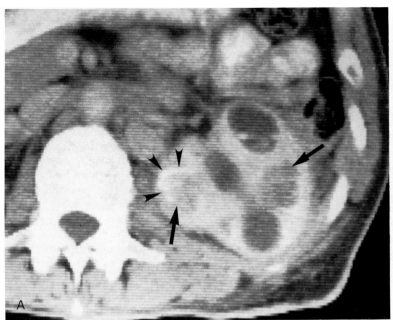

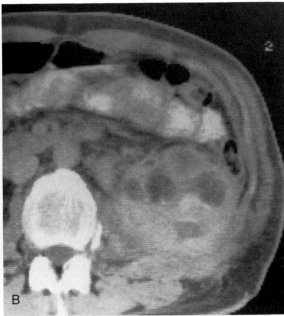

Figure 21–58. Pyonephrosis—chronic. Fever developed in this quadriplegic patient with a long history of urinary tract calculi. *A*, CT reveals left hydronephrosis with dense material in some calyces (*arrows*) and renal pelvis, as well as poor excretion. Note contrast layering (rims) over the dense material (*arrowheads*). *B*, CT scan more caudal than *A*. There is infiltration of the perinephric fat and obscuration of psoas margins with streaky density extending into the flank. This indicates perinephric extension.

Definitive cultures of the offending organism can be obtained to assure proper antibiotic choice. If pyonephrosis remains a consideration because of inadequate or nonspecific ultrasonographic or CT findings, percutaneous aspiration is a quick and relatively noninvasive means of diagnosis or exclusion of pyonephrosis. It does not require anesthesia, which may cause great risk, depending on the patient's status. In either case, after the initial percutaneous aspirate (if pus is obtained), a percutaneous nephrostomy tube can be inserted. Drainage in conjunction with appropriate antibiotics may be definitive therapy. Even if patients may require eventual surgery, percutaneous nephrostomy can improve their status and thus, one hopes, reduce surgical morbidity and mortality. Although they are rarely indicated, percutaneous techniques also allow clear definition of the site of obstruction by antegrade pyelography.

The key elements in the management of pyonephrosis are appropriate antibiotics and adequate drainage. In addition to percutaneous nephrostomy, operative nephrostomy, and retrograde ureteral catheterization/stenting may be used. In most cases in which adequate therapy is provided, fever and symptoms resolve in 24 hours.[3] Overall mortality of pyonephrosis is about 2.5% (including surgically and nonsurgical treated cases).[3] Although about two-thirds of patients may eventually undergo nephrectomy, the kidney can be salvaged in many cases, if it has not been severely damaged before presentation. Yoder and colleagues report that at least 14% of cases in the world literature have retained significant renal func-

tion after conservative therapy.[3] This is especially appropriate for patients with solitary kidney or in whom the opposite kidney has previously been severely damaged.

References

1. Robbins SL: Pathologic Basis of Disease. Philadelphia, WB Saunders Company, 1974, p 1121.
2. Yoder IC, Pfister RC, Lindfors KK, Newhouse JH: Pyonephrosis: Imaging and intervention. AJR 141:735–740, 1983.
3. Yoder IC, Lindfors KK, Pfister RC: Diagnosis and treatment of pyonephrosis. Radiol Clin North Am 22:407–414, 1984.
4. Subramanyam BR, Raghavendra BN, Bosniak MA, et al: Sonography of pyonephrosis: A prospective study. AJR 140:991–993, 1983.
5. Coleman BG, Arger PH, Mulhern CB Jr, et al: Pyonephrosis: Sonography in the diagnosis and management. AJR 137:939–943, 1981.
6. Talner LB, Scheible W, Ellenbogen PH, et al: How accurate is ultrasonography in detecting hydronephrosis in azotemic patients? Urol Radiol 3:1–6, 1981.
7. Jeffrey RB, Laing FC, Wing VW, Hoddick W: Sensitivity of sonography in pyonephrosis: A re-evaluation. AJR 144:71–73, 1985.
8. Morehouse JT, Weiner SN, Hoffman-Tretic JC: Inflammatory disease of the kidney. Semin Ultrasound CT MR 7:246–258, 1986.
9. Bosniak MA, Megibow AJ, Ambos MA, et al: Computed tomography of ureteral obstruction. AJR 138:1107–1113, 1982.
10. Morehouse HT, Weiner SN, Hoffman JC: Imaging in inflammatory disease of the kidney. AJR 143:135–141, 1984.
11. Parienty RA, Ducellier R, Pradel J, et al: Diagnostic value of CT numbers in pelvocalyceal filling defects. Radiology 145:743–747, 1982.
12. Elkin M: Radiology of the Urinary System. Boston, Little, Brown & Company, 1980, p 209.

REFLUX NEPHROPATHY

ROBERT L. LEBOWITZ

Happy is he who has been able to learn the causes of things.

Virgil

Happy is the one who finds wisdom, the one who gains understanding; For its fruits are better than silver, its yield than fine gold. It is more precious than rubies; No treasure can match it.

Proverbs 3:13

The term reflux nephropathy (RN) was introduced by Bailey[1] and Heale and associates[2] in 1973 to serve as both a more precise and a more descriptive name for the condition that had previously been known as chronic atrophic (nonobstructive) pyelonephritis.[3] RN was thought to better portray the relationship between acquired focal inflammatory renal abnormalities and vesicoureteral reflux. RN has become a common term[4–12] and *is* more descriptive than its predecessor; however, it falls short in precision because it does not stress the crucial role of infection in this pathological process. (Unless sterile reflux is very severe or occurs in the presence of elevated pressure in the bladder, it seems to have no significant deleterious effect on the kidney, except for reversible inhibition of renal growth.[13])

RN describes a constellation of phenomena that begin in infancy and childhood, are more common in females, and include (1) infection of the kidney by pathogenic bacteria from the patient's own fecal reservoir—the bacteria usually reach the kidney in an ascending fashion by vesicoureteral reflux (VUR) through an incompetent ureteral orifice; (2) lobar distribution of these acute infections (lobar nephronia)—the bacteria-laden urine reaches the individual renal lobes by intrarenal reflux (IRR) through incompetent papillary duct orifices; (3) destruction of tubules and eventually of entire nephrons, and even of populations of nephrons (if repeated infections occur and are unrecognized or untreated, or if they are treated after a significant delay); and (4) sequelae of the destruction of renal tissue, such as a significant decrease in the amount of functional renal tissue remaining (resulting in varying degrees of renal insufficiency) and physiological stresses on the remaining intact nephrons, such as hyperfiltration (resulting in focal glomerular sclerosis and secondary systemic hypertension and *its* sequelae).

The inciting bacterial infection of the kidney in RN occurs because of an imbalance in host defense mechanisms, on the one hand, and bacterial virulence factors on the other.

HOST DEFENSES

Many specific and nonspecific host resistance factors or defense mechanisms protect the child's kidney from bacterial infection. Some children are susceptible to colonization of their feces by pathogenic or virulent* bacteria,

*The term virulent is not used to imply that the bacteria are extremely poisonous, or that they cause a disease that has an unusually rapid, severe, or malignant course. Virulence here simply describes bacteria that possess properties that can overcome host defenses.

and others are not;[14] the former are at greater risk of urinary infection. The reasons for individual differences in susceptibility to colonization are not clear.

The unimpeded unidirectional flow of urine out of the urinary tract, including complete emptying of the bladder, is an extremely important nonspecific host defense mechanism,[15] because the urine washes unattached bacteria out of the system. Its effectiveness is compromised whenever there is obstruction, VUR, or infrequent or incomplete emptying of the bladder from any cause.

VUR is often a familial condition, is seen more frequently than expected in children with dysfunctional voiding,[16] and is uncommon in black children.[17] VUR not only provides a ready-made pathway for bacteria in the bladder to reach the kidney but is also associated with aberrant micturition,[18] that is, each time the patient with reflux voids, only part of the urine passes out through the urethra. The rest refluxes into the ureter(s) and pyelocalyceal system(s). As the wave of reflux recedes, the refluxed urine rapidly refills the bladder, resulting in a volume of stagnant urine that remains until the next voiding, when aberrant micturition will occur again.

IRR is the phenomenon that occurs when the refluxed urine reaches the pyelocalyceal system and then travels further cephalad into the distal collecting ducts and collecting tubules. This happens because the papillary duct orifices are incompetent, which is frequently the case in papillae that are compound (complex). Compound papillae tend to be found at the poles of the kidney, which explains why scars (in the child, the sequelae of the IRR of infected urine) tend to be seen most often in the polar regions of the kidney.[5] The orifices of the papillary ducts of the very young infant tend to be more susceptible to IRR than the orifices of older children and adults.[19] Without VUR, the competence of the papillary duct orifices is irrelevant.

All individuals have receptors on their epithelial cells. In the urinary tract, the receptors that enable bacteria to attach to the cells and prevent them from washing away are glycolipids of the globoseries.[20, 21] A spectrum of receptor molecule densities is found on the uroepithelium, and patients with more receptors (higher receptor density) may be at greater risk of colonization of the urinary tract by bacteria than those with fewer receptors. Experimental infections have been prevented by pretreating bacteria with synthetic receptor analogues.[22] The clinical relevance of this latter approach is not yet clear.

Specific antibodies to the bacterium or its adhesins (see following discussion) serve to protect the host against bacterial colonization or invasion. There may be a spectrum of the host's ability to mount an antibody response. Some children who have had repeated urinary tract infections have been shown to have lower levels of vaginal immunoglobulin A (IgA) than other children who have not had infections.[21, 23] In the young infant the immune defense system is immature, which may, in part, explain the susceptibility of the infant and young child to bacterial infection and scarring of the kidney.

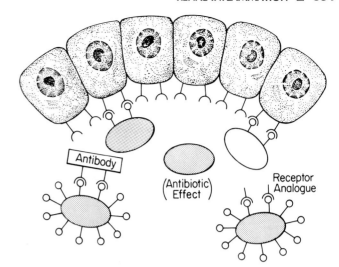

Figure 21–59. Diagrammatic representation of methods for interfering with bacterial adherence to host epithelial cells. Adherence of pathogenic bacterium (*shaded*) to host epithelial cell receptor can be blocked by antibody, competing nonpathogenic bacteria (*not shaded*) synthetic receptor analogues, or interference with synthesis of fimbria (antibiotic affect). (From Lebowitz RL, Mandell J: Urinary tract infection in children: Putting radiology in its place. Radiology 165(1):1–9, 1987.)

BACTERIAL VIRULENCE

Bacterial virulence factors are also myriad. There are general survival mechanisms, such as the ability to rapidly generate (33 minutes for some species of *E. coli*)[24] and the ability to sequester iron.[25, 26] Bacteria that reproduce more rapidly and are hardier in the environment of the host urinary tract are more likely to be of pathological significance.

The ability of bacteria to adhere to host uroepithelial cells in order to avoid being washed away by urine and thus to colonize the region, depends on their having the "correct" adhesins. These adhesins are often fimbria (pili),[21, 26] which are filamentous proteinaceous appendages of the bacterial cell wall. The greater the match between the bacterial adhesins and the host epithelial cell receptors, the greater the likelihood that colonization (and potential invasion of the mucosa) will occur. The crossover between adhesion of bacteria to receptors on the epithelial cell and adhesion to receptors on the white blood cell is not well understood.

Bacterial endotoxins (lipopolysaccharides) can paralyze the ureteral musculature,[21] thereby impeding the unidirectional flow of urine and permitting more bacteria to remain in the area, even when there are fewer adhesin-receptor linkages. Endotoxins may also play a role in tissue damage or systemic toxicity, once invasion has taken place.

HOST–BACTERIAL INTERACTION

The above phenomena suggest that RN is a biological system in which the host and his or her bacterial environment are in constant competition, and in which the degree of balance between the two prevents disease or enables it to become manifest.[27] Deficient host defenses compensate for fewer bacterial virulence factors, and the most virulent bacteria cause disease in the least-compromised host. For example, the resistant host (older child with no VUR, high levels of IgA, and low receptor density), who has primarily nonvirulent colonic bacteria, is not at risk. On the other hand, the severely compromised host (infant with VUR, IRR, low levels of IgA, high receptor density) is at great risk of developing infection of the kidney and

RN, even from bacteria with few virulence factors. The partially compromised host (infant with high receptor density, *no VUR*) may develop renal infection, but only when colonized by a virulent strain of bacteria.

Practical and theoretical methods exist for interfering with this natural model at many levels. The most important one is treatment of the acute urinary tract infection with an appropriate antibiotic in therapeutic doses and for an appropriate length of time. Treatment beginning soon after the onset of symptoms appears to abort the scarring process in the kidney. Conversely, treatment delayed for more than several days, although sterilizing the urine, will not prevent scars.[28]

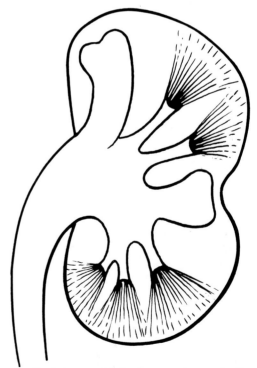

Figure 21–60. Diagram of infectious renal scars. In the middle portion of the kidney, eversion (clubbing) of the compound calyces and thinning of the overlying renal parenchyma results in a groove or valley when the adjacent renal lobes are unaffected. When the process affects the uppermost (or lowermost) renal lobes, the parenchyma over the distorted calyx is thinned, but no groove or valley is present since only one side has an adjacent renal lobe.

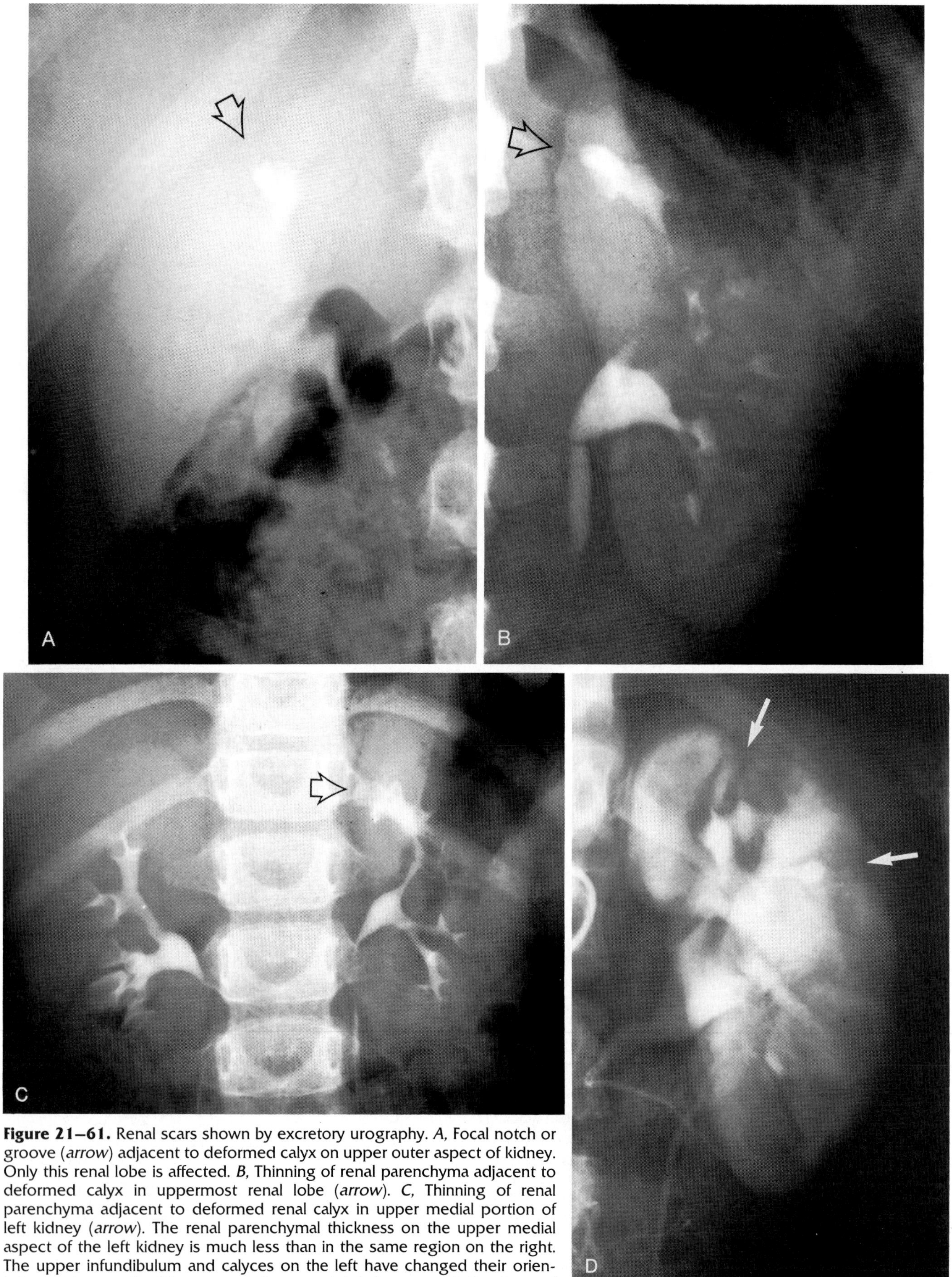

Figure 21–61. Renal scars shown by excretory urography. *A,* Focal notch or groove (*arrow*) adjacent to deformed calyx on upper outer aspect of kidney. Only this renal lobe is affected. *B,* Thinning of renal parenchyma adjacent to deformed calyx in uppermost renal lobe (*arrow*). *C,* Thinning of renal parenchyma adjacent to deformed renal calyx in upper medial portion of left kidney (*arrow*). The renal parenchymal thickness on the upper medial aspect of the left kidney is much less than in the same region on the right. The upper infundibulum and calyces on the left have changed their orientation (compared with same region on right) because of the loss of surrounding renal tissue and fibrous retraction of the scar, accounting for the so-called medial drift. *D,* Focal (lobar) scars (thinning of parenchyma) resulting in grooves or notches and adjacent deformed (clubbed) calyces as shown on nephrogram phase of renal arteriogram (*arrows*).

Methods for interfering with bacterial adherence (Fig. 21–59) include the following: (1) Host antibody (IgA). Antibody molecules seem to be able to block the adhesin-receptor linkage in vivo, and synthetic receptor analogues have been shown to block the process in vitro (see earlier discussion).[22] The practical therapeutic implications of the latter approach remain to be seen. (2) Competing non-virulent bacteria. These may attach to the epithelial cell receptor sites and thus prevent virulent bacteria from attaching.[29] It is not known whether in some circumstances so-called asymptomatic bacteriuria is protective. (3) Subtherapeutic doses of some antibiotics seem to interfere with the adhesion process. This may be due to inhibition of the synthesis of bacterial adhesins.[30, 31]

URORADIOLOGY

The Kidney

The scars of RN develop in 4 to 6 months and when uncomplicated are characteristic (Fig. 21–60). They can be shown by excretory urography (EU) (Fig. 21–61), ultrasonography (Fig. 21–62), nuclear scintigraphic renal imaging (Fig. 21–63), or computed tomography (CT). The latter is almost never necessary for either diagnosis or follow-up. The typical EU image shows a deformed (clubbed) calyx in association with thinning of the adjacent renal parenchyma.[3] This produces a notch or valley in the surface of the kidney immediately opposite the affected calyx, except in the extreme polar regions. In these latter areas—the most medial upper and lower renal lobes—a notch does not develop because there is only one adjacent normal renal lobe (Fig. 21–61B). The scars are lobar in distribution because of the ascending nature of the infection and are focal; that is, normal renal lobes are usually found immediately adjacent to the affected lobes (Figs. 21–60 to 21–63).

In the past, scars were often seen when a child was being investigated for the first time by uroradiological methods because the recent infection, which prompted the evaluation, was actually not the child's first. The resulting confusion explains why scars were once thought to be congenital. It is now clear, however, that scars are acquired. Countless examples of normal kidneys becoming scarred have been seen, often in children as old as 7 years of age (Figs. 21–64 to 21–66).[32] Without infection, focal scarring does not occur (Fig. 21–67). Once the scarring process begins, several years may pass before fibrous retraction becomes complete (Figs. 21–64 to 21–66). Maturation of a scar should not be mistaken for

Text continued on page 858

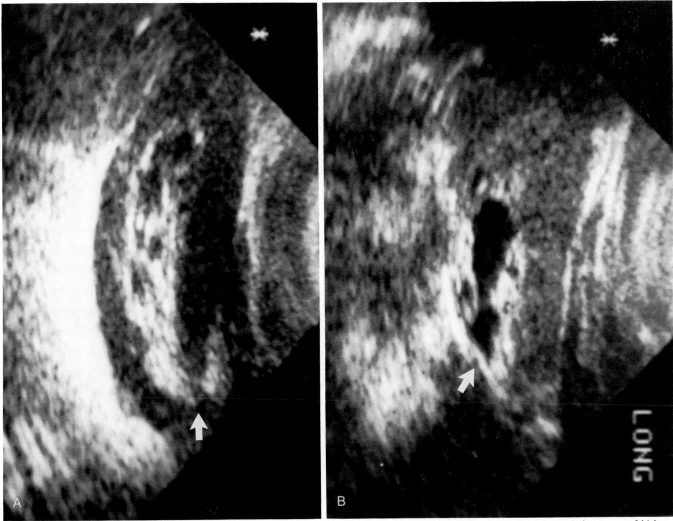

Figure 21–62. Scars shown by ultrasonography. *A,* Marked decrease in parenchymal thickness in lower medial aspect of kidney (*arrow*). (Kidney vertically oriented for comparison with Fig. 21–61). *B,* In another patient there is mild dilatation of the pyelocalyceal system and marked thinning of renal parenchyma over dilated calyx in the lower pole of kidney (*arrow*).

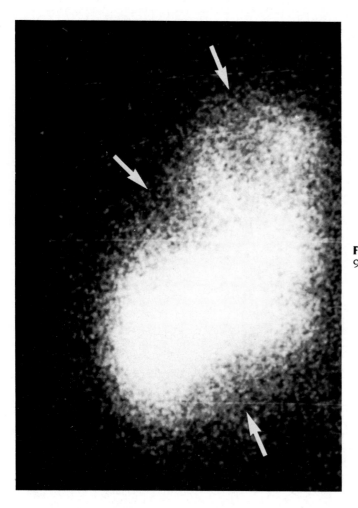

Figure 21–63. Scars shown by renal scintigraphy (technetium-99m DMSA). There are several focal photopenic areas (*arrows*).

Figure 21–64. Development of scars. *A,* Voiding cystourethrography (VCU). Right Grade 4/5 reflux with intrarenal reflux (IRR) into upper renal lobes (*arrows*). *B,* Intravenous urography (IVU). Kidney normal; renal parenchymal thickness and calyceal configuration normal in upper renal lobes. *C,* IVU 2 years later. There is thinning of renal parenchyma and clubbing of calyces in renal lobes into which infected IRR previously flowed (*arrow*). *D,* IVU 4 years later shows progression (maturation) of scarring process (*arrow*). The urine was sterile during the interval.

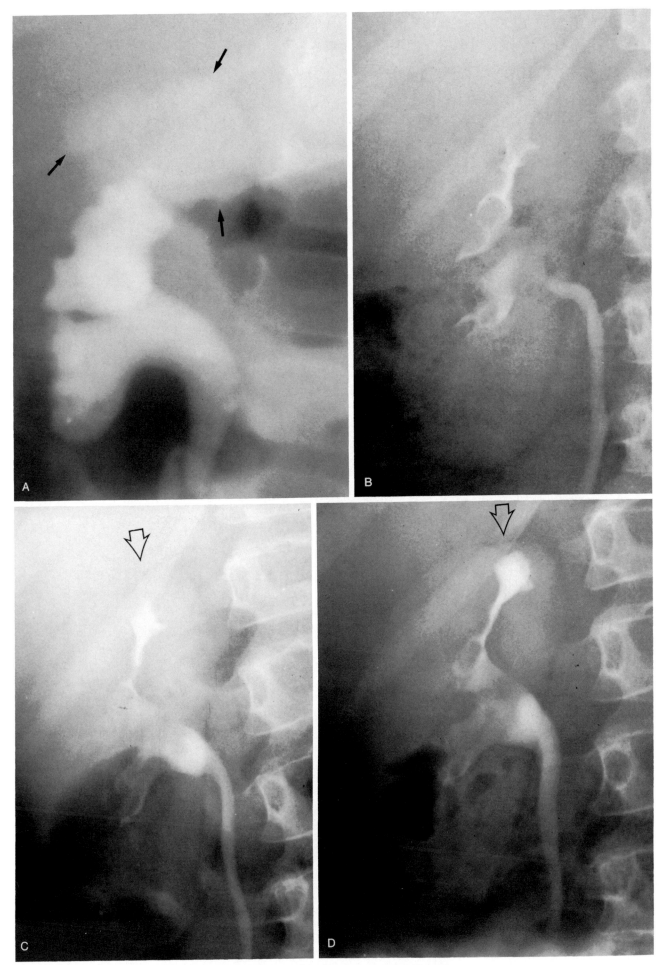

Figure 21–64 See legend on opposite page

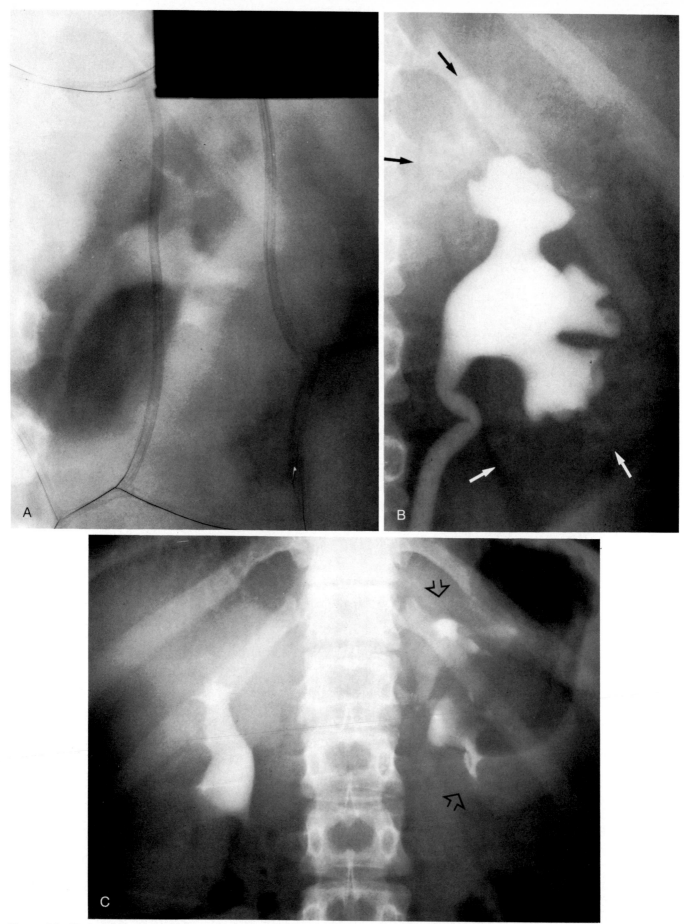

Figure 21–65. Development of scars. *A,* IVU. Normal kidney. The lines result from film emulsion degradation. *B,* VCU 1 year later. Film shows IRR in upper and lower renal lobes (*arrows*). *C,* IVU 8 years later. The patient was lost to follow-up and had several urinary infections. The right kidney remains normal. On the left are several focal areas of renal scarring, corresponding to the renal lobes into which infected IRR flowed (*arrows*).

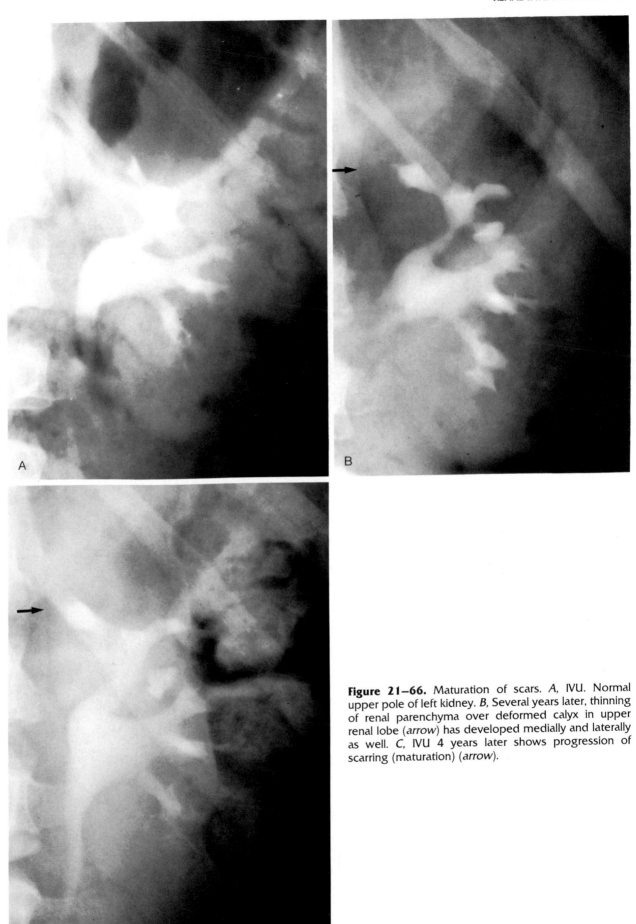

Figure 21–66. Maturation of scars. *A*, IVU. Normal upper pole of left kidney. *B*, Several years later, thinning of renal parenchyma over deformed calyx in upper renal lobe (*arrow*) has developed medially and laterally as well. *C*, IVU 4 years later shows progression of scarring (maturation) (*arrow*).

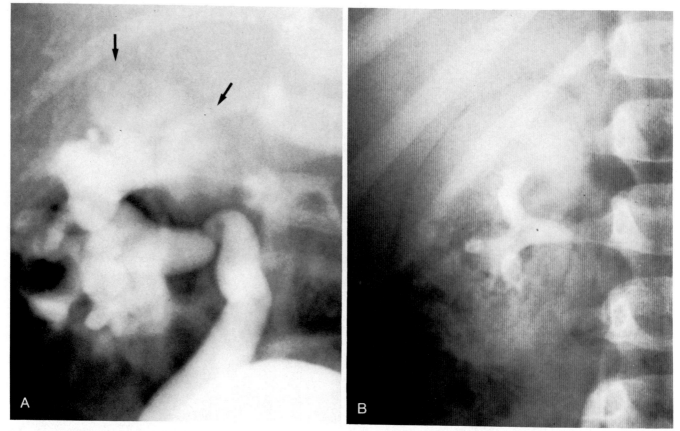

Figure 21–67. IRR without infection. *A,* VCU done to evaluate appearance of urethra in infant with ambiguous genitalia. The child never had urinary infection. Right Grade 4/5 reflux with IRR into upper renal lobes (*arrows*) (compare with Fig. 21–64). *B,* IVU 4 years later. The right kidney remains normal in spite of IRR because the patient never had urinary infection.

continuing infection. Histological examination of the mature scar, of course, will show no sign of inflammatory reaction.

The so-called Ask-Upmark kidney was thought to be a specific type of congenital segmental renal hypoplasia, seen in young women with renal insufficiency and hypertension, when it was first described by Ask-Upmark in 1929 (Fig. 21–68).[33] It probably simply represents the late stage of RN.[34–36]

In acute renal parenchymal infection, before scars develop, the findings are (1) occult on EU, although they can be seen as focal (lobar) regions of decreased enhancement on CT; (2) focal (lobar) areas of abnormal echogenicity on sonograms, and (3) most reliably shown by nuclear medicine techniques, using a radionuclide that binds to the tubules such as Tc-99m-DMSA. A focal (lobar) area of decreased uptake is seen.[37–39] These abnormal areas of the kidney usually progress to frank scars.

Vesicoureteral Reflux

VUR is most effectively and efficiently shown by either conventional (fluoroscopically monitored) voiding cystourethrography (VCU)[40, 41] or by radionuclide cystography.[42, 43] Nuclear cystography, because it is both more sensitive in detecting fleeting episodes of reflux and exposes the child's gonads to a lower dose of radiation, is favored for screening and follow-up. VCU is favored for

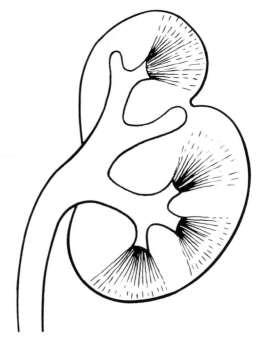

Figure 21–68. Drawing of left kidney. The abnormal areas of the kidney bear a striking resemblance to focal renal scars of RN caused by IRR of infected urine (compare with Fig. 21–60). (Modified from Ask-Upmark E: Uberjuvenile maligne nephrosclerose und ihr verhaltuis zer storungen in der nierenentwicklung. Acta Path Microbiol Scan 6:383, 1929.)

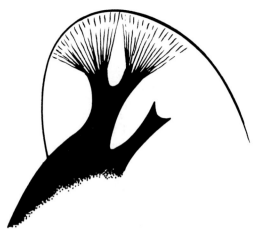

Figure 21–69. Diagrammatic representation of IRR into upper renal lobes.

characterizing reflux and for showing the detailed anatomy of the child's lower urinary tract.

Intrarenal Reflux (Fig. 21–69)

For practical purposes, IRR can be shown only by VCU, and even then its depiction is unpredictable. The stated incidence of IRR is probably a gross underestimate of the actual incidence, since its occurrence is usually fleeting (Figs. 21–70, 21–71).[13, 19, 41] Visualizing IRR depends on meticulous filming of the entire kidney at the peak of the reflux—it also requires luck. The recognition of IRR has been crucial to understanding the pathophysiology of RN, but showing that it occurs in an individual child is not of much practical importance for management.

Imaging Recommendations

When a young child has a well-documented urinary infection, it is important to ascertain whether the child's defenses are compromised by obstruction or reflux, or both. The first imaging study should usually be evaluation of the lower urinary tract by VCU (or nuclear cystography).[40, 44] Signs of bladder/sphincter dyssynergia should be sought.[45] If results are normal, or if only mild, uncomplicated reflux is shown, renal imaging can then be performed using ultrasonography.[46] If the kidneys and collecting systems are normal, no other uroradiological imaging tests are necessary. If the child has subsequent upper tract infections, a repeat VCU may be indicated, if the initial one was negative. With a second lower tract infection, repeated imaging tests may be unnecessary. If

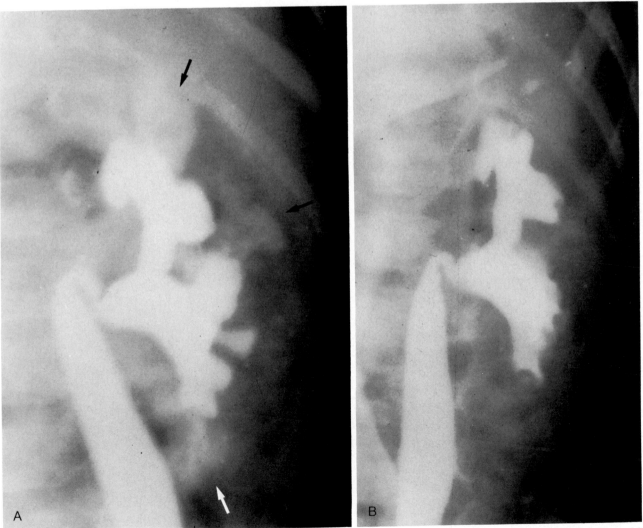

Figure 21–70. Fleeting nature of IRR. *A,* VCU. IRR into several renal lobes (*arrows*) during voiding. *B,* Immediately after voiding ceases, IRR is no longer visible.

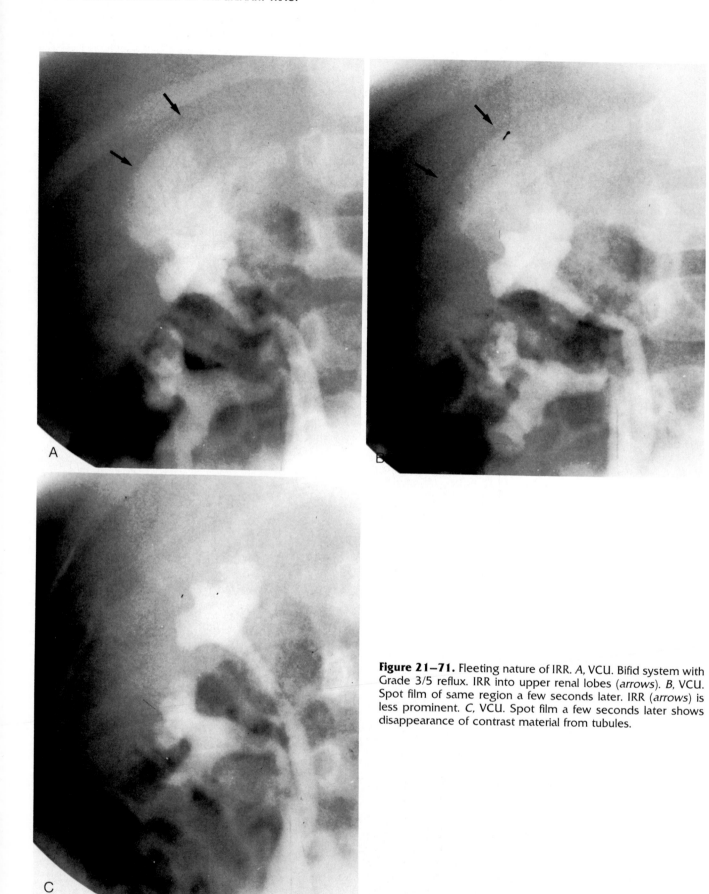

Figure 21–71. Fleeting nature of IRR. *A*, VCU. Bifid system with Grade 3/5 reflux. IRR into upper renal lobes (*arrows*). *B*, VCU. Spot film of same region a few seconds later. IRR (*arrows*) is less prominent. *C*, VCU. Spot film a few seconds later shows disappearance of contrast material from tubules.

the nuclear cystogram is the first imaging examination and shows reflux, VCU may be performed to further characterize the reflux. If VCU is markedly abnormal, EU is usually performed to assess the functional implications of the reflux.

If VCU and ultrasonography are normal but the child has signs and symptoms that strongly suggest renal infection, renal scintigraphy with a tubule-labeling agent such as Tc-99m-DMSA will occasionally show a photopenic area.[37-39] In this situation, treatment with antibiotic may be intensified or prolonged.

In the older child or teenager, and especially if only lower urinary tract signs and symptoms are found, a normal renal sonographic examination alone provides reassurance that (1) the child does not have RN and (2) the child (by this age) is not at much risk of developing it in the future.

THE SEQUELAE OF RENAL SCARRING

RN is thought to be responsible for 10% to 30% of all cases of end-stage renal disease.[47] The pathogenesis seems to be that the nephrons *not* damaged by the inflammation/scarring process (the so-called remnant nephron population) must filter more than the usual amount of blood per nephron.[11, 47-49] This increase in the single nephron glomerular filtration rate results in damage to these remnant nephrons in the form of focal or segmental glomerular sclerosis. This acquired glomerulopathy coincides with the onset of proteinuria and the subsequent decrease in the clearance of creatinine.

The combination of (1) damage to one population of nephrons by inflammation/scarring and, in theory, (2) damage to the remaining population by hyperfiltration-induced glomerular sclerosis, can result in end-stage renal disease.

The greater the initial magnitude of infection-induced scarring, the smaller the population of remaining normal nephrons. This leads to a greater magnitude of hyperfiltration by each of these remnant nephrons and, it seems, a greater likelihood of glomerular sclerosis.

CONCLUSIONS

The diagnostic and therapeutic challenges in this disease are (1) prompt, accurate diagnosis of urinary infection in infants and young children, who are at special risk for renal scarring because of their age; (2) appropriate antibiotic treatment, without delay, in order to abort the scarring process; (3) diagnostic uroradiological evaluation, beginning with voiding cystography, to determine which children are at risk because of VUR; and (4) protecting from infection the child who is found to have reflux, by administering "prophylactic" antibiotics until the reflux disappears spontaneously or is corrected surgically, or until the child grows older.

References

1. Bailey RR: The relationship of vesico-ureteric reflux to urinary tract infection and chronic pyelonephritis—reflux nephropathy. Clin Nephrol 1:132, 1973.
2. Heale WF, Weldon AP, Hewstone AS: Reflux nephropathy. Presentation of urinary infection in childhood. Med J Aust 1:1138–1140, 1973.
3. Hodson CJ: The radiological contribution toward the diagnosis of chronic pyelonephritis. Radiology 88:857, 1967.
4. Hodson CJ: Reflux nephropathy: A personal historical review. AJR 137:451, 1981.
5. Risdon RA: Reflux nephropathy. Diagn Histopathol 4:61, 1981.
6. Hodson CJ, Cotran RS: Reflux nephropathy. Hosp Pract 17:133, 1982.
7. Senekjian HO, Suki WN: Vesicoureteral reflux and reflux nephropathy. Am J Nephrol 2:245, 1982.
8. Thomsen HS: Vesicoureteral reflux and reflux nephropathy. Acta Radiol Diagn 26:3, 1985.
9. Davidson A: Radiology of the Kidney. Philadelphia, WB Saunders Company, 1985.
10. Johnston JH (ed): Management of Vesicoureteric Reflux. Baltimore, Williams & Wilkins, 1984.
11. Steinhardt GF: Reflux nephropathy. J Urol 134:855, 1985.
12. Leavitt SB, Weiss RA: Vesicoureteral reflux. Natural history, classification and reflux nephropathy. In Kelalis PP, King LR, Belman AB: Clinical Pediatric Urology. Philadelphia, WB Saunders Company, 1985.
13. Fowler R: The many faces of vesico-ureteric reflux: Factors contributing to renal damage. Aust NZ J Surg, 54:417, 1984.
14. Winberg J, Bollgren I, Kallenius G, et al: Clinical pyelonephritis and focal renal scarring. Pediatr Clin North Am 29:801, 1982.
15. Mackowiak PA: The normal microbial flora. N Engl J Med 307:83, 1982.
16. Allen TD: Vesicoureteral reflux and the unstable bladder. J Urol 134:1180, 1985.
17. Bailey RR, Janus E, McLoughlin K, et al: Familial and genetic data in reflux nephropathy. In Hodson CJ, Heptinstall RH, Winberg J (eds): Reflux Nephropathy Update: 1983. New York, Karger, 1984.
18. Willi U, Lebowitz RL: The so-called megaureter-megacystis syndrome. AJR 133:409, 1979.
19. Cremin BJ: Observations on vesico-ureteric reflux and intrarenal reflux: A review and survey of material. Clin Radiol 30:607, 1979.
20. Lomberg H, Hanson LA, Jacobsson B, et al: Correlation of p blood group, vesicoureteral reflux, and bacterial attachment in patients with recurrent pyelonephritis. N Engl J Med 308:1189, 1983.
21. Roberts JA: Urinary tract infections. Am J Kidney Dis 4:103, 1984.
22. Svanborg Eden C, Freter R, Hagberg L, et al: Inhibition of experimental ascending urinary tract infection by an epithelial cell-surface receptor analogue. Nature 298:560, 1982.
23. Cohen MS, Black JR, Proctor RA, Sparling PF: Host defenses and the vaginal mucosa. Scand J Urol Nephrol 86(suppl):13, 1984.
24. Hooke AM, Sordelli DO, Erguetti MC, Vogt AJ: Quantitative determination of bacterial replication in vivo. Infect Immun 49:424, 1985.
25. Bullen JJ: The significance of iron in infection. Rev Infect Dis 3:1127, 1981.
26. Ogata RT: Factors determining bacterial pathogenicity. Clin Physiol Biochem 1:145, 1983.
27. Torres VE, Kramer SA, Holley KE, et al: Interaction of multiple risk factors in the pathogenesis of experimental reflux nephropathy in the pig. J Urol 133:131, 1985.
28. Ransley PG, Risdon RA: Reflux nephropathy: Effects of antimicrobial therapy on the evolution of the early pyelonephritic scar. Kidney Int 20:733, 1981.
29. Chan RC, Reid G, Irvin RT, et al: Competitive exclusion of uropathogens from human uroepithelial cells by Lactobacillus whole cells and cell wall fragments. Infect Immun 47:84, 1985.
30. Vosbeck K, Handschin H, Menge E-B, Zak O: Effects of subminimal inhibitory concentrations of antibiotics on adhesiveness of Escherichia coli in vitro. Rev Infect Dis 1:845, 1979.
31. Eisenstein BI, Ofek I, Beachey EH: Interference with the mannose binding and epithelial cell adherence of Escherichia coli by sublethal concentrations of streptomycin. J Clin Invest 63:1219, 1979.
32. Smellie JM, Ransley PG, Normand ICS, et al: Development of new renal scars: A collaborative study. Br Med J 290:1957–60, 1985.
33. Ask-Upmark E: Uber juvenile maligne nephrosclerose und ihr verhaltuis zer storungen in der nierenentwicklung. Acta Pathol Microbiol Scand 6:383, 1929.
34. Arant BS, Sotelo-Avila C, Bernstein J: Segmental "hypoplasia" of the kidney (Ask-Upmark). J Pediatr 95:931, 1979.

35. Johnston JH, Mix LW: The Ask-Upmark kidney: A form of ascending pyelonephritis? Br J Urol 48:393, 1976.
36. Stamey TA: Pathogenesis and Treatment of Urinary Tract Infections. Baltimore, Williams & Wilkins, 1980.
37. Conway JJ: Radionuclide imaging of a acute bacterial nephritis. *In* Hodson CJ, Heptinstall RH, Winberg J, (eds): Reflux Nephropathy Update: 1983. New York, Karger, 1984.
38. Treves ST, Lebowitz RL, Kuruc A, et al: Kidney. *In* Treves ST: Pediatric Nuclear Medicine. New York, Springer-Verlag, 1985.
39. Majd M: Nuclear medicine. *In* Kelalis P, King L, Belman AB (eds): Clinical Pediatric Urology, 2nd Ed. Philadelphia, WB Saunders Company, 1985.
40. Blickman JG, Taylor GA, Lebowitz RL: Voiding cystourethrography: The initial radiologic study in children with urinary tract infection. Radiology 156:659, 1985.
41. Lebowitz RL: The detection of vesicoureteral reflux in the child. Invest Radiol 21:519–531, 1986.
42. Willi UV, Treves ST: Radionuclide voiding cystography. *In* Treves ST: Pediatric Nuclear Medicine. New York, Springer-Verlag, 1985.
43. Conway JJ: Radionuclide cystography. *In* Hodson CT, Heptinstall RH, Winberg J (eds): Reflux Nephropathy Update: 1983. New York, Karger, 1984.
44. Cohen HL, Haller JO: Diagnostic sonography of the fetal genitourinary tract. Urol Radiol 9:88, 1987.
45. Fotter R, Kopp W, Skein E, et al: Unstable bladder in children: Functional evaluation by modified voiding cystourethrography. Radiology 161:811–813, 1986.
46. Lebowitz RL, Mandell J: Urinary tract infection in children: Putting radiology in its place. Radiology 165:1, 1987.
47. Bhathena DB, Weiss JH, Holland NH, et al: Focal and segmental glomerular sclerosis in reflux nephropathy. Am J Med 68:886, 1980.
48. Torres VE, Velosa JA, Holley KE, et al: The progression of vesicoureteral reflux nephropathy. Ann Intern Med 92:776, 1980.
49. Cotran RS: Glomerulosclerosis in reflux nephropathy. Kidney Int 21:528, 1982.
50. Westra SJ, Verbeeten B, Bots TC, et al: Urinary tract malacoplakia with extension into the retroperitoneum with secondary gastrointestinal involvement. Urol Radiol 10:181–185, 1988.

22

Perinephric Inflammation

JOSEPH K. T. LEE □ RANDOLPH J. KNIFIC

Inflammation of the perinephric space presents an extremely difficult and often frustrating diagnostic problem for the clinician and radiologist. This is particularly disturbing because delayed diagnosis is associated with high morbidity and mortality[1] and frequently leads to removal or loss of an irreversibly damaged kidney. However, early and accurate diagnosis allows prompt treatment that may result in complete morphological and functional recovery of the kidney. Several noninvasive imaging techniques, particularly ultrasonography and computed tomography (CT), allow the radiologist to directly image the retroperitoneal spaces and often provides an early and accurate diagnosis of perinephric infection.[2]

ANATOMICAL CONSIDERATIONS

Knowledge of the retroperitoneal compartments is essential to an understanding of the development and spread of perinephric infection. This information has been discussed in detail in earlier chapters (Chapters 6 and 13), but is briefly summarized here for the reader's convenience. At the level of the kidneys, the retroperitoneum is anatomically divided into three extraperitoneal compartments by well-defined anterior and posterior layers of the renal fascia.[3] They are (1) the anterior paranephric space, which extends from the posterior parietal peritoneum to the anterior renal fascia; (2) the perinephric space, which lies between the two layers of the renal fascia; and (3) the posterior paranephric space, which extends from the posterior renal fascia to the fascia overlying the quadratus lumborum and psoas muscles (Fig. 22–1).

The renal fascia is a collagenous yet elastic connective tissue sheath of medium-to-hard consistency that surrounds the kidney and adrenal gland. Between the renal capsule and its fascial envelope lies a variable amount of perinephric fat, which is most abundant posteriorly and laterally. This fatty space is traversed by connective tissue septa containing blood vessels and lymphatics.[4, 5] Superiorly, the two layers are firmly fixed to each other above the adrenal glands to the diaphragmatic fascia. Laterally, the two renal fasciae fuse to form the lateroconal fascia, which relates to the posterior aspect of the colon and continues anterolaterally to fuse with the parietal peritoneum. Medially, the posterior renal fascia fuses with the psoas or quadratus lumborum fascia, and the anterior renal fascia blends with the dense mass of connective tissue surrounding the great vessels in the root of the mesentery and behind the pancreas and the duodenum.[6]

The perinephric space narrows as it extends inferiorly and medially so that it has been likened to an inverted cone.[7] Inferiorly, the layers fuse weakly or blend with the iliac fascia; as they narrow medially, the layers also blend loosely with the periureteral connective tissue. It has been shown that the weakest point, through which perinephric fluid collections escape most easily, is at the inferomedial angle of the perinephric space adjacent to the ureter.[8] At this level, fluid may extend through the midline to the opposite side or into the pelvis. With greatly increased pressure in the perinephric space, transperitoneal rupture may occur in the region of the renal hilus.[9]

ETIOLOGY AND BACTERIOLOGY

Most cases of perinephric abscess in the adult are thought to arise from renal extension of ascending urinary infections. A renal cortical abscess, perhaps associated with pyonephrosis, may perforate the capsule and contaminate the perinephric space. Extensions of chronic renal inflammation, for example, xanthogranulomatous pyelonephritis or tuberculosis, may be a cause.

Perforation of the ureter or a calyceal fornix with discharge of infected urine may lead to a smoldering perinephric abscess. At times, the underlying site of renal communication is difficult to identify, even at surgery. Some have thought that the rich vascular and lymphatic network existing in the kidney and perinephric fat facilitates the spread of infection. The offending organism is usually *Escherichia coli*, *Proteus*, or a streptococcus.[1, 10]

Extraperitoneal sites of infection may occasionally spread to the perinephric space. These include colonic diverticulitis, perforated carcinoma of the colon, retroperitoneal appendicitis, pancreatitis, or pelvic inflammatory conditions.[11–13]

Hematogenous spread from remote sites of infection, such as furunculosis, wound infection, or upper respiratory disease also occurs.[14, 15] More common in children, it is usually caused by *Staphylococcus aureus*. A fourth cause of perinephric abscess is pursuant to surgery. Any

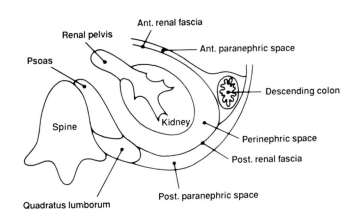

LEFT KIDNEY PLUS PARANEPHRIC SPACES AND FASCIAL BOUNDARIES

Figure 22–1. Diagram of retroperitoneal compartments. Anterior paranephric space, perinephric space, and posterior paranephric space.

operation on the kidney, for example, partial nephrectomy, can result in a post-operative abscess.

Thorley and associates,[1] in their review of perinephric abscesses, found that the relevant literature had changed since the introduction of antimicrobial agents in the 1940s. They reported that the percentage of cases caused by *S. aureus* decreased from 45% before 1940 to 6% after 1940 and that those attributable to *E. coli* and *Proteus* rose from 8% to 30% and 4% to 44%, respectively. This change was attributed to the expeditious use of antibiotics to treat skin and wound infections, thereby decreasing the chance of hematogenous seeding from the infection.

CLINICAL FEATURES

Few patients with acute perinephric infection present with classic signs and symptoms of fever, chills, flank pain, a tender bulging flank, and leukocytosis. More commonly, the clinical picture is nonspecific. Malaise, weight loss, and low-grade fever may be present for weeks or months before localizing signs develop. Pleuritic pain may be present, owing to diaphragmatic irritation. A mass is palpable only if it is large or localizes inferiorly below the costal margin. With pressure on the extraperitoneal nerves, pain may be referred to the groin, thigh, or knee.[16] Because a portion of the ascending and descending colon lies very close to the perinephric space, a perinephric abscess may erode into the colon resulting in a nephrocolonic fistula. If that occurs, patients may complain of diarrhea, bloody stools, passage of urine per rectum, and fecaluria. If the abscess also forms a connection with the skin, a nephrocolonic-cutaneous fistula is formed. With such a fistula, urine and feces are discharged from the skin track.[17]

Laboratory tests are seldom helpful in ascertaining the specific diagnosis, since 25% of infected patients have a normal urinalysis, 60% have pyuria and 30% have hematuria.[1] Leukocytosis is usually present, but only 24% of infected patients have a total leukocyte count greater than 15,000. In as many as 36% of patients, the leukocyte count is less than 10,000.[18] Anemia, which is defined as hemoglobin less than 10 gm%, is found in as many as 42%. The erythrocyte sedimentation rate is uniformly elevated.[1]

Perinephric abscesses show no sex predilection. Predisposing factors such as renal calculi, neurogenic bladder, urinary tract infection, and intravenous drug abuse are very common.[19–21] Diabetes was found in 67% of the patients in one series.[22]

IMAGING

The radiological evaluation of patients with suspected perinephric inflammation/abscess has undergone drastic changes in recent years. Because the diagnosis of perinephric involvement by plain radiography and excretory urography often relies on indirect signs, and because diagnosis by retrograde pyelography and renal arteriography is invasive, renal ultrasonography and CT have become the methods of choice because of their high accuracy and the ease with which they delineate the perinephric space. A particular advantage of CT is its ability to frequently localize retroperitoneal effusions to a specific compartment. This is not always of great clinical importance; in numerous instances, however, the precise anatomical localization of an effusion provided a key observation leading to definitive diagnosis and treatment. Anterior paranephric space collections, for example, usually originate in the gastrointestinal tract. Therefore, recognition of an abscess residing in the anterior paranephric space should prompt consideration of such underlying diseases as perforated ulcer of the second part of the duodenum, diverticulitis of the retroperitoneal surfaces of the colon, retrocecal appendicitis, and pancreatitis. Posterior paranephric effusions usually result from disease of the psoas muscle, spine, lymph nodes, or penetrating injuries; however, abscesses can also extend from one compartment to another. Subcapsular renal abscesses are seen occasionally. Meyers[3] and Whalen[23] have established elaborate criteria to differentiate perinephric from paranephric effusions on plain abdominal radiographs. With the advent of cross-sectional imaging, these characteristics are no longer as vital to diagnosis as they once were, but they remain as a landmark in anatomicoradiological investigation.

Plain Radiographs

In patients with perinephric abscesses, many abnormalities may be seen on the plain radiograph of the abdomen. In approximately 50% of patients, however, the abdominal film is normal.[24] These findings are often nonspecific, and similar changes can result from duodenal perforation or emphysematous pancreatitis, as well as from a lesser sac abscess. Nevertheless, a correct diagnosis can be made if these findings are correlated with the clinical data. Abnormalities that may be seen on the affected side include the following:

1. *Loss of renal outline with increased density in region of kidney* (Figs. 22–2 and 22–3). However, according to one report the renal outline was preserved in 50% of patients with perinephric abscess.[9] The usual appearance is of a large elliptical soft-tissue density in the flank, owing to distention of the perinephric space with fluid. Care must be taken not to mistakenly attribute this to an enlarged kidney.

2. *Displacement and rotation of the kidney.* Perinephric fluid usually localizes in the rich dorsolateral perinephric fat near the lower pole, because the infection follows the path of least resistance, abetted by gravity in the supine position. The kidney is therefore usually displaced medially and upward and may be rotated about its vertical axis (Figs. 22–4 and 22–5). As the exudate increases, it tends to seek the infrahilar area, extending inferiorly along the ureter. Loss of definition with lateral displacement of the inferior renal pole results. Loculations in other parts of the perinephric space may produce renal displacement and rotation in other axes.

3. *Perinephric gas.* Gas-producing infection secondary to *E. coli, Aerobacter aerogenes,* or very rarely *Clostridia* occurs, especially among diabetics. The gas may encircle the kidney or present as a mottled, localized collection of radiolucencies within the shadows of the perinephric fat (Figs. 22–3 and 22–6).[25] Fluid levels may be identified in the upright position and may mimic dilated bowel.[26, 27]

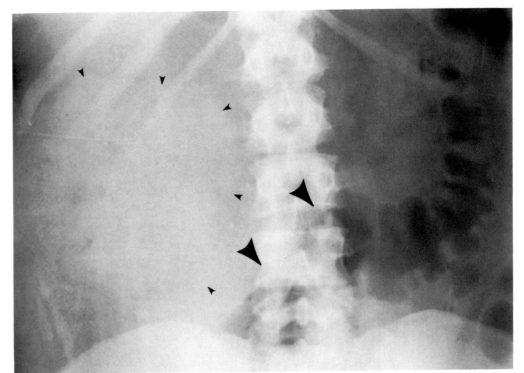

Figure 22–2. Plain radiograph of perinephric abscess. The right renal outline is lost. Density *(small arrowheads)* is increased, and a paucity of bowel gas is in the expected region of the right kidney. The hepatic flexure *(large arrowheads)* is displaced medially and inferiorly, and lumbar scoliosis, concave toward the abscess, is present.

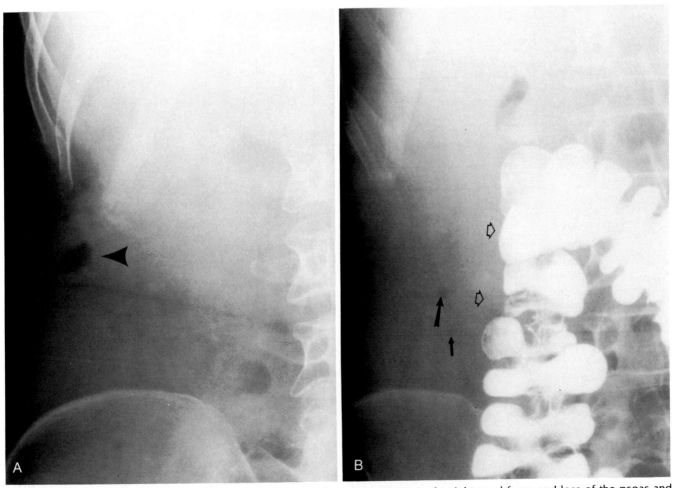

Figure 22–3. Perinephric abscess. *A,* Plain radiograph shows increased density in the right renal fossa and loss of the psoas and right renal margins. The flank stripe is obliterated and a perinephric gas collection is seen *(arrowhead). B,* Barium enema demonstrates medial displacement of the ascending colon *(open arrows).* Again noted are perinephric gas collections *(arrows).*

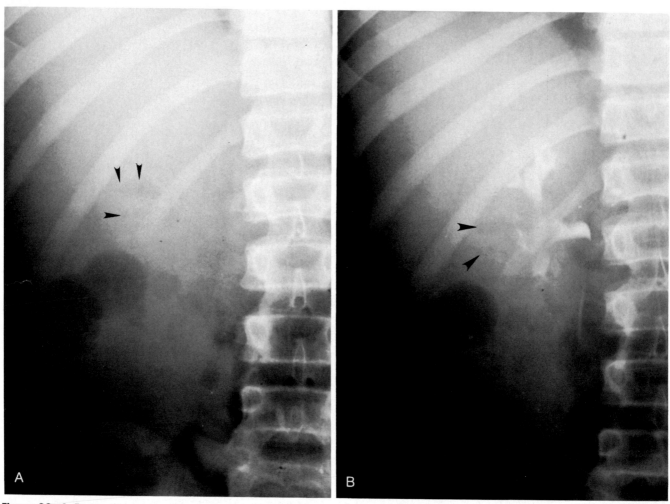

Figure 22–4. Perinephric abscess in a 15-year-old patient 1 week after surgical drainage of a periappendiceal abscess. *A*, Scout film shows obliteration of psoas margin and gas collections over right kidney area *(arrowheads)*. *B*, Excretory urogram (IVU) shows medial displacement of the right kidney. Numerous small perinephric gas collections are also seen *(arrowheads)*. Incidentally noted is spondyloepiphyseal dysplasia tarda.

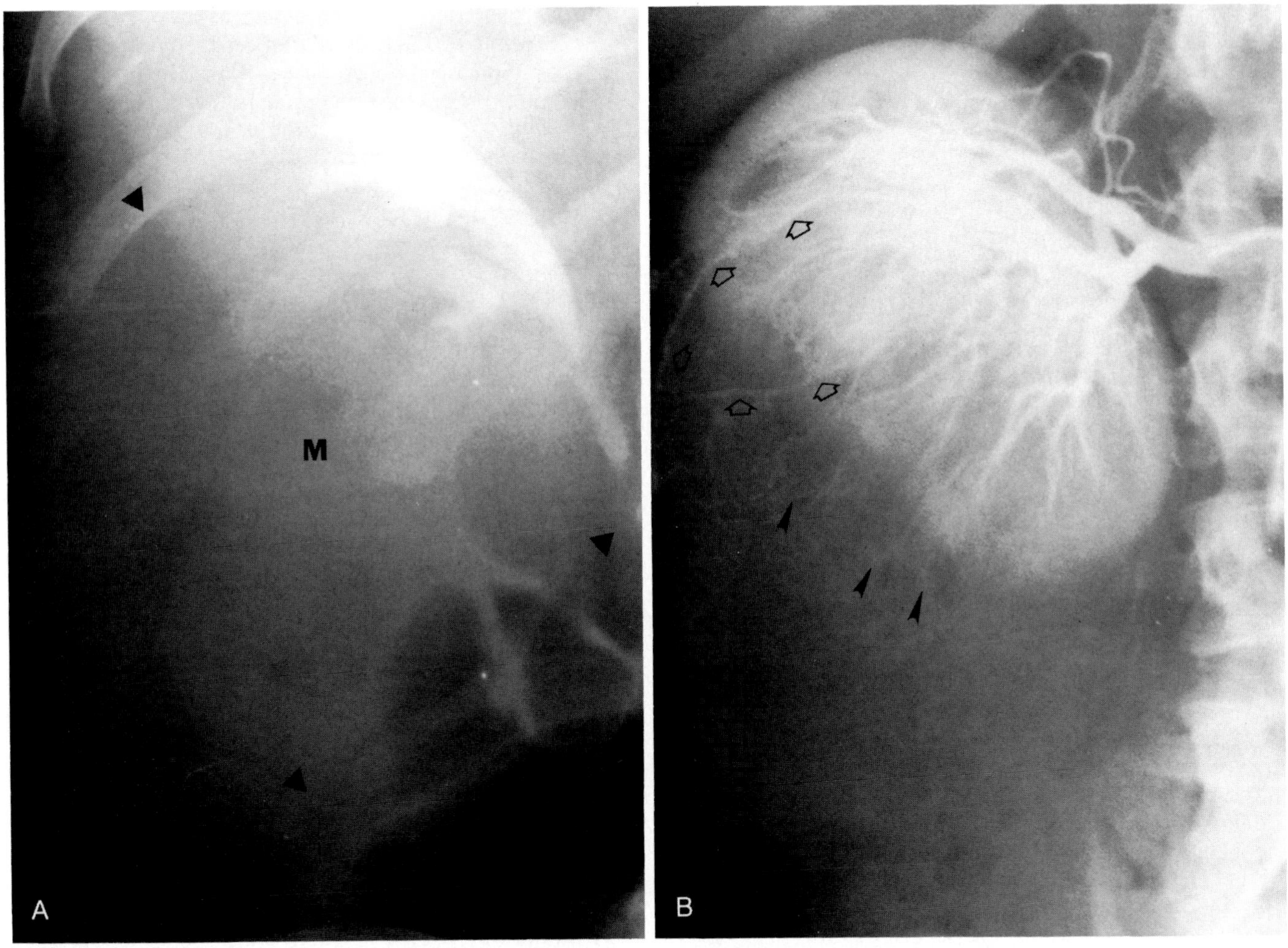

Figure 22–5. Perinephric abscess *(Klebsiella)*, surgically proven. *A,* Excretory urogram demonstrates marked compression and displacement of the pyelocalyceal system by a soft-tissue mass (M). Bowel gas is also displaced. The lower renal outline and psoas margin are obliterated. Arrowheads define perimeter of mass. *B,* Renal arteriogram shows prominence of perforating capsular vessels along the lateral aspect of the kidney *(open arrows).* Note stretching and displacement of the intrarenal arterial branches. Fine, reticular neovascularity is present in perinephric space *(arrowheads).*

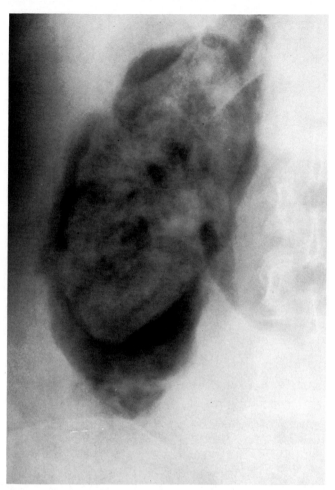

Figure 22–6. Plain radiograph showing gas in the perinephric space secondary to emphysematous pyelonephritis and perinephritis in a diabetic patient with *E. coli* in urine and blood. Gas throughout the right perinephric space outlines the kidney. Extensive gas formation is present within the renal interstitium.

4. *Displacement of bowel gas.* A perinephric abscess may be large enough to produce a mass effect upon adjacent intestine. On the right, the descending duodenum may be displaced medially and anteriorly, and the hepatic flexure of the colon may be displaced downward (Figs. 22–2 and 22–3).[4] On the left, the descending colon, the duodenal jejunal junction, and the stomach may be displaced medially.[28, 29]

5. *Absence of a segment of the psoas muscle margin* (Figs. 22–2 and 22–3). The psoas margin may also be absent in extremely emaciated patients or in patients with slight rotation of the lumbar spine. In one study, the psoas margin was absent bilaterally in 3% of normal patients and unilaterally in 10% of normal patients, leading to a high false-positive rate.[30]

6. *Scoliosis.* Curvature of the lumbar spine with the concavity pointing toward the side with the lesion may indicate spasm of the paraspinal muscle secondary to irritation by abscess (Fig. 22–2). This occurs in less than half the patients with perinephric abscess.[31]

7. *Limited diaphragmatic excursion.* Nesbit and Dick showed that of 85 patients with perinephric abscesses, 14 (16.5%) had supraphrenic complications.[32] These include pleural effusion, atelectasis, pneumonia, and nephrobronchial fistula.[32, 33]

8. *Infiltration of flank stripe.* Blurring and widening of the extraperitoneal flank fat indicates spread of the perinephric infection into the paranephric spaces (Fig. 22–3).

Excretory Urography

Specific abnormalities seen on plain abdominal radiographs, such as indistinct renal outline and renal displacement, are more easily recognized when contrast opacification of the renal parenchyma and collecting system is coupled with linear tomography (Fig. 22–4). The following may also be found:

1. *Diminution in concentration and volume of the contrast medium excreted by the affected kidney.* This is a manifestation of reduced urine flow. Complete nonvisualization of the collecting system may occur.

2. *Compression and distortion of the pyelocalyceal system.* Calyces may be stretched, partially filled, or amputated (Fig. 22–5). The proximal ureter may be compressed and displaced anteriorly and medially by the perinephric effusion. Compression may be severe enough to cause dilatation of the upper collecting system.

3. *Opacification of a thickened Gerota's fascia as a result of inflammation and hypervascularity.*

4. *Fixation of the kidney.* Normally, renal mobility of 2 to 6 cm can be shown on erect films or with respiratory excursions.[34] A perinephric process tends to fix the kidney in the majority of patients.[9] However, prior infection, tumor, previous surgery, diaphragmatic immobility, or subphrenic abscess may lead to a false-positive result. Renal mobility may be assessed by fluoroscopy or by the technique of Mathe.[35] This involves doubly exposing an abdominal film during inspiration and expiration. The normally mobile kidney will reveal a blurred renal silhouette, while the outline of the fixed kidney will remain sharp (Fig. 22–7).

5. *Extravasation of contrast material from the collecting system to the perinephric space.* This is a highly specific sign for perinephric abscess, although it rarely is seen.[36] The extravasation may be demonstrated by retrograde pyelography or fistulography (Figs. 22–8 and 22–9).

Radionuclide Imaging

Gallium-67 (Ga-67) citrate, initially introduced as a tumor-scanning agent in 1950, has been helpful in the diagnosis of intrarenal, perinephric, and other abscesses when more conventional radiographic studies have failed (Fig. 22–10).[37, 38] It is particularly useful when the normal anatomy is distorted by previous surgery, polycystic kidney disease, congenital anomalies, or chronic pyelonephritis.[39] The accuracy of Ga-67 in detecting perinephric abscess has not been firmly established, however. Experiences with abdominal abscesses suggest a true positive rate of 90% and an even higher true negative rate.[40] Abnormal uptake of Ga-67 is nonspecific and may be due to infection (i.e., pyelonephritis), neoplastic infiltration, acute tubular necrosis, or vasculitis.[41] Other disadvantages of Ga-67 imaging are the long time delay for adequate tracer accumulation—sometimes up to 72 hours—and a relatively high radiation dose. Ga-67 is normally taken up by the colon and sites of postoperative healing, making

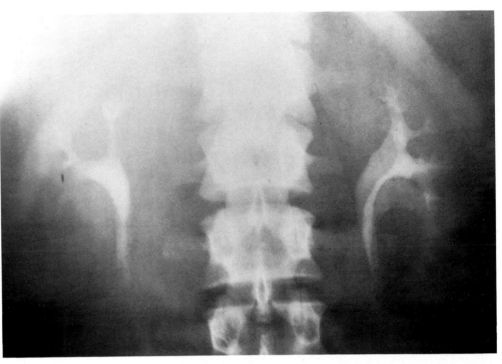

Figure 22–7. Double-exposure breathing film of right perinephric abscess in an elderly male. Inspiration-expiration double-exposure radiograph of kidneys during IVU reveals fixation of right kidney by perinephric inflammation. This is a nonspecific finding that may also be seen in any case of limited diaphragmatic excursion.

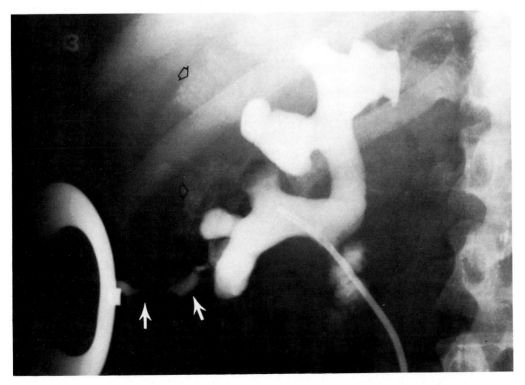

Figure 22–8. Pyelocutaneous fistula secondary to perinephric abscess. Retrograde pyelogram demonstrates hydronephrosis and a fistulous communication *(arrows)* between a lower-pole calyx and the flank, secondary to a perinephric abscess. Pyelointerstitial backflow is present *(open arrows)*. Note extravasation around ureteropelvic junction.

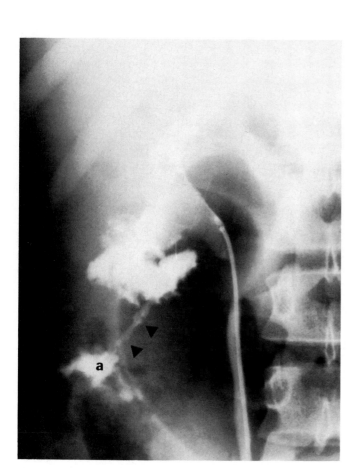

Figure 22–9. Sinus track formation secondary to perinephric abscess. Retrograde pyelogram shows irregularity and distortion of the right renal collecting system and a lower-pole sinus track *(arrowheads)* to an abscess cavity (a) in the perinephric space.

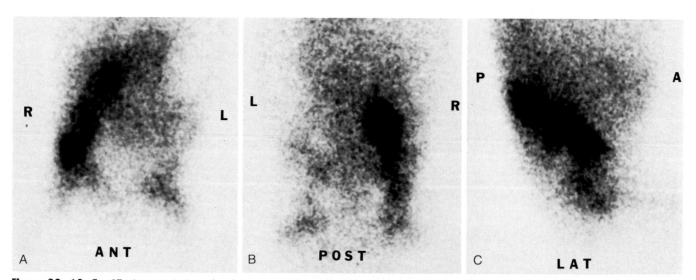

Figure 22–10. Ga-67-citrate scintigraphy. Four-year-old female with right psoas abscess. Images obtained 41 hours after injection Ga-67-citrate. Note an intense accumulation of radiopharmaceutical in the right psoas region. *A,* Anterior view. *B,* Posterior view. *C,* Right lateral view. (A = anterior, P = posterior.)

interpretation of studies difficult in these cases. The lack of anatomical detail provided by Ga-67 images makes it difficult, at times, to determine whether one is dealing with primary renal or perinephric inflammation.

Indium-111–labeled leukocytes have recently been proposed as a more sensitive means of localizing inflammatory foci.[42] However, the effectiveness of this technique with perinephric abscess has not yet been established.

Angiography

Since the advent of ultrasonography and CT, renal angiography has rarely been performed in cases of suspected perinephric abscesses. Renal vessels have a unique vasoconstrictive response to inflammation, in contrast to other areas that respond with vasodilatation.[43] Because of vasospasm in the area of inflammation, angiography (if performed) reveals persistent arterial filling ("staining") after the surrounding kidney has reached the nephrogram phase.[44] However, the differentiation between renal inflammatory lesions and hypovascular necrotic malignancies is often difficult, if not impossible.[45]

Arteriographic findings that suggest perinephric involvement include the increased number and size of the perforating arteries extending from the kidney, stretching of tortuous and prominent capsular and perhaps pelvic arteries around the abscess margin, and a tissue blush (Fig. 22–7).[46] The nephrogram phase may show a localized or diffuse loss of sharpness of the renal outline due to the inflammatory edema involving the perinephric fat.

Ultrasonography

Ultrasonography provides a clear anatomical display of the kidney and its adjacent structures. Fluid collections anterior and posterior to the kidney that are poorly seen with conventional radiographs are clearly visualized by ultrasonography. The sonographic signs of abscess vary with the homogeneity of the abscess contents. Perinephric abscesses present a complex sonographic pattern (Figs. 22–11 and 22–12). They transmit sound well, but usually contain multiple low-level echoes. The wall of the abscess may be smooth or irregular. Occasionally, internal organized exudate may layer dependently, creating a debris-fluid level within the abscess. Internal septations may also be present. A perinephric abscess may be highly echogenic if it contains numerous small gas bubbles (Fig. 22–13).[47]

The sonographic features of a perinephric abscess are by no means tissue specific. Urinomas, lymphoceles, and hematomas may present with similar sonographic findings. Percutaneous needle aspiration under sonographic guidance to obtain fluid and/or tissue for culture and laboratory analysis is often necessary to establish a definitive diagnosis.[48, 49] Once a diagnosis of perinephric abscess is confirmed, a drainage catheter can be placed into the cavity, using a needle-wire exchange method under combined sonographic and fluoroscopic guidance. Successful percutaneous drainage of perinephric abscesses have been reported by several groups.[50, 51] Successful therapy demands prompt and thorough drainage, preferably by percutaneous techniques, where possible, or by operative intervention if percutaneous techniques fail.

Computed Tomography

The introduction of CT has made possible the direct visualization of the retroperitoneum with a level of clarity unsurpassed by any other imaging method. Sub-5-second scanners coupled with improvement of software technology have made it possible to evaluate even lean and

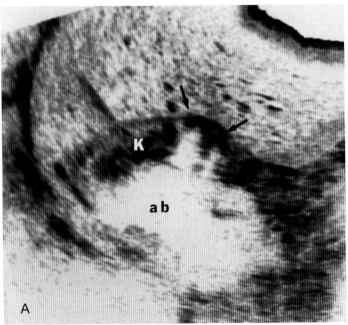
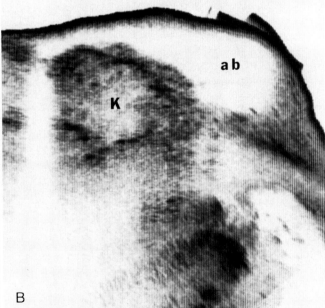

Figure 22–11. Large perinephric abscess. Sonogram shows abscess with posterior extension to subcutaneous tissues. Patient presented with long history of a right flank mass and low-grade fever. *A,* Sagittal scan through right kidney (K) demonstrates a large hypoechoic abscess (ab) extending posteriorly and inferiorly. Note renal calculi *(arrows)* causing acoustic shadowing. *B,* Transverse sonogram through lower pole of right kidney (K) in a prone patient shows the abscess (ab) extending from the perinephric space into the subcutaneous tissues.

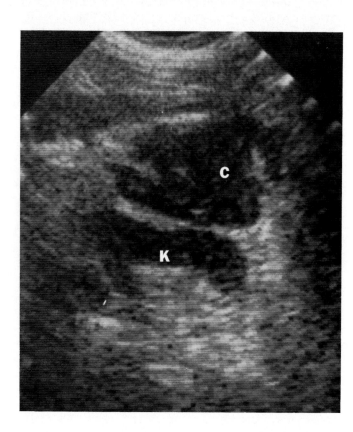

Figure 22–12. Perinephric abscess. Coronal oblique sonogram demonstrates a complex fluid collection with multiple internal echoes (C) located lateral to the right kidney (K). (Courtesy Michael Hill, M.D., Washington, D.C.)

Figure 22–13. Gas-containing perinephric abscess. Sonogram reveals extremely echogenic mass in the perinephric space apposing the posterior surface of the kidney. The innumerable echoes are attributable to microair bubbles within the abscess. (From Kressel HY, Filly RA: Ultrasonic appearance of gas-containing abscesses in the abdomen. AJR 130(1):71–73, 1978. © by Am Roentgen Ray Soc.)

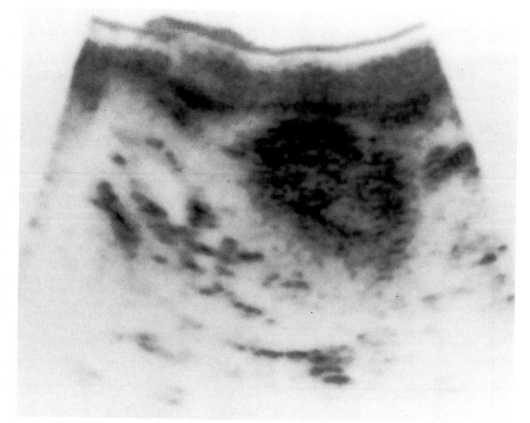

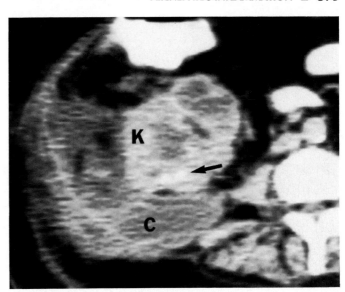

Figure 22–14. Sixty-three-year-old female presenting with perinephric abscess after a right percutaneous nephrostomy. There is a history of left nephrectomy. Noncontrast CT scan demonstrates an irregular low-attenuation collection (C) involving the dorsal aspect of the right perinephric and posterior paranephric spaces. There is infiltration of the subcutaneous fat and anteromedial displacement of the severely hydronephrotic kidney (K). Two renal calculi (arrow) are also present. Extension into the right flank tissues can also be seen.

critically ill patients. CT is more accurate than ultrasonography in detecting perinephric infections,[52] and is superior to it in delineating the extent of perinephric and paranephric fluid collections. Because of its high accuracy and the precision with which retroperitoneal anatomy can be displayed, CT is now the procedure of choice for evaluating patients with suspected perinephric abscess.[53, 54] Ultrasonography, because of its flexibility and mobility, is reserved for patients who are too ill to come to the radiology department for a CT examination and guiding percutaneous aspiration/drainage procedures. Ultrasonography has the added advantage of ready availability and in most hospitals is more quickly obtainable than CT. Initial screening for perinephric abscess with ultrasonography, therefore, seems reasonable, with CT to follow if the results are equivocal.

Although a diagnosis of perinephric abscess can be made on noncontrast CT scans, delineation of the disease extent and separation between the renal and perinephric components is often much easier on contrast-enhanced scans. On CT, a perinephric abscess has characteristics similar to a renal abscess; it is a well-defined collection with thick, irregular walls of soft-tissue density (Figs. 22–14 to 22–18). The center of the process often has an intermediate attenuation value between that of water and nonenhanced renal parenchyma. After intravenous administration of water-soluble iodinated contrast medium, the walls or fascial borders of the abscess may enhance, whereas the center of the abscess remains of low density, creating a so-called rind sign (Fig. 22–17).[51] Gas bubbles or a gas-fluid level may exist within the lesion, which assure the diagnosis of a perinephric abscess (assuming an iatrogenic source of gas has been excluded). In the absence of gas bubbles, a perinephric abscess may be confused with a hematoma or a urinoma. Percutaneous needle aspiration of the suspected abnormality under radiological guidance is often necessary for differentiation of these entities.

In patients with perinephric abscesses, the ipsilateral kidney may be focally or diffusely enlarged. Discrete hypodense lesion(s) representing abscesses may be seen within the renal parenchyma. This characteristic can be best appreciated on postcontrast scans. Other CT findings include asymmetrical ipsilateral enlargement of the psoas muscle, focal ipsilateral thickening of the Gerota's fascia, and obliteration of normal adjacent tissue planes.[55] However, the latter findings are nonspecific and can be seen in patients with pancreatitis and following colectomy.

Magnetic Resonance Imaging

The experience in using magnetic resonance (MR) imaging for the detection and diagnosis of perinephric abscess is limited. However, MR does have several theoretical advantages, which make it an ideal imaging technique. It does not use ionizing radiation, has a superior contrast sensitivity, is not hampered by bone, gas or nonferrous metallic clips, and has a direct multiplanar imaging capability. The disadvantages of MR include insensitivity to calcifications, long imaging time, more stringent patient requirements (patients with intracranial aneurysm clips, pacemakers, and severe claustrophobia are excluded from MR examinations) and high cost. Because of these limitations, MR is reserved for cases in which ultrasound and CT findings are equivocal. Preliminary data suggest that MR is superior to CT in delineating involvement of psoas muscle and other adjacent soft-tissue structures.[56–58]

The signal intensity of a perinephric abscess is variable and depends upon its fluid composition. The presence of proteinaceous material in an abscess shortens its T1 value and leads to a relatively high signal intensity on T1-weighted images.[57] In general, the signal intensity of the abscess is intermediate between that of urine (or pure water) and that of a soft-tissue tumor on T1-weighted images. On T2-weighted images, the central portion of an abscess has a very high signal intensity, whereas the wall has a medium to low signal intensity (Fig. 22–19). Debris-fluid levels are easily appreciated. If a perinephric abscess is entirely surrounded by retroperitoneal fat, it is best seen on a T1-weighted image. In contrast, if a perinephric abscess has extended into adjacent soft-tissue structures, its border is best delineated on a T2-weighted image. As in the case of CT, a definitive diagnosis of a perinephric abscess by MR depends on the demonstration of gas bubbles within the mass. Unfortunately, MR is not as sensitive as CT in detecting small gas collections.

Text continued on page 879

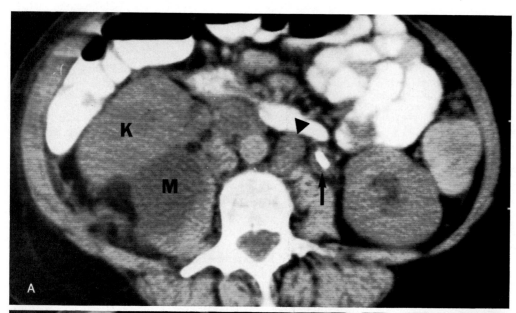

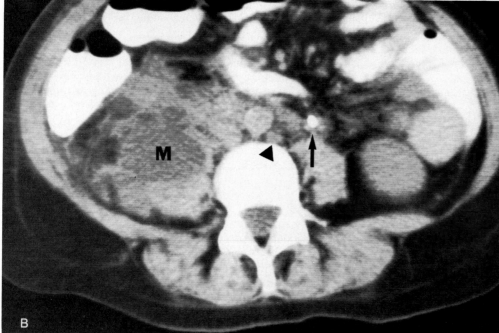

Figure 22–15. Right perinephric abscess secondary to perforation of the proximal ureter. *A,* CT scan shows large extrarenal collection (M) extending posteriorly and inferiorly to the right kidney (K). A left ureteral stent *(arrow)* and retroperitoneal adenopathy *(arrowhead)* are also seen. *B,* A CT scan caudad to *A* shows extension of perinephric abscess (M) inferiorly involving the right psoas, perinephric space, and anterior paranephric space. The inferior vena cava is obliterated by the inflammatory process. Note the thickened posterior abdominal wall muscles.

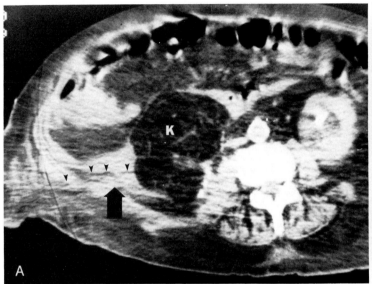

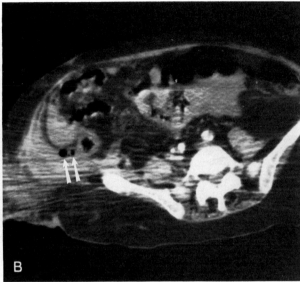

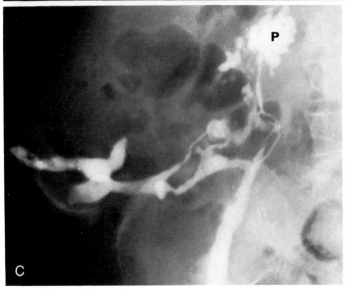

Figure 22–16. Perinephric abscess in 94-year-old female with chronic drainage from the right flank. *A*, CT scan shows mixed attenuation process (infection) *(large arrow)* in the right perinephric and posterior paranephric spaces. The overlying abdominal wall and subcutaneous tissues are also involved. There is total fatty replacement of the nonfunctioning kidney (K). Extension of the process into subcutaneous and flank tissues is noted *(arrowheads)*. *B*, The abscess extends inferiorly to the level of the iliac crest. Gas bubbles are seen within the collection *(arrows)*. *C*, Injection of the tract demonstrates a network of fistulae communicating with the pyelocalyceal system (P) of this functionless kidney.

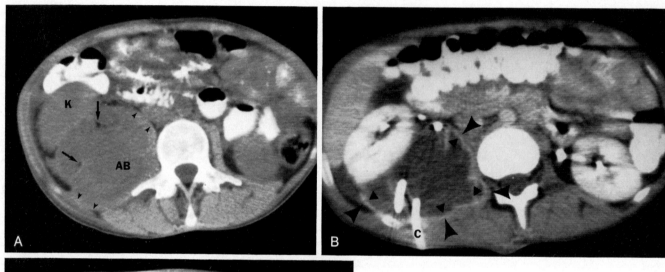

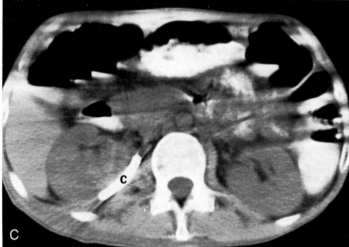

Figure 22–17. "Rind sign"—CT scan. *A,* Large, septated perinephric abscess (AB) displaces right kidney (K) antero-laterally and has a faint rind *(arrowheads)* of slightly increased attenuation. A few gas collections are seen *(arrows).* *B,* After administration of intravenous contrast material, there is enhancement of the wall ("rind-sign") *(arrowheads).* A drainage catheter (C) has been placed percutaneously. *C,* Follow-up scan at 8 days shows complete resolution after percutaneous drainage and antibiotic treatment. Kidney has returned to anatomical position. (C = catheter.)

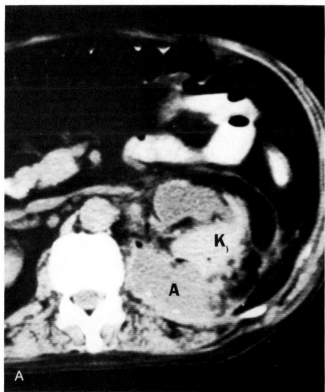

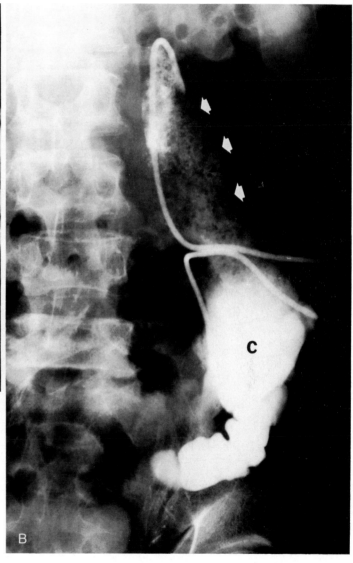

Figure 22–18. Colonic involvement by a left perinephric abscess. *A,* CT scan. A large perinephric abscess (A) causes slight anterior displacement of the hydronephrotic left kidney (K). This collection was subsequently drained under CT guidance. *B,* Tube injection. Injection of drainage catheter with contrast demonstrates fistulous communication between descending colon (C) and abscess *(arrows).*

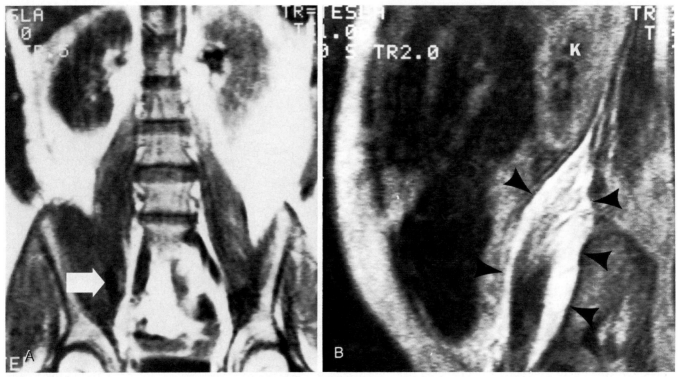

Figure 22–19. Magnetic resonance imaging. Iliopsoas abscess in a 40-year-old male with right flank pain. *A,* On the T1-weighted coronal image, the abscess *(arrow)* has a very low signal intensity, similar to that of the normal psoas muscle. *B,* The high signal intensity on the sagittal spin-echo T2-weighted image allows the abscess and surrounding inflammatory reaction *(arrowheads)* to be easily distinguished from normal muscle. (K = kidney.) (Courtesy RJ Lorig, M.D., Cleveland, Ohio.)

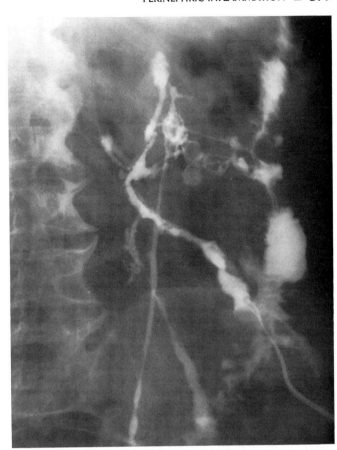

Figure 22–20. Nephrocolocutaneous fistula secondary to perinephric abscess. Patient with long-standing calculous pyelonephritis and perinephric abscess. Contrast injection of draining fistula in flank fills renal collecting system, ureter, and left colon from multiple sites. Note left renal calculus.

COMPLICATIONS

The potential complications of perinephric abscess are numerous. Inadequately treated, the abscess may spread extensively into the retroperitoneum and pelvis, producing increasingly severe sepsis, and even death. Rarely, the abscess may rupture into the peritoneum, or it may cross the diaphragm and spread into the chest. Spontaneous decompression may occur, resulting in fistulas to the skin, colon, small bowel, duodenum, stomach, bladder, or even the lung (Figs. 22–20 and 22–21).[24] Empyema, atelectasis, and pneumonia are serious and potentially lethal complications.

Figure 22–21. Nephrobronchial fistula secondary to perinephric abscess. In the case of this long-standing calculous perinephric abscess, there were eventual erosion through left hemidiaphragm and extrusion of stones into lung and bronchial tree. The patient complained of "coughing up stones." (From Gordonson J, Sargent EN: Nephrobroncholithiasis: Report of a case secondary to renal lithiasis with a nephrobronchial fistula. AJR 110:701–703, 1970, © by Am Roentgen Ray Soc.)

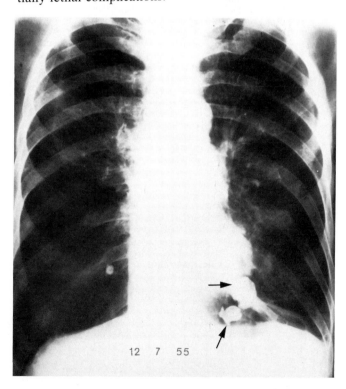

TREATMENT

Until recently, the morbidity and mortality of patients with perinephric abscess was relatively high. The main reason for this, undoubtedly, was delay in recognizing the lesion. Because of the availability of CT and ultrasonography, in addition to an imposing antibiotic armamentarium, the outcome is no longer fearsome; however, the need for prompt diagnosis and vigorous treatment remains critical. Percutaneous abscess drainage, which has been a boon in many other areas, has been slow to gain

acceptance in the treatment of perinephric abscess. Perhaps this is due to the fear that these abscesses are too large or compartmented to be drained efficiently without surgery. Whatever the case, it now appears that almost all of these purulent collections can be managed nicely by percutaneous drainage.[59] This in no way mitigates the need to search out and treat—often by nephrectomy—the underlying renal disease; nevertheless, preliminary percutaneous abscess drainage may be life saving as a temporary holding maneuver, permitting an otherwise dangerously ill patient to recover sufficiently to allow anesthesia and surgery to be performed safely. De-

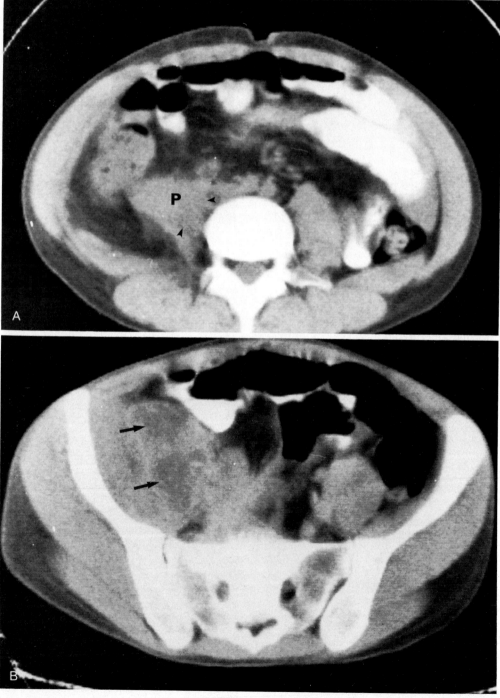

Figure 22–22. Iliopsoas abscess—Noncontrast CT scans. *A,* The right psoas muscle (P) is enlarged and contains, medially, poorly defined areas of decreased attenuation *(arrowheads).* Inflammatory response causes poor definition of the muscle margins and increased attenuation of the adjacent fat. *B,* Inferior extension of inflammatory process involves iliopsoas muscle *(arrows).*

compression of the abscess also renders later renal surgery less difficult.

PSOAS ABSCESS

The psoas muscle originates from fibers of the transverse processes of the T12 vertebra as well as all lumbar vertebrae. The muscle fibers fuse into the psoas muscle proper, which passes inferiorly in a paraspinal location. As it exits from the pelvis, the psoas proceeds in a more anterior direction, merging with the iliac muscle to become the iliopsoas. The iliopsoas passes beneath the inguinal ligament to insert on the lesser trochanter of the femur. At its superior attachment, the psoas muscle passes beneath the arcuate ligament of the diaphragm. Owing to differences in the medial attachment site for the posterior renal fascia, the psoas muscle is separated from the perinephric space above the renal hilus, whereas it is in direct contact with the perinephric space below the renal hilus.[60, 61] Infection within the psoas muscle is commonly due to direct extension from contiguous structures such as the spine, kidney, bowel loops, and pancreas.[62] In one series, 8 out of 10 cases of nontuberculous psoas abscess in adults resulted from direct extension of adjacent bowel lesions.[63] These included appendicitis, diverticulitis, Crohn's disease, and perforated colon carcinoma. With the decreasing incidence of tuberculous

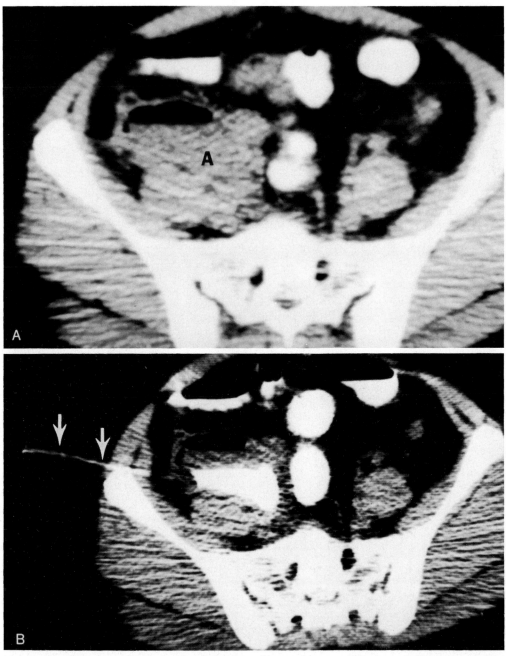

Figure 22–23. Psoas muscle abscess arising as a complication of hysterectomy—CT scans. *A,* Noncontrast CT scan shows a gas-containing abscess (A) involving the right psoas muscle. *B,* Repeat scan after percutaneous placement of a drainage catheter *(arrows).* Iodinated contrast material has been injected into the cavity.

spondylitis, the majority of psoas abscesses now encountered are of pyogenic origin.

The most common offending organisms are *Staphylococcus aureus* and *E. coli*.[64, 65] Fungal agents such as *Nocardia* and *Candida* as well as coccidioidomycosis also have been cultured from patients on immunosuppressive therapy.[65]

Patients with psoas abscess most often complain of unilateral flank, hip, or back pain, particularly upon extension of the ipsilateral leg.[65] Other signs include fever, a tender mass in the abdomen or in the iliac fossa, and scoliosis. If there is extensive inferior dissection of the inflammatory process, a psoas abscess may present as an inflammatory mass in the proximal thigh.

Conventional radiographic findings in psoas abscesses include bone destruction from either osteomyelitis or disc space infection and adjacent paraspinal widening. Gas bubbles dissecting along the psoas shadow are a useful finding. By urography, the kidney and proximal ureter are often displaced laterally if the psoas abscess is in the abdomen, whereas the urinary bladder and distal ureter are usually displaced medially if the abscess is in the pelvis. Ureteral obstruction with hydronephrosis also may occur.[64–66]

Ga-67-citrate imaging and ultrasonography can provide helpful information (Fig. 22–10).[67–68] However, Ga-67 imaging is time-consuming, and ultrasonography is often hampered by bowel gas and bone. As in the case of perinephric abscess, CT has become the procedure of choice for evaluating patients with suspected psoas abnormality.[60] MR has been shown to provide better contrast between the normal and abnormal psoas than CT in some patients.[56, 69] However, CT scanning is still a better screening procedure at the present time, because it requires a shorter imaging time and is more readily available.

On CT scans, the involved psoas muscle is often diffusely enlarged, usually with central areas of low attenuation value (0 to 30 H) (Fig. 22–22).[70, 71] Visualization of the abscess can frequently be improved on the contrast-enhanced scans. Uniform enlargement of the psoas can also be seen in patients with hemorrhage and neoplastic involvement of the muscle. However, demonstration of gas bubbles within the psoas is virtually pathognomonic of an abscess. In cases in which the CT findings are nonspecific, CT can be used to guide percutaneous needle aspiration of the observed abnormality to obtain tissue for microbiological culture (Fig. 22–23). In cases in which the diagnosis of psoas abscess is certain, CT can be used to guide percutaneous drainage.

References

1. Thorley JD, Jones SR, Sanford JP: Perinephric abscess. Medicine, 53:541, 1974.
2. Sheinfeld J, Erturk E, Spataro RF, Cockett ATK: Perinephric abscess—Current concepts. J Urol 137:191, 1987.
3. Meyers MA: Dynamic Radiology of the Abdomen: Normal and Pathologic Anatomy, 2nd Ed. New York, Springer Verlag, 1982.
4. Evans JA, Meyers MA, Bosniak MA: Acute renal perirenal infections. Semin Roentgenol 6:274, 1971.
5. Kunin M: Bridging septa of the perinephric space: Anatomic, pathologic and diagnostic considerations. Radiology 158:361, 1986.
6. Mitchell GAG: The renal fascia. Br J Surg 37:257, 1950.
7. Congdon ED, Edson JN: The cone of renal fascia in the adult white male. Anat Rec 80:289, 1941.
8. Mitchell GAG: The spread of retroperitoneal effusions arising in the renal regions. Br Med J 2:1134, 1939.
9. Parks RE: The radiographic diagnosis of perinephric abscess. Urology 64:555, 1950.
10. Salvatierra O, Bucklew WB, Morrow JW: Perinephric abscess: A report of 71 cases. J Urol 98:296, 1967.
11. McGahan JP: Perinephric abscess secondary to ruptured retrocecal appendix diagnosed by computerized tomography. Urology 19:217, 1982.
12. Childs GJ, Pickleman J, Churchill RJ, et al: Renal cell carcinoma complicated by perinephric abscess and colon perforation. Urol Radiol 4:37, 1982.
13. Maglinte D, Pollack HM: Retroperitoneal abscess: A presentation of colon carcinoma. Gastrointest Radiol 8:177, 1983.
14. Atcheson DW: Perinephric abscess with a review of 17 cases. J Urol 46:201, 1941.
15. Vermooten V: The mechanism of perinephric and perinephritic abscesses: A clinical and pathological study. J Urol 30:181, 1933.
16. Le Comte RM: Perinephritis and perirenal abscess. J Urol 56:636, 1946.
17. Elkin M: Infections of the urinary tract. *In* Elkin M (ed): Radiology of the Urinary System. Boston, Little, Brown & Company, p 148, 1980.
18. Truesdale BH, Rous SN, Nelson RP: Perinephric abscess: A review of 26 cases. J Urol 118:910, 1977.
19. Malgieri JJ, Kursh ED, Persky L: The changing clinicopathological pattern of abscesses in or adjacent to the kidney. J Urol 118:230, 1977.
20. Anderson KA, McAninch JW: Renal abscesses: Classification and review of 40 cases. Urology 16:333, 1980.
21. Merimsky E, Feldman C: Perinephric abscess: Report of 19 cases. Int Surg 66:79, 1981.
22. Cotran RS: Experimental pyelonephritis. *In* Rouiller C, Muller AF (eds): The Kidney, Vol II. New York, Academic Press, 1969, p 269.
23. Whalen J: Radiation Risks in Medical Imaging. Chicago, Year Book Medical Publishers, 1984.
24. Doughney KB, Dineen MK, Venable, DD: Nephrobronchial colonic fistula complicating perinephric abscess. J Urol 135:765, 1986.
25. Love L, Baker D, Ramsey R: Gas producing perinephric abscess. AJR 119:783, 1973.
26. Braman R, Cross RR: Perinephric abscess producing a pneumonephrogram. J Urol 75:194, 1956.
27. Rudy CD, Woodside JR: Perinephric abscess radiologically mimicking dilated bowel. JAMA 249:401, 1983.
28. Meyers MA: Colonic changes secondary to left perinephritis: New observations. Radiology 11:525, 1974.
29. Morgan WR, Nyberg LM: Perinephric and intrarenal abscesses. Urology 26:529, 1985.
30. Shane JH, Harris M: Roentgenologic diagnosis of perinephric abscess. J Urol 32:19, 1934.
31. Rigler LG, Marrson MH: Perinephric abscess: A roentgenological and clinical study. Am J Surg 13:459, 1931.
32. Nesbit RM, Dick VS: Pulmonary complications of acute renal and perirenal suppuration. AJR 44:161, 1940.
33. Hampel N, Sidor TA, Persky L: Nephrobronchial fistula. Urology 16:608, 1980.
34. Baron RD: Respiratory pyelography: A study of renal motion in health and disease. AJR 44:71, 1940.
35. Mathe CP: Diagnosis and treatment of perinephric abscess: Renal fixation, a new roentgenographic sign. Am J Surg 38:35, 1937.
36. Hotchkiss RS: Perinephric abscess. Am J Surg 85:471, 1953.
37. Hopkins GB, Hall RL, Mende CW: Gallium-67 scintigraphy for the diagnosis and localization of perinephric abscess. J Urol 115:126, 1976.
38. Sweet R, Keane WF: Perinephric abscess in patients with polycystic kidney disease undergoing chronic hemodialysis. Nephron 23:237, 1979.
39. Hempel N, Class RN, Persky L: Value of gallium-67 scintigraphy in the diagnosis of localized renal and perirenal inflammation. J Urol 124:311, 1980.
40. Hauser MF, Alderson PO: Gallium-67 imaging in abdominal disease. Semin Nucl Med 8:251, 1978.
41. Patel R, Tanaka T, Mishkin F, et al: Gallium-67 scan: Aid to diagnosis and treatment of renal and perirenal infections. Urology 16:225, 1980.
42. Coleman RE, Brock RE, Welch DM, Maxwell JG: Indium-111 labeled leukocyte in the evaluation of suspected abdominal abscesses. Am J Surg 139:99, 1980.

43. Zweifach BW, Rolewenstin BE, Chambers R: Response of blood capillaries to acute hemorrhage in the rat. Am Physiol 142:80, 1944.
44. Becker JA, Kanter IE, Perl S: Rapid intrarenal circulation. AJR 109:167, 1970.
45. Koehler PR: The roentgen diagnosis of renal inflammatory masses—special emphasis on angiographic changes. Radiology 112:247, 1974.
46. Caplan LH, Siegelman SS, Bosniak MA: Angiography and inflammatory space occupying lesions of the kidney. Radiology 88:14, 1967.
47. Kressel HY, Filly RA: Ultrasonographic appearance of gas-containing abscesses in the abdomen. AJR 130:71, 1978.
48. Conrad MR, Sanders RC, Mascrado AD: Perinephric abscess aspiration using ultrasound guidance. AJR 128:459, 1977.
49. Schneider M, Becker JA, Staiano S, Campos E: Sonographic-radiographic correlation of renal and perirenal infections. AJR 127:1007, 1976.
50. Elyaderani MK, Subramanian VP, Burgess JE: Diagnosis and percutaneous drainage of a perinephric abscess by ultrasound and fluoroscopy. J Urol 125:405, 1981.
51. Gerzof SG: Percutaneous drainage of renal and perirenal abscess. Urol Radiol 2:171, 1981.
52. Hoddick W, Jeffrey RB, Goldberg HI, et al: CT and sonography of severe renal and perirenal infections. AJR 140:517, 1983.
53. Mendez G, Isikoff MB, Morillo G: The role of computed tomography in the diagnosis of renal and perirenal abscesses. J Urol 122:582, 1979.
54. Saksouk FA, Tipton-Donovan A, Amis ES, Goldman SM: Computed tomography of perirenal and pararenal inflammatory disease complicating renal calculi. Urology 24:200, 1984.
55. Bova JG, Potter JL, Arevalos E, et al: Renal and perirenal infection: The role of computerized tomography. J Urol 133:375, 1985.
56. Lee JKT, Glazer HS: Psoas muscle disorders: MR imaging. Radiology 160:683, 1986.
57. Terrier F, Didier R, Hannu P, et al: MR imaging of body fluid collections. J Comput Assist Tomogr 10:953, 1986.
58. Totty W, Murphy WA, Lee JKT: Soft-tissue tumors: MR imaging. Radiology 160:135, 1986.
59. Gerzoff SG, Gale ME: Computed tomography and ultrasonography for diagnosis and treatment of renal and retroperitoneal abscesses. Urol Clin North Am 9:185, 1982.
60. Feldberg MAM, Koehler PR, van Waes FGM: Psoas compartment disease studied by computed tomography. Radiology 148:505, 1983.
61. Raptopoulous V, Kleinman PK, Marks S Jr: Renal fascial pathway: Posterior extension of pancreatic effusions within the anterior pararenal space. Radiology 158:367, 1986.
62. Kyle J: Psoas abscess in Crohn's disease. Gastroenterology 61:149, 1971.
63. Hardcastle JD: Acute nontuberculous psoas abscess. Br J Surg 57:103, 1970.
64. Firor HV: Acute psoas abscess in children. Clin Pediatr 4:228, 1972.
65. Lam SF, Hodgson AR: Non-spinal pyogenic psoas abscess. J Bone Joint Surg 48:867, 1966.
66. Oliff M, Chuang VP: Retroperitoneal iliac fossa pyogenic abscess. Radiology 126:647, 1978.
67. Shimshak RR, Korobkin M, Hoffer PB: Complementary role of Gallium citrate imaging in computed tomography and the evaluation of suspected abdominal infection. J Nucl Med 19:262, 1978.
68. Laing FC, Jacob RP: Value of ultrasonography in the detection of retroperitoneal inflammatory masses. Radiology 123:169, 1972.
69. Weinreb JC, Cohen JM, Maravilla KR: Iliopsoas muscles: MR study of normal anatomy and disease. Radiology 156:435, 1985.
70. Ralls PW, Boswell W, Henderson R, et al: CT of inflammatory disease of the psoas muscle. AJR 134:767, 1980.
71. Jeffrey RB, Callen PW, Federle MP: Computed tomography of psoas abscesses. J Comput Assist Tomogr 4:639, 1980.

23

Inflammatory Conditions of the Renal Pelvis and Ureter

ROBERT F. SPATARO

Ascending infection of the lower urinary tract may lead to infection of the ureter, renal pelvis, and intrarenal collecting system. This and the resulting inflammation of the renal pelvis and ureter may cause dynamic changes that lead to abnormalities of size and function of the ureter, such as ureteral hypotonia or atony, abnormal ureteral peristalsis, and ureteral dilatation.[1-8] These are the most common abnormalities of the renal pelvis and ureter associated with infection and inflammation and are usually reversible after appropriate treatment.

Acute infection of the renal pelvis and ureter may also cause changes in the appearance of the ureter, such as mucosal striations, edema, and severe infection that can lead to the formation of gas in the wall of the ureter—ureteritis emphysematosa.[9, 10]

Infection and inflammation uncommonly lead to chronic and more permanent histopathological changes in the renal pelvis and ureter, such as inflammatory stricture formation (obliterative pyelitis),[88] eosinophilic pyeloureteritis,[11] pyeloureteritis cystica,[12] ureteral diverticulosis (pseudodiverticulosis),[13] plasma cell granuloma,[14] xanthogranulomatous pyeloureteritis,[15] malacoplakia,[16] and keratinizing desquamative squamous metaplasia (KDSM), including leukoplakia and cholesteatoma.[17] These lesions are all uncommon, but they may have characteristic clinical and diagnostic imaging features that allow a presumptive diagnosis.

URETERAL DILATATION: NONOBSTRUCTIVE HYDRONEPHROSIS OF INFECTION; PSEUDO-OBSTRUCTION OF INFECTION

Infection may lead to acute changes in the ureter and pelvis, even in the absence of reflux. Among the many such abnormalities is dilatation of the calyces, renal pelvis, and ureter.[3, 7, 8] Dilatation of the collecting system may occur in up to 12.5% of patients with acute pyelonephritis.[7] Shopfner described dilatation of the calyces, pelves, and ureter—the nonobstructive hydronephrosis and hydroureter of infection— and ascribed it to "ileus," caused by bacteria (endotoxins) reducing ureteral peristalsis and resulting in poor emptying and consequent dilatation.[5, 6] This nonobstructive dilatation of the collecting system, not associated with reflux, was shown to completely resolve after appropriate antibiotic therapy and resolution of the infection.[4-6] Such dilatation of the collecting system may appear as mild segmental or generalized dilatation of the ureter; it must be differentiated from true obstruction, which it may mimic, particularly when appearance of contrast in the calyces is delayed (Fig. 23–1). Segmental dilatation of the renal pelvis or calyces may also occur, presumably by the same mechanism.

The ureteral ileus postulated by Shopfner as the cause of the nonobstructive dilatation of the collecting system with infection has been experimentally proven by a number of investigators.[18-23] Teague and Boyarsky, and Boyarsky and colleagues,[20, 23] using a dog model, and King and Cox,[22] using a perfused isolated ureteral strip model of both animal and human ureters, have shown suppression of ureteral peristaltic activity after instillation of live *Escherichia coli* bacteria into the ureter. Peristaltic activity ceased soon after introduction of the bacteria and could be reversed by removing the bacteria. Distention of the renal pelves, calyces, and ureter accompanied the cessation of ureteral activity.[20] The same effect was observed using a heat-killed *E. coli* suspension and also *E. coli* endotoxin. *Klebsiella, Proteus, Pseudomonas* and *Staphylococcus aureus* caused similar ureteral smooth-muscle inhibitory effects. It must be kept in mind that these changes may be so profound that they can closely mimic the changes of ureteral obstruction.

STRIATED URETER AND RENAL PELVIS RESULTING FROM ACUTE INFECTION

Mucosal striations of the renal pelvis and ureter due to mucosal redundancy from distention may result from vesicoureteral reflux (VUR) or obstruction[24, 25] and occasionally occur as a normal variant.[26] Longitudinal mucosal striations also have been described as being caused by urinary tract infection.[9, 27, 28] The longitudinal mucosal striations accompanying infection that are unassociated with VUR or obstruction may be attributed to either of two factors: (1) mucosal and submucosal edema or (2) ureteral dilatation due to bacterial endotoxic ileus. Mucosal and submucosal edema is probably the cause in many cases. An example of mucosal striations in an elderly adult with severe pyelonephritis without obstruction or VUR is shown in Figure 23–2. Mucosal striations due to infection are much less common than those resulting from VUR or ureteral dilatation from previous obstruction. The mucosal striations associated with upper urinary tract infection disappear with resolution of the infection and may be confused with submucosal hemorrhage (Fig. 23–3). Isolated longitudinal mucosal striations may occasionally be seen in the nearly empty normal ureter.

URETERITIS EMPHYSEMATOSA

Ureteritis emphysematosa, or intramural ureteral gas, is a rare manifestation of acute infection.[10, 29, 30] It may be seen in conjunction with cystitis emphysematosa and extension into the ureter[29] or may occur as an isolated involvement of the ureter without affecting the blad-

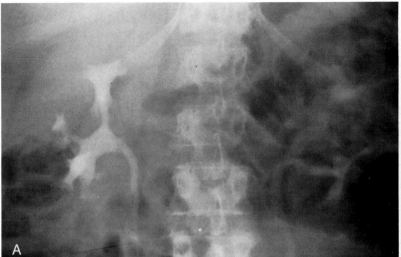

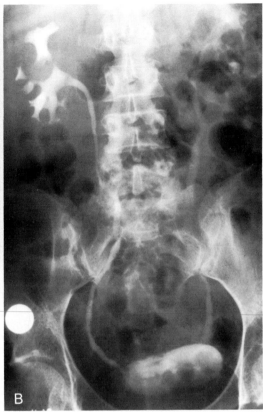

Figure 23–1. Nonobstructive hydronephrosis of infection (pseudo-obstruction of infection). A 45-year-old woman presented with left flank pain, fever, pyuria, microscopic hematuria, and bacteriuria. An excretory urogram was performed because of the severity of the left flank pain. *A,* A coned view of the kidneys and upper collecting system shows a normal right kidney. The left kidney is enlarged. There are decreased concentration of contrast material and dilatation of the pelvis and upper ureter. *B,* There is dilatation of the left ureter throughout its course, due to acute bacterial infection with ileus of the collecting system from bacterial endotoxins. No obstruction is present. *E. coli* was cultured from the urine. After appropriate antibiotic therapy, the dilated left collecting system returned to normal.

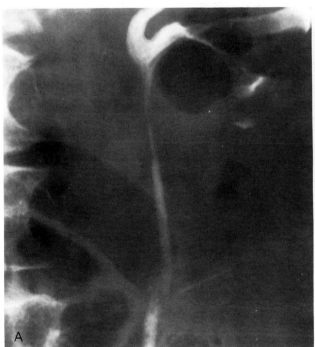

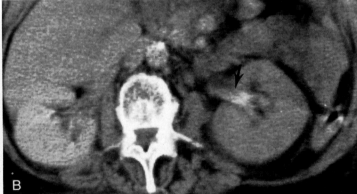

Figure 23–2. Mucosal striations of the renal pelvis and ureter due to urinary tract infection in a 77-year-old woman presenting with fever, pyuria, and left flank pain. An excretory urogram showed an enlarged left kidney with delayed excretion and decreased concentrating ability, but no evidence of obstruction. Because of the poor response to antibiotic treatment, a retrograde pyelogram was performed to rule out partial ureteral obstruction. *A,* A film from the retrograde pyelogram shows linear mucosal striations of the renal pelvis and ureter. No obstruction was present. These mucosal striations result from mucosal and submucosal edema caused by acute pyelonephritis. *B,* A CT scan performed to rule out renal or perinephric abscess shows an edematous enlarged left kidney with decreased enhancement after injection of contrast material. Irregularity *(arrow)* and thickening of the wall of the renal pelvis and ureter were noted. These changes were due to acute pyelonephritis.

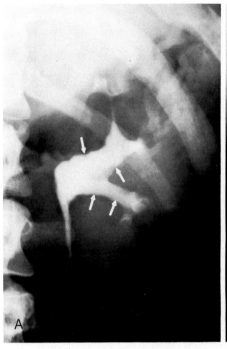
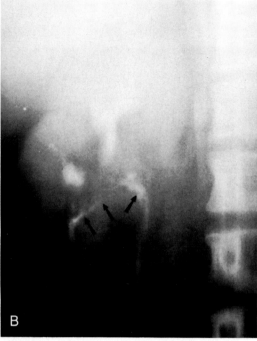
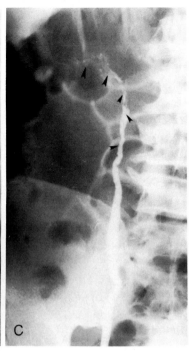

Figure 23–3. Causes of mucosal striations. *A,* Acute pyelonephritis (pyelitis). A 30-year-old man had clinical evidence of left pyelonephritis. Mucosal irregularity in left renal pelvis and infundibula *(arrows)* was evident on otherwise unremarkable urogram. Follow-up IVU was normal after treatment. *B,* Tomogram from urography performed on a 31-year-old man with gross hematuria who had been taking anticoagulants. Right lower-pole infundibulum and renal pelvis show marked mucosal irregularity *(arrow)*. The coarse striations extend into the proximal ureter. These findings cleared, as shown by follow-up urography, after adjustment of anticoagulant therapy. Diagnosis was submucosal hemorrhage. *C,* Nonvisualization of the right kidney in this 35-year-old female prompted this retrograde pyeloureterogram. Coarse mucosal striations *(arrows)* correspond to submucosal edema or hemorrhage due to proven right renal vein thrombosis.

der.[10, 30] In the condition, gas may be seen in the lumen of the ureter, as well as within the ureteral wall (Fig. 23–4). In the reported cases of isolated ureteritis emphysematosa, the patients were all diabetic and had ureteral obstruction. Ureteritis and pyelitis emphysematosa may also be seen in association with emphysematous pyelonephritis.[31] As in cystitis emphysematosa, the usual infecting bacteria are *E. coli* and *Aerobacter aerogenes.* Antimicrobial therapy alone can treat the infection and cause the gas to disappear,[10, 29] although it is necessary to relieve obstruction, if it is present. Other sources of gas within the ureter must be excluded, including ureterocolic or ureteroileal fistulas. Ureteritis emphysematosa can simulate pneumatosis intestinalis clinically and radiographically.[30]

CHANGES IN THE RENAL PELVIS AND URETER ASSOCIATED WITH VESICOURETERAL REFLUX AND/OR INFECTION

The relationship between VUR and infections is close and complicated, and some disagreement about the topic still exists. It is now well established that VUR of infected urine is the major cause of upper urinary tract infection in children. VUR may cause dilatation of the ureter and collecting system, increased distensibility of the collecting system, decreased ureteral motility and emptying, and mucosal striations.[1, 2, 5, 6, 24, 32] The issue of whether infection can produce VUR without some underlying abnormality has been a point of contention.[33, 34] Reflux in childhood is usually found during the investigation of a urinary tract infection. The role of VUR of infected urine in producing pyelonephritic scarring and reflux nephropathy is well documented by Hodson and colleagues[1, 2, 35] and is discussed in a separate section (Chapter 21, Reflux Nephropathy).

VUR is of two types. The most common cause of reflux (primary reflux) is a congenital abnormality of ureterovesical junction, manifested by a lateral superior ectopia of the ureteral orifice, a perpendicular (rather than oblique) course of the ureter through the bladder wall, and a short or otherwise abnormal intramural segment of the ureter. Incompetence of the ureterovesical junction results, allowing reflux of urine from the bladder into the ureter and pyelocalyceal system. This occurs with all degrees of severity.[36-38] Secondary reflux is caused by or associated with another abnormality that produces changes in the ureterovesical junction, rendering it incompetent. Secondary VUR is most often caused by a paraureteral or Hutch-type diverticulum of the bladder.[85, 86] It can also result from iatrogenic trauma to the ureterovesical junction or from prolonged obstruction (e.g., posterior urethral valves or neuropathic bladder disease). Although lower urinary tract infection was once thought to cause secondary reflux by causing inelasticity of the ureterovesical junction,[1, 34, 36, 37, 39] this cause is now known to be infrequent.[33] Similarly, the belief that most reflux is due to "bladder outlet obstruction" is no longer widely held.[38, 40-42] Bladder neck obstruction in children is, in fact, a rarity.

Because reflux leads to incomplete bladder emptying

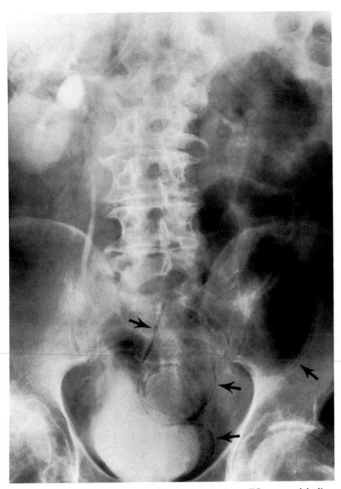

Figure 23–4. Ureteritis emphysematosa in a 79-year-old diabetic man presenting with left-sided abdominal pain, fever, and nausea. Three years earlier, excretory urography had shown the patient to have a nonvisualizing left kidney. An intravenous urogram (IVU) shows a dilated left ureter *(arrows)*. Intramural ureteral gas is seen as linear lucencies paralleling the dilated gas-filled ureteral lumen. There is no contrast excretion from the left kidney. Note the indentation of the bladder by the gas-filled left ureter. The right kidney is normal. (From Imray TJ, Huberty LH: Isolated ureteritis emphysematosa simulating pneumatosis intestinalis. AJR 135(5):1082, 1980, © by Am Roentgen Ray Soc.)

and persistence of a significant postvoid residual urine, reflux and infection often coexist. The major cause of nonobstructive hydronephrosis and hydroureter in children is VUR (Fig. 23–5). Fortunately, most vesicoureteral reflux is self limited. Mild or moderate reflux disappears spontaneously in many children as they grow and mature.[33, 39, 45] Edwards and colleagues showed in long-term follow-up that reflux disappeared in 79% of ureters (the children were on long-term prophylaxis with antibiotics).[45] The initial severity of reflux was the most important factor affecting its outcome. Reflux disappeared from only 41% of ureters with Grade-4 reflux with dilated ureters, but from 85% of those with less severe grades of reflux and no ureteral dilatation. Reflux was just as likely to disappear in children who had recurrent urinary tract infections as in those with isolated infections, and there was no objective evidence that antibacterial treatment cured reflux.[43–47] As a child grows older, the intramural ureter increases in length, reaching adult length at about age 12.[38] Ureteroneocystotomy maintains a role in the treatment of severe reflux.[48]

VESICOURETERAL REFLUX IN ADULTS

Sterile VUR in adult patients with normal upper tracts and no evidence of urinary obstruction is of uncertain significance.[49] Reflux in the presence of benign prostatic hypertrophy, neuropathic bladder, bladder carcinoma, drug-induced cystitis, granulomatous cystitis, or iatrogenic ureteral orifice injury is occasionally evident. In the presence of lower urinary tract infection, however, reflux may predispose to pyelonephritis. Cattolica reported 20 adults with primary VUR, 12% of whom had urographic features of pyelonephritis.[50] Six of the 12 had *no* history of childhood urinary tract infections. Berquist and associates detected VUR in 200 adult patients over a 4-year period.[51] A group of 172 had positive signs or symptoms that were suggestive of urinary tract infection. Eighteen patients had sterile reflux and no history of urinary infection. Excretory urograms were positive in the vast majority of patients. Adults with VUR require careful scrutiny. Findings of parenchymal scarring, ureteral dilatation, mucosal striations, or calyceal clubbing should prompt consideration of performing voiding cystourethrography (VCU) (Fig. 23–6). The surgical correction of VUR in adults must be individualized, and the subject remains controversial.[49]

MUCOSAL STRIATIONS

Fine longitudinal striations of the renal pelvis and ureter are frequently seen in patients with VUR (Fig. 23–7). Friedland and Forsberg reported that all patients with renal pelvic striations in their study had reflux of Grades 2 to 3 on the side of the reflux, and no pelvic striations were seen in nonrefluxing ureters.[24] Striations were found in 15% of all renal pelves drained by refluxing ureters. Renal pelvic and ureteral striations should alert the clinician to the fact that VUR of a severe grade is probably present.[25] Striations of the renal pelvis and ureter may also be seen after obstruction with dilatation of the ureter and pelvis,[24] but they are rare in the normal renal pelvis without reflux.[26] Linear mucosal striations may be seen in refluxing ureteroenteric conduits. In most of these cases, the mucosal striations are due to redundancy of the mucosa and submucosa resulting from renal pelvic dilatation; the striations are apparent when the renal pelvis empties, and inapparent with a filled, distended renal pelvis and ureter. These are distinguished from mucosal striations caused by infection (see Figs. 23–2 and 23–3).[9, 27, 28]

Longitudinal striations of the renal pelvis and ureter must be differentiated from submucosal hemorrhage (Fig. 23–3) and from transverse folds in the proximal ureter. These are normal variants in infants, probably representing persistence of the fetal "corkscrew" ureter (Fig. 23–8).[55a]

INFLAMMATORY URETERAL EDEMA AND STRICTURES

Severe edema may cause stenosis of the ureter and temporary obstruction. Examples include ureteral obstruction caused by acute bacterial infection with bullous

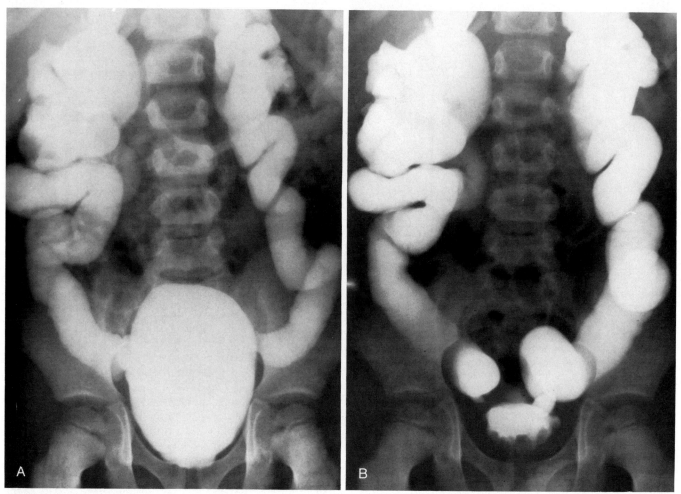

Figure 23–5. Vesicoureteral reflux in a child. Voiding cystourethrogram shows a child with severe vesicoureteral reflux causing hydronephrosis and hydroureter. *A,* A cystogram shows Grade-4 vesicoureteral reflux with marked dilatation of right and left ureters and renal pelves, and severe blunting of the calyces. The bladder is smooth walled, there is no evidence of neurogenic bladder, and the urethra was normal during voiding. *B,* Immediately after voiding, distention of the ureters and upper renal collecting systems is even more marked. The bladder shows some mucosal redundancy. The bladder refills soon after voiding, as a result of emptying of the ureters and upper collecting systems. This urinary stasis may predispose to recurrent urinary tract infection and subsequent reflux nephropathy.

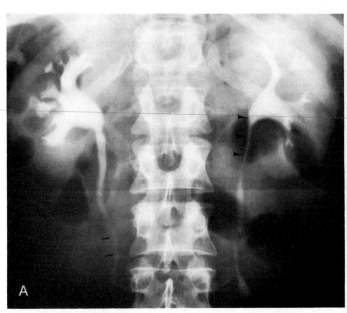

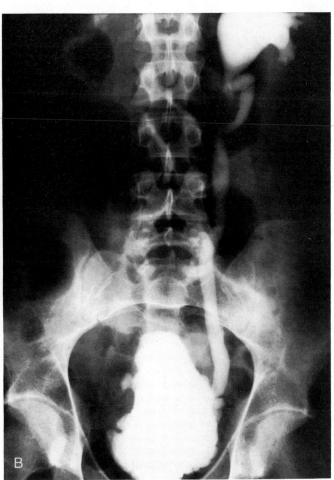

Figure 23–6. Vesicoureteral reflux in adult. A 39-year-old male has neuropathic bladder and recurrent urinary tract infections. *A,* IVU shows normal upper tracts, but bilateral ureteral striations *(arrows). B,* Cystography reveals Grade 4/5 reflux on the left. Note marked tortuosity of proximal ureter and dilatation throughout. Ureteral striations are the only clue on the urogram that reflux was present.

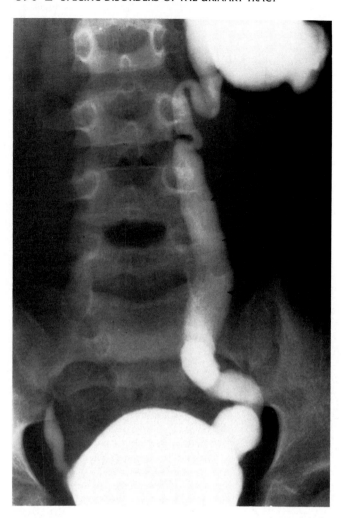

Figure 23–7. A 6-year-old boy presenting with urinary tract infection. Voiding cystourethrogram showed bilateral vesico-ureteral reflux, Grade 1 on the right and Grade 4 on the left. Fine linear striations of the ureter are seen in this patient *(arrowheads)*. Although more commonly seen in the proximal ureter, renal pelvis, and renal infundibula, mucosal striations may also be seen elsewhere in the ureter, owing to vesicoure-teral reflux. (Courtesy Dr. Beverly Wood, Rochester, New York.)

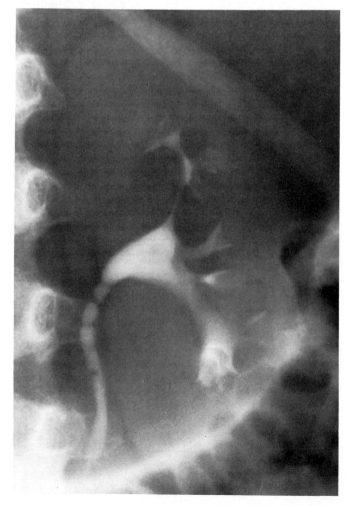

Figure 23–8. Transverse folds in the proximal ureter. Transverse folds in the upper ureter, giving the upper ureter a "corkscrew" appearance, are a normal variant in infants. They represent a persistence of normal fetal tortuosity of the ureter and must be differentiated from the abnormal longitudinal folds (striations) of the renal pelvis and upper ureter. (From Kirks DR, Gurrarino G, Weinberg AG: Transverse folds in the proximal ureter: A normal variant in infants. AJR 130(3):463–464, 1978, © by Am Roentgen Ray Soc.)

cystitis of the trigone,[53] ureteral stenting,[54, 55b] and retrograde ureteral catheterization.[56] Ureteritis due to schistosomiasis (bilharziasis)[57] and tuberculosis[58, 59] may cause both acute and chronic ureteral obstruction and can lead to permanent ureteral stricture. Both idiopathic segmental ureteritis, and nonspecific granulomatous ureteritis may mimic malignant strictures by their focal nature and worrisome signs (e.g., hematuria).[60]

Inflammatory obstruction of the ureter often occurs at the narrowest points of the collecting system (i.e., the ureteropelvic and ureterovesical junctions) but may occur in any portion of the ureter. Acute obstructive ureteritis is reversible, in general, if appropriate antibiotic treatment is provided.

Chronic bacterial ureteritis, on the other hand, may go on to produce ureteral and/or periureteral fibrosis with stricture formation. Considering the frequency of urinary tract infections, ureteral stricture due to bacterial infection is rare. Ureteral and periureteral fibrosis may appear as a smooth or slightly irregular stenosis of the distal ureter (Fig. 23–9), often accompanied by significant obstruction.[61]

Infection in the periureteral tissues of the pelvis or retroperitoneum, resulting from abscess or pelvic inflammatory disease, may lead to ureteral strictures. This differs from retroperitoneal fibrosis, in which a dense fibrotic plaque involves the retroperitoneum, aorta, vena cava, and ureter, causing ureteral obstruction—usually in the middle third of the ureter. Localized ureteral or periureteral fibrosis occurs in any portion of the ureter. Computed tomography (CT) can differentiate ureteral obstruction due to localized ureteral and periureteral fibrosis from retroperitoneal fibrosis. In ureteral and periureteral fibrosis, CT reveals a normal or thickened ureter in the region of the obstruction, sometimes with periureteral soft-tissue thickening, but without significant surrounding mass (Fig. 23–9). The appearance is similar to that of direct metastases to the ureter, radiation fibrosis, and amyloidosis of the ureter.[61] Retroperitoneal fibrosis, on the other hand, demonstrates a dense plaque-like fibrotic mass involving the retroperitoneum and surrounding the ureter. Ureteral and periureteral fibrosis due to inflammatory lesions must be differentiated from early primary and metastatic carcinoma, which may induce a desmoplastic response resulting in fibrosis and may mimic benign inflammatory periureteral fibrosis.[62]

RADIATION URETERITIS AND FIBROSIS OF THE URETER

Paradoxically, although the normal ureter is relatively resistant to radiation-induced injury, periureteral fibrosis and obstruction are occasionally seen in women irradiated for carcinoma of the uterine cervix.[63, 64] It is seen much less often after irradiation for other pelvic malignancies. The explanation for this phenomenon probably lies in the fact that the fibrosis is related to necrosis and fibrosis in pre-existing periureteral cancer tissue.[65] It is not surprising, therefore, that most cases of postirradiation ureteral obstruction occur in patients with residual or recurrent neoplasm, although 3% to 5% of cases are seen in tumor-free patients.[66] Pre-existing diseases and trauma such as previous surgery, which compromise the vitality or blood supply of the ureter, may render it more susceptible to postirradiation stricture.

The radiographic appearance of irradiation stricture of the ureter is nonspecific. The strictures may be long or short and, in the vast majority of cases, are located in the distal third. The strictures are fusiform and tapering, with preservation of a normal mucosal pattern. On CT scans, a normal or thickened ureter is seen (Fig. 23–10). Recurrent tumor cannot be ruled out by the radiographic appearance alone, and fine-needle biopsy and/or operative exploration may be necessary for final diagnosis.

EOSINOPHILIC PYELOURETERITIS

Ureteral stricture and obstruction due to ureteral and periureteral fibrosis, with either mild or massive eosinophilic infiltrate, have been reported and termed eosinophilic pyeloureteritis.[11, 15, 67] The etiology is unknown, but the disease has a predilection for patients with a strong history of food and medication allergies. It may also be seen as a reaction to parasites, but cases have been encountered in patients with no history of allergies or parasitic infection. The histopathological findings resemble eosinophilic granuloma (histiocytosis X)[67] and are similar to those occurring in eosinophilic cystitis.[68, 69]

Eosinophilic ureteritis is a rare cause of ureteral stricture and presents a nondescript radiological appearance (Fig. 23–11).

XANTHOGRANULOMATOUS PYELOURETERITIS

Ureteropelvic junction obstruction due to localized isolated xanthogranulomatous pyeloureteritis confined to the ureteropelvic junction without xanthogranulomatous pyelonephritis has been reported (Fig. 23–12).[15] The area of stricture is characterized by chronic inflammation and fibrosis with fat necrosis and lipid-containing macrophages, consistent with the pathological appearance of xanthogranulomatous inflammation.

Nonspecific ureteral granulomas with inflammatory infiltrates and fibrosis with obstruction of unknown etiology are reported; however, they are rare.[70] Ureteral granuloma due to surgical glove talc leading to ureteral stricture and obstruction has also been described.[71]

PYELOURETERITIS CYSTICA

Pyeloureteritis cystica is an uncommon abnormality, in which subepithelial cysts form and project into the lumen of the renal pelvis and/or ureter.[72] The cystic changes in the wall of the ureter may have an adverse effect on ureteral peristalsis.[73] The cysts contain a clear proteinaceous fluid, and their walls are made up of immature epithelium, which may be single or multilayered (see Fig. 23–15C). There is usually a surrounding inflammatory infiltrate that includes lymphocytes and plasma cells. The exact evolution of the cysts in pyeloureteritis cystica is uncertain, but most authors agree that they are associated with chronic urinary tract infection and are probably the end result of chronic mucosal irritation secondary to inflammation.[12] The cysts are thought to be formed from

Text continued on page 896

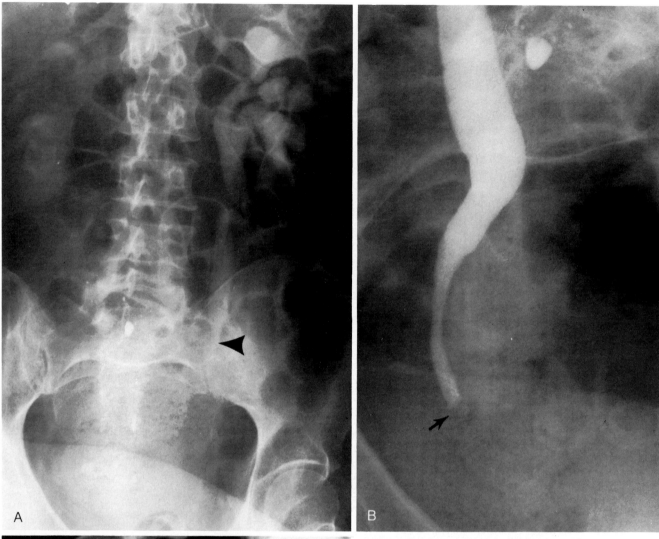

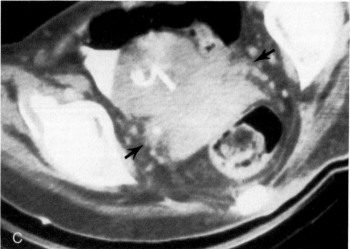

Figure 23–9. Ureteral stricture due to ureteritis; ureteral and periureteral fibrosis from chronic bacterial infection. A 43-year-old woman with longstanding severe multiple sclerosis, requiring long-term indwelling catheterization of the bladder, had a history of chronic recurrent urinary tract infection. During an episode of infection, the creatinine was noted to be elevated. *A,* IVU shows bilateral ureteral obstruction, greater on the right than on the left, on this 2-hour delayed radiograph. The distal left ureter smoothly tapers at the point of obstruction at the pelvic brim *(arrowhead). B,* An antegrade pyelogram of the right ureter shows gradual narrowing and irregularity causing a high-grade obstruction of the distal right ureter *(arrow)* several centimeters proximal to the insertion into the bladder. *C,* CT section 2 cm above the bladder shows irregular periureteral soft-tissue thickening about both right and left ureters *(arrows).* The right ureter is opacified with contrast material. The smooth, tapering stricture of the pelvic ureter, with thickened ureteral wall and with periureteral fibrosis due to bacterial infection, is the most common appearance of ureteritis. The patient underwent resection of the distal ureters and ileal conduit diversion. The surgical specimen showed bilateral thickened ureters with submucosal edema, and chronic inflammation with focal transmural chronic inflammation and serosal fibrosis.

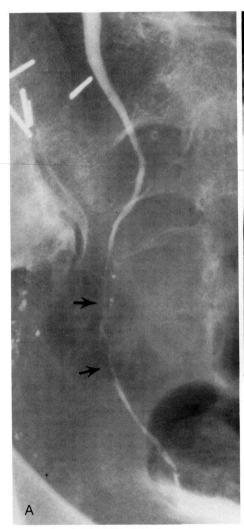

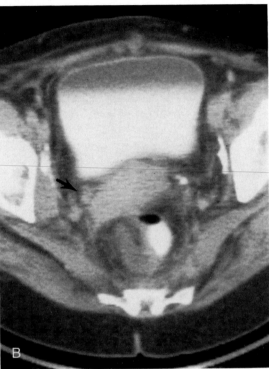

Figure 23–10. Radiation ureteritis and fibrosis of the ureter. A 46-year-old woman who received intracavitary radiation therapy for carcinoma of the cervix presented with right flank pain and high-grade ureteral obstruction on excretory urography. A right percutaneous nephrostomy was performed. *A,* An antegrade pyelogram shows a narrowed, slightly irregular pelvic ureter *(arrows).* This appearance could be secondary to either recurrent metastatic tumor or radiation ureteritis and fibrosis. *B,* A CT scan shows a thickened ureter *(arrow)* with no evidence of a significant periureteral mass. There is no contrast excretion from the right kidney. The patient underwent surgical exploration and ileal conduit diversion. There was no evidence of recurrent tumor, and the pathological diagnosis was radiation fibrosis of the ureter.

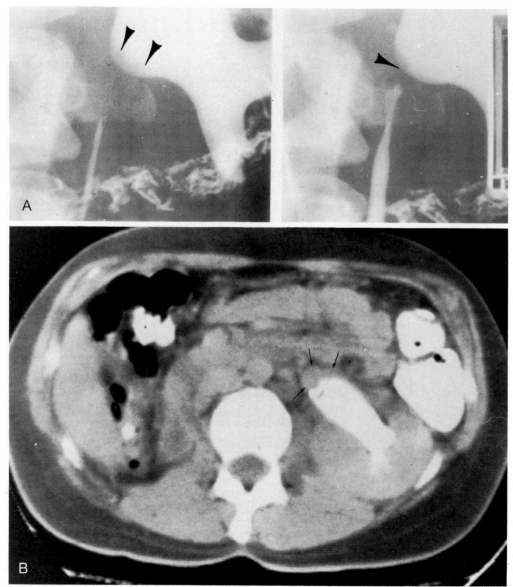

Figure 23–11. Eosinophilic pyeloureteritis in a 37-year-old woman with 1-week history of abdominal pain followed by anuria. She had a solitary left kidney. *A,* A retrograde pyelogram shows irregularity and mass effect *(arrowheads)* involving the left ureteropelvic junction (UPJ). A retrograde drainage catheter was placed in the renal pelvis. *B,* A CT scan after contrast material was injected through the ureteral catheter shows thickening of the wall of the proximal ureter and UPJ *(arrows).* A preoperative diagnosis of transitional cell carcinoma was made. At surgery the UPJ was thickened. The removed tissue showed acute and chronic inflammation with infiltration of eosinophils. (From Wadsworth DE, McClennan BL: Benign causes of acquired ureteropelvic junction obstruction: A uroradiologic spectrum. Urol Radiol 5:77, 1983.)

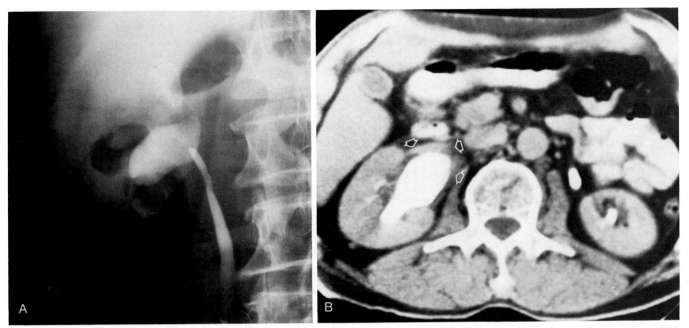

Figure 23-12. Xanthogranulomatous pyeloureteritis. A 69-year-old man presenting with acute onset of right flank pain. An IVU showed partial right UPJ obstruction; previous urograms had been normal. A, A right retrograde pyelogram shows a narrowed, strictured ureteropelvic junction with no intraluminal filling defect. B, A CT scan shows a soft-tissue density and thickening of the right ureteropelvic junction *(open arrowheads).* Inflammation was considered to be likely because of the history of infection. (From Wadsworth DE, McClennan BL: Benign causes of acquired ureteropelvis junction obstruction: A uroradiologic spectrum. Urol Radiol 5:77, 1983.)

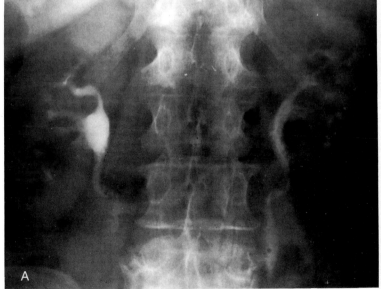

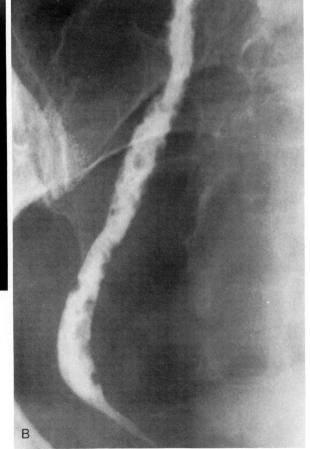

Figure 23-13. Ureteritis cystica. A, A 63-year-old female with history of chronic urinary tract infections had an IVU. Some diminished concentration was evident on the left, along with multiple filling defects within both ureters. B, A right retrograde ureterogram shows the ureteritis cystica to better advantage.

degeneration and cavitation of metaplastic surface urothelium or submucosal Brunn's cell nests. The cysts may vary from 1 mm to 2 cm in diameter but usually are only a few millimeters in diameter. Once formed, the cysts may persist for the lifetime of the patient.

The appearance of pyeloureteritis cystica by excretory urography, antegrade pyelography, or retrograde pyelography is usually characteristic; multiple, smooth, well-rounded or oval filling defects with sharp borders that protrude into the lumen are seen (Fig. 23–13). They may vary from a few scattered cysts to innumerable cysts that involve the entire pelvis and ureter. They tend to persist for long periods of time, and sometimes indefinitely. Pyeloureteritis cystica may also be associated with cystitis cystica. The main differential diagnosis includes distinguishing the condition from multiple papillary transitional cell tumors, vascular ureteral impressions, ureteral pseudodiverticula, submucosal (suburothelial) hemorrhage, and tuberculosis (subepithelial tubercles).[74] Cystic blebs similar to pyeloureteritis cystica may be seen with the Stevens-Johnson syndrome, but this is usually a reversible finding.[75]

MULTIPLE URETERAL DIVERTICULA; URETERAL PSEUDODIVERTICULOSIS

Small 2- to 4-mm outpouchings of the ureter have been referred to as ureteral diverticula (Fig. 23–14).[75] Ureteral diverticula are nearly always multiple, usually numbering three to eight per ureter, and most are bilateral (70%).[13, 76] The radiological diagnosis of multiple ureteral diverticula (pseudodiverticula) is made by demonstrating the typical small invaginations of contrast into the ureteral wall. They occur predominantly in the upper and middle ureter and are usually demonstrated more clearly on retrograde or antegrade studies, as opposed to intravenous urography. Sometimes, they are associated with narrowing of the ureter. Their appearance may remain unchanged over many years.

The pathology of ureteral pseudodiverticula has recently been reviewed by Wasserman and coworkers.[87] Histopathologically, ureteral diverticula are associated with widespread hyperplasia of the transitional epithelium and buds of epithelial tissue projecting into the lamina propria of the ureter (Fig. 23–15).[13] The epithelium may be increased to twice its normal thickness of epithelial cell layers. Because these multiple ureteral diverticula are a downward proliferation of epithelium into the loose connective tissue of the lamina propria, they create a pouchlike intramural invagination. They are neither congenital (true) nor acquired (false) diverticula, but are actually pseudodiverticula.[77] A true (congenital) diverticulum, or bud, is formed by an outpouching of the entire ureteral wall and is usually much longer than it is wide. An acquired false diverticulum is caused by protrusion of the mucosa through a defect—usually traumatic in origin—in the muscularis of the ureter and protrudes from its external surface. Both true and false diverticula are usually single, unilateral, and larger than multiple ureteral diverticula.[77] Multiple ureteral pseudodiverticula are believed to be a manifestation of chronic infection or inflammation of the ureter leading to reactive hyperplasia of the urothelium, similar in its etiology and histology to pyeloureteritis cystica (see Fig. 23–13), but with a different result. Some of the pseudodiverticula may result from rupture of suburothelial cysts into the ureteral lumen.

An association of multiple ureteral diverticula with

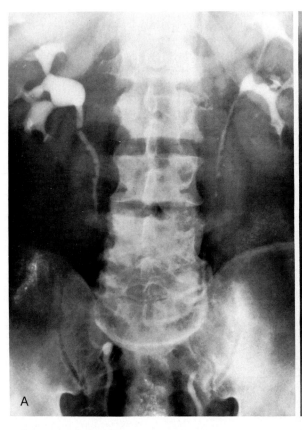
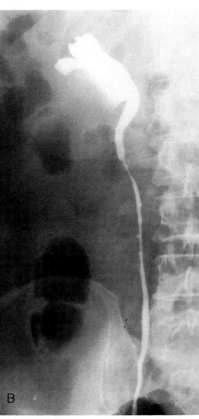

Figure 23–14. Ureteral pseudodiverticulosis. *A,* 58-year-old male with benign prostatic hyperplasia. No definite history of prior urinary tract infection. Urogram reveals bilateral ureteral outpouchings limited to the upper half. *B,* 40-year-old male with right flank pain. Retrograde pyeloureterogram reveals multiple pseudodiverticula in right ureter. Note the right lower-pole renal mass.

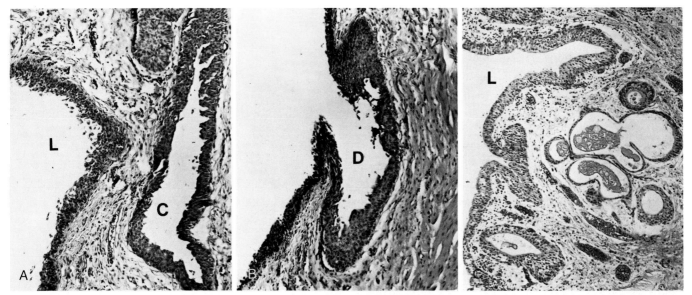

Figure 23–15. Histopathological appearance of ureteral diverticula (pseudodiverticula). *A,* There is widespread hyperplasia of the transitional epithelium of the left ureter with buds of epithelial tissue (Brunn's nests) projecting into the lamina propria; some are solid and round, and others are tubular or microcystic. There are several inclusions in the lamina propria, one of which is cystic (C). L = lumen. (H & E × 100.) *B,* This is a rare example of a cystic cavity that is connected with the lumen and corresponds to a small diverticulum (D) in the left ureter. (H & E × 100.) *C,* Dilated left ureter with its lumen (L) to the left demonstrating hyperplastic transitional epithelium with pronounced ureteritis cystica. (H & E × 100.) (From Cochran ST, Waisman J, Barbaric ZL: Radiographic and microscopic findings in multiple ureteral diverticula. Radiology 137:631, 1980).

urinary tract infection, obstruction, and urinary stones has been reported, frequently leading to the hypothesis that they are a response to infection or inflammation. In a high proportion of patients with ureteral pseudodiverticula, urine cytologic findings show cellular atypia. An increased incidence of transitional cell carcinoma (TCC) of the bladder and ureter has been alleged in male patients who have multiple ureteral diverticula.[13, 77] Because of this association, patients with multiple ureteral diverticula should be closely screened for the presence or development of transitional cell carcinoma.[77] More than 25% of patients with multiple diverticula may have or may develop transitional cell carcinoma of the bladder. Ureteral pseudodiverticula need to be radiographically distinguished from pyeloureteritis cystica, tuberculous ureteritis, multiple polyposis, multicentric TCC, schistosomiasis, ureteral notching, and polyarteritis nodosa.[78] When the appearance is typical, however, it is usually diagnostic.

PLASMA CELL GRANULOMA OF THE RENAL PELVIS

Plasma cell granuloma is a very rare cause of a radiolucent filling defect of the renal pelvis (Fig. 23–16).[79] Radiographically, plasma cell granuloma appears as a round, well-demarcated radiolucent filling defect of the renal pelvis, which must be differentiated from a urothelial neoplasm. Macroscopically, the lesion is a homogeneous solid white-yellow mass with no hemorrhage or necrosis. Histologically, the plasma cell granuloma is composed of collagenous fibrous tissue with numerous mature plasma cells (Fig. 23–16). The etiology of this

unusual lesion of the renal pelvis is uncertain. The lesion is benign, and only local surgical excision is required for its treatment, if a preoperative differentiation from carcinoma is possible.

MALACOPLAKIA OF THE URETER

Malacoplakia may involve the renal pelvis and ureter as well as the renal parenchyma.[16, 80–82] Malacoplakia of the ureter has most often been reported in association with bladder and renal pelvis involvement but may rarely present with the primary (or only) finding of a solitary lesion causing ureteral obstruction.[16, 80, 83]

The radiological appearances of malacoplakia of the ureter and renal pelvis are varied.[80–83] Malacoplakia may be solitary but more commonly is multifocal. Multiple smooth nodular filling defects are a common appearance (Fig. 23–17), but strictures may be seen as well (Fig. 23–18). Malacoplakia must be differentiated from pyeloureteritis cystica, tuberculous ureteritis, multiple papillary transitional cell tumors, malignant melanoma, and vascular ureteral notching. When a large plaquelike deposit causes ureteral obstruction without demonstrable involvement elsewhere, the differential diagnosis includes primary ureteral cancer or ureteral metastases from lung, breast, gastrointestinal, and other malignancies. The diagnosis may be made preoperatively by urinary sediment cytology or ureteral biopsy.[84] When malacoplakia involves the renal pelvis or ureter, the primary differential diagnosis involves ruling out transitional cell carcinoma. Malacoplakia is discussed in more detail in Chapter 21.

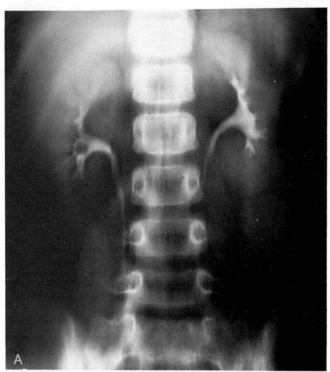

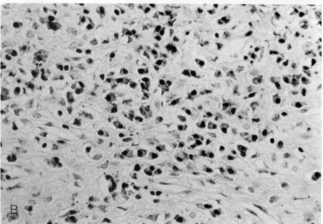

Figure 23–16. Plasma cell granuloma of the renal pelvis. *A,* Nephrotomogram in a 12-year-old boy presenting with painless hematuria shows a clear, well-circumscribed filling defect in the right renal pelvis. A localized resection was performed. *B,* Microscopically, the lesion consisted of fibrous granulomatous tissue rich in mature plasma cells, with no neoplastic features. The histological diagnosis was plasma cell granuloma. (H & E reduced from × 400.) (From Itoh H, Namiki M, Yoshioka T, Itantani H: Plasma cell granuloma of the renal pelvis. J Urol 127(6):1177–1178, © Williams & Wilkins, 1982.)

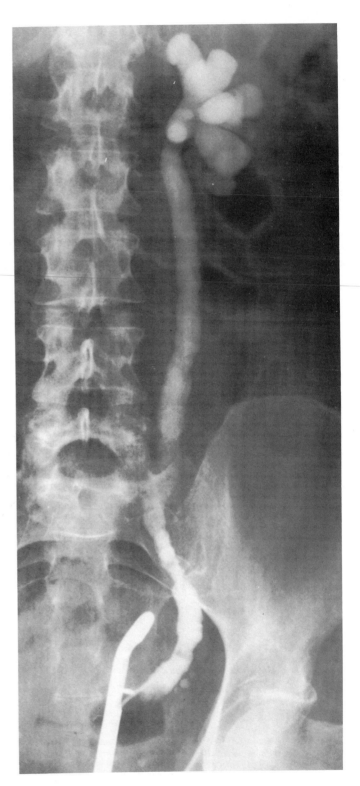

Figure 23–17. Malacoplakia of the ureter. Left retrograde pyelogram reveals multiple nodular defects in the wall of the ureter. The lesions are smooth and protrude slightly into the ureteral lumen. (Courtesy Richard Pfister, M.D.)

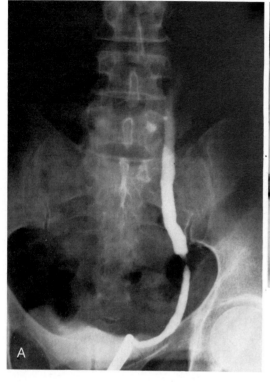

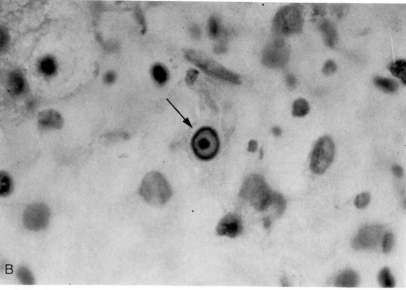

Figure 23–18. Malacoplakia of the ureter. Fifty-year-old woman with a solitary left kidney presenting with left flank pain and pyuria. *A,* A retrograde pyelogram shows a smooth circumferential stricture of the distal left ureter. A segmental ureterectomy was performed. *B,* High-power photomicrograph shows characteristic Michaelis-Gutmann body within a histiocyte in the center of the field. H & E reduced from × 1000 oil immersion. (From Nieh PT, Althausen AF: Malacoplakia of the ureter. J Urol 122(5):701–702, © by Williams & Wilkins, 1979.)

SQUAMOUS METAPLASIA; CHOLESTEATOMA; LEUKOPLAKIA

This subject has been previously described (Chapter 21, Chronic Inflammation of the Renal Parenchyma).

References

1. Hodson CJ, Edwards D: Chronic pyelonephritis and vesico-ureteric reflux. Clin Radiol 11:219–231, 1960.
2. Hodson CJ, Wilson S: Natural history of chronic pyelonephritic scarring. Br Med J 2:191–194, 1965.
3. Little PJ, McPherson DR, deWardener HE: The appearance of the intravenous pyelogram during and after acute pyelonephritis. Lancet 1 June 5:1186–1188, 1965.
4. Kass EJ, Silver TM, Konnak JW, et al: The urographic findings in acute pyelonephritis: Non-obstructive hydronephrosis. J Urol 116:544–546, 1976.
5. Shopfner CE: Nonobstructive hydronephrosis and hydroureter. AJR 98:172–180, 1966.
6. Shopfner CE: Urinary tract pathology with sepsis. AJR 108:632–640, 1970.
7. Silver TM, Kass EJ, Thornbury JR, et al: The radiological spectrum of acute pyelonephritis in adults and adolescents. Radiology 118:65–71, 1976.
8. Wicks JD, Thornbury JR: Acute renal infections in adults. Radiol Clin North Am 17:245–260, 1979.
9. Gwinn JL, Barnes GR Jr: Striated ureters and renal pelves. AJR 91:666–668, 1964.
10. Harrow BR, Sloane JA: Ureteritis emphysematosa: Spontaneous ureteral pneumogram; renal and perirenal emphysema. J Urol 89:43–48, 1963.
11. Hellstrom HR, Davis BK, Shonnard JW, MacPherson TA: Eosinophilic pyeloureteritis: Report of a case. J Urol 122:833–834, 1979.
12. Limburg D, Zuidema BJJ: Pyeloureteritis cystica. Diagn Imag 49:141–144, 1980.
13. Cochran ST, Waisman J, Barbaric ZL: Radiographic and microscopic findings in multiple ureteral diverticula. Radiology 137:631–636, 1980.
14. Davides KC, Johnson SH III, Marshall M Jr, Price SE Jr, Stavrides A: Plasma cell granuloma of the renal pelvis. J Urol 107:938–939, 1972.
15. Wadsworth DE, McClennan BL: Benign causes of acquired ureteropelvic junction obstruction: A uroradiologic spectrum. Urol Radiol 5:77, 1983.
16. Sexton CC, Lowman RM, Nyongo AO, Baskin AM: Malacoplakia presenting as complete unilateral ureteral obstruction. J Urol 128:139–141, 1982.
17. Hertle L, Androulakakis P: Keratinizing desquamative squamous metaplasia of the upper urinary tract: Leukoplakia–cholesteatoma. J Urol 127:631–635, 1982.
18. Swenson O, Fisher JH, Smyth BT: Studies of normal and abnormal ureteral peristalsis. Med J Aust 46:805, 1959.
19. Teague N, Boyarsky S: Further effects of coliform bacteria on ureteral peristalsis. J Urol 99:720, 1968.
20. Teague N, Boyarsky S: The effects of coliform bacilli upon ureteral peristalsis. Invest Urol 5:423, 1968.
21. Grana L, Donnellen WL, Swenson O: Effects of gram negative bacteria on ureteral stricture and function. J Urol 99:539, 1968.
22. King WW, Cox CE: Bacterial inhibition of ureteral smooth muscle contractility. I. The effect of common urinary pathogens and endotoxin in an in vitro system. J Urol 108:700–705, 1972.
23. Boyarsky S, Labay P, Teague N: Aperistaltic ureter in upper urinary tract infection—cause or effect? Urology 12:134–138, 1978.
24. Friedland GW, Forsberg L: Striation of the renal pelvis in children. Clin Radiol 23:58–60, 1972.
25. Silber I, McAlister WH: Longitudinal folds as an indirect sign of vesicoureteral reflux. J Urol 103:89, 1970.
26. Daughtridge TG: Mucosal folds in the upper urinary tract. AJR 107:743, 1969.
27. Vezina JA, Leger LP, Raymond O, Guy R: Les réplis muqueux de l'arbre urinaire supérieur. J Can Assoc Radiol 14:10, 1963.
28. Wright FW: Mucosal oedema of the ureter and renal pelvis. Radiology 93:1309, 1969.
29. Soteropoulos C, Kawashima E, Gilmore JH: Cystitis and ureteritis emphysematosa. Radiology 68:866–868, 1957.
30. Imray TJ, Huberty LH: Isolated ureteritis emphysematosa simulating pneumatosis intestinalis. AJR 135:1082–1083, 1980.
31. McLelland R: Ureteritis, pyelitis and pyelonephritis emphysematosa. Acta Radiol 57:97, 1962.
32. Hutch JA, Hinman F Jr, Miller ER: Reflux as a cause of hydronephrosis and chronic pyelonephritis. J Urol 88:169–175, 1962.
33. Shopfner CE: Vesicoureteral reflux. Five-year re-evaluation. Radiology 95:637–648, 1970.

34. Gross GW, Lebowitz RL: Infection does not cause reflux. AJR 137:929–932, 1981.
35. Hodson CJ, Maling TMJ, McManamon LM: The pathogenesis of reflux nephropathy. Br J Radiol (Suppl):13, 1975.
36. Ambrose SS, Nicholson WP III: The causes of vesicoureteral reflux in children. J Urol 87:688–694, 1962.
37. Ambrose SS, Nicholson WP III: Vesicoureteral reflux secondary to anomalies of the ureterovesical junction: Management and results. J Urol 87:695–700, 1962.
38. Hutch JA: Theory of maturation of the intravesical ureter. J Urol 86:534, 1961.
39. Stephens FD: Urologic aspects of recurrent urinary tract infection in children. J Pediatr 80:725, 1971.
40. Shopfner CE: Roentgenologic evaluation of bladder neck obstruction. AJR 101:162, 1967.
41. Hinman F Jr, Hutch JA: Atrophic pyelonephritis from ureteral reflux without obstructive signs (reflux pyelonephritis). J Urol 87:230, 1962.
42. Harrow BR, Sloane JA, Witus WS: A critical examination of bladder neck obstruction. J Urol 98:613, 1967.
43. Jeffs RD, Allen MS: The relationship between ureterovesical reflux and infection. J Urol 88:691, 1962.
44. Haverton LW, Lich RJR: The cause and correction of ureteral reflux. J Urol 89:672, 1963.
45. Edwards D, Normand ICS, Prescod N, Smellie JM: Disappearance of vesicoureteric reflux during long-term prophylaxis of urinary tract infection in children. Br Med J 2:285–288, 1977.
46. Govan DE, Friedland DW, Fair WR, et al: Management of children with urinary tract infections: The Stanford experience. Urology 6:273, 1975.
47. Asscher AW, Fletcher EWI, Johnston HH, et al: Cardiff-Oxford bacteriuria study group. Sequelae of covert bacteriuria in school girls: A four year follow-up study. Lancet 2:889, 1978.
48. Wikstad I, Aperia A, Broberger O, Löhr G: Long-term effect of large vesicoureteral reflux with or without urinary tract infection. Acta Radiol (Diagn) 22:325–330, 1981.
49. Senoh K, Iwatsubo E, Momose S, et al: Non-obstructive vesicoureteral reflux in adults: Value of conservative treatment. J Urol 117:566–570, 1977.
50. Cattolica EV: Renal scarring and primary reflux in adults. Urology 4:397–401, 1974.
51. Berquist TH, Hattery RR, Hartman GW, et al: Vesicoureteral reflux in adults. AJR 125:314–321, 1975.
52. Amar AD, Hutch JA, Katz I: Coexistence of urinary calculi and vesicoureteral reflux. JAMA 206:2312–2313, 1968.
53. Shackelford GD, Manley CB: Acute ureteral obstruction secondary to bullous cystitis of the trigone. Radiology 132:351, 1979.
54. Levine RS, Pollack HM, Banner MP: Transient ureteral obstruction after ureteral stenting. AJR 138:323, 1982.
55a. Kirks DR, Currarino G, Weinberg AG: Transverse folds in the proximal ureter: A normal variant in infants. AJR 130:463–464, 1978.
55b. Gibbons RP, Correa RJ, Cummings KB, et al: Experience with indwelling ureteral stent catheters. J Urol 115:22, 1976.
56. Kauffman JJ, Maloney PJ, Maxwell MH: Urinary blockade after bilateral catheterization. N Engl J Med 275:412, 1966.
57. Young SW, Khalid KH, Forid Z, et al: Urinary tract lesions of *Schistosoma haematobium*. Radiology 111:81, 1974.
58. Friedenberg RM, Ney C, Stachenfed RA: Roentgenographic manifestations of tuberculosis of the ureter. J Urol 99:25, 1968.
59. Murphy DM, Fallon B, Lane V, O'Flynn JD: Tuberculous stricture of ureter. Urology 20:382–384, 1962.
60. Das S, Taylor RS, Javaheri P: Inflammatory ureteral strictures after ureteroileal diversion. J Urol 129:820–822, 1983.

61. Bosniak MA, Megibow AJ, Ambos MA, et al: Computed tomography of ureteral obstruction. AJR 139:1107–1113, 1982.
62. Mieza M, Rotstein JM, Geffen A: CT demonstration of periureteral fibrosis of malignant etiology. J Comput Assist Tomogr 6:290–293, 1982.
63. Sklaroff DM, Gnaneswaran P, Sklaroff RB: Postirradiation ureteric stricture. Gynecol Oncol 6:538–545, 1978.
64. Goodman M, Dalton JR: Ureteral strictures following radiotherapy: Incidence, etiology and treatment guidelines. J Urol 128:21–24, 1982.
65. Aron BS, Schlesinger A: Complications of radiation therapy: The genitourinary system. Semin Roentgenol 9:65, 1974.
66. Pearse HD, Hodges CV: Surgical and traumatic ureteral injuries. *In* Smith RD, Skinner DG: Complications of Urologic Surgery. Philadelphia, WB Saunders Company, 1974.
67. Uyama T, Moriwaki S, Aga Y, Yamamoto A: Eosinophilic ureteritis? Regional ureteritis with marked infiltration of eosinophils. Urology 18:615–617, 1981.
68. Mitas JA II, Thompson T: Ureteral involvement complicating eosinophilic cystitis. Urology 26:6770, 1985.
69. Hellstrom HR, Davis BK, Shonnord JW: Eosinophilic cystitis: A study of 16 cases. Am J Clin Pathol 72:777, 1979.
70. O'Flynn WF, Sandrey JG: Nonspecific granulomata of the ureter and bladder. Br J Urol 35:267, 1963.
71. Joannides JI: Talc granuloma of the ureter: A case report. Br J Surg 65:883–885, 1978.
72. Loitman BS, Chiat H: Ureteritis cystica and pyelitis cystica. A review of cases and roentgenologic criteria. Radiology 68:345, 1957.
73. Meesmann D: Pyeloureteritis cystica. Munch Med Wochenschr 118:1243, 1976.
74. Malek RS, Aguilo JJ, Hattery RR: Radiolucent filling defects of the renal pelvis: Classification and report of unusual cases. J Urol 114:508–513, 1975.
75. Ney C, Friedenberg RM: Diseases of the Ureter. *In* Ney C, Friedenberg RM (eds): Radiographic Atlas of the Genitourinary System, 2nd Ed. Philadelphia, JB Lippincott Company, 1981.
76. Holly LE, Sumcad B: Diverticular ureteral changes. A report of four cases. AJR 78:1053, 1957.
77. Wasserman NF, LaPointe S, Posalaky IP: Ureteral pseudodiverticulosis. Radiology 155:561–566, 1985.
78. Glanz I, Grünebaum M: Ureteral changes in polyarteritis nodosa as seen during excretory urography. J Urol 116:731–733, 1976.
79. Itoh H, Namiki M, Yoshioka T, Itatani H: Plasma cell granuloma of the renal pelvis. J Urol 128:1177–1178, 1982.
80. Nieh PT, Althausen AF: Malacoplakia of the ureter. J Urol 122:701–702, 1979.
81. O'Dea MJ, Malek RS, Farrow GM: Malacoplakia of the urinary tract: Challenges and frustrations with 10 cases. J Urol 118:739–742, 1977.
82. Elliott GB, Moloney PJ, Clement JG: Malacoplakia of the urinary tract. AJR 116:830–837, 1972.
83. Rudd EG, Matthews MD: Malacoplakia: An unusual etiology of ureteral obstruction. Obstet Gynecol 60:134–136, 1982.
84. Tsung SH: Urinary sediment cytology: Potential diagnostic tool for malakoplakia. Urology 20:546–547, 1982.
85. Hutch JA, Tanagho EA: Etiology of non-occlusive ureteral dilatation. J Urol 93:177, 1965.
86. Hutch JA, Smith DR: Sterile reflux: Report of 24 cases. Urol Int 24:460–465, 1969.
87. Wasserman NF, Posalaky IP, Dykoski R: The pathology of ureteral pseudodiverticulosis. Invest Radiol 23:592, 1988.
88. Nino-Murcia M, Friedland GW: Obliterative pyelitis. Urol Radiol 10:100, 1988.

24

Inflammation of the Bladder

RALPH V. CLAYMAN □ PHILIP J. WEYMAN □ ROBERT R. BAHNSON

For each of the nontuberculous inflammatory lesions affecting the bladder, a cause-and-effect relationship exists. The causes of bladder inflammation, which are diverse, can be categorized as either infectious (i.e., bacterial, viral, and fungal/parasitic) or noninfectious (i.e., congenital, acquired, and iatrogenic). In contrast, the effect of bladder inflammation is predictable and often follows a course progressing from mild to severe changes in the bladder urothelium.

BACTERIAL INFECTIONS

Bacterial infections of the urinary tract in *children* are second in frequency only to bacterial infections of the upper respiratory tract. In neonates, symptomatic bacteriuria is more common in males than in females, with reported ratios ranging from 2:1 to 5:1.[1, 2] However, the sex ratio reverses within the first year of life, and infections occur nearly ten times as frequently in girls who are 1 to 11 years of age.[3] At least 5% of school-age girls will acquire bacteriuria; recurrent bacteriuria will occur in over half of these girls within 5 years.[4] *Escherichia coli* is the responsible pathogen in the majority of pediatric urinary tract infections; the remaining infections are primarily due to *Proteus, Klebsiella,* and *Pseudomonas.*[5]

Symptomatology varies with the age of the child. The neonate or newborn with urinary tract infection may fail to thrive as a result of poor feeding, vomiting, and diarrhea. In the toddler, fever becomes a more prominent sign and may be accompanied by urinary urgency, frequency, hematuria, enuresis, and dysuria. Older children and adults may complain of suprapubic discomfort, urgency, frequency, hematuria, and incontinence. Fever is less commonly noted.[5] When hematuria is unusually prominent, the term *hemorrhagic cystitis* is sometimes used. This is not a separate type of cystitis, but merely a particularly severe form of the disease. Most often it is associated with *E. coli* but it may also be of viral origin.

The radiological evaluation of infants and children with urinary tract infection should be directed at defining predisposing anatomical or pathological conditions, rather than diagnosing bacterial cystitis. Ultrasonography and radionuclide imaging are helpful in identifying upper urinary tract pathology in the neonate and may confirm lower urinary tract problems. In the older child, an intravenous urogram supplies similar information.[5, 78] Radionuclide or contrast voiding cystourethrography may be helpful in diagnosing vesicoureteral reflux, vesical diverticula, ureteroceles, or male posterior urethral valves. However, urography and cystography are of limited value in diagnosing acute cystitis. The bladder is most often normal on the urogram. Pertinent findings are related to edema caused by inflammation. In the male child with an initial infection or the female child with recurrent infections, cystoscopy is helpful in identifying congenital conditions predisposing to infection (such as

diverticula or urethral valves) or in evaluating the ureteral tunnel in patients with ureteral reflux. Among patients with ureteral reflux or changes of cystitis cystica or cystitis follicularis, long-term suppressive antibiotics are indicated.[79] With appropriate therapy, recurrent infections can be reduced, and any cystic changes or milder forms of ureteral reflux will usually resolve.

In *adults,* cystitis is primarily a disease of females. It usually results from colonization of the vaginal and urethral mucosa with Enterobacteriaceae from the rectal flora. Recent studies have demonstrated that increased adherence of pathogenic bacteria to vaginal epithelial cells is the only demonstrable biological change that can be demonstrated in women susceptible to urinary tract infections.[6] In the male population, cystitis is usually associated with lower urinary tract obstruction (i.e., prostatic hyperplasia, urethral stricture, etc.) or acute and chronic bacterial prostatitis. The most common pathogen in both adult males and females is *E. coli.*

Urographic evaluation of women with lower urinary tract infection is usually unrewarding and rarely provides information helpful for management.[7, 8] In the absence of a history of childhood infection, calculi, or acute pyelonephritis, radiographic evaluation should be reserved for women with recurrent urinary tract infection caused by the same organism (true recurrent versus reinfection)[8] and is directed at detecting underlying pathology. Since cystitis in males is often associated with lower urinary tract obstruction, evaluation should be directed at detecting underlying prostatic or urethral pathology.

Diffuse irregularity and thickening of mucosal folds may be seen with severe inflammation and thickening of the bladder wall (Fig. 24–1). Decreased capacity due to edema and irritative symptoms is common. Findings are often more prominent at the bladder base and trigone; irregularity and enlargement of the trigone (trigonitis) (Fig. 24–2) or irregularity of the bladder neck (Fig. 24–3) is seen, with or without more generalized changes elsewhere (Fig. 24–4). Because these findings may be obscured by dense contrast or bladder distention, they are often most evident with the bladder partially filled or on postvoid radiographs (Figs. 24–1 and 24–3).

Bullous edema, consisting of fluid-filled cystic collections in the lamina propria of the bladder mucosa, may produce discrete rounded filling defects or clusters of such defects (Fig. 24–5). These are most often seen at the floor of the bladder and may produce ureteral obstruction (Fig. 24–6).[9] Differentiation from neoplastic processes may be difficult to achieve radiographically,[10] but these entities are more easily distinguished cystoscopically. The changes of bullous edema should also be distinguished from the chronic inflammatory disorders cystitis cystica and cystitis glandularis, as discussed later. Bullous edema is a nonspecific inflammatory reaction to bladder irritation of any cause. Thus, it may result from such diverse causes as infection and an indwelling catheter. It usually resolves

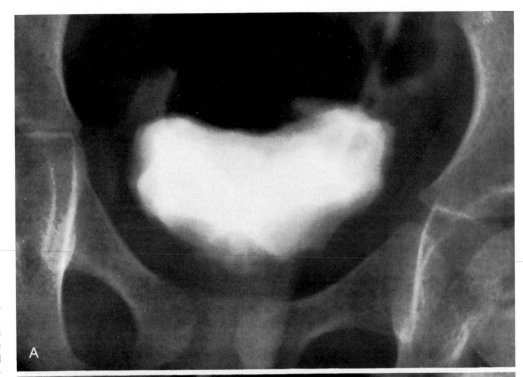

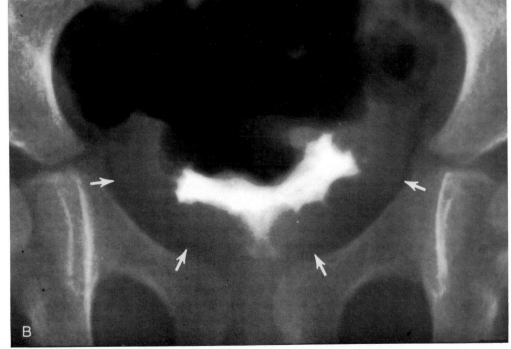

Figure 24–1. Severe bacterial cystitis with diffuse edema in a child. *A,* A partially filled view of the bladder from an intravenous urogram (IVU) demonstrates generalized mucosal fold thickening producing a scalloped, irregular contour. *B,* The diffuse fold thickening is readily apparent on postvoid radiographs with a markedly thickened bladder wall *(arrows).*

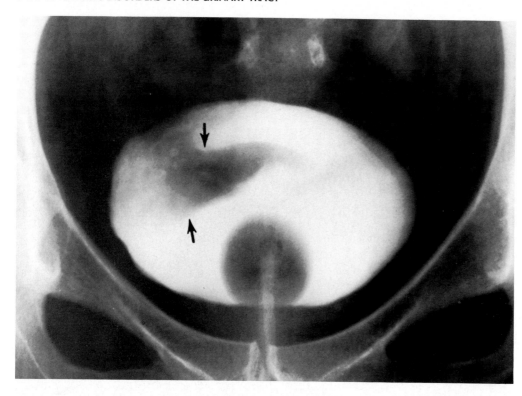

Figure 24–2. Trigonitis. Asymmetrical thickening of the right portion of the bladder floor *(arrows)* can be seen in this 40-year-old woman with bacterial cystitis.

promptly with treatment. The sonographic appearance of bullous cystitis has been described as hypoechoic areas of bladder wall thickening with a gradual transition to the normal bladder wall. This may be useful in distinguishing these changes from tumors, which are usually more echogenic with an abrupt transition.[11] In the usual forms of cystitis, ultrasonography usually shows diffuse bladder involvement (Fig. 24–7A). The less common focal forms, especially when polypoid (inflammatory pseudotumor [pseudosarcoma]), are difficult to differentiate from malignancy (Fig. 24–8).[12, 81] Computed tomography (CT) has not proved to be especially valuable, or often necessary, in patients with cystitis (Fig. 24–7B).

Alkaline Encrustation Cystitis

The term alkaline encrustation cystitis was first coined by Francois in 1914.[13] It describes a form of chronic cystitis in which the inflamed bladder mucosa is covered by a layer of calcium phosphate, often dense enough to be appreciated radiographically. Two conditions appear to be necessary for the development of this disorder. First, the bladder mucosa is usually inherently abnormal, even before the deposition of calcium salts. Thus, alkaline encrustation cystitis is a form of dystrophic calcification in which the underlying mucosa is likely to have been the site of irradiation,[15] fulguration, neoplasm, or other processes leading to devitalization of tissue. Cyclophosphamide (Cytoxan) administration may have the same effect. (Fig. 24–9).[16] Second, because precipitation of calcium salts is enhanced in an alkaline medium, the pH of urine in patients with alkaline encrustation cystitis is usually very high.[17] Urea-splitting organisms such as *Proteus mirabilis* are usually found in the urine where the degradation of urea by enzyme urease produces sufficient ammonia to maintain an alkaline urine.[14]

The radiographic appearance of alkaline encrustation cystitis, including the findings by CT, has recently been pointed out.[12] Although calcification is the dominant feature, the bladder wall itself is strikingly abnormal, being thick and irregular, and even necrotic in places (Fig. 24–9). The bladder lumen may be filled with debris. With proper treatment of the underlying defects, the disease may be reversible.

Three other forms of bacterial cystitis that have remarkably distinct presentations include malacoplakia, emphysematous/gangrenous cystitis, and pyocystis.

Malacoplakia

A detailed discussion of malacoplakia is presented in Chapter 21 (p. 835). In the bladder, the lesions of malacoplakia may produce single or multiple smooth round filling defects, most commonly near the base (Fig. 24–10).[18] As is found with malacoplakia elsewhere, the lesion may be locally invasive and may extend from the bladder to the pelvic musculature, and even to adjacent bowel loops.[19]

Emphysematous Cystitis

Emphysematous cystitis is an unusual condition most commonly seen in patients with longstanding and poorly controlled diabetes mellitus.[20, 21] In these patients, bacterial fermentation of excessive glucose within the urothelium produces carbon dioxide in the bladder wall. Intraluminal gas is also present in many patients. Usually, patients present with symptoms of cystitis, and occasionally with pneumaturia. Although *E. coli* is the causative organism in most of these patients, emphysematous cystitis due to *Aerobacter aerogenes* has been reported; other bacteria[21] and *Candida albicans* are also reported causes.[22] Urinary stasis resulting from diabetic neuropathy and from other causes in nondiabetic patients has been implicated.[21, 23] Infection with gas formation in the bladder

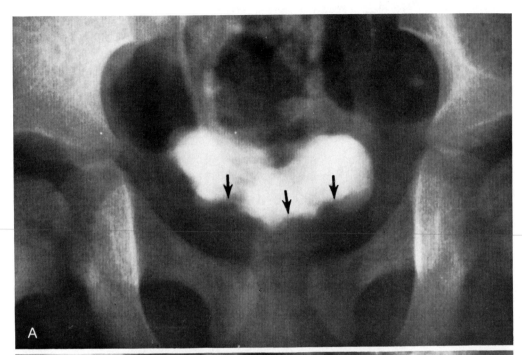

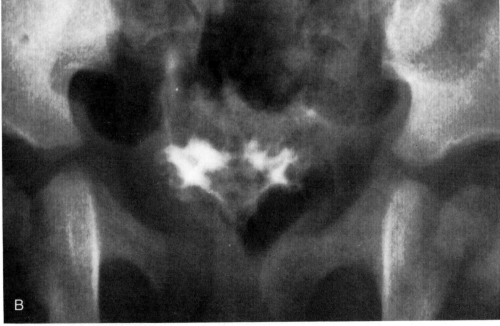

Figure 24–3. IVU in a child with acute hemorrhagic cystitis. *A,* Edema and fold thickening *(arrows)* are more apparent at the bladder base and trigone. *B,* Marked irregularity and thickened folds are readily apparent on a postvoid radiograph.

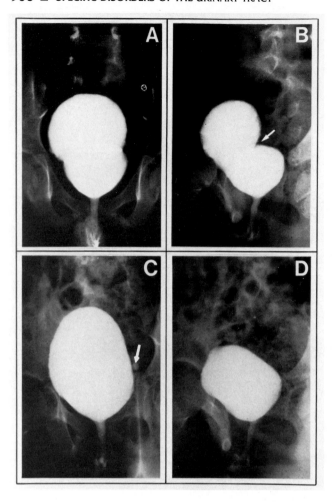

Figure 24—4. Bladder spasm simulating diverticulum or urachal cyst in a 4-year-old female with suspected adenovirus cystitis. A, Frontal, B, oblique view from voiding cystourethrogram (VCU) performed during acute phase of illness (clinical cystitis). Anterior "diverticulum-like" deformity *(arrow)* involving superior portion of bladder. C, Frontal, D, oblique view from VCU 6 weeks later shows return to normal appearance. Small diverticulum on left is noted *(arrow)*. No reflux was present. (Courtesy Ellen Shapiro, M.D., Washington University School of Medicine, St. Louis, Missouri.)

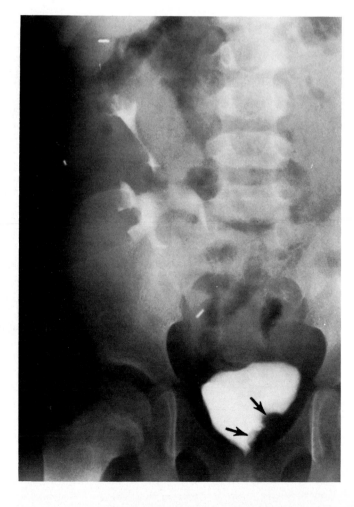

Figure 24—5. Bullous edema of the bladder in a renal transplant patient. Discrete rounded filling defects *(arrows)* are present in the bladder. These were due to bullous edema from cystitis and were not related to the operative site.

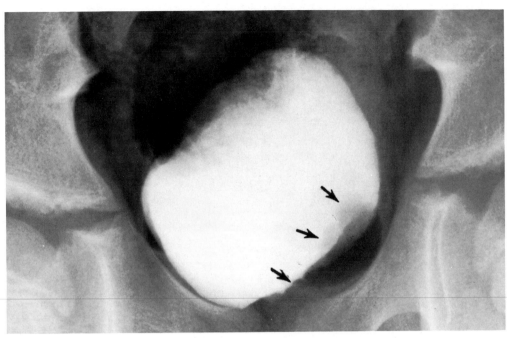

Figure 24–6. Bullous edema in a 9-year-old child with cystitis. Radiographic findings on IVU are confined to the left side of the bladder base and hemitrigone. Irregularity of the contour and rounded nodular filling defects *(arrows)* can be seen. These changes produced left ureteral obstruction, which resolved following therapy.

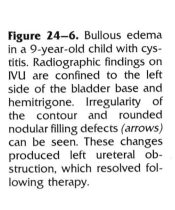

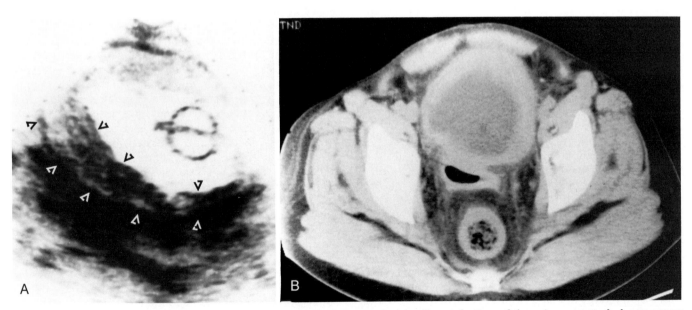

Figure 24–7. Chronic cystitis. A 49-year-old woman with a longstanding bacillary infection of the urinary tract. *A,* A sonogram through the urinary bladder reveals diffuse thickening of the bladder wall *(arrowheads).* While the bladder mucosa is not smooth, it demonstrates no evidence of focal nodularity. Note the urethral catheter's balloon within the bladder. *B,* A CT study emphasizes the marked thickening of the bladder wall. There is also slight prominence of layers of the endopelvic fascia posterior to the bladder and lateral to the vagina and rectum. Gas outlines the vagina.

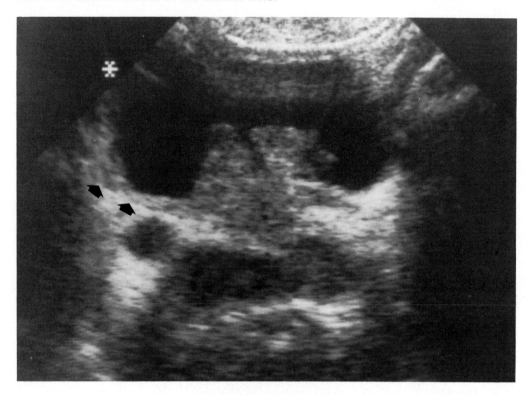

Figure 24–8. Polypoid cystitis in a 38-year-old male with recurrent urinary tract infections secondary to repeated self-insertion of foreign bodies into bladder. Transverse sonogram reveals thickened bladder wall *(arrowheads)* and large polypoid mass projecting into bladder lumen. Biopsy revealed chronic cystitis. This picture is difficult to distinguish from malignancy.

lumen, but without gas in the bladder wall, is often described as a separate entity (primary pneumaturia or pneumocystis)[21] (Fig. 24–11). These infections, too, are most common in diabetics and in nondiabetics with urinary stasis and, like cystitis emphysematosis, are also usually due to *E. coli* or *A. aerogenes*. Gas gangrene of the bladder with clostridial infection is rare, and patients who have this condition present with severe sepsis.

At cystoscopy, the urothelium is markedly hyperemic and redundant. Within the clefts of the redundant urothelium are hundreds of tiny transparent glistening gas-filled cysts. Treatment depends on the underlying condition: For diabetics, the hyperglycemia must be controlled and antibiotic therapy instituted, whereas the patient with gas gangrene requires aggressive management with penicillin G and surgical débridement of other affected areas.[20, 25] Bladder outlet obstruction must be relieved.

The radiographic diagnosis of emphysematous cystitis is based on detection of gas within the bladder wall. This may have the appearance of localized clusters of gas-filled vesicles early in the process. This appearance may be difficult to distinguish from bowel gas or an adjacent abscess, but urography will confirm the location of this gas within the bladder wall (Fig. 24–12). Overlying contrast can obscure the characteristic radiolucency of the gas-filled vesicles, which may then have an appearance similar to that of submucosal filling defects produced by tumors or other inflammatory changes. A comparison with radiographs obtained without contrast should reveal the correct diagnosis. As the process progresses, a ring of gas can often be seen partially or completely surrounding the bladder and separated from the bladder lumen (Fig. 24–13). The bladder wall may have a thickened irregular or nodular appearance, owing to the gas collections and edema. Intravesical gas may develop and perivesical gas extension has been seen (Fig. 24–14). The process may also involve the ureters and (rarely) the renal pelvis. Differential diagnosis of cystitis emphysematosum

is straightforward—the radiographic and/or CT appearance is characteristic.[24] Intraluminal gas, however, must be differentiated from gas entering the bladder iatrogenically or from an enteric fistula.

Gangrenous Cystitis

The normally abundant vesical circulation may be compromised by a number of factors, including virulent bladder infections, immunocompromise, arterial ischemia, trauma, pressure necrosis from prolonged labor or chronic vesical overdistention, and instillation of intravesical corrosive agents, which may lead to gangrenous cystitis. Rare today because of the widespread availability of antibiotics, this disease was once associated with a 60% mortality rate.[26] In gangrenous cystitis, the bladder epithelium is necrotic and ulcerated and forms a membranous cast of the bladder lumen, which may detach completely.[27] The necrosis may involve the muscular layers of the bladder wall, sometimes leading to perforation. No specific radiographic signs are identified with gangrenous cystitis. A correct diagnosis is made by considering the gravity of the symptoms in conjunction with the patient's history, physical and laboratory findings, and (if feasible) cystoscopy.

Pyocystis (Empyema of the Bladder)

Following supravesical urinary diversion, the defunctionalized bladder may become infected in up to 15% of patients.[28] This condition, termed *pyocystis*, or empyema of the bladder, is associated with increased muscle spasticity, fever, and, at times, generalized septicemia. If the bladder is neurogenically incapable of emptying or if the bladder neck is obstructed, any infection of the bladder becomes essentially a closed-space infection. Diagnosis is

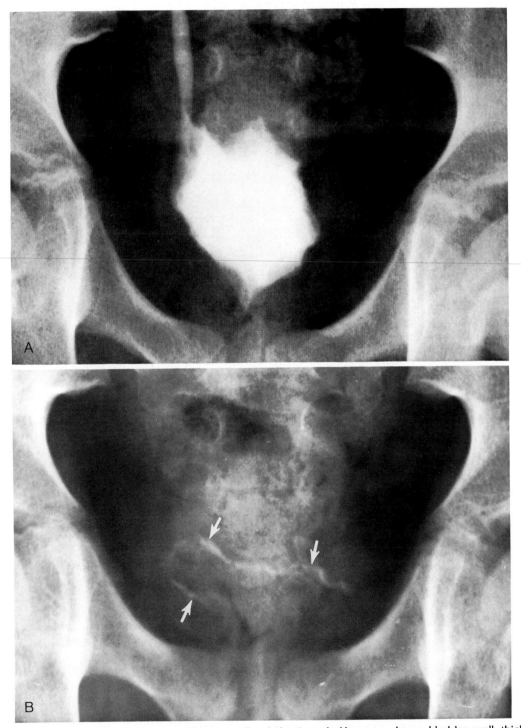

Figure 24–9. Cyclophosphamide cystitis with bladder wall calcification. *A,* Urogram shows bladder wall thickening due to hemorrhage and edema, producing diffuse irregularity, decreased bladder capacity, and altered bladder contour. *B,* Plain film 4 months later shows calcification *(arrows)* within the bladder wall.

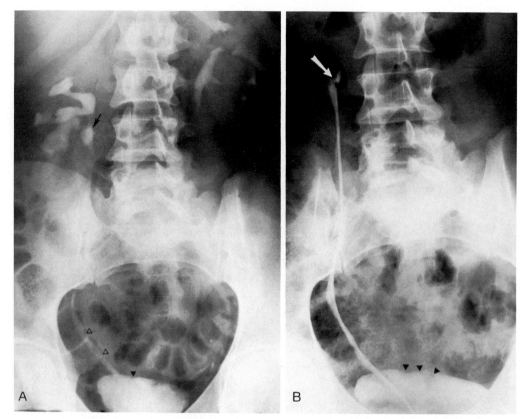

Figure 24–10. Malacoplakia of the bladder. *A,* IVU shows dilatation of right collecting system. Area of dilatation *(arrow)* in right proximal ureter. Distal right ureter also dilated *(open arrowheads).* The bladder shows numerous mural lesions *(solid arrowhead).* *B,* A retrograde ureterogram on the right shows mass *(arrow)* that partially obstructed the right kidney. Bladder lesions of malacoplakia again noted *(arrowheads).* A right nephrectomy was performed and the diagnosis of malacoplakia of the ureter with obstruction of the kidney was made.

usually made by catheterization of the bladder; radiographic and cystoscopic evaluation are usually of little value. However, evidence of this process may be detected by other imaging techniques such as CT or ultrasonography, and pyocystis must be considered when imaging the symptomatic patient who has a defunctionalized bladder. The treatment consists of bladder drainage and intermittent bladder irrigations with antibiotics. In refractory cases, cystectomy may be necessary.

VIRAL CYSTITIS

Viral cystitis occurs predominantly in children. The male-to-female ratio is 2:1. The etiological agent is most often adenovirus Type 11 or, less commonly, Type 21.[29] Rarely, varicella may cause a viral cystitis. Urinary tract involvement is likely to follow a viremia. In the typical case, the clinical picture begins with a 12- to 24-hour prodrome of dysuria and frequency, followed by gross hematuria. Should cystoscopy be performed, the urothelium will appear hemorrhagic and congested. The urographic picture varies with the extent of the inflammation. In mild cases no abnormalities are seen, whereas in severe cases the capacity of the bladder may be markedly reduced and may demonstrate large bullae and a polypoid mucosal appearance (Fig. 24–15). Care must be taken not to confuse the small polypoid bladder of viral cystitis with the normal-volume polypoid bladder harboring em-

bryonal rhabdomyosarcoma. The process is self limited and usually resolves within 4 to 5 days without antibiotic therapy.[30] In adults, the only case reports of virus-associated cystitis have been secondary to an influenza Type A[31] virus, and more recently to a BK polyamine virus.[32]

FUNGAL CYSTITIS

Mycotic infections of the bladder have been discussed in detail in Chapter 29. *C. albicans* is the most common fungal pathogen in the bladder. Usually, it affects patients who are immunosuppressed, patients on long-term broad-spectrum antibiotics who have indwelling urinary catheters, or patients with diabetes mellitus. Although often normal, urographic findings may reveal nonspecific inflammatory changes. An unusual feature of fungal urinary tract infections is the formation of bezoars or "fungus balls." These are localized collections or clusters of pseudomycelia, which may become quite large[33] and appear radiographically as nonopaque laminated spheres within the bladder (Fig. 29–6). Since *Candida* can ferment sugar, this appearance may be accentuated by gas trapped within the laminated mass.[12] Other fungal infections can affect the bladder, but they usually do so only after first involving the upper urinary tract.[34] These infections include aspergillosis, actinomycosis, cryptococcosis, coccidioidomycosis, blastomycosis, and mucormycosis, as discussed elsewhere.

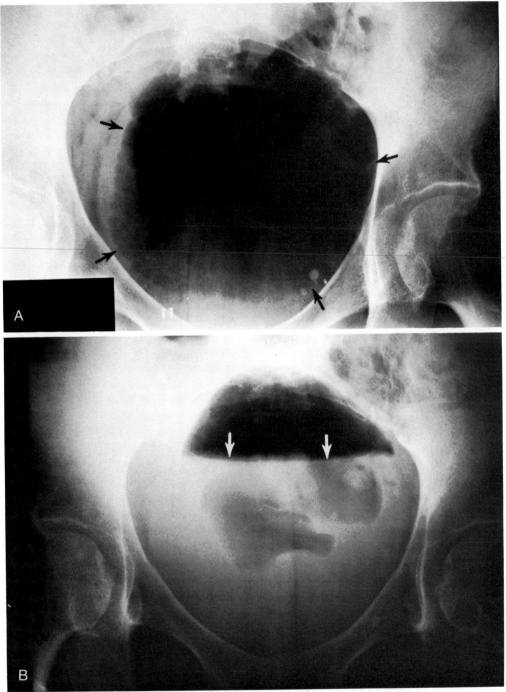

Figure 24–11. Primary pneumaturia (pneumocystis) in an elderly diabetic with *E. coli* urinary tract infection. *A,* Supine radiograph shows a large gas shadow *(arrows)* overlying the bladder. *B,* On an erect radiograph the intraluminal gas produces an air-fluid level *(arrows)* with urine. There is no detectable intramural gas. A diabetic neuropathic bladder was responsible for the large residual urine.

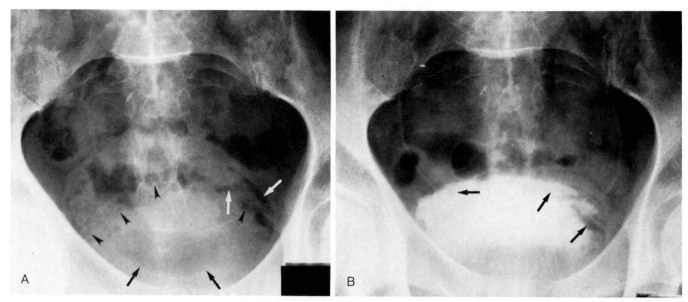

Figure 24–12. Emphysematous cystitis in a 54-year-old diabetic with urinary tract infection. *A,* Radiograph of the abdomen demonstrates a gas collection overlying the bladder. Both linear *(white arrows)* and more rounded or vesicular-appearing collections *(arrowheads)* can be seen. Intraluminal gas *(black arrows)* is also apparent. *B,* IVU shows that the gas collections *(arrows)* lie within the bladder wall, with irregularity of the bladder contour and filling defects produced by the intramural gas and edema.

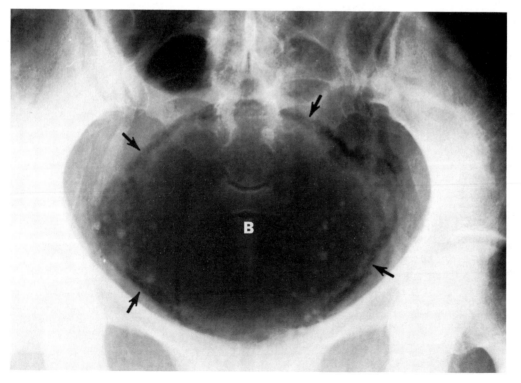

Figure 24–13. Emphysematous cystitis in an elderly diabetic. A ring of gas *(arrows)* completely surrounds the bladder. A large gas collection is also seen within the bladder lumen (B). The intramural gas is clearly separated from the intraluminal gas.

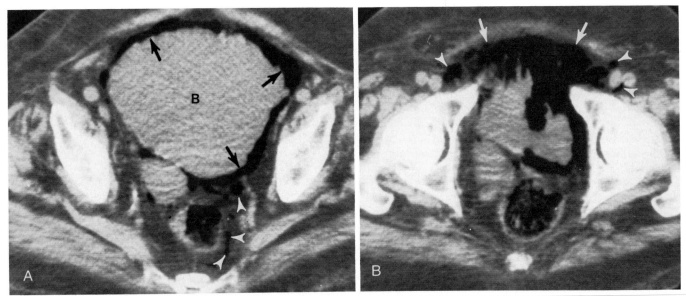

Figure 24–14. Emphysematous cystitis with perivesical extension demonstrated by computed tomography (CT). *A,* CT scan demonstrates a ring of gas *(arrows)* surrounding the bladder. Gas can be seen extending into the perivesical and perirectal fat posteriorly *(arrowheads). B,* Slightly lower, gas is seen in the bladder wall and perivesical space *(arrows)* from which it has dissected into the femoral canal and along the femoral vessels *(arrowheads).*

Figure 24–15. Viral cystitis. A 6-year-old male with urgency, frequency, dysuria and hematuria following shortly after episode of varicella. The capacity of the bladder, as visualized on an IVU, is extremely reduced. There are multiple mucosal nodules protruding into the bladder lumen. 1n rhabdomyosarcoma, the bladder volume is rarely affected to this degree. (Courtesy Robert Lebowitz, M.D., Boston, Massachusetts.)

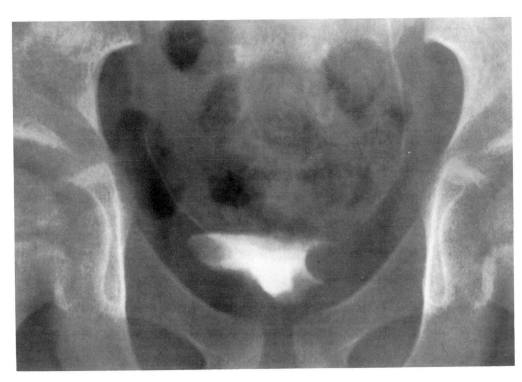

CONDYLOMA ACUMINATUM

This subject is covered more fully in the discussion of urethral inflammation (Chapter 25). Rarely, condyloma may extend to involve the urinary bladder. Keating and associates were able to compile only nine recorded cases.[35] Almost always, a primary urethral lesion is the focus. The cystoscopic and radiographic appearances of intravesical condyloma are similar to those seen in the urethra.

PARASITIC CYSTITIS

Parasitic infestation of the bladder is most often due to the blood fluke, *Schistosoma haematobium*,[36] as described in Chapter 30. Patients develop irritative voiding symptoms, suprapubic pain, and hematuria. Radiographically, the hallmark of vesical schistosomiasis is curvilinear, eggshell calcification in the wall of the bladder, which is readily evident on conventional radiographs. Early in the course of the disease, however, only mucosal edema may be observed. Later, intravenous urography and cystography may reveal a contracted bladder, ureteral reflux, hydroureter, hydronephrosis, and rarely ureteral stenosis or an intravesical filling defect secondary to squamous cell carcinoma. Histologically, marked changes are found in the urothelium, including Brunn's nests, cystitis cystica, cystitis follicularis, cystitis cystica calcinosa, and the development of squamous cell carcinoma.

NONINFECTIOUS CYSTITIS

The various forms of noninfectious cystitis represent both congenital and acquired causes. An example of a *congenital* disorder associated with chronic irritative changes is exstrophy of the bladder. In this anomaly, the urothelium of the posterior bladder wall lies exposed.[39] This altered environment causes irritation of the mucosa and eventually the development of cystitis cystica and cystitis glandularis—lesions that are considered to be forms of chronic cystitis.

The *acquired* forms of noninfectious cystitis include lupus erythematosus, eosinophilic cystitis, interstitial cystitis, pelvic lipomatosis, and inflammation secondary to extravesical processes producing a "herald lesion" within the bladder. Patients with systemic *lupus erythematosus* may at times develop a severe cystitis marked by urgency, frequency, and dysuria. Histologically, a marked vasculitis of the bladder wall is found; histological stains reveal immune-complex deposition along small vessels and smooth muscle within the lamina propria of the bladder. There are no distinguishing radiographic or cystoscopic features. Effective therapy consists of treatment with intravesical instillation of dimethyl sulfoxide on a biweekly or monthly basis. Systemic prednisone or azathioprine is of little benefit.[40]

Eosinophilic cystitis is a relatively rare form of bladder inflammation that affects both children and adults. Since the initial reports of this condition by Palubinskas[41] in 1960, about 40 more cases have been added to the literature.[42, 43] Predisposing factors include asthma, past or present bladder trauma, food allergies, and a history of eosinophilic gastroenteritis. Males are affected more commonly than females. The presenting symptoms are dysuria, urinary frequency, and urgency to void; signs include terminal hematuria, pyuria, and occasional proteinuria. Systemic eosinophilia is present in half of the patients. At cystoscopy, slightly elevated glistening velvety red globules 2 to 5 mm in diameter are noted, primarily along the trigone. The rest of the bladder appears hyperemic; ulcers are rarely present. Bladder biopsy reveals pancystitis and the presence of eosinophils, as well as mast cells and lymphocytes within the tunica propria and bladder muscle. At times, muscle necrosis and fibrosis are present.

Radiographic findings by intravenous urography or cystography include bladder wall thickening, which at times may be marked, and a nodular mucosa (Fig. 24–16). Both ureteral obstruction and vesicoureteral reflux

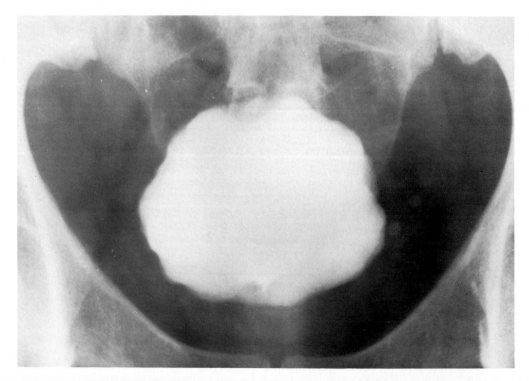

Figure 24–16. Eosinophilic cystitis. The bladder capacity is reduced. Marked thickening and edema can be seen in the irregular and nodular-appearing contour of the bladder.

have been seen.[44, 45] Eosinophilic cystitis follows a self-limited course, with 90% of cases resolving over a 2- to 12-week period. Steroids, antihistamines, and antibiotics are of little benefit. Surgical intervention by fulguration of focal lesions or by cystectomy and diversion is rarely needed. Overall, it is believed that eosinophilic cystitis may represent a milder, more self-limited form of interstitial cystitis.

Interstitial cystitis is a chronic nonspecific pancystitis of unknown cause, which predominantly affects middle-aged females.[46, 47] It was first recognized by Nitze in 1907, but not until 1915 did Hunner fully describe the urothelial ulcers seen in the more severe cases. Interstitial cystitis has often been associated with other systemic diseases, including lupus erythematosus, rheumatoid arthritis, and polyarteritis. More than 30% of patients with interstitial cystitis have a history of an allergic condition. The diagnostic triad is (1) sterile urine, (2) chronic unexplained irritative voiding symptoms (often associated with pre-micturitional suprapubic pain and a history of dyspareunia), and (3) at cystoscopy, urothelial glomerulations or ulcerative disruption of the urothelium (Hunner's ulcer).

More recently, the disease entity has been subdivided into early and late phases. In the early phase, the bladder capacity is greater than 450 cc, irritative voiding symptoms are moderate, and cystoscopy reveals only glomerulations (pinpoint petechial hemorrhagic lesions within the urothelium). These patients are usually young (average 38 years of age). In the late classic phase, the bladder capacity is reduced (i.e., is less than 450 cc), voiding symptoms are severe, and cystoscopy reveals Hunner's ulcer and urothelial fissures. These patients are older (average 57 years of age).[48, 49] Biopsy of the bladder reveals pancystitis with transmural inflammation and fibrosis. Marked submucosal edema and vasodilation are evident. Mast cells in the submucosa, and especially in the muscle layers, are strongly suggestive of interstitial cystitis.

Radiographic findings are usually absent in the early phase before bladder capacity is reduced. In the later phase, urography reveals a small contracted bladder, which may be smooth or irregular (Figs. 24–17 and 24–18). Either vesicoureteral reflux or ureteral obstruction may occur as a consequence of bladder wall fibrosis (Fig. 24–18), and, paradoxically, both may occur together.

Pelvic lipomatosis is characterized by the benign overgrowth of perivesical and pericolonic retroperitoneal fatty tissue.[50, 51] Its relationship to cystitis glandularis now appears well established, with some workers reporting such changes in as many as 80% of patients with pelvic lipomatosis.[52, 75] However, the pathogenesis of this relationship is unclear. A fuller discussion of pelvic lipomatosis and its imaging characteristics may be found in Chapter 94.

EXTRINSIC PROCESSES

The *herald lesion* of the bladder, described by Melicow and colleagues in 1961, refers to the bladder's response to neoplastic or inflammatory disease arising in a nearby perivesical organ.[53] The lesion may be the result of cancer (of the uterus, cervix, prostate, vagina, or colon), diverticulitis with or without abscess formation, regional enteritis (Crohn's disease)—occasionally with fistula formation, endometriosis, or a variety of other less common diseases. The herald lesion has three degrees of severity, each corresponding to a stage of the continuous process in which the extravesical lesion encroaches, penetrates, and perforates the bladder wall. Patients usually present with symptoms from the primary disease process and with associated irritative voiding complaints. A bowel fistula results in fecaluria and pneumaturia.[54] The intravenous urogram and cystogram may show localized inflammatory changes in the bladder wall with bullous edema, thickening, or nodularity. The bladder wall may be flattened, the ureters may be displaced or obstructed, and rarely a fistulous tract to the bowel may be demonstrated (Fig. 24–19). Reactions encroaching upon the ureteral orifice may result in a pseudoureterocele.[55] Cystoscopy reveals a localized area of inflammation that, depending on the stage of the lesion, may be ulcerated. In addition, the location of the lesion is helpful. A herald lesion at the bladder neck in males suggests prostate disease (infection or cancer), whereas a midline lesion, behind the trigone, in females is generally associated with a uterine or cervical process. Disease affecting the rectosigmoid involves the left lateral wall or dome of the bladder in both sexes. Histological evaluation of the herald lesions shows an infiltrating inflammatory process more marked in the adventitial and outer muscular layers of the bladder. The process may be associated with metaplasia and cystic changes in the urothelial and submucosal layers of the bladder, respectively.

IATROGENIC INFLAMMATION

Common causes of *iatrogenic* bladder inflammation include foreign bodies (causing catheter cystitis), drug reaction, radiation therapy, and postoperative changes. The most common *foreign-body* reaction is due to an indwelling urethral catheter. Catheter cystitis usually results from the prolonged catheterization of the bladder with associated mechanical irritation and the development of discrete areas of cystitis, usually along the posterior wall or floor of the bladder.[11] In some patients, the changes develop with surprising rapidity. This lesion develops in approximately 80% of patients with a chronic indwelling urethral catheter. Although bacteriuria is often associated with catheter cystitis, it is not an acknowledged cause. The radiographic changes in catheter-induced cystitis are a manifestation of inflammation from chronic contact with indwelling catheters, and possibly of a sensitivity to the catheter material itself. These changes are usually localized posteriorly along the floor of the bladder or at the trigone. Radiographic findings are those of nonspecific inflammation or bullous edema, as previously discussed.

Endoscopic evaluation reveals a red, elevated area 2 to 5 cm in diameter, with surrounding bullous edema. Microscopic examination is remarkable for evidence of mucosal and lamina propria involvement with dilated vessels and occasional fibrosis. Neither metaplasia nor muscle involvement is found. The problem is directly related to catheterization and resolves within a few weeks of removing the catheter. Of greater concern is the development of squamous cell cancer in patients with chronic indwelling urethral catheters. The occurrence of malig-

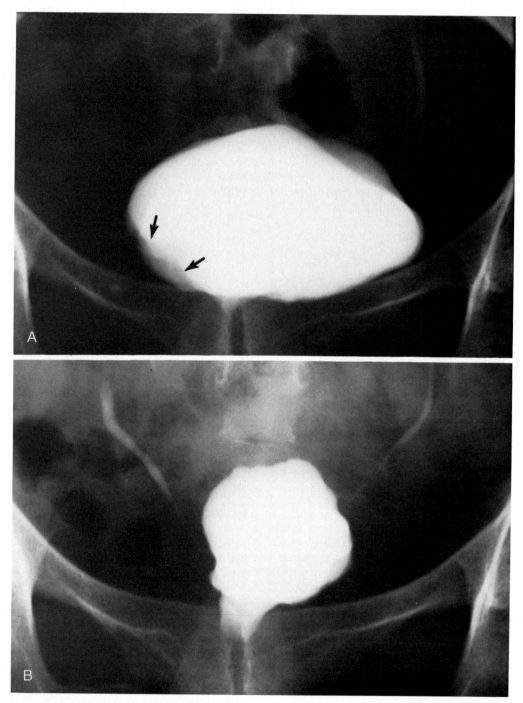

Figure 24–17. Chronic interstitial cystitis. *A,* In the early stages bladder capacity is nearly normal, although the patient complained of severe frequency. Mild irregularity *(arrows)* is noted at the right bladder base. *B,* Several months later the bladder appears markedly contracted and irregular.

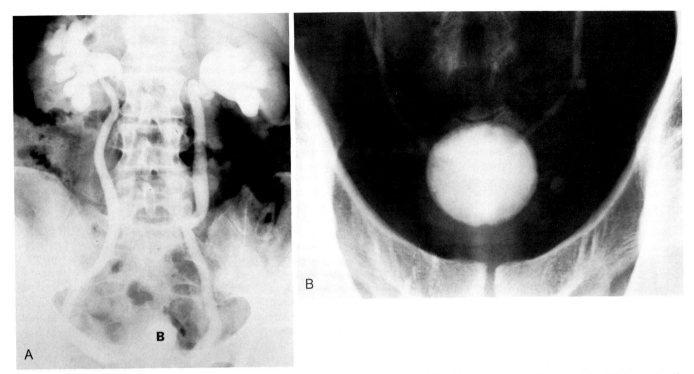

Figure 24–18. *A,* Chronic interstitial cystitis in a patient with a long history of bladder symptoms. The bladder (B) is markedly contracted and smooth-walled. Bladder capacity was 75 cc. Ureteral obstruction with bilateral hydronephrosis secondary to the bladder fibrosis is evident. *B,* In a different patient, chronic interstitial cystitis with contracted smooth-walled bladder is seen. The ureters are not dilated.

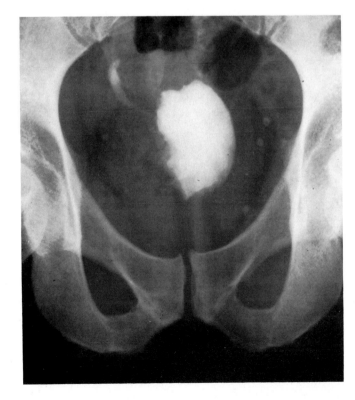

Figure 24–19. Perivesical abscess secondary to infected inguinal herniorrhaphy. Bladder film from an IVU reveals flattening of right vesicle wall from a right-sided perivesical mass. The bladder is poorly distensible, and the mucosa lining the right side exhibits prominent bullous edema. Ten days previously, the patient had a right inguinal herniorrhaphy. All changes were promptly reversed following drainage of perivesical abscess.

nancy is directly related to the duration of catheterization; 5% at more than 10 years.[56] In many cases, prophylactic urinary diversion without cystectomy is recommended as preventive therapy, because catheter cystitis and the risk of malignancy usually resolve upon removal of the catheter.

Other types of foreign bodies within the bladder may also induce a generalized cystitis. Such articles may become encrusted and eventually present as a bladder stone. Owing to psychopathic conditions, sexual misadventures, or problems encountered during therapeutic procedures, various foreign bodies have been reported. These include pieces of urethral catheter balloons, wires from stone baskets, safety pins, thermometers, toothpicks, suppositories and sutures, among others. Radiographically, the metallic foreign bodies are readily identified.[57, 57a, 80] Likewise, encrustation or stone formation can unmask radiolucent foreign bodies, which appear as a lucent center within the calculus. A mass effect, associated with the cystitis, may be appreciated on intravenous urography or cystography. Diagnosis and treatment are both usually accomplished cystoscopically. However, urethral injury is best avoided, and at times, therefore, a suprapubic cystotomy may be necessary to remove an iatrogenic intruder.[57]

Drug-induced cystitis, although usually a self-limited condition, is sometimes life threatening. It is most often associated with antibiotics (methicillin, piperacillin sodium, penicillin G, carbenicillin, ticarcillin) or chemotherapeutic agents (cyclophosphamide [Cytoxan], busulfan, mercaptopurine, cytarabine, mitomycin C, 1-asparaginase, intravesical bacille Calmette-Guérin [BCG]). Other drugs associated with cystitis include aniline dyes, chlordimeform hydrochloride (a pesticide), methaqualone, turpentine, misdirected vaginal suppositories containing 9-nonoxynol (a powerful spermicide)[80] (Fig. 24–20), and intravesical formalin or ether.[57a, 77] The development of cystitis is secondary to either (1) a direct toxic effect of drug metabolites on the urothelium or (2) an allergic-type reaction with the deposition of immunoglobulins (IgG, IgM) and complement (C3) within the bladder wall. Special note should be made of two agents commonly used in the bladder, which, when employed in unduly high concentrations, may be quite irritative and possibly quite harmful: contrast agents in very young patients[59] and silver nitrate.[60] Pancreatic exocrine secretions, which are secreted directly into the bladder by means of duodenocystostomy in patients undergoing pancreatic transplantation, may also be irritating to the bladder mucosa.

Cyclophosphamide cystitis is a prime example of drug-induced cystitis of the direct toxic variety.[58] Hydroxylation of cyclophosphamide by hepatic microsomes releases both the active metabolite, phosphoramide mustard, and the toxic metabolite, acrolein. Although the urothelium of the entire urinary tract may be affected, lower tract symptoms are usual, because bladder epithelium is in contact with the toxic substances, the longest of any part of the urinary tract. Nevertheless, upper tract involvement has been reported.[61] In the acute phase, which usually occurs within days of drug administration, the patient presents with irritative voiding symptoms and gross hematuria. A more chronic and intractable phase may develop after several months of therapy and is characterized by fibrosis, decreased capacity, and unremitting hemorrhage.[62] The hemorrhagic aspect of the process may progress to passage of blood clots and strangury; on rare occasion, it is life threatening. More than 40% of patients receiving cyclophosphamide may develop cystitis, and there appears to be a linear relationship between the likelihood of developing symptoms and the total amount of drug administered (usually more than 6 gm/m² is required in order to produce symptoms). Cytoscopy is notable for severe mucosal hyperemia with associated ulceration and active hemorrhage. Biopsies reveal predominantly a fibroblastic proliferation with associated atypia. In rare circumstances, the urothelial changes progress to cancer. Overall, it is estimated that

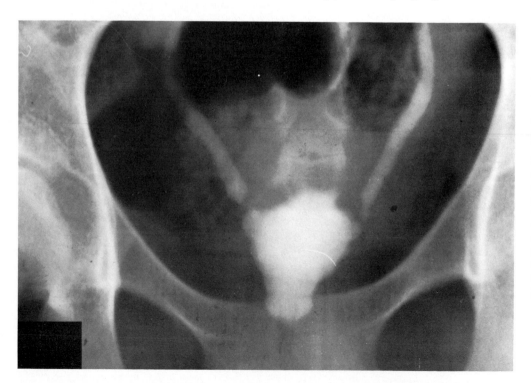

Figure 24–20. Chemical cystitis secondary to misdirected contraceptive suppository. A 19-year-old female with severe strangury and hematuria. Several days previously the patient had inadvertently inserted a contraceptive vaginal suppository into her urethra. The bladder film from an IVU reveals an extremely reduced capacity with nodular mucosal changes. Both ureters are slightly dilated as a result of trigonal edema, and possibly, vesicoureteral reflux. The active spermicidal ingredient was 9-nonoxynol, a powerful vesical irritant.[80] (Courtesy Gerald Goodman, M.D., Reading, Pennsylvania.)

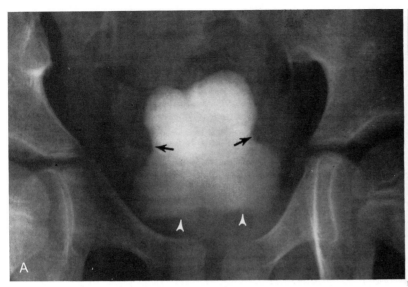

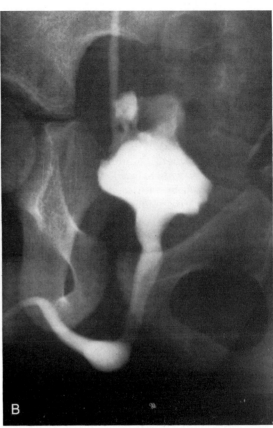

Figure 24–21. Cyclophosphamide cystitis in a 6-year-old leukemic. *A,* In the acute hemorrhagic phase, marked deformity of the bladder wall due to hemorrhage and edema is noted. The intraureteral ridge *(arrowheads)* is thickened and large scalloped defects *(arrows)* in the bladder wall are present. *B,* Voiding film from the IVU shows the severe diffuse deformity to better advantage.

patients receiving cyclophosphamide therapy have a 45-fold increased risk of developing bladder carcinoma.[62] Unfortunately, the bladder wall fibrosis seen following cyclophosphamide therapy tends to be irreversible.

The radiographic findings reflect the severity of the hemorrhagic cystitis. Bladder-wall thickening and nodular defects due to hemorrhage and edema (Fig. 24–21)[63] are prominent and may be severe enough to simulate neoplasia. In the chronic phase, a small contracted bladder resembling that seen in interstitial cystitis (Figs. 24–17 and 24–18) may occur. Either ureteral obstruction and/or vesicoureteral reflux may complicate the bladder changes.[64] Calcifications of the bladder wall have also been reported (Fig. 24–9).[16]

Concurrent parenteral administration of cyclophosphamide and 2-mercaptoethanesulfonate (Mesna) will usually prevent the vesical complications associated with administration of cyclophosphamide alone. Mesna acts directly on acrolein and renders it harmless. When troublesome hematuria does occur, it can be treated by intravesical irrigations with alum, silver nitrate, formalin, or phenol. Angiographic interventional procedures such as intravenous vasopressin or hypogastric artery embolization have usually been unsuccessful. In rare circumstances, emergency cystectomy and urinary diversion are required.[62]

Methicillin cystitis is a prime example of an allergic type of drug-induced cystitis. Approximately 12% of patients treated with this drug develop hemorrhagic cystitis. Interestingly, cystitis may presage the later occurrence of interstitial nephritis or agranulocytosis, both of which are recognized complications of methicillin. Laboratory studies reveal a peripheral eosinophilia. Cystoscopic findings are of an erythematous diffusely inflamed urothelium, which is microscopically shown to be due to infiltration of the tunica propria with eosinophils and lymphoreticular cells. The entire process is self limited and usually resolves within 5 days of cessation of the drug.[65, 66] Similar reactions have been noted with ticarcillin, disodium carbenicillin, and penicillin G potassium.[66]

External or intracavitary radiation therapy may result in either immediate or delayed *radiation cystitis.*[67] The use of external-beam radiation therapy for prostate and bladder cancer or of intravesical or intravaginal brachytherapy for carcinomas of the bladder or uterine cervix may result in the development of marked irritative voiding symptoms (frequency, nocturia, and dysuria) sometimes in association with gross hematuria. This is most commonly seen when the radiation absorbed dose exceeds 4000 rad, but the severity of the symptoms is related to the methods of dose fractionation. In many cases, symptoms are due to superinfection following radiation injury. Cystoscopically, multiple punctate erythematous lesions are seen amid patches of pale urothelium. Microscopically, there is evidence of both mucosal ulcerations and panvesical fibrosis. In the acute phase of radiation cystitis, radiography is normal or may show varying degrees of nonspecific inflammatory changes, such as bullous edema. The later effects, which are due to vasculitis and fibrosis, usually become evident 1 to 4 years after treatment but may develop earlier with high doses. With progressive fibrosis, bladder capacity may be reduced to less than 50 cc and a small contracted bladder, which is either smooth or irregular, may be noted. Vesicoureteral reflux is common.[68] Calcification of the bladder wall due to an alkaline encrusting cystitis has been reported, usually in association with a *Proteus* infection.[15] Chronic radiation changes in the blood vessels of the bladder wall may lead to persistent and severe hematuria troublesome enough to require the use of intravesical cauterizing agents such as formalin or hypogastric artery embolization.

A FINAL COMMON PATHWAY—CHRONIC PROLIFERATIVE EFFECTS

The effect of chronic inflammation on the bladder is often predictable, following a well-defined evolutionary histological pattern, regardless of the cause. These changes include Brunn's nests, cystitis cystica, cystitis follicularis, cystitis glandularis, and squamous metaplasia. *Brunn's nests* are the most common pathological change seen in the chronically inflamed bladder; they are found in 90% of bladders at autopsy. The lesion consists of solid nests of urothelial cells lying in the lamina propria beneath the surface urothelium.[69] If the central portion of the nest of cells undergoes degeneration, then a fluid-filled cyst results (cystitis cystica). This development is seen in more than 60% of bladders at autopsy. The cysts are lined by a nonsecretory epithelium and are covered by a thin layer of mucosa. Cystitis cystica is more frequent in women and children with chronic urinary tract infection and is most common at the trigone and base of the bladder.[70, 71, 72] At times, the surface of the cyst may become calcified, leading to the designation *cystitis cystica calcinosa,* a lesion commonly associated with schistosomiasis. At other times, particularly in children with chronic urinary tract infections, the cysts are associated with submucosal lymphoid aggregates (cystitis follicularis). These small lesions have a pearly or tan-to-yellow appearance and are usually located on the trigone or along the bladder neck.[71]

With further chronic irritation, the Brunn's nests develop into glandular structures (*cystitis glandularis*) of either an intestinal (thick mucus, goblet-like cells) or subtrigonal (thin mucus, columnar cell lining) nature.[52, 75] These changes are also seen in patients with exstrophy of the bladder and pelvic lipomatosis, and may be precursors of adenocarcinoma of the bladder. Rarely, the glandular lesions may obstruct the ureters and cause hydronephrosis.

Lastly, *squamous metaplasia* of the urothelium may occur. Unlike the previously described conditions, this is unrelated to the development of Brunn's nests. It is quite common in females and has been noted to be a normal epithelial variant, which occurs secondary to hormonal changes. One reason for its occurrence is the fact that the trigone and the upper third of the vagina are of similar embryological origin. With the development of squamous metaplasia, the urothelium in this area is replaced by nonkeratinizing squamous epithelium.[69] At times, the affected area may extend beyond the trigone and affect the entire bladder epithelium. This occurs predominantly in patients with a history of chronic inflammation. In males, the lesions may progress to leukoplakia, with the development of thick white plaques. Although leukoplakia of the bladder is generally regarded as benign, cases of malignant transformation to squamous cell carcinoma are known.[73, 74]

Any of these chronic inflammatory foci may become large enough to produce radiographically discrete nodular defects in the bladder on urography or ultrasonography.[75] These may take the form of single rounded nodules, clusters of nodules producing a "cobblestone" appearance (Fig. 24–22), or a more papillary appearance (Fig. 24–23). They are often indistinguishable from the changes of bullous edema or neoplastic processes, particularly bladder carcinoma, or extrinsically invading malignancies of the cervix or prostate.

An interesting bladder lesion of controversial etiology is the nephrogenic adenoma. Although some classify it as a benign neoplasm, others view it primarily as another in the list of metaplastic responses of bladder epithelium to chronic irritation.[76] The lesion arises in the bladder epithelium and may attain considerable size. Microscopically, it is composed of tubules that superficially resemble renal proximal tubules, located predominantly in the tunica propria. The symptoms usually are those of vesical irritation, accompanied in some cases by hematuria. The radiographic findings are nonspecific and are those of an intravesical or mural mass.

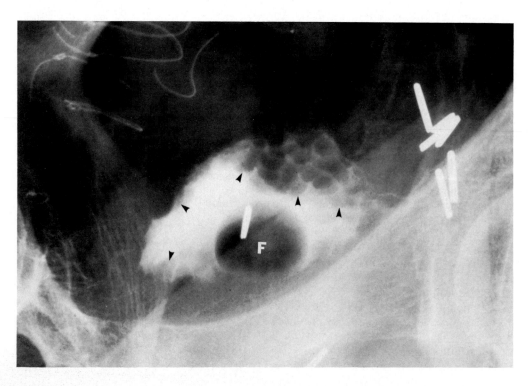

Figure 24–22. Cystitis cystica. Numerous smooth rounded defects are seen in the bladder (*arrowheads*) giving a "cobblestone" appearance. A Foley urethral catheter (F) is present.

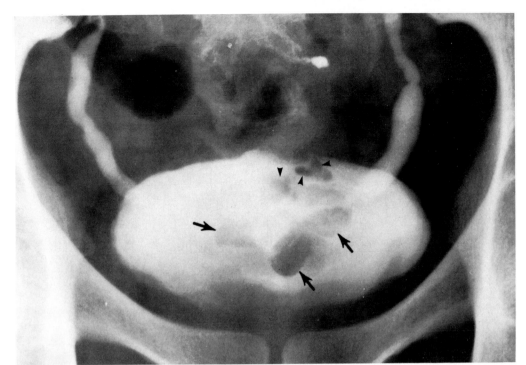

Figure 24–23. Cystitis glandularis. Discrete filling defects *(arrows)* are present within the bladder. Some of these *(arrowheads)* have a lobulated or papillary appearance. Biopsy revealed cystitis glandularis.

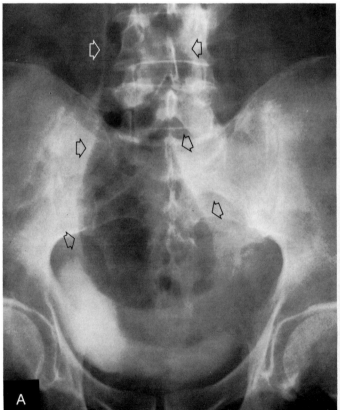

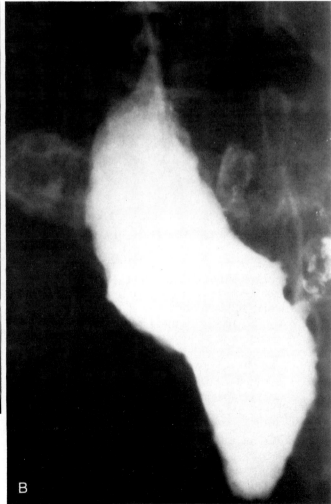

Figure 24–24. Infected urachal cyst in a 31-year-old male with suprapubic and periumbilical pain. There was purulent drainage from the umbilicus. *A,* IVU reveals gourd-shaped gas collection in lower abdomen *(arrowheads).* The urinary bladder is impressed by a supravesical mass. *B,* Film taken following catheterization of umbilical fistula and injection of contrast medium reveals opacification of the cyst. There is some irregularity of the cyst lining. A large infected urachal cyst was discovered at surgery. No evidence of malignancy was found. (Courtesy Leon Love, M.D., Chicago, Illinois.)

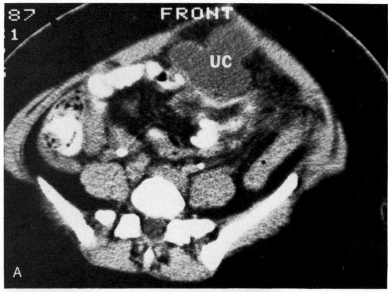

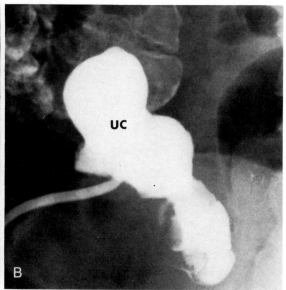

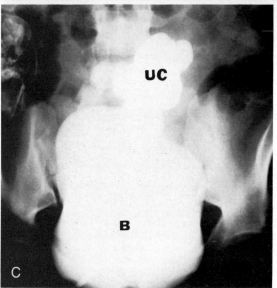

Figure 24–25. Infected urachal cyst. A 29-year-old female, 2 weeks postpartum, presented with diffuse abdominal pain, fever, and leukocytosis. *A,* CT scan through lower abdomen shows urachal cyst (UC) prior to drainage. The patient improved with percutaneous drainage and antibiotics. *B,* Contrast injection fills urachal cyst (UC) via percutaneous catheter previously placed for drainage of infected cyst. The bowel is opacified from oral contrast for CT. *C,* Cystogram was performed after percutaneous drainage of infected urachal cyst. Contrast material did not fill urachal cyst (UC) from cystography, but rather from direct injection. B = bladder.

INFLAMMATIONS OF THE URACHUS

In the fetus, the urachus is a patent canal that connects the bladder with the allantois. Some time before birth, the urachus becomes obliterated and is thereafter known as the medial umbilical ligament. Persistence of the urachus is of little concern, unless it becomes infected.[37, 38] The infected cyst is usually colonized by *Staphylococcus aureus;* it may drain either via the umbilicus or transvesically. Rarely, the cyst may rupture into the preperitoneal tissues, peritoneal cavity, or involved adjacent organs. Symptoms include midline abdominal pain, fever, dysuria, and a palpable suprapubic mass. The urine culture may be positive. At cystoscopy, a bulging mass may be seen at the dome of the bladder. The overlying epithelium may be intact, but more often the surface is ulcerated. Cystography may show a mass impression at the dome of the bladder. Inflammation from an infected cyst may produce thickening and irregularity of the adjacent bladder wall. Communication between the bladder and an infected urachal cyst is rarely demonstrated, but the cyst may contain gas, which is readily evident (Fig. 24–24). Ultrasonography and CT may both be useful in a number of ways, especially in revealing the full extent of the supravesical component of the mass[30] (Fig. 24–25). Definitive treatment consists of excision of the cyst, along with a cuff of bladder, and the umbilicus, while temporary relief may be obtained by percutaneous drainage (Fig. 24–25). Urachal anomalies are described in more detail in Chapter 19.

References

1. Bergstrom T, Larson K, Lincoln K, et al: Studies of urinary tract infections in infancy and childhood. J Pediatr 80:858, 1972.
2. Drew, JH, Acton CM: Radiological findings in newborn infants with urinary tract infection. Arch Dis Child 51:628, 1976.
3. Winberg J, Anderson HJ, Bergstrom T, et al: Epidemiology of syptomatic urinary tract infection in childhood. Acta Pediatr Scand 252(suppl): 1, 1974.
4. Kunin CM: The natural history of recurrent bacteriuria in schoolgirls. N Engl J Med 282:1443, 1970.

5. Woodard JR: Urinary tract infections. *In* Kelalis PP and King LR (eds): Clinical Pediatric Urology. Philadelphia, WB Saunders Company, 1976, pp 182–213.

6. Schaeffer AJ, Jones JM, Dunn JK: Association of in vitro *Escherichia coli* adherence to vaginal and buccal epithelial cells with susceptibility of women to recurrent urinary tract infections. N Engl J Med 304:1062, 1981.

7. Fowler JE Jr, Pulaski ET: Excretory urography, cystography and cystoscopy in the evaluation of women with urinary tract infection. N Engl J Med 304:462, 1981.

8. Fair WR, McClennan BL, Jost RG: Are excretory urograms necessary in evaluating women with urinary tract infection? J Urol 121:313, 1979.

9. Shackelford GD, Manley CB: Acute ureteral obstruction secondary to bullous cystitis of the trigone. Radiology 132:351, 1979.

10. Pittari JJ, May RE: Bullous edema of the bladder simulating tumor. AJR 86:863, 1961.

11. Abs-Yousef MM, Narayana AS, Brown RC: Catheter-induced cystitis: Evaluation by cystosonography. Radiology 151:471, 1984.

12. Verguts L, Deconinck K, Mortelmans LL: Alkaline encrusting cystitis. Urol Radiol 4:53, 1981.

13. Rifkin MD, Kurtz AB, Pastome, Goldberg BB: Unusual presentations of cystitis. J Ultrasound Med 2:25, 1983.

14. Harrison RB, Stier FM, Cochrane JA: Alkaline encrusting cystitis. AJR 130:575, 1978.

15. Jameson RM: The treatment of phosphatic encrusted cystitis (alkaline cystitis) with nalidixic acid. Br J Urol 38:89, 1966.

16. Francis RS, Shackelford GD: Cyclophosphamide cystitis with bladder wall calcification. J Can Assoc Radiol 25:324, 1974.

17. Pollack HM, Banner MP, Martinez LO, Hodson CJ: Diagnostic considerations in bladder wall calcification. AJR 136:791, 1981.

18. Stanton MJ, Maxted W: Malacoplakia: A study of the literature and current concepts of pathogenesis, diagnosis, and treatment. J Urol 125:139, 1981.

19. Bidwell JK, Dunne MG: Computed tomography of bladder malacoplakia. J Comput Assist Tomogr 11:909, 1987.

20. Teasley GH: Cystitis emphysematosa: Case report with a review of literature. J Urol 62:48, 1949.

21. Bailey H: Cystitis emphysematosa: 19 cases with intramural and interstitial collections of gas. AJR 86:850, 1961.

22. Singh CR, Lytle WF: Cystitis emphysematosa caused by *Candida albicans*. J Urol 130:1171, 1983.

23. Hawtrey CE, Williams JJ, Schmidt JD: Cystitis emphysematosa. Urology 3:612, 1974.

24. Ney C, Kumar M, Billah K, Doerr J: CT Demonstration of cystitis emphysematosa. J Comput Assist Tomogr 11:552, 1987.

25. Weinstein L, Barga M: Gas gangrene. N Engl J Med 289:1129, 1972.

26. Busse K, Altwein JE: Catheter-induced bladder gangrene. J Urol 112:461, 1974.

27. Peterson RO: Urologic Pathology. Philadelphia, JB Lippincott, 1986, p 306.

28. Duckett JW Jr, Raezer DM: Neuromuscular dysfunction of the lower urinary tract. *In* Kelalis PP, King LR (eds): Clinical Pediatric Urology. Philadelphia, WB Saunders Company, 1976, p 421.

29. Numazaki Y, Shigota S, Kumasaka T, et al: Acute hemorrhagic cystitis in children: Isolation of adenovirus type II. N Engl J Med 278:700, 1968.

30. Mufson MA, Belshe RB: A review of adenoviruses in the etiology of acute hemorrhagic cystitis. J Urol 115:191, 1976.

31. Kharpour M, Nik-Akhtar B: Epidemic of hemorrhagic cystitis due to influenza A virus. Postgrad Med J 53:251, 1977.

32. Arthur RR, Shah KV, Baust SJ, et al: Association of BK viruria with hemorrhagic cystitis in recipients of bone marrow transplants. N Engl J Med 315:230–234, 1986.

33. Harold DL, Koff SA, Kass EJ: *Candida albicans* "fungus ball" in bladder. Urol 9:662, 1977.

34. Wise GJ, Kozinn J, Goldberg P: Amphotericin B as a urologic irrigant in the management of noninvasive candiduria. J Urol 128:82, 1982.

35. Keating MA, Young RH, Carr CP, et al: Condyloma acuminatum of the bladder and ureter: Case report and review of literature. J Urol 133:465, 1985.

36. Lehman JS Jr, Fariz S, Smith JH, et al: Urinary schistosomiasis in Egypt: Clinical radiological, bacteriological, and parasitological correlations. Trans R Soc Trop Med Hyg 67:384, 1973.

37. MacMillan RW, Schullinger JN, Santulli VT: Pyourachus: An unusual surgical problem. J Pediatr Surg 8:87, 1973.

38. Sanders RC, Oh KS, Dorst JP: B-Scan ultrasound: Positive and negative contrast material evaluation of congenital urachal anomaly. AJR 120:448, 1973.

39. Duckett JW, Caldamone AA: Anomalies of the urinary tract: Bladder and urachus. *In* Kelalis PP, King LR, Belman AB (eds): Clinical Pediatric Urology. Philadelphia, WB Saunders Company, 1985, pp 726–751.

40. Orth RW, Weisman MH, Cohen AH, et al: Lupus cystitis: Primary bladder manifestations of systemic lupus erythematosus. Ann Intern Med 98:323, 1983.

41. Palubinskas AJ: Eosinophilic cystitis: Case report of eosinophilic infiltration of the urinary bladder. Radiology 75:589, 1960.

42. Sutphin M, Middleton AW Jr: Eosinophilic cystitis in children: A self-limited process. J Urol 132:117, 1984.

43. Nkposong EO, Attah EB: Eosinophilic cystitis. Eur Urol 4:274, 1978.

44. Goldstein M: Eosinophilic cystitis. J Urol 106:854f, 1971.

45. Marshall FF, Middleton AW Jr: Eosinophilic cystitis. J Urol 112:335, 1974.

46. Rosin RD, Griffiths T, Sofras F, et al: Interstitial cystitis. Br J Urol 51:524, 1979.

47. Larsen SA, Thompson T, Hald T, et al: Mast cells in interstitial cystitis. Br J Urol 54:283, 1982.

48. Messing EM, Stamey TA: Interstitial cystitis. Urology 12:381, 1978.

49. Messing EM: The diagnosis of interstitial cystitis. *In* Interstitial Cystitis—1987. Urology 24(suppl):4, 1987.

50. O'Dea MJ, Malek RS: Foreign body in bladder and perivesical inflammation masquerading as pelvic lipomatosis. J Urol 116:669, 1976.

51. Davies G, Osborn DE, Castro JE: Pelvic lipomatosis with associated cystitis glandularis. Urol 2:494, 1978.

52. Navarro JE, Huggins TJ: Cystitis glandularis: An unusual cause of ureteral obstruction. Urol Radiol 6:27, 1984.

53. Melicow MM, Uson AC, Stams U: Herald lesion of urinary bladder. Urology 3:140, 1974.

54. Nielson K, Orholm M, Anderson SP, et al: Herald lesion of the urinary bladder. Scand J Urol Nephrol 18:173, 1984.

55. Mitty HA, Schapira HE: Ureterocele and pseudoureterocele cobra versus cancer. J Urol 117:557, 1977.

56. Broecher BH, Klein FA, Hackler RH: Cancer of the bladder in spinal cord injury patients. J Urol 125:196, 1981.

57. Aycinema JF: Foreign bodies in the urinary bladder and urethra. *In* Kauffman JM (ed): Current Urologic Therapy. Philadelphia, WB Saunders Company, 1986, p 252.

57a. Gattegno B, Michel F, Thibault Ph: A serious complication of vesical ether instillation: Ether cystitis. J Urol 139:357, 1988.

58. Klein FA, Smith MJ: Urinary complications of cyclophosphamide therapy: Etiology, prevention and management. South Med J 76:1413, 1983.

59. McAllister WH, Cacciarelli A, Shackleford GD: Complications associated with cystography in children. Radiology 111:167, 1974.

60. Jerkins GR, Noe HN, Hill DE: An unusual complication of silver nitrate treatment of hemorrhagic cystitis: Case report. J Urol 136:456, 1986.

61. Texter JH Jr, Koontz WW Jr, McWilliams NB: Hemorrhagic cystitis as a complication of the management of pediatric neoplasms. Urol Surg 29:47, 1979.

62. Ehrlich RM, Freedman A, Goldsobel AB, et al: The use of sodium 2-mercaptoethane sulfonate to prevent cyclophosphamide cystitis. J Urol 131:960, 1984.

63. Revert WA, Berdon WE, Baker DH: Hemorrhagic cystitis and vesicoureteral reflux secondary to cytoxan therapy for childhood malignancies. AJR 117:664, 1973.

64. Gellman E, Kissane J, Frech R, et al: Cyclophosphamide cystitis. J Can Assoc Radiol 20:99, 1969.

65. Godin M, Deshayes P, Ducastelle T, et al: Agranulocytosis, hemorrhagic cystitis and acute interstitial nephritis during methicillin therapy. J Antimicrobiol Ther 6:296, 1980.

66. Marx CM, Alpert SE: Ticarcillin-induced cystitis. Am J Dis Child 138:670, 1984.

67. Maatman TJ, Novick AC, Montague DK, Levin HS: Radiation-induced cystitis following intracavitary irradiation for superficial bladder cancer. J Urol 130:338, 1983.

68. Aron BS, Schlesinger AS: Complications of radiation therapy: The genito-urinary tract. Semin Roentgenol 9:65, 1974.

69. Weiner, DP, Koss LG, Sablay B, et al: The prevalence and significance of Brunn's nests, cystitis cystica, and squamous metaplasia in normal bladders. J Urol 122:317, 1977.

70. Kaplan GW, King LR: Cystitis cystica in childhood. J Urol 103:657, 1970.
71. Mostofi FK: Potentialities of bladder epithelium. J Urol 71:705–714, 1954.
72. Sarma KP: Cystitis cystica (cystosis) with bladder cancer. J Urol 120:169, 1978.
73. Connery PB: Leukoplakia of the urinary bladder and its association with carcinoma. J Urol 69:121, 1953.
74. Mueller SC, Thueroff JW, Rumpelt HJ: Urothelial leukoplakia: New aspects of etiology and therapy. J Urol 137:979–983, 1987.
75. Kauzlaric D, Barmeir E, Campana A: Diagnosis of cystitis glandularis. Urol Radiol 9:50, 1987.
76. Stilmant MM, Siroky MB: Nephrogenic adenoma associated with intravesical bacille Calmette-Guérin treatment: A report of two cases. J Urol 135:359, 1986.
77. Alter AA, Malek GH: Bladder wall calcification after topical mitomycin C. J Urol 138:1239, 1987.
78. Redman JF, Seibert JJ: The role of excretory urography in the evaluation of girls with urinary tract infection. J Urol 132:953, 1984.
79. Vlatkovic G, Bradic I, Batinic D: Cystitis cystica: Characteristics of the disease in children. Br J Urol 49:57, 1977.
80. Pliskin MJ, Dresner ML: Inadvertent urethral insertion of contraceptive suppository. J Urol 139:1049, 1988.
81. Stark GL, Feddersen R, Lowe BA, et al: Inflammatory pseudotumor (pseudosarcoma) of the bladder. J Urol 141:610–612, 1989.

Despite the availability of urethroscopy, radiographic assessment of the urethra continues to play an important role in evaluation of urethral inflammatory processes and their sequelae. No longer limited simply to the detailed anatomical information provided by urethrography, newer imaging methods such as ultrasonography, computed tomography (CT), and magnetic resonance imaging (MRI) more completely depict periurethral tissues, supplying data that are often key in therapeutic decision making. Detailed in this section are the various forms of infectious and noninfectious inflammatory processes of the urethra (Table 25–1), with emphasis on the contribution of uroradiology to diagnosis and management.

INFLAMMATORY CONDITIONS OF THE URETHRA

Infectious Urethritides

Gonorrhea

Gonorrhea has ranked as the most common reportable infectious disease in the United States, with more than one million cases reported in 1980.[1] For both gonococcal and nongonococcal urethritis, the age group most frequently affected is the 20- to 24-year-old group.[2] Classically, dysuria with thick, purulent urethral discharge is the hallmark of acute gonococcal urethritis in the male; however, symptoms are not always present. Some surveys have shown the prevalence of infection to be 40% to 60% in selected groups of asymptomatic males.[1]

Urethral gonorrhea is acquired through sexual contact, and the risk of infection for a male is approximately 17% from a single intercourse with an infected partner.[3] In the distal urethra, the gonococci adhere to and proliferate on the mucosa, and the periurethral Littre's glands fill with bacteria and leukocytes. The infection proceeds proximally into the bulb, where the external urethral sphincter retards more proximal spread.[4] In the acute phase, both periurethral and parafrenular gland abscesses may complicate the urethritis.[5, 6] The acute inflammatory symptoms may subside without therapy. Frequently, however, the submucosa remains inflamed, the Littre's glands harbor organisms, and a thin urethral discharge persists.[4]

The etiology of postgonococcal strictures remains debatable, and several pathogenetic mechanisms are thought to be possible. With an aggressive initial infection, spread to the corpus spongiosum may cause venous thrombosis, and scars may result. Conversely, a mild initial attack, with delayed or inadequate therapy, may result in chronic low-grade infection; years of granulation tissue deposition and scar formation may follow.[4] An alternative theory indicts infection-induced metaplasia of the urethral columnar mucosa, becoming poorly distensible stratified squamous epithelium. Voiding pressure produces multiple small rents, with extravasation of urine engendering periurethral scar formation.[7]

Antibiotic therapy has led to a lower incidence of postgonorrheal strictures. In North America, the disease accounts for only about 40% of urethral strictures, whereas in underdeveloped nations it is responsible for up to 90%.[8] Although postgonococcal strictures may involve any portion of the urethra, 70% occur in the bulb. Not only is this the most dependent part of the urethra, but it also contains the greatest number of paraurethral glands.[9] In contrast, strictures secondary to instrumentation are found, characteristically, where the urethral lumen is narrowest (urethral meatus, fossa navicularis, bladder neck) or where the urethra is fixed (penile/scrotal junction, membranous urethra). Strictures caused by iatrogenic or other trauma usually involve only the mucosa and submucosa, whereas inflammatory strictures frequently extend into the subjacent corpus spongiosum.[10] Ultrasonography may help to assess the extent of periurethral fibrosis.

Postgonorrheal strictures may cause obstructive symptoms, usually after a delay ranging from months to years.[11] At that point, urethrography may aid in defining the site and extent of narrowing. Both antegrade and retrograde studies show filling of Littre's glands as a result of damaged patulous ostia. Because of the spreading nature of the infection, postgonorrheal strictures are often multiple and may involve several centimeters of urethra (Figs. 25–1 and 25–2).[4] In severe instances, virtually the entire anterior urethra may become narrow (Fig. 25–3). This is in contrast to traumatic strictures, which are most often short and flanked by normal-caliber lumen. Often the urethra proximal to a tight stricture will appear normal or dilated on initial voiding studies, as a result of increased voiding pressure (Fig. 25–4). These regions are nearly always involved by fibrosis to some extent, and these more proximal strictures become apparent on studies

Table 25–1. Inflammatory Conditions of the Urethra

Infectious urethritides
  Gonococcal urethritis and stricture
  Nongonococcal urethritis
  Condylomata acuminata
  "Urethral syndrome"
  Urethritis and strictures in children
  Tuberculosis

Other inflammatory and stricture-inducing conditions
  Chemical urethritis
  Reiter's syndrome
  Wegener's granulomatosis
  Balanitis xerotica obliterans
  Epidermolysis bullosa
  Amyloidosis
  Malacoplakia
  Acquired urethral fistulas

Acquired urethral diverticula

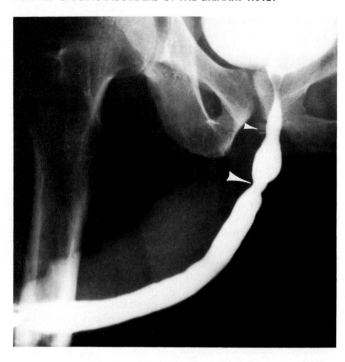

Figure 25–1. Bulbar urethral stricture (soft). A 37-year-old male with known history of gonococcal urethritis presented with urethral discharge. Retrograde urethrogram (RUG) demonstrates proximal bulbar urethral stricture *(large arrowhead)*. Reflux into Cowpers' gland is noted *(small arrowhead)*. The verumontanum is well demonstrated.

performed after repair of the tightest lesion.[4] Gonorrhea may involve the posterior urethra by ascending infection, resulting in some scarring of the membranous portion. Distortion of the normal cone shape of the proximal bulbous urethra shown by retrograde urethrography provides a clue to membranous urethral involvement (Fig. 25–4).[12] Urethrography is an important adjunct to the evaluation of urethral strictures of all types, especially when surgery is contemplated. It defines the location, size, length, and number of strictures in the urethra and discloses periurethral communications that may be present. It is also valuable in postoperative assessment (Fig. 25–5), especially in detecting residual or recurrent stenoses. Ultrasonography has been used to visualize urethral strictures.[12a, 72, 73] Sonourethrography of the anterior urethra can determine stricture length and the degree of

periurethral fibrosis with more accuracy than is possible using retrograde urethrography.[12a] Satisfactory images of the posterior urethra, however, have not yet been obtained with ultrasonography.

COMPLICATIONS AND SEQUELAE

As described by McCallum and Colapinto, urethrography frequently demonstrates complications resulting from postinflammatory strictures. Urethral false passages are the complications most commonly seen, resulting from attempts at urethroscopy or dilation. Urethrography depicts them as short channels, usually paralleling the bulbous urethra, occasionally re-entering the lumen proximally. Generally, false passages are not symptomatically significant.[4]

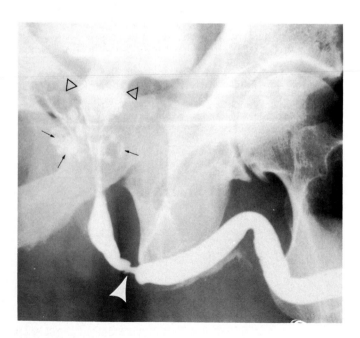

Figure 25–2. Midbulbar urethral stricture (hard). A 64-year-old male (status post-transurethral resection of the prostate [post–TURP]) with a history of venereal disease. RUG demonstrates midbulbar urethral stricture *(arrowhead)*. Irregularity at site of stricture is from previous instrumentation. Slight amount of periurethral extravasation is noted. Reflux into the prostatic acini has occurred *(arrows)*. The prostatic fossa is excavated from TURP *(open arrowheads)*.

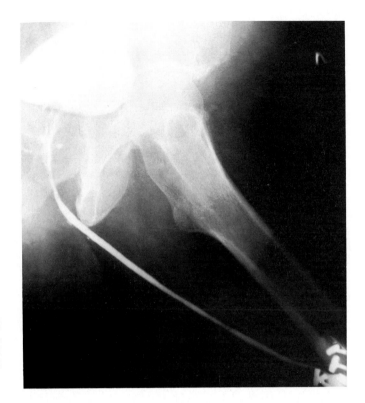

Figure 25–3. Uniformly narrowed urethra. RUG in 71-year-old male with long history of infectious urethritis demonstrates marked diminution in caliber of the entire urethra (anterior and bulbar). Reflux into the prostate is seen. Treatment required extensive internal urethrotomy.

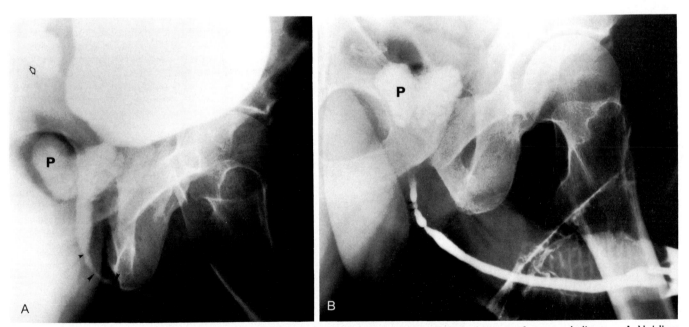

Figure 25–4. Bulbar and membranous urethral strictures in 58-year-old male with long history of venereal disease. *A,* Voiding cystourethrogram (VCU) prior to RUG shows bulbous and membranous urethral strictures *(arrowheads)* but fails to demonstrate adequately the penile urethra. The posterior (prostatic) urethra is well filled, and extensive reflux into the prostate (P) gland is noted. A dilated right distal ureter was present on the urogram *(open arrowhead). B,* RUG demonstrates diffuse urethral narrowing with several small strictures in the bulbar and membranous urethra *(arrowheads).* The cone of the bulbous urethra cannot be seen. Reflux into the prostate (P) is from previous VCU. The prostatic acini are well outlined by the contrast material. RUG clearly reveals the anterior urethra, but VCU is necessary to evaluate the posterior urethra.

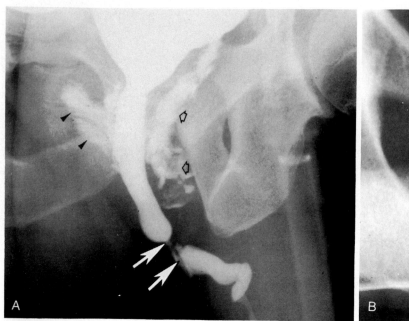

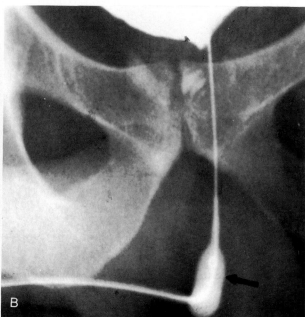

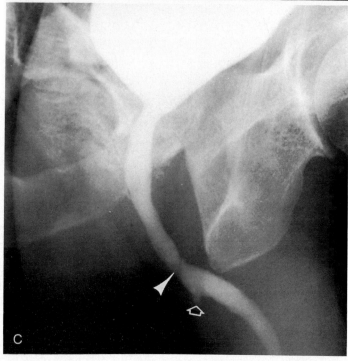

Figure 25–5. Midbulbar urethral stricture in 24-year-old man. *A,* VCU demonstrates midbulbar urethral stricture with marked irregularity *(arrows).* Patient had known inflammatory strictures and had undergone previous instrumentation and dilatation. Reflux into the prostate gland *(arrowheads)* and residual barium in the rectum *(open arrowheads)* are noted. Significant obstruction at the level of the stricture is shown on the VCU, as evidenced by a dilated posterior urethra. *B,* Balloon dilatation using angioplasty balloon *(arrow)* was performed after antegrade and retrograde catheterization had bypassed the stricture with a guide wire. *C,* Follow-up VCU 6 months later shows successful dilatation of the bulbar urethral stricture *(arrowhead)* and return to normal caliber of posterior urethra. A small diverticulum *(open arrowhead)* is at the site of the balloon dilatation, and reflux persists into the prostate gland. The patient's symptoms had abated. (Courtesy Dr. Barry Katzen.)

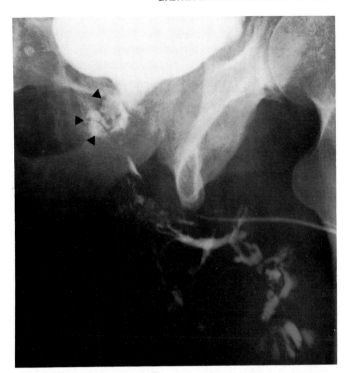

Figure 25–6. "Watering-can perineum." A 71-year-old male with long history of urethral stricture presented with scrotal and perineal fistulae. RUG outlines urethra and numerous scrotal and perineal fistulae. Reflux into the prostate gland is present *(arrowheads)* at the level of the verumontanum.

Many complications are related to secondary infection in the distended and inflamed urethra proximal to the stricture. The damaged Littre's glands provide ready abscess sites and a route for spread of infection into the periurethral tissues. If a periurethral abscess drains into the urethra, urethrography may demonstrate a narrow-mouthed, irregular cavity adjacent to the lumen, or possibly a wide-mouthed, smooth urethral diverticulum. If the abscess drains to the skin, a perineal or scrotal sinus results. The abscess cavity may connect with both the urethra and the skin, resulting in a fistula.[4] Such tracts may be delineated by urethrography or by catheter injection of the perineal ostium. Longstanding cases may result in networks of periurethral fistulas ("watering-can" perineum) (Fig. 25–6).[13]

Although the prevalence of periurethral phlegmon has decreased, stricture-induced extravasation of infected urine beneath Colles' and Scarpa's fascia does remain a cause of this form of cellulitis.[14] An extreme example is so-called Fournier's gangrene.[15] Urethrography can demonstrate the underlying urethral stricture and extravasation but should be avoided in acute disease.[4]

Additional complications that may result from the inflammation and stasis engendered by urethral strictures include urinary tract calculi, hydronephrosis,[4] cystitis, pyelonephritis, prostatitis, and epididymitis, as well as strictures of the ejaculatory ducts and vas deferens.[16]

Nongonococcal Urethritis

Although the incidence of gonorrhea has somewhat reached a plateau in recent years, nongonococcal urethritis (NGU) continues to increase.[2] Characterized by mild dysuria and scant mucoid discharge, NGU now accounts for most cases of urethritis in nonindigent male populations. *Chlamydia trachomatis* and *Ureaplasma urealyticum* are believed to be the agents most frequently responsible, isolated from 70% to 80% of men with acute NGU.[2, 17] They may also cause coinfection in patients with gonorrhea and might underlie the "postgonococcal urethritis" sometimes seen after penicillin therapy.[2, 18] Additional agents suspected of occasionally causing NGU are *Mycoplasma hominis,* herpes simplex virus, *Trichomonas vaginalis,* and *Candida* species.[2, 17, 19]

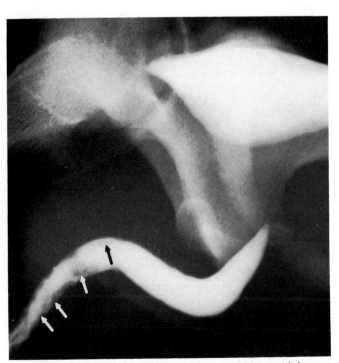

Figure 25–7. Anterior urethritis. A 13-year-old boy with known sexual contact and positive cultures for gonococcus. RUG demonstrates marked anterior urethral irregularity. Nodular mucosal lesions are present *(arrows)*.

The prevalence of post–NGU strictures is uncertain. Although it has been estimated to be 0.5% to 5.0%, the frequent inability to exclude pre-existing gonorrhea raises doubt about these figures.[20] If adequate antimicrobial treatment is provided, post–NGU stricture is believed to be exceedingly rare.[2] No specific urethrographic features are known to distinguish post–NGU strictures from other postinflammatory strictures. Urethral inflammation from any cause may produce polypoid urethritis or urethritis cystica, with mucosal changes that can be seen on urethrography (Fig. 25–7).

Condyloma Acuminatum

Venereal warts, or condylomata acuminata, are caused by DNA–containing viruses of the papilloma species. Sexual contact is their mode of transmission. Squamous papillomas appear most commonly on the skin of the perineal, genital, and perianal regions, and they may spread to the urethral meatus, vagina, and anus.[21] It is estimated that 0.5% to 5.0% of patients with penile condylomata may also have urethral involvement.[22] The meatus and fossa navicularis are sites of predilection; however, virtually the entire urethra may be involved, and bladder lesions have been reported.[23, 24]

Clinically, urethral involvement is suspected when pyuria or urethral discharge appears in a patient with genital verrucae or when the lesions occur at the urethral meatus.[23] Both urethroscopy[21] and urethrography[25] have been suggested for assessment of the urethral mucosa. On urethrography, the lesions appear as sessile filling defects, ranging from 1 to 10 mm, with smooth mucosa covering them and normal mucosa between them (Fig. 25–8). Generally, strictures and ulcerations are absent.[25] In ad-

dition to standard retrograde urethrography, double-contrast studies reportedly have been useful in detecting small papillary lesions in the anterior urethra.[26] After therapy, urethrography is valuable in evaluating the degree of response and identifying residual lesions.[23]

Because of the risk of urothelial seeding with condylomata, retrograde urethrography may theoretically be preferred to urethroscopy, since it causes less urothelial trauma. This risk can be minimized by prophylactically instilling agents such as 5-fluorouracil after the examination, or by performing an antegrade study as part of an intravenous urogram.[25]

Differential diagnostic considerations for the urethrographic appearance of condylomata acuminata include benign and malignant primary urethral neoplasms and urethral metastases,[25] as well as polypoid urethritis and urethritis cystica.[27]

In addition, both malacoplakia[28] and leukoplakia[29] can occur in the urethra, with resultant plaquelike mucosal irregularity. Urethral amyloidosis also causes a papillary eruption of the mucosa, which is visible on urethrography.[30] Although anterior urethral condylomata have been described in the absence of penile lesions,[31] the presence of genital verrucae generally points toward the correct diagnosis.

Urethral Syndrome

The term *urethral syndrome* has typically been applied to women with urgency, frequency, dysuria, and/or dyspareunia who do not fulfill objective clinical criteria for urinary tract infection. Although some would include in this group symptomatic patients with less than 10^5 microorganisms/ml voided urine,[32] others limit the group to

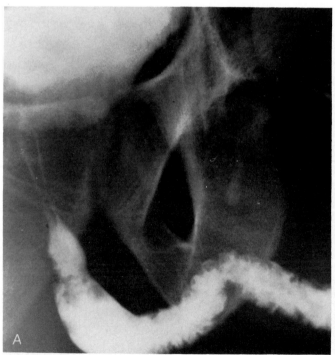
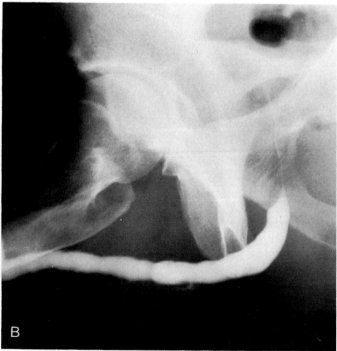

Figure 25–8. Condylomata acuminata. *A*, RUG demonstrates that the entire anterior urethra is carpeted with multiple small round mucosal filling defects. Patient had external condylomata removed several months earlier. Polypoid urethritis, urethritis cystica, and squamous cell carcinoma could mimic this appearance. *B*, After 8 weeks of topical therapy with thiotepa and 5-fluorouracil, repeat urethrography reveals no residual polypoid defects in the urethra. (From Sawczuk I, Badillo F, Olsson CA: Condylomata acuminata: Diagnosis and follow-up by retrograde urethrography. Urol Radiol 5:273, 1983.)

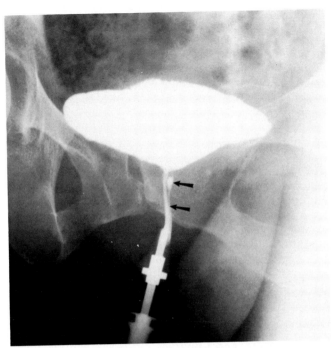

Figure 25–9. Long-necked urethral diverticulum. A 55-year-old female with symptoms of the urethral syndrome. RUG shows a normal urethra, but a long-necked urethral diverticulum is noted (arrows).

those with sterile urine and negative urinalyses.[33] Urinary tract infection with less than 10^5 bacteria/ml voided urine is now believed to be the cause of symptoms in a portion of patients with urethral syndrome, especially those with pyuria.[34] In addition, both chlamydia and gonococci have been implicated in some cases.[35] Data supporting the contributory role of relative urethral stenosis and external sphincter spasm are not thought to be conclusive.[33]

Although the yield from uroradiological studies is low in patients with urethral syndrome, the studies may be warranted to exclude conditions that mimic the symptoms, such as an occult urethral diverticulum (Fig. 25–9).[33] Intravenous urography, with a postvoid film including the urethral region, has been suggested.[33] Urography may also demonstrate changes secondary to periurethral inflammation. When edema and proliferative changes are evident cystoscopically, irregularity and crenation of the bladder base may be seen by cystography.[36] With more extensive periurethral inflammation, indentation and elevation of the bladder floor may occur, resembling changes of prostate hypertrophy in the male.[37] Periurethral calcifications, possibly related to paraurethral gland hyperplasia, are occasionally seen.[36]

Urethritis and Strictures in Children

In girls, the short urethra is believed not only to provide bacteria with an access route to the bladder, but also to act as a reservoir for potential pathogens, resulting in repeated infections.[38] During the evaluation of these children with recurrent lower urinary tract infections, voiding cystourethrography (VCU) should be performed. Radiological findings reportedly associated with inflammation include intermittent stream, narrowed urethral lumen, and prominence of longitudinal linear mucosal urethral folds (Fig. 25–10).[38] Even in cases of repeated infection, urographically demonstrable strictures are rare.

The significance of distal urethral and meatal stenosis as a causative factor of chronic urinary tract infection in girls has been an area of uncertainty. Anatomical studies have demonstrated that the striated muscle layer of the female urethra ends in a collagenous ring constituting the distal 0.5 to 1.0 cm.[38] In some symptomatic patients, bougie-à-boule calibration has shown this segment to be relatively narrow and rigid, and voiding urethrography has demonstrated diminished caliber of the distal urethra with proximal dilation ("spinning-top" configuration).[39] This morphological change seen during voiding is, likely, a normal variant, reflecting the response of the various urethral segments to voiding pressure. Consequently, in the absence of confirmatory findings such as bladder trabeculation, urethral uroradiological evaluation is not considered a reliable means of diagnosing urodynamically significant lesions in the young female.[38, 39, 40]

Radiographic evidence of urethritis in boys is not frequently seen, but irregular narrowing of the prostatic urethra, accompanied by thickening of mucosal folds below the bladder outlet, has been reported. These changes are said to regress after antibiotic therapy.[38] Chronic nonspecific urethritis may give rise to proliferative inflammatory changes in the bulbous urethra, characterized by small filling defects as shown by urethrography.[41]

In adolescent males, in most regions of the United States,[42] urethritis due to C. trachomatis is more common than gonorrhea but, usually because of child molestation, gonorrhea may be seen in males of any age—even infants. Urethrography is rarely performed in the acute phase, but it may be expected to show edematous mucosal folds indenting the urethral lumen in the affected segment (Fig. 25–7). Urethral condylomata acuminata also may be seen in adolescents, as well as in children as young as 2 years old.[43]

Urethral strictures in the pediatric age group are seen almost exclusively in males.[39] Most of these cases result from iatrogenic or spontaneous trauma,[39, 44, 45] and infection is an uncommon cause, except in older adolescents. Urethral strictures of unknown etiology are not unusual

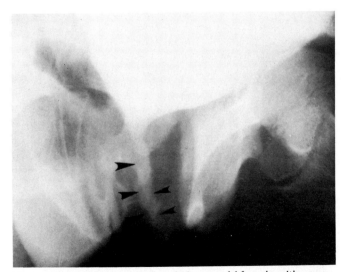

Figure 25–10. Acute urethritis. A 6-year-old female with symptoms of dysuria, urgency, and frequency. VCU demonstrates marked irregularity of the urethral mucosa (arrowheads).

in symptomatic boys,[39] in whom VCU often shows a short area of narrowing in the bulbous segment.

Other Inflammatory and Stricture-Inducing Conditions of the Urethra

Chemical Urethritis

Therapeutic instillation of potentially damaging chemical solutions into the urethra was once a common practice. Potassium permanganate, for example, was used to treat gonococcal urethritis, whereas podophyllin and dilute silver nitrate were used for venereal warts or refractory nonspecific urethritis.[4] Although they were once common, strictures related to such measures, are now almost never seen (see Chapter 54, Injuries of the Urethra). Chemical urethritis due to deliberate[46] or accidental[47] misplacement of medication is occasionally encountered. Urethroscopy is the preferred means of diagnosis for this condition because it may allow removal of the causative agent.

The administration of high-dose oral estrogen was reported by Yokoyama and coworkers to cause reversible anterior urethral strictures in 17 of 33 men receiving relatively large doses of estrogens for prostate carcinoma.[48, 49] At urethrography, the strictures appeared long and smooth, progressing proximally over time. Interestingly, the cessation of therapy has been followed by the return to normal caliber in several patients. The pathogenesis of this phenomenon is uncertain, but it may be related to the epithelial changes in the urethra and the atrophy of the corporal bodies known to accompany estrogen administration.

Reiter's Syndrome

Characterized by urethritis, balanitis, conjunctivitis, keratoderma blennorrhagicum, and polyarthritis, Reiter's syndrome predominantly affects males in the 15- to 35-year-old age group.[50] The urethritis may progress to inflammatory necrosis of the mucosa and may involve the entire urethra.[10] Because extensive reconstruction is often necessary in such cases, urethrography may be used in the postinflammatory phase to define the extent of scarring.

Wegener's Granulomatosis

Although this nerotizing vasculitis classically involves the respiratory tract and kidney, it may involve the urethra as well.[51, 52] Purulent periurethral inflammatory

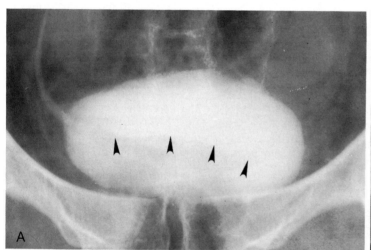

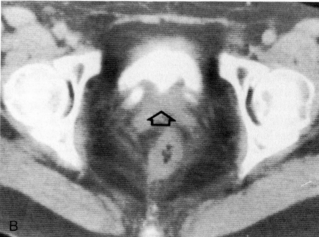

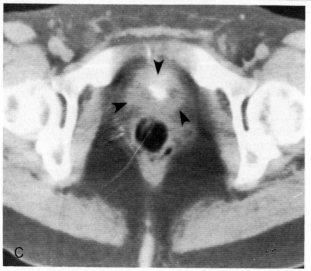

Figure 25–11. A 56-year-old female complained of hematuria, dysuria, and urethral discharge for 10 years; recently it had become worse. Cytoscopy revealed periurethral inflammation and urethral necrosis, and biopsies showed necrotizing granulomatosis with plasma cells and eosinophils. The patient was treated with prednisone and cyclophosphamide. The periurethral inflammatory mass regressed, and an IVU 4 years later showed a normal bladder. *A,* Coned view of bladder from initial urogram shows a mass indenting the base of the bladder ("female prostate" sign) *(arrowheads). B,* Computed tomography (CT) scan shows irregular mass in subtrigonal region, *(arrowhead).* Distal ureterectasis is present. *C,* CT scan, more caudal than *B,* shows paraurethral soft-tissue mass *(arrowheads)* compressing contrast-filled bladder neck. (*A–C* from St. Amour TE, Miller D: CPC—voiding symptoms and periurethral mass. Urol Radiol 8:219–221, 1986. With permission.)

masses occur, with necrosis of the urethral mucosa, and sometimes the formation of fistulas. Acutely, intravenous urography may show elevation of the bladder base due to the adjacent inflammatory masses (Fig. 25–11A). CT and MRI aid in defining the size and distribution of inflammation (Fig. 25–11B, C), as well as in assessing response to steroid therapy. In the postinflammatory stage, urethrography may be useful in identifying fistulas and assessing urethral caliber.

Balanitis Xerotica Obliterans

A skin disease of uncertain etiology, balanitis xerotica obliterans is characterized by white thickened plaques involving the glans, prepuce, and urethral meatus of adult males. The fossa navicularis and distal urethra may also be involved.[10] Urethrography may demonstrate a smooth, uniform decrease in urethral caliber, ranging from a few centimeters long to the entire length of the penile urethra.[53] Treatment often includes meatotomy and urethroplasty.

Epidermolysis Bullosa

Characterized by scar-inducing cutaneous blistering in response to minor trauma, epidermolysis bullosa (dystrophic form) may involve the male and female genitalia. This sometimes causes narrowing or distortion of the urethral meatus, with resultant urinary obstruction or alteration of the urinary stream. (Fig. 25–12).[54, 55] Intravenous urography is useful to assess the degree of obstruction, whereas VCU aids in defining and quantifying the meatal narrowing.

Amyloidosis

A description of urethral amyloidosis is to be found in Chapter 97.

Tuberculosis

Tuberculosis of the urethra is discussed in Chapter 31.

Acquired Urethral Fistulas

As the prevalence of postgonococcal strictures and resultant fistulas has fallen, other causes of urethral fistulas have assumed greater importance. Trauma in men, including iatrogenic trauma is now a leading cause of urethrocutaneous fistulas.[56] Malignancy, such as urethral carcinoma, and radiation therapy are other causes.[57] Similarly, urethrorectal fistulas may be seen following transurethral or perineal surgical procedures on the prostate gland,[56] and usually arise from the prostatic or membranous portions.[57] Prostatic abscess, rectal or prostatic malignancy,[57] and rectal inflammatory disease[58] also may give rise to these fistulas. In women, urethrovaginal fistula is often the result of obstetrical injury, a complication of gynecological surgery, or irradiation. In addition, inflammation or surgery related to urethral diverticula,[59] vaginal/cervical or urethral neoplasm, and radiation therapy can result in fistula formation.

Retrograde urethrography and VCU provide information regarding location and number of urethrocutaneous fistulas. Concurrent injection of the perineal ostia may aid in filling all the tracts (Fig. 25–13).[60] Although ure-

Figure 25–12. A 10-year-old female patient with epidermolysis bullosa. VCU shows dilatation of the proximal urethra with distal tapering *(arrowheads)*. There are filling of the vagina *(curved arrow)* and uterine cavity *(open arrowhead)* and narrowing of the distal vagina with proximal dilatation. Patient had a history of three previous urinary tract infections. Distal urethral and introital scarring was the cause of the urethral dilatation and reflux of urine into the vagina. (From Shackelford G, Bauer EA, Graviss EA, McAlister WH: Upper airway and external genital involvement in epidermolysis bullosa dystrophica. Radiology 143:429–432, 1982. With permission.)

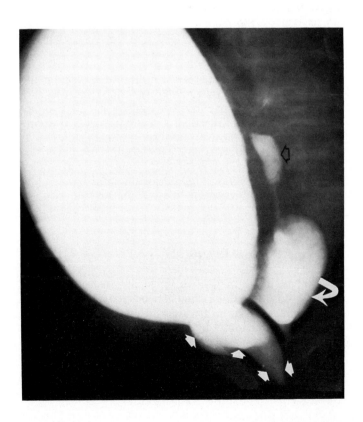

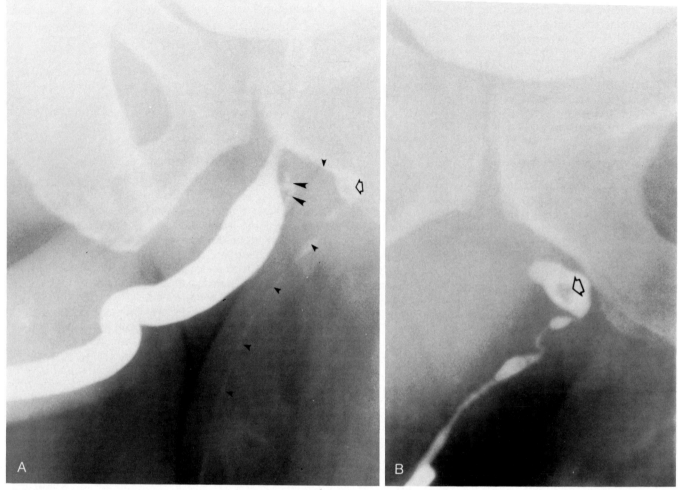

Figure 25–13. Urethroperineal fistula with calculus in fistula tract. RUG in 49-year-old male who complained of dysuria and perineal leakage of urine. *A,* RUG shows normal urethra with reflux into Cowper's gland *(large arrowheads).* Perineal fistula *(small arrowheads)* is demonstrated with scrotal opening in or near the midline. Filling defect *(open arrowhead)* in fistula tract was a calculus. *B,* Retrograde injection of midline perineal fistulous opening with vacuum suction cannula shows the fistula in more detail. Numerous air bubbles are present in the fistula. The precise communication with the urethra was not demonstrated well on either study. Subsequent surgical resection of the fistula and tract was curative. This fistula is thought to result from secondary infection of congenital midline scrotal (perineal) cyst. Again seen is the calculus *(arrowhead).*

throscopy is usually diagnostic, urethrorectal fistulas are demonstrable by urethrography as well.[56] Because contrast material may pass more readily from the urethral side than from the intestinal side, urethrography is important in the diagnosis of urethrointestinal fistulas.[57]

Cystourethroscopy is the chief means of diagnosing urethrovaginal fistulas, with VCU generally not adding significant information.[61] Occasionally, retrograde double-balloon urethrography may delineate the connection.[62]

Acquired Urethral Diverticula

Thought to be present in up to 3% of asymptomatic women,[62] urethral diverticula may be an overlooked cause of frequency, dysuria, postvoid dribbling, frequent urinary tract infections, and dyspareunia. Occasionally, a sizable diverticulum is clinically evident as a bulging mass in the anterior vaginal wall that when compressed, may cause expression of pus or cloudy urine from the urethral meatus (Fig. 25–14).[63] More often, however, the results of physical examination are normal.

Most female urethral diverticula are thought to result from infection and abscess formation within the periurethral glands, which then rupture into the urethral lumen and remain as outpouchings. Although diverticula may occur anywhere along the length of the urethra, most are found posteriorly in the midurethra, correlated with the position of the urethral glands.[64] The size of the diverticula and number of openings into the urethra vary, and multilocular diverticula may occur.[61] Urethroscopy alone is not believed to be adequate for diagnosis of diverticula, because up to 60% of lesions may be overlooked. Consequently, both VCU and positive-pressure retrograde urethrography have been utilized, with some authors advocating both.[64] Retrograde urethrography utilizing a double-balloon catheter or a vacuum-suction cannula is a particularly effective means of demonstrating diverticula.[65]

Because intravenous urography is frequently performed in women with chronic urinary tract symptoms, an appropriately positioned postvoid film has been suggested as a screening measure for diverticula. In one study, small collections of contrast material along the course of the urethra on postvoid films correctly diagnosed 77% of them.[66]

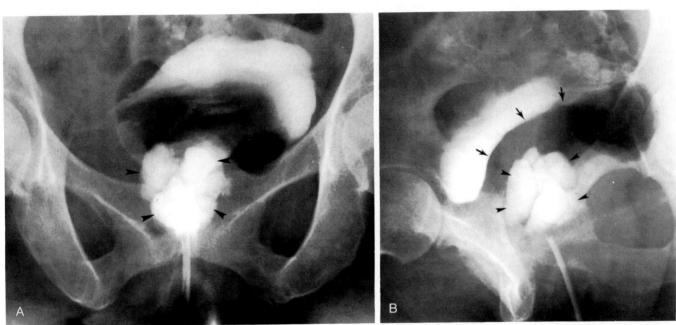

Figure 25–14. Very large urethral diverticulum. A 55-year-old female with recurrent urinary tract infections and "urethral syndrome." *A,* Frontal film from RUG performed with straight urethral catheter demonstrates elevation of the bladder base and large multiloculated urethral diverticulum *(arrowheads). B,* Right posterior oblique view of RUG with straight catheter shows multiloculated urethral diverticulum *(arrowheads)* and marked elevation of the bladder base *(arrows).* This diverticulum and periurethral edema cause large "female prostate" sign.

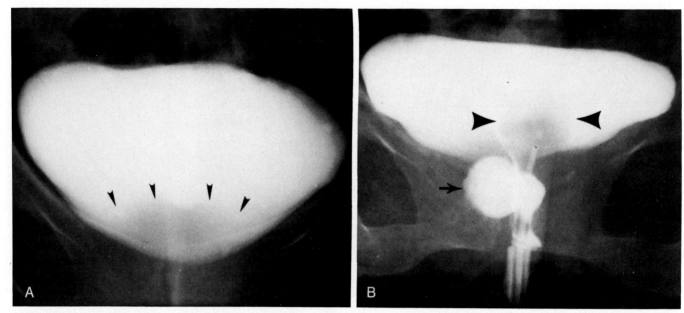

Figure 25–15. Urethral diverticulum in female. *A,* Coned bladder view from IVU shows "female prostate" sign *(arrowheads).* The slight elevation of the base of the bladder was suggestive of urethral diverticulum. *B,* RUG was obtained, using double-balloon technique. Injection of contrast material after placement of the double balloon with the proximal balloon in the bladder *(large arrowheads)* demonstrates a diverticulum off the right posterior aspect of the urethra *(small arrow).* Double-balloon technique requires instrumentation of the usually irritated urethra. The vacuum suction cannula provides adequate detail without instrumentation of the urethra (see Fig. 25–16).

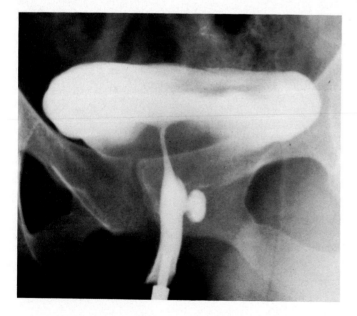

Figure 25–16. RUG using vacuum-suction cannula shows urethral diverticulum in 35-year-old female with urinary tract infection. Elevation of the bladder base causes "female prostate" sign.

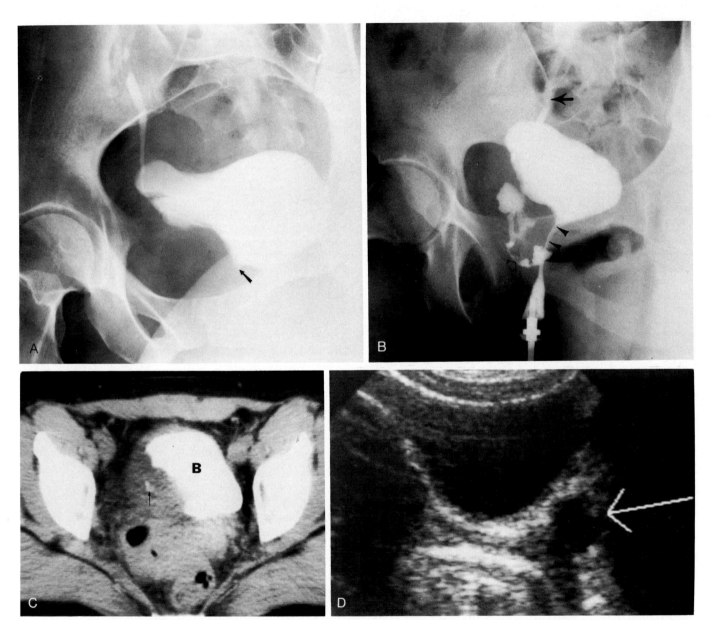

Figure 25–17. Urethral diverticulum in a 35-year-old female, which was repaired 4 years ago, presenting with recurrent symptoms. *A,* IVU shows large mass elevating right side of the bladder base. A right posterior oblique view coned to the bladder shows deviation of bladder neck *(arrow)* to the left. The distal portion of the right ureter is elevated along with the bladder. *B,* RUG using vacuum-suction cannula shows marked deviation of urethra *(arrowheads)* and bladder neck to the left. There is recurrence of the urethral diverticulum with fistula *(open arrowhead)* to a perivesical abscess. Deviation of urethra and bladder is due to abscess and inflammatory reaction. A suprapubic tube *(arrow)* is in place. *C,* CT scan through pelvis shows contrast in bladder (B). Mass (abscess) indents right bladder wall and contains contrast material *(arrow)* from previous RUG. Gas collection represents vagina, distended from air trapped in tampon. *D,* Longitudinal sonogram of 45-year-old woman with urethral diverticulum. This was obtained with the transducer held just above the symphysis pubis and angled downward and demonstrates the urethral diverticulum *(arrow)* just distal to and beneath the urinary bladder.

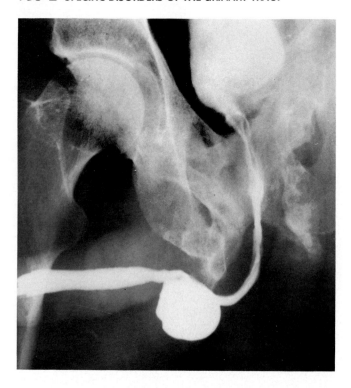

Figure 25–18. Acquired urethral diverticulum in 17-year-old male. Previous pelvic trauma resulted in multiple fractures and injury to the urethra. RUG demonstrates urethral diverticulum near the penile/scrotal junction. Patient complained of postvoid dribbling secondary to pooling of urine in the large urethral diverticulum.

At urethrography, diverticula appear as rounded or elongated sacs, with a short or long neck connecting them with the urethral lumen (Fig. 25–15).[67] When filling defects appear within a diverticulum, calculi as well as benign and malignant neoplasms should be considered. In some patients who have urethral diverticula, cystography or the bladder view from an intravenous urogram may reveal elevation of the bladder base, simulating the appearance of prostatic hypertrophy in the male (Fig. 25–16).[37] This occurs only with diverticula arising from the posterior third of the urethra, because the anterior two-thirds of the urethra and vagina are fused by interdigitation of their surrounding muscle layers, precluding cephalad extension of the diverticulum.[37, 68]

In addition to urographic studies, both ultrasonography[69, 70] and CT may aid in the assessment of urethral diverticula. The extent of periurethral inflammation is often more clearly demonstrated (Fig. 25–17), and the actual size of the lesion (especially those laden with inflammatory debris) more accurately judged, by these techniques.[69] These factors may be important in preoperative planning.

Acquired Diverticula in Males

Although they are much more common in women, acquired urethral diverticula are occasionally encountered in men. In general, they are thought to result from trauma and infection of the urethra, associated with transurethral surgery or other instrumentation, and from catheterization; the penile/scrotal junction is the most common site.[71] Paraplegics, in particular, are prone to develop anterior urethral diverticula as a consequence of prolonged catheterization.[68, 72] Urethral diverticula may be seen in incontinent men as the result of chronic use of a penile clamp, such as the Cunningham clamp.

Anterior urethral diverticula also may result from periurethral abscess, when sloughing of a portion of the urethral wall yields a wide communication with the urethral lumen.[4] In the posterior urethra, rupture of a prostatic abscess into the urethra accounts for most acquired diverticula.[67] The urethrographic appearance of diverticula in males is variable. Lesions may be single or multiple, round or elongated, and unilocular or multilocular. Both wide-neck and narrow-neck types occur, and the walls of the lesions may be either smooth or irregular (Fig. 25–18)[67].

References

1. Harrison WO: Gonococcal urethritis. Urol Clin North Am 11:45, 1984.
2. Bowie WR: Nongonococcal urethritis. Urol Clin North Am 11:55, 1984.
3. Hooper RR, Weisner PJ, Harrison WO, et al: Cohort study of venereal diseases: I. Risk of transmission from infected women to men. Am J Epidemiol 107:235, 1978.
4. McCallum RW, Colapinto V: The anterior urethra. *In* Urologic Radiology of the Adult Male Lower Urinary Tract. Springfield, Illinois, Charles C Thomas, 1976.
5. Subramanian S: Gonococcal urethritis with bilateral tysonitis and periurethral abscess. Sex Transm Dis 8:77, 1981.
6. Pattman RS, McMillan A: Parafraenal gland inflammation as a complication of urethritis. Br J Clin Pract 32:25, 1978.
7. Chambers RM, Baitera B: The anatomy of the urethral stricture. Br J Urol 49:545, 1977.
8. McCallum RW: The adult male urethra. Radiol Clin North Am 17:227, 1979.
9. Singh M, Blandy JP: The pathology of urethral stricture. J Urol 115:673, 1976.
10. Devine CJ Jr: Surgery of the urethra. *In* Walsh P, Gittes R, Perlmutter A, Stamey T (eds): Campbell's Urology, 5th Ed. Philadelphia, WB Saunders Company, 1986.
11. Osegbe DN, Amaku EO: Gonococcal strictures in young patients. Urology 18:37, 1981.

12. McCallum RW, Colapinto V: The membranous urethra. *In* Urologic Radiology of the Adult Male Lower Urinary Tract. Springfield, Illinois, Charles C Thomas, 1976.

12a. McAninch JW, Laing FC, Jeffrey RB: Sonourethrography in the evaluation of urethral strictures: A preliminary report. J Urol 139:294, 1988.

13. Osoba AO, Alausa O: Gonococcal urethral stricture and watering can perineum. Br J Vener Dis 52:387, 1976.

14. Luria S, Evans AT: Periurethral phlegmon. J Urol 106:384, 1971.

15. Walker L, Cassidy MT, Hutchison AG, et al: Fournier's gangrene and urethral problems. Br J Urol 56:509, 1984.

16. Greenberg SH: Male reproductive tract sequelae of gonococcal and nongonococcal urethritis. Arch Androl 3:317, 1979.

17. Rapp CE: Nonspecific urethritis: Its current status. J Am Coll Health Assoc 27:87, 1978.

18. Jahn G, Bialasiewicz AA, Jenisch A, Blenk H: The importance and frequency of mixed infections with chlamydia trachomatis and mycoplasmas in acute gonococcal urethritis. S Afr Med J 65:462, 1984.

19. Protapnev FV, Voskresenskaya GA: Mycotic urethritis in men. Vestn Dermatol Venerol 11:34, 1976.

20. Imray TJ, Kaplan P: Lower urinary tract infections and calculi in the adult. Semin Roentgenol 18:276, 1983.

21. Berger RE: Sexually transmitted diseases. *In* Walsh P, Gittes R, Perlmutter A, Stamey T (eds): Campbell's Urology, 5th Ed. Philadelphia, WB Saunders Company, 1986.

22. Wein AJ, Benson GS: Treatment of urethral condyloma acuminatum with 5-fluorouracil cream. Urology 9:413, 1977.

23. Sawczuk I, Badillo F, Olsson CA: Condylomata acuminata: Diagnosis and follow-up by retrograde urethrography. Urol Radiol 5:273, 1983.

24. Bissada NK, Cole AT, Fried FA: Extensive condylomas acuminata of the entire male urethra and bladder. J Urol 112:201, 1974.

25. Pollack HM, Debenedictis TJ, Marmar JL, Praiss DE: Urethrographic manifestations of venereal warts (condyloma acuminata). Radiology 126:643, 1978.

26. Yokoyama M, Watanabe K, Iwata H, et al: Double-contrast urethrography by visualizing small lesions in distal urethra. Urology 19:440, 1982.

27. Mostofi FK, Price EB: Tumors and tumor-like conditions of the male urethra. *In* Mostofi FK, Price EB (eds): Tumors of the Male Genital System. Washington, DC, Armed Forces Institute of Pathology, 1973.

28. Sharma TC, Kagan HN, Sheils JP: Malacoplakia of the male urethra. J Urol 125:885, 1981.

29. Reece RW, Koontz WW: Leukoplakia of the urinary tract: A review. J Urol 114:165, 1975.

30. Walzer Y, Bear RA, McCallum R, Lang A: Localized amyloidosis of the urethra. Urology 21:406, 1983.

31. Hopkins SC, Grabstald H: Benign and malignant tumors in the male and female urethra. *In* Walsh P, Gittes R, Perlmutter A, Stamey T (eds): Campbell's Urology, 5th Ed. Philadelphia, WB Saunders Company, 1986.

32. Marchant DJ: Sensory urgency (urethral syndrome). *In* Slate WG (ed): Disorders of the Female Urethra and Urinary incontinence, 2nd Ed. Baltimore, Williams & Wilkins, 1982.

33. Messing EM: Urethral syndrome. *In* Walsh P, Gittes R, Perlmutter A, Stamey T (eds): Campbell's Urology, 5th Ed. Philadelphia, WB Saunders Company, 1986.

34. Stamm WE, Wagner KF, Amsel R, et al: Causes of the acute urethral syndrome in women. N Engl J Med 303:409, 1980.

35. Latham RH, Stamm WE: Urethral syndrome in women. Urol Clin North Am 11:95, 1984.

36. Jackson EA: Urethral syndrome in women. Radiology 119:287, 1976.

37. Amis ES, Cronan JJ, Yoder IC, Pfister RC: Impressions on floor of female bladder: "The female prostate." Urology 19:441, 1982.

38. Allen RP: The lower urinary tract. *In* Kaufman HJ (ed): Progress in Pediatric Radiology, Vol 3. Basel, Karger, 1970.

39. Currarino G: The genitourinary tract. *In* Silverman FN (ed): Caffey's Pediatric X-ray Diagnosis, 8th Ed. Chicago, Year Book Medical Publishers, 1985.

40. Weiss RM: Obstructive uropathy. *In* Kelalis PP, King LR, Belman AR (eds): Clinical Pediatric Urology, 2nd Ed. Philadelphia, WB Saunders Company, 1985.

41. Barton E, Whitaker RH: Abnormal urethrogram in bulbar urethritis of male childhood. Br J Radiol 56:760, 1983.

42. McGregor JA: Adolescent misadventures with urethritis and cervicitis. J Adolesc Health Care 6:286, 1985.

43. Mininberg DT, Rudick DH: Urethral condyloma acuminata in male children. Pediatrics 57:571, 1976.

44. Kaplan GW, Brock WA: Urethral strictures in children. J Urol 129:1200, 1983.

45. Harshman MW, Cromie WJ, Wein AJ, Duckett JW: Urethral stricture disease in children. J Urol 126:650, 1981.

46. Ellison JM, Dobies DF: Methamphetamine abuse presenting as dysuria following urethral insertion of tablets. Ann Emerg Med 13:198, 1984.

47. Cattolica EV: Chemical cystourethritis: The errant contraceptive. Urology 20:293, 1982.

48. Yokoyama M, Fukutani K, Kawamura T, et al: Urethral stricture following antiandrogen therapy. J Urol 127:342, 1982.

49. Yokoyama M, Fukutani K, Kawamura T, et al: Stricture of the anterior urethra following estrogen therapy in patients with prostatic cancer. Urol Int 38:247, 1983.

50. Resnick D: Reiter's syndrome. *In* Resnick D, Niwayama G (eds): Diagnosis of Bone and Joint Disorders. Philadelphia, WB Saunders Company, 1981.

51. Fowler M, Martin SA, Bowles WT, et al: Wegener granulomatosis—unusual cause of necrotizing urethritis. Urology 14:66, 1979.

52. Jensen K, Nielsen KK, Kock K: Necrotising urethritis in Wegener's granulomatosis. Br J Urol 54:434, 1982.

53. Staff WG: Urethral involvement in balanitis xerotica obliterans. Br J Urol 47:234, 1970.

54. Shackelford GD, Bauer EA, Graviss ER, McAlister WH: Upper airway and external genital involvement by epidermolysis bullosa dystrophica. Radiology 143:429, 1982.

55. Kretkowski RC: Urinary tract involvement in epidermolysis bullosa. Pediatrics 51:938, 1973.

56. Witten DM, Myers GH, Utz DC (eds): Trauma to the urinary system: Urinary fistulas. *In* Emmett's Clinical Urography, 4th Ed. Philadelphia, WB Saunders Company, 1977.

57. Ney C, Friedenberg RM (eds): Miscellaneous conditions of the urethra. *In* Radiographic Atlas of the Genitourinary System, 2nd Ed. Philadelphia, JB Lippincott, 1981.

58. Stamler JS, Bauer JJ, Janowitz HD: Rectourethroperineal fistula in Crohn's disease. Am J Gastroenterol 80:111, 1985.

59. Gray LA: Urethrovaginal fistulas and fistulas of the urethrovesical junction. *In* Slate WG (ed): Disorders of the Female Urethra and Urinary Incontinence, 2nd Ed. Baltimore, Williams & Wilkins, 1982.

60. Oshin DR, Bowles WT: Congenital cysts and canals of the scrotal and perineal raphe. J Urol 88:406, 1962.

61. ten Cate HW: Gynecologic problems related to the urinary tract. *In* Witten DM, Myers GH, Utz DC (eds): Emmett's Clinical Urography, 4th Ed. Philadelphia, WB Saunders Company, 1977.

62. Anderson MJF: The incidence of diverticula in the female urethra. J Urol 98:96, 1967.

63. Pratt JH, Malek RS: Lesions of the female urethra. *In* Slate WG (ed): Disorders of the Female Urethra and Urinary Incontinence, 2nd Ed. Baltimore, Williams & Wilkins, 1982.

64. Greenberg M, Stone D, Cochran ST, et al: Female urethral diverticula: Double-balloon catheter study. AJR 136:259, 1981.

65. Becker JA, Gregoire A: Retrograde urethrography. J Urol 100:92, 1968.

66. Houser LM II, VonEschenbach AC: Diverticula of female urethra—diagnostic importance of post-voiding film. Urology 3:453, 1974.

67. Ney C, Friedenberg RM (eds): Diverticula of the urethra. *In* Radiographic Atlas of the Genitourinary System, 2nd Ed. Philadelphia, JB Lippincott, 1981.

68. Dretler SP, Vermillion CD, McCullough DL: The roentgenographic diagnosis of female urethral diverticula. J Urol 107:72, 1972.

69. Wexler JS, McGovern TP: Ultrasonography of female urethral diverticula. AJR 134:737, 1980.

70. Lee TG, Keller FS: Urethral diverticulum: Diagnosis by ultrasound. AJR 128:690, 1977.

71. Utz DC, Barrett DM: Stasis involving the lower part of the urinary tract. *In* Witten DM, Myers GH, Utz DC (eds): Emmett's Clinical Urography, 4th Ed. Philadelphia, WB Saunders Company, 1977.

72. Merkle W, Wagner W: Sonography of the distal male urethra—a new diagnostic procedure for urethral strictures: Results of a retrospective study. J Urol 140:1409, 1988.

73. Gluck CD, Bundy AL, Fine C, et al: Sonographic urethrogram: Comparison of roentgenographic techniques in 22 patients. J Urol 140:1404, 1988.

26

Inflammation of the Lower Genitourinary Tract: The Prostate, Seminal Vesicles, and Scrotum

MATTHEW D. RIFKIN

PROSTATITIS

Inflammation of the prostate is difficult to diagnose and to treat. There are a number of inciting causes, but nonbacterial causes of prostatitis predominate.[1] The condition is currently grouped into three categories based on rectal examination and features of the expressed prostate secretion (EPS):[1] (1) bacterial prostatitis, (acute and chronic), (2) nonbacterial prostatitis, and (3) prostadynia (negative EPS and rectal examination). Bacterial prostatitis is usually caused by the same gram-negative organisms that cause urinary tract infections. Eighty per cent of bacterial prostatitis is attributable to *Escherichia coli,* whereas 10% to 15% is associated with *Klebsiella, Serratia, Proteus, Pseudomonas* and *Enterobacter.* In approximately 5% of cases, gram-positive organisms, such as *enterococcus, Staphylococcus,* and *Streptococcus* may be the causative agents. Anaerobic bacteria such as *Bacteroides fragilis* or *Clostridium perfringens* may cause a fulminant prostatitis after transrectal or transperineal biopsy.[1, 2] Even *Salmonella* and *Candida* have been found to be capable of causing prostatitis.[1, 2] When tuberculosis, blastomycosis, coccidioidomycosis and cryptococcosis are ruled out, "granulomatous" prostatitis is thought to represent a histological stage of resolving, acute bacterial prostatitis.[1, 2] Eosinophilic prostatitis and malacoplakia are other forms of chronic granulomatous prostatitis. Chronic prostatitis may refer to a variety of disease, from chronic bacterial or nonbacterial prostatitis to prostadynia. Unfortunately, all too often it is used as a "wastebasket" term to describe vague or nonspecific symptoms that are not readily classifiable. Clinical differentiation between bacterial and nonbacterial inflammation may be important for determining treatment options, but imaging cannot effectively differentiate among various etiological categories. The morphological features of the inflammatory process or abscess formation are best depicted with cross-sectional imaging techniques (e.g., ultrasonography computed tomography [CT], magnetic resonance imaging [MRI]).

At one time, prostatitis was thought to affect the entire prostate. However, more recent studies have shown that instead of diffuse involvement, more often a focal inflammatory process of the peripheral acinar glandular tissue is found.[3] In acute baterial prostatitis, the gland is usually diffusely and symmetrically edematous. In chronic prostatitis however, either diffuse or focal involvement may occur. The size of the chronically inflamed prostate varies. The gland may be enlarged; however, the increase in size may be secondary to concurrent noninflammatory benign hypertrophy, since both processes can occur in the same individual (although neither predisposes the patient to the occurrence of the other). Often the gland is small and fibrotic. Prostatic calculi are suspected as one sequela of prostatitis, although they may occur in men with no history of glandular inflammation as a result of calcification of naturally sloughed acini or calcification of corpora amylacea (Fig. 26–1). The role of prostatic calculi in perpetuating prostatitis is a controversial topic.

Imaging studies used to diagnose acute or chronic prostatitis are limited and often performed late in the course of the disease or in problem cases. In the acute process, plain radiography is of little use. In the chronic stage, prostatic calculi may be identified, although it bears repeating that this finding is not pathognomonic of prostate inflammation.

The findings of intravenous urography (IVU) are usually normal but may show an enlarged prostate. On occasion, acute inflammation of the prostate is manifested as edema of the interureteral ridge seen on the cystogram phase of IVU (Fig. 26–2). Retrograde urethrography (RUG) or voiding cystourethrography (VCU) may reveal elongation of the prostatic urethra, along with compression and narrowing. Displacement of the verumontanum or utricle can occur. Reflux into the prostate gland occurs with chronic prostatitis, especially when the prostatic ducts are dilated, as is found in longstanding urethral stricture. However, this finding is nonspecific, because it may also be seen in patients with no history of prostatitis (see Chapter 25, Urethral Inflammation).

Radionuclide scintigraphy with gallium-67 citrate (Ga-67-citrate) has been described by Sullivan and colleagues in two patients with prostatitis, but neither the sensitivity nor the specificity of the method is well understood at this time.[4] Similar limitations are noted with CT, except when prostatic abscess is suspected.

The transabdominal suprapubic sonogram may delineate and identify the prostate gland. Both radiopaque and nonradiopaque prostate calculi may be identified as acoustically bright foci with shadowing. Endorectal ultrasonography of the prostate delineates the gland much more clearly. Studies have reported that in patients with acute prostatitis, the following three main characteristics may be identified: (1) a hypoechoic rim surrounding the entire prostate gland (Fig. 26–3), (2) a low-level or echo-free halo surrounding the periurethral zone (Fig. 26–4), or (3) low-level echogenic areas within the prostate.[5]

In chronic prostatitis, the endorectal sonogram may demonstrate diffuse inhomogeneous echogenicity of the prostate (Fig. 26–5), with areas of fluid and/or decreased acoustic reflectivity. Similar sonographic characteristics may also be seen in noninflammatory, nonmalignant conditions of the prostate (i.e., prostate hypertrophy).[6] Although prostatic calculi may be identified by conventional suprapubic ultrasonography, they are more accu-

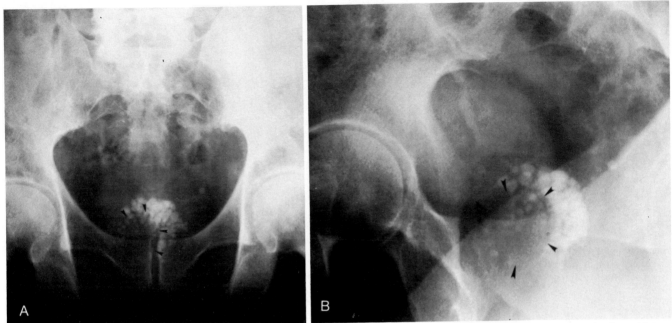

Figure 26–1. Prostatic calcifications in an elderly male, with recent onset of frequency, nocturia, and dysuria, and a long history of urinary tract infections. *A,* Plain film of pelvis shows extensive prostatic calculi with focal area *(arrowheads)* devoid of concretions. *B,* Film from an intravenous urogram demonstrates prostatic enlargement with focal area devoid of calculi, corresponding to area of prostatic hyperplasia with infection. Areas of benign prostatic hyperplasia (BPH), chronic prostatitis and focal abscess were found in prostatectomy specimen.

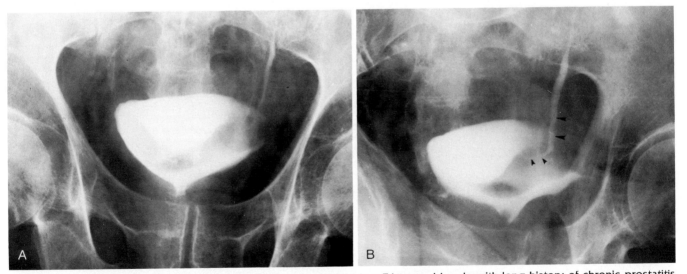

Figure 26–2. Swollen interureteral ridge in prostatitis. The patient is a 71-year-old male with long history of chronic prostatitis. Previous transurethral resection of prostate was performed. Cystoscopy revealed edematous hyperemic trigone and interureteral ridge. *A,* Frontal view. Urogram confirms swollen interureteral ridge. *B,* Oblique view confirms large interureteral ridge. Note normal distal ureter *(arrowheads).*

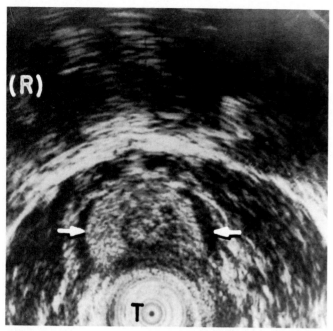

Figure 26–3. Acute prostatitis, endorectal sonogram. A hypoechoic rim is noted *(arrows)* surrounding the peripheral aspect of the prostate. This is clearly identified on this radially oriented transrectal endosonogram of the prostate. R = patient's right side, T = transducer in rectum. (From Griffiths GJ, Crooks AJR, Roberts EE, et al: Ultrasonic appearances associated with prostatic inflammation: A preliminary study. Clin Radiol 35:343–345, 1984. With permission.)

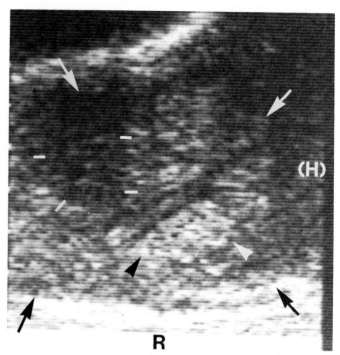

Figure 26–5. Chronic prostatitis. A linear array longitudinally oriented endorectal sonogram demonstrates diffuse areas of abnormality of the prostate *(arrows)*. No normal-appearing prostatic tissue is identified. There are hyperechoic *(arrowheads)* and hypoechoic *(slashes)* areas in the prostate consistent with chronic inflammation of the gland. This may also be due in part to benign hypertrophic changes. R = rectum. H = toward patient's head. (From Rifkin MD, Kurtz AB, Choi HY, Goldberg BB: Endoscopic ultrasonic evaluation of the prostate using a transrectal probe: Prospective evaluation and acoustic characterization. Radiology 149:265–271, 1983.)

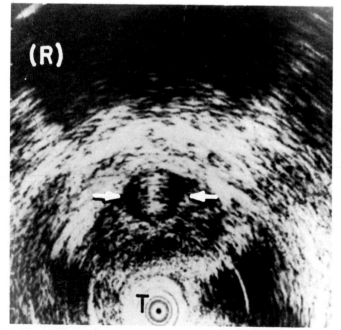

Figure 26–4. Acute prostatitis, endorectal sonogram. Hypoechoic rim *(arrows)* surrounds the periurethral zone of this transversely oriented radial scan obtained by the transrectal approach. R = patient's right side, T = transducer in rectum. (From Griffiths GJ, Crooks, AJR, Roberts EE, et al: Ultrasonic appearances associated with prostatic inflammation: A preliminary study. Clin Radiol 35:343–345, 1984. With permission.)

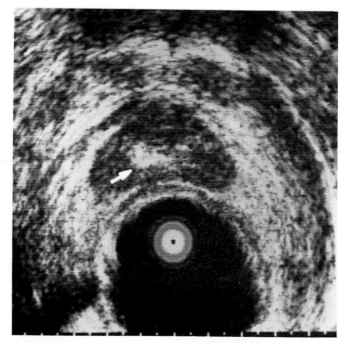

Figure 26–6. Prostatic calculi, axial endorectal sonogram of the prostate demonstrates a bright echogenic area *(arrow)*, attributable to calculus. This is a nonspecific finding of chronic prostatitis. Subtle calculi can also be clearly defined by the endorectal approach. (From Rifkin MD: Diagnostic Imaging of the Lower Genitourinary Tract. New York, Raven Press, 1985.)

rately delineated on the endorectal sonograms (Fig. 26–6).[6]

MRI has shown limited utility differentiating prostatitis from neoplastic processes.[7, 8] Acute prostatitis visualized by MRI shows homogeneous signals from the entire prostate, which has an appearance similar to normal noninflamed tissue.[8, 9] Chronic prostatitis may show inhomogeneous areas containing high-and/or low-signal intensity. This is similar to, and may mimic, prostate cancer or benign prostatic hypertrophy.[8, 9]

Baert and associates have performed seminal vesiculography on patients with chronic bacterial prostatitis and have found that a high percentage (87%) have stenotic or atrophic seminal vesicles.[31] They believe that the entire prostatovesicular complex is involved in chronic prostatitis.

Prostatic Abscess

Abscesses are usually secondary to prostatitis but can develop from hematogenous spread.[10, 11] Reflux of infected urine into the prostate with concurrent urethral obstruction is thought to be a contributory factor.[12, 13] E. coli is typically the offending bacterium, and predisposing causes include diabetes mellitus, hemodialysis, immunosuppression, urethral trauma (instrumentation), and carcinoma of the prostate.[1, 2, 12–14] The differential diagnosis includes fulminant acute prostatitis without abscess. Although conventional imaging has limited benefit in the diagnosis of abscesses, CT and MRI may be definitive.[12–14] Endorectal ultrasonography can show areas of irregularity and abnormal echogenicity within the prostate, as well as differences in size of the gland (Fig. 26–7).[15] The abnormal focus is usually slightly hypoechoic, suggesting the liquefied components of the abscess. Thick septa may be identified.[32] The sonographic characteristics may be nonspecific. Nevertheless, if they are considered in conjunction with clinical presentation, the diagnosis can be suggested. Additionally, endorectal ultrasonography permits accurate ultrasound-guided transperineal aspiration for diagnosis and drainage.[15]

The CT appearance of prostatic and periprostatic abscess is that of a unilocular or multilocular collection, limited to the prostate gland.[32] If the abscess ruptures through the dense prostatic capsule, the periprostatic soft tissues and venous plexus are engulfed or displaced. The seminal vesicles may become secondarily involved, and direct peritoneal extension (peritonitis) may occur.[14] The urogenital diaphragm prevents caudal migration to the perineum. CT scanning clearly depicts the extent of the disease and provides detailed cross-sectional information sufficient for diagnosis, percutaneous/surgical drainage, and follow-up (Figs. 26–8 to 26–10). Prostatic abscesses are readily identifiable on MR scans as localized areas of high-signal intensity on T2-weighted images (Fig. 26–11).

SEMINAL VESICLE INFLAMMATION

Seminal vesiculitis or seminal vesicle inflammation is usually a secondary inflammatory process associated with prostatitis.[16] Inflammation of the seminal vesicle in the absence of an inflamed prostate is unusual, although it may occur.

Imaging studies have produced limited diagnostic benefit. The plain film and excretory urogram are usually not useful, except when mesonephric duct abnormalities exist (e.g., seminal vesicle cyst; ectopic ureter entering the seminal vesicle).[17] In these cases, epididymitis or seminal vesiculitis may be the initial presenting complaint (Fig. 26–12).[17] Ultrasonography may show enlarged and less echogenic seminal vesicles. This appearance is best appreciated by endorectal ultrasonography (Fig. 26–13), which may also demonstrate seminal vesicle or ejaculatory duct calculi.[39] The CT demonstration of cystic dilatation of inflamed seminal vesicles has been reported.[34, 37]

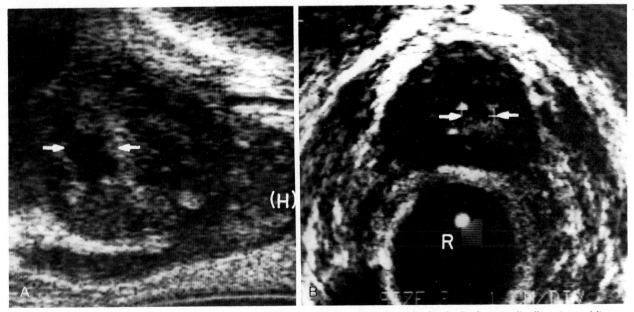

Figure 26–7. Prostatic abscess, endorectal sonogram. Prostate abscess is defined by both the longitudinally oriented linear array (A) and transverse scans (B). The endorectal approach clearly defines an irregularly marginated hypoechoic area (arrows) seen in the middle portion of the gland. Although this is not pathognomonic for prostatic abscess, with clinical correlation it is highly suggestive. R = rectum. H indicates direction of patient's head. (Courtesy Dr. Fred Lee.)

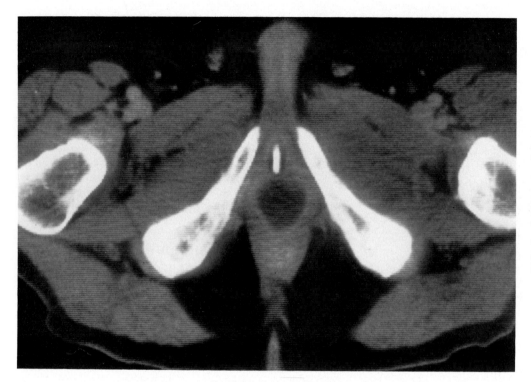

Figure 26–8. Prostatic abscess in a 70-year-old male with fever, chills, and urinary retention. Rectal examination revealed fluctuant prostatic mass. CT scan demonstrates large, low-attenuation mass that is highly suggestive of abscess within the prostate gland. A urethral catheter is present.

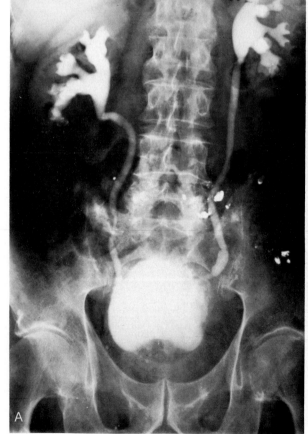

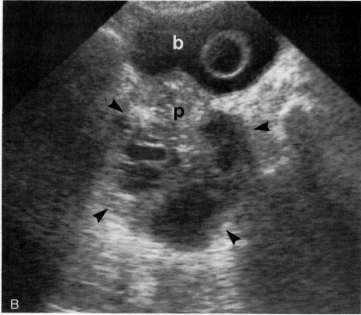

Figure 26–9. Prostatic abscess. An 83-year-old man presented with urinary retention and findings suggestive of prostatic abscess. Concurrent carcinoma of the prostate was found when the prostatic abscess was drained. *A,* Marked elevation of the bladder base is noted on IVU. Mild ureterectasis and pyelocaliectasis are also seen. *B,* Longitudinal transabdominal sonogram of the pelvis shows a complex mass *(arrowheads)* representing prostatic abscess, arising from posterior aspect of prostate (p), rupturing into pelvic soft tissues. Note cephalad displacement of prostate by extraprostatic component of abscess. A catheter has been placed within urinary bladder (b). (From Washecka R, Rumancik WM: Prostatic abscess evaluation by serial computed tomography. Urol Radiol 7(1):54–56, 1985. © Springer-Verlag 1985. With permission.)

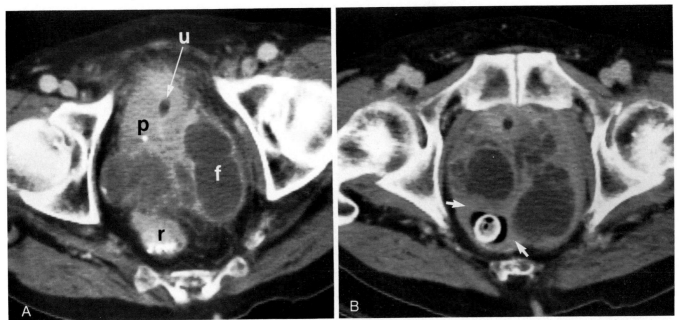

Figure 26–10. CT scans of prostate and prostatic fossa at initial evaluation of prostatic abscess (same as in Fig. 26–9). *A,* Prostate (p) is asymmetrically distorted and anteriorly displaced by complex inflammatory mass, which arises within prostate and extends into the posterior periprostatic space. Areas of low attenuation within abscess (f) correspond to multilocular fluid collections. Prostatic urethra (u) is identified. There is oral contrast in the rectum (r). *B,* Scan 2 cm caudal to *A.* Rectal tube has been inserted; full extraprostatic extent of abscess is visible. Note perirectal involvement *(arrows).* (From Washecka R, Rumancik WM: Prostatic abscess evaluation by serial computed tomography. Urol Radiol 7(1):54–56, 1985. © Springer-Verlag 1985. With permission.)

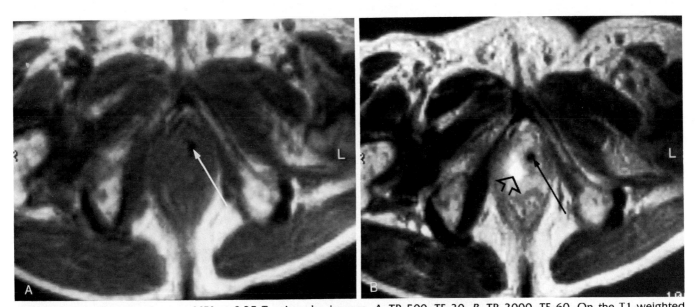

Figure 26–11. Prostate abscess. MRI at 0.35-T spin-echo images. *A,* TR-500, TE-30; *B,* TR-2000, TE-60. On the T1-weighted image *(A),* the prostate is of homogeneous signal intensity. *B,* On the T2-weighted image, an ill-defined high-signal intensity area *(open arrow)* is seen along the right posterior aspect. At surgery, this was found to be an abscess. Urethra *(long arrow)* is indicated. (Courtesy Dr. Hedvig Hricak.)

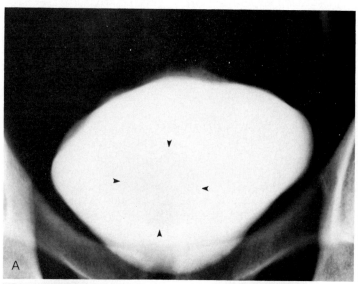

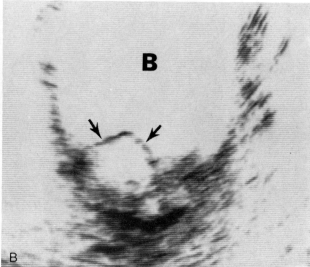

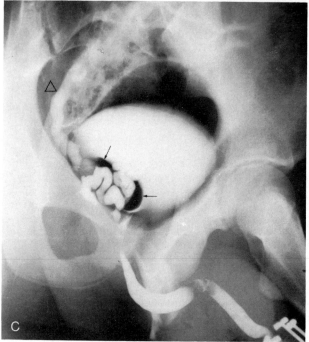

Figure 26–12. "Cystic" seminal vesicle with ureterocele and single ectopic ureter (mesonephric duct abnormality). *A,* Filled bladder film from IVU shows extrinsic mass effect represented by lucent filling defect *(arrowheads)* in contrast-filled bladder. *B,* Transabdominal transverse-view sonogram shows 2 × 2 × 4 cm cystic mass *(arrows)* posterior to and indenting urine-filled bladder (B). *C,* Seminal vesiculography was performed endoscopically, and air was injected into ureterocele *(arrows).* The right (blind-ending) ureter also filled with injection of dilated seminal vesicle *(open arrowhead).* At surgery, excision of the cystlike right seminal vesicle and the ureter was performed. No right ureteral orifice was present in the bladder. (From Weyman PJ, McClennan BL: Computed tomography and ultrasonography in the evaluation of mesonephric duct anomalies. Urol Radiol 1(1):29–37, 1979. © Springer-Verlag 1985. With permission.)

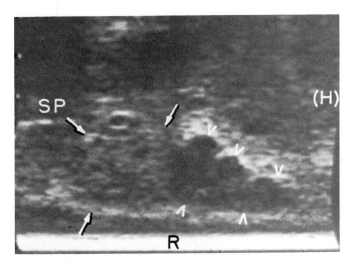

Figure 26–13. Seminal vesiculitis. A longitudinally oriented linear endorectal sonogram of the normal-sized prostate *(arrows)* demonstrates an enlarged hypoechoic seminal vesicle *(arrowheads)*. This is consistent with diffuse seminal vesicle inflammation. SP = symphysis pubis, R = rectum. H indicates direction of patient's head. (From Rifkin MD: Diagnostic Imaging of the Lower Genitourinary Tract. New York, Raven Press, 1985. With permission.)

Seminal vesiculitis may lead to seminal vesicle abscess.[16] In these cases, asymmetrical enlargement of one seminal vesicle may be seen by MRI (Fig. 26–14), CT (Fig. 26–15),[33, 36] or ultrasonography (Fig. 26–16). Endorectal ultrasonography may show an anechoic or hypoechoic, partially fluid-filled lesion.[16, 33]

Seminal vesicle abscesses may be due to congenital mesonephric duct anomalies (Fig. 26–12), the most common being ectopic ureteral insertion into the seminal vesicles.[17, 38] In these cases, as the seminal vesicle enlarges, a mass may be seen on the urogram, impressing upon the fluid-filled bladder (Fig. 26–17A). An ectopic positioning of the kidney and/or renal agenesis may also be noted. The mass and partial fluid contents of the abscessed stricture may be seen by CT (Fig. 26–17B), ultrasonography (Fig. 26–17C), or direct puncture (Fig. 26–18). MRI may show high- or low-signal intensity, depending on the imaging sequence used. Seminal vesiculography may show changes in patients with chronic seminal vesiculitis (Fig. 26–19). Stenoses, fibroses, and dilatation of the seminal vesicles have been described[31] but in view of the nonspecificity of the findings[18] and the availability of less invasive imaging modalities, vesiculography is rarely indicated in the evaluation of such patients.

In general, inflammatory conditions of the prostate and seminal vesicles are usually diagnosed by clinical symptomatology and the physical examination. Imaging studies are often complementary and may guide appropriate intervention.

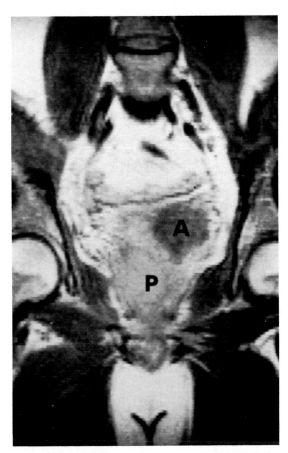

Figure 26–14. MR scan of left seminal vesicle abscess. Field strength 0.35 T, coronal image SE: TR = 1000, TE = 30. The left seminal vesicle is enlarged and shows lower signal intensity than the adjacent right seminal vesicle. Abscess (A) was present at surgery. P = prostate gland. (From Higgins CB, Hricak H: Magnetic Resonance Imaging of the Body. New York, Raven Press Ltd., 1987. With permission.)

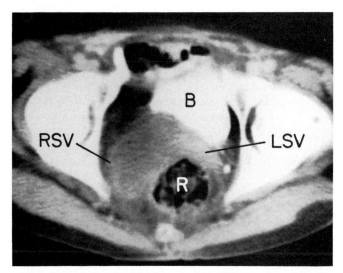

Figure 26–15. Seminal vesicle abscess. CT scan demonstrates an inhomogeneous, enlarged right seminal vesicle (RSV) compared with the normal left seminal vesicle (LSV). This contrast-enhanced study demonstrates contrast material in the bladder (B) and a normal-appearing rectum (R). (Courtesy Dr. Fred Lee.)

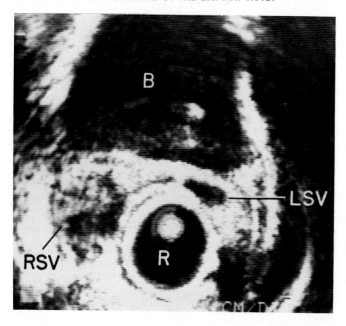

Figure 26–16. Seminal vesicle abscess (Same patient as in Fig. 26–15). Transrectal sonogram with a transversely oriented radial approach demonstrates the right seminal vesicle (RSV) to be enlarged with mixed hypoechoic and anechoic areas, but relatively good acoustic through transmission. Given the patient's history, the findings are most consistent with a seminal vesicle abscess. LSV = left seminal vesical, R = rectum, B = bladder. (Courtesy Dr. Fred Lee.)

SCROTAL INFLAMMATION

Inflammation of the scrotum may be due to a number of causes and may affect various components of the scrotal sac. Scrotal wall abscesses are usually due to infection of the hair follicles, sweat glands, or open cuts of the skin. They may also be attributable to previous surgical intervention, (i.e., vasectomy). Imaging may aid in the diagnosis, especially when underlying orchitis or epididymitis causes the scrotal wall infection.

Clinically, the most frequently encountered inflammatory process is epididymitis. This common entity, in which the clinical presentation includes scrotal tenderness, erythema, and occasionally shooting pain, usually affects the adolescent or adult male,[19-21] often without demonstrable bacteriuria. However, epididymitis may be seen in infants and young children. Elderly males may be affected, but usually in the presence of lower urinary tract infection. The inciting cause may be traumatic, resulting from specific bacterial infections or from nonspecific inflammatory causes.[19-22]

The most frequent cause is retrograde spread of bacteria from the prostate or urethra to the vas deferens and then to the epididymis. Reflux of sterile urine may cause a chemical or noninfectious form of epididymitis.[19-21] Nonspecific epididymitis refers to infectious causes, including nonbacterial, viral, granulomatous, and bacterial inflammation.[21-22] The most common isolated infectious agents, *E. coli, Pseudomonas, Aerobacter, Mycobacterium tuberculosis*, and *Schistosoma haematobium*, are common causes of epididymitis in underdeveloped areas of the world.[23]

Specific epididymitis refers to metastatic infection from the genitourinary or other systems. In many cases (nonspecific ones), no inciting agent is identified. Regardless of the cause, patients may experience sepsis and leukocytosis, usually of a low-grade severity. The physical examination may demonstrate enlargement and/or pain in the inflamed epididymis. Frequently, however, the scrotal skin is swollen and edematous, and therefore the physical examination may be inconclusive.

Clinically, it is important to differentiate acute epididymitis from acute torsion of the spermatic cord, torsion of the testicular or epididymal appendages, orchitis, and intrascrotal hematoma. It may be difficult to exclude a neoplasm, particularly when it is infarcted. Usually, marked swelling and edema of the scrotum are associated with acute epididymitis. When edema of scrotal contents is severe, testicular blood flow may be compromised, resulting in focal or diffuse infarction of the testis and/or epididymis. This may occur without torsion of the spermatic cord.

Sonographic features of acute epididymitis include enlargement and a primarily inhomogeneous echo texture (Fig. 26–20 to 26–22). Echogenic areas within the swollen epididymis may be seen along with reactive hydrocele formation.[20] In chronic epididymitis, increased echogenicity of the head and body of the epididymis may develop. Discrete hypoechoic or anechoic areas suggest suppuration and/or early abscess formation (Figs. 26–21 and 26–22).[24, 25]

Scrotal abscesses and scrotal gangrene are complications or epididymitis and/or orchitis. However, they have also been reported to follow scrotal surgery, trauma, urethritis, perianal abscess, vasectomy, and hemorrhoidectomy.

With the exception of mumps orchitis, acute infection involving only the testis is rare. Although a variety of infections have been reported to be capable of hematogenous spread to the testis, by far, the vast majority of testicular infection occurs in association with epididymitis (epididymo-orchitis).

Orchitis is most commonly a diffuse process,[24] focal inflammation being rare. Clinically, orchitis presents with sudden onset of pain, testicular swelling, scrotal edema, and erythema. Pain radiates to the inguinal canal, and nausea or vomiting is associated. Fever, septicemia, and

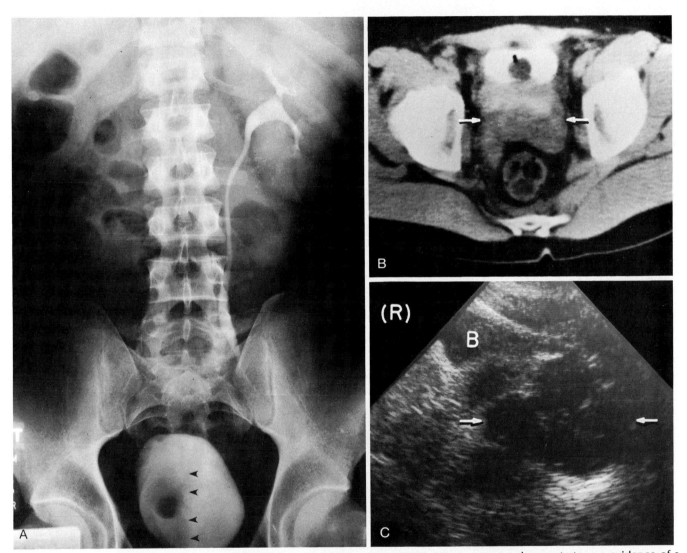

Figure 26–17. Seminal vesicle abscess due to ectopic ureteral insertion. *A,* Intravenous urogram demonstrates no evidence of a right kidney, and a large left kidney. There is a soft-tissue mass posterior to the bladder causing extrinsic compression *(arrowheads). B,* The CT scan demonstrates an inhomogeneous soft-tissue mass *(arrows)* posterior to the contrast-filled urinary bladder. *C,* The abdominal sonogram through an almost empty urinary bladder (B) demonstrates a complex septated but mostly fluid-filled mass *(arrows).*

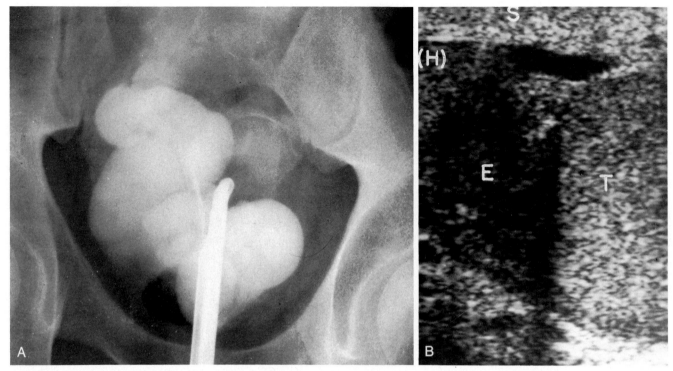

Figure 26–18. Seminal vesicle abscess due to ectopic ureteral insertion (same case as in Fig. 26–17). *A,* Transcystoscopic insertion of catheter into bulging cystic mass on the right side of the trigone. Contrast fills a huge ureter emptying into a massively dilated right seminal vesicle. *B,* Retrograde flow into the epididymis causing epididymitis was confirmed by ultrasonic evaluation of the scrotum where the head of the epididymis (E) is markedly enlarged and hypoechoic. The testis (T) was normal. The skin (S) was slightly thickened due to chronic inflammation. H points toward patient's head.

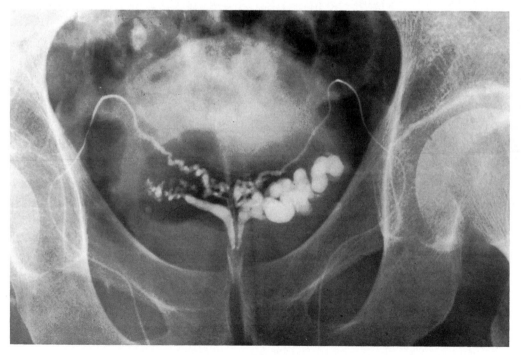

Figure 26–19. Chronic right seminal vesiculitis. A 63-year-old man with chronic bacterial prostatitis had a recent episode of right-sided epididymo-orchitis. Seminal vesiculogram reveals shrunken right seminal vesicle. The left seminal vesicle appears marginally dilated. (From Baert L, Leonard A, D'Hoedt M, Vandeursen R: Seminal vesiculography in chronic bacterial prostatitis. J Urol 136(4):844–845, © by Williams & Wilkins, 1986.)

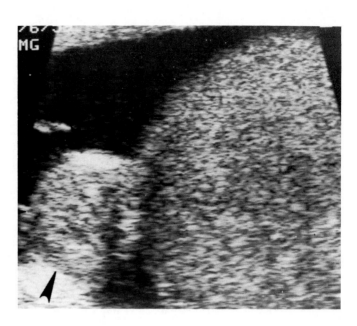

Figure 26–20. Acute epididymitis. Longitudinal ultrasound image shows enlarged, diffusely echogenic head of the epididymis *(arrowheads).* An associated hydrocele is also present. The visualized testis is normal.

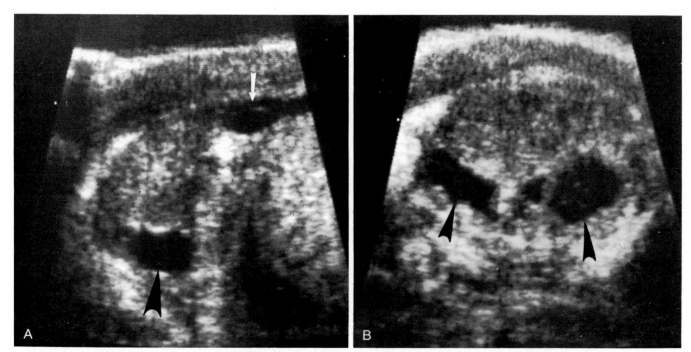

Figure 26–21. Diffuse epididymitis with epididymal abscess. *A,* Longitudinal ultrasound image of right testis. Focal anechoic area *(arrowhead)* in swollen epididymis represents surgically proven abscess. Small hydrocele can be seen anteriorly *(arrow). B,* Transverse view reveals abscess formation in body of epididymis as well *(arrowheads).*

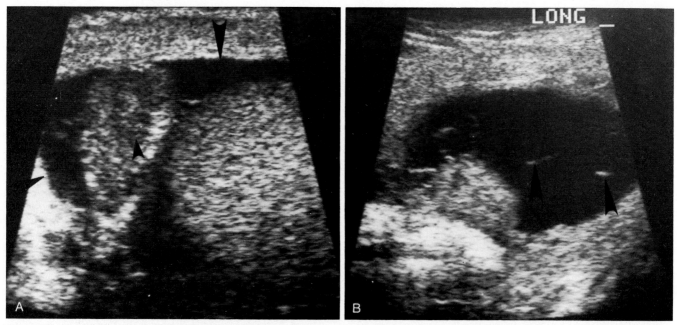

Figure 26–22. Epididymitis with infected septated hydrocele. A, Longitudinal sonogram of left testis. Diffusely enlarged epididymal head and associated hydrocele *(arrowheads)* are present. Focal area of decreased echogenicity *(small arrowhead)* may represent early abscess formation. B, Longitudinal view shows septations *(arrowheads)* in hydrocele.

scrotal wall erythema usually ensue. One complication of orchitis is testicular rupture. Infected hydroceles (pyocele) occur and are usually due to a pyogenic abscess.[25, 26]

Diffuse inflammation of the testes usually causes a sonographic picture of mild to moderate enlargement with preservation of the testicular oval shape and smooth contour.[24] The internal testicular echo texture is generally homogeneous, and the epididymis is frequently enlarged.[24] In distinction, neoplasms usually cause more eccentric testicular enlargement, with lobular contours and a heterogeneous echo texture. The epididymis and scrotal skin are normal in most patients with malignancy.[24]

The diagnosis of inflammation of the scrotal sac is usually made by clinical examination and appropriate symptomatology. Imaging of the past, using conventional radiographic techniques, has been of limited value. Radiography and CT have little utility in the diagnosis, unless a pyogenic, gas-producing infection occurs (see Fig. 26–34). Radionuclide studies often demonstrate increased flow to the affected side in inflammatory processes, especially early in the course of the disease. Unilateral uptake is usually linear or curvilinear in epididymitis, corresponding to the inflamed epididymis.[18] Focal inflammation of the structure may result in a discrete "hot" area (Fig. 26–23 and 26–24). In epididymitis, the delayed static images may show a central or medial displacement of the epididymis. In orchitis, there may be increased flow to the involved testis (Fig. 26–25) or a diffuse, but subtle, uptake in the hemiscrotum. Because of the close proximity of the epididymis to the testis, the nuclear medicine studies may, on occasion, be unable to demonstrate or differentiate between epididymitis and orchitis.

Ultrasonography delineates enlargement and either decreased (Fig. 26–22) or normal echogenicity (Fig. 26–21) of the epididymis. Focal inflammation may be identified by a localized lesion, which is also enlarged and hypo-

echoic or of mixed echogenicity, compared with the normal epididymis (Fig. 26–22). A hydrocele is a frequent accompaniment—occasionally with echogenic exudate. Echogenic bands due to fibrin strands may be seen following treatment (see Fig. 26–26).

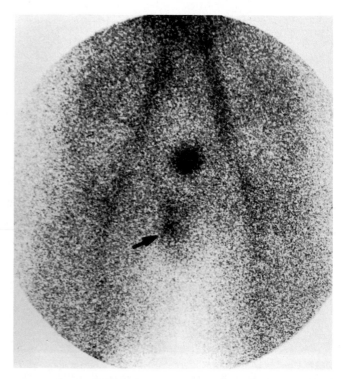

Figure 26–23. Epididymitis. A static radionuclide technetium-99m (Tc-99m) DTPA scintiscan demonstrates an area of increased uptake attributable to an inflamed right epididymis *(arrow)*. (From Rifkin MD: Diagnostic Imaging of the Lower Genitourinary Tract. New York, Raven Press Ltd., 1985. With permission.)

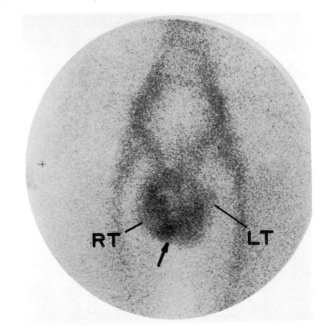

Figure 26–24. Focal epididymitis Tc-99m-DPTA radionuclide study demonstrates diffuse increased uptake in the scrotum, secondary to hyperemia. In addition there is a focally "hot" area on the right *(arrow)* corresponding to a focal epididymitis. (RT = right testis, LT = left testis.) (From Rifkin MD: Diagnostic Imaging of the Lower Genitourinary Tract. New York, Raven Press Ltd., 1985. With permission.)

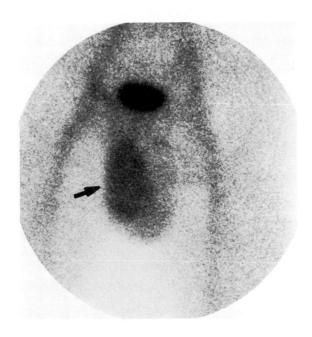

Figure 26–25. Orchitis. A radionuclide study with Tc-99m-DTPA demonstrates a focal area of increased radioactivity *(arrow)* in the right testicle in comparison with the left in this patient with diffuse orchitis. (From Rifkin MD: Diagnostic Imaging of the Lower Genitourinary Tract. New York, Raven Press Ltd., 1985. With permission.)

Figure 26–26. Multiseptated infected hydrocele following epididymo-orchitis. Longitudinal sonogram shows extensive septation formation within the hydrocele *(arrowheads),* secondary to infection.

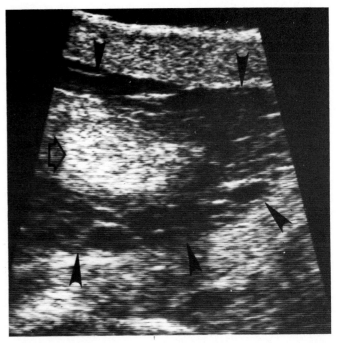

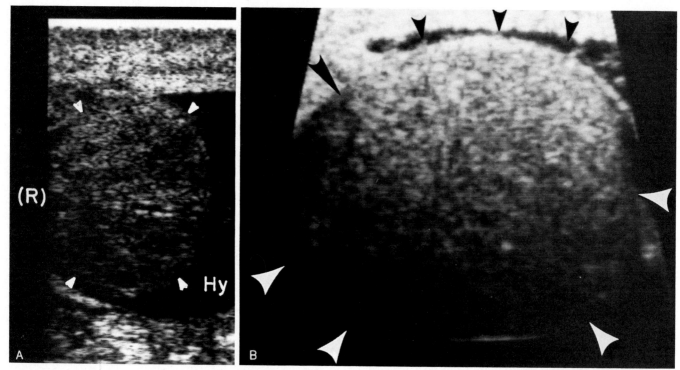

Figure 26–27. Orchitis. *A,* High-resolution sonogram of the scrotum, transverse orientation, demonstrates the testis *(arrowheads)* to have diffuse abnormal echogenicity, with no residual normal tissue. A hydrocele (Hy) is noted. Of importance, is that the superficial skin is thickened, a classic finding in inflammation of the scrotal contents. R = patient's right side. *B,* Transverse scan of a different patient with right-sided orchitis; enlarged testis *(large arrowheads)* with some skin thickening is noted. Diffuse homogeneous hypoechoic patterns like this can occur. Small septated hydrocele is present *(small arrowheads, top).*

The ultrasound examination in orchitis generally demonstrates diffuse sonographic abnormalities of the testis.[24] Decreased testicular echogenicity (Fig. 26–27) is most common, although the appearance may be inhomogeneous. Focal orchitis may show a localized area of decreased echogenicity (Figs. 26–28 and 26–29). This is usually secondary to inflammation of the epididymis and is usually adjacent to the inflamed epididymis. Differentiation from malignancy based on imaging characteristics alone may be difficult to achieve (Fig. 26–29). Scrotal wall thickening is usually not seen in neoplastic processes but is often identified in inflammatory processes (Figs. 26–27 and 26–28).

CT has not proved to be of great value in examining patients with intrascrotal inflammation. In view of this fact and the gonadal irradiation involved, it is infrequently used to evaluate such conditions. MRI, however, adds a new dimension to scrotal imaging. MR images demonstrate, in elegant anatomical detail, the entire scrotum and inguinal region. In epididymo-orchitis MRI clearly delineates the disease and is sensitive to slight changes in testicular and epididymal integrity. The affected areas, in general, show, a decreased signal intensity in acute inflammation.[28, 30] The size, shape, and location of both the epididymis and testis are visible, and the two structures can usually be individually identified (Fig. 26–30). Inflam-

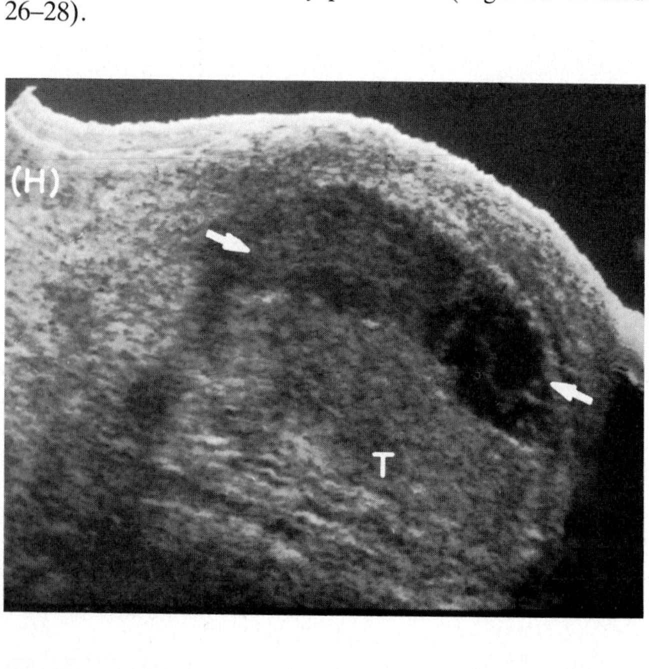

Figure 26–28. Focal orchitis. A longitudinally oriented sonogram demonstrates a normal-appearing testis (T) posteriorly, but a hypoechoic infiltrative area *(arrows)* anteriorly. The diagnosis of focal orchitis, which is usually situated posteriorly but in this case is situated anteriorly, can be suggested, because the scrotal skin anterior to the inflamed area is thickened. The presence of skin thickening and some fibrous septae separating multiple hypoechoic areas, raises the possibility of testicular abscess. H indicates direction of patient's head. (From Rifkin MD: Diagnostic Imaging of the Lower Genitourinary Tract. New York, Raven Press Ltd., 1985. With permission.)

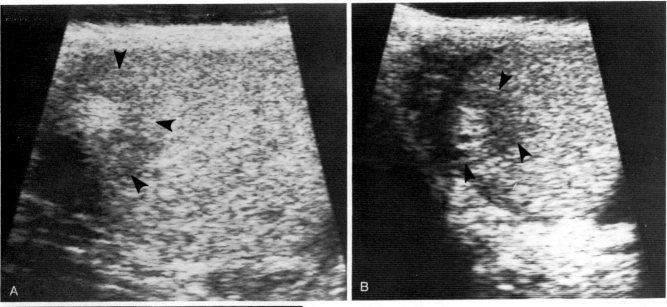

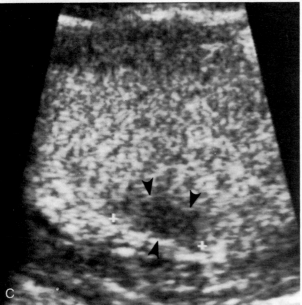

Figure 26–29. Focal orchitis. *A*, Longitudinal view shows left testis in patient, at initial presentation with testicular pain; testis was normal to palpation. A focal hyperechoic area with surrounding hypoechoic rim *(arrowheads)* is seen. *B*, Similar view as *A*, 10 months later. Allowing for difference in scan technique, area has similar appearance but has increased very slightly in size. Because of this, surgery was performed (orchiectomy). Diagnosis was focal orchitis. *C*, Focal orchitis in a different patient *(arrowheads)* was biopsied after intraoperative sonographic localization. Sonographic guidance enabled both accurate diagnosis and local excision.

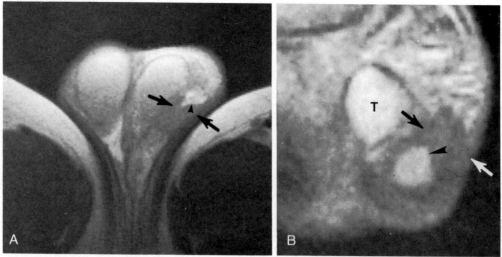

Figure 26–30. Acute epididymitis. MRI at 0.5 T field strength. *A*, T2-weighted coronal image (TR-2100 msec, TE-90 msec). A discrete fluid collection *(arrowhead)* is seen within the enlarged low-intensity epididymis *(arrows)*. Note that the testis (T) is displaced superiorly and medially. A prior sonogram showed essentially the same findings. *B*, T1-weighted transverse image (TR-500 msec, TE-35 msec) of another patient with post-traumatic epididymitis. The inflamed epididymis *(arrows)* is of lower-than-normal signal intensity, and contains within it a high intensity focus *(arrowhead)* believed to represent an area of hemorrhage. However, the left epididymis was found to be definitely enlarged on physical examination. (From Rholl KS, Lee JKT, Ling D, et al: MR imaging of the scrotum with a high-resolution surface coil. Radiology 163:99–1003, 1987.)

matory hydroceles are prominently displayed and can be differentiated from simple hydroceles by their increased signal (Fig. 26–31).[28] T2-weighted images in the coronal plane, obtained by means of surface coils are usually the most informative.

Testicular infarction may occur secondarily to epididymitis and/or epididymo-orchitis (Fig. 26–32). It is usually due to compromise of testicular blood flow from edema and swelling.[25, 26] In these cases, the clinical course may

be more severe than with simple epidymo-orchitis.[27] Early diagnosis of vascular compromise to the testis is important because a prompt epididymotomy at the onset of scrotal fixation may avert testicular necrosis (Fig. 26–33; see also Fig. 26–29).[2, 26] Untreated orchitis may advance to abscess formation. Testicular abscesses may be recognized sonographically by the presence of hypoechoic compartments separated by echogenic septa.[35]

The differentiation of subacute testicular torsion from

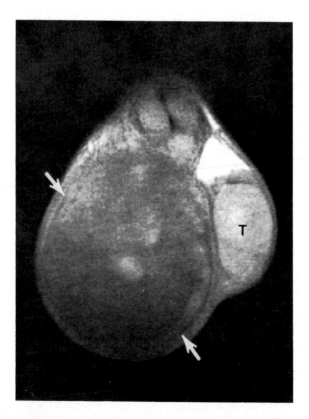

Figure 26–31. Infected hydrocele. MRI at a 0.5 T Spin-echo image with receive-only surface coil. T1-weighted coronal image (TR-500, TE-35 msec) shows large nonuniform low-signal mass within right hemiscrotum *(arrow)*. Areas of high-signal intensity within the collection differentiate it from a simple hydrocele. Testis (T) appears normal. (From Rholl KS, Lee JKT, Ling D, et al: MR imaging of the scrotum with a high-resolution surface coil. Radiology 163:99–1003, 1987.)

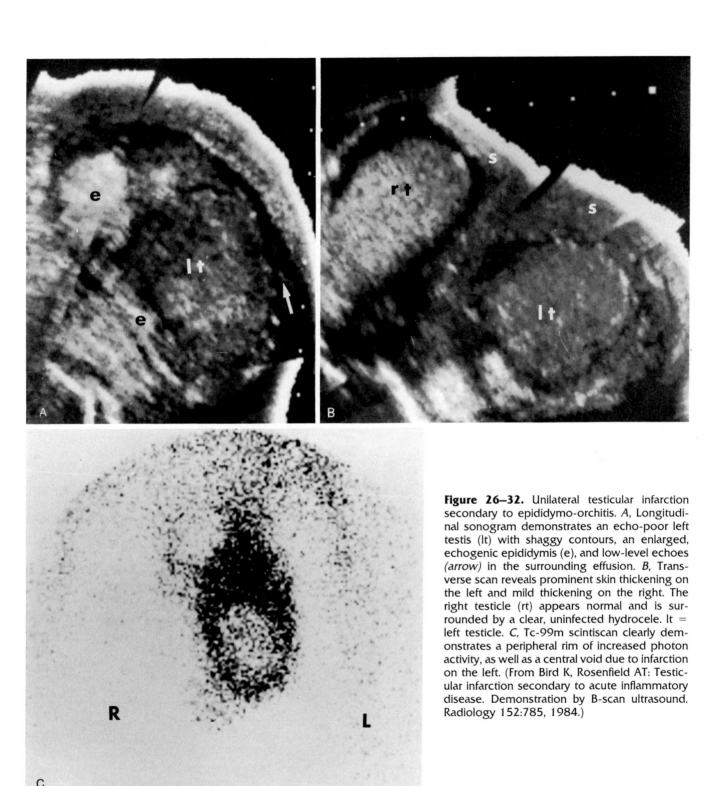

Figure 26–32. Unilateral testicular infarction secondary to epididymo-orchitis. *A,* Longitudinal sonogram demonstrates an echo-poor left testis (lt) with shaggy contours, an enlarged, echogenic epididymis (e), and low-level echoes *(arrow)* in the surrounding effusion. *B,* Transverse scan reveals prominent skin thickening on the left and mild thickening on the right. The right testicle (rt) appears normal and is surrounded by a clear, uninfected hydrocele. lt = left testicle. *C,* Tc-99m scintiscan clearly demonstrates a peripheral rim of increased photon activity, as well as a central void due to infarction on the left. (From Bird K, Rosenfield AT: Testicular infarction secondary to acute inflammatory disease. Demonstration by B-scan ultrasound. Radiology 152:785, 1984.)

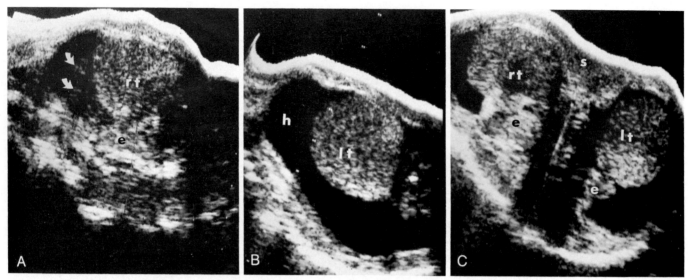

Figure 26–33. Bilateral epididymo-orchitis with testicular infarction. *A,* longitudinal sonogram demonstrates a hypoechoic right testis (rt). A complex hydrocele is noted containing purulent debris *(curved arrows).* The epididymis (e) is slightly enlarged and echogenic. *B,* Longitudinal image of the left hemiscrotum demonstrates an inhomogeneous testicle (lt) and a clear hydrocele (h). *C,* Transverse sonogram demonstrates bilateral skin thickening (s) and epididymal enlargement (e) with inhomogeneous testicular echogenicity. Pathological findings reveal bilateral testicular necrosis and infarction with acute and chronic inflammation (rt = right testicle, lt = left testicle). (From Bird K, Rosenfield AT: Testicular infarction secondary to acute inflammatory disease. Demonstration by B-scan ultrasound. Radiology 152:785, 1984.)

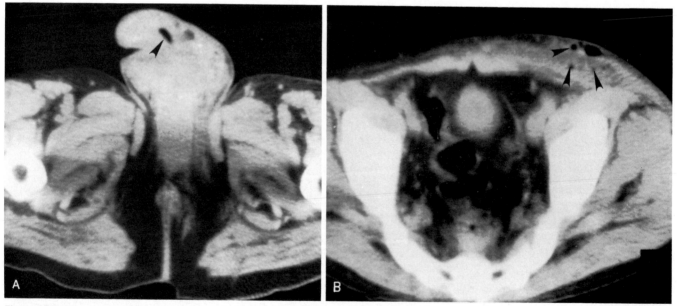

Figure 26–34. Gas-containing abscess. *A,* Computed tomogram at the level of the penis and high scrotal region. *B,* More cephalad at the level of the inguinal canal demonstrates gas-containing areas *(arrowheads)* in the soft tissues from dissection of an abscess from the scrotum.

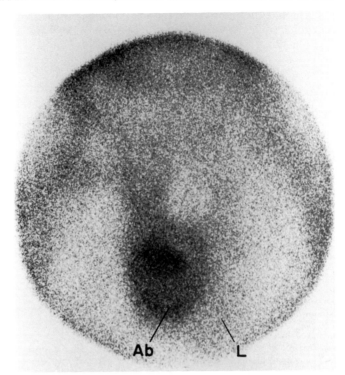

Figure 26–35. Scrotal abscess. A radioisotope study demonstrates the entire right side of the scrotum to be diffusely increased in radioactivity. (Ab) in comparison to the normal left hemiscrotum (L). This diffuse increase in radioactivity is due to diffuse abscess formation. (From Rifkin MD: Diagnostic Imaging of the Lower Genitourinary Tract. New York, Raven Press Ltd., 1986. With permission.)

testicular infarction secondary to acute inflammatory processes of the scrotum may be difficult.[27] Decreased echogenicity of the testis with increased or decreased echogenicity of the epididymis is a typical presentation. Increased echogenicity may be due to hemorrhage, whereas decreased echogenicity may result from inflammation without hemorrhage (Figs. 26–32 and 26–33).

If the inflammatory process extends to the testicular tunics and scrotal wall, purulent fluid (or gas) may dissect through the fascia of the scrotum and spread into the subcutaneous tissues of the perineum, abdominal wall, or thigh. In these cases, a plain film or CT may show the gas (Fig. 26–34). The radionuclide examination may demonstrate a diffusely hot hemiscrotum (Fig. 26–35). The

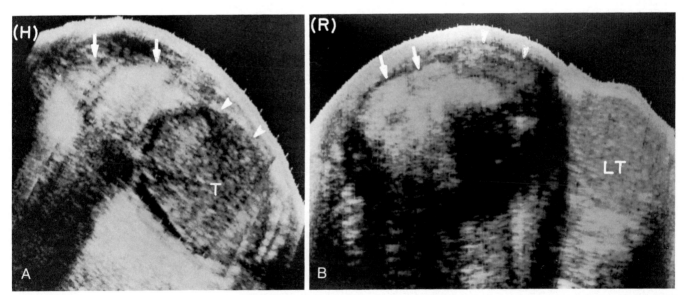

Figure 26–36. Sonography of scrotal abscess: testicular involvement. *A,* The longitudinal image demonstrates the right testis (T) to be sonographically inhomogeneous *(arrowheads).* There are areas of bright acoustic reflectivity with shadowing extending superior to the testis *(arrows),* which on the transverse orientation, *B,* is quite extensive. The left testis (LT) is unremarkable. This was a scrotal abscess that caused secondary inflammation of the right testis. R = patient's right side. H indicates direction of patient's head. (From Rifkin MD: Diagnostic Imaging of the Lower Genitourinary Tract. New York, Raven Press Ltd., 1985. With permission.)

sonographic findings may be pathognomonic, with bright echogenic reflectors (gas) causing acoustic shadowing (Fig. 26–36).

References

1. PFAV A: Prostatitis: A continuing enigma. Urol Clin North Am 13:695–715, 1986.
2. Meares EM: Prostatitis and related disorders. In Walsh PL, Gittes RE, Perlmutter AD, Stamey TA (eds): Campbell's Urology, 5th Ed. Philadelphia, WB Saunders, 1986.
3. McNeal JE: Regional morphology and pathology of the prostate. Am J Clin Pathol 49:347–357, 1968.
4. Sullivan WT, Rosen PR, Kleiland RL Ritchey ML: Prostatitis update of Ga-67. Radiology 152:537, 1984.
5. Griffiths GJ, Crooks AJR, Roberts EE, et al: Ultrasonic appearances associated with prostatic inflammation: A preliminary study. Clin Radiol 35:343–345, 1984.
6. Rifkin MD, Kurtz AB, Choi Hy, Goldberg BB: Endoscopic ultrasonic evaluation of the prostate using a transrectal probe: Prospective evaluation and acoustic characterization. Radiology 149:265–271, 1983.
7. Hricak H, Williams RD, Spring DB, et al: Anatomy and pathology of the male pelvis by magnetic resonance imaging. AJR 141:1101–1110, 1983.
8. Bryan DJ, Butler HE, Nelson AO, et al: Magnetic resonance imaging of the prostate. AJR 146:543–548, 1986.
9. Lee JKT, Rholl KS: MRI of the bladder and prostate. AJR 147:732–736, 1986.
10. Becker LE, Harrin WR: Prostatic abscess: A diagnostic and therapeutic approach. J Urol 91:582–584, 1964.
11. Dajani AM, O'Flynn JD: Prostatic abscess. Br J Urol 40:736–739, 1968.
12. Davidson KC, Garlow WB, Brewer J: Computerized tomography of prostatic and periurethral abscesses: 2 case reports. J Urol 135:1257–1258, 1986.
13. Kadmon D, Ling D, Lee JKT: Percutaneous drainage of prostatic abscesses. J Urol 135:1259–1260, 1986.
14. Washecka R, Rumancik WM: Prostatic abscess evaluation by serial computed tomography. Urol Radiol 7:54–56, 1985.
15. Lee F Jr, Lee F, Solomon MH, et al: Ultrasonic demonstration of prostatic abscess. J Ultrasound Med 5:101, 1986.
16. Lee SB, Lee F, Solomon MH, et al: Seminal vesical abscess: Diagnosis by transrectal ultrasound. J Clin Ultrasound 14:546, 1986.
17. Weyman PJ, McClennan BL: Computed tomography and ultrasonography in the evaluation of mesonephric duct anomalies. Urol Radiol 1:29–37, 1979.
18. Dunnick NR, Ford K, Osborne D, et al: Seminal vesiculography: Limited value in vesiculitis. Urology 20:454, 1982.
19. Mittemeyer BT, Lennox KW, Borski AA: Epididymis: A review of 610 cases. J Urol 95:390–392, 1966.
20. Hricak H, Hoddick WK: Scrotal ultrasound. In Hricak H (ed): Clinic in Diagnostic Ultrasound: Genitourinary Ultrasound. New York, Churchill Livingstone, 1986.
21. Berger RE, Alexander ER, Harnisch JP, et al: Etiology, manifestations and therapy of acute epididymitis: Prospective study of 50 cases. J Urol 121:750–754, 1979.
22. Wolin LH: On the etiology of epididymitis. J Urol 105:531–533, 1971.
23. Reeve HR, Weinerth JL, Peterson LJ: Tuberculosis of epididymis and testicle presenting as hydrocele. Urology 4:329–331, 1974.
24. Subramanyam BR, Horii SC, Hilton S: Diffuse testicular disease: Sonographic features and significance. AJR 145:1221–1224, 1985.
25. Eltayeh AA: Schistosomiasis of the epididymis. Br J Surg 56:522–553, 1969.
26. Witherington R, Harper WM: The surgical management of acute bacterial epididymitis with emphasis on epididymotomy. J Urol 128:722–725, 1982.
27. Vordermark JS, Favila MQ: Testicular necrosis: A preventable complication of epididymitis. J Urol 128:1322–1324, 1982.
28. Rholl K, Lee JKT, Ling D, et al: MR imaging of the scrotum with a high-resolution surface coil. Radiology 163:99–1003, 1987.
29. Rifkin MD: Diagnostic Imaging of the Lower Genitourinary Tract. New York, Raven Press, 1985.
30. Baker LL, Hajek PC, Burkhard TK, et al: MR imaging of the scrotum: Pathologic conditions. Radiology 163:93, 1987.
31. Baert L, Leonard A, D'Hoedt M, Vandeursen R: Seminal vesiculography in chronic bacterial prostatitis. J Urol 136:844, 1986.
32. Thornhill BA, Morehouse HT, Coleman P, Hoffman-Tretin JC: Prostatic abscess: CT and sonographic findings. AJR 148:899, 1987.
33. Zagoria RJ, Papanicolaou N, Pfister RC, et al: Seminal vesicle abscess after vasectomy: Evaluation by transrectal sonography and CT. AJR 149:137, 1987.
34. Patel PS, Wilbur AC: Cystic seminal vesiculitis: CT demonstration. J Comput Assist Tomgr 11:1103, 1987.
35. Mevorach RA, Lerner RM, Dvoretsky PM, Rabinowitz R: Testicular abscess: Diagnosis by ultrasonography. J Urol 136:1213, 1986.
36. Fox CW Jr, Vaccaro JA, Kiesling VJ Jr, Belville WD: Seminal vesicle abscess: The use of computerized coaxial tomography for diagnosis and therapy. J Urol 139:384, 1988.
37. Rifkin MD: Ultrasound of the Prostate. New York, Raven Press, 1988.
38. Squadrito Jr, JF, Rifkin MD, Mulholland SG: Ureteral ectopia presenting as epididymitis and infertility. Urology 30:67, 1987.
39. Littrup PJ, Lee F, McLeary RD, et al: Transrectal US of the seminal vesicles and ejaculatory ducts: Clinical correlation. Radiology 168:625, 1988.

27

Genitourinary Manifestations of Gastrointestinal Disease

DENNIS M. BALFE ☐ JAMES G. BOVA

The genitourinary tract is developmentally separate from the gastrointestinal tract, except for a brief connection at the cloaca that normally disappears by the end of the seventh intrauterine week.[1] Therefore, in the adult, communications between the two systems are, with rare exception, acquired and are governed by anatomical rather than embryological considerations. In multiple anatomical regions, the urinary tract and portions of the gastrointestinal tract are contiguous or in close proximity. The importance of these anatomical relationships has been stressed repeatedly in more recent years, particularly by Meyers (Fig. 27–1).[2]

ANATOMICAL RELATIONSHIPS OF THE RIGHT KIDNEY

The right kidney is surrounded by an envelope of perinephric fat. Although its volume and distribution vary, most of this fat lies posterolateral to the kidney. Anteriorly, the kidney and perinephric fat are covered by the posterior parietal peritoneum and by anterior renal (Gerota's) fascia. Two communications are potentially present between the perinephric space and the anterior paranephric space (see Chapter 22, Fig. 22–1). The larger of these is in the area of the renal hilus, which is related anteriorly to the descending duodenum. The perinephric fat near the hilus is greatly thinned and may be absent,

diminishing the distance between the renal pelvis and the midportion of the descending duodenum; these structures lie even closer together in the case of an extrarenal pelvis. The second, smaller area of potential communication overlies the anterior portion of the lower pole and is due to the reflection of parietal peritoneum over the ascending colon.[2]

ANATOMICAL RELATIONSHIPS OF THE LEFT KIDNEY

The left kidney, like the right, has two surfaces that are related to mesenteric structures in the anterior paranephric space. An oblique nonperitonealized stripe crosses the medial portion of the upper pole and extends toward the lateral margin of the midpolar region. This thin area of kidney and the overlying perinephric fat are related to the lienorenal ligament, which contains the pancreatic tail and the short gastric vessels. Another thin horizontal nonperitonealized stripe represents the posterior insertion of the transverse mesocolon and is related to the lower pole of the left kidney. The confluence of these two surfaces occurs where the transverse colon mesentery fuses with the posterior body wall. This fusion, which marks the origin of the descending colon, is usually close to the anterolateral surface of the left kidney near the junction of the middle and lower thirds.[2]

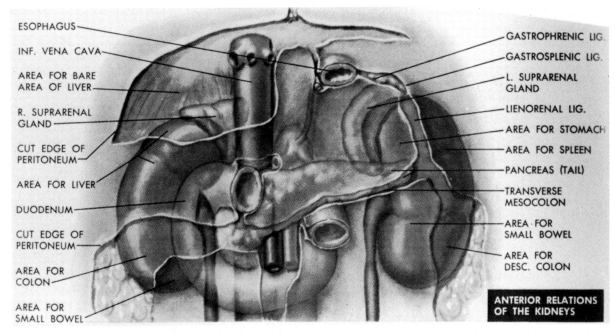

Figure 27–1. Anterior anatomical relationships of the kidneys. (Copyright 1973. CIBA-GEIGY Corporation. Reproduced with permission from the CIBA COLLECTION OF MEDICAL ILLUSTRATIONS by Frank H. Netter, MD. All rights reserved.)

URETERS

The *right ureter* exits the perinephric space and enters a fat-containing region on the anterolateral surface of the right psoas muscle. As the ureter descends, it crosses medial to the common iliac artery and vein at the pelvic inlet. As it enters the true pelvis, the ureter passes medial to the internal obturator muscle before eventually coursing anteriorly and medially to enter the posterior aspect of the urinary bladder. During the abdominal portion of its course, it is related to loops of distal ileum, the cecum, and the appendix, especially if the latter is retrocecal. Low-lying ileal loops accompany the right ureter into the pelvis, as does an occasional rightward-directed segment of the sigmoid colon. In the region of the ureterovesical junction, the retroperitoneal portion of the rectum may lie in close apposition to the ureters but is usually separated from it by perirectal fat.

Anatomically, the *left ureter* follows a course along the psoas, which is similar to that described for the right. The abdominal segment of the left ureter passes behind mesenteric loops of jejunum and proximal ileum. Its superior pelvic course is related to the proximal portion of the sigmoid colon at its junction with the descending colon.[3]

ANATOMICAL RELATIONSHIPS OF THE URINARY BLADDER IN MALES

In males, the posterior aspect of the bladder is separated from the rectum by a fold of peritoneum, the rectovesical pouch, or the pouch of Douglas. This peritoneal recess may contain pelvic loops of ileum and is a common site of abscesses that may arise from a lower abdominal or pelvic source. The dome and left lateral wall of the bladder are adjacent to the descending and sigmoid colons; the right lateral aspect of the bladder is related to peritonealized loops of ileum, and occasionally the cecum or appendix. The posterior aspect of the bladder base is retroperitoneal, and this portion of the bladder is separated from the rectum by the seminal vesicles and prostate.[3]

ANATOMICAL RELATIONSHIPS OF THE URINARY BLADDER IN FEMALES

In females, the peritoneal surface behind the superior aspect of the bladder covers the uterus, and laterally the fallopian tubes and the ovaries. More caudally, the extraperitoneal surface of the bladder base is separated from the rectum by the lower uterine segment and cervix, and laterally by the parametrial and paracervical tissues. The most caudal portion of the bladder is separated from the rectum by the vaginal canal.

ANATOMICAL SUMMARY

It is evident, based on the foregoing discussion, that the factor most influencing genitourinary tract involvement from primary gastrointestinal disease is the anatomical relationship of the gastrointestinal and genitourinary tracts. In rare cases, ectopic positioning of gastrointestinal or urinary structures (e.g., pelvic kidney) may lead to unusual sites of communication with the alimentary tract (Fig. 27–2).

The remainder of this chapter will describe specific gastrointestinal disease processes that can extend to involve the genitourinary system and induce secondary inflammatory changes.[4, 31]

CROHN'S DISEASE

Crohn's disease (granulomatous ileocolitis) is a chronic inflammatory disorder that may affect any portion of the gastrointestinal tract. Pathologically, ulcerations involving alimentary mucosa extend through the full thickness of the bowel wall, thus exposing adjacent structures to the granulomatous process. Because the genitourinary and gastrointestinal tract are neighbors, transmural Crohn's disease can secondarily affect the genitourinary system; estimates of the incidence of such involvement vary.[5–7, 31] In the report by Shield and coworkers of 233 patients with granulomatous ileitis, urological complications occurred in 54 (23%).[6]

Urinary tract complications of Crohn's disease may occur by either of two general mechanisms:[7, 31] (1) direct extension of an active inflammation or (2) production of a metabolic disorder that secondarily affects the urinary tract.

Direct Extension of Active Inflammatory Disease

Abscess

The chronic granulomatous process may produce a focal perforation of the bowel wall, leading to extraluminal soilage of the adjacent peritoneal or retroperitoneal spaces. If the purulent material enters the peritoneal space, it will tend to gravitate toward the most dependent portion of the peritoneal cavity—namely, the pouch of Douglas. Anteriorly, the peritoneal space surrounds the dome of the bladder, and localized collections of pus may therefore produce secondary inflammatory reaction in the bladder wall. This bullous change, which can be seen at cystoscopy, has been described by Melicow and coworkers as a "herald" lesion.[8, 9] Pathologically, this herald patch represents focal cystitis (Fig. 27–3). However, in contrast to the usual distribution of inflammatory cells in primary cystitides, the intensity of the inflammatory reaction increases in deeper layers of the bladder and is relatively low at the point closest to the transitional urothelium. Despite the fact that the origin of the inciting inflammatory process is gastrointestinal, patients often present with complaints related to their secondary cystitis.

Retroperitoneal abscesses may occur within the psoas compartment on either the right or the left side. Because Crohn's disease has a predilection for involving the terminal ileum, right-sided psoas abscesses predominate (Fig. 27–4). The right ureter courses along the psoas margin throughout most of its abdominal path; thus, it may be obstructed at any level. Most commonly, the site of obstruction is near the terminal ileum (at the pelvic brim).

Duodenal involvement with Crohn's disease may cause secondary inflammation of the anterior paranephric space; this space is anatomically close to the perinephric

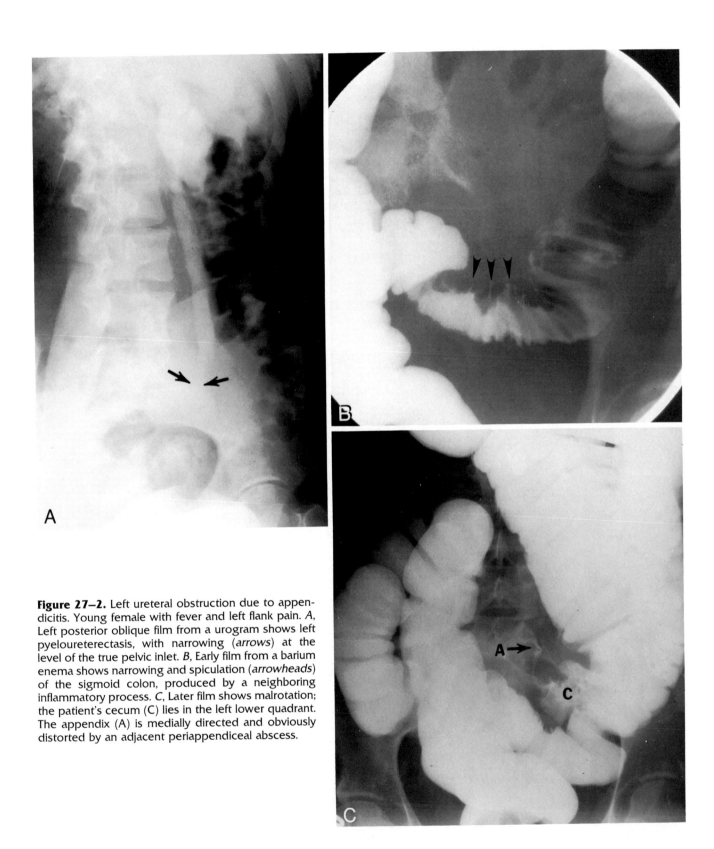

Figure 27–2. Left ureteral obstruction due to appendicitis. Young female with fever and left flank pain. *A,* Left posterior oblique film from a urogram shows left pyeloureterectasis, with narrowing (*arrows*) at the level of the true pelvic inlet. *B,* Early film from a barium enema shows narrowing and spiculation (*arrowheads*) of the sigmoid colon, produced by a neighboring inflammatory process. *C,* Later film shows malrotation; the patient's cecum (C) lies in the left lower quadrant. The appendix (A) is medially directed and obviously distorted by an adjacent periappendiceal abscess.

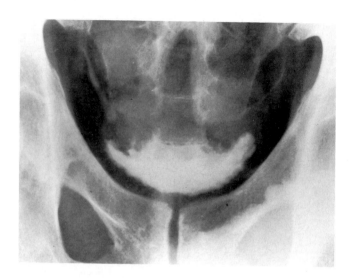

Figure 27–3. Crohn's disease involving the urinary bladder. A 22-year-old college student presented with symptoms of urgency, frequency, and dysuria. The intravenous urogram reveals marked bullous edema of the entire superior surface of the urinary bladder, attributable to a peri-ileal abscess complicating Crohn's disease. The patient later went on to develop an ileovesical fistula.

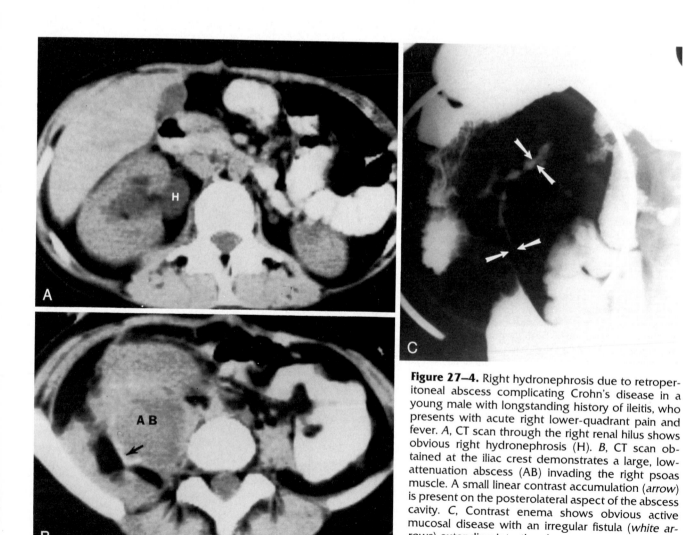

Figure 27–4. Right hydronephrosis due to retroperitoneal abscess complicating Crohn's disease in a young male with longstanding history of ileitis, who presents with acute right lower-quadrant pain and fever. *A,* CT scan through the right renal hilus shows obvious right hydronephrosis (H). *B,* CT scan obtained at the iliac crest demonstrates a large, low-attenuation abscess (AB) invading the right psoas muscle. A small linear contrast accumulation (*arrow*) is present on the posterolateral aspect of the abscess cavity. *C,* Contrast enema shows obvious active mucosal disease with an irregular fistula (*white arrows*) extending into the abscess.

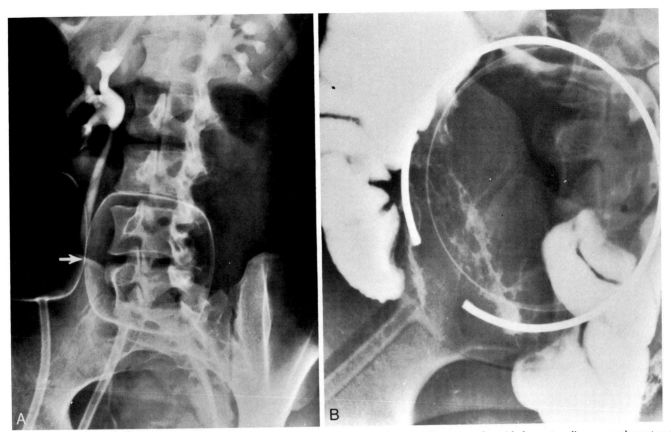

Figure 27–5. Crohn's disease producing right hydronephrosis *without* abscess. Young male with longstanding granulomatous enteritis and no urinary symptoms. *A*, Right posterior oblique film from a urogram shows slight narrowing (*arrow*) of the right midureter, with minimal dilatation of the proximal system. *B*, Film from a small-bowel contrast examination shows marked irregularity of the entire distal ileum, without sinus tract formation. It is postulated that chronic retroperitoneal inflammation produces a fibrotic response that results in the right ureteral narrowing. (Case courtesy Armed Forces Institute of Pathology.)

spaces; thus, a perinephric abscess may result from primary duodenal disease. Because a long segment of duodenum lies close to the right kidney, the right perinephric space is the most commonly affected.

Retroperitoneal Fibrosis

Ureteral obstruction may occur from inflammatory retroperitoneal fibrosis in the absence of frank infection. This phenomenon has been reported frequently in patients with Crohn's disease, and it occurs almost exclusively in the right ureter at the pelvic brim (Fig. 27–5). In one report,[10] 10 of 150 patients who were studied for Crohn's disease had obstructive uropathy in this specific anatomical distribution. Such patients complain of chronic dull right flank pain; urography may demonstrate right hydronephrosis with smooth tapering of the affected ureter at the pelvic brim.

Fistulas

One of the most serious complications of Crohn's disease is the formation of fistulous tracts between the inflamed bowel and its adjacent organs or spaces. Enterovesical fistulas are the most common, with an incidence in one series of 3.9%.[6] Usually, the distal ileum is the involved segment of bowel; however, in patients with Crohn's colitis, the sigmoid colon may also contribute to enterovesical fistulas. Barium studies of the gastrointestinal tract are generally not helpful in demonstrating the

fistulas; cystoscopy allows inspection of the mucosa for focal inflammatory disease but may not demonstrate the fistulous opening. Enteroclysis (or small-bowel enema) is probably the most sensitive radiographic means of demonstrating small fistulous communications arising from the small intestine in patients with granulomatous ileitis. Although ultrasonography cannot reliably demonstrate small enterovesical fistulas, it can be helpful in detecting the relationships of inflammatory bowel masses to the urinary bladder and in depicting the bladder-wall involvement.[40] CT is a sensitive and important method of evaluating the bladder and can be used to identify patients in the prodromal stage who are at risk of developing enterovesical fistulae.[41]

Rectovaginal or ileovaginal fistulas are common in patients with Crohn's disease. These individuals present with chronic vaginal discharge. Rectovaginal fistulas are easily demonstrated by contrast enemas (Fig. 27–6), but demonstrating an ileovaginal fistula by any radiographic means may be difficult. Rectovesical and rectourethral fistulas are also encountered in granulomatous disease of the colon.[32]

Metabolic Processes Secondarily Affecting the Genitourinary Tract

Calculi

The incidence of this common complication has been reported to be as high as 9% in patients without ileosto-

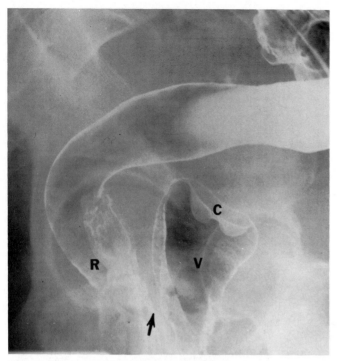

Figure 27–6. Crohn's disease: rectovaginal fistula in a young woman with a feculent vaginal discharge. Air-contrast enema demonstrates narrowing and irregularity of the anterior rectum (R). A fistula (*arrow*) arising near the anorectal junction connects to the vagina (V), allowing it to be coated with barium. (C = uterine cervix.)

mies and up to 18% in those with ileostomies.[11] The stones are most frequently composed of uric acid and calcium oxalate. Although the latter composition predominates, the incidence of uric acid stones is higher in patients with Crohn's disease, especially after ileostomy, than in the general population. The occurrence of nephrolithiasis is roughly proportional to the amount of distal small-bowel involvement or resection and degree of malabsorption.[12]

Urinary tract calculi in patients with Crohn's disease is a consequence of two mechanisms:[6] (1) Dehydration, acid urine, and excess urate excretion promote the formation of uric acid stones in ileostomy patients. (2) Calcium oxalate stones occur because patients with active enteritis malabsorb fat. Free intraluminal fatty acids are available to form complexes with calcium ions. As a result, fewer calcium ions are available to combine with oxalate to form insoluble calcium oxalate crystals. The end result is excessive absorption of dietary oxalate, hyperoxaluria, and subsequent precipitation of calcium oxalate crystals in the urine.[6]

Amyloidosis

Any chronic disease can eventually lead to amyloidosis, in which abnormal immunoglobulin products are deposited within endothelial submucosa; these deposits resemble starch in regard to their histological staining properties, giving rise to the term *amyloid*. Such deposition may occur within the skin, gastrointestinal tract, or rarely in the genitourinary tract.[7] The radiographic findings are no different from those observed in secondary amyloidosis of any cause.

Glomerulitis

Mild, histologically nonspecific glomerular inflammation without clinical manifestations has been reported in association with Crohn's disease. Degeneration of the proximal convoluted tubule has been described in both Crohn's disease and chronic ulcerative colitis.[7]

Aside from Crohn's disease, the small bowel is a rare source of urinary bladder disease. Small bowel neoplasms may invade the bladder. Both adenocarcinoma and leiomyosarcoma have been associated with ileovesical fistulae. Meckel's diverticulum may involve the bladder producing bullous edema or even a fistula. Stones in a Meckels' diverticulum may be mistaken for bladder or ureteral calculi.

DIVERTICULITIS

Diverticulitis is an acute inflammatory disorder of the colon, resulting from the perforation of an obstructed colonic diverticula and pericolonic abscess formation. Because the most common location for diverticula is in the sigmoid colon, two urinary structures are most likely to be affected by the process: (1) the left lateral and superior portion of the dome of the urinary bladder and (2) the left distal ureter. In the series of Hafner and coworkers,[13] studying 500 patients with diverticulitis, 178 (35.6%) had genitourinary symptoms, 104 of whom had symptoms definitely related to the diverticular process; eight of these patients had symptoms referable only to the genitourinary tract, despite the gastrointestinal origin of their disease. Frequency, nocturia, and dysuria were the most commonly reported complaints. Symptoms suggestive or diagnostic of a fistulous complication of diverticulitis were less common, but they included pneumaturia and feculent vaginal discharge. Bladder involvement is more common in males, presumably because of the protective effect of the uterus in the female.

The diagnosis of genitourinary complications of diverticulitis may be difficult. Intravesical gas may be present on an erect abdominal radiograph. Cystography rarely demonstrates a fistulous communication; more frequently, a raised irregular patch on the left lateral portion of the bladder dome is the only finding.[9] Contrast colon examination occasionally shows extraluminal accumulation of contrast material within the abscess or fistula. Often, the rectally administered contrast is not clearly shown to enter the bladder (Fig. 27–7), even when clinical symptoms are highly suggestive of a fistulous communication. In such instances, concentrated urinary sediment may show barium sulfate crystals on in vitro radiography—the so-called Bourne test—confirming the diagnosis.[14] Suspicious-looking areas at cystoscopy may be probed with a small ureteral catheter, and contrast material may be injected.

Radiographic diagnosis of a vesicoenteric fistula is probably best accomplished using computed tomography (CT). Scans obtained by means of alimentary contrast, but in the absence of intravenous contrast, are the most sensitive; CT findings include demonstration of extraluminal (including intravesical) gas or barium, focal bladder-wall thickening, and adherence of perivesical bowel loops (Fig. 27–8). At least one of these was found in all 20 patients studied by Goldman and associates.[15] CT may

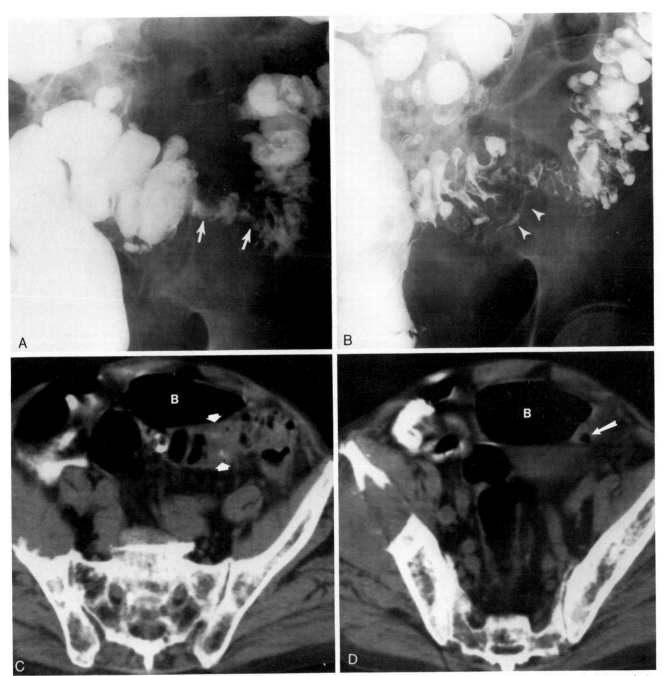

Figure 27–7. Diverticulitis producing colovesical fistula. *A*, Filled film of the colon obtained during contrast enema shows obvious segmental narrowing (*arrows*) of the horizontal portion of the sigmoid. *B*, On the postevacuation film, a sinus track (*arrowheads*) exits the inferior surface of the sigmoid and courses medially. Apparently, no contrast enters the bladder. *C*, CT section through the sigmoid shows diffuse thickening (*white arrows*) of its transverse segment. The gas-filled bladder dome (B) is anatomically contiguous with the sigmoid. *D*, Two centimeters lower than in *C*, a sinus track (*arrow*) adjacent to the thick-walled bladder (B) extends from the area of diverticulitis and accounts for the intravesical gas.

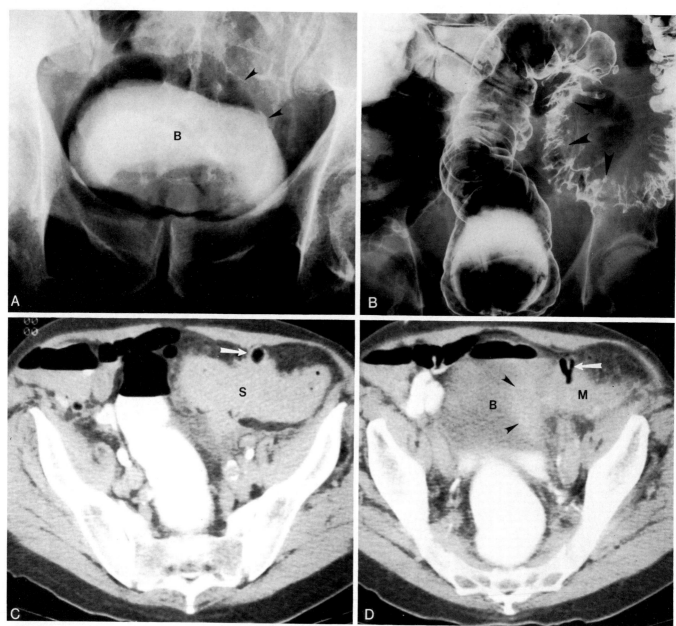

Figure 27–8. Colovesical fistula secondary to sigmoid diverticulitis in a patient with symptoms of urinary tract infection and pneumaturia. *A,* Film from a urogram shows gas distending the urinary bladder (B), which contains contrast as well. Slight flattening (*arrowheads*) of the left superior bladder dome is seen. *B,* Film from an air-contrast enema demonstrates irregular narrowing (*arrowheads*) of the sigmoid without abscess or fistula. *C,* CT scan demonstrates thickening of the transverse segment of the sigmoid colon (S). Gas is present in a sinus track (*white arrow*) on its anterior surface. *D,* Two centimeters caudal to view in C, the sinus track (*white arrow*), accompanied by a soft-tissue mass (M) courses adjacent to the bladder (B). Focal thickening of the left bladder wall (*arrowheads*) is seen. Note gas-fluid level within the bladder lumen.

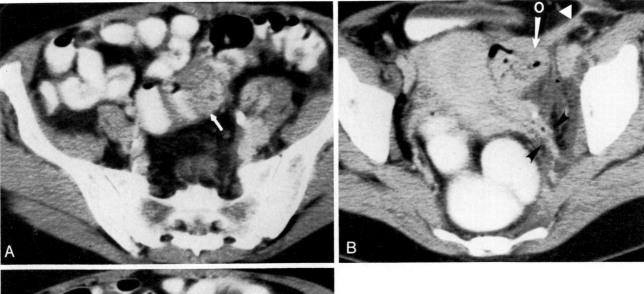

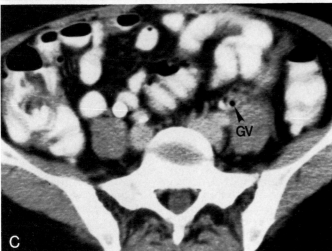

Figure 27–9. Diverticulitis producing tubo-ovarian abscess. Middle-aged woman with left lower-quadrant pain and fever. Gynecological examination detected a tender left adnexal mass. *A,* CT section through transverse segment of the sigmoid colon shows luminal narrowing due to thickening of the wall (*arrow*). *B,* Four centimeters caudal to *A,* a gas-containing mass appears in the region of the left ovary (O), extending anteriorly along the round ligament (*white arrowhead*) and posteriorly along the recto-uterine fold (*black arrowheads*). *C,* Two centimeters cephalad to *A,* gas is seen within the left ovarian (gonadal) vein (GV), coursing just lateral to the left ureter.

also be useful in documenting genital inflammations that are due to diverticulitis (Fig. 27–9). Carcinomas of the rectum and sigmoid colon may invade the urinary bladder, mimicking a primary urothelial neoplasm. A diagnosis of adenocarcinoma of the urinary bladder should always prompt a search for an adjacent malignancy.

PANCREATITIS AND PANCREATIC CANCER

The pancreas lies in the anterior paranephric space. Its body and tail cross anterior to the left perinephric space; the splenic vessels course particularly close to the left adrenal gland. Normally, no portion of the pancreatic head extends to the right far enough to anatomically contact the right kidney. However, the fascial boundaries of the anterior paranephric space, into which pancreatic effusions extend, lie close to the anterior margin of the upper right renal pole. Furthermore, inflammatory processes extending posteriorly from the pancreatic head will contact the right renal vein, producing secondary renal effects. Pancreatic effusions primarily affect the left kidney. Fluid in the left paranephric space can produce a dramatic appearance when it contrasts with the lucent perinephric fat, resulting in the so-called halo sign (Fig. 27–10).[36]

Pancreatic effusions or pseudocysts are capable of producing perinephric or (if they are extensive) intrinsic renal disease (Fig. 27–11).[16, 17] Pancreatic pseudocysts may extend posteriorly in the retroperitoneum to displace, or otherwise involve, the kidney and/or perinephric space (Fig. 27–12).[37] The left kidney or its fascia may form the floor of the pseudocyst owing to pressure necrosis on, and enzymatic digestion of, renal and perinephric tissues. Pseudocysts may actually invade the renal parenchyma, thereby mimicking an upper-pole renal mass or a perinephric abscess with inferior renal displacement, renal deformity, or extrinsic pressure on the renal artery or vein.[37] A pseudocyst may also extend far beyond the renal bed, displacing or obstructing either ureter (Fig. 27–12). Often, thickening of the renal fascia can be identified, especially by CT.[38] Because pseudocysts may occur in the retroperitoneum far from their pancreatic origin, it is possible for ureteral or even bladder involvement to complicate extensive pancreatitis. (See Chapter 94, Pelvic Lipomatosis.)

Radiological findings vary, depending on the form of the pathological extension. Pancreatitis usually produces widespread infiltration of the anterior paranephric space (Fig. 27–13); this may be a helpful clue to the nature of a cystic renal mass.[39] Pseudocysts may displace the left kidney, and the distance of displacement is variable. If a

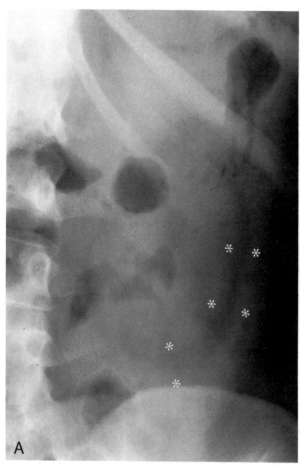

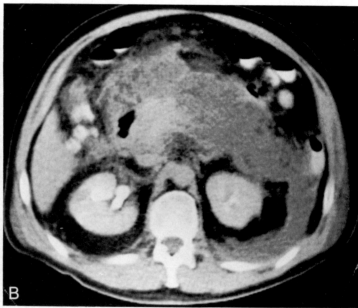

Figure 27–10. Halo sign of acute pancreatitis. *A*, A plain abdominal radiograph demonstrates marked radiolucency outlining the left kidney ("halo effect") (*asterisks*). *B*, A CT examination (patient different from one in *A*) in acute pancreatitis demonstrates an extensive pancreatic effusion dissecting posteriorly to involve the anterior and posterior paranephric spaces on the left. The sharp contrast in the densities of the paranephric and perinephric fat explain the halo effect.

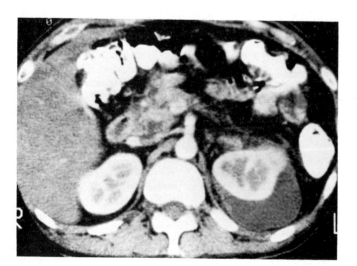

Figure 27–11. Pancreatic pseudocyst invading the perinephric space in a young male with a history of alcoholism and chronic pancreatitis. CT examination reveals a left perinephric fluid collection that originated in the pancreas. This pancreatic pseudocyst had digested its way through Gerota's fascia and insinuated itself directly into the perinephric space. Some pancreatic pseudocysts have been known to digest renal tissue, presumably owing to action of the pancreatic enzymes. (From Master's Film Interpretation Panel: 72nd Scientific Assembly and Annual Meeting, Radiological Society of North America, 1986. RadioGraphics 7:465, 1987.)

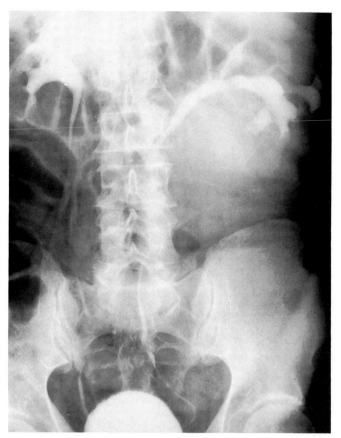

Figure 27–12. Pancreatic pseudocyst displacing left kidney. Excretory urography demonstrates a large abdominal mass displacing the left kidney inferiorly and laterally. The pseudocyst dissects below the kidney, resulting in medial displacement of most of the left ureter.

OTHER PROCESSES PRODUCING ABSCESSES OR FISTULAS

Abscess

Abscesses that arise within or extend into the peritoneal cavity follow well-defined pathways. The most dependent portion of the peritoneal space in a supine individual is the rectovesical pouch (or pouch of Douglas). Fluid collections tend to collect in several "saddle points" (regionally dependent areas)—these include the sigmoid mesentery, the midportion of the transverse mesocolon, and the insertion of the small bowel mesentery near the ileocecal valve.[20] Collections in the sigmoid mesentery may produce secondary effects on the bladder dome, whereas those near the ileocecal valve may cause irritative urinary symptoms owing to their proximity to the right ureter.

Retroperitoneal abscesses are less likely to extend far from their site of origin; they may be expected to arise from a segment of bowel anatomically adjacent to the involved portion of the genitourinary tract. The best-known example of this is retrocecal appendicitis, which may actually lie on the ureter, producing ureterectasis (Fig. 27–15). Symptomatically, appendicitis may mimic renal colic with flank pain and hematuria, especially if an appendicolith is seen. Appendiceal abscess may cause hydronephrosis, a defect on the urinary bladder, or an appendicovesical fistula.

Peritoneal abscesses may arise from perforated appendicitis, colonic carcinoma, or any spontaneous perforation of a viscus (Fig. 27–16). Many peritoneal abscesses that extend to involve the bladder have postoperative or post-traumatic origins, and they probably reflect secondarily infected hematomas.

pancreatic pseudocyst is being considered in the differential diagnosis of a thick-walled cystic renal mass, percutaneous puncture should successfully retrieve fluid for an analysis of the pancreatic enzyme content.

Carcinomas of the pancreas may extend directly into the left kidney from a primary source in the tail, or they may infiltrate the retroperitoneum diffusely from any site, secondarily invading either kidney (see Fig. 27–14).[18, 19]

Patients with primary pancreatic carcinoma generally have systemic signs of their disease: weight loss, celiac ganglion pain syndrome, and jaundice are common symptoms. Radiographic identification of the primary pancreatic mass is most easily accomplished with CT (Fig. 27–14).

Pancreatic tail carcinoma may displace the left kidney inferiorly or laterally, may grow directly into the kidney (usually into the left upper pole, simulating a primary renal mass), or may compress the renal artery and/or renal vein, thereby causing the findings typical of renal vein occlusion (Fig. 27–14). Venous notching of the renal pelvis or proximal ureter may call attention to the primary pancreatic disease. Occasionally, a left varicocele may result and bring the patient to medical attention. Ureteral obstruction, especially at the pelvic brim, suggests a malignant retroperitoneal fibrosis caused by the pancreatic carcinoma. Malignancy of the head and body of the pancreas rarely affects the urinary tract.

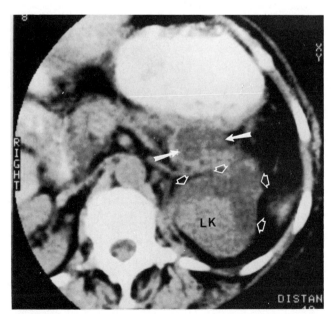

Figure 27–13. Pancreatitis presents as a left renal abnormality in a young man with left flank pain. CT scan shows a large effusion (*arrows*) in the pancreatic tail. A similar collection (*open arrows*) is observed adjacent to the left renal margin. Both fluid collections were due to pancreatitis. (LK = left kidney.) (Case courtesy Gaston Morillo, M.D., Miami, Florida.)

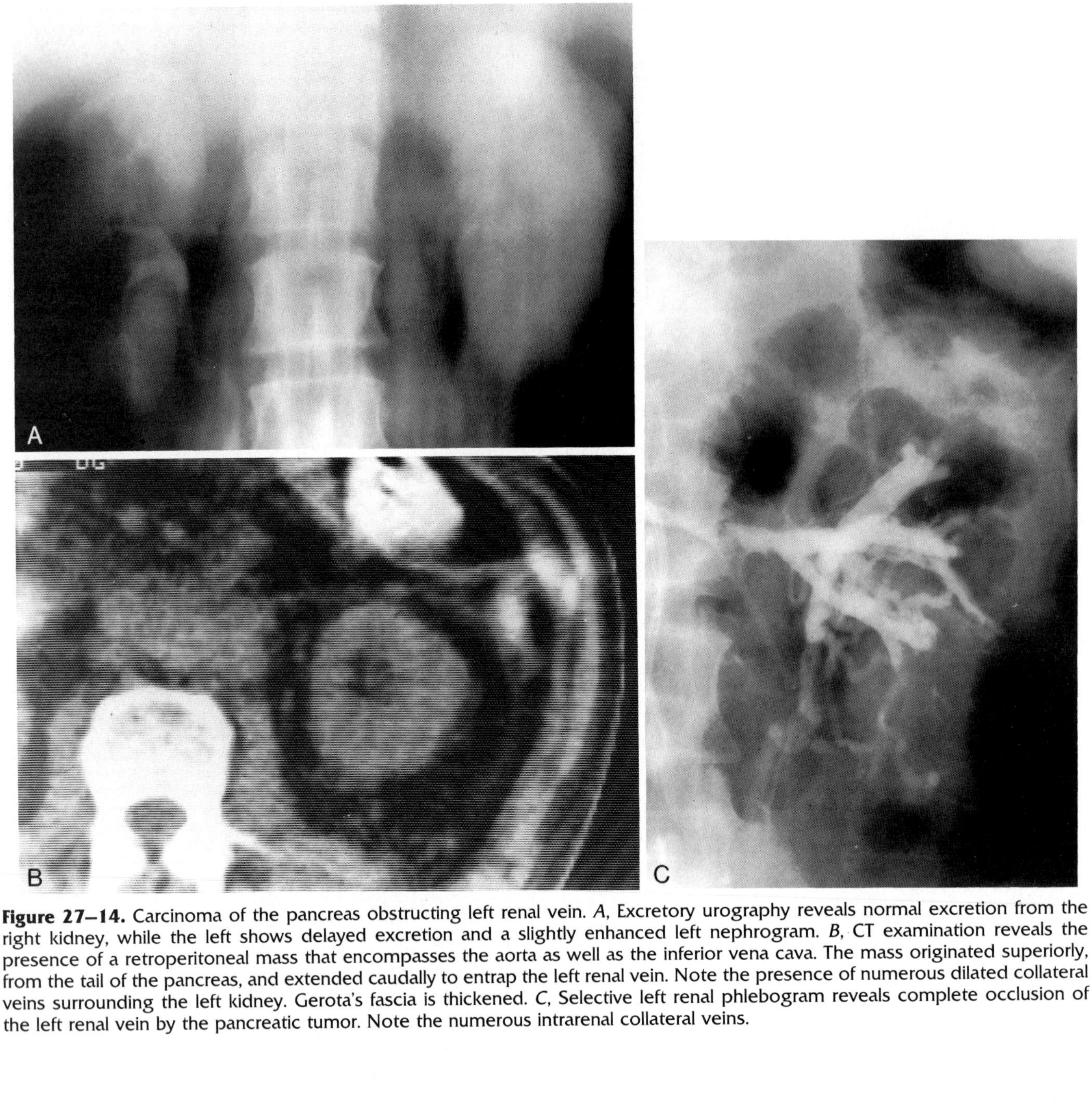

Figure 27–14. Carcinoma of the pancreas obstructing left renal vein. *A,* Excretory urography reveals normal excretion from the right kidney, while the left shows delayed excretion and a slightly enhanced left nephrogram. *B,* CT examination reveals the presence of a retroperitoneal mass that encompasses the aorta as well as the inferior vena cava. The mass originated superiorly, from the tail of the pancreas, and extended caudally to entrap the left renal vein. Note the presence of numerous dilated collateral veins surrounding the left kidney. Gerota's fascia is thickened. *C,* Selective left renal phlebogram reveals complete occlusion of the left renal vein by the pancreatic tumor. Note the numerous intrarenal collateral veins.

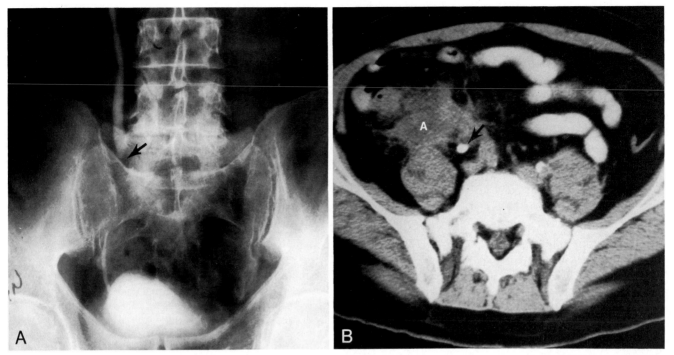

Figure 27–15. Retrocecal appendicitis producing right ureteral obstruction in a middle-aged man with right flank pain and fever, but no gastrointestinal symptoms. *A,* Urogram shows right ureterectasis with focal narrowing (*arrow*) at the level of the sacrum. *B,* CT section shows the dilated ureter (*arrow*) immediately posterior to a large abscess (A). Retrocecal appendicitis was surgically proved.

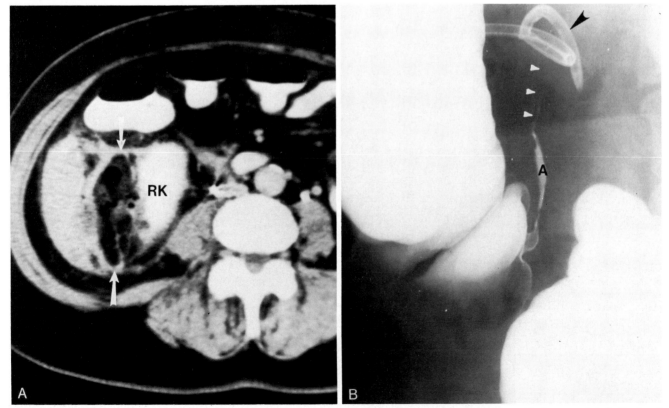

Figure 27–16. Right perinephric abscess caused by appendicitis in a middle-aged diabetic woman with fever and right flank pain. *A,* CT section through inferior pole of the right kidney (RK) shows a large gas-containing collection (*arrows*) within the perinephric space. *B,* Contrast enema obtained after percutaneous catheter drainage of the abscess shows filling of the appendix (A) and subsequent leakage of contrast material into a sinus track (*white arrowheads*) in the direction of the catheter (*arrowhead*). Appendiceal abscess with extension to the perinephric space was surgically confirmed.

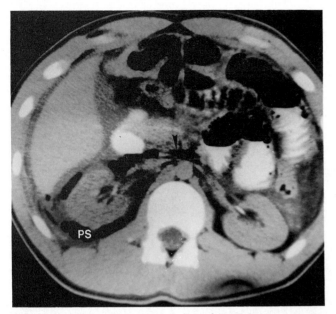

Figure 27–17. Traumatic perinephric abscess in a young man with recent severe blunt trauma. CT section at the level of the renal hila shows gas and fluid within the right perinephric space (PS). Some gas (*arrowhead*) has dissected along the renal vessels into the space anterior to the aorta. Traumatic rupture of the ascending colon was surgically proved.

Retroperitoneal abscesses may also stem from penetrating trauma (Fig. 27–17), inflammatory bowel disease, duodenal ulcer with penetration (Fig. 27–18), or perforating colonic carcinoma (Fig. 27–19).

Fistula (See also Chapter 101)

Nephrointestinal fistulas are uncommon.[21, 22] Several nephroduodenal fistulas have been described; all but one have arisen between the right renal pelvis and the first or second portion of the duodenum.[23, 24] Primary chronic renal inflammatory disease is the usual cause, but large pelvic calculi may erode directly into the duodenum.[34] Peptic ulcer disease with posterior penetration, penetrating trauma, or foreign bodies, may produce the same connection (Fig. 27–18).

Nephrocolic fistulas are the most common kidney–intestinal communication. In these cases, primary renal inflammation is also the most likely cause.[21] Fistulas between the stomach and the kidney or ureter have also been described.[35]

Ureterointestinal fistulas may occur in Crohn's disease, in colonic carcinoma, or after surgical resection of the intestinal tract, particularly after irradiation of the operative field.

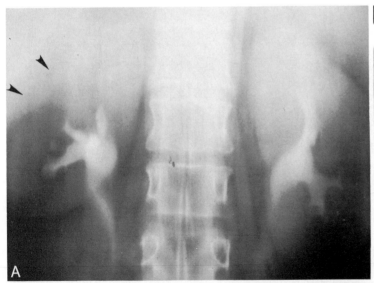

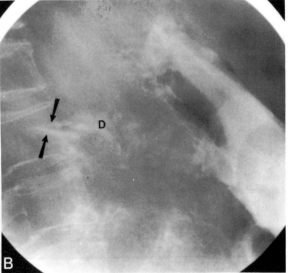

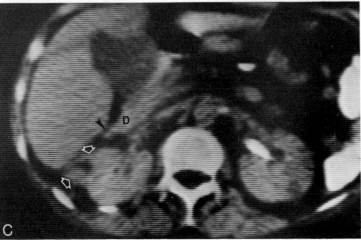

Figure 27–18. Duodenal ulcer perforating into right perinephric space in a middle-aged woman with fever and right flank pain. *A*, Tomogram obtained during urography shows mottled gas collection adjacent to the right upper pole (*arrowheads*). *B*, Water-soluble contrast examination shows angulation of the proximal segment of the descending duodenum (D) (*arrows*). No extravasation is evident. *C*, CT section shows thin line of contrast material (*arrowhead*) extending from duodenum (D) into perinephric space collection (*open arrows*). Endoscopic examination confirmed a small perforating ulcer in the postbulbar duodenum.

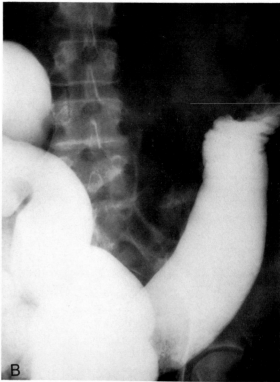

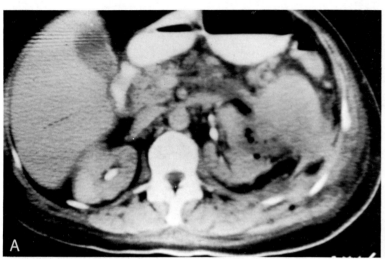

Figure 27–19. Paranephric abscess secondary to perforating carcinoma of the colon. *A,* CT examination reveals a large inflammatory mass involving the left perinephric and paranephric spaces and seemingly extending within the renal parenchyma. The kidney is displaced medially, and numerous gas bubbles can be seen at the interface between the kidney and the mass. There are thickening of the retrofascial structures dorsal to the kidney, edema of the abdominal wall musculature, and evidence of gas forming infection in the lumbodorsal area of the abdominal wall. *B,* Barium enema examination reveals complete obstruction in the descending colon, attributable to an adenocarcinoma. The malignancy had caused a retroperitoneal perforation of the colon with extension into the left anterior paranephric space. From there the abscess eroded through Gerota's fascia into the perinephric space to involve the kidney as well as the posterior abdominal wall structures.

Vesicointestinal fistulas frequently arise from inflammatory masses in the rectovesical space, or from the proximity of the appendix to the right anterior dome of the bladder.

The urethra may rarely receive a fistula from the ileum in patients who have undergone cystectomy,[25] or from the rectum in patients with Crohn's disease. Most urethral fistulas connect to the rectum and may be traumatic or postsurgical in origin.[26]

INFILTRATING TUMORS

Many abdominal neoplasms undergo dissemination in the subperitoneal retroperitoneum.[27] Diffusely infiltrating tumors typically extend along ligaments or fascial planes as sheets of neoplastic cells. Such spread can cause urinary tract obstruction at sites anatomically quite distant from the primary source. Scirrhous cancers of the colon (Fig. 27–21),[28] stomach, or duodenum (Fig. 27–20) and poorly differentiated tumors of the pancreas are the gastrointestinal sources likely to produce urinary obstruction. Stein and Kendall state that the stomach is the second most frequent primary site (ranking behind melanoma) of all metastatic tumors in the urinary bladder.[33]

UNCOMMON ENTITIES

Gastrointestinal tuberculosis is no longer common in the United States. Tuberculous bowel involvement creates caseous inflammatory masses that cause a predisposition to fistulas to the adjacent bladder or ureter. From a radiographic standpoint, the urinary tract diseases stemming from intestinal tuberculosis are similar to those produced by Crohn's disease.

Either of the kidneys may be seeded with *Echinococcus granulosus* via a primary cyst in the liver or spleen. Rupture of the cyst into the peritoneal space may lead to infestation of organs adjacent to the pouch of Douglas: the seminal vesicles, prostate, and vas deferens in males; or the ovaries, fallopian tubes, and uterus in females.[29, 30]

BILIARY TRACT

Gallbladder enlargement may occasionally displace the right kidney. Adenocarcinoma of the gallbladder may deviate and obstruct the ureters as a result of either malignant retroperitoneal fibrosis or metastatic adenopathy in the porta hepatis, which may be contiguous with

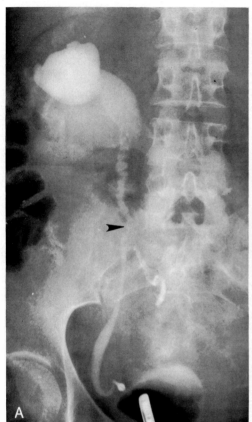

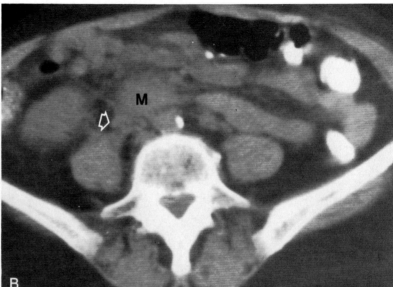

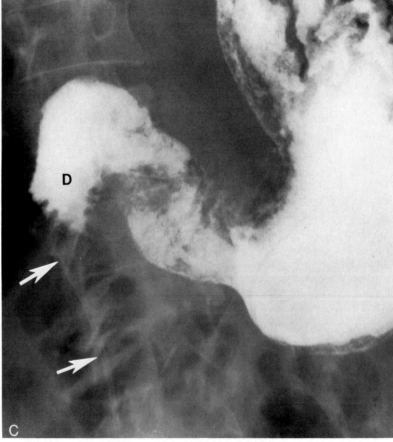

Figure 27–20. Invasive duodenal carcinoma producing obstructive uropathy in a middle-aged woman with right flank pain and early satiety. *A,* Retrograde pyeloureterogram demonstrates segmental ureteral narrowing (*arrowhead*) at the level of L5 to S1. *B,* CT scan shows the right ureter (*open arrow*) adjacent to large infiltrating tumor mass (M). *C,* Barium examination (performed after right ureteral stent was placed) shows high-grade obstruction of the descending duodenum (D) near the course of the right ureteral stent (*arrows*). Surgery confirmed invasive duodenal adenocarcinoma.

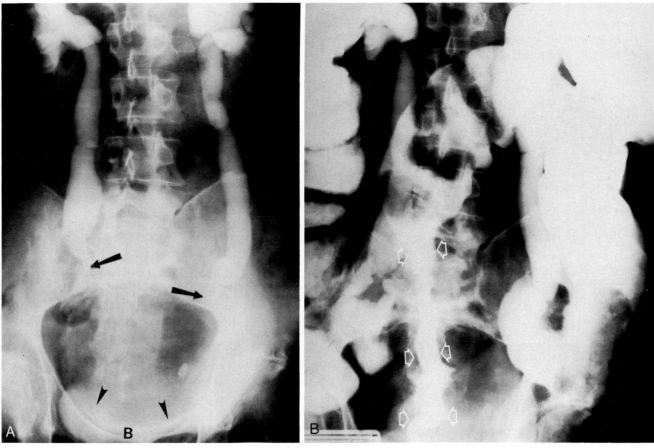

Figure 27–21. Bilateral ureteral obstruction due to scirrhous carcinoma of the rectum. *A,* Anteroposterior (AP) film from intravenous urogram shows dilatation of the ureters with bilateral narrowings at the level of the pelvic brim (*arrows*). Inferior displacement (*arrowheads*) of the bladder dome (B) is shown. *B,* AP film from a barium enema performed the same day shows marked irregularity and narrowing of the rectal contour (*open arrows*). At surgical exploration, a scirrhous carcinoma, 25 cm in diameter and arising from the rectum, had extended along peritoneal surfaces to obstruct the ureters.

the right renal pelvis and the proximal ureter. Rarely, gallbladder calculi mimic renal calculi.

LIVER

Masses in the posterior portion of the liver may compress and displace the right kidney. Thus, metastases to the liver may suggest the presence of a not-yet-appreciated primary genitourinary malignancy, such as a renal neoplasm. Cysts of the liver may accompany polycystic kidney disease, and at times they may be much more apparent than their renal counterparts. Hepatic fibrosis may accompany infantile polycystic disease and some of the more severe cases of tubular ectasia. A congenitally enlarged caudate lobe, or one enlarged because of a mass, can inferiorly displace the right kidney. Cranial retraction of the right kidney is occasionally seen in patients with hepatic atrophy secondary to cirrhosis.

SPLEEN

Because it is primarily an intraperitoneal structure, the enlarged spleen usually does not cause renal displace-

ment. Exceptions do occur, however, with a resultant displacement (usually caudal) of the left kidney (Fig. 27–22).

CONGENITAL LESIONS

Imperforate Anus

Approximately 50% of children with an imperforate anus or anorectal atresia have associated genitourinary anomalies. The incidence of genitourinary malformations is approximately 3.5 times greater for anorectal anomalies of the high (supralevator) type than for those of the low (infralevator) type. In the former type, agenesis of one kidney is the most common single anomaly, others being renal fusion anomalies, duplication anomalies, and polycystic kidneys. Vesicoureteral reflux has been noted in many cases. It is usually pronounced and is particularly common in females and in infants with urinary tract infections. Dilated ureters with no reflux may be seen, attributable to ureteral compression by the dilated distal colonic segment. In approximately 10% of patients with an imperforate anus, a neurogenic bladder is found. Congenital malformation of the sacrum with associated

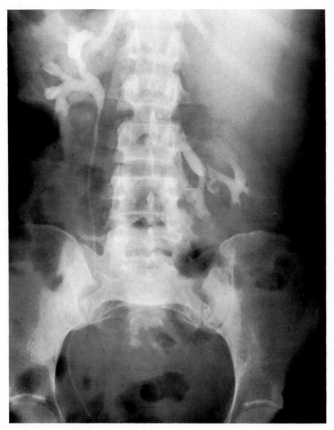

Figure 27–22. Displacement of the left kidney, secondary to splenomegaly. An intravenous urogram demonstrates marked caudal displacement of the left kidney, attributable to a markedly enlarged spleen. The patient had malaria.

spinal cord abnormalities may be the primary cause; however, excessively vigorous perineal dissection at the time of rectal pull-through, with secondary bladder denervation, may also be a factor.

Fistulas between the blind rectal pouch and the bladder neck or prostatic urethra exist in more than half of male patients with the supralevator type of imperforate anus. The diagnosis is confirmed by the appearance of gas in the urinary bladder on an erect film. However, a voiding cystourethrogram is necessary to establish the anatomical features of the fistula. In females, fistulous communication between the rectum and vagina may be present. After surgery, a remnant of the tract may persist. If this is large enough, it can simulate a urethral diverticulum.

Hirschsprung's Disease

Massive fecal impactions, especially in children, may deviate the ureters laterally and even cause partial obstruction of the ureters at the ureteral, ureterovesical, or urethral levels. Although this deviation may be seen with fecal impaction from any cause, it is especially likely to occur with Hirschsprung's disease.

MISCELLANEOUS

Displacement of the distal ureters into the scrotum and groin has been seen in patients with a large sliding inguinal or femoral hernia.

References

1. Moore KL: The Developing Human, 3rd Ed. Philadelphia, WB Saunders Company, 1982, pp 249, 256–260.
2. Meyers M: Dynamic Radiology of the Abdomen, 2nd Ed. New York, Springer-Verlag, 1982, pp 186–222.
3. Eycleshymer AC, Schoemaker DM: A Cross-Section Anatomy. New York, D Appleton & Company, 1922, pp 151–191, 211–219.
4. Demos TC, Moncada R: Inflammatory gastrointestinal disease presenting as genitourinary disease. Urology 13:115–121, 1979.
5. McManamon P, Reddy R, MacLaughlin E: Urological complications in Crohn's disease. J L'Assoc Can Radiol 36:230–233, 1985.
6. Shield DE, Lytton B, Weiss RM, Schiff M Jr: Urologic complications of inflammatory bowel disease. J Urol 115:701–706, 1976.
7. Bagby RJ, Clements JL Jr, Patrick JW, et al: Genitourinary complications of granulomatous bowel disease. AJR 117:297, 1973.
8. Melicow MM, Uson AC: The "Herald" lesion of the bladder: A lesion which portends the approach of cancer or inflammation from outside the bladder. J Urol 85:543, 1961.
9. Melicow MM, Uson AC, Stams U: Herald lesion of urinary bladder: A nonspecific but significant pathologic process. Urology 3:140, 1974.
10. Present DH, Rabinowitz JG, Banks PA: Obstructive hydronephrosis: Frequent but seldom recognized complication of granulomatous disease of the bowel. N Engl J Med 280:523, 1969.
11. Gelzayd EA, Breuer RI, Kirsner JB: Nephrolithiasis in inflammatory bowel disease. Am J Dig Dis 13:1027, 1968.
12. Deren JJ, Pouish JG, Levitt MF, Khilnami MT: Nephrolithiasis as a complication of ulcerative colitis and regional enteritis. Ann Intern Med 56:843, 1962.
13. Hafner CD, Ponka JL, Brush BE: Genitourinary manifestations of diverticulitis of the colon: A study of 500 cases. JAMA 179:174, 1962.
14. Amendola MA, Agha FP, Dent TL, et al: Detection of occult colovesical fistula by the Bourne Test. AJR 142:715, 1984.
15. Goldman SM, Fishman EK, Gatewood OMB, et al: CT in the diagnosis of enterovesical fistulae. AJR 144:1229, 1985.
16. Lilienfeld RM, Lande A: Pancreatic pseudocysts presenting as thick-walled renal and perinephric cysts. J Urol 115:123, 1976.
17. Gorder JL, Stargardter FL: Pancreatic pseudocysts simulating intrarenal masses. AJR 107:65, 1969.
18. Marshall S, Lapp M, Schulte JW: Lesions of the pancreas mimicking renal disease. J Urol 93:41, 1965.
19. Guerrier K, Persky L: Pancreatic disease simulating renal abnormality. Am J Surg 120:46, 1970.
20. Meyers M: Dynamic Radiology of the Abdomen, 2nd Ed. New York, Springer-Verlag, 1982, pp 20–54.
21. Arthur GW, Morris DG: Reno-alimentary fistulae. Br J Surg 53:396, 1966.
22. Bissada NK, Cole AT, Fried FA: Reno-alimentary fistula: An unusual urological problem. J Urol 110:273, 1973.
23. Pickard LR, Tepas JJ III, Agarwal BL, Haller JA Jr: Duodeno-renal fistula: An uncommon complication of an ingested foreign body. J Pediatr Surg 15:337, 1980.
24. Rodney K, Maxted WC, Pahira JJ: Pyeloduodenal fistula. Urology 22:536, 1983.
25. Hertz M, Goldwasser B, Rubinstein ZJ, et al: Ileourethral fistula following cystectomy: A rare complication. Urol Radiol 6:187, 1984.
26. Wesolowski S, Bulinski W: Vesico-intestinal fistulae and recto-urethral fistulae. Br J Urol 45:34, 1973.
27. Oliphant M, Berne AS, Meyers MA: Subperitoneal spread of intra-abdominal disease. In Meyers M (ed): Computed Tomography of the Gastrointestinal Tract. New York, Springer-Verlag, 1986, pp 95–137.
28. Greenfield SM, Seedor JW, Nack SL, Sohn M: Obstructive uropathy: An unusual presentation of primary linitis plastica of the colon. Dig Dis Sci 30:689, 1985.
29. Kirkland K: Urological aspects of hydatid disease. Br J Urol 38:241, 1966.
30. Birkhof J, McClennan BL: Echinococcus cyst of the pelvis—urologic complications and treatment. J Urol 109:473, 1973.
31. Banner MP: Genitourinary complications of inflammatory bowel disease. Rad Clin North Am 25:199, 1987.
32. Stein EJ, Banner MP, Pollack HM: Rectourethrocutaneous fistula in Crohn's disease. Urol Radiol 5:103, 1983.
33. Stein BS, Kendall AR: Malignant melanoma of the genitourinary tract. J Urol 132:859, 1984.
34. Bahn DK, Brown RKJ, Reidinger AA, et al: Renal stone ileus. AJR 150:145, 1988.

35. Dunn M, Kurt D: Renogastric fistula: Case report and review of the literature. J Urol 109:785, 1973.
36. Susman N, Hammerman AM, Cohen E: The renal halo sign in pancreatitis. Radiology 142:323, 1982.
37. Master's Film Interpretation Panel: 72nd Scientific Assembly and Annual Meeting, Radiological Society of North America, 1986. Radiographics 7:465, 1987.
38. Nicholson RL: Abnormalities of the perinephric fascia and fat in pancreatitis. Radiology 139:125, 1981.
39. Raptopoulos V, Kleinman PK, Marks S Jr, et al: Renal fascial pathway: Posterior extension of pancreatic effusions. Radiology 158:367, 1986.
40. Boag GS, Nolan RL: Sonographic features of urinary bladder involvement in regional enteritis. J Ultrasound Med 7:125, 1988.
41. Merine D, Fishman EK, Kuhlman JE, et al: Bladder involvement in Crohn disease: Role of CT in detection and evaluation. J Comp Assist Tomogr 13:90, 1989.

28 Gynecological Inflammatory Disease

MARK SCHWIMMER

Inflammation of the female genital tract may result from any of a variety of genital or extragenital (e.g., diverticulitis) conditions. Bacterial pathogens—gonococcus, staphylococcus, and enteric bacteria—enter the true pelvis via the vagina and lead to inflammatory responses in the cervix, uterus, fallopian tubes, or ovaries. Direct peritoneal spread may occur, accompanied by clinically evident peritoneal irritative signs or symptoms that can mimic those of intraperitoneal disease or endometriosis. If purulent material forms, adhesions or obstruction within the uterus or tubes, or about the ovaries, may cause an obstructive pyometria, cervical infection, or tubo-ovarian abscesses (see Figs. 28–5 and 28–6).

Vaginitis, common in girls or young women, may also be secondary to frank infection with bacteria, parasites (*Trichomonas*), fungi (*Candida*), instrumentation, or foreign bodies.[1, 2] Emphysematous vaginitis (cervicocolpitis) is an unusual condition in which multiple gas vacuoles occur within the subepithelial layers of the vagina (Fig. 28–1). It occurs primarily in gravid women and is usually transitory, disappearing spontaneously after delivery. *Trichomonas* infestation has been implicated.[1] The condition is often asymptomatic, but radiologically it may mimic gas gangrene of the uterus and cervix or a large necrotizing fibroid tumor of the uterus (Fig. 28–2). Lateral radiographs of the vagina or lower pelvis will show gas collections posterior to the bladder and anterior to the rectum. Pneumotosis intestinalis and emphysematous cystitis are considerations in the differential diagnosis.

Gangrenous infections of the uterus are rare, but they may follow a septic abortion or a complicated delivery. *Clostridium* may be cultured from the uterine specimen or the blood. The gas within the uterus may be manifested on the plain abdominal radiograph as linear or "onion-skin" collections throughout, or as more globular, discrete collections.[4] Poppel and Silverman described a patient with such an infection in 1941, for whom the outcome was fatal.[4] In 1960, Holly and coworkers described a case of mural uterine emphysema in the postpartum uterus of a 27-year-old prima gravida,[5] who survived after surgery. Occasionally, gas may dissect into the parametrial tissues and into the retroperitoneum. Computed tomography (CT) and/or ultrasonography may be able to stage the extent of gas accumulation and distribution. Prompt diagnosis and treatment (usually surgical) should be provided, because otherwise this condition is usually fatal.

The cervix may be the site of an inflammatory process, which is usually an external, erosive cervicitis. Endocervical infection of nabothian glands may occur. Hysterosalpingography or ultrasonography are usually normal in such cases. The outpouchings or invaginations into the cervical wall that are seen on the hysterogram are nonspecific. They may rarely represent adenomyosis or may be the sequelae of previous infections in the endocervical canal.

Anatomically and embryologically, a close relationship exists between the female urinary and genital tracts. Owing to the anatomical proximity of these adjacent

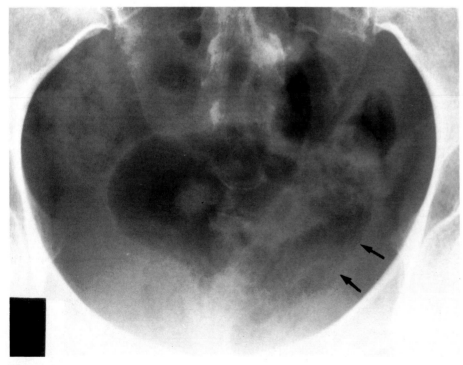

Figure 28–1. Vaginitis emphysematosum in a 37-year-old female 4 weeks after a spontaneous abortion. Numerous small, discrete radiolucencies overlie the upper part of the vagina and extend well out into the left vaginal fornix *(arrows)*. The appearance is typical of the small blebs of gas seen in vaginitis emphysematosum. The large collection of gas just above the vagina is in the rectum.

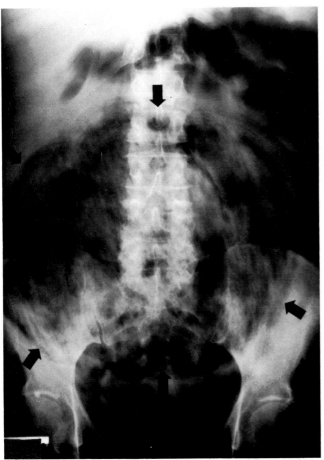

Figure 28–2. Necrotizing infection in a large fibroid uterus. Plain abdominal radiograph of a 69-year-old patient in septic shock. A large gas-filled abdominal mass (*arrows*) is present. It appeared to arise from the true pelvis. Linear collections of gas create a whorled (onion-skin) pattern within the mass. A diagnosis of uterine gangrene was made, but the patient expired in the emergency room. In addition to gram-negative gas-forming bacilli such as *Escherichia coli*, uterine fibroids may be infected with other organisms such as streptococci or staphylococci.

organs, inflammatory changes in the genital tract commonly have an effect on adjacent organs of the urinary system. Pelvic inflammatory disease (PID) and genital tuberculosis are two such inflammatory diseases of the gynecological tract. The incidence of pelvic actinomycosis, a disease that has previously been only rarely reported, has significantly increased during the past decade owing to the increased use of intrauterine devices for contraception. It has been observed to cause simultaneous inflammatory changes in the female pelvis and the urinary tract.[6]

PELVIC INFLAMMATORY DISEASE

In the heterosexual population, upper genital tract infection (i.e., PID) is the major complication of sexually transmitted diseases. The economic impact of hospitalization, treatment, and appropriate follow-up approaches $700 million annually.[7] The impact of PID on the childbearing capacity of the affected population is also significant. Ectopic pregnancy and infertility are the major

sequelae of chronic or poorly treated infections. A tenfold increase in the incidence of ectopic pregnancy as well as infertility rates between 6% and 60% have been reported.[8] Surgical correction of infertility caused by PID has a success rate of less than 25%.[9]

The pathophysiology of PID is, in most cases, characterized by the proximal migration of pathogens acquired through sexual contact. Rarely, contiguous spread of infection from an extragenital source in the pelvis occurs. The organisms most responsible are *Neisseria gonorrhoeae* and *Chlamydia trachomatis*,[10] but a number of anaerobic and aerobic organisms have been isolated from cervical cultures of patients with PID.[11] The mechanism most widely accepted to explain upper genital tract infection involves initial colonization of the cervix by the offending organism, which then extends to involve the endometrium and fallopian tubes, occasionally involving the ovaries. Extension from the parametrium to the peritoneal cavity is a well-recognized complication of PID. Within the fallopian tubes, an inflammatory purulent exudate is produced, often resulting in secondary stenosis or occlusion (pyosalpinx). Extension of purulent material to involve the ovary or peritoneal cavity produces tubo-ovarian or pelvic intraperitoneal abscesses (Fig. 28–3).

The radiological examination of choice for evaluating patients with PID is ultrasonography. Early PID may show no sonographic abnormality. Later, when inflammation causes swelling of the lumen of the fallopian tube, ultrasonography may demonstrate sonolucent tubular adnexal masses (Fig. 28–4). When extension involves the ovaries and peritoneal cavity, well-defined masses or indistinct anechoic or hypoechoic masses can be seen. The associated free fluid in the pelvis may indicate peritonitis. The masses may not always appear to be cystic, depending on the amount of necrotic debris within them. The distinction between an infection confined to the tube and ovary and one that has extended into the peritoneal cavity can be difficult to establish. Pelvic abscesses may tend to localize in more dependent regions of the pelvis, such as the cul-de-sac, whereas tubo-ovarian abscesses may be found more superiorly in the pelvis (see Fig. 28–3).[12]

Ultrasonography is commonly used to monitor a patient's response to antibiotic therapy once the diagnosis is made. In most cases, adequately treated PID will resolve rapidly with appropriate antibiotic therapy (Fig. 28–5). If that therapy fails, ultrasonography can be used to localize an abscess cavity prior to surgery or percutaneous drainage.

CT can also be used to diagnose PID. Often CT is performed when the clinical impression is of something other than PID. Bilateral cystic-appearing adnexal masses are characteristic of primary pelvic inflammation. Additional findings of free fluid with ill-defined low-density masses in the pelvis suggest peritonitis with associated abscess formation (Figs. 28–6 and 28–7).

In poorly treated or severe infections, pelvic or tubo-ovarian abscesses can cause a ureteral obstruction and a resulting unilateral or bilateral hydronephrosis (Figs. 28–7 and 28–8). Reports published in the preantibiotic era that evaluated the incidence of hydronephrosis in large series of patients who had various pelvic diseases state the incidence of obstruction from inflammatory processes to be in the range of 50%.[13, 14] At the present time,

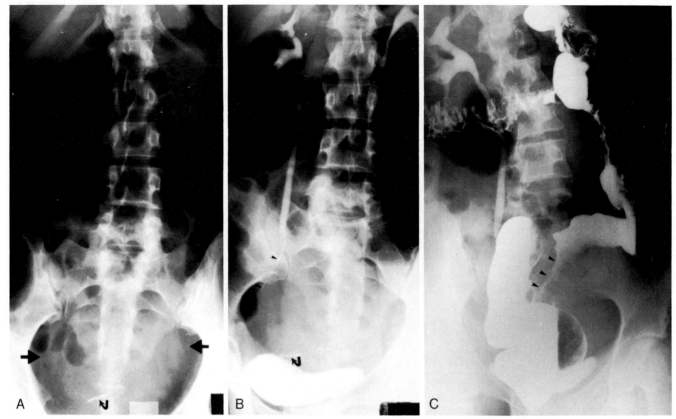

Figure 28–3. Bilateral tubo-ovarian abscesses, secondary to intrauterine contraceptive device (IUCD) (Dalkon Shield). *A,* A 21-year-old nurse complained of pelvic pain, fullness, and low-grade fever. A plain radiograph (scout film prior to urography) showed a large pelvic soft-tissue mass (*arrows*). An IUCD is noted (*curved arrow*). *B,* Urography (RPO view) shows right ureteral narrowing and compression (*arrowhead*) from right-sided mass (abscess). IUCD is again noted in uterus (*curved arrow*). *C,* Barium enema shows spiculation (irritation) of sigmoid colon (*arrowheads*) secondary to pelvic inflammation (tubo-ovarian abscess). Laparotomy revealed bilateral tubo-ovarian abscesses caused by *Bacteroides*; IUCD was removed.

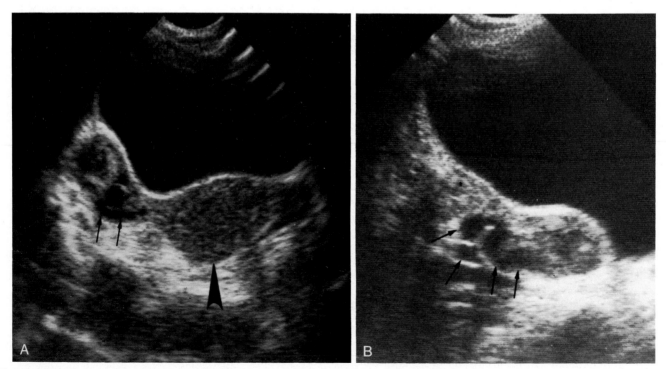

Figure 28–4. Pelvic inflammatory disease (PID) (gonococcal). *A,* Pelvic sonogram in the transverse plane demonstrates a right-sided hypoechoic, tubular adnexal mass (*arrows*) in a patient with gonococcal pelvic inflammatory disease (*arrowhead* = uterus). *B,* Longitudinal view shows tubular structure (*arrows*) corresponding to the hydrosalpinx.

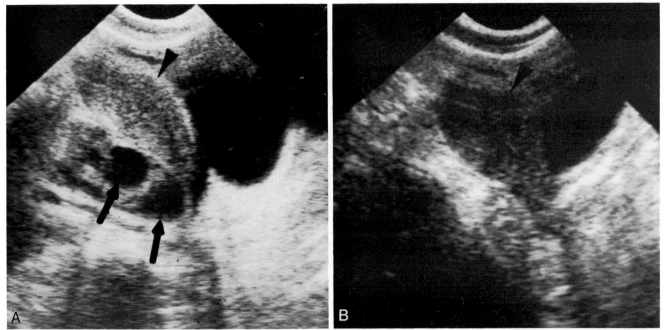

Figure 28–5. PID: response to treatment. *A,* Longitudinal sonogram shows the uterus (*arrowhead*) and fluid collections in the cul-de-sac (*arrows*). *B,* Follow-up scan at same level, taken 2 weeks later, demonstrates complete resolution of the masses. The patient was treated with antibiotics alone (*arrowhead* = uterus).

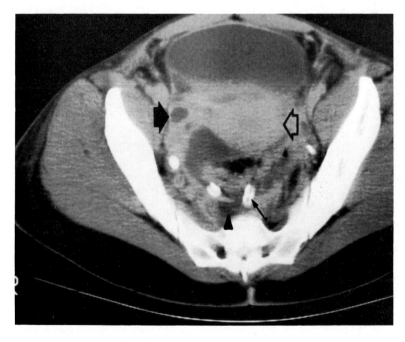

Figure 28–6. CT scan of a patient with gonococcal PID and pelvic abscesses. The uterus is prominent (*large open arrow*) and free fluid is in the pelvis (*small arrowhead*). Right adnexal mass represents tubo-ovarian abscess (*large solid arrow*). Drainage catheter is in place (*small arrow*).

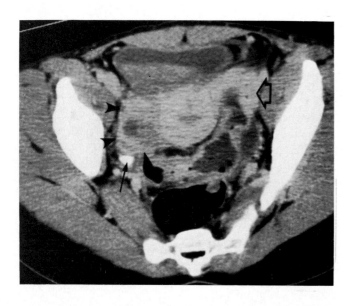

Figure 28–7. CT scan in a patient with gonococcal PID. Contrast-enhanced scan at the level of the uterine body. Ureteral dilatation is noted on right (*small arrow*) with a tubo-ovarian abscess seen adjacent to the ureter at this level (*arrowheads*). A left tubo-ovarian abscess is present also (*open arrow*).

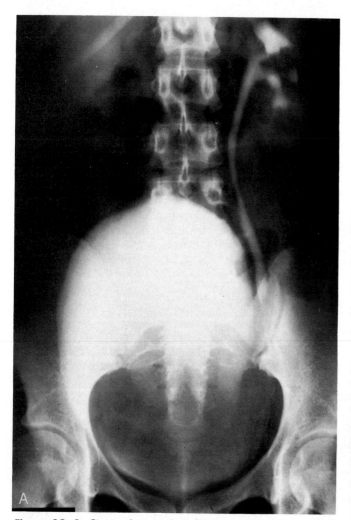

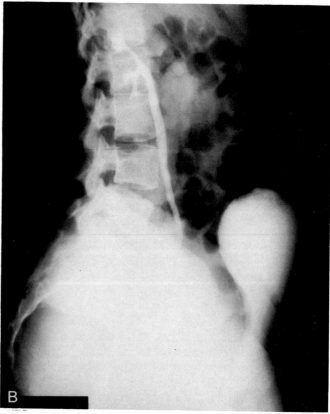

Figure 28–8. Giant tubo-ovarian abscess. *A*, An AP view from an intravenous urogram demonstrates marked deformity on the urinary bladder by a large abdominal mass. Minimal dilatation of the left ureter is seen, whereas the right kidney shows delayed excretion and hydronephrosis. *B*, A film in the lateral projection more accurately discloses the full dimensions of the mass, which fills the entire pelvis and markedly compresses the urinary bladder from behind.

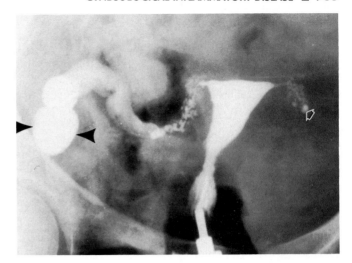

Figure 28–9. Salpingitis isthmica nodosa (SIN) in a 25-year-old female with secondary infertility and history of left ectopic pregnancy. Distal left fallopian tube (*open arrow*) was surgically removed 2 years previously. Large right hydrosalpinx (*arrowheads*) presents along with bilateral hysterosalpingographic changes of salpingitis (numerous nodular outpouchings into the hyperplastic tubal wall).

hydronephrosis complicating PID is thought to be distinctly uncommon. This may be due to more effective therapy coupled with more rapid clinical detection in the modern antibiotic era. Tubo-ovarian abscesses may become exceedingly large, producing marked deformity of the bladder, as well as ureteral obstruction (Fig. 28–8).

Other reported complications of PID affecting the urinary tract include the formation of tubovesical fistulas[15] and a transmural effect on the urinary bladder, simulating the clinical and radiographic appearance of bullous cystitis.[16]

SALPINGITIS ISTHMICA NODOSA

Salpingitis isthmica nodosa (SIN) is an uncommon condition that unilaterally or bilaterally affects the fallopian tubes.[17] Typically, several small diverticular outpouchings are seen in the midportion of the tubes, although the entire extrauterine tube extending to the ampulla may be involved (Fig. 28–9). The precise cause is unknown in most cases—hence, the designation *nodosa*—but in most instances an infectious etiology or history exists. A very high incidence of infertility and

ectopic pregnancy occurs in patients with this condition. Tuberculous salpingitis can cause a hysterographic appearance similar to SIN.

GENITAL TUBERCULOSIS

Genital tuberculosis, although a relatively rare entity in the United States, is still a well-recognized disease in many areas of the world.[18, 19] In the United States, the incidence of genital tuberculosis among infertile women is less than 1%.[20] For that reason, the disease is rarely suspected and can progress for long periods of time before diagnosis and appropriate treatment are instituted.

Genital tuberculosis is almost always acquired from an extragenital source. The most common site of primary infection is the lung; however, direct extension from an adjacent affected organ, such as the urinary tract, may occur. The site of the primary disease is often inactive at the time the secondary genital tract disease is discovered. Rarely, tuberculosis may be acquired by coitus, if the male partner suffers from tuberculosis of the seminal tract.

Unlike gonococcal salpingitis, which is the result of an

Figure 28–10. Hysterosalpingogram. Tuberculous salpingitis causes cornual occlusion on the left, and marked irregularity of the right tube (*small arrows*) and tubal diverticula (*open arrows*). Spillage of contrast material from the right tube is shown (*arrowheads*). The uterus appears normal, but the lower uterine segment (internal os) is widened. No evidence of calcifications or ossification of the tubes or ovaries was found. (Courtesy Z. Steven Kiss, M.D., Melbourne, Australia.)

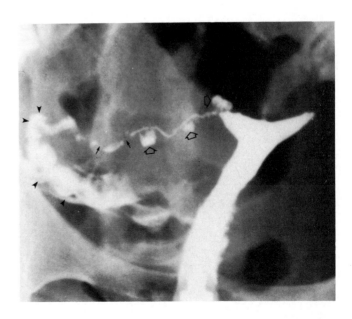

ascending infection acquired through sexual contact, the primary focus of genital tuberculosis is the fallopian tube. Spread from the fallopian tube to the uterus can occur in up to 50% of patients with tubal infections (Fig. 28–10).[21] Tuberculous salpingitis causes the same pathological changes in the fallopian tube that are seen in chronic pelvic inflammatory disease or salpingitis isthmica nodosa (Fig. 28–8).

Radiologically, the hysterosalpingogram is the study most helpful for suggesting the diagnosis of genital tuberculosis in a patient being examined for infertility. Although the examination is contraindicated in the patient with acute infection, a number of findings have been reported in patients with chronic infection. Fallopian tube narrowing, occlusion, and fistula formation have all been observed.[20] A club-shaped appearance caused by eversion of the fimbriated portion of the fallopian tube has been described in pathological specimens[21] and correlated with hysterosalpingographic findings of distal tubal dilatation and diverticula formation. Tuberculous salpingitis may rarely lead to calcification, producing a "string-of-pearls" appearance, which must be differentiated from salpingolithiasis as well as from calcification in the uterine artery.[23]

Tuberculous involvement of the endometrium has a nonspecific appearance on hysterosalpingography, commonly characterized by synechiae, distorted uterine contours, and lymphatic intravasation.[22]

References

1. Whitehouse GH: Inflammatory disease of the female genital tract. *In* Gynaecological Radiology. London, Blackwell Scientific Publications, 1981, pp 73–86.
2. Wepfer JF, Sinsky JE: Roentgen manifestations of vaginitis emphysematosum. AJR 102:946, 1968.
3. Winfield AC, Wentz AC: Diagnostic Imaging of Infertility. Baltimore, Williams & Wilkins, 1987, p 112.
4. Poppel MH, Silverman M: Gas gangrene of the uterus. Radiology 37:491–492, 1941.
5. Holly LE, Hartwell SW, McNair JN, Lowry RA: Mural emphysema of the uterus. AJR 84:913–922, 1960.
6. Fulton IC, Paterson WG, Crucioli V: Pelvic actinomycosis causing ureteric obstruction. Br J Obstet Gynaecol 88:1044, 1981.
7. Curran JW: Economic consequences of pelvic inflammatory disease in the United States. Am J Obstet Gynecol 138:848, 1980.
8. Westrom L: Incidence, prevalence and trends of acute pelvic inflammatory disease and its consequences in industrialized countries. Am J Obstet Gynecol 138:880, 1980.
9. Schwimmer M, Heiken JP, McClennan BL, Friedrich ERF: Postoperative hysterosalpingogram: Radiographic surgical correlation. Radiology 157:313, 1985.
10. Chow AW, Marshall JR, Guze LB: Anaerobic infections of the female genital tract: Prospects and perspectives. Obstet Gynecol Surg 30:477, 1975.
11. Sweet RI: Diagnosis and treatment of acute salpingitis. J Reprod Med 19:21, 1977.
12. Berland LL, Lawson TL, Foley WD, Albarelli JN: Ultrasound evaluation of pelvic infections. Radiol Clin North Am 20:367, 1982.
13. Everette HS, Sturgis WJ: The effect of some common gynecologic disorders upon the urinary tract. Urol Cut Rev 44:638, 1940.
14. Long JP, Montgomery JB: The incidence of ureteral obstruction in benign and malignant gynecologic lesions. Am J Obstet Gynecol 59:552, 1950.
15. London AM, Burkman RT: Tubovarian abscess with associated rupture and fistula formation into the urinary bladder: Report of two cases. Am J Obstet Gynecol 133:1113, 1979.
16. Blight EM: Case profile: Gonorrheal pelvic inflammatory disease presenting as bullous cystitis. Urology 11:196, 1978.
17. Creasy JL, Clark RL, Cuttino JT, Groff TR: Salpingitis isthmica nodosa: Radiologic and clinical correlates. Radiology 154:597, 1985.
18. Sharman A: Endometrial tuberculosis in sterility. Fertil Steril 3:144, 1952.
19. Ylinen O: Genital tuberculosis in women: Clinical experience with 348 proved cases. Acta Obstet Scand 40(Suppl)2:1–213, 1961.
20. Siegler AM, Koutopoulos V: Female genital tract tuberculosis and the role of hysterosalpingography. Semin Roentgenol 14:295, 1979.
21. Greenberg JP: Tuberculous salpingitis: A clinical study of 200 cases. Johns Hopkins Hosp Rep 21:97, 1921.
22. Polishuk WZ, Sadovsky B, Aviad I: Clinical significance of organic hypomenorrhea. Am J Obstet Gynecol 116:1058, 1973.
23. McAfee JG, Donner MW: Differential diagnosis of calcifications encountered in abdominal radiographs. Am J Med Sci 243:609, 1962.

29 Fungal Diseases of the Urinary Tract

DAVID B. SPRING

Of the approximately 100,000 fungal species, about 175 cause disease in humans.[1-3] Fewer than 10% cause urinary tract disease (Table 29–1). The most common fungus invading the urinary tract is *Candida albicans*. Other fungal agents, also, invade the urinary tract, most often in patients with diabetes mellitus, indwelling catheters, hematopoietic disorders, underlying malignancies, chronic antibiotic or steroid therapy, renal transplants (including immunosuppression), acquired immunodeficiency syndrome (AIDS), premature birth,[4] or a history of intravenous drug abuse.

FUNGI

Candidosis (Candidiasis)

Candida albicans is a frequently encountered commensal (an organism deriving benefit from the host without causing benefit or harm to it) and is often present on the skin, in the gastrointestinal tract, and in the lower genitourinary tract.[5-9] *C. albicans* has been demonstrated in the pharynx, colon, or vagina of as many as 50% of normal individuals.[9] Other common *Candida* species that may cause significant urinary tract disease include *C. krusei, C. parakrusei, C. parapsilosis*. Mycologists prefer the term *candidosis*, in order to be consistent with the form for other mycotic infections (e.g., histoplasmosis, coccidioidomycosis), whereas the term *candidiasis* has been used more commonly in the uroradiological literature.[5, 11, 12] Statements concerning *C. albicans* infections generally apply to infections by other species of *Candida* and to *Torulopsis* species as well. *Candida* is dimorphic, existing at body temperature in two phases: (1) unicellular yeasts (the Y-form) and (2) as apparent multicellular filaments in a mycelium or masses of pseudohyphae (the M-form). Microscopically, both yeasts and mycelial elements may be seen in the same specimen.

In the immunocompromised or debilitated host, *Candida albicans* may become a pathogen, causing considerable tissue destruction. Renal parenchymal, renal pelvic, ureteral, bladder, prostatic, and vaginal infections may occur in the genitourinary tract. The clinical presentation of the infection depends on the site and severity of the infection.

In urinary candidosis, the urinary sediment contains characteristic yeasts, pseudohyphae, and necrotic debris, regardless of the level of the infection.[6] The diagnosis may be made most simply with a standard Gram's stain. Special staining and culture techniques are necessary to confirm and subcategorize the various *Candida* species.

Because *benign candiduria* is frequently encountered, debate has surrounded the question of what constitutes significant candiduria. Kozinn and Taschdjian[13] found a useful cutoff point, separating colonization and infection, to be 15,000 colonies/ml of catheterized urine specimen. Vaginal, fecal, or skin contamination may produce misleading results. Indwelling bladder catheters similarly produce misleading results, as they almost always are associated with high colony counts.

Renal parenchymal candidosis most often follows systemic candidemia. Microscopic parenchymal and subcapsular abscesses develop in the kidney in the region of the glomeruli. The kidney is particularly susceptible to *Candida* sepsis and is the organ most commonly involved at autopsy in patients dying of systemic candidemia.

Depending on the number of viable organisms in the kidney and upon patient susceptibility, several events may occur. If the low-grade fungemic episode has been brief, no recognizable parenchymal disease may develop. Lowrie and colleagues noted that *Candida* yeasts, however, after being filtered by the glomerulus, seem to evade host immunological defenses by becoming confined within the tubules.[14] In less resistant individuals who have greater numbers of organisms, numerous microabscesses develop in the cortex, medulla, and subcapsular areas of the kidney. Such fungal microabscesses in the kidney behave in a manner similar to bacterial infections (Fig. 29–1). On computed tomography (CT), these lesions appear as multiple low-attenuation rounded parenchymal defects (see Fig. 29–3). When healed, they may calcify.[76]

Candida pyelonephritis probably occurs more frequently than is recognized, rarely presenting a specific clinical picture. The clinical setting, urinary sediment, and culture characteristics contribute to the diagnosis. In the appropriate setting (e.g., sterile pyuria) one should consider *Candida* pyelonephritis.[15, 16]

If the inflammatory process extends through the renal capsule and outside the kidney, a *perinephric abscess* may develop. The abscess is usually limited to the perinephric space by the perinephric (Gerota's) fascia. Jeffrey and Federle, and Hoddick and associates, note that CT dem-

Table 29–1. Genitourinary Tract Fungal Diseases and Common Agents

Disease	Agent
Fungal	
Candidosis (candidiasis)*	*Candida albicans* and other *C.* spp
Torulopsosis	*Torulopsis glabrata*
Cryptococcosis (torulosis)*	*Cryptococcus neoformans*
Aspergillosis	*Aspergillus fumigatus*
Coccidioidomycosis	*Coccidioides immitis*
North American blastomycosis	*Blastomyces dermatitidis*
South American blastomycosis (Paracoccidioidomycosis)*	*Paracoccidioides brasiliensis*
Penicilliosis	*Penicillium* sp
Sporotrichosis	*Sporothrix schenckii*
Histoplasmosis	*Histoplasma capsulatum*
Phycomycosis (Zygomycosis)*	*Absidia* sp
	Rhizopus sp
	Mucor sp
Fungus-like bacterial (*Schizomycetes*)	
Actinomycosis	*Actinomyces israelii*
Nocardiosis	*Nocardia asteroides*

*Alternative disease names appear in parentheses.

987

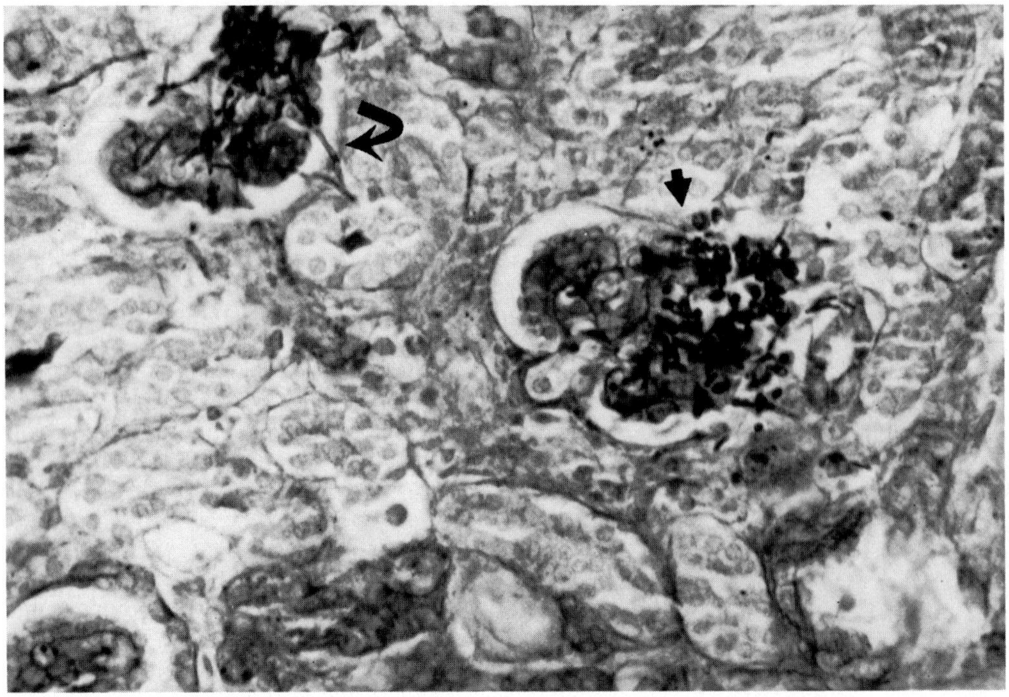

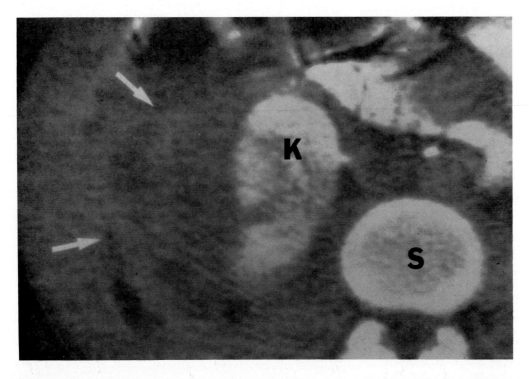

Figure 29–1. Renal cortical microabscesses of *C. albicans.* Both spores *(arrow)* and pseudohyphae *(curved arrow)* can be seen in glomeruli. The microabscesses reflect dissemination by fungemia.

onstrates perinephric inflammatory processes much more clearly than conventional urography (Fig. 29–2).[17, 18]

Papillary necrosis sometimes develops from infections involving the inner medulla. Tomashefski and Abramowsky, in a series of patients dying with systemic candidosis, noted that 21% had renal papillary necrosis, associated in every instance with fungal invasion of the kidney.[19] Most patients in this series were premature infants. Only 2 of 16 patients with candidosis and papillary necrosis appeared to have diabetes mellitus.

The papilla may also be involved by an indolent infection that results in infundibular *stenosis* and a *Candida*

pyocalyx, as reported by Sonda and Amendola.[20] Such processes are traditionally associated with tuberculous pyelonephritis, but they may be caused by *Candida* infections, as well.

Primary renal candidosis refers to an infection developing in the kidney without a recognized candidemia and without involvement of other organs.[21, 22] Because there is no recognized sepsis, mild candidemia[23] and an ascending lower urinary tract infection[24] have been offered as explanations for the origins of primary renal candidosis. This infection is probably far less common than disseminated candidosis. The clinical settings for primary renal

Figure 29–2. Perinephric *Candida* abscess—CT scan. Extension of an aggressive *Candida* renal infection into the perinephric space *(arrows)* occurs with fungal infections, as it does with bacterial abscesses. K = right kidney, S = spine. (From Jeffrey RB, Federle MP: CT and ultrasonography of acute renal abnormalities. Radiol Clin North Am 21:515–525, 1983).

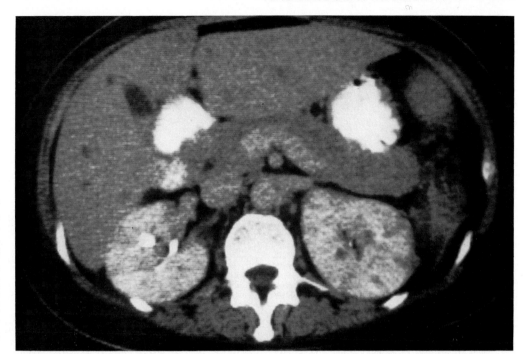

Figure 29–3. Bilateral multiple renal abscesses—CT scan. Disseminated neonatal *Candida* abscesses are indistinguishable from abscesses of other etiologies. (From Hoddick W, Jeffrey RB, Goldberg HI, et al: CT and sonography of severe renal and perirenal infections. AJR 140(3):517–520, 1983, © by American Roentgen Ray Society.)

candidosis are the same as for disseminated disease (Fig. 29–3).

Neonates, especially if premature, appear to be at increased risk for the development of renal candidosis.[78, 79] Patriquin and associates described 14 infants with *neonatal renal candidosis*.[25] All patients were receiving broad-spectrum antibiotics, and most were premature infants presenting with bradycardia and apnea. Candiduria was coexistent in some patients (12 of 14 cases). Urographic findings included ureteropelvic junction obstruction and fungus ball in the renal pelvis (8 of 12 cases). A hematogenous origin of the infection was considered, because most patients had positive-culture intravascular catheters (Fig. 29–4). The disease can be fulminant with rapid destruction of renal parenchyma.[78]

Invasion of the renal pelvis and ureter by *Candida albicans* results in a superficial mat of fungal growth on the pyelocalyceal mucosal surface (*urothelial thrush*). Fragmented bits of fungi and mucoid debris coexist freely within the renal pelvis and become molded to its contours as *fungus balls* (mycetomas, urobezoars). These fungus balls contain many living organisms. Mindell and Pollack[26] described the fungus balls as forming irregularly margined or shaggy-contoured casts of the collecting system, extending downward as a serpiginous tube into the ureter, like a "cat's tail." These living sheets of mycelial threads may be intermixed with gas and proteinaceous debris (Fig. 29–5).[27]

A renal pelvic fungus ball may lead to mechanical urinary tract obstruction with hydronephrosis, obstructive uropathy, and even anuria.[28, 29, 79] Fungus balls may resemble other filling defects in the renal pelvis or ureter and must be differentiated from blood clots, nonopaque urinary calculi, transitional cell or squamous cell carcinoma, air bubbles, inflammatory debris, fibroepithelial polyps, cholesteatoma (keratin debris), and leukoplakia.[26, 30] They may often be treated successfully by topical irrigation with amphotericin B. If this treatment fails, fungus balls may be extracted percutaneously[81] (Fig. 29–5).

Sonographically, a fungus ball in the urinary collecting system appears echogenic, usually without shadowing.[31] The finding is nonspecific, inasmuch as tumor, blood clot, and cellular debris, also, may appear echogenic (Fig. 29–4). Thickening of the renal pelvic mucosa may be demonstrable,[80] as may echogenic foci in the renal medullae.[78]

Fungal cystitis has become increasingly common during the past 2 decades.[32] Presenting symptoms include urgency, frequency, nocturia, dysuria, hematuria, and suprapubic pain. Cystoscopic examination may confirm a diffusely erythematous bladder mucosa. Urographic findings are nonspecific and include bladder wall thickening and irregularity, which may mimic neoplasia or other inflammations. On CT scans, the thickened bladder wall is apparent, but, here again, it lacks specificity.[77]

In poorly controlled diabetic patients bladder fungus balls may develop. Other possible symptoms include the passage of whitish particulate matter and difficulty voiding, with strangury and dribbling. When gas has been present, bladder fungus balls have been described as having a characteristic laminated appearance[27]; this may produce the so-called "double-fungus-ball wall sign." The diameters of bladder fungus balls have ranged between 2 and 10 cm (Fig. 29–6).

Rarely, *C. albicans* infects the prostate gland, according to Lentino and colleagues.[33] In diabetic males of any age who have prostatitis, *Candida* species should be carefully considered as the causal agent. CT has been helpful in identifying low-attenuation foci within the prostate; however, the findings are nonspecific.

In urinary diversions, para- and periloopal infections may develop in susceptible patients. Poorly vascularized tissues in the region of the diversion or cystectomy bed are sites where *C. albicans* abscesses may develop (Fig. 29–7).

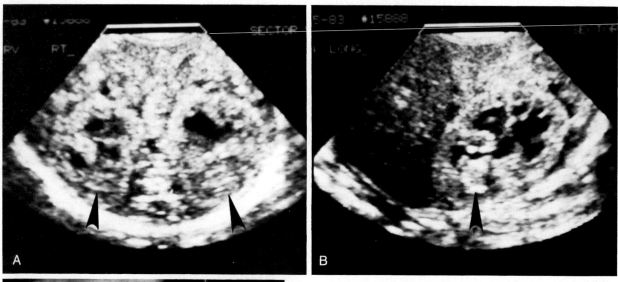

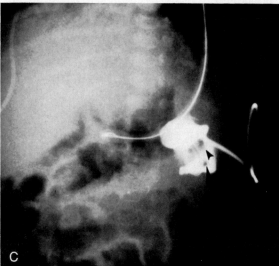

Figure 29–4. Premature 1-month-old infant with bilateral *Candida* fungus balls of the kidneys. *A*, Transverse sonogram shows mild to moderate hydronephrosis bilaterally and echogenic balls of material in dependent calyces *(arrowheads)*. *B*, Longitudinal sonogram shows hydronephrosis and fungus ball *(arrowhead)* in posterior upper-pole calyx of right kidney. *C*, A left percutaneous nephrostomy was performed for irrigation with amphotericin B. The patient was successfully treated for renal candidiasis. Small filling defect is attributable to fungus ball *(large arrowhead)*; large defect to Foley catheter *(small arrowhead)*.

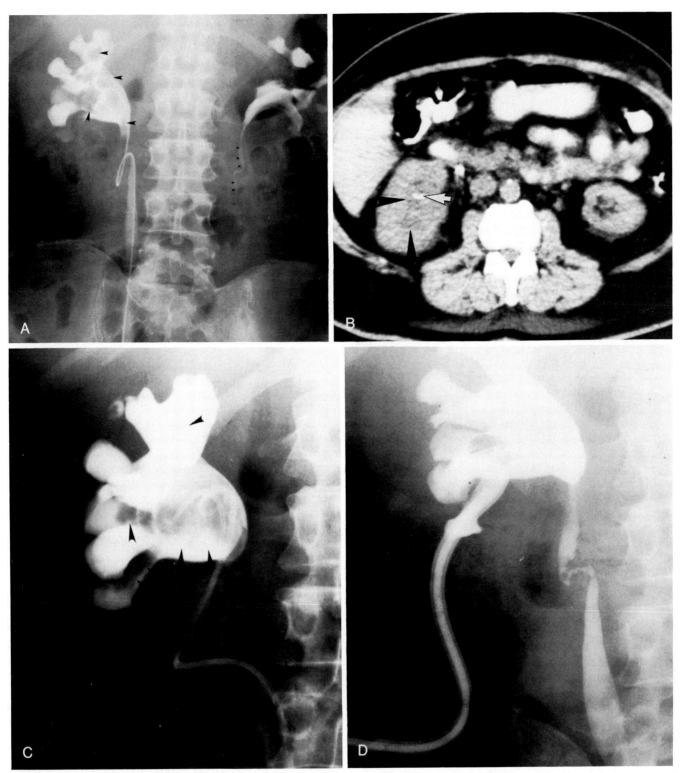

Figure 29–5. Fungus ball in collecting system. A 55-year-old man with insulin-dependent diabetes mellitus had a long history of urinary tract infection. One month before, a fungus ball had been removed from his bladder. He presented at this examination with acute urosepsis and hyphae in his urine. *A*, Bilateral retrograde pyelogram shows pelvic filling defects (fungus balls) on the right *(arrowheads)*, extending into the ureter. Left ureteral striation *(small arrowheads)* is consistent with previous dilatation and infection. *B*, CT scan shows high-density material *(arrowheads)* in dilated right collecting system. Ureteral catheter is noted *(arrow)*. *C*, A second ureteral catheter was passed on the right for better irrigation, but fungus balls *(arrowheads)* persisted. *D*, A percutaneous nephrostomy with endoscopic removal of fungus balls and irrigation was performed. Collecting system is patent after treatment.

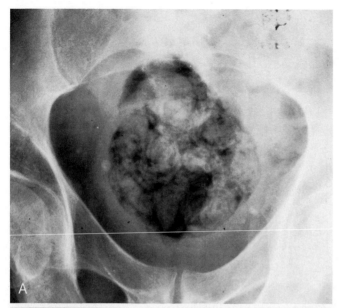

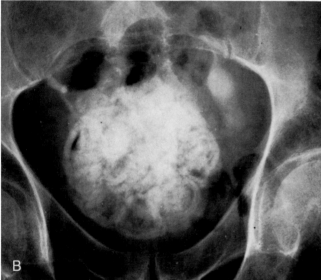

Figure 29–6. Fungus balls in bladder *(Candida)*. *A*, A 61-year-old diabetic man presented with stranguria and passage of white material in urine. Scout film for cystogram shows gas within the bladder outlining laminated fungus balls. *B*, Contrast from intravenous urogram outlines numerous filling defects in bladder (fungus balls). The left ureter was dilated. Suprapubic cystotomy was performed, and the fungus balls were removed. The bladder was irrigated with amphotericin B. (From McDonald DF, Fagan CJ: Fungus balls in the urinary bladder. Case report. AJR 114:753–757, 1972, © by American Roentgen Ray Society.)

Torulopsosis

Torulopsis species, like those of *Candida*, are classified as asexual, or imperfect, fungi *(Deuteromycetes)*. Unlike *Candida* species, however, *Torulopsis* species occur only as unicellular yeasts. No mycelial form has been identified, and hyphae or pseudohyphae are not seen. *Torulopsis* species have in the past been grouped with *Candida* species because of their strong similarities. Cultures appear quite similar to those of *Candida*. The most common species colonizing and infecting the urinary tract is *T. glabrata*.[7, 34, 35]

Like *Candida*, *Torulopsis* often colonizes the gastrointestinal tract of normal individuals. Urine cultures, how-

ever, are positive in only about 2% to 4% of normal individuals. Among fungi, *Torulopsis* is second only to *Candida* in its frequency of isolation from the urinary tract. As with *Candida*, the likelihood of culturing *Torulopsis* from the urinary tract correlates with the degree of glycosuria.

There are two main forms of renal *torulopsosis: disseminated* and *primary*. Clinically apparent fungemia or involvement of other organs is necessary for the diagnosis of the more common *disseminated* form. This form of renal torulopsosis urinary tract infection is likely to result in multiple renal microabscesses, much as one sees with *Candida*. Both disseminated and primary renal torulopsosis may produce pyelonephritis, which urographically is indistinguishable from other forms of the disease. Because sheets of mycelia do not develop, torulopsosis does not cause fungus balls, although yeast may grow in necrotic debris, resembling fungus balls (Fig. 29–8). *Torulopsis* has rarely infected simple cysts.[36]

The uroradiographic diagnosis of *Torulopsis* urinary tract infections is the same as for *Candida*. Interventional techniques, including percutaneous nephrostomy and stent placement, have proved helpful in both diagnosis and treatment (see Figs. 29–4 and 29–5).[37–39]

Cryptococcosis

Primary renal *Cryptococcus* pyelonephritis has been described. *Disseminated* renal disease is far more common. Up to 50% of patients who have disseminated

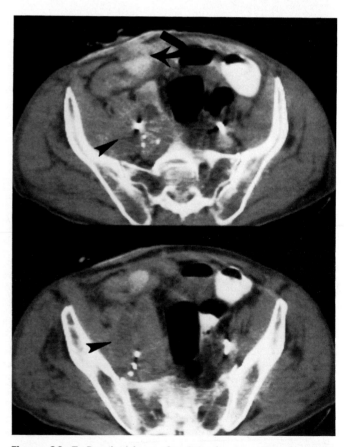

Figure 29–7. Paraileal loop *Candida* abscess. CT scan shows an abscess *(arrowhead)* extending into the true pelvis from the region of an ileal loop. The ileal loop itself passes through the right anterior abdominal wall *(curved arrow)*.

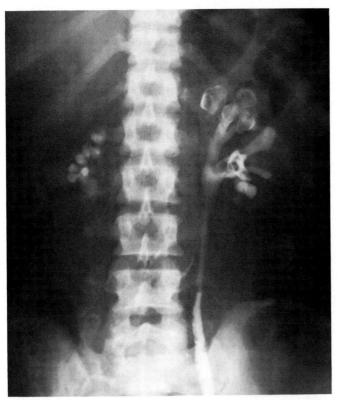

Figure 29–8. Filling defects in the collecting system of the left kidney are from *Torulopsis glabrata* infection. *Torulopsis* does not have a mycelial phase; nevertheless, large numbers of yeast forms may be present within a mass of cellular debris in the collecting system. Incidentally noted is ureteritis cystica of the left ureter. (Courtesy Alan C. Winfield, M.D.)

cryptococcosis show renal involvement. Blood-borne *C. neoformans* usually reaches the kidney from a preceding respiratory infection.[40] Although prostatic infection is described in specific settings, it is uncommon. Lief and Sarfarazi more recently described recurrent dysuria and urinary obstruction in a 36-year-old man with AIDS and cryptococcal prostatitis.[41] No radiographic signs have been described.

Aspergillosis

Although *Aspergillus* is the second most common fungal invader in humans, it is relatively uncommon in the kidney.[42] *A. fumigatus* most often causes urinary tract involvement. *Aspergillus* species have relatively low pathogenicity for human tissues, unless resistance is overcome by an underlying debilitating illness or there is an overwhelming inoculum. Both primary and disseminated forms of renal involvement occur with microabscesses, pyelonephritis, macroabscesses, and papillary necrosis. Renal pelvic involvement may include the development of fungus balls (mycetomas) and urinary tract obstruction.[43–45]

Primary renal aspergillosis may occur in patients with renal transplants and in patients with altered host resistance. The *disseminated* form of renal aspergillosis occurs most commonly in patients who have leukemia, in patients with renal transplants, and in individuals with chronic debilitating diseases. In a series reported by

Meyer and colleagues, as many as 41% of patients dying with acute leukemia had incidental renal aspergillosis.[46]

Aspergillus species may produce a nephrotoxic mycelial endotoxin. Comings and associates reported a fatal epidemic among penguins in the Chicago Zoo and confirmed experimentally that such a mycelial nephrotoxin could produce renal cortical necrosis.[43]

Coccidioidomycosis

Coccidioides immitis is a noncontagious, highly infectious fungus found most frequently in the dry, warm climates of the Southwestern United States. The arthrospores become airborne and are inhaled, producing a respiratory infection; about 60% of these infections are subclinical, and about 40% are mild to severe. Fewer than 1% of patients develop severe, disseminated disease, which may be fatal in up to 50% of these patients.[47, 48]

About 60% of patients dying of disseminated disease show renal lesions at autopsy. The findings and extent of disease are variable and may radiographically mimic other granulomatous infections of the kidney. Infundibular stenosis and hydrocalyx formation may mimic renal candidosis or tuberculosis. Scarring and focal dystrophic calcification may develop.[47, 49]

Renal transplant recipients appear to be at a particular risk.[50] About 5% of renal transplant recipients at the University of Arizona developed urinary tract coccidioidomycosis. Diagnosis may be made from urine cultures; because colony counts are so low, centrifuged urinary specimens should be used. Urographic findings are nonspecific.

Prostate coccidioidomycosis has been reported.[51] It may mimic carcinoma because of the formation of hard granulomas. The symptoms are nonspecific and include prostatic enlargement and nodules. Prostatic involvement may be diagnosed by culture from expressed prostatic secretions (EPS).[48]

North American Blastomycosis

North American blastomycosis involving the urinary tract is caused by the dimorphic fungus *Blastomyces dermatitidis*. The organism has been found naturally in the soil, and recently from a beaver lodge and nearby soil.[52, 53] Oval conidia are inhaled from the environment and are converted to yeast forms at body temperature. Although the pneumonitis usually resolves, other organ systems may become involved. The skin, bones, joints, and prostate glands are the most common extrapulmonary sites of infection.[52, 54]

South American Blastomycosis (Paracoccidioidomycosis)

Ureteral involvement in South American blastomycosis has rarely been reported. In each instance, this has been part of a systemic infection. Two of the cases had unilateral ureteral involvement with hydronephrosis. Three had bilateral ureteral involvement. Findings were not clinically suspected and were discovered at autopsy. Where appropriate, imaging studies may confirm clinical suspicions.[55-57]

Penicillosis

Schonebeck cites three reports of *Penicillium* species involving the urinary tract.[60] The most recent report was more than one-quarter of a century ago and involved a 65-year-old man with back pain who passed mycelial fragments that, on culture, proved to be *Penicillium citrinum*.[58] In another case involving a 61-year-old woman with chronic cystitis and bladder bezoars,[59] masses removed from the bladder proved to be *Penicillium glaucum*.

Sporotrichosis

Schonebeck cites one instance of renal sporotrichosis reported by Rochard in 1909.[60] A renal abscess was removed from a 29-year-old woman with pyelonephritis and a palpable mass over three-quarters of a century ago; *Sporotrichum Schenk de Beurmann* was cultured.

Phycomycosis (Zygomycosis)

Phycomycosis is an infection caused by fungi of the class *Phycomycetes*.[61, 62] The fungi genera *Mucor*, *Absidia*, and *Rhizopus*, which constitute this group, are present in soil, manure, decaying vegetation, and fruit with high sugar content. Rhinocerebral infections are seen most often with these organisms; insulin-dependent diabetics are at particular risk. Most often, renal involvement occurs, as part of an overwhelming systemic infection. Focal renal involvement has previously been described.[61, 63]

BACTERIA (SCHIZOMYCETES)

The bacterial class *Schizomycetes* resembles fungi in tissue and in some culture characteristics. In the vegetative state, these bacteria consist of very fine filaments and are usually less than 1 μm in diameter; in contrast, most true fungi have hyphae of 5–10 μm in diameter. Also, the *Actinomycetales* lack the chitin or cellulose normally found in fungal cell walls. Antifungal agents are ineffective against the *Actinomycetales*, whereas they are susceptible to antibiotics that are effective against gram-positive bacteria.[3] The two most notable bacteria in this group are *Actinomycetex* and *Nocardia*. Their role in the genitourinary tract is described below. This group of bacteria produces cells that branch in filaments and sometimes produce spores.[1]

Actinomycosis

Israel described the anaerobic "fungus" *Actinomyces* in 1885.[64] *A. israelii*, which is indigenous to the oral cavity and the gastrointestinal tract, has never been found free in nature. The organism grows in conglomerates of filamentous branching cells by direct extension. The so-called sulfur granules often associated with *A. israelii* infections are bacterial conglomerates in abscessed and necrotic tissue. The organisms appear as gram-positive bacteria closely resembling fungi. They may appear "acid fast." Other bacteria may coexist in infections of *A. israelii* in up to two-thirds of cases.[65-67]

Within the urinary tract, renal involvement is the most common presentation (Fig. 29–9).[68-71] The subclinical infection in another organ system, which is frequently found, is analogous to that seen in renal tuberculosis. The infection rarely spreads within the urinary tract and is likely to remain localized. The presentation of renal actinomycosis includes pyelonephritis, pyonephrosis, and renal abscess. A slow-growing abscess may penetrate into the perinephric space and develop a sinus tract. Both ultrasonography and radionuclide imaging have proved helpful in managing renal actinomycosis.[65]

Female genital tract actinomycosis may mimic lower urinary tract infection. *Actinomycetes* are an important factor in the development of salpingitis. Intrauterine contraceptive devices are frequently associated with such infections (Fig. 29–10).[72-74]

Nocardiosis

Nocardia asteroides most often infects the urinary tract in association with systemic involvement. This bacterial agent has led to the development of renal masses, renal abscesses, and bacterial "mycetomas" (Fig. 29–11). *N. asteroides* resembles *A. israelii* on smear. The aerobic *Nocardia* is easily cultured on Sabouraud's agar or blood agar, whereas the anaerobic *A. israelii* is not.[75]

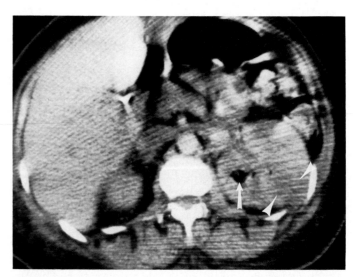

Figure 29–9. Renal actinomycosis with perinephric extension—CT scan. A 45-year-old female with urosepsis from actinomycosis. Gas in both kidneys *(arrow)* is from ureteral catheters. Obliteration of renal sinus fat on left, with enlargement of kidney and intrarenal mass effect *(arrowheads)* (low attenuation) is seen. There is extension to the perinephric space.

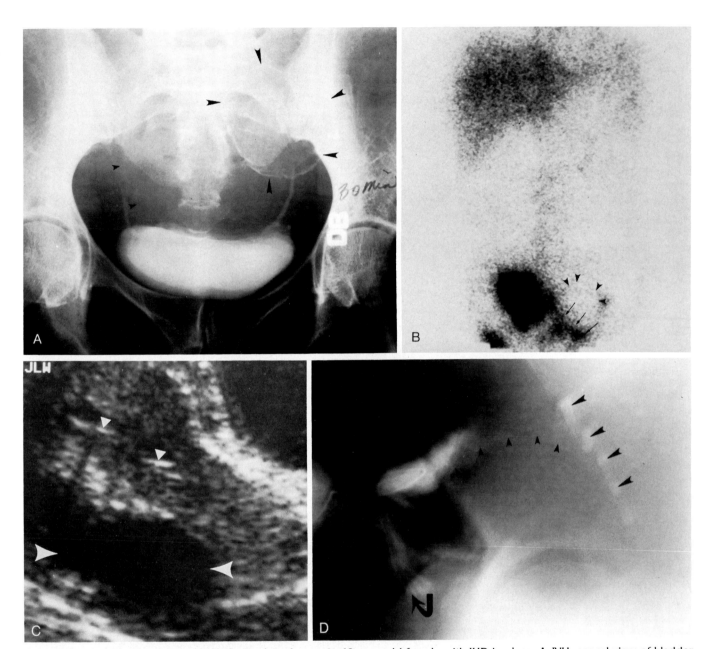

Figure 29–10. Actinomycosis and calcified pelvic abscess in 43-year-old female with IUD in place. *A,* IVU, coned view of bladder at 30 minutes, shows calcified pelvic mass *(arrowheads)* and soft-tissue supravesical mass *(small arrowheads)* indenting bladder superiorly. *B,* Gallium-67-citrate radionuclide scan shows "hot" area on right corresponding to infected parauterine collections with fistulous tract to the skin *(arrows).* Cold area *(arrowheads)* was due to calcified mass. *C,* Sonogram, longitudinal view through uterus, shows IUD in place *(small arrowheads).* Retrouterine collection of fluid corresponds to actinomycotic abscess *(large arrowheads).* *D,* Fistulogram performed with catheter *(curved arrow)* in sinus tract in left lower-quadrant outlines sinus tract connecting to the uterus *(small arrowheads);* IUD *(large arrowheads)* is still in place. Surgery revealed a calcified left lower-quadrant abscess (etiology unknown) and actinomycosis with uterocutaneous fistula.

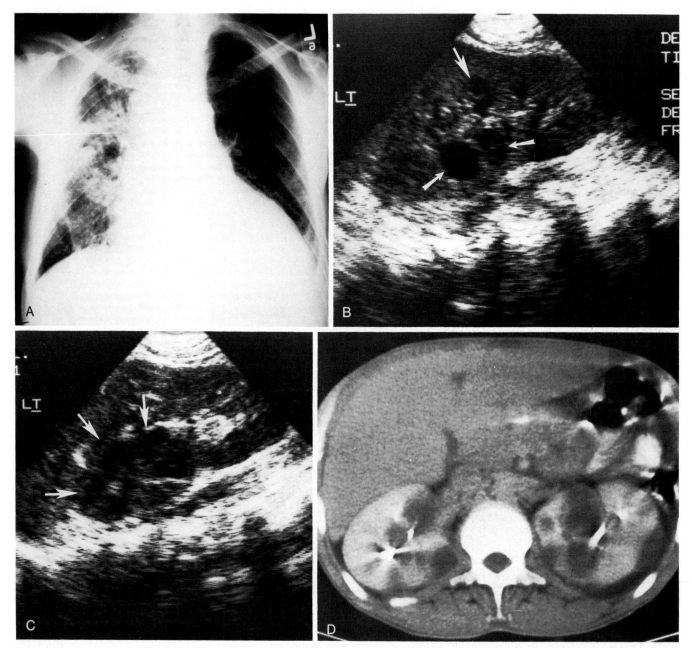

Figure 29–11. Nocardia renal abscess. A 32-year-old black man with necrotizing pneumonia and abnormal liver function. The patient was positive for HTLV III. *A,* Chest film reveals necrotizing diffuse right-sided pneumonia. *B,* Longitudinal sonogram through left kidney at time of ultrasound evaluation of liver shows several hypoechoic areas *(arrows)* throughout posterior upper-pole region, corresponding to abscesses. *C,* Another view of same kidney shows isoechoic mass *(arrows)* corresponding to focal renal inflammatory process. Nocardia cultured from sputum and renal aspiration. *D,* CT scan through both kidneys after contrast administration. Numerous round, nonenhancing masses (nocardia renal abscesses) are present in both kidneys. *(A–D courtesy Gaston Morillo, M.D., Miami, Florida.)*

References

1. Rippon JW: Medical Mycology. The Pathogenic Fungi and the Pathogenic Actinomycetes. Philadelphia, WB Saunders Company, 1982.
2. Jawetz E, Melnick JL, Adelberg EA: Medical mycology. In Jawetz E, et al (eds): Review of Medical Microbiology, 16th Ed. Los Altos, Lange Medical Publications, 1984, pp 295.
3. Bulmer GS: Introduction to Medical Mycology. Chicago, Yearbook Medical Publishers, 1979.
4. Taber WA, Taber RA: Growth and multiplication of fungi. In The Impact of Fungi on Man. Chicago, Rand McNally, 1967, p 7.
5. Odds FC: Candida and Candidosis. Baltimore, University Park Press, 1979.
6. Fisher JF, Chew WH, Shadomy S, et al: Urinary infections due to Candida albicans. Rev Infect Dis 4:1107, 1982.
7. Michigan S: Genitourinary fungal infections (review article). J Urol 116:390, 1976.
8. Roy JB, Geyer JR, Mohr JA: Urinary tract candidiasis: An update. Urology 23:533, 1984.
9. Ellenbogen PH, Talner LB: Uroradiology of diabetes mellitus. Urology 8:413, 1976.
10. Kozinn PJ, Taschdjian CL, Goldberg PK, et al: Advances in the diagnosis of renal candidiasis. J Urol 119:184, 1978.
11. Dolan CT, Funkhouser JW, Koneman EW, et al: Atlas of Clinical Mycology I. Chicago, American Society of Clinical Pathologists, 1975.
12. Roberts SOB, Hay RJ, Mackenzie DWR: A Clinician's Guide to Fungal Disease. New York, Marcel Dekker, 1984.
13. Kozinn PJ, Taschdjian CL: Candida albicans: Saprophyte or pathogen? A diagnostic guideline. JAMA 198:170–172, 1966.
14. Louria DB, Brayton RG, Finkel G: Studies on the pathogenesis of experimental Candida albicans infections in mice. Sabouraudia 2:271, 1963.
15. Tennant FS Jr, Remmers AR Jr, Perry JE: Primary renal candidiasis. Arch Intern Med 122:435, 1968.
16. Gerle RD: Roentgenographic features of primary renal candidiasis. AJR 119:731, 1973.
17. Jeffrey RB Jr, Federle MP: CT and ultrasonography of acute renal abnormalities. Radiol Clin North Am 21:515, 1983.
18. Hoddick W, Jeffrey RB, Goldberg HI, et al: CT and sonography of severe renal and perirenal infections. AJR 140:517, 1983.
19. Tomashefski JF Jr, Abramowsky CR: Candida-associated renal papillary necrosis. Am J Clin Pathol 75:190, 1981.
20. Sonda LP, Amendola MA: Candida pyocalix: Unusual complication of prolonged nephrostomy drainage. J Urol 134:722–724, 1985.
21. Albers DD: Monilial infection of the kidney: Case reports. J Urol 69:32, 1953.
22. Clark RE, Minagi H, Palubinskas AJ: Renal candidiasis. Radiology 101:567, 1971.
23. Hurley R, Winner HI: Experimental renal moniliasis in the mouse. J Path Bact 86:75, 1963.
24. Parkash C, Chugh T, Gupta S, et al: Candida infection of urinary tract: An experimental study. J Assoc Physicians India 18:497, 1970.
25. Patriquin H, Lebowitz R, Perreault G, et al: Neonatal candidiasis: Renal and pulmonary manifestations. AJR 135:1205, 1980.
26. Mindell HJ, Pollack HM: Fungal disease of the ureter. Radiology 146:46, 1983.
27. McDonald DF, Fagan CJ: Fungus balls in the urinary bladder. AJR 114:753, 1972.
28. Cohen GH: Obstructive uropathy caused by ureteral candidiasis. J Urol 110:285, 1973.
29. Turner RW, Grigsby TH, Enright JR, et al: Anuria secondary to mechanical obstruction caused by Candida fungus ball. J Urol 109:938, 1973.
30. Boldus RA, Brown RC, Culp DA: Fungus balls in the renal pelvis. Radiology 102:555, 1972.
31. Stuck KJ, Silver TM, Jaffe MH, et al: Sonographic demonstration of renal fungus balls. Radiology 142:473, 1981.
32. Rohner TJ Jr, Tuliszewski RM: Fungal cystitis: Awareness, diagnosis and treatment. J Urol 124:142, 1980.
33. Lentino JR, Zielinski A, Stachowski M, et al: Prostatic abscess due to Candida albicans. J Infect Dis 149:282, 1984.
34. Marks MI, Langston C, Eickhoff TC: Torulopsis glabrata—an opportunistic pathogen in man. N Engl J Med 283:1131, 1970.
35. Kauffman CA, Tan JS: Torulopsis glabrata renal infection. Am J Med 57:217, 1974.
36. Cho KJ, Maklad N, Curran J, et al: Angiographic and ultrasonic findings in infected simple cysts of the kidney. AJR 127:1015, 1976.
37. Mazer MJ, Bartone FF: Percutaneous antegrade diagnosis and management of candidiasis of the upper urinary tract. Urol Clin North Am 9:157, 1982.
38. Wise GJ: Ureteral stent in management of fungal pyonephrosis due to Torulopsis glabrata. Urology 24:128, 1984.
39. Dembner AG, Pfister RC: Fungal infection of the urinary tract: Demonstration by antegrade pyelography and drainage by percutaneous nephrostomy. AJR 129:415, 1977.
40. Salyer WR, Salyer DC: Involvement of the kidney and prostate in cryptococcosis. J Urol 109:695, 1973.
41. Lief M, Sarfarazi F: Prostatic cryptococcosis in acquired immune deficiency syndrome. Urology 28:318, 1986.
42. Myerson DA, Rosenfield AT: Renal aspergillosis: A report of two cases. J Can Assoc Radiol 28:214, 1977.
43. Comings DE, Turbow BA, Callahan DH, et al: Obstructing Aspergillus cast of the renal pelvis. Arch Intern Med 110:255, 1962.
44. Melchior J, Mebust WK, Valk WL: Ureteral colic from a fungus ball: Unusual presentation of systemic aspergillosis. J Urol 108:698, 1972.
45. Warshawsky AB, Keiller D, Gittes RF: Bilateral renal aspergillosis. J Urol 113:8, 1975.
46. Meyer RD, Young LS, Armstrong D, et al: Aspergillosis complicating neoplastic disease. Am J Med 54:6, 1973.
47. Conner WT, Drach GW, Bucher WC Jr: Genitourinary aspects of disseminated coccidioidomycosis. J Urol 113:82, 1975.
48. Petersen EA: Genitourinary coccidioidomycosis. In Stevens DA (ed): Coccidioidomycosis: A Text. New York, Plenum, 1980, p 225.
49. McGahan JP, Graves DS, Palmer PES, et al: Classic and contemporary imaging of coccidioidomycosis. AJR 136:393, 1981.
50. Schröter GPJ, Bakshandeh K, Husberg BS, Weil R: Coccidioidomycosis and renal transplantation. Transplantation 23:485, 1977.
51. Chen KTK, Schiff JJ: Coccidioidomycosis of prostate. Urology 25:82, 1985.
52. Klein BS, Vegeront JM, Weeks RJ, et al: Isolation of Blastomyces dermatitidis in soil associated with a large outbreak of blastomycosis in Wisconsin. N Engl J Med 314:529, 1986.
53. Dismukes WE: Blastomycosis: Leave it to beaver. N Engl J Med 314:575, 1986.
54. Eickenberg HU, Amin M, Lich R Jr: Blastomycosis of the genitourinary tract. J Urol 113:650, 1975.
55. Silveira E, Billis A, Trevisan MS, Viera RJ: South American blastomycosis of the ureter. Am J Trop Med Hyg 25:530, 1976.
56. Silva WB: Registro de um caso de blastomicose sul-americana generalizada com comprometimento cardiaco. Ann Fac Med Univ Recife 16:235, 1956.
57. Billis A, Silveira E: Blastomicose sul-americana do ureter. Rev Assoc Med Bras 19:463, 1973.
58. Gilliam JS Jr, Vest SA: Penicillium infection of the urinary tract. J Urol 65:484, 1951.
59. Chute AL: An infection of the bladder with Penicillium glaucum. Boston Med Surg J 144:420, 1911.
60. Schonebeck J: Fungal infections of the urinary tract. In Walsh P, Gittes RF, Perlmutter AD, Stamey TA (eds): Campbell's Urology, Vol I. Philadelphia, WB Saunders Company, 1986, p 1025.
61. Langston C, Roberts DA, Porter GA, et al: Renal phycomycosis. J Urol 109:941, 1973.
62. Low AI, Tulloch AGS, England EJ: Phycomycosis of the kidney associated with a transient immune defect and treated with clotrimazole. J Urol 111:732, 1974.
63. Prout GR, Goddard AR: Renal mucormycosis. N Engl J Med 263:1246, 1960.
64. Abbott DP: Primary actinomycosis of the kidney. JAMA 82:1414, 1979.
65. Ellis LR, Kenny GM, Nellans RE: Urogenital aspects of actinomycosis. J Urol 122:132, 1979.
66. Levin SL, Andrew LB: The clinical features of renal actinomycosis. Report of a case. Med Bull Vet Admin 19:153, 1942.
67. Weese WC, Smith IM: A study of 57 cases of actinomycosis over a 36-year period. Arch Intern Med 135:1562, 1975.
68. Hunt VE, Mayo CW: Actinomycosis of the kidney. Ann Surg 93:501, 1932.
69. Cross JEW, Soderdahl DW, Schamber DT: Renal actinomycosis. Urol 7:309, 1976.
70. Anhalt M, Scott R Jr: Primary unilateral renal actinomycosis: Case report. J Urol 103:126, 1970.

71. Baron E, Arduino LT: Primary renal actinomycosis. J Urol 62:410, 1949.
72. Yoonessi M, Crickard K, Cellino IS, et al: Association of *Actinomyces* and intrauterine contraceptive devices. J Reprod Med 30:48, 1985.
73. Schiffer MA, Elguezabel A, Sultana M, et al: Actinomycosis infections associated with intrauterine contraceptive devices. Obstet Gynecol 45:67, 1975.
74. Piper JV, Stoner BA, Mitra SK, et al: Ileo-vesical fistula associated with pelvic actinomycosis. Br J Clin Pract 23:341, 1969.
75. Palmer DL, Harvey RL, Wheeler JK: Diagnostic and therapeutic considerations in *Nocardia asteroides* infection. Baltimore, Medicine, 53:391, 1974.
76. Shirkhoda A: CT findings in hepatosplenic and renal candidiasis. J Comput Assist Tomogr 11:795, 1987.
77. Trinh TD, Gatewood OMB, Fishman EK: Candida of the bladder wall: Computerized tomography demonstration. J Urol 135:1008, 1986.
78. Kintanar C, Cramer BC, Reid WD, Andrews WL: Neonatal renal candidiasis: Sonographic diagnosis. AJR 147:801, 1986.
79. Robinson PJ, Pocock RD, Frank JD: The management of obstructive renal candidiasis in the neonate. Br J Urol 59:380, 1987.
80. Bick RJ, Bryan PJ: Sonographic demonstration of thickened renal pelvic mucosa/submucosa in mixed candida infection. J Clin Ultrasound 15:333, 1987.
81. Doemeny JM, Banner MP, Shapiro MJ, et al: Percutaneous extraction of renal fungus ball. AJR 150:1331–1332, 1988.

30 Parasitic Disease of the Urinary Tract

PHILIP E. S. PALMER □ MAURICE M. REEDER

Throughout the world, hundreds of millions of people of all ages suffer from parasitic infection. Worms, flukes, and other organisms are often so much a part of normal life that anyone without them may be regarded by family and friends as abnormal. Seldom are these infestations the cause of the illness that sends patients to the doctor; rather they form a constant background and cause the poor health that makes the carrier increasingly liable to other illnesses. Practically speaking, the urinary tract contains only three kinds of parasites that need to be considered. However, they account for a great deal of chronic, and occasionally acute, ill health. One basic principle must be recognized: Those who have lived with parasites all their lives often present a clinical picture different from those who are infected for the first time.

SCHISTOSOMIASIS (BILHARZIA)

This is one of the most common parasitic infections in the world, affecting over 200 million people.[34] While other schistosomes can affect the urinary tract, *Schistosoma haematobium* infection is by far the most likely to present with urinary symptoms. Although hematuria is the most frequent initial complaint, evidence of the disease may well exist long before bleeding has occurred; the patient's history is important.

The Katayama Syndrome

Children or adults who have not been previously exposed to schistosomiasis but who have returned, for example, from a vacation in Africa or the Caribbean may suspect that they are sick with the "flu" about 3 weeks after swimming in fresh water.[12] They can usually remember that they felt ill for a day or two after bathing and often ascribe it to too much sun, which caused "sunburn" and unusual skin irritation. They probably recovered quickly from that and developed the symptoms of flu 3 or 4 weeks later. They subsequently complain of an irritating cough, general feeling of malaise, and sometimes of tender and swollen lymph nodes. Almost invariably, peripheral eosinophilia is present, and it may provide the first indication that the illness is not a common cold or bronchitis. The chest radiograph may show mild hilar and mediastinal lymphadenopathy with faintly increased vascular markings throughout both lungs. The findings are subtle and nonspecific.[12] As larvae pass through the lungs, soft patchy nodular densities that fluctuate in position and size may be seen on either side. By the time the patient first has urinary symptoms, the chest radiograph is normal, although some eosinophilia may persist. However, it must be remembered that the Katayama syndrome (which can be caused by any of the schistosomes) does not usually occur in those who live where the disease is endemic and who have been previously exposed.

Active Schistosomiasis

Schistosomiasis is primarily an infection of the vascular system, from which it spreads to damage a number of organs. The worms (blood flukes) live and copulate in the portal vein and its mesenteric tributaries or, as in the case of *S. haematobium* in particular, in the perivesical venous plexus. The worms first enter the human host as cercariae, which penetrate the skin and eventually are carried to the liver, where they mature into their adult form. Access from the portal into the systemic venous system in the case of *S. haematobium* is probably through the hemorrhoidal plexus. The life cycle is perpetuated by the passage of egg-containing urine into freshwater localities where the intermediate snail host (*Bulinus* species) resides. Miracidia, which are released when the egg hatches, penetrate the snail; there, they eventually develop into cercariae, completing the cycle.[19] The flukes are intravenous parasites attached to the wall of the vein by two suckers, with which they migrate upstream along the vessel wall. If they are swept away, they become emboli. The female deposits eggs in the smallest venules of the wall of the urinary bladder or ureters and may produce several thousand eggs a day. *S. haematobium* is found throughout Africa, around the southern shores of the Mediterranean, and in Arabia and southwest Asia. Although it primarily causes urinary tract infection, it may also affect the portal system, the colon, and the lungs. *Schistosoma japonicum*, which usually involves the small intestine, is the common schistosome of China, Japan, Taiwan, and other western Pacific countries. *Schistosoma mansoni* is found in the Caribbean and northern South America, as well as throughout Africa. It affects the rectum and large intestine in particular, but rarely the urinary tract.

The pathological process underlying schistosomiasis is the formation of granulomas and obliterative endarteritis. In *S. haematobium* infection, the ureters and bladder are chiefly affected; however, schistosomal granulomas may also be found in the testes, seminal vesicles, and not infrequently in the female genitalia (e.g., cervix, ovary, and endometrium). Individual responses to the infection vary considerably: bladder neck obstruction, for example, is frequently found in Egypt but is seldom seen in southern Africa.[16, 17]

The laboratory diagnosis depends on the identification of the ova and on serological tests. Rectal biopsy may be necessary if the urine is normal, and may in fact be more efficient and rapid than examination of the urine. The rectal biopsy should be taken from the region of the first rectal valve and immediately pressed between two glass slides for histological examination. Serological tests are useful, although they may be misleading because avian schistosomes can produce antibody formation. Other nonviable eggs, such as those of *Schistosoma mattheei* or other nonhuman schistosomes, can cause diagnostic problems.

Examination of the urine was once thought to be essential in the diagnosis of *S. haematobium* infection, but its accuracy is limited, even if multiple specimens are collected over a period of 24 hours.[27] The release of ova follows a diurnal pattern, controlled by sunlight. Therefore, a single specimen collected in the early afternoon near the end of micturition may be more important than several samples. The daily ova load varies considerably; even during active cystitis, urinalysis may be positive in as few as 20% of patients. Although positive results are useful, the absence of ova does not exclude either active or chronic infection. The presence of pus or other cells does not help the diagnosis. As the disease progresses, bladder calcification seen on radiographs may be a much more accurate indicator.

Clinical Findings

Although schistosomiasis is generally a chronic low-grade infection, severe infestations in those who have never been exposed to the disease may be life threatening. Headache, neck stiffness, and even severe neurological symptoms may be present. The invasion of the hepatic and portal veins and of the mesenteric vessels and lymphatics may cause abdominal pain and nausea. In the less acute pattern, children may simply complain of fatigue, and, if they are in school, the standard of their work may decline. Similarly, adults may experience ill health, fatigue, and lack of energy as the only generalized symptoms, while gross hematuria and symptoms of frequency and urgency call attention to the urinary tract. It should be emphasized that the worms cannot multiply within the body and that most of the clinical manifestations result from dead worms or ova. Consequently, many infected individuals are asymptomatic.

Radiological Findings

Plain radiography of the abdomen is not helpful until calcification has developed in the ureters and bladder (Fig. 30–1).[10]

Intravenous urography is the most useful examination; all the early findings are in the ureters and bladder.[10, 24] The kidneys remain normal until late in the disease. In the ureters, the earliest change is persistent filling of the lower segment, seen throughout the urogram (Fig. 30–2).[32] The next finding is dilated ureters, but it is not present in every case. The dilatation may be slight or severe, and there may be no visible stenosis.[26] The ureteral constriction first occurs within the bladder wall and at this stage may still be reversible. Hypertrophy of the ureteral mucosa, producing striations in the renal pelvis or ureter, may be observed.[37, 38]

As the disease progresses, the lower ureters appear beaded, and irregular dilatation resulting from acute pseudotubercles in the submucosa may be seen.[10] The ureteral changes may then progress in several ways. Dilatation may affect the entire ureter, owing to extensive involvement of the ureteral wall, or local stenosis and irregular dilatation may occur, above and below the stenotic segment (Fig. 30–3).[5] Eighty per cent of the early stricturing occurs in the bladder wall. Next in frequency

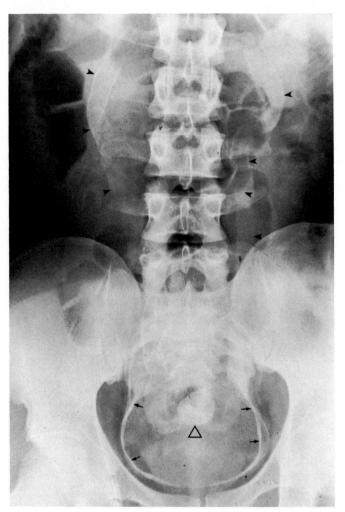

Figure 30–1. Schistosomiasis in an African patient with dilated, calcified ureters (black *arrowheads*) and heavy calcification in a thick bladder wall *(arrows)* (plain abdominal film). Note also a large bladder calculus *(open arrowhead)*. Recurrent infection with *Schistosoma haematobium* is common, but the incidence of calculi varies considerably throughout the tropics.

are strictures 5 cm above the ureteral orifice[8] and strictures in the midureter, approximately at the level of L3 ("Makar's" stricture).[35] The number of strictures then increases, and muscular hypertrophy may develop above the obstruction; gross irregularity and sacculation occur throughout the length of the ureter. This development is almost always bilateral but is very seldom symmetrical. At this stage, fine calcification may be seen, beginning with scattered areas that eventually coalesce, until the ureters are calcified throughout their length and are easily seen on plain radiographs (Fig. 30–4). Ureteral aperistalsis,[25] calculi, bilharzial papillomas,[21] ureteritis cystica,[22] and hydronephrosis may occur in advanced cases with ureteral stricture. In many cases, however, ureteral dilatation, presumably as a result of impaired peristalsis, mimics an absent stricture.[26] The fluid in the ureteral cysts may be bloody, predisposing to calcification in the cyst walls. This gives rise to a distinctive type of punctate calcification that is unique to bilharziasis, termed *ureteritis calcinosa*.[36] These small calcifications may predispose to subsequent calculus formation.

The thickening of the ureters may be demonstrated by ultrasonography. In the early stages, this may be a useful

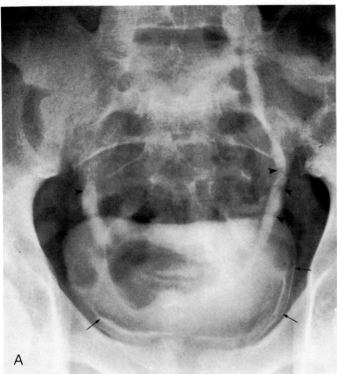

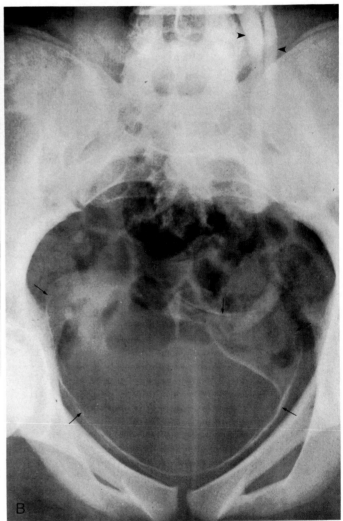

Figure 30–2. The early changes in schistosomiasis of the ureter (excretory urography). *A,* Persistent filling of the lower segments with beading, slight irregularity, and dilatation bilaterally *(arrowheads).* There is also calcium within the bladder wall *(arrows).* (From Reeder MM, Palmer PES: The Radiology of Tropical Diseases [with Epidemiological, Pathological and Clinical Correlation]. Baltimore, Williams & Wilkins Company, 1981.) *B,* Similar changes are seen in the duplicated left ureter of another patient, together with ringlike calcification of the entire bladder wall *(arrows).* The right ureter is not dilated and was found to be normal. Note the thin, delicate nature of the bladder calcification.

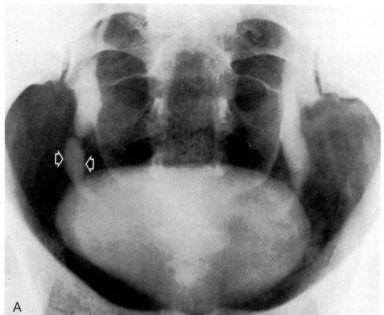

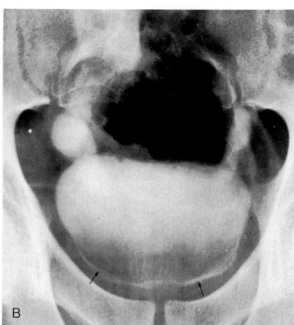

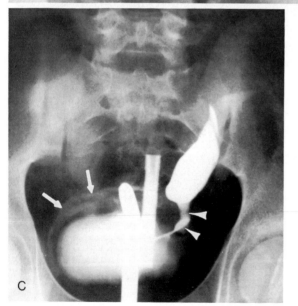

Figure 30–3. Progressive ureteral schistosomiasis. *A,* Dilatation and stenosis of both ureters is shown. In the right ureter, a segment of dilatation is between two areas of stenosis *(arrows)* (excretory urogram). *B,* Dilatation of both ureters is more marked on the right side, and stenosis is at the ureteral orifices. Bladder wall calcification is present *(arrows)*. *C,* Retrograde urography in another patient shows stenosis of the distal segment of the left ureter down to and including the bladder wall *(arrowhead),* and a markedly dilated ureter above the stenosis. Note also the marked calcification and thickening of the bladder wall *(arrows)*. (From Reeder MM, Palmer PES: The Radiology of Tropical Diseases [with Epidemiological, Pathological and Clinical Correlation]. Baltimore, Williams & Wilkins Company, 1981.)

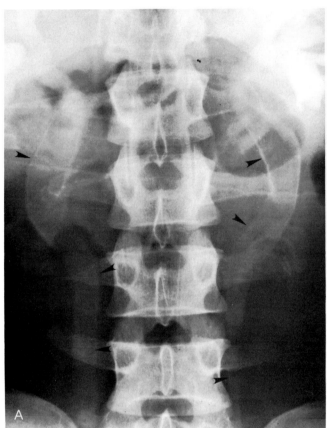

Figure 30–4. Calcification of the ureters in schistosomiasis. *A*, Calcification and dilatation of both ureters *(arrowheads)* is present throughout the entire course from the uretero-pelvic junction to the ureterovesical junction. Despite this, only moderate hydronephrosis is seen. *B*, Heavily calcified ureters (L > R) *(arrowheads)* in an Egyptian patient with heavy calcification of the bladder. The obstructed left kidney has become a hydronephrotic sac outlined with calcium. The lower left ureter, in particular, shows very thick calcification with obliteration of its lumen. On intravenous urography, the left kidney was nonvisualizing, and there was slight hydronephrosis of the right kidney, which contained two renal calculi *(arrow)*. (From Reeder MM, Palmer PES: The Radiology of Tropical Diseases [with Epidemiological, Pathological and Clinical Correlation]. Baltimore, Williams & Wilkins Company, 1981.)

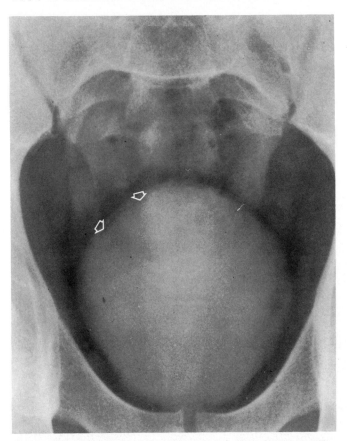

Figure 30–5. Early bladder changes in schistosomiasis. The outline of the bladder is hazy, and edema of the wall is apparent. In the right side of the dome, the mucosa separates the contrast medium within the bladder lumen from the calcification in the tunica propria. The mucosa is the negative linear shadow *(open arrowheads).* (From Reeder MM, Palmer PES: The Radiology of Tropical Diseases [with Epidemiological, Pathological and Clinical Correlation]. Baltimore, Williams & Wilkins Company, 1981.)

means of monitoring the progress of the disease after treatment.[28, 40] The thick ureter and calcification may also be documented by computed tomographic (CT) scanning, but this is rarely available in Africa and has little advantage over contrast urography.[31] Bilharzial ureteral strictures may be successfully treated by balloon dilatation.[40]

The changes in the bladder are similar. Early in the infection, the bladder outline becomes hazy and indistinct as a result of submucosal edema and pseudotubercles (Fig. 30–5). As the granulomas become more fibrotic, the bladder wall shows calcification. However, this is not within fibrous tissue; it is entirely submucosal and is due to calcified ova (Fig. 30–6).[7] A calcified area usually contains between 500,000 and 1 million eggs/gm.[9] It is necessary to have 100,000 eggs/ml in order to detect them on a radiograph.[9] Of course the thickened bladder can be seen by ultrasonography[28] or CT scanning,[31] but is not of much diagnostic assistance, although ultrasound has been used to screen populations at risk and to monitor therapeutic response, especially in children.[39] The extent of bladder calcification is roughly correlated with the number of calcified eggs within the bladder lumen. However, the excretion of eggs in the urine depends on the activity of the infection and is not affected by bladder calcification. Partial or complete resolution of bladder calcification can

result from reabsorption or shedding of the eggs. The excretion rate must be about 2 million eggs/year, if decalcification is to occur.[9] Thus, calcified bladders are less common during old age.

The pattern of calcification is widely variable.[7] It may be fine and granular, fine and linear, or thick and irregular and may involve the whole bladder or occasionally only segments (Figs. 30–7 and 30–8). The calcification has little or no effect on bladder capacity or emptying, because it is not an indication of the degree of fibrosis (Figs. 30–7E, 30–8D and 30–9). Later, however, as a result of repeated schistosomal and secondary infections, the bladder does become fibrosed, shrunken, and contracted with restricted capacity.[4] At this stage, the wall may contain less calcification. Ureteral and bladder calculi are relatively common, with some geographic variation.

The incidence of squamous cell bladder carcinoma is higher in chronic cases, but this is not a simple cause-and-effect relationship (Fig. 30–10).[14] Asymmetry of the calcification in the bladder wall may indicate that carcinoma is locally destroying the calcification, and cystoscopy should be performed. Generally, the intraluminal filling defects caused by bilharzial granulomas or carcinoma are better seen by cystoscopy than by intravenous urography.

Some important geographic variations exist. In Egypt, a syndrome of "bladder neck obstruction" is found. The trigone is the structure that is most affected, and it hypertrophies to form a prominence bulging into the vesical lumen between the ureteral orifices.[16] Eventually, this fibroses and atrophies, leaving the mucosa and muscularis as a mass, which is pushed forward over the internal urethral orifice. Trigonal fibrosis may cause the ureters to retract medially and to bow upward ("cow-horn" deformity).[26] Infiltration of the bladder neck by the schistosomes causes obstruction, dilatation, and finally atrophy of the detrusor muscle, resulting in gross dilatation of the bladder. It is rare to find such marked bladder changes outside Egypt.[23]

In those who have been reinfected after a period of freedom from the disease, a marked urticarial edematous reaction in the bladder wall sometimes occurs (Fig. 30–11A). This is unlikely to be seen in endemic areas. Large circular filling defects are observed, both radiologically and cystoscopically, which may be mistaken for sarcoma botryoides.[13] In adults, there are often a number of small, rather flat papillomas ("bilharzial polyps") that require cystoscopy to distinguish them from malignancy (Fig. 11B,C). When schistosomiasis is known or suspected, a therapeutic trial should often be the first procedure in the presence of papillomas, ulcerations, or thickening of the bladder wall.

Complications

In addition to carcinoma of the bladder and urolithiasis, other complications of bilharziasis exist. Reflux from the bladder up the ureters is common, but it does not occur in the early stages because of the ureteral stenosis. It may be expected only as the fibrosis replaces the granulomas and the ureters become aperistaltic. Ascending urinary tract infection does occur at this stage. A voiding cysto-urethrogram provides valuable information about reflux, which occurs in about 30% of patients who have signifi-

Text continued on page 1009

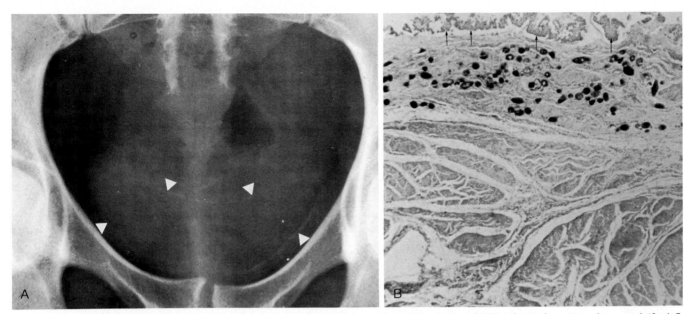

Figure 30–6. *A*, Early faint calcification of the entire bladder wall *(arrowheads)* is shown. *B*, Histological section shows calcified *S. haematobium* (black spots, *top*) in the tunica propria of the bladder wall. This amount of bladder calcification might be invisible radiologically, because at least 100,000 eggs/cm² must be present for calcification to appear on plain radiographs. The normal bladder epithelium has been replaced by squamous cell metaplasia in this case *(arrows)*. (From Reeder MM, Palmer PES: The Radiology of Tropical Diseases [with Epidemiological, Pathological and Clinical Correlation]. Baltimore, Williams & Wilkins Company, 1981.)

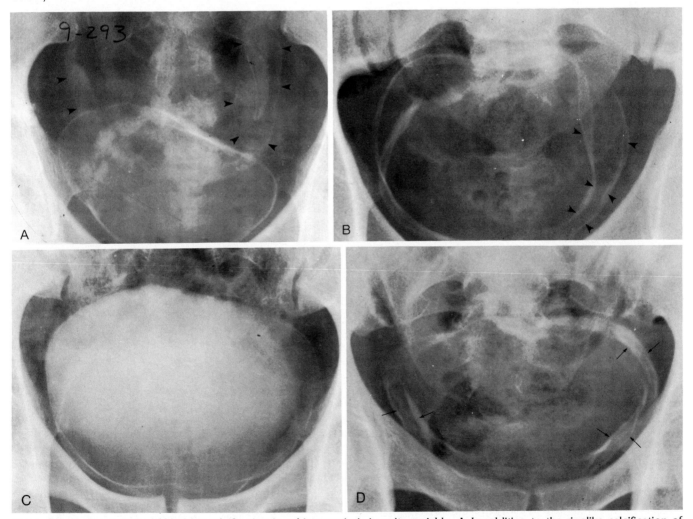

Figure 30–7. The pattern of bladder calcification in schistosomiasis is quite variable. *A*, In addition to the ringlike calcification of the bladder wall, there is calcification within dilated tortuous distal ureters *(arrowheads)*. *B*, A thin double-contoured calcification is seen in the bladder wall *(arrowheads)*. *C*, Despite the presence of considerable calcification, a normal capacity of the bladder is noted on the urogram. *(A to C from Reeder MM, Palmer PES: The Radiology of Tropical Diseases [with Epidemiological, Pathological and Clinical Correlation]. Baltimore, Williams & Wilkins Company, 1981.) D*, Thicker, multilayered calcification of the entire bladder wall *(arrows)*.

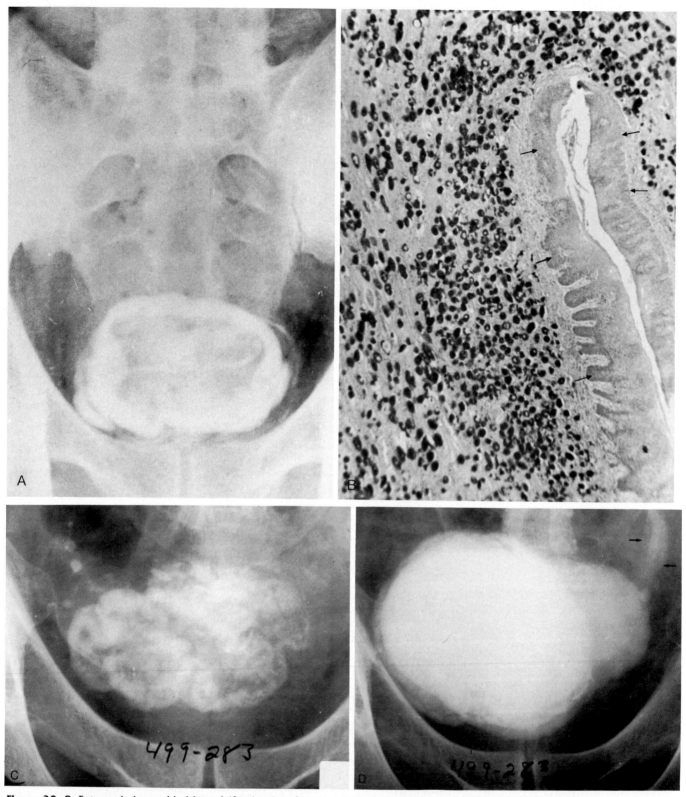

Figure 30–8. Extremely heavy bladder calcification in schistosomiasis. *A,* Dense, wavy calcification in the submucosa and bladder wall is seen on plain radiograph of the pelvis of an African patient. *B,* Histological section shows innumerable calcified *S. haematobium* eggs (black spots) within the bladder wall, and marked squamous metaplasia of the mucosa has replaced the normal bladder epithelium *(arrows).* The narrow open space on the right is the bladder lumen. *C,* In this Egyptian patient, dense serpiginous calcification is seen throughout the distorted bladder wall. *D,* A relatively normal bladder capacity is seen on intravenous urography, despite heavy calcification within the bladder submucosa and wall. The left ureter is dilated as well in this patient *(arrows).* (From Reeder MM, Palmer PES: The Radiology of Tropical Diseases [with Epidemiological, Pathological and Clinical Correlation]. Baltimore, Williams & Wilkins Company, 1981.)

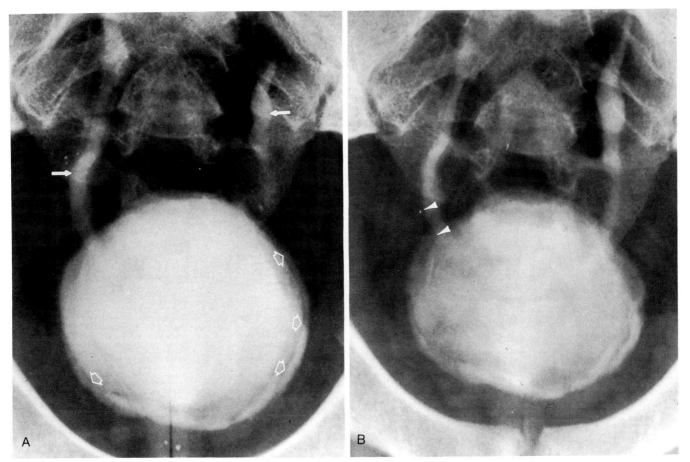

Figure 30–9. Bladder calcification in schistosomiasis. *A,* This young African male has heavy bladder calcification. On this radiograph from an intravenous urogram, the bladder capacity and shape appear relatively normal. Slight dilatation of the ureters *(arrows)* can be seen. The bladder mucosa is well delineated as a radiolucent line *(arrowheads)* between the heavily calcified submucosa and the contrast medium in the bladder lumen. Bladder calcification alone does not cause problems in micturition. *B,* At the start of micturition, the bladder wall becomes irregular and folds in the normal way. Some reflux was noted, particularly up the left ureter. Because the calcification is in the eggs, it is not until the stage of fibrosis and contraction that there is any significant difficulty in bladder emptying. Note also in *B* the lucent line *(arrowheads)* on either side of the right ureter representing the mucosa, separating the contrast medium from the calcification in the submucosa of the ureter. (From Reeder MM, Palmer PES: The Radiology of Tropical Diseases [with Epidemiological, Pathological and Clinical Correlation]. Baltimore, Williams & Wilkins Company, 1981.)

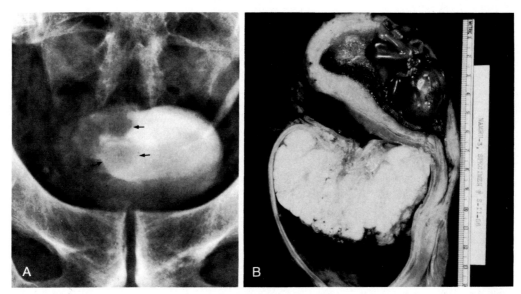

Figure 30–10. There is a significantly increased incidence of squamous cell carcinoma of the urinary bladder associated with chronic schistosomiasis. *A,* An irregular mass representing a complicating carcinoma fills the right side of the urinary bladder *(arrows)* in this Egyptian patient. *B,* Large carcinoma of the bladder is shown in a case of urinary schistosomiasis in a pregnant woman. Note the fetus in the uterus above the bladder. *(B,* from Reeder MM, Palmer PES: The Radiology of Tropical Diseases [with Epidemiological, Pathological and Clinical Correlation]. Baltimore, Williams & Wilkins Company, 1981.)

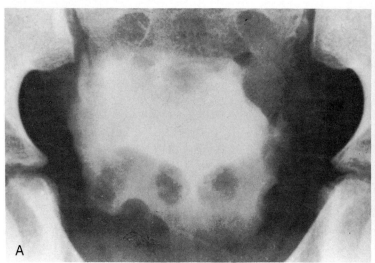

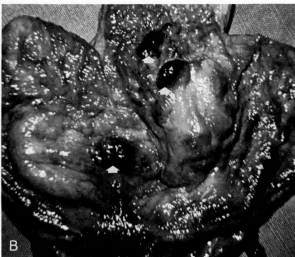

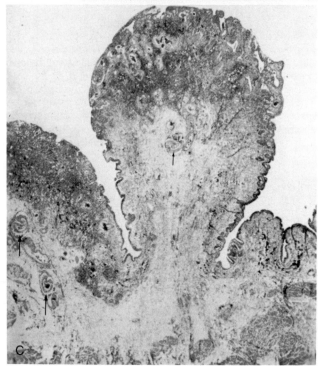

Figure 30–11. *A,* Severe, acute bladder reaction in this Nigerian child was due to urticarial edema of the bladder wall and mucosa. It is probable that these changes occur when there has been reinfection with *S. haematobium* after a disease-free period. As shown on the intravenous urogram, there are large round filling defects within the bladder, distorting its outline and somewhat resembling a sarcoma botryoides. These respond rapidly to appropriate treatment, after which the bladder usually returns to normal. *B,* The bladder is opened to show three schistosomal polyps *(arrows)* as well as a nodular, edematous and inflamed mucosal surface. *C,* This histologic study of inflammatory polyps is from the urinary bladder of a patient with *S. haematobium* infestation. Adult schistosomes are present in the venules of the large polyp *(arrows)* and in the veins of the lamina propria. There are multiple calcified schistosome eggs in the submucosa and lamina propria *(black dots).* (From Reeder MM, Palmer PES: The Radiology of Tropical Diseases [with Epidemiological, Pathological and Clinical Correlation]. Baltimore, Williams & Wilkins Company, 1981.)

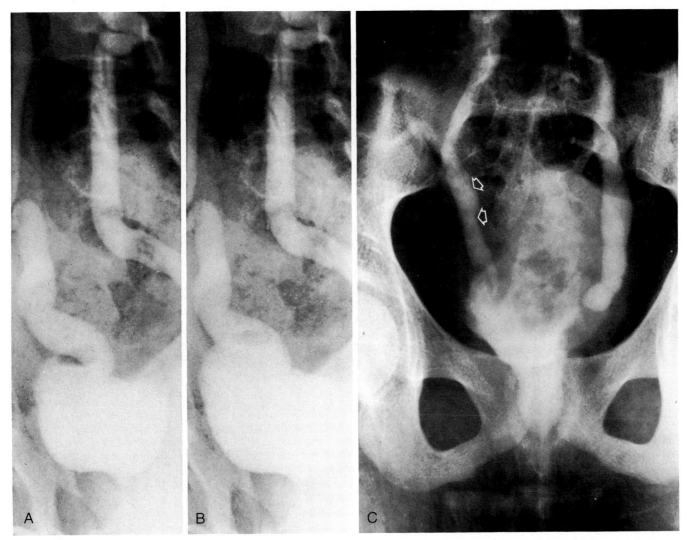

Figure 30–12. A, B, Marked reflux into both ureters is seen during voiding cystourethrography in a patient with advanced schistosomiasis. The ureters are dilated, smooth, and aperistaltic. The bladder is somewhat small and fibrotic, and cannot expand to a normal capacity. The urethra in this male patient is normal. C, Reflux into both ureters from a contracted, nodular bladder is shown in a different patient. Both ureters show beading (arrowheads), irregularity, and dilatation, and the prostatic urethra is dilated, possibly as a result of urethral stricture. (From Reeder MM, Palmer PES: The Radiology of Tropical Diseases [with Epidemiological, Pathological and Clinical Correlation]. Baltimore, Williams & Wilkins Company, 1981.)

cantly calcified bladders (Fig. 30–12). However, even when reflux has existed for many years, renal disease develops slowly, regardless of the presence of hydroureter and hydronephrosis (Fig. 30–13). Children, in particular, often respond very well to treatment and show a surprising improvement in post-therapy urograms. There is no evidence that this reflux contributes to hypertension.

Some schistosomal infections show evidence of glomerular disease, which is almost certainly of immunological origin. Renal biopsy may then be useful to establish the cause of nephrosis in either S. haematobium or S. mansoni infections. Electron-dense deposits are found in the basement membranes of the glomeruli, with laminated bodies near mesangial cells, particularly in S. mansoni infections.

Urethral stricture secondary to schistosomiasis does rarely occur, but in most countries gonorrhea remains the most common inflammatory cause of such a stricture. In males, a voiding cystourethrogram or retrograde ure-

throgram may show a narrow bladder neck, a sacculated prostatic urethra, fistulas involving the bulbar urethra, long strictures of the penile urethra, urethritis cystica, or calculi.[26, 32] The prostate gland may be enlarged, owing to a bilharzial prostatitis, and may protrude into the bladder base. Calcification may be seen in the seminal vesicles (Fig. 30–14) and may rarely be found in the spermatic cord. In women, the fallopian tubes may be infected and blocked, but they are not usually calcified.

It is important, when managing a case of schistosomiasis of the urinary tract, to remember that the liver will almost certainly be affected, although usually without the profound portal hypertension and splenomegaly often seen in severe S. mansoni and S. japonicum infections.[20] In spite of the presence of the parasite in the lungs, the chest radiograph is almost always normal (except for the Katayama stage). Occasionally, generalized interstitial fibrosis and, rarely, pulmonary hypertension are found.

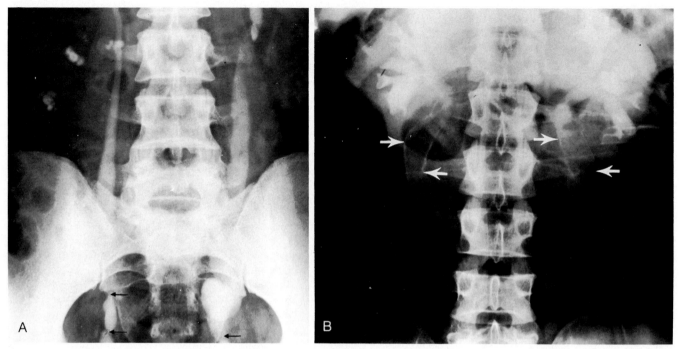

Figure 30–13. Renal disease follows late in the course of schistosomiasis. *A,* An intravenous urogram in a Caucasian shows dilated ureters throughout their length with stenotic areas *(arrows)* at or above the ureterovesical junctions. Despite this, the kidneys are within normal limits with no dilatation or blunting of the renal pyelocalyceal systems. (From Reeder MM, Palmer PES: The Radiology of Tropical Diseases [with Epidemiological, Pathological and Clinical Correlation]. Baltimore, Williams & Wilkins Company, 1981.) *B,* Marked calcification of tortuous dilated ureters *(arrows)* occurs throughout their entire course, with resultant moderate hydronephrosis late in the disease. However, most of the calyces still retain their normal cupping. End-stage hydronephrosis and renal destruction can occur in very advanced cases (see Fig. 30–4*B*).

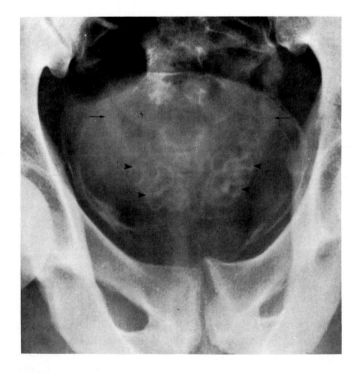

Figure 30–14. Calcification in the seminal vesicles *(arrowheads)* behind a calcified bladder. Ureters are also calcified *(arrows).* (From Reeder MM, Palmer PES: The Radiology of Tropical Diseases [with Epidemiological, Pathological and Clinical Correlation]. Baltimore, Williams & Wilkins Company, 1981.)

S. haematobium infection of the colon, particularly in combination with *S. mansoni*, may occur, causing a granulomatous type of colitis and proctitis.

Differential Diagnosis

The most important urinary tract disease to be excluded is tuberculosis. It usually starts in the kidney and progresses toward the lower urinary tract—a pattern the *reverse* of that found in schistosomiasis. The renal cavitary changes of tuberculosis have no counterpart in schistosomiasis. Therefore, ureteral calcification in tuberculosis first occurs in the proximal ureter, whereas in schistosomiasis it begins in the distal ureter. The bladder calcification of tuberculosis is patchy but is seldom extensive. Malignant tumors may calcify, but these are nearly always localized; following radiotherapy, the scar may also show calcification. However, neither is likely to be mistaken for the ring calcification of schistosomiasis. In any case, the most common cause of bladder calcification, by far, is *S. haematobium*.

In travelers, it is important to recognize the early urographic signs of prolonged ureteral filling followed by irregularity and beading of the ureter; at this stage the bladder may still be entirely normal, and the disease may be reversible after treatment with agents such as trichlorophone or praziquantel. Nevertheless, when such an infection is diagnosed, a repeat urogram 3 months after treatment and again 12 months later may be helpful to make sure that stenosis has not occurred. In order to decrease ionizing radiation in children, follow-up using ultrasonography[28] or radionuclide studies may be satisfactory.[30, 33]

HYDATID DISEASE (ECHINOCOCCOSIS)

Hydatid disease is predominantly found in sheep- and cattle-raising areas, worldwide. It is divided into two major varieties: the less common multilocular or alveolar variety (*Echinococcus multilocularis*) and the more common unilocular or cystic hydatid disease (*Echinococcus granulosus*). Either species can affect the urinary tract—the former only rarely. The larvae of *E. multilocularis* primarily involve the liver, where they behave like a malignant neoplasm with a poorly demarcated invasion, resembling a bunch of grapes. They can be seen on plain radiographs as multiple calcifications in small spheres with central radiolucency, ranging in diameter from 2 to 4 mm.[51]

In the more common form of hydatid disease, caused by *E. granulosus*, humans become infected by contact with sheep or dogs or by ingesting food, water, or soil containing the ova.[44] Adult tapeworms are found in the intestine of dogs, the primary host. Eggs are excreted in the feces and are ingested by humans, sheep, cattle, or pigs, which act as intermediate hosts; the cycle is completed when dogs ingest infected meat. Once the eggs are swallowed by humans or another intermediate host, they hatch in the duodenum and the oncospheres migrate through the intestinal mucosa and into the portal system, mesenteric venules, and lymphatics, where they can be spread to any part of the body. If the larvae are not trapped in the liver or lungs, they may be deposited anywhere. Tiny cysts, which are filled with clear fluid, develop and grow slowly over the years. In the kidney, they are often clinically silent until very large. The rate of growth varies with the particular organ, being more rapid in the lungs than in the solid organs, and slowest in bone.

Each cyst consists of the following elements: (1) a pericyst or fibrous adventitial layer contributed by the host, (2) an outer laminated membrane (the ectocyst), and (3) an inner, delicate endocyst with a germinal membrane responsible for the growth of the cyst and from which develop the brood capsules containing the scolices. As these separate from the germinal layer, they precipitate to the bottom of the hydatid fluid to become "hydatid sand," which can be recognized by ultrasonography or CT.

Daughter cysts form within the mother cyst, which until recently has been thought to be an abnormal part of the parasite's life, occurring only when the cyst is threatened by mechanical, chemical, or bacterial insult. However, CT and ultrasonography have demonstrated that most hydatid cysts have multiple daughter cysts, particularly as they grow larger.[46, 58] Eventually, the cysts die and frequently undergo calcification to become visible on plain radiographs (the exception to this is lung hydatids, which do not calcify) (see Fig. 30–17).[43] Total calcification of the cyst wall is an indication of quiescence, or perhaps death, but a partially calcified cyst is not always harmless. The liver is the organ most commonly infected, being involved in 50% to 70% of all cases; the lungs are the organ next most frequently infected.[51] Kidney cysts are found, in most series, in 2% to 5% of patients.[49]

Laboratory tests are more accurate when hydatids are in the liver than when they are in other organs, in which false negatives may result. The complement fixation test is positive in over 70% of cases but often remains positive for 2 or 3 years after surgical removal of the cyst; therefore, it is a somewhat unreliable indicator of the existence of cysts elsewhere. The intradermal skin test (Casoni's test) serves only to reflect the overall state of sensitivity to the hydatid antigen and does not necessarily correlate with the pathological state of genitourinary hydatid disease. The various flocculation, precipitation, and agglutination tests, together with serological confirmation, can lead to an accurate diagnosis; however, a demonstration of the cyst by ultrasonography or CT—or by radiography, when the cyst is calcified—is also reliable. In older patients, the differential diagnosis, ruling out simple cysts of the kidneys, is not easy.[41] The discovery of hooklets, fragments of laminated membrane, or daughter cysts in the urine, is always diagnostic.

Clinical symptoms are rare, until the cyst has grown large enough to cause pressure or distortion, or until it is ruptured. Even in the kidney, a huge cyst may exist in the absence of clinical evidence, until some acute event, such as a blow, causes symptoms.

As in other organs, hydatids in the kidney usually develop as the result of vascular spread, rather than as a result of direct invasion from a cyst in the liver or spleen. They are usually solitary and most commonly develop in the upper or lower poles of the kidney; they seldom develop centrally (Fig. 30–15).[45, 47, 48, 50] The cysts may grow outward and rupture into the perinephric tissues or

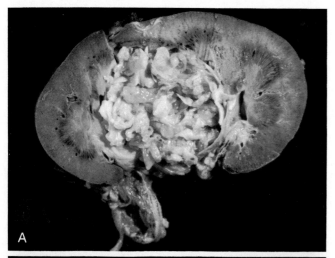

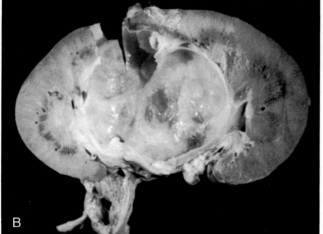

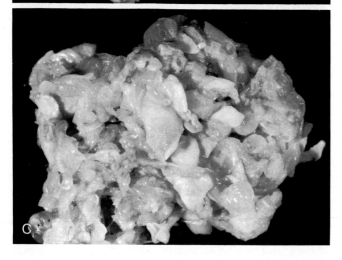

Figure 30–15. Large unilocular hydatid cyst involving the central portion of the kidney in the region of the renal pelvis. *A,* The kidney has been opened to show the large hydatid in the renal pelvis containing numerous daughter cysts. *B,* The daughter cysts have been removed revealing the glistening inner surface of the cyst. *C,* The removed cyst contents show numerous daughter cysts. (From Reeder MM, Palmer PES: The Radiology of Tropical Diseases [with Epidemiological, Pathological and Clinical Correlation]. Baltimore, Williams & Wilkins Company, 1981.)

retroperitoneum, or may grow anteriorly into the peritoneum and adjacent organs. Alternatively, a cyst may rupture into the renal pelvis with accompanying renal colic, and portions of the cyst contents, as well as blood, will be present in the urine. Secondary infection of the cyst and kidney are usual if this occurs.

Radiological Findings

A plain film of the abdomen may demonstrate a localized bulge on the renal contour, which is often in the anterior region because it is the area of least resistance.

The cyst may or may not be calcified and is more often found by chance on urography, causing distortion of the renal calyces, infundibula, or pelvis.[42] Angiographically, there is no neovascularity or intrinsic abnormality of the renal vessels, and the lesion may be indistinguishable from a simple serous cyst or avascular tumor.[1, 41, 52] If a vascular rim is found during the capillary or venous phase, a hydatid cyst should be seriously suspected. The pattern of calcification in renal hydatids is nonspecific, ranging from a delicate eggshell appearance to dense, reticular calcification (Fig. 30–16). Multiple ringshaped calcifications within a larger calcified lesion suggest the presence of daughter cysts. If a calcified hydatid cyst has collapsed,

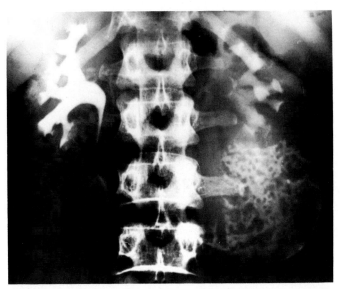

Figure 30–16. *Echinococcus* cyst of the kidney. An excretory urogram reveals a calcified mass occupying the lower pole of the left kidney. The lacy pattern of calcification is often encountered in hydatid disease.

it will have the typical "crushed eggshell" or "sunburst" appearance, which at times may be confused with neoplastic or tuberculous calcification (Fig. 30–17).

Basically, three types of hydatid cysts can be recognized on intravenous or retrograde urography. Closed hydatids have an intact cyst lining and adventitia and do not communicate with the renal collecting system. The outline of the kidney may be enlarged, with a rounded mass (with or without calcification) causing elongation and splaying of the infundibula and calyces and, occasionally, obliteration of one or more calyces because of pressure. These cysts, expecially if not calcified, may be impossible to differentiate from other renal masses by pyelography, urography, or angiography, as already noted (Fig. 30–18). Nephrotomography may show a thick cyst wall with an inhomogeneous lucent center. Ultrasonography, however, is very accurate in demonstrating renal hydatid disease, and if the "sand" can be demonstrated, the differential diagnosis, ruling out a simple cyst, can be established.[46, 58] Similarly, CT scanning clearly demonstrates renal cysts but does not provide an absolute diagnosis. Biopsy of the renal cyst with a fine needle has proved harmless, but cyst rupture may lead to acute "toxic" shock and may be a major catastrophe. Dissemination of fertile hydatid bodies into the perinephric and retroperitoneal tissues is an added hazard.[54]

The pseudoclosed type of hydatid cyst shows resorption of the adventitia of the cyst wall (pericyst) and the calyceal epithelium. This permits contrast medium to interpose itself in crescent-like fashion in the space between the laminated ectocyst and the adventitia, producing the "goblet" or "wine-glass" sign (Surraco's Sign) (Fig. 30–19).[53]

In the open type of hydatid cyst, an intermittent or permanent communication exists between the hydatid and the pyelocalyceal system, so that contrast medium flows directly into the cyst. Usually, the contrast medium has a typical mottled appearance and insinuates itself among a mass of daughter cysts. However, occasionally, if the cyst contents are tightly packed, the contrast is compressed between the contents and cyst wall to produce an extensive false crescent sign.[47, 55]

Multiple hydatid cysts may occur along the ureter, and single or multiple hydatid cysts can occur in the urinary bladder, with or without calcification of the cyst walls.

The CT and sonographic appearances of renal hydatidosis have been amply described, both studies yielding important and often quite similar information.[46, 58] It is not, however, pathognomonic in most cases. In its earliest stages of development, a round anechoic cyst is identifiable, and its wall may be somewhat thicker than that seen with simple serous cysts.[46] Mural irregularity, if seen, suggests the presence of scolices. Calcification is frequent, and "sand" may be encountered. Such cysts may visibly enhance by CT, following contrast administration.[47] Later, when daughter cysts are produced, ultrasonography will reveal a multilocular structure with curvilinear septa within the cysts (Fig. 30–20).[60] Parallel echogenic "stripes," formed when the membranes of dead daughter cysts become adherent, are very suggestive of an echinococcal origin.[46] Hydatid cysts tend to have a low CT attenuation value when unilocular,[60] but as daughter cysts are formed, the CT appearance becomes heterogenous. The daughter cysts, however, which usually arrange themselves peripherally around the mother cyst, almost invariably exhibit a lower CT attenuation value than does the parent cyst,[60] resulting in a rosette appearance (Fig. 30–21). Ultrasonography has been used to monitor the progress of hydatic cysts undergoing medical therapy. During treatment, the cyst may be seen to undergo a metamorphosis, changing from an anechoic pattern, to a complex, and finally a "pseudosolid" pattern, owing to detachments of the cyst membrane and the appearance of an echogenic matrix in its center.[61] Under the effects of therapy, cysts may shrink notably, and may calcify.

FILARIASIS

Filarial infections are widespread in various parts of the world, and probably 200 million people are infected with different filariae in the tropical and subtropical countries of Africa, Asia, the Pacific Islands, and Central and South America. Although present in some islands of the Caribbean, filariasis is not seen in the United States. There is a fairly strict geographic distribution and a variable incidence of infection. The peak ages of infection are from 10 to 12 years, but the symptoms and signs may not develop for many years thereafter. Although the most common clinical findings are those related to elephantiasis, the urinary tract may be involved with resultant chyluria.

Chyluria is the passage of lymphatic fluid in the urine associated with lymphatic abnormalities, and it may be either tropical or nontropical in nature.[72] The tropical form is by far the most common and is almost always due to *Wuchereria bancrofti* infection. Filariasis results when the larvae of *W. bancrofti* are transmitted to the human by mosquitoes, after which they migrate in the lymphatics and nodes where they mature. The worms have been known to survive for 10 years in humans. The pathological findings depend on the cycle of filariae and are due to the presence of living or dead larvae or adult worms in the lymphatics, particularly in the afferent channels of

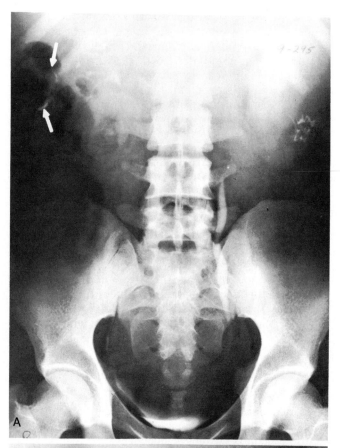

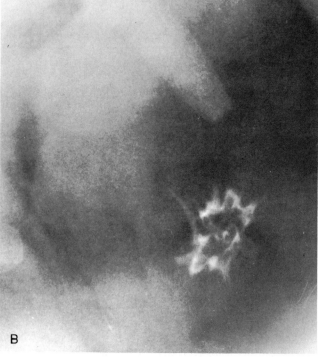

Figure 30–17. *A*, Calcified hydatid cysts in both kidneys. A supine radiograph taken during intravenous urography shows a mass with crescent-shaped calcification in its wall, arising from the lateral margin *(arrows)* of the right kidney. There is a ruptured hydatid cyst in the lower pole of the left kidney with typical "crushed eggshell" or "sunburst appearance." The right renal pyelocalyceal system appears relatively undisturbed by the hydatid cyst arising from the periphery of the renal cortex. The left renal pyelocalyceal system does not fill out well, although contrast in the left ureter is considerable, indicating a functioning kidney. *B*, Close-up of the crushed eggshell or sunburst calcification, which is virtually pathognomonic for a collapsed hydatid cyst. (From Reeder MM, Palmer PES: The Radiology of Tropical Diseases [with Epidemiological, Pathological and Clinical Correlation]. Baltimore, Williams & Wilkins Company, 1981.)

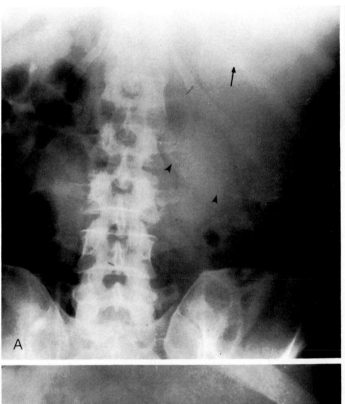

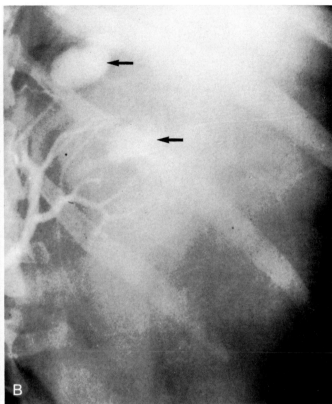

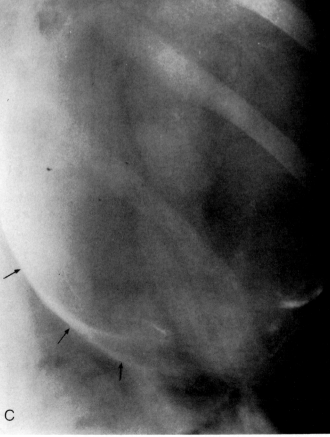

Figure 30–18. Huge communicating hydatid cyst of the left ureter. *A,* An intravenous urogram shows a large mass *(arrowheads)* arising in the left kidney. The right kidney appears normal. Contrast medium is minimal in distorted calyces in the upper pole of the left kidney *(arrow). B,* Left renal arteriogram shows stretching of intrarenal branches around the large avascular mass. Some contrast medium is noted in blunt distorted calyces in the upper pole *(arrow). C,* Contrast medium has spread around the large communicating hydatid cyst, outlining its contour *(arrows).* This may occur during intravenous or retrograde urography or during renal arteriography, when the cyst has ruptured and is communicating. At times, the contrast medium may fill the cyst rather than surround it. (From Reeder MM, Palmer PES: The Radiology of Tropical Diseases [with Epidemiological, Pathological and Clinical Correlation]. Baltimore, Williams & Wilkins Company, 1981.)

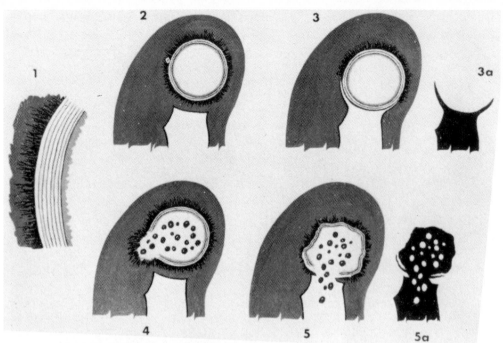

Figure 30–19. The three layers of a renal hydatid cyst, and its relationship to the collecting system are represented: *1,* endocyst, ectocyst, and pericyst constituting the wall of a hydatid cyst; *2,* closed cyst with all three membranes intact, overlying a calyx; *3,* exposed cyst with absence of adventitial layer or pericyst—cyst is in close contact with urine. Note "goblet sign"; *4, 5, and 5a,* open cysts resulting from rupture and discharge of daughter cysts. (From Kirkland K: Urological aspects of hydatid disease. Br J Urol 38:241–254, 1966.)

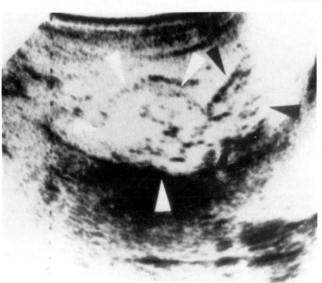

Figure 30–20. Sonogram of renal and hepatic hydatid cysts. Longitudinal ultrasound scan of right kidney shows loculated cystic mass within kidney *(white arrows)* and second similar mass above kidney *(black arrows)* and beneath right lobe of liver. At surgery, the upper mass was found to be in the liver. (From Babcock DS, Kaufman L, Cosnow I: Ultrasound diagnosis of hydatid disease (echinococcosis) in two cases. AJR 131(5):895–897, 1978, © by Am Roentgen Ray Soc.)

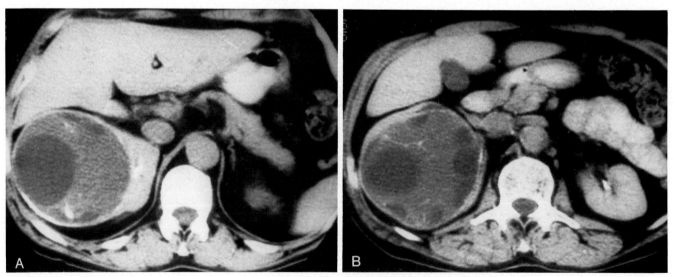

Figure 30–21. Hydatid cyst of the kidney. CT appearance. *A,* A 64-year-old man with palpable right flank mass. Contrast-enhanced CT reveals large right renal mass. The wall is densely calcified, and discrete low-attenuation cysts are noted within a somewhat higher attenuation matrix. *B,* A more caudal CT section reveals multiple daughter cysts arranged in rosette formation around the periphery of the mother cyst. Fine, delicate internal calcifications can be seen. Surgery revealed large hydatid cysts. No other intra-abdominal manifestations of hydatid disease were encountered. (Courtesy Drs. Jose and Felix Lerborgne, Montevideo, Uruguay.)

the pelvis. The living worm causes lymphadenitis and lymphangitis, with edema, eosinophilic infiltration, and fibroblastic reaction. Fever occurs during this stage. When the disease becomes more chronic and the worms die and disintegrate, the walls of the lymphatics thicken and a marked granulomatous reaction occurs around the dead filariae; eventually the adult worm may calcify. In spite of an inflammatory reaction in the walls of the veins, capillaries, and especially the lymphatics (which are selectively involved), many patients will be clinically normal and quite asymptomatic.

The chronic complications of filariasis occur from 5 to 20 years after the primary infection and include elephantiasis, chyluria, and chylous ascites. The thickening of the soft tissues is often enormous. The elephantiasis is not only due to fibrosis and obliteration of the lymphatics and lymph nodes but also to the reaction in the small blood vessels, particularly the veins. Enlargement of the penis, scrotum, and breast may be spectacular, in addition to the gross enlargement of one or more extremities.[64, 70]

Radiological examination of the soft tissues shows gross thickening with loss or blurring of the fat planes. Although technically very difficult, lymphangiography should be attempted. It will show an increase in the number of small lymphatic channels, which have a redundant and tortuous course.[68, 70] Dermal backflow is often present. Occasionally, contrast material flows from the lymphatics into the kidney and outlines the calyces, infundibula, renal pelves, and even the urinary bladder (Fig. 30–22).

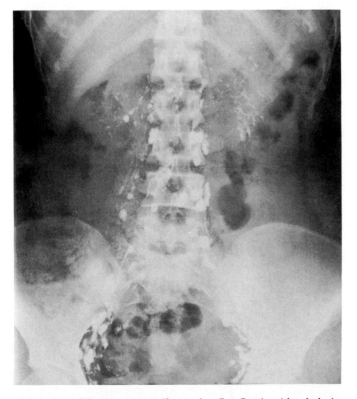

Figure 30–22. A patient (from the Far East) with chyluria. Following lymphography, the contrast medium is seen in a few iliac nodes, presacral nodes, and para-aortic nodes. Contrast medium has gained access to the perinephric and pericalyceal lymphatics, which fill in a retrograde fashion. (From Reeder MM, Palmer PES: The Radiology of Tropical Diseases [with Epidemiological, Pathological and Clinical Correlation]. Baltimore, Williams & Wilkins Company, 1981.)

Intravenous urography is usually normal, but pyelolymphatic reflux may be noted. Dilated renal lymphatics may be clearly demonstrated, particularly when ureteral pressure is applied (there is no reason to perform this examination unless lymphuria is present). When ureteral pressure is adequate, or on retrograde urography, backflow may be dramatic and may extend as far as the major para-aortic lymph nodes. Occasionally, saccular collections of contrast material are seen in the para-aortic region and in renal hila on lymphangiography. Whereas the lymphatics normally empty in a few hours, this process may be markedly delayed for several days in patients with filariasis. The retroperitoneal and pelvic lymph nodes may be enlarged with a mottled appearance early in the course of the disease, whereas multiple small round granular nodes can be seen in advanced disease.[68] Apparently, there are no direct effects on the kidneys, although they may be enlarged in the presence of severe lymphatic disease, a situation that may be mistaken for renal vein thrombosis. Contrast medium may remain within the intrarenal lymphatics for a long time (Fig. 30–18).[62, 63, 65–69, 71] In the usual case of chyluria caused by filariasis, the contrast medium may pass from the kidney to the bladder as evidenced by the fact that it is seen simultaneously in the renal pelvis and in the urinary bladder. It has been shown that obstruction of the thoracic duct does not cause chyluria.

Filariasis in India and other Asian countries usually follows the same pattern as that seen in most patients elsewhere, often eventuating in elephantiasis. In India, however, a number of patients present with chyluria, which is always associated with filariasis, but without any lymphedema. Most of these patients have hydroceles or lymphoceles in the groin, but elephantiasis is not present. The patient has a history of fever and chills, or occasionally of painful lymphangitis of the legs or groin, and transient swelling. A marked loss of lymph occurs in the urine, which may "set" like jelly if left standing in a test tube. The patients are malnourished, and pyelonephritis is always present.

Routine plain radiographs are normal. Intravenous urography without compression shows pyelonephritis and varying degrees of pyelosinus reflux. Lymphangiography shows normal or dilated lymphatics in the leg as far as the groin.

A characteristic rapid transit of the contrast media occurs, and numerous dilated and tortuous lymphatics are found in the inguinal region, with varices and collaterals extending to the retroperitoneum. The inguinal nodes do not fill; the para-aortic nodes are also bypassed by the lymphatic varices, which cross the midline and enter the perinephric lymphatics on both sides.

The perinephric and intrarenal lymphatics are dilated, and they surround and often outline the major and minor calyces (Fig. 30–23). Contrast material often enters the renal collecting system and can be followed into the bladder. The lymph varices connect with the cisterna chyli, which is also dilated.[2]

The entire lymphangiogram may be accomplished within 30 minutes, and the thoracic duct is often visualized in its entirety. In a large series of cases, no obstructions have been demonstrated, and delayed radiographs do not show the usual accumulation of contrast medium in the lymph nodes. It seems probable that this group of patients from India has a congenital scarcity of groin and para-

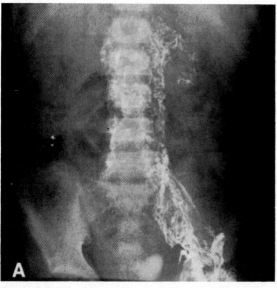
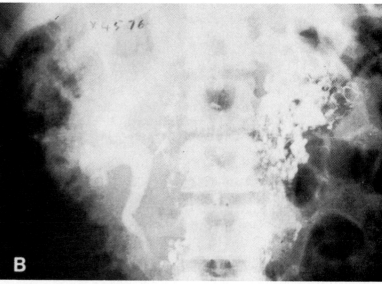

Figure 30–23. *A,* Lymphogram shows chyluria in an Indian. An abundance of dilated left inguinal and para-aortic lymph varices are noted, but the inguinal nodes are not visualized. The contrast enters the perinephric lymphatic varices and the renal calyces. There is cross filling of the right renal lymph varices. Some of the contrast medium (Ethiodol) is seen in the urinary bladder, having traveled down the ureter. *B,* In a chyluric patient from South India, this lymphangiogram was followed by an intravenous urogram. Within one-half hour of injecting contrast medium into a lymphatic channel of the left foot, it is in multiple dilated lymph varices near both renal hila, mainly on the left side. The calyces are outlined by dilated pericalyceal lymphatics. The urogram showed bilateral hydronephrotic changes with calyceal clubbing and also delayed renal function on the left side. Chyluria was more severe from the left kidney. (From Reeder MM, Palmer PES: The Radiology of Tropical Diseases [with Epidemiological, Pathological and Clinical Correlation]. Baltimore, Williams & Wilkins Company, 1981.)

aortic lymph nodes, but an excess of lymphatics in the variceal form. This would explain the absence of lymphedema and the poor filling or absence of contrast medium in the lymph nodes, as well as the rapid transit of contrast to the level of the kidneys. The inflammatory changes in the renal pelvis that result from pyelonephritis alter the interface between the lymphatics and the calyces, thus allowing lymph to leak through microruptures from the intrarenal lymphatics into the renal calyces and pelvis. An alternative explanation for these findings suggests that the filariae can pass freely up the lymphatics without causing irritation or fibrosis in these patients. Possibly, elephantiasis does not develop in filariasis without secondary infection or other precipitating factors, a hypothesis that would explain why only a very small percentage of patients with filariasis eventually develop lymphatic blockage—not only in India, but among other populations in which filariasis is common. This problem obviously requires further study.

MISCELLANEOUS PARASITES AFFECTING THE URINARY TRACT

Other parasites may also infest the genitourinary system. The resulting infections include dracunculosis (guinea worm infestation), trichomoniasis, amebiasis, and Chaga's disease. Infection can also result from the tiny catfish *Candiru*, which can migrate up the urethra of natives who swim in the Amazon. With rare exception, however, these parasites do not give rise to uroradiological manifestations.[3]

References

General References

1. Binford CH, Connor DH: Pathology of Tropical and Extraordinary Diseases. Washington DC, Armed Forces Institute of Pathology, 1976.
2. Reeder MM, Palmer PES: The Radiology of Tropical Diseases (with Epidemiological, Pathological and Clinical Correlation). Baltimore, Williams & Wilkins Company, 1981.
3. Husain I: Tropical Urology and Renal Disease. London, Churchill Livingstone, 1984.

Schistosomiasis

4. Al-Ghorab MM, El-Rifaie M, Abou El Azm T, et al: Radiologic findings of bilharzial (schistosomal) contracted bladder. Urology 11:303–305, 1978.
5. Alvarez SA: Urogenital bilharziasis (apropos of 28 cases). J Trop Med Hyg 48:154–181, 1972.
6. Bhagwandeen SB: The pathology of ureteric bilharziasis. S Afr Med J 41:950–955, 1967.
7. Buchanan WM, Gelfand M: Calcification of the bladder in urinary schistosomiasis. Trans R Soc Trop Med Hyg 64:593–596, 1970.
8. Chatelain C, et al: The schistosomoid ureteral stenosis at the lumbo-iliac level. J Urol Nephrol 79:276–279, 1973.
9. Cheever AW, Young SW, Shohata A: Calcification of *Schistosoma haematobium* eggs: Relation of radiologically demonstrable calcification to eggs in tissues and passage of eggs in urine. Trans R Soc Trop Med Hyg 69:410–414, 1975.
10. Cheynet M: Radiological study of urinary bilharziasis. J Urol Med Chir 66:237–253, 1960.
11. El-Badawi AA: Bilharzial polypi of the urinary bladder. Br J Urol 38:24–35, 1966.
12. Gelfand M: Pulmonary schistosomiasis in the early "Katayama" phase of the disease. J Trop Med Hyg 69:143–144, 1966.
13. Gelfand M, Gilles HM: Filling defects of the bladder on intravenous pyelography in children passing schistosome ova in the urine. J Trop Med Hyg 69:4–6, 1966.
14. Ghoneim MA, Awaad HK: Results of treatment in carcinoma of the bilharzial bladder. J Urol 123:850, 1980.

15. Gilles HM, Lucas A, Adenyi-Jones C, et al: *Schistosoma haematobium* infection in Nigeria. II. Infection at a primary school in Ibadan. Ann Trop Med Parasitol 59:451–450, 1965.
16. Girges MR: The syndrome of bladder-neck obstruction and ureteric fibrosis in *Schistosoma haematobium* infection. J Trop Med Hyg 69:187–188, 1966.
17. Honey RM, Gelfand M: The urological aspects of bilharziasis in Rhodesia. Cent Afr J Med 6:199–212, 1960.
18. Iarotskii LS, Medvedev VF, Zal'Nova NS: Urogenital schistosomiasis in the People's Democratic Republic of Yemen and its clinicoroentgenological characteristics. Med Parazitol 46:485–487, 1977.
19. Mahmoud AA: Schistosomiasis. N Engl J Med 297:1329, 1977.
20. Rocha H, Cruz T, Brito E, et al: Renal involvement in patients with hepatosplenic schistosomiasis mansoni. Am J Trop Med Hyg 25:108–115, 1976.
21. Saad SM, Hanafy HM: Bilharzial (schistosomal) polypi of ureter. Urology 4:85, 1974.
22. Saad SM, Hanafy HM: Bilharzial (schistosomal) ureteritis cystica. Urology 4:261, 1974.
23. Shokeir AA, Ibrahim AM, Hamid MY, et al: Urinary bilharziasis in upper Egypt (I and II). East Afr Med J 49:298–326, 1972.
24. Stepanov EP: X-ray data in schistosomiasis of the urinary tracts. Vestn Roentgenol Radiol 4:72–76, 1976.
25. Umerah BC: Evaluation of the physiological function of the ureter by fluoroscopy in bilharziasis. Radiology 124:645–647, 1977.
26. Umerah BC: Less familiar manifestations of schistosomiasis of the urinary tract. Br J Radiol 40:105, 1977.
27. Weber MC, Blair DM, Clark VV de: The distribution of viable and non-viable eggs of *Schistosoma haematobium* in the urine. Cent Afr J Med 15:27–30, 1969.
28. Degremont A, Burnier E, Meudt R, et al: Value of ultrasonography in investigating morbidity due to *Schistosoma haematobium* infection. Lancet 1:662–665, 1985.
29. Gentile JM: Schistosome-related cancers: A possible role of genotoxins. Environ mutagen 7:775–785, 1985.
30. Genseke R, Hofs R, Otto HJ, Meinhard F: X-ray and nuclear medicine studies in children with urinary bilharziasis (German with English abstract). Radiol Diagn (Berlin) 26:575–580, 1985.
31. Jorulf H, et al: Urogenital schistosomiasis: CT evaluation. Radiology 157:745–749, 1985.
32. Sewcz C, et al: X-ray findings in urogenital bilharziosis. Radiol Diagn (Berlin) 26:213–219, 1985.
33. Wilkins HA, et al: Isotope renography and urinary schistosomiasis: A study in a Gambian community. Trans R Soc Trop Med Hyg 79:306–313, 1985.
34. World Health Statistics: Global distribution of schistosomiasis: CEGET/WHO atlas (English and French). WHO Stat Q 37:186–199, 1984.
35. Makar N: The bilharzial ureter. Br J Surg 36:148, 1958.
36. Al-Ghorab MM: Ureteritis calcinosa. A complication of bilharzial ureteritis and its relation to primary ureteric stone formation. Br J Urol 34:33, 1962.
37. Hugosson C, Olsen P: Early ureteric changes in schistosomiasis haematobia infection. Clin Radiol 37:501, 1986.
38. Hugosson C: Striation of the renal pelvis and ureter in bilharziasis. Clin Radiol 38:407, 1987.
39. Dittrich M, Doering E: Ultrasonic aspects of urinary schistosomiasis: Assessment of morphologic lesions in the upper and lower urinary tract. Pediatr Radiol 16:225, 1986.
40. Jacobsson B, Linstedt E, Narasimham DL, et al: Balloon dilatation of bilharzial ureteric strictures. Br J Urol 60:28, 1987.

Hydatid Disease

41. Baltaxe HA, Fleming RJ: The angiographic appearance of hydatid disease. Radiology 97:559–604, 1970.

42. Begg RC: Pyelography in renal hydatids. Br J Surg 24:691–701, 1937.
43. Bloomfield JA: Protean radiological manifestations of hydatid infestation. Aust Radiol 10:330–343, 1966.
44. Bonakdarpour A: *Echinococcus* disease. Report of 112 cases from Iran and a review of 611 cases from the United States. AJR 99:660–667, 1967.
45. Diamond HM, et al: Echinococcal disease of the kidney. J Urol 115:742–744, 1976.
46. King DL: Ultrasonography of echinococcal cysts. J Clin Ultrasound 1:64–67, 1976.
47. Kirkland K: Urological aspects of hydatid disease. Br J Urol 38:241–254, 1966.
48. Musacchio F, et al: Primary renal echinococcosis—a case report. Am J Trop Med Hyg 15:168–171, 1966.
49. O'Leary P: A five-year study of human hydatid disease in Turkana district—Kenya. East Afr Med J 53:540–544, 1976.
50. Reay ER, Polleston GL: Diagnosis of hydatid cyst of the kidney. J Urol 64:26–52, 1950.
51. Reeder MM: Tropical diseases of the liver and bile ducts. Semin Roentgenol 10:229–243, 1975.
52. Shawket IN, et al: Hydatid cysts of the kidney simulating similar kidney lesions. Br J Urol 46:371–376, 1974.
53. Surraco LA: Renal hydatidosis. Am J Surg 44:581–586, 1939.
54. Roylance J, Davies ER, Alexander WD: Translumbar puncture of a renal hydatid cyst. Br J Radiol 46:960, 1973.
55. Beggs I: The radiology of hydatid disease. AJR 145:639, 1985.
56. Aragona F, DiCandio G, Seretta V, Florentini L: Renal hydatid disease: Report of 9 cases and discussion of urologic diagnostic procedures. Urol Radiol 6:182, 1984.
57. Gilsanz V, Lozano F, Jiminez J: Renal hydatid cysts: Communicating with collecting system. AJR 135:357, 1980.
58. Babcock DS, Kaufman L, Cosnow I: Ultrasound diagnosis of hydatid disease (echinococcosis) in two cases. AJR 131:895, 1978.
59. Hertz M, Zissin R, Dresnik Z, et al: Echinococcus of the urinary tract: Radiologic findings. Urol Radiol 6:175, 1984.
60. Kalovidouris A, Pissiotis C, Pontifex G, et al: CT characterization of multivesicular hydatid cysts. J Comput Assist Tomogr 10:428, 1986.
61. Bezzi M, Teggi A, DeRosa F, et al: Abdominal hydatid disease. Ultrasound findings during medical treatment. Radiology 162:91, 1987.

Filariasis

62. Bernageau J, et al: Lymphography in chyluria. J Radiol Electrol 45:529–540, 1964.
63. Chen KC: Lymphatic abnormalities in patients with chyluria. Urology 106:111–114, 1971.
64. Davey WW: Chronic lymphoedema. Companion to Surgery in Africa. London, E & S Livingstone Ltd, 1968, pp 37–48.
65. Kittredge RD, Hashim S, et al: Demonstration of lymphatic abnormalities in a patient with chyluria. AJR 90:159–165, 1963.
66. Koehler PR, Chiang TC, et al: Lymphography in chyluria. AJR 102:455–465, 1968.
67. Legre J: Radiological aspects of urinary bilharziasis and filariasis. J Radiol Electrol Med Nucl 40:816–818, 1959.
68. Montangerand Y, et al: Lymphographic aspects of filarian adenopathy. J Radiol Electrol Med Nucl 50:135–142, 1969.
69. Ortiz F, Walzak MP, et al: Chyluria: Lymphaticourinary fistula demonstrated by lymphangiography. J Urol 91:608–612, 1964.
70. Reeder MM: Tropical diseases of the soft tissues. Semin Roentgenol 8:47–71, 1973.
71. Swanson GE: Lymphangiography in chyluria. Radiology 81:473–478, 1963.
72. Klousia JW, McClennan BL, Semerjian HS: Chyluria: A case report and brief literature review. J Urol 117:393, 1977.

31

Urogenital Tuberculosis

MILTON ELKIN

In the United States, about 30,000 new cases of tuberculosis occur annually, of which 10% to 15% are in extrapulmonary sites.[1, 2] Urogenital tuberculosis is the third most common extrapulmonary site, after lymphatic tissue and pleura, and constitutes 3% to 4% of all new cases of tuberculosis or about 30% of new extrapulmonary cases.[3]

The initial symptoms of genitourinary tuberculosis become manifest most commonly in the 20- to 50-year age group,[4, 5] and about twice as often in males as in females.[6–9] Urinary tract tuberculosis is uncommon in children, possibly as a result of the time lag (average 8 years) between an initial pulmonary infection and the clinical appearance of genitourinary tuberculosis.[10]

In symptomatic patients, lower urinary tract symptoms are the most common, consisting of dysuria, frequency of urination, nocturia, and urgency.[4, 6–9] Gross hematuria occurs in about 20% to 25%, with microscopic hematuria being found in most patients (75%). In a series of 127 male patients with renal tuberculosis, the initial symptom was related to tuberculous epididymitis for 36%.[4] However, 10% to 20% of patients with urogenital tuberculosis—even advanced disease—may have no urinary tract symptoms.[4, 6]

Sterile pyuria, microscopic hematuria, and acid pH are the features of urinalysis that suggest the diagnosis of urogenital tuberculosis. The diagnosis should also be considered in patients with recurrent urinary tract infections or urinary tract infection that is unresponsive to therapy for the usual pathogens. Definitive diagnosis is made by the demonstration of acid-fast tubercle bacilli in a Ziehl-Neelsen's preparation of urine or culture of the urine on a special medium (Lowenstein-Jensen). At present, guinea pig inoculation is only occasionally needed. Diagnosis can also rest on positive tissue biopsy or needle aspiration (e.g., from bladder, prostate, kidney).

Tuberculous infection of the kidney is most commonly the result of hematogenous seeding by *Myobacterium tuberculosis* from the lung, with the urinary tract involvement not becoming clinically evident until many years after the clinical manifestations of active pulmonary disease appear. The skeletal or the gastrointestinal system can also be the site of the primary infection. Clinically silent renal granulomas containing tubercle bacilli can remain stable for as long as 15 to 20 years before breaking down. The peak age incidence of urinary tract tuberculosis is, on the average, 5 to 10 years later than that of the initial manifestations of active pulmonary tuberculosis. Analyses of chest films in patients with urogenital tuberculosis have shown widely varying results in reported series. As expected, evidence of active pulmonary tuberculosis is frequent (about 40%) in patients of hospitals specializing in tuberculosis.[7, 11] In the general hospital population, about 10% of patients with urogenital tuberculosis show radiological evidence of active pulmonary disease; 35% to 50% have normal lungs, and 40% to 55% have radiological evidence of inactive or healed

pulmonary tuberculosis.[6, 8, 12] About 2% to 5% of patients presenting with active pulmonary tuberculosis also show evidence of urogenital tuberculosis. In a series of 5000 autopsies of patients who died of tuberculosis in a large New York City municipal hospital, genitourinary lesions were found in 26%, almost half of whom had generalized miliary tuberculosis. This contrasts with an incidence of only 3% of generalized miliary tuberculosis in the other 74% of the total group who had no autopsy evidence of genitourinary tuberculosis.[13]

KIDNEY

Discharge of *Myobacterium tuberculosis* into the blood stream from an active site of infection (most often pulmonary) leads to the formation of miliary tuberculomas in the kidneys. Most of the granulomas occur in the renal

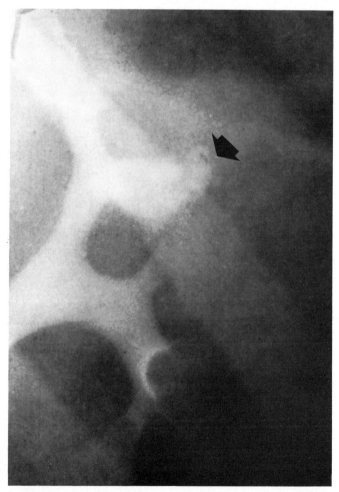

Figure 31–1. Early cavitation in renal tuberculosis. Urography shows caseation into a calyx with formation of an irregular cavity (*arrow*), simulating the appearance of renal papillary necrosis, in a 30-year-old woman with microscopic hematuria. Urine culture was positive for tuberculosis.

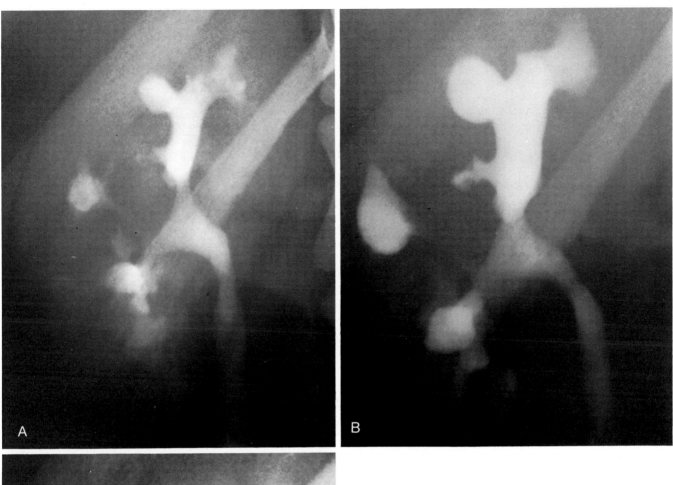

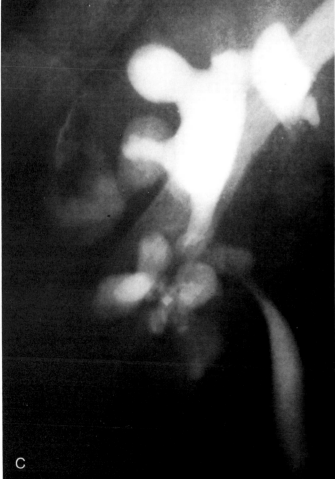

Figure 31–2. Progressing radiological findings during treatment in a 27-year-old man with gross hematuria and frequent urination. Urinary tuberculosis proved by positive bladder biopsy. *A,* Initial urogram shows caseation into several calyces with irregular cavitations. Patient was placed on triple chemotherapy. *B,* Repeat urogram obtained 3 months later shows calyceal dilatations, likely due to strictures of infundibula. *C,* Urogram obtained 6 months after *B* shows fibrotic narrowing of the renal pelvis, as well as progressive calyceal dilatation and several communicating parenchymal cavities.

cortices. No doubt, their location is related to the distribution of blood flow in the kidney. Usually, these multiple minute tubercles heal, either spontaneously or as a result of antituberculous chemotherapy administered to control the clinically active primary focus. Nevertheless, one or more tubercles may enlarge after years of inactivity. An enlarging focus in the cortex can break into the renal tubular system, allowing the *M. tuberculosis* organism to be carried to the pyramid, where an active tuberculoma develops. Such foci may eventually rupture into a calyx, even after years of dormancy. Similarly, the calyx can be involved by enlargement of one or a coalescence of the miliary tuberculomas that had been seeded in the pyramid from the initial hematogenous focus in the cortex.

Even though the miliary tubercles involve both kidneys, the progression to clinical activity usually occurs unilaterally. The stage of parenchymal miliary tubercles, before calyceal involvement, produces no radiological findings. When a calyx is involved, urography becomes positive, although the result is initially subtle—a slight loss of sharpness of the calyx, which very likely represents mucosal edema. Progressive enlargement of the tuberculoma and its caseation into the adjacent calyx result in a cavity that is irregular, and that resembles renal papillary necrosis on an intravenous urogram or retrograde pyelogram (Figs. 31–1, 31–2*A* and 31–3). This appearance has led

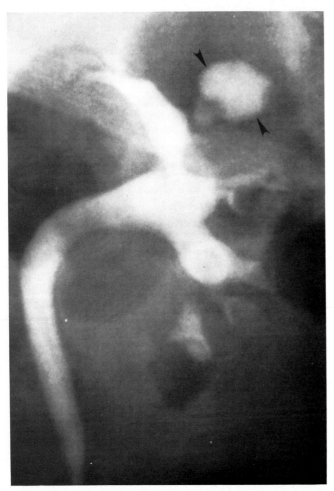

Figure 31–3. Cavitation into a calyx. Urogram shows relatively smooth cavitation *(arrowheads)* into a single calyx in a 12-year-old boy with urine culture positive for tuberculosis. (From Elkin M: Radiology of the Urinary System. Boston, Little, Brown & Company, 1980.)

some authors to include tuberculosis as a cause of renal papillary necrosis. Strictly speaking, this is incorrect, because the mechanism of tissue destruction by tuberculosis is very different from that of ischemia, which is the basis of the changes in renal papillary necrosis. Following the establishment of the cavity draining into the calyceal system, pronounced *M. tuberculosis* bacilluria results, introducing the likelihood that renal infection will spread to other parts of the urogenital system.

Renal involvement is common in patients with disseminated miliary tuberculosis. In one autopsy study, over 60% of patients who died of miliary tuberculosis had renal involvement.[13] Pathologically, small granulomas, most of which are in the renal cortices, result from the bacillemia of the miliary tuberculosis. They are similar to the miliary renal granulomas seen in hematogenous seeding with *M. tuberculosis* from an active pulmonary focus. Although these miliary tuberculomas, in their preulcerative stage, do not communicate directly with the pyelocalyceal system, tubercle bacilli may appear in the urine. In a series of 24 patients with miliary tuberculosis, urine cultures were performed in 20, and 5 were positive for *M. tuberculosis*.[6] Other studies have shown similar results.[14, 15]

Although dilatations of the urinary tract in tuberculosis are commonly related to fibrotic strictures, an early and potentially reversible ureteropyelocaliectasis has been attributed to spasm or mucosal edema at the terminal portion of the ureter. Other causes of nonstrictural dilatation could be (1) ureteral atony due to the bacilluria or (2) vesicoureteral reflux, a late manifestation related to bladder changes. Antituberculous chemotherapy can cause regression of an obstruction due to mucosal edema, although the process may take several weeks, or even months. This dilatation must be differentiated from that attributable to a fibrous stricture, which actually might develop and be exaggerated by the fibrosis of healing during chemotherapy.

The abnormalities outlined so far—edema of the calyceal mucosa, initial cavitation of the calyces, and spasm or edema at the terminal portion of the ureter—are the early changes of renal tuberculosis. The late or advanced manifestations include fibrotic stricture, extensive cavitation, mass lesion, calcification, perinephric abscess, and fistula.

Stricture

Renal damage resulting from changes secondary to strictures is greater than that resulting directly from tuberculomas seeded in the renal parenchyma. The fibrosis causing the strictures represents healing of tuberculous ulcerations, and thus may develop during appropriate chemotherapy (Fig. 31–4). In the kidney, stricture of a calyceal neck may occur (resulting in hydrocalyx), of an infundibulum (resulting in focal or regional hydrocalycosis), or of the renal pelvis (resulting in generalized dilatation of calyces and infundibula) (Figs. 31–2*B*, 31–5, and 31–6). Commonly, a number of strictures are present. In addition, deformity of the pyelocalyceal system caused by the traction of a strictured infundibulum and parenchymal fibrosis can kink the pelvis so as to produce obstruction of areas not directly affected by tuberculous ulcerations (Fig. 31–7). Known as Kerr's kinks, these

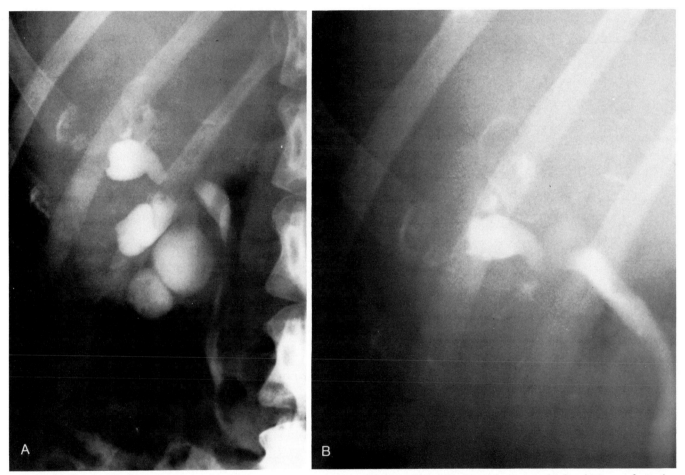

Figure 31—4. Progressive fibrotic strictures in a patient receiving therapy. This 38-year-old woman had a history of ovarian tuberculosis 17 years ago, proved by pelvic laparotomy and biopsy. For the past year she experienced frequency of urination and nocturia. Several urine cultures were positive for tuberculosis. *A,* Intravenous urogram (IVU) shows calyceal dilatations secondary to infundibular strictures. The superior calyces do not visualize, most likely owing to complete block of the superior infundibulum. (From Elkin M: Radiology of the Urinary System. Boston, Little, Brown & Company, 1980.) *B,* This repeat urogram was obtained 15 months after *A.* The patient had antituberculous chemotherapy. Now only very few calyces visualize, most likely due to progressive fibrotic strictures of the infundibula.

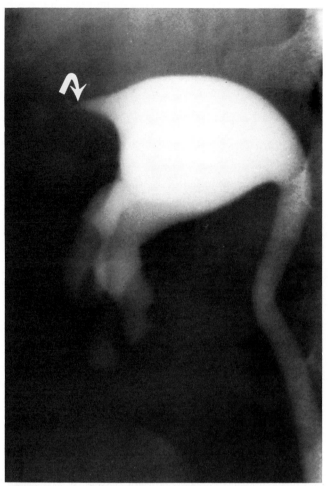

Figure 31–5. Stricture of infundibulum. This 53-year-old man had dysuria and frequent urination. Urinary tuberculosis was proved by bladder biopsy. Retrograde opacification shows a well-defined stricture of the superior (*curved arrow*) infundibulum in a distorted, scarred kidney. Urography had shown poor visualization of the pyelocalyceal system.

cause functional destruction of more of the kidney than had been directly infected by tuberculosis.[16] The mechanical effects of obstructing strictures lead to dilatation of the pyelocalyceal system, with pressure atrophy of the renal tissue. Tuberculous infection in the dilated calyces, resulting in closed pyocalyces, leads to caseation of the surrounding renal tissue (Fig. 31–8). A completely stenosed infundibulum or calyx may lead to the complete failure of contrast excretion by the involved renal parenchyma ("phantom calyx"). If such an area is small and represents the only abnormal focus within the kidney, the urogram may erroneously be interpreted as normal (Fig. 31–6).[17]

Cavitation

Renal cavitations result from caseation of enlarging tuberculomas or conglomerations of tuberculomas. These cavities, if they communicate with the pyelocalyceal system, can be visualized radiographically by urography in functioning kidneys or by retrograde pyelography (Fig. 31–2C and 31–8). Extensive cavitations are referred to as ulcerocavernous; such kidneys usually do not excrete contrast medium at urography.

Mass Lesion

Renal tuberculosis may present radiographically as a mass lesion, representing either a conglomeration of tuberculomas in the renal parenchyma (Fig. 31–9) or a collection of hydrocalyces secondary to an infundibular stricture (Fig. 31–10).

Calcification

Calcification in areas of caseation can be divided into various types, which in most cases are not specifically diagnostic of tuberculosis. The calcification may be homogeneous and only faintly calcified and may have indistinct borders (smudgy), or it may be speckled, with sharply defined calcific densities of varying size; or it may be sharp and curvilinear (Figs. 31–11 to 31–14). A combination of these various types may occur (Fig. 31–15). One type of distribution may be specific for renal tuberculosis. The configuration of the calcification defines the renal lobes. This appearance, which can be referred to as lobar calcification, occurs in far advanced renal tuberculosis in which the kidney shows no evidence of function (Figs. 31–16 and 31–17). Inasmuch as tuberculosis often independently involves each lobe of the kidney, renal destruction takes place lobe by lobe, which accounts for the distribution of the calcification. Likely, the curvilinear calcification is deposited between the central mass of caseation in the kidney lobe and the rim of remaining renal parenchyma.

Calcification demonstrable by urography has been reported in various series, in 10% to 50% of patients with renal tuberculosis, usually in advanced stages of the disease.[8, 9, 11] Computed tomography (CT) detects calcifications with greater accuracy, precision, and sensitivity.

Hydronephrosis

In tuberculosis, dilatation of the pyelocalyceal system along with a segment of the ureter can result from a temporary or a fixed ureteral obstruction, most frequently at the lower end of the ureter (Figs. 31–18 and 31–19). Temporary obstruction can result from edema of ureteral or bladder mucosa, ureteral spasm, or ureteral atony. Fixed obstruction is most commonly due to a ureteral fibrous stricture. If the obstruction is not relieved, destruction and caseation of the kidney result, often being associated with calcification. Even if *M. tuberculosis* is in the destroyed kidney, often no bacteria are found in the urine, because the ureteral lumen is obliterated at the site of the stricture. This condition of isolation of the kidney is referred to as *autonephrectomy* and the caseated kidney, which is often calcified, is called *putty kidney* (Fig. 31–20).

Perinephric Abscess

As already noted, in urinary tuberculosis, several mechanisms lead to obstruction and resulting tuberculous pyocalyces, parenchymal abscesses, or pyonephrosis, any of which may perforate into the perinephric spaces and tissues to cause perinephric abscesses. Secondary infec-

Text continued on page 1035

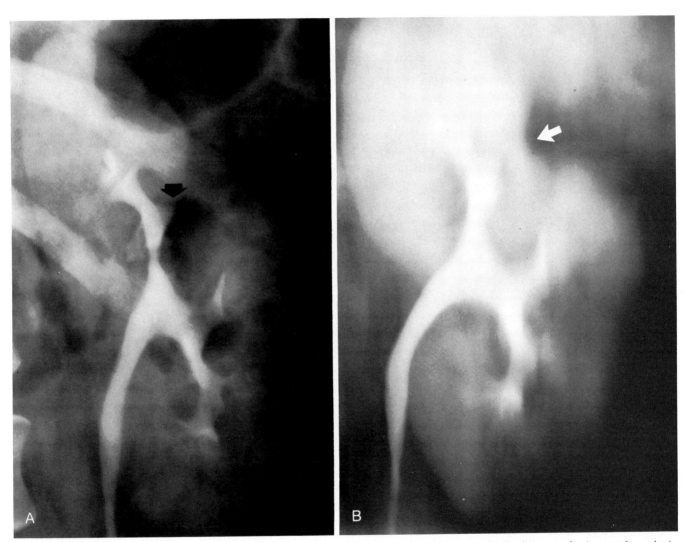

Figure 31–6. Parenchymal scar associated with stricture of calyx. This 37-year-old woman had a history of urinary tuberculosis; urine culture had been positive 15 years ago. At this examination, the right kidney was functionless. *A,* IVU in left posterior oblique projection shows stricture of a calyceal neck (*arrow*). *B,* Tomogram demonstrates a wide parenchymal scar (*arrow*) in the region of the stricture.

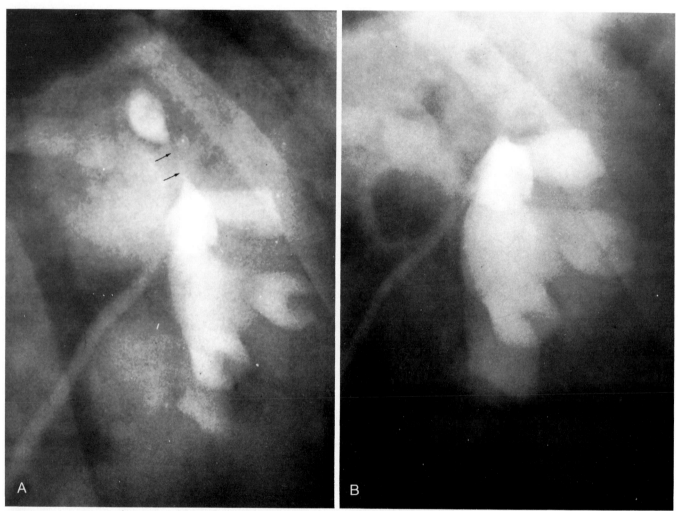

Figure 31–7. Obstruction due to kinking of the renal pelvis. This 35-year-old man had a small calcified nonfunctioning right kidney and urine culture that was positive for tuberculosis. *A,* Urogram at onset of antituberculosis chemotherapy shows a stricture of the superior infundibulum of the left kidney *(arrows)* with kinking of the pelvis superiorly, resulting in dilatation of the middle and inferior groups of calyces (Kerr's kink). *B,* Repeat urogram obtained 15 months after *A* shows nonvisualization of the superior calyces and a greater degree of dilatation of the remaining calyces. (From Elkin M: Radiology of the Urinary System. Boston, Little, Brown & Company, 1980.)

Figure 31–8. Tuberculous pyonephrosis. This 35-year-old woman had dysuria, frequent urination, pyuria, and microscopic hematuria. Usual urine cultures were negative, and no response to antibiotics occurred. Urine cultures were positive for tuberculosis. IVU had demonstrated narrowing of the lower portion of the right ureter with proximal dilatation. Retrograde pyelogram shows marked right hydronephrosis with shaggy borders of the upper calyces due to caseation of surrounding renal parenchyma.

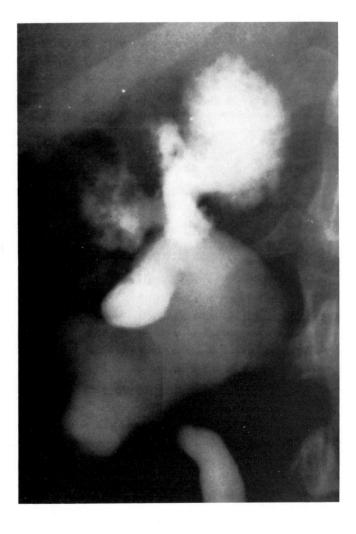

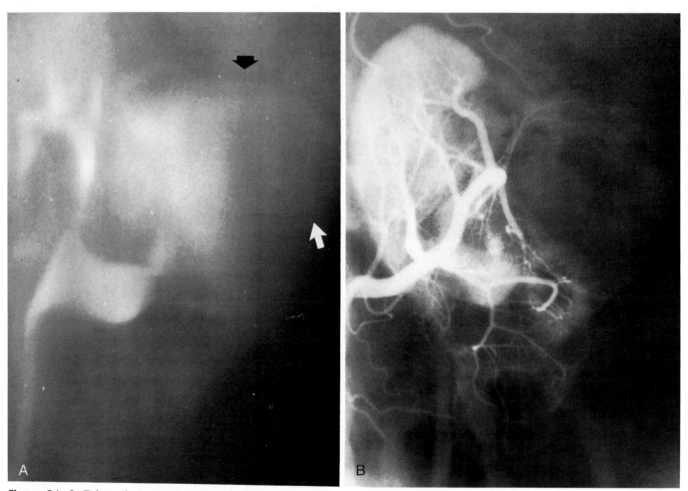

Figure 31–9. Tuberculomas presenting as a large renal mass. This 68-year-old man experienced several months of frequent urination and nocturia. Microscopic hematuria was found. *A,* IVU shows a mass (*arrows*) at the lateral aspect of the left kidney, displacing calyces. *B,* Selective renal arteriogram shows the mass to be hypovascular, representing a conglomeration of tuberculomas. The lower pole of the kidney is scarred and hydronephrotic, owing to tuberculosis.

Figure 31–10. Renal mass due to hydrocalyces. This 37-year-old man complained of left flank pain. Urine culture was positive for tuberculosis. The patient was given triple antituberculosis chemotherapy. *A,* Initial IVU shows stricture of superior infundibulum (*arrow*) with dilatation of the superior calyces. *B,* Urogram 7 years later shows an upper-pole mass and poor opacification of the superior calyces. *C,* Tomogram during urography 4 years after *B* again shows the upper-pole mass and the stricture of the superior infundibulum (*arrow*). *D,* Later in the same study as *C,* it is demonstrated that the mass consists chiefly of marked dilatation of the upper calyces.

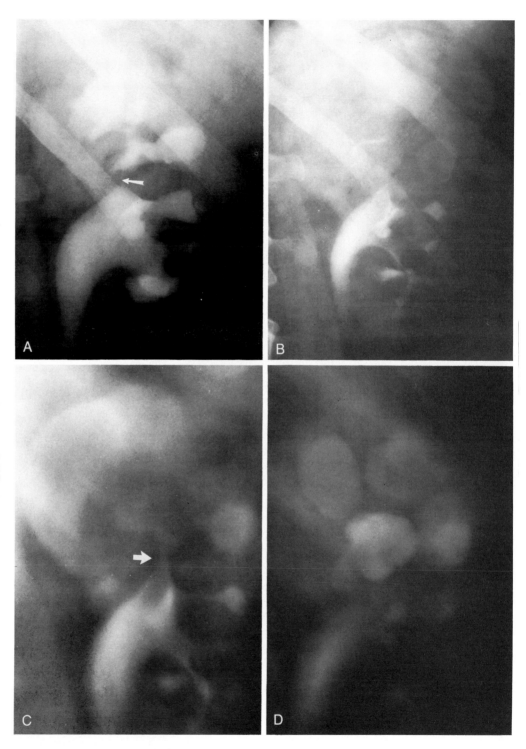

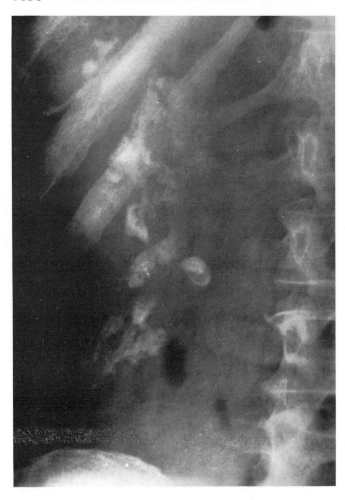

Figure 31–11. Amorphous, smudgy calcification. This 71-year-old woman had a diagnosis of urinary tuberculosis 28 years ago. She had received several courses of antituberculosis medication. Abdominal radiograph shows several collections of calcification in the right kidney, which are largely amorphous and poorly defined. Urography showed no visualization of the collecting system.

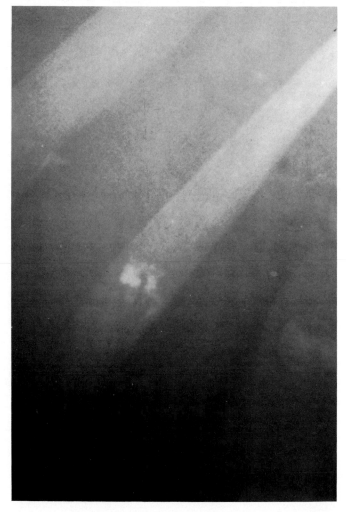

Figure 31–12. Speckled calcification. Scout film of the right kidney shows the speckled type of calcification seen in renal tuberculosis.

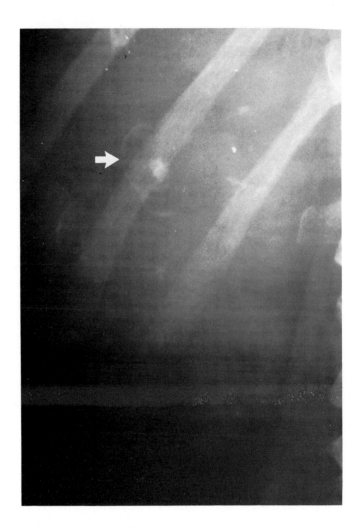

Figure 31–13. Curvilinear calcification (*arrow*) in renal tuberculosis. Scout film is of the same patient as in Figure 31–4. The other small calcifications are in overlying costal cartilages.

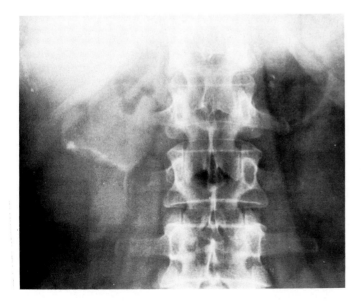

Figure 31–14. Rims of calcification around tuberculomas. This 45-year-old woman had a history of pulmonary and urinary tract tuberculosis. Scout radiograph of the abdomen shows enlargement of the upper pole of the right kidney. Density of the upper pole is also increased, owing to peripheral rims of calcification, which are most likely located around caseated tuberculomas. Subsequent urography showed no excretion of contrast material by the right kidney.

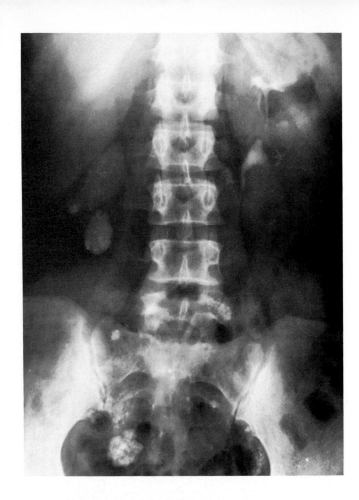

Figure 31–15. Abdominal calcifications due to tuberculosis. This 62-year-old woman presented with no urinary tract symptoms. IVU shows several findings typical of tuberculosis. The right kidney is small and nonexcreting, with calcifications of various types—amorphous, speckled, and curvilinear. The left kidney is enlarged, owing to compensatory hypertrophy resulting from the right autonephrectomy lasting many years. The irregular, rounded calcifications in the pelvis represent old calcified ovarian tuberculosis. Scattered, calcified abdominal and pelvic lymph nodes are also due to tuberculosis.

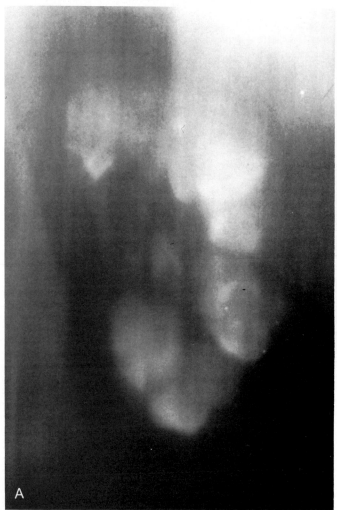

Figure 31–16. Lobar calcification in advanced renal tuberculosis. *A,* Tomogram shows a small left kidney with areas of calcification in lobar distribution. The calcifications are most dense at the periphery of the lobes. Urography demonstrated no excretion of contrast material by the left kidney. *B,* In another patient with a small nonvisualizing right kidney and lobar calcification, a nonenhanced CT scan also shows the calcifications to be most dense at the periphery of the lobes.

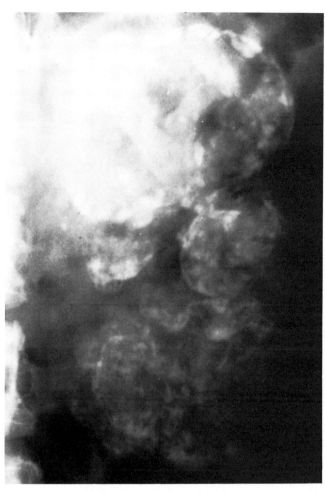

Figure 31–17. Lobar calcification in a large, destroyed kidney. This 86-year-old man with prostatism supplied no history of tuberculosis. Abdominal radiograph shows a large left kidney with irregularly curvilinear and speckled calcifications, generally with a lobar distribution. IVU showed no excretion of contrast medium from the left kidney. Advanced renal tuberculosis was proved at autopsy.

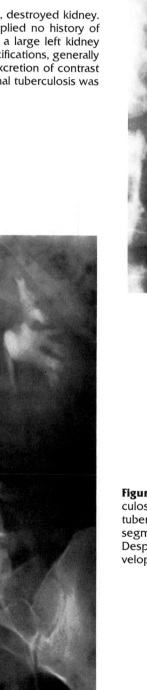

Figure 31–18. Pyeloureterectasis secondary to ureteral tuberculosis. This 35-year-old woman had newly diagnosed urinary tuberculosis. IVU shows irregular narrowing of the terminal segment of the right ureter, with marked dilatation proximally. Despite antituberculosis chemotherapy, a fibrous stricture developed with persistence of the pyeloureterectasis.

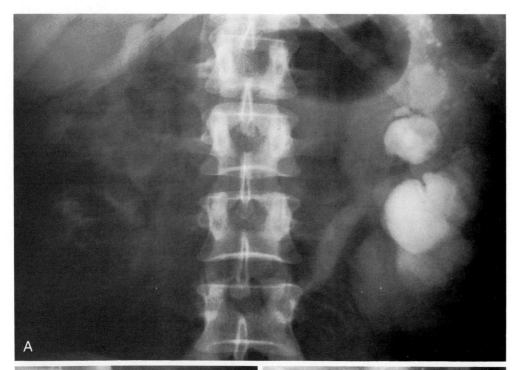

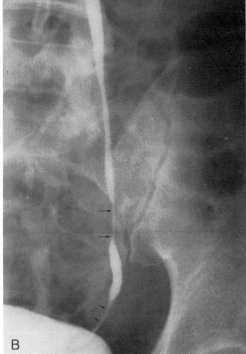

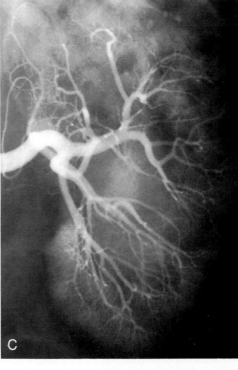

Figure 31–19. Renal tuberculosis and ureteral strictures. This 53-year-old man had bilateral urinary tuberculosis and evidence of renal insufficiency; serum creatinine was 2.5 mg/dl. *A,* IVU shows very poor excretion of the contrast medium by the right kidney. On the left is marked dilatation of the calyces but no corresponding dilatation of the renal pelvis, probably due to fibrosis of the pelvis. The poorly opacified upper segment of the left ureter is dilated. The overlying nodular calcifications represent old granulomas in the spleen. *B,* Left retrograde ureterography shows several long smooth strictures (*arrows*), which account for the dilatation of the proximal ureter. *C,* Selective left renal angiography defines, much better than urography, the extent of renal parenchymal involvement. In the lower pole, the arteries and their branches appear normal. Elsewhere, the arteries are pruned (lack of branches); the nephrogram is inhomogeneous and of diminished intensity. (From Elkin M: Radiology of the Urinary System. Boston, Little, Brown & Company, 1980.)

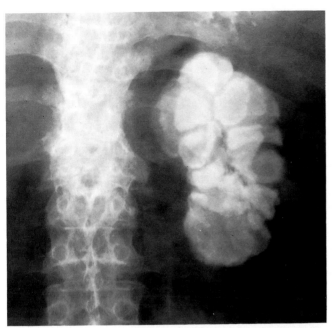

Figure 31–20. "Putty kidney." Abdominal plain radiograph. The large round-to-elliptical calcifications represent calcified caseating material within medullary cavities and dilated calyces. This occurs when an already severely affected tuberculous kidney is further damaged by superimposed ureteral obstruction. Note also the changes of tuberculous spondylitis at the levels of T10 to L1.

tion of the renal lesions with extension into the perinephric tissues can produce superimposed nontuberculous perinephric abscesses.

Fistulas and Sinus Tracts

Extension of perinephric abscesses to adjacent viscera or tissues results in fistulas or sinus tracts, such as nephrogastric, pyeloduodenal, nephrocolonic (Fig. 31–21), and nephrocutaneous.

Pyonephrosis with associated perinephric abscess is the most common cause of fistulas between the kidney and the gastrointestinal tract, resulting more often from nontuberculous than from tuberculous infection. A fistula leading to the stomach is from the left kidney; to the duodenum it is almost always from the right kidney, to the ascending colon from the right kidney, and to the descending colon from the left kidney. Less commonly, such fistulas result from trauma, inflammatory lesions of the gastrointestinal tract, or a primary renal or gastrointestinal neoplasm.

All these fistulas are uncommon, the least common being that between kidney and stomach.[18] A review of 31 cases of pyeloduodenal fistula showed that five were due to renal tuberculosis, and 23 to chronic nontuberculous infection.[19] Almost always, urography shows no excretion of contrast medium from the affected kidney. The diagnosis is established by retrograde pyelography.

URETER

Ureteral involvement is almost always secondary to renal tuberculosis (usually advanced), with spread of

infection by the bacilluria. Occasionally, mycobacteria may hematogenously be carried to the ureter from a distant site, or may gain entry to the ureter from disease in a contiguous site, such as the ovary.[20]

Early manifestations are mucosal edema and ulcerations. The ulcers are linear and found at any level of the ureter, although they are most commonly seen at its distal portion (Fig. 31–22). The sites of ulceration may be numerous. Antituberculous chemotherapy may lead to the ulcers healing completely. However, healing in tuberculosis, with or without chemotherapy, is often accompanied by fibrosis, which leads to strictures, most commonly found in the lower third of the ureter (see Figs. 31–19B and 31–23 to 31–25). Multiple ureteral strictures result in the corkscrew or beaded ureter (Fig. 31–26). Diffuse fibrosis of the entire ureter produces shortening, a thickened rigid wall, and luminal narrowing, known as the pipe-stem ureter (Figs. 31–21 and 31–27). Calcification in the ureteral wall is uncommon (Fig. 31–28).

Ulcerations produce an irregular ureteral lumen, as seen radiologically, sometimes with multiple serrations representing the ulcers (Figs. 31–22 and 31–25). As the ulcers and fibrosis heal, the strictures are demonstrated as smooth narrowings of the ureteral lumen. Ureteral strictures have been reported in about 10% to 20% of patients with urinary tuberculosis.[7, 21]

Tuberculous involvement of the ureter has been classified into three stages of severity: early, chronic, and late terminal disease.[22] (1) Early disease, which may resolve completely without stricture formation, includes ureteral dilatation, due to edema at the ureterovesical junction or due to ureteral atony, and ulcerative ureteritis. (2) Fibrotic strictures make up the chronic disease stage. They may be single or multiple, and include the beaded and corkscrew ureters. (3) The late terminal stage includes the pipe-stem ureter and the ureter showing evidence of calcification in its wall.

BLADDER

Bladder involvement is frequent. The infection is usually carried there from the kidney via the urine. The changes in the bladder are responsible for dysuria and frequency, common initial complaints of patients with urogenital tuberculosis.

A number of sites in the bladder are affected simultaneously. The earliest manifestations are mucosal edema and ulcerations (Fig. 31–29), predominantly surrounding the ureteral orifices. Edema of the trigonal mucosa can produce ureteral obstruction. Tuberculomas in the vesical wall can be large, being manifested radiologically as filling defects, simulating carcinoma (Figs. 31–30 and 31–31). With multiple vesical tuberculomas, cystography shows filling defects simulating the appearance of multiple polypoid neoplasms (Fig. 31–32). Fibrotic healing typically results in the thick-walled, small, symmetrical bladder (Fig. 31–33). However, bands of fibrosis can cause an irregular luminal contour or marked asymmetry (Fig. 31–34). The tuberculous bladder may contract to minute proportions (Fig. 31–35). Dilatation of the upper tracts can result from the bladder abnormalities, due to either the small vesical capacity or constriction of the intramural portion of the ureters by the thick vesical wall. Fibrosis in the region of the trigone produces gaping ureteral

Text continued on page 1046

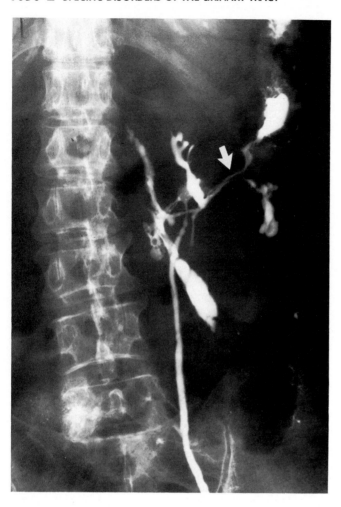

Figure 31–21. Nephrocolonic fistulas due to tuberculosis. Intravenous urography had shown no excretion of contrast medium by the left kidney. Retrograde pyelography demonstrates marked distortion of the pyelocalyceal system with several fistulas (*arrow*) to the descending colon. The ureter is straight and its lumen narrowed, owing to diffuse fibrosis of its wall (pipe-stem ureter).

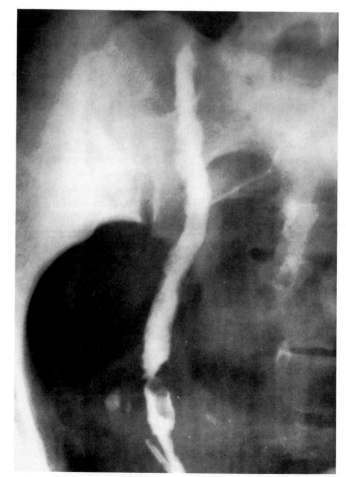

Figure 31–22. Ulcerations of the ureter due to tuberculosis. This 38-year-old woman presented with dysuria and gross hematuria. IVU showed poor excretion of contrast medium on the right, with dilatation of the right renal pelvis and ureter to the region of the bladder. The left kidney appeared normal. Diagnosis of urinary tuberculosis was made by bladder biopsy. Retrograde ureterogram shows narrowing and serrations of the distal portion of the ureter; the serrations represent multiple mucosal ulcerations. The filling defect probably represents a hematoma.

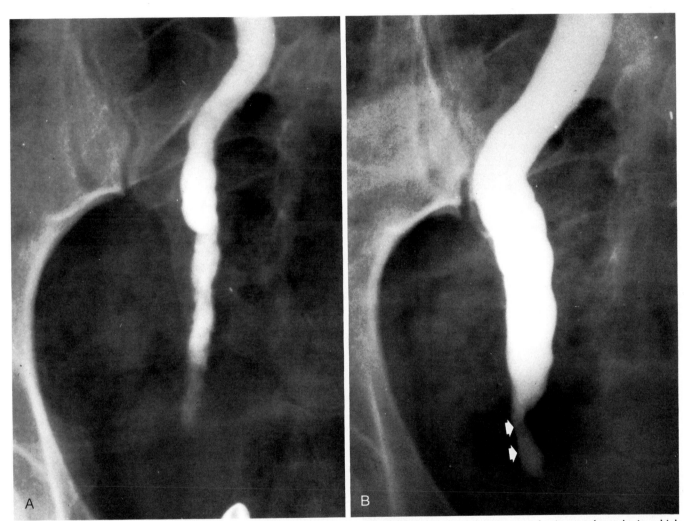

Figure 31–23. Tuberculosis of the ureter. This 35-year-old woman presented with recently diagnosed urinary tuberculosis, which had not been treated. *A*, Retrograde pyelogram shows the lower segment of the right ureter to be of irregular caliber, with peripheral serrations representing ulcerations. *B*, Repeat retrograde pyelogram after 3.5 months of treatment with antituberculosis chemotherapy now shows the lowermost segment of the ureter to be narrow and smooth in outline (*arrows*), the result of a fibrotic stricture. Proximal dilatation is more pronounced than in *A*.

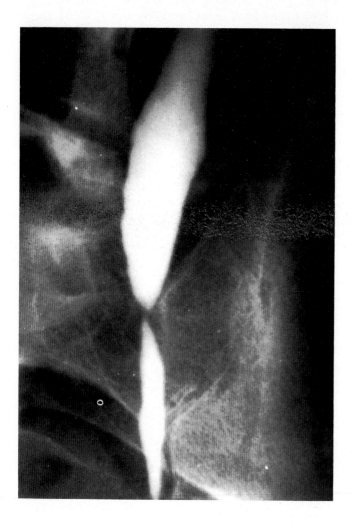

Figure 31–24. Short fibrotic stricture of ureter. This 39-year-old man was being treated for cavitary tuberculosis of the upper lobes of both lungs. There were no urinary symptoms. Urography showed a small left kidney that was not excreting contrast medium. Retrograde pyelogram demonstrates a very short stricture of the ureter at about the junction of its middle and lower thirds, with marked proximal dilatation.

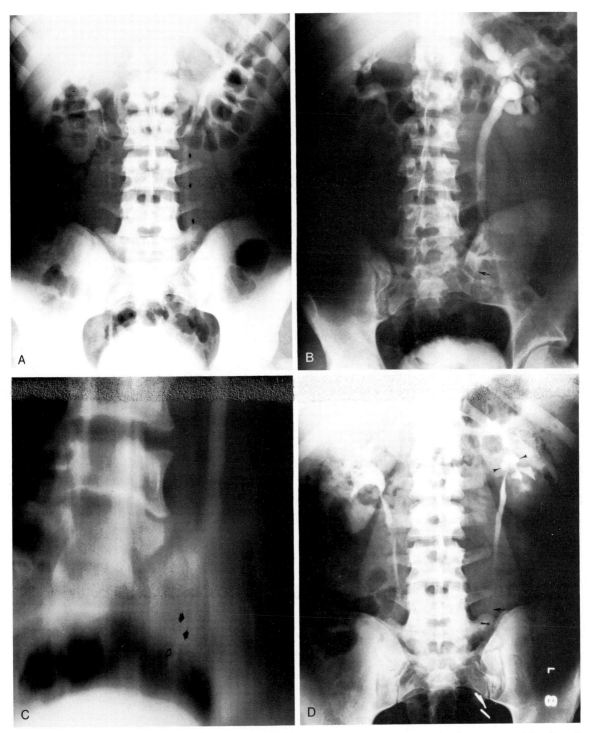

Figure 31–25. An 18-year-old male presents with a scrotal abscess. Chest film, skin test, and culture are positive for tuberculosis. *A,* IVU was obtained 1.5 years before patient's admission. Left kidney visualization is poorer than right, and slight ureteral dilatation is seen on the left (*arrows*). *B,* Urogram at time of admission shows typical urographic features of tuberculosis of the left kidney. Patient was on antituberculosis medication. Note ureteral dilatation and early stricture formation (*arrow*). Ureteropelvic and infundibulopelvic stricturing has caused diffuse pyelocaliectasis on the left. *C,* Tomogram of left ureter shows stricture (*solid arrowheads*) and ureteral ulceration (*open arrowhead*). *D,* Follow-up urogram 1 year after successful medical therapy and left ureteral stricture repair shows normal-caliber left ureter (*arrows*). Residual infundibulopelvic stricture on left resulted in hydrocalycosis of midpolar group on that side (*arrowheads*). Upper-pole and lower-pole calyces are nearly normal.

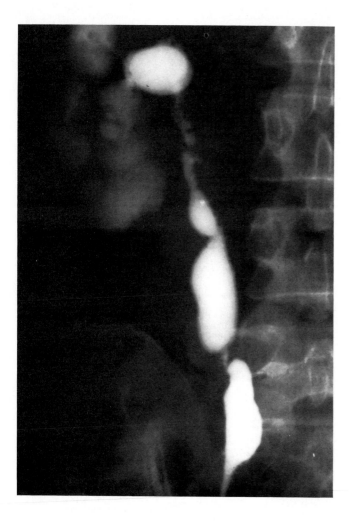

Figure 31–26. Multiple ureteral fibrotic strictures. Retrograde pyelogram shows multiple ureteral strictures in advanced urinary tuberculosis with destruction of the right kidney. The appearance is that of a beaded ureter.

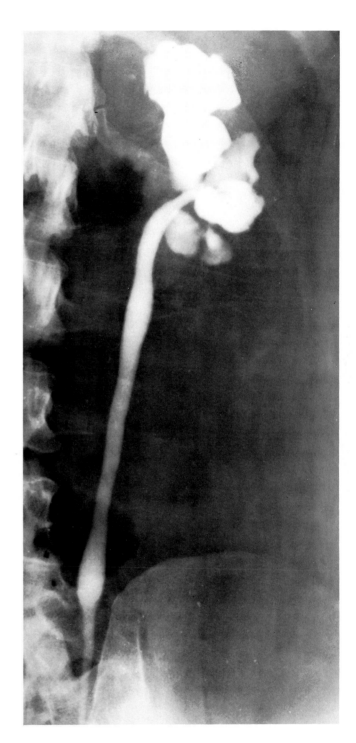

Figure 31–27. Pipe-stem ureter. Retrograde pyelogram shows dilated and destroyed calyces. The renal pelvis is not dilated and is probably fibrotic. The ureter is straight and appears rigid, owing to diffuse fibrosis of its wall. (From Elkin M: Radiology of the Urinary System. Boston, Little, Brown & Company, 1980.)

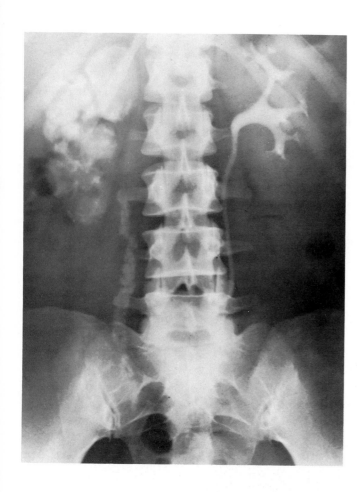

Figure 31–28. Tuberculous calcification of kidney and ureter. IVU shows no excretion from extensively calcified right putty kidney. The diffuse calcification in the right ureter is probably attributable to both mural calcification and calcified intraluminal debris.

Figure 31–29. Tuberculosis of the bladder. This 35-year-old woman, with newly discovered urinary tuberculosis, complained of dysuria and frequent urination. Urinalysis revealed microscopic hematuria and pyuria. Cystoscopy showed the bladder mucosa to be edematous and inflamed, with areas of ulceration. Cystogram shows marked irregularity of the bladder lumen, resulting from the edema and ulcerations.

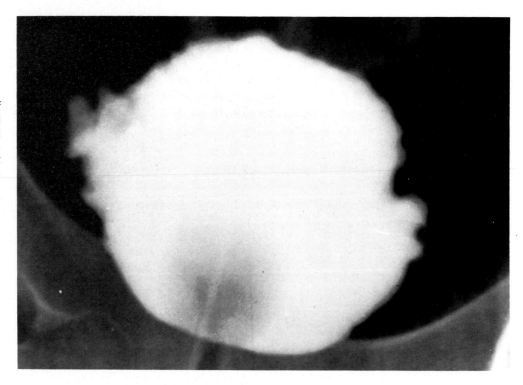

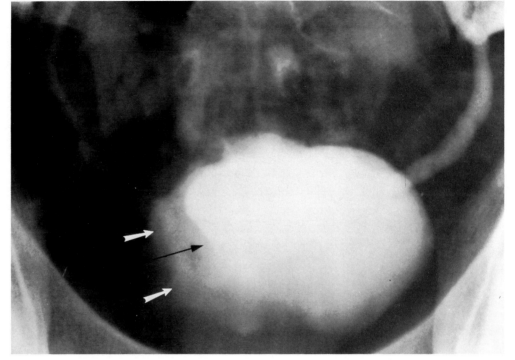

Figure 31–30. Tuberculosis of the bladder, mass effect. A 27-year-old man with frequency of urination and gross hematuria. IVU revealed cavitary lesions of the right kidney and dilatation of the right ureter. The bladder shows an irregular filling defect on the right, proved by biopsy to represent a tuberculoma (*arrows*).

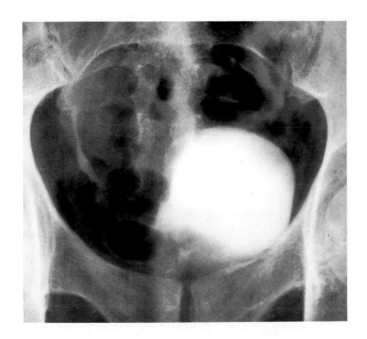

Figure 31–31. Tuberculosis of the bladder, mass effect. A 54-year-old man, with urinary tuberculosis diagnosed 10 months earlier, is treated with antituberculosis chemotherapy. Cystogram shows a large filling defect of the right lateral wall of the bladder, due to tuberculomas. (From Elkin M: Radiology of the Urinary System. Boston. Little, Brown & Company, 1980.)

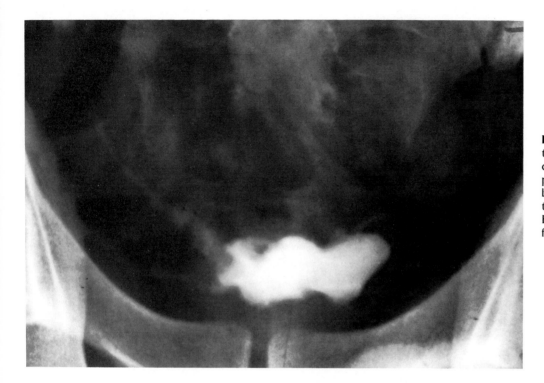

Figure 31–32. Tuberculosis of the bladder, multiple filling defects. IVU shows multiple polypoid filling defects of the bladder in a patient with untreated urinary tuberculosis. Bladder biopsy was positive for tuberculosis.

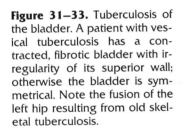
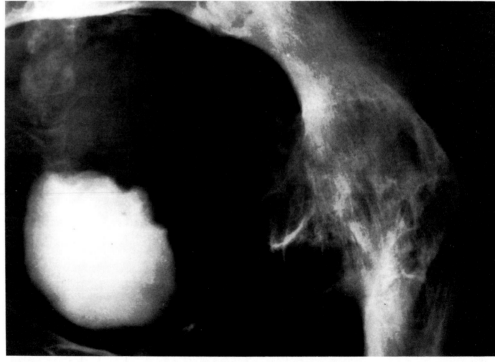

Figure 31–33. Tuberculosis of the bladder. A patient with vesical tuberculosis has a contracted, fibrotic bladder with irregularity of its superior wall; otherwise the bladder is symmetrical. Note the fusion of the left hip resulting from old skeletal tuberculosis.

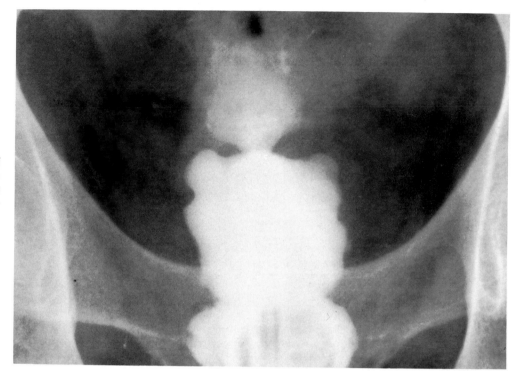

Figure 31–34. Tuberculosis of the bladder. Cystogram in a patient with vesical tuberculosis shows that the bladder is contracted asymmetrically.

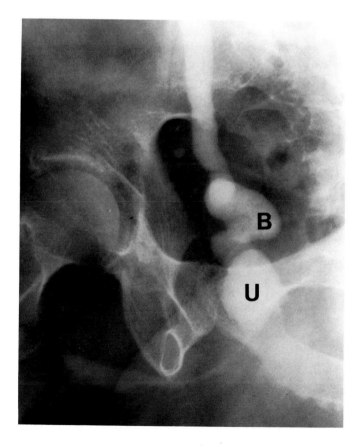

Figure 31–35. Severely contracted tuberculous bladder. A 42-year-old man who underwent a left nephrectomy for tuberculosis complained of severely frequent and urgent urination, bordering on incontinence. Film of the pelvis taken during an IVU shows involuntary filling of the dilated posterior urethra (U). The bladder (B) is irregularly contracted and reduced to a capacity of 5 to 10 cc, and the right ureter is dilated.

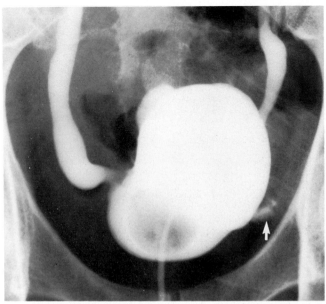

Figure 31—36. Vesicouretereal reflux in urinary tuberculosis. This 54-year-old man was receiving antituberculosis medication for urinary tuberculosis that was diagnosed 6 months earlier. Cystography shows bilateral reflux. Note the ulcer (*arrow*) at the left lateral wall of the bladder. (From Elkin M: Radiology of the Urinary System. Boston, Little, Brown, & Company, 1980.)

orifices and vesicoureteral reflux (Fig. 31–36). Calcification of the bladder wall is rare;[23] it presents as multiple speckled or curvilinear areas of calcification (Fig. 31–37).

URETHRA

The male urethra is uncommonly involved by tuberculosis (less than 2% of patients with genitourinary tuberculosis). The infection is transmitted via infected urine or by direct spread of infection from the prostate.[24, 25] A review of the literature during a 21-year period yielded only 21 male patients with urethral tuberculosis; the majority were younger than 35 years of age.[26] The usual manifestation is a stricture, almost always in the bulbomembranous urethra, that is indistinguishable on radio-

logical examination from strictures of other causes. Often, the urethral stricture is associated with periurethral abscesses and multiple fistulas from the urethra to the perineum, known as the "watering-can" perineum. Diagnosis is made by isolation of *M. tuberculosis* from the urine and from the exudate of the perineal ulcers or by positive biopsy of perineal lesions. Tuberculosis of the female urethra is extremely rare.

FEMALE GENITAL TRACT

See Chapter 28 for a discussion of tuberculosis of the female genital tract.

MALE GENITAL TRACT

Over 50% of male patients with urogenital tuberculosis have genital involvement.[27] The epididymis is most commonly affected (42%). Other involved sites are as follows: seminal vesicle (23%), prostate (21%), testis (15%), vas deferens (12%), and penis (less than 1%).

Tuberculous epididymo-orchitis presents as swelling of the testis or epididymis. There are no specific radiological findings. Seminal vesicle involvement, usually bilateral, consists of tuberculous abscesses and calcification (Fig. 31–38). Obstruction of the vas deferens can be caused by tuberculosis and may be demonstrable by vasovesiculography, although it may be indistinguishable from obstruction due to other causes. Vas deferens calcifications resulting from tuberculousis are characteristically intraluminal concretions, but intramural calcification has also been reported, radiologically indistinguishable from that seen in diabetes mellitus or in aging. In a review of 61 male patients with urinary tract tuberculosis, calcification was radiologically demonstrated in the seminal vesicle in two patients, and in the vas deferens in three patients.[8]

The prostate may be infected by hematogenous spread of tubercle bacilli from a distant active site (usually the lung) or by organisms carried in the urine from active tuberculosis in the upper urinary tract.[28, 29] Tuberculous abscesses and excavations are produced in the prostate (Fig. 31–39). The cavities communicating with the urethra

Figure 31—37. Bladder calcification. Scout radiograph shows speckled calcifications in tuberculosis of the bladder.

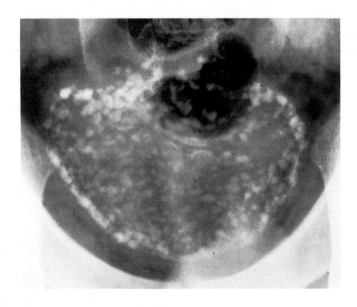

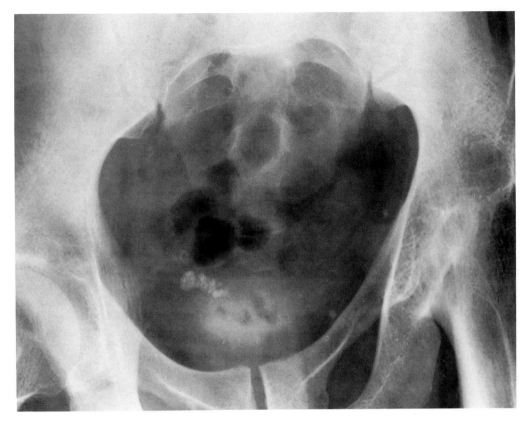

Figure 31—38. Tuberculous seminal vesicle calcification. Note the intraluminal calcification in the right seminal vesicle, as opposed to the mural calcification seen in diabetes mellitus (see Fig. 5–69). There is fusion of the left hip, also secondary to tuberculosis.

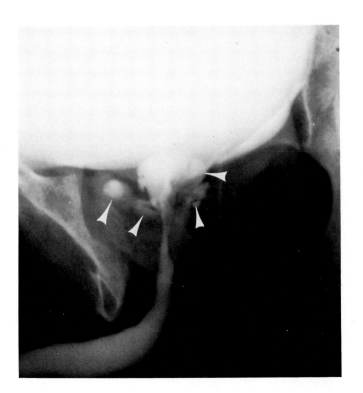

Figure 31—39. Tuberculosis of the prostate. A 39-year-old man with active pulmonary tuberculosis had been treated with chemotherapy for several weeks. Retrograde urethrography shows opacification of several prostatic cavitations (*arrowheads*), also seen at subsequent endoscopic examination. The patient also has a ureteral stricture with cavitations of the left kidney, demonstrable by retrograde pyelography (not illustrated here).

are radiologically demonstrable by voiding cystourethrography or retrograde urethrography.[30] Tuberculosis can also cause calcifications in the prostate, but the radiological appearance cannot be differentiated from other types of prostatic calculi or calcific prostatitis (Fig. 31–40).

Tuberculosis of the penis is very rare, presenting as a painless, although sometimes tender, ulcer on the glans penis. The diagnosis is usually made by biopsy. Radiological findings are absent. Penile involvement may be secondary to coexisting urinary tract tuberculosis, in which case the transmission occurs by bacilluria; or infection may occur by direct contact at time of intercourse with a partner having urogenital tuberculosis.

THE ADRENAL GLAND

The adrenal gland is an important site of involvement in hematogenous tuberculosis. The subject is discussed in Chapter 86, Diseases of the Adrenal Cortex Causing Hypofunction.

RADIOLOGIC IMAGING

The urinary tract abnormalities that are due to tuberculosis result from combinations of different pathological events, including tissue destruction with cavitations and ulcerations, dystrophic calcifications, fibrotic strictures and scars, mass effects of granulomas or conglomerations of granulomas, and the many changes secondary to obstructions in multiple locations of the urinary tract. The radiological findings can be widely variable, simulating appearances seen in other conditions, including carcinoma, nontuberculous infections, reflux nephropathy with renal scars, and renal cysts (Fig. 31–41). This has led to tuberculosis being designated "the great imitator" in its involvement of the urinary tract.

Urography and, when needed, retrograde pyelography are still the most informative radiological examinations for the diagnosis of urinary tract tuberculosis. Urography in patients with genitourinary tuberculosis is usually abnormal in 60% to over 90% of patients.[6, 7, 11] Cystography is helpful in the study of vesical tuberculosis and for the investigation of vesicoureteral reflux. Voiding cystourethrography or retrograde urethrography is necessary for the study of the strictures of urethral tuberculosis and for the cavitations in prostatic tuberculosis. Genital tuberculosis in the female is best demonstrated by hysterosalpingography and ultrasonography.

Ultrasonography typically reveals less morphological information than does conventional urography or CT scanning.[31, 32] Gross pathological changes, especially in advanced renal tuberculosis, can be depicted with ultrasonography. However, early in the course of the disease the sonogram may be normal, since early tuberculous renal involvement is focal. Even when tuberculosis is diffuse, the echo texture of the kidney may be normal. Calcification causes shadowing or merely diffuse specular echoes throughout the kidney. Hydronephrosis secondary to ureteropelvic junction or ureteral strictures is readily detected by ultrasonography, but lower urinary tract involvement may escape detection until late in its course. Bladder-wall thickening, with or without calcification, prostatic abscess, and distal ureteral strictures with proximal hydroureter can be seen, often to best advantage, with transrectal sonography in males or transvaginal sonography in females. Ultrasonography has effectively been used to monitor the progress of renal and vesical tuberculosis in children.[51]

CT reveals the full spectrum of changes of urinary tract tuberculosis, often in more detail than urography.[52] As on urograms, early focal calyceal changes are manifested on CT scans as calyceal enlargement, pericalyceal areas of early caseation, and infundibular strictures with loss of renal sinus fat planes. Late or more advanced tuberculosis may present CT features of hydronephrosis (focal or

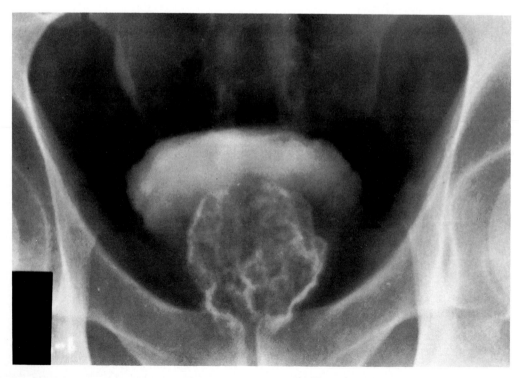

Figure 31–40. Tuberculous calcification of the prostate. Bladder film from an IVU shows diffuse calcification in the prostatic fossa of a 44-year-old man with known urinary tract tuberculosis. At cystoscopic examination, no prostatic tissue was seen; presumably, the glandular portions of the gland had sloughed and passed. The calcification lined the surface of the remaining excavated prostatic fossa.

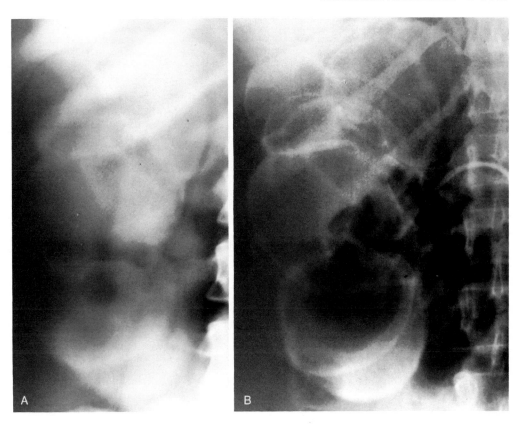

Figure 31–41. Advanced renal tuberculosis with radiological appearance simulating that of multiple renal cysts. This 34-year-old woman had a history of "kidney infection" 7 years ago, associated with hematuria, right hydronephrosis, and dilatation of the right ureter. The condition was diagnosed as urinary tuberculosis. *A,* Urogram shows curvilinear rims of renal parenchyma, simulating the appearance of multiple cysts. Later films showed no opacification of the pyelocalyceal system. *B,* Selective right renal angiography, late phase, shows rims of opacification, apparently in rims of remaining renal lobes around areas of calyceal dilatation and parenchymal destruction.

diffuse), calcification (specular, curvilinear, or solid), and usually asymmetrical renal involvement.[29, 30] Nonvisualization on contrast-enhanced CT scans of an autonephrectomized (partially or completely) kidney is more clearly represented on CT than on either intravenous urography or ultrasonography (Fig. 31–42). In cases of contralateral compensatory hypertrophy, the marked diminution in size of the more severely involved kidney can be seen. Calcifications may occur in up to 38% or more cases in one series (Fig. 31–16*B*).[29] An overall better assessment of the extent of renal, perinephric, and ureteral involvement from tuberculosis is achieved with CT scanning,[32, 33] and enhanced visualization of tuberculous seminal vesicles is obtained.[53]

Angiography is of no specific help in the diagnosis of urinary tract tuberculosis, although it is superior to urography for demonstrating the extent of involvement of the renal parenchyma (see Fig. 31–19). Renal tuberculosis is usually hypovascular, with irregular and pruned arteries, and produces a generally diminished and inhomogeneous nephrogram. In bladder tuberculosis the areas of involvement are poorly vascularized; the changes are not specific and are similar to the angiographic findings in cystitis of other etiologies or even to some instances of vesical neoplasm.[34]

In summary, the radiological findings in renal, ureteral, and vesical tuberculosis are summarized in Tables 31–1, 31–2, and 31–3, respectively.

Figure 31–42. Elderly female with history of tuberculosis, treated successfully. Contrast-enhanced CT scan shows nonfunctioning autonephrectomized putty kidney on right. Milk of calcium layered out posteriorly (*open arrowhead*). Left kidney is compensatorily enlarged, and distorted calyx is noted (*arrows*). Prominent hilar veins (*arrowheads*) proved to be ureteropelvic varices on left.

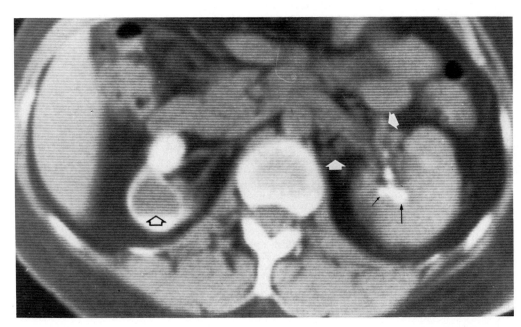

Table 31–1. Radiological Findings in Renal Tuberculosis

1. Poor excretion of contrast medium: focal or global.
2. Poor definition (loss of sharpness) of one or more calyces.
3. Irregular parenchymal cavitations, often communicating with the pyelocalyceal system.
4. Cortical scarring with distortion or dilatation of adjacent calyces.
5. Mass lesions representing conglomerations of tuberculomas or closed pyocalyces.
6. Strictures of the pyelocalyceal system, producing luminal narrowings directly and sometimes by kinking of the renal pelvis (Kerr's kinks).
7. Dilatation of segments of the pyelocalyceal system due to parenchymal destruction or strictures.
8. Calcification in the renal parenchyma, of various types: amorphous (smudgy), granular, speckled, curvilinear. The calcification of lobar distribution is unique, and its presence should suggest the diagnosis of renal tuberculosis ("putty kidney").
9. Autonephrectomy. The nonfunctioning kidney, often with areas of calcification; it is usually small, but is sometimes enlarged.
10. Evidence of tuberculosis in other systems, such as pulmonary and skeletal.

In a review of 52 consecutive patients with urinary tract tuberculosis, dilatation of all or part of the pyelocalyceal system was the most common radiological abnormality, seen in 70% of the patients.[9] Of the 52 patients, ureteral abnormalities occurred in 43%, and vesical abnormalities in 33%.

TREATMENT

Urinary tract tuberculosis, if untreated, progresses to involve and destroy both kidneys by caseation as well as by obstructive uropathy secondary to the development of strictures of the pyelocalyceal systems and ureters. Before the introduction of effective drugs, initially streptomycin in 1944, the 5-year mortality rate was greater than 80%. Now the mortality rate is less than 10%.

Because effective antituberculous drug therapy is available, it is especially important that urogenital tuberculosis be diagnosed early so that prompt chemotherapy can limit the destruction of renal tissue. A period of 18 to 24 months of drug treatment is the usual recommendation, although effective 6- to 9-month courses have been reported. Combinations of drugs are advised, usually three for the first few months and two for the continuation of the treatment.[35] If tuberculosis therapy is limited to a single drug, the organism often develops resistance to it. Isoniazid, rifampin, and ethambutol are the commonly used drugs; the older agents, streptomycin and para-

Table 31–2. Radiological Findings in Ureteral Tuberculosis

1. Ulcerations of long or (more often) short segments, usually at the lower portion of the ureter, but sometimes in a number of areas.
2. Obstruction, usually in the distal third, and especially at the ureterovesical region, sometimes due to spasm or mucosal edema. More often it is due to strictures that are initially irregular but that, with continuing fibrosis, become smooth.
3. Ureteral dilatation secondary to the obstructions or to ureteral atony or to vesicoureteral reflux.
4. The beaded or corkscrew ureter resulting from multiple fibrotic strictures.
5. The pipe-stem ureter, resulting from diffuse fibrosis of the wall. It is short and rigid with a narrow lumen.
6. Single or multiple filling defects representing tuberculomas.
7. Wall calcification (infrequently).

Table 31–3. Radiological Findings in Tuberculosis of the Bladder

1. Luminal irregularities due to ulcerations.
2. Uniformly thick-walled bladder, due to the fibrosis of healing.
3. Diminutive ("thimble") bladder.
4. Markedly irregular bladder, due to asymmetrical band of fibrosis.
5. Filling defects representing granulomas in the bladder wall.
6. Reflux from the bladder, due to gaping ureteral orifices secondary to trigonal fibrosis.
7. Calcification (rare).

aminosalicylic acid, are used occasionally. Patients are followed carefully, every 4 to 6 months for 2 years, and then annually for another 3 years. Follow-up examinations include bacteriological checks of the urine and radiological studies, most commonly by urography and sometimes by ultrasonography, to determine the possible appearance or increase of dilatation.

Nephrectomy, a frequent procedure in the prechemotherapy era, is performed less often in the treatment of renal tuberculosis. However, it still has an important, if infrequent, role.[36] Urologists disagree about the necessity for removal of a symptomless, nonfunctioning tuberculous kidney.[37, 38] Generally accepted indications for removal of a destroyed kidney include flank pain, draining sinus tract in the flank, recurrent urinary tract infections, suspicion of an associated renal malignancy, severe hematuria, drug resistance, and drug intolerance.[5, 39]

Even in patients for whom the diagnosis of urinary tract tuberculosis has been made at a relatively early stage, rapid deterioration can occur during treatment, owing to the fibrosis of healing that results in intrarenal scars and pyelocalyceal distortion, strictures, vesicoureteral reflux, and progressive hydronephrosis. Kerr and colleagues reported a constant annual nephrectomy rate of about 25% in renal tuberculosis in the period of 1956 to 1967.[40] They recommended close supervision of the patient during the early period of chemotherapy, in order to detect the development or increase of dilatation due to strictures, and prompt surgical intervention to relieve such obstruction. Intrarenal scars, most commonly found at the superior infundibulum, can sharply kink the renal pelvis, consequently obstructing the rest of the collecting system, which is not directly infected by the tubercle bacilli. Such patients have been treated by heminephrectomy for removal of tuberculous abscesses and infected parenchyma, and by lysis of the scars for alleviation of the kinks. Surgical procedures are performed only after the patient has had several weeks to a few months of antituberculous drug treatment.

Obstruction is common at the necks of the calyces. In the acute phase, the obstruction is due to edema, which often resolves with appropriate antituberculous chemotherapy, thereby allowing the calyx to drain. In that instance, the previously sterile urine may now contain tubercle bacilli, clearing again with continued drug treatment. However, a large pyocalyx closed off by a fibrotic stricture does not drain. Instead, it increases in size or remains unaltered, producing a mass in the kidney. Deroofing of the abscess (also called cavernotomy) has been recommended to remove the purulent content.[41] Possibly, abscesses with liquid contents could also be drained percutaneously. Cavernotomy is not performed if a cavity openly communicates with the pyelocalyceal system in the presence of obstruction of the lower urinary tract.

A ureteral fibrous stricture, which is most common at or near the lower end of the ureter and is often multiple, may develop or become more severe during effective chemotherapy. Failure to relieve the obstruction results in progressive renal destruction. Administration of steroids has been recommended to reduce the fibrosis and to prevent stricture formation; this is usually ineffective.[35, 42, 43] Dilatation of the stricture has been accomplished by an indwelling ureteral catheter, with reported immediate success rates of 65% to 85%, but the stricture recurred in some of the patients.[20, 40, 42, 44] Successful transluminal balloon dilatation of a short stricture at the juxtavesical portion of the ureter has also been reported.[45] Transurethral dilatation should be attempted before turning to open surgery. For a stricture at the lower end of the ureter, the operation is excision or bypass of the stricture, and reimplantation of the ureter into the bladder. For obstructing short strictures at sites other than at the lower end, excision and end-to-end anastomosis may be feasible.

On occasion, enterocystoplasty, using ileum or colon, is beneficial for treatment of tuberculous contracture of the urinary bladder. The indications for this procedure are frequency of micturition and vesicoureteral reflux with progressive hydronephrosis secondary to the small capacity bladder. Under unusual conditions, ureteral diversion to an ileal conduit may be required.

Tuberculous urethral stricture, often associated with multiple sinus tracts to the perineum, is treated with antituberculous drugs and repeated urethral dilatations, as needed.

NONTUBERCULOUS MYCOBACTERIA

Nontuberculous mycobacterial infection of the urinary tract is very uncommon. *Mycobacterium bovis* may involve the urinary tract,[46] but it is generally limited to countries in which infected cattle are prevalent. The clinical, pathological, and radiological changes produced by the nontuberculous organisms are indistinguishable from those produced by *M. tuberculosis*. They are often more resistant, however, to standard antituberculous therapy. Infections resulting from *Mycobacterium kansasii*,[47] *Mycobacterium avium-intracellulare* (formerly Battey bacillus),[48] and *Mycobacterium fortuitum*[49] have been reported. These infections are often seen in patients who have impaired cellular immunity (Fig. 31–43).

BACILLE CALMETTE-GUÉRIN (BCG)

Bacille Calmette-Guérin, an attenuated strain of *M. tuberculosis,* is effective in the treatment of superficial bladder cancer, when it is administered intravesically or intracutaneously. Clinically significant infection secondary to the administration of BCG is rare, but occasional cases of genitourinary granulomas are reported. Stanisic and colleagues noted the development of caseating renal granulomas in the kidney of a patient 7 months after BCG therapy.[50] They also called attention to previously reported cases of granulomatous prostatitis, epididymitis, cystitis, and ureteral stricture (in a patient with vesicoureteral reflux) in patients treated with BCG.

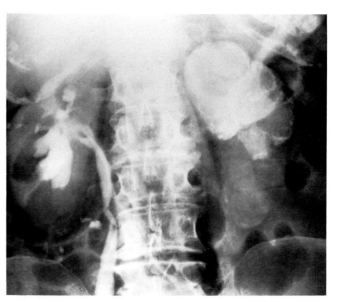

Figure 31–43. *Mycobacterium avium-intracellulare* infection mimicking *Mycobacterium tuberculosis.* The urinary changes, which included left putty kidney, strictured right renal pelvis, calcification of the left ureter, and contracted bladder, are those of classic urinary tract tuberculosis. However, the organism was *M. avium-intracellulare.* (From Pergament M, Gonzalez R, Fraley EE: Atypical mycobacteriosis of the urinary tract: A case report of extensive disease caused by the Battey bacillus. JAMA 229:816, 1974. Copyright 1974, American Medical Association.)

References

1. Kearns TJ, Russo, PK: The control and eradication of tuberculosis. N Engl J Med 303:813, 1980.
2. Glassroth J, Robins AG, Snider DE Jr: Tuberculosis in the 1980s. N Engl J Med 302:1441, 1980.
3. Cinman AC: Genitourinary tuberculosis. Urology 20:353, 1982.
4. Wechsler H, Westfall M, Lattimer JK: The earliest signs and symptoms in 127 male patients with genitourinary tuberculosis. J Urol 83:801, 1960.
5. Narayana AS: Overview of renal tuberculosis. Urology 19:231, 1982.
6. Simon HB, Weinstein AJ, Pasternak MS, et al: Genitourinary tuberculosis: Clinical features in a general hospital population. Am J Med 63:410, 1977.
7. Teklu B, Ostrow JH: Urinary tuberculosis: A review of 44 cases treated since 1963. J Urol 115:507, 1976.
8. Kollins SA, Hartman GW, Carr DT, et al: Roentgenographic findings in urinary tract tuberculosis: A 10 year review. AJR 121:487, 1974.
9. Roylance J, Penry JB, Davies ER, Roberts M: The radiology of tuberculosis of the urinary tract. Clin Radiol 21:163, 1970.
10. Ehrlich RM, Lattimer JK: Urogenital tuberculosis in children. J Urol 105:461, 1971.
11. Christensen WI: Genitourinary tuberculosis: Review of 102 cases. Medicine 53:377, 1974.
12. Gregory PG, Seki M, Sawada H, Johnson KG: Renal tuberculosis in the Japanese. J Chron Dis 20:225, 1967.
13. Medlar EM, Spain DM, Holliday RW: Post-mortem compared with clinical diagnosis of genito-urinary tuberculosis in adult males. J Urol 61:1078, 1949.
14. Munt PW: Miliary tuberculosis in the chemotherapy era: With a clinical review in 69 American adults. Medicine 51:139, 1971.
15. Gelb AF, Leffler C, Brewin A, et al: Miliary tuberculosis. Am Rev Respir Dis 108:1327, 1971.
16. Barrie HJ, Kerr WK, Gale GL: The incidence and pathogenesis of tuberculous strictures of the renal pelvis. J Urol 98:584, 1967.
17. Brennan RE, Pollack HM: Nonvisualized ("phantom") renal calyx: Causes and radiological approach to diagnosis. Urol Radiol 1:17–23, 1979.
18. Dunn M, Kirk D: Renogastric fistula: Case report and review of the literature. J Urol 109:785, 1973.

19. Batch AJG, Amery AH, Reddy ER: Pyeloduodenal fistula: A case report and review of the literature. Br J Surg 66:31, 1979.
20. Friedenberg RM: Tuberculosis of the genitourinary system. Semin Roentgenol 6:310, 1971.
21. Murphy DM, Fallon B, Lane V, O'Flynn JD: Tuberculous stricture of ureter. Urology 20:382, 1982.
22. Friedenberg RM, Ney C, Stachenfeld RA: Roentgenographic manifestations of tuberculosis of ureter. J Urol 99:25, 1968.
23. Pollack HM, Banner MP, Martinez LO, Hodson CJ: Diagnostic considerations in urinary bladder wall calcification. AJR 136:791, 1981.
24. Symes JM, Blandy JP: Tuberculosis of the male urethra. Br J Urol 45:432, 1973.
25. LeBrun HI: Tuberculous urethral stricture. Br J Urol 30:82, 1958.
26. Raghavaiah NV: Tuberculosis of the male urethra. J Urol 122:417, 1979.
27. Ross JC: Renal tuberculosis. Br J Urol 25:277, 1953.
28. Sporer A, Auerbach O: Tuberculosis of prostate. Urology 11:362, 1978.
29. Moore RA: Tuberculosis of the prostate gland. J Urol 37:372, 1937.
30. Tonkin AK, Witten DM: Genitourinary tuberculosis. Semin Roentgenol 14:305, 1979.
31. Schaffer R, Becker JA, Goodman J: Sonography of tuberculous kidney. Urology 22:209, 1983.
32. Goldman SM, Fishman EK, Hartman DS, et al: Computed tomography of renal tuerculosis and its pathological correlates. J Comput Assist Tomogr 9:771, 1985.
33. Premkumar A, Lattimer J, Newhouse JH: CT and sonography of advanced urinary tract tuberculosis. AJR 148:65, 1987.
34. Heitala SO, Duchek M: Angiography in urinary bladder tuberculosis. Acta Radiol 16:297, 1975.
35. Gow JG: Genitourinary tuberculosis: A 7-year review. Br J Urol 51:239, 1979.
36. Wong SH, Lau WY, Poon GP, et al: The treatment of urinary tuberculosis. J Urol 131:297, 1984.
37. Flechner SM, Gow JG: Role of nephrectomy in the treatment of non-functioning and very poorly functioning unilateral tuberculous kidney. J Urol 123:822, 1980.
38. Wechsler M, Lattimer JK: An evaluation of the current therapeutic regimen for renal tuberculosis. J Urol 113:760, 1975.
39. Bloom S, Wechsler H, and Lattimer JK: Results of a long-term study of non-functioning tuberculous kidneys. J Urol 104:654, 1970.
40. Kerr WK, Gale GL, Peterson SS: Reconstructive surgery for genitourinary tuberculosis. Trans Am Assoc Genitourin Surg 60:93, 1968.
41. Hanley HG: Cavernotomy and partial nephrectomy in renal tuberculosis. Br J Urol 42:661, 1970.
42. Clardige M: Ureteric obstruction in tuberculosis. Br J Urol 42:688, 1970.
43. Horne NW, Tulloch WS: Conservative management of renal tuberculosis. Br J Urol 47:481, 1975.
44. Cavalli A, Bianchi G, Franzdin N, Tallarigo C: Molding catheterism in the treatment of TB ureter stenoses: A ten-year experiment. Endoscopy 12:175, 1980.
45. Waller RM III, Finnerty DP, Casarella WJ: Transluminal balloon dilatation of a tuberculous ureteral stricture. J Urol 129:1225, 1983.
46. Stoller JK: Late recurrences of *Mycobacterium bovis* genitourinary tuberculosis: Case report and review of literature. J Urol 134:565, 1985.
47. Listwan WJ, Roth DA, Tsung SH, et al: Disseminated *Mycobaterium kansasii* infection with pancytopenia and interstitial nephritis. Ann Intern Med 83:70, 1975.
48. Pergament M, Gonzalez R, Fraley EE: Atypical mycobacteriosis of the urinary tract. A case report of extensive disease caused by the Battey bacillus. JAMA 229:816, 1974.
49. Rosen DI: Mycobacteria fortuitum in the urinary tract. A case report. J Urol 114:951, 1975.
50. Stanisic TH, Brewer ML, Graham AR: Intravesical bacillus Calmette-Guérin therapy and associated granulomatous renal masses. J Urol 135:356, 1986.
51. Cremin BJ: Radiological imaging of urogenital tuberculosis in children with special emphasis on ultrasound. Pediatr Radiol 17:34, 1987.
52. Becker JA: Renal tuberculosis. Urol Radiol 10:25, 1988.
53. Premkumar A, Newhouse JH: Seminal vesicle tuberculosis: CT appearance. J Comput Assist Tomogr 12:676, 1988.

32

Brucellosis

ANDREW J. LEROY

Brucellosis is a disease of considerable worldwide medical and economic importance. Although the records of the Center for Disease Control list only 131 cases in the United States in 1984, this zoonosis is considered to be widely underdiagnosed and underreported.[1] Thousands of cases still occur annually in the countries bordering the Mediterranean and in the Middle East, the Soviet Union, North America, and South America.

Sir David Bruce, after whom the disease is named, isolated and described the responsible organism on Malta in 1866. Thirty years later in Copenhagen, Bang described the bacillus responsible for bovine abortion. In 1918, Evans noted the similarity of the two organisms, introduced the generic name *Brucella*, and suggested that the term *brucellosis* be used, instead of "Malta fever" or "undulant fever." The *Brucella* organisms that affect humans include the *abortus* (cattle), *suis* (swine), *melitensis* (goats), and rarely the *canis* (dogs) species. The primary modes of transmission to humans are direct contact with infected animals such as occurs in the meat-processing industry and by the ingestion of unpasteurized dairy products, most popularly goat-milk cheese.

Brucellosis is a systemic disease that can affect nearly every human organ, owing to hematological spread. *Brucella* organisms have been recovered from the urine in 4% to 50% of cases. Despite this finding, documented cases of symptomatic urinary tract brucellosis are rare. *Brucella* prostatitis and epididymitis have been described.[5]

Brucella orchitis is a rare cause of human sterility and impaired sexual potency. The bladder wall may be involved, with resultant thickening and, possibly, bladder contraction.

Human brucellosis may be divided into acute or chronic phases. The acute bacteremic febrile form may be associated with positive urine cultures. An acute interstitial nephritis, including azotemia, proteinuria, and hypertension, has been described in this stage. Chronic brucellosis is a poorly defined systemic illness that may include interstitial nephritis or renal abscess formation, although both are rare. More common are renal granulomas, which may calcify. Culture of the *Brucella* organism may be difficult, and measurement of agglutination titers is extremely helpful. The prognosis of human brucellosis is excellent, when appropriate antibiotic therapy is carried out.

RADIOLOGICAL FINDINGS IN ACUTE BRUCELLOSIS

The excretory urogram is normal in most cases of acute brucellosis for which urinary tract symptoms are absent. Sonographic evaluation of acute brucellosis in a child showed bilaterally enlarged kidneys resulting from interstitial nephritis. Resolution to a normal appearance occurred in 6 weeks.[2]

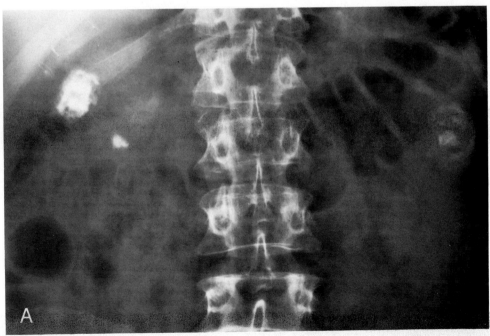

Figure 32–1. Renal brucellosis. *A*, Plain radiographs showing two calcified renal masses (brucellomas) in the upper portion of the right kidney and a single lesion on the left.

Illustration continued on following page

1053

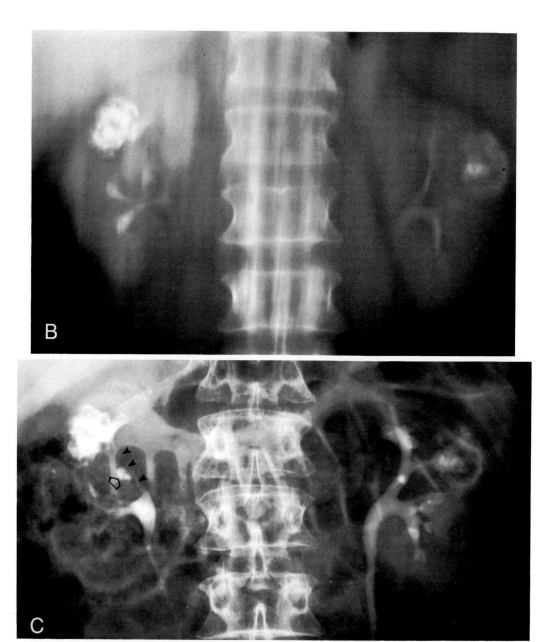

Figure 32–1 *Continued B,* Urogram documents the intrarenal location of the brucellomas. *C,* Urogram shows slight narrowing of the right upper-pole infundibulum (*arrowheads*) near the smaller (*open arrowhead*) of the right-sided calcifications. These granulomas do not communicate with the collecting system, and the remainder of the urogram is normal.

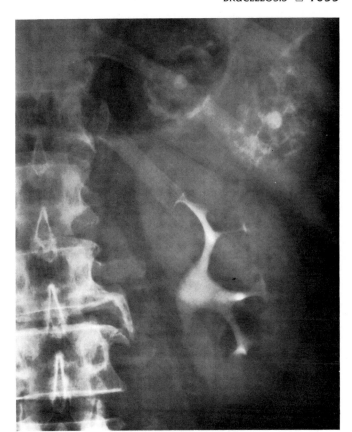

Figure 32–2. Urogram shows calcified "target" lesions in the spleen due to brucellosis. The left kidney is normal.

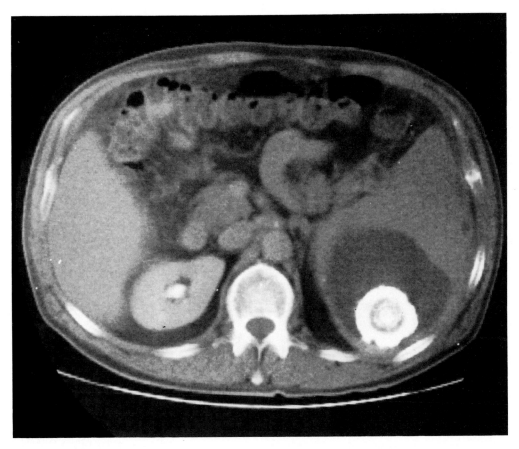

Figure 32–3. Computed tomographic scan, obtained prior to splenectomy for recurrent fever, shows a calcified splenic brucelloma within an area of acute reactivation in the spleen.

RADIOLOGICAL FINDINGS
IN CHRONIC BRUCELLOSIS

The urographic descriptions of chronic renal brucellosis have repeatedly stressed the similarity to tuberculosis.[3, 4] As in tuberculosis, cicatricial deformity of the infundibula may result in dilatation of the renal pelvis and calyces. However, cavities are not usually encountered in brucellosis, and the pattern of calcification is dissimilar to that of tuberculosis. Calcification of granulomatous *Brucella* lesions is common within the kidneys. These may be punctate and randomly distributed throughout the kidneys, or they may be solitary or bilateral densely calcified "bull's-eye" or "target" lesions (Fig. 32–1). The bull's-eye appearance is very suggestive of brucellosis. Although marked thickening of the wall of the renal pelvis and ureter have been described pathologically, ureteral calcification has not been reported.

Because brucellosis is a systemic disease, other intra-abdominal involvement may be documented during the course of a urogram. Calcified splenic brucellomas are the most common finding (Figs. 32–2 and 32–3). Rarely, similar lesions may be seen in the liver. Brucellar spondylitis may also be noted, but is radiographically indistinguishable from other forms.

References

1. Young EJ: Human brucellosis. Rev Infect Dis 5:821, 1983.
2. Fattah HA, Khuffash FA: Reversible renal failure in a child with brucellosis: A case report. Ann Trop Paediatr 4:247, 1984.
3. Kelalis PP, Greene LF, Weed LA: Brucellosis of the urogenital tract: A mimic of tuberculosis. J Urol 88:347, 1962.
4. Petereit MF: Chronic renal brucellosis: A simulator of tuberculosis, Case Report. Radiology 96:85, 1970.
5. Ibrahim AIA, Awad R, Shetty SD, et al: Genitourinary complications of brucellosis. Br J Urol 61:294, 1988.

33 Genitourinary Involvement in AIDS

ALLEN J. ROVNER

Acquired immunodeficiency syndrome (AIDS) is characterized by infection with human T-cell lymphotropic virus Type III/lymphadenopathy-associated virus (HTLV-III/LAV) and a concurrent illness indicative of the underlying cellular immune deficiency.[1] The manifestations of this syndrome are protean, and virtually any organ system or anatomical region can be affected by the ravages of this disease. The lungs, lymph nodes, brain, and gastrointestinal tract are the most commonly involved organ systems,[2–4] but alterations of the urinary tract can be the most lethal.[5, 6]

The clinical spectrum for AIDS patients with urinary tract disease includes proteinuria, pyuria, hematuria, urinary tract infection, renal insufficiency, acute tubular necrosis, and electrolyte abnormalities.[5, 7–9] Pathological changes usually reflect the primary agent of the renal disease (e.g., opportunistic infection, primary or contiguous tumor invasion, sepsis, and shock).[2, 4, 6, 8, 10] Because of the diversity of these agents, the pathological changes are not specific for AIDS. Focal and segmental glomerular sclerosis (FSS) and diffuse glomerular mesangial hyperplasia (MH) were observed in 35 and 15 of 139 patients, respectively, in one series,[11] but these findings are not pathognomonic. The etiology of these changes is not clear, although intravenous drug abuse was a significant risk factor for renal disease, compared with homosexuality.[11]

Autopsy series[2, 4] demonstrate cytomegalic virus (CMV) infection in the kidneys, bladder, and most commonly the adrenals. The adrenal is the most common extrapulmonary site of CMV infection, with 40% of patients involved in one series.[4] The adrenals were involved in 8 of 9 patients in another series,[2] and two patients had suspected Waterhouse-Friderichsen syndrome. Whenever CMV was found in the adrenal, it was also present in the lung. In the kidney, characteristic inclusion cells are found in the glomerular tufts, rather than the collecting system and distal tubules (a more typical distribution). Other renal lesions include proliferative glomerulonephritis with deposits of IgM, IgG, and C3. Even testicular tissue may be susceptible. Testicular fibrosis with partial to complete spermatic maturation arrest may also be associated with CMV infection. One patient had CMV inclusions in the small blood vessels of the seminiferous tubules.

AIDS-related lymphoma, Kaposi's sarcoma, and lymphadenopathy syndrome are the tumors most commonly found, and they are typically more aggressive and poorly differentiated in AIDS patients.[10, 12, 13] Patients with Hodgkin's disease and AIDS did not have renal involvement. Non–Hodgkin's lymphoma involved the kidneys in 11% of patients.[10] Abdominal adenopathy, including para-aortic, mesenteric, and pelvic nodes, was more prevalent in these AIDS variants. The differential diagnosis of adenopathy in these patients also includes disseminated infection. Hydronephrosis may result from ureteral obstruction by the enlarged nodes.[20]

No pathognomonic findings have been imaged in the urinary tract, but several articles have described abnormalities in AIDS patients.[10, 12–17] Urinary tract involvement by malignancy or infection is indistinguishable in appearance from that in patients without AIDS. The distribution or extent of disease, however, may be unusually severe in these patients. There is one case report of cortical and medullary nephrocalcinosis in AIDS-associated Mycobacterium avium intracellulare (MAI) infection.[17] The increased echogenicity was due to diffuse calcification, rather than to chronic renal disease. In a series of 10 patients with AIDS and proteinuria, azotemia, or uremia who were examined with ultrasonography, all had some evidence of altered renal echogenicity (Fig. 33–1).[16] There was no direct correlation between the degree of echogenicity and the clinical severity of renal disease, and the biopsy finding of focal segmental glomerulosclerosis was not pathognomonic for AIDS. The authors did suggest that renal sonographic screening may, nevertheless, be useful as an early sign of impending renal dysfunction. Further studies are obviously required. Hamper and coworkers suggested that the altered echogenicity may be due to tubular changes, distinctive for AIDS (see Fig. 102–9).[19]

An important group at risk for AIDS are renal hemodialysis patients and transplant patients.[5, 18] The progression of disease in these patients is more rapid, and the virus can be more virulent than for other AIDS patients. Documented transmission of HIV infection from renal transplantation (but not cornea transplantation) was found within 12 days of the transplant. This transmission

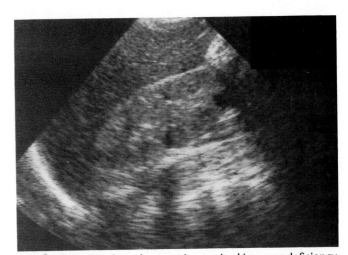

Figure 33–1. Renal involvement in acquired immunodeficiency syndrome (AIDS). Sonogram of the right kidney (sagittal view) demonstrates a diffuse increase in echogenicity in the cortex and the medulla. This results in a loss of corticomedullary demarcation. The echogenicity of the kidney exceeds that of the liver and parallels that of the renal sinus fat. The size of the kidney is normal. Renal biopsy revealed focal glomerulosclerosis, one of the known renal manifestations of AIDS. The left kidney showed similar changes. (Courtesy Nagesh Raghavendra, M.D., New York).

occurred in spite of cold storage of the transplanted organ. Frozen sperm has also been documented as a vector of disease.[18]

At present, the urinary tract imaging changes are not characteristic for AIDS infection. As imaging procedures are more extensively applied to this group of patients, those at risk for the lethal complications of HIV infection may be discovered earlier.

References

1. Solinger AM, Hess EV: Acquired immune deficiency syndrome—An overview. Semin Roentgenol 21:9–13, 1987.
2. Reichert CM, O'Leary TJ, Levens DL, et al: Autopsy pathology in the acquired immune deficiency syndrome. Am J Pathol 112:357–382, 1983.
3. Federle MP: A radiologist looks at AIDS: Imaging evaluation based on symptom complexes. Radiology 166:553–562, 1988.
4. Welch K, Finkbeiner W, Alpers CE, et al: Autopsy findings in the acquired immune deficiency syndrome. JAMA 252:1152–1159, 1984.
5. Gardenswartz MH, Lerner CW, Seligson GR, et al: Renal disease in patients with AIDS: A clinicopathologic study. Clin Nephrol 21:197–204, 1984.
6. Sreepada Rao TK, Friedman EA, Nicastri AD: The types of renal disease in the acquired immunodeficiency syndrome. N Engl J Med 316:1062–1068, 1987.
7. Vaziri ND, Barbari A, Licorish K, Gupta S: Spectrum of renal abnormalities in acquired immune-deficiency syndrome. J Nat Med Assoc 77:369–375, 1985.
8. Chander P, Soni A, Suri A, et al: Renal ultrastructural markers in AIDS–associated nephropathy. Am J Pathol 126:513–526, 1987.
9. Kaplan MS, Wechsler M, Benson MC: Urologic manifestations of AIDS. Urology 30:441–443, 1987.
10. Nyberg DA, Jeffrey RB, Federle MP, et al: AIDS–related lymphomas: Evaluation by abdominal CT. Radiology 159:59–63, 1986.
11. Pardo AV, Meneses R, Ossa L, et al: AIDS–related glomerulopathy: Occurrence in specific risk groups. Kidney Internat 31:1167–1173, 1987.
12. Moon KL, Federle MP, Abrams DI, et al: Kaposi sarcoma and lymphadenopathy syndrome: Limitations of abdominal CT in acquired immunodeficiency syndrome. Radiology 150:479–483, 1984.
13. Nyberg DA, Federle MP: AIDS–related Kaposi sarcoma and lymphomas. Semin Roentgenol 22:54–65, 1987.
14. Jeffrey RB, Nyberg DA, Bottles K, et al: Abdominal CT in acquired immunodeficiency syndrome. AJR 146:7, 1986.
15. Hill CA, Harle TS, Mansell PWA: The prodrome, Kaposi sarcoma, and infections associated with acquired immunodeficiency syndrome: Radiologic findings in 39 patients. Radiology 149:393–399, 1983.
16. Schaffer RM, Schwartz GE, Becker JA, et al: Renal ultrasound in acquired immune deficiency syndrome. Radiology 153:511–513, 1984.
17. Falkoff GE, Rigsby CM, Rosenfield AT: Partial, combined cortical and medullary nephrocalcinosis: US and CT patterns in AIDS–associated MAI infection. Radiology 162:343–344, 1987.
18. Schwarz A, Hoffman F, L'age-Stehr J, et al: Human immunodeficiency virus transmission by organ donation. Transplantation 44:21–24, 1987.
19. Hamper U, Goldblum L, Hutchins G, et al: Renal involvement in AIDS: Sonographic-Pathologic correlation. AJR 150:1321, 1988.
20. Mohler JL, Jarow JP, Marshall FF: Unusual urological presentations of acquired immune deficiency syndrome: Large cell lymphoma. J Urol 138:627, 1987.

Index

Note: Page numbers in *italics* refer to illustrations; page numbers followed by t refer to tables.
Vol. I, 1–1058; Vol. II, 1059–2075; Vol. III, 2076–3051

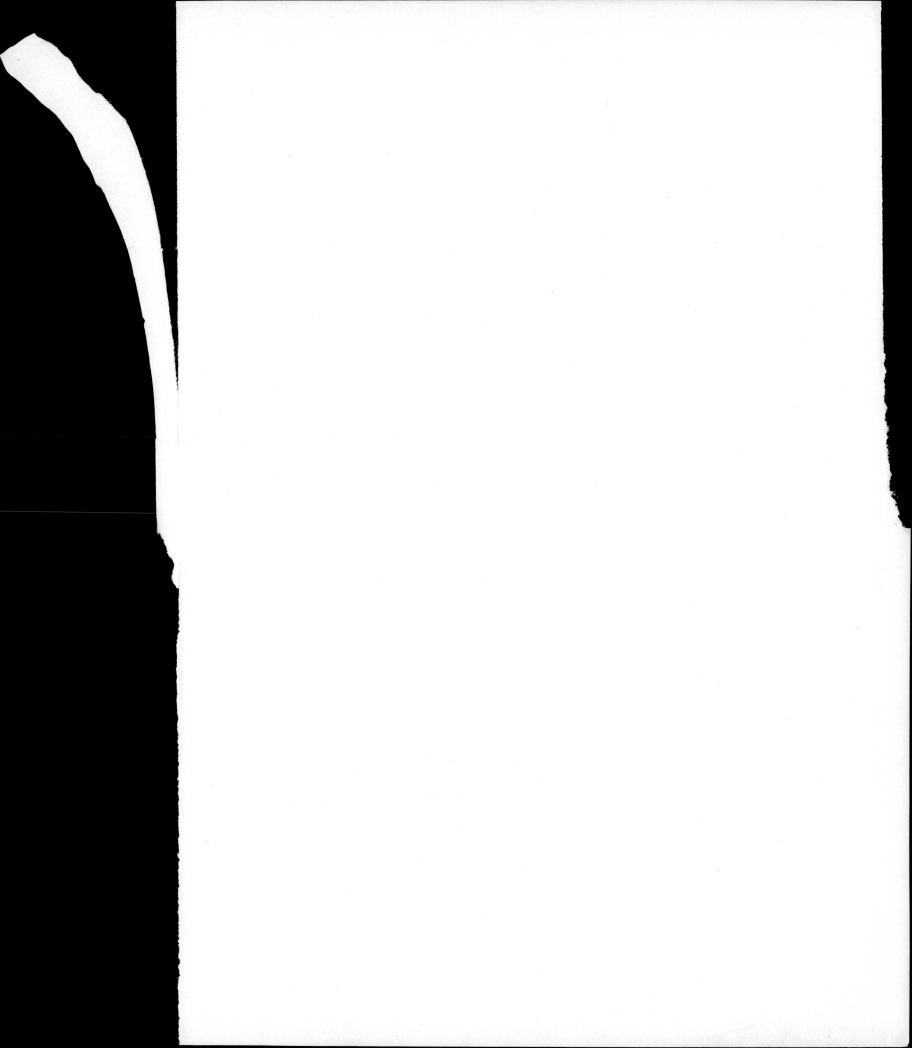